W9-ABH-611

SALEM HEALTH

MAGILL'S MEDICAL GUIDE

SALEM HEALTH

MAGILL'S MEDICAL GUIDE

Seventh Edition

Volume III

Growth – Nervous system

Medical Editors

Bryan C. Auday, Ph.D.
Gordon College

Michael A. Buratovich, Ph.D.
Spring Arbor University

Geraldine F. Marrocco, Ed.D., APRN, CNS, ANP-BC
Yale University School of Nursing

Paul Moglia, Ph.D.
South Nassau Communities Hospital

SALEM PRESS
A Division of EBSCO Information Services, Inc.
Ipswich, Massachusetts

GREY HOUSE PUBLISHING

Magill's Medical Guide: Health and Illness, 1995
Supplement, 1996
Magill's Medical Guide, revised edition, 1998
Second revised edition, 2002
Third revised edition, 2005
Fourth revised edition, 2008
Sixth edition, 2011
Seventh edition, 2014

∞ The paper used in these volumes conforms to the American National Standard for Permanence of Paper for Printed Library Materials, Z39.48-1992 (R1997).

Note to Readers

The material presented in *Magill's Medical Guide* is intended for broad informational and educational purposes. Readers who suspect that they suffer from any of the physical or psychological disorders, diseases, or conditions described in this set should contact a physician without delay; this work should not be used as a substitute for professional medical diagnosis or treatment. This set is not to be considered definitive on the covered topics, and readers should remember that the field of health care is characterized by a diversity of medical opinions and constant expansion in knowledge and understanding.

Library of Congress Cataloging-in-Publication Data

Magill's medical guide / medical editors: Bryan C. Auday, Ph.D., Gordon College [and three others].
— Seventh Edition.

5 volumes : illustrations ; cm. — (Salem health)

Title page verso indicates: Seventh Revised Edition, 2014.
Includes bibliographical references and index.
ISBN: 978-1-61925-214-1 (set)
ISBN: 978-1-61925-503-6 (v.1)
ISBN: 978-1-61925-504-3 (v.2)
ISBN: 978-1-61925-505-0 (v.3)
ISBN: 978-1-61925-506-7 (v.4)
ISBN: 978-1-61925-507-4 (v.5)

1. Medicine--Encyclopedias. I. Auday, Bryan C., editor. II. Series: Salem health (Pasadena, Calif.)

RC41 .M345 2014
610.3

First Printing

COMPLETE TABLE OF CONTENTS

VOLUME I

VOLUME II

VOLUME III

Shading indicates current volume.

Shading indicates current volume.

Shading indicates current volume.

Shading indicates current volume.

VOLUME IV

Volume V

SALEM HEALTH

MAGILL'S MEDICAL GUIDE

GROWTH

Biology

Anatomy or system affected: All

Specialties and related fields: Embryology, endocrinology, obstetrics, orthopedics, pediatrics

Definition: The development of the human body from conception to adulthood; growth occurs at different rates for different systems over this period, and varies by sex and individual as well.

Key terms:

accretion: a type of growth in which new, nongrowing material is simply added to the surface

allometric growth: unequal rates of growth of different body parts, or in different directions

developmental biology: broadly, the study of ontogeny; narrowly, the study of how gene action is controlled

embryonic stage: that part of ontogeny during which organs are formed

fetal stage: that part of ontogeny after the organs are formed but before birth takes place

interstitial growth: growth throughout a structure, usually in all directions

isometric growth: equal rates of growth of all parts, or in all directions

ontogeny: the entire developmental sequence, from conception through the various embryonic stages, birth, childhood, maturity, senescence, and death; also, the study of this sequence

ossification: the formation of bone tissue

Process and Effects

The human body grows from conception until adult size is reached. Adult size is reached in females around the age of eighteen and in males around twenty or twenty-one, but there is considerable variation in either direction. (Nearly all numerical measurements of growth and development are subject to much variation.) On the average, males end up with a somewhat larger body size than females because of these two or three extra years of growth.

Growth begins after conception. The first phase of growth, including approximately the first month after conception, is called embryonic growth, and the growing organism is called an embryo. During embryonic growth, the most important developmental process is differentiation, the formation of the various organs and tissues. After the organs and tissues are formed, the rest of prenatal growth is called fetal growth and the developing organism is called a fetus. Respiratory movements begin around the eighteenth week of gestation, during the fetal stage; limb movements (such as kicking) begin to be felt by the mother around the twenty-fourth week, with a considerable range of variation. At birth, the average infant weighs about 3.4 kilograms (7.5 pounds) and measures about 50 centimeters (20 inches) in length.

Growth continues after birth and throughout childhood and adolescence. From the perspective of developmental biology, childhood is defined as the period from birth to puberty, which generally begins at twelve years of age, and adolescence continues from that point to the cessation of skeletal growth at around the age of eighteen in females and twenty or twenty-one in males. The long period of adulthood that follows is marked by a stable body size, with little or no growth except for the repair and maintenance of the body, including the healing of wounds. After about age sixty, there may be a slight decline in body height and in a few other dimensions.

By one year of age, the average baby is seventy-five centimeters (thirty inches) long and weighs ten kilograms (twenty-two pounds). (There is actually a slight decline in weight in the first week of postnatal life, but this is usually regained by age three weeks.) For ages one to six, the average weight (in kilograms) can be approximated by the equation "weight = age × 2 + 8." For ages seven to twelve, growth takes place more rapidly: Average weight (in kilograms) can be approximated by "weight = age × 3.5 - 2.5," while average height (in centimeters) can be approximated for ages two to twelve by the equation "height = age × 6 + 77." Head circumference has a median value of about 34.5 centimeters at birth, 46.3 centimeters at an age of one year, 48.6 centimeters at age two, and 49.9 centimeters at age three. All these figures are about one centimeter larger in boys than in girls, with considerable individual variation. Median heights and weights, when differentiated by sex, reveal that boys and girls are generally similar until age fourteen, after which boys continue to gain in both dimensions.

Growth of the teeth takes place episodically. In most children, the first teeth erupt between five and nine months of age, beginning with the central incisors, the lower pair generally preceding the upper pair. The lateral incisors (with the upper pair first), the first premolars, the canines, and the second premolars follow, in that order. All these teeth are deciduous teeth ("baby teeth") that will eventually be shed, to be replaced during late childhood by the permanent teeth. At one year of age, most children have between six and eight teeth.

Growth takes place in several directions. Growth at the same rate in all directions is called isometric growth, which maintains similar proportions throughout the growth process. Isometric growth occurs in nautilus shells and a variety of other invertebrates. Most of human growth, however, is allometric growth, which takes place at different rates in different directions. Allometric growth results in changes in shape as growth proceeds. Moreover, different parts of the body grow at different rates and in different directions. During fetal development, for example, the head develops in advance of the fore and hind limbs, and the fetus at about six months of age has a head which is about half its length. The head of a newborn baby is about one-third of its body length, compared to about one-seventh for an adult. In contrast, the legs make up only a small part of the body length in either the six-month-old fetus or the newborn baby, and their absolute length and proportionate length both increase throughout childhood and adolescence.

Growth of the skeleton sets the pace for growth of the majority of the body, except for the nervous system and reproductive organs. Most parts of the skeleton begin as fast-growing cartilage. The process in which cartilage tissue turns into bone tissue is called ossification, which begins at various centers in the bone. The first center of ossification within each bone is called the diaphysis; in long bones, this ossification usually takes place in the center of the bone, forming the shaft. Secondary centers of ossification form at the ends of long bones and at certain other specified places; each secondary center of ossification is called an epiphysis. In a typical long bone, two epiphyses form, one at either end. Capping the end of the bone, beyond the epiphysis, lies an articular cartilage. Between the epiphysis and the diaphysis, the cartilage that persists is called the epiphyseal cartilage; this becomes the most rapidly growing region of the bone. During most of the growth of a long bone, the increase in width occurs by accretion, a gradual process in which material is added at a slow rate only along a surface. In the case of a bone shaft, increase in width takes place only at the surface, beneath the surrounding membrane known as the periosteum. By contrast, the epiphyseal cartilage grows much more rapidly, and it also grows by interstitial growth, meaning that growth takes place throughout the growing tissue in all directions at once. As the epiphyseal cartilage grows, parts of it slowly become bony, and those bony portions grow more slowly.

During the first seven or eight years of postnatal life, the growth of the epiphyseal cartilage takes place faster than its replacement by bone tissue, causing the size of the epiphyseal cartilage to increase. Starting around age seven, the interstitial growth of the epiphyseal cartilage slows down, while the replacement of cartilage by bone speeds up, so that the epiphyseal cartilage is not growing as fast as it turns into bone tissue; the size of the epiphyseal cartilage therefore starts to decrease. At the time of puberty, the hormonal influences cre-

ate an adolescent growth spurt during which the individual's bone growth increases for about a one-year period. In girls, the adolescent growth spurt takes place about two years earlier than it does in boys—the average age is around twelve in girls, versus about fifteen in boys—but there are tremendous individual variations both in the extent of the growth spurt and in its timing. By age fourteen, most girls have already experienced most of their adolescent growth spurt, while most boys are barely beginning theirs. Consequently, the average fourteen-year-old girl is a bit taller than the average fourteen-year-old boy.

At around eighteen years of age in females and twenty or twenty-one years of age in males, the replacement of the epiphyseal cartilage by bone is finally complete, and bone growth ceases. The age at which this occurs and the resulting adult size both vary considerably from one individual to another. For the rest of adult life, the skeleton remains more or less constant in size, diminishing only slightly in old age.

Most of the other organs of the body grow in harmonious proportion with the growth of the skeleton, reaching a maximum growth rate during the growth spurt of early adolescence and reaching a stable adult size at around age eighteen in women and age twenty or twenty-one in men. The nervous system and reproductive system, however, constitute major exceptions to this rule. The nervous system and brain grow faster at an earlier age, reaching about 90 to 95 percent of their adult size by one year of age. The shape of the head, including the shape of the skull, keeps pace with the development of the brain and nervous system. For this reason, babies and young children have heads that constitute a larger proportion of their body size than do the heads of adults.

The growth of the reproductive system also follows its

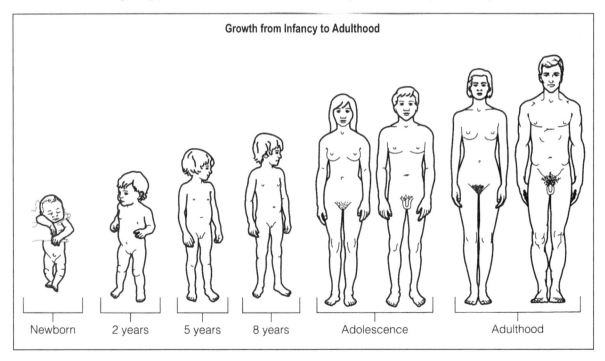

Growth from Infancy to Adulthood

Newborn   2 years   5 years   8 years   Adolescence   Adulthood

Median Heights and Weights from Childhood to Adulthood

	Boys			Girls	
Age	Height (cm)	Weight (kg)		Height (cm)	Weight (kg)
2	87	12		87	12
3	95	15		94	14
4	103	17		102	16
5	110	19		108	18
6	117	21		115	20
7	122	23		121	22
8	127	25		127	25
9	132	28		132	28
10	138	31		138	33
11	143	35		145	37
12	150	40		152	42
13	157	45		157	46
14	163	51		160	50
15	169	57		162	54
16	174	62		162	56
17	176	66		163	57
18	177	69		164	57

own pattern. Most reproductive development is delayed until puberty. The reproductive organs of the embryo form slowly and remain small. The reproductive organs of children, though present, do not reach their mature size until adolescence. These organs, both the internal ones and the external ones, remain small throughout childhood. Their period of most rapid growth marks the time of puberty, which spans ages eleven through thirteen, with a wide range of variation. At this time, the pituitary gland begins secreting increased amounts of the follicle-stimulating hormone (FSH), which stimulates the growth and maturation of the gonads (the ovaries of females and the testes of males). The ovaries or testes then respond by producing increased amounts of the sex hormones testosterone (in males) or estrogen (in females), which stimulate the further development of both primary and secondary sexual characteristics. Primary sexual characteristics are those which are functionally necessary for reproduction, such as the presence of a uterus and ovaries in females or the presence of testes and sperm ducts in males. Secondary sexual characteristics are those which distinguish one sex from another, but which are not functionally necessary for reproduction. Examples of secondary sexual characteristics include the growth of breasts or the widening of the hips in females, the growth of the beard and deepening of the voice in males, and the growth of hair in the armpits and pubic regions of both sexes.

Growth takes place psychologically and socially as well as physically. Newborn babies, though able to respond to changes in their environment, seem to pay attention to such stimuli only on occasion. At a few weeks of age, the baby will respond to social stimuli (such as the sound of the mother's voice) by smiling. Babies usually can grasp objects by five months of age, depending on the size and shape of the object. By six months, most babies will show definite signs of pleasure in response to social stimulation; this may include an open-mouth giggle or laugh. At seven months of age, most babies will respond to adult facial expressions and will show different responses to familiar adults as opposed to strangers. The age at which babies learn to crawl varies greatly, but most infants learn the technique by nine or ten months of age. Social imitation begins late in the first year of life. Also, by this time, children learn object permanence, meaning that they will search for a missing object if they have watched it being hidden. Walking generally develops around eighteen months of age, but the time of development varies greatly.

Jean Piaget (1896–1980) was a pioneer in the study of the social and cognitive development of children. Piaget identified four stages of cognitive and social growth, which he called sensorimotor, preoperational, concrete operational, and formal operational. In the sensorimotor stage, from birth to about two years of age, infants begin with reflexes such as sucking or finger curling (in response to touching their palms). Starting with these reflexes, they gradually learn to understand their senses and apply the resulting information in order to acquire important adaptive motor skills that can be used to manipulate the world (as in picking up things) or to navigate about and explore the world (as in walking). Socially, infants develop ways to make desirable stimuli last by such acts as smiling. In the preoperational stage, which lasts from about two to six years of age, children acquire a functional use of their native language. Their imagination flourishes, and pretending becomes an important and frequent activity. Most of the thinking at the preoperational stage is egocentric, however, which means that the child perceives the world only from his or her own point of view and has difficulty seeing other points of view.

The concrete operational stage spans the years from about seven to eleven years of age. This is the stage at which children learn to apply logic to concrete objects. For example, they realize that liquid does not change volume when poured into a taller glass, and they develop the ability to arrange objects in order (for example, by size) or to classify them into groups (for example, by color or shape). The final stage is called the formal operational stage, beginning around age twelve. This is the stage of adolescence and adulthood, when the person learns to manipulate abstract concepts in such areas as ethical, legal, or mathematical reasoning. This is also the stage at which people develop the ability to construct hypothetical situations and to use them in arguments.

Complications and Disorders

Disorders of growth include dwarfism, gigantism, and several other disorders such as achondroplasia (chondrodystrophy). Dwarfism often results from an insufficiency of the pituitary growth hormone, also called somatostatin or somatotrophic hormone. Some short-statured individuals are normally proportioned, while others have proportions differing from those of most other people. An overabundance of growth hormone causes gigantism, a condition marked by unusually rapid growth, especially during adolescence. In some individuals, the amount of growth hormone remains normal during childhood but increases to excessive amounts during the teenage years; these individuals are marked by acromegaly, a greater than normal growth which affects primarily the hands, feet, and face.

Achondroplasia, also called chondrodystrophy, is a genetically controlled condition caused by a dominant gene. In people having this condition, the epiphyseal cartilages of the body's long bones turn bony too soon, so that growth ceases before it should. Those exhibiting chondrodystrophy therefore have short stature and childlike proportions but rugged faces that look older than they really are.

Inadequate growth can often result from childhood malnutrition, particularly from insufficient amounts of protein. If a child is considerably shorter or skinnier than those of the same age, that child's diet should be examined for the presence of malnutrition. Intentional malnutrition is one of the characteristic features of anorexia nervosa. The opposite problem, overeating, can lead to obesity, although obesity can also result from many other causes, including diabetes and other metabolic problems.

By the late twentieth century, human growth hormone, a drug used since the 1950s to help very short children grow, was being used for "off-label" purposes that included antiaging and body building. In 2002, researchers suggested an apparent link between the use of the hormone and cancer, specifically Hodgkin's disease and colorectal cancer.

Perspective and Prospects

As a phenomenon, growth of both wild and domestic animals was well known to ancient peoples. Hippocrates (ca. 460–ca. 370 BCE), considered the founder of medicine, wrote a treatise on embryological growth, and Aristotle (384–322 BCE) wrote a longer and more complete work on the subject. During the Renaissance, Galileo Galilei (1564–1642) studied growth mathematically and distinguished between isometric and allometric forms of growth, arguing that the bones of giants would be too weak to support their weight.

The most important era in the study of human embryonic development was ushered in by the Estonian naturalist Karl Ernst von Baer (1792–1876), who discovered the human ovum. From this point on, detailed studies of human embryonic and postnatal development proceeded at a rapid pace, especially in Germany. Much of the modern understanding of growth in more general or mathematical terms derives from the classic studies of the British anatomist D'Arcy Wentworth Thomson (1860–1948). In the twentieth century,

Piaget became a leader in the study of childhood social and cognitive growth phases.

—*Eli C. Minkoff, Ph.D.*

See also Aging; Childbirth; Conception; Dwarfism; Embryology; Endocrine disorders; Endocrinology; Endocrinology, pediatric; Failure to thrive; Gigantism; Glands; Hormones; Hypertrophy; Malnutrition; Menopause; Menstruation; Nutrition; Prader-Willi syndrome; Pregnancy and gestation; Puberty and adolescence; Sexuality; Vitamins and minerals; Weight loss and gain.

For Further Information:

Bar, Robert S., ed. *Early Diagnosis and Treatment of Endocrine Disorders*. Totowa, N.J.: Humana Press, 2003.

Behrman, Richard E., Robert M. Kliegman, and Hal B. Jenson, eds. *Nelson Textbook of Pediatrics*. 18th ed. Philadelphia: Saunders/Elsevier, 2007.

Bukatko, Danuta, and Marvin W. Daehler. *Child Development: A Thematic Approach*. Belmont, Calif.: Wadsworth, 2012.

"Facts About Child Development." *Centers for Disease Control and Prevention*, September 12, 2011.

Galotti, Kathleen M. *Cognitive Development: Infancy through Adolescence*. Thousand Oaks, Calif.: SAGE Publications, 2011.

Goodman, H. Maurice. *Basic Medical Endocrinology*. 4th ed. Boston: Academic Press/Elsevier, 2009.

Kail, Robert V., and John C. Cavanaugh. *Human Development: A Life-Span View*. Belmont, Calif.: Wadsworth, 2013.

McMillan, Julia A., et al., eds. *Oski's Pediatrics: Principles and Practice*. 4th ed. Philadelphia: Lippincott Williams & Wilkins, 2006.

Marieb, Elaine N. *Essentials of Human Anatomy and Physiology*. 9th ed. San Francisco: Pearson/Benjamin Cummings, 2009.

Moore, Keith L., and T. V. N. Persaud. *The Developing Human*. 8th ed. Philadelphia: Saunders/Elsevier, 2008.

Rosse, Cornelius, and Penelope Gaddum-Rosse. *Hollinshead's Textbook of Anatomy*. 5th ed. Philadelphia: Lippincott-Raven, 1997.

Standring, Susan, et al., eds. *Gray's Anatomy*. 40th ed. New York: Churchill Livingstone/Elsevier, 2008.

Tsiaras, Alexander, and Barry Werth. *From Conception to Birth: A Life Unfolds*. New York: Doubleday, 2002.

GUILLAIN-BARRÉ SYNDROME
Disease/Disorder

Also known as: Acute inflammatory demyelinating polyneuropathy

Anatomy or system affected: Immune system, muscles, musculoskeletal system, nerves, nervous system

Specialties and related fields: Internal medicine, neurology

Definition: An acute degeneration of peripheral motor and sensory nerves, known to physicians as acute inflammatory demyelinating polyneuropathy, a common cause of acute generalized paralysis.

Key terms:

antibody: a substance produced by plasma cells which usually binds to a foreign particle; in Guillain-Barré syndrome, antibodies bind to myelin protein

antigen: any substance that stimulates white blood cells to mount an immune response

areflexia: loss of reflex

autoimmune disorder: a condition in which the immune system attacks the body's own tissue instead of foreign tissue

B cell: a type of white blood cell that produces antibodies

CSF protein: a protein in the cerebrospinal fluid which is usually very low

demyelination: a loss of the myelin coating of nerves

electromyogram: the external recording of electrical impulses from muscles

macrophage: a white blood cell that engulfs foreign protein; in Guillain-Barré syndrome, it also attacks myelin

motor weakness: muscle weakness resulting from the failure of motor nerves

nerve conduction velocity: the speed at which a nerve impulse travels along a nerve

neurogenic atrophy: shrinkage of muscle caused by a loss of nervous stimulation

neuropathy: a condition in which nerves are diseased, are inflamed, or show abnormal degeneration

phagocytosis: the process of engulfing particles

polyneuropathy: neuropathy found in many areas

Causes and Symptoms

Guillain-Barré syndrome (GBS) is an acute disease of the peripheral nerves, especially those that connect to muscles. It causes weakness, areflexia (loss of reflex), ataxia (difficulty in maintaining balance), and sometimes ophthalmoplegia (eye muscle paralysis). GBS demonstrates a variable, multifocal pattern of inflammation and demyelination of the spinal roots and the cranial nerves, although the brain itself is not obviously affected. By the 1990s and early 2000s, it was the most common cause of generalized paralysis in the United States, averaging one to two cases per 100,000 people per year. The disease was first described in the early twentieth century by Georges Guillain and Jean-Alexander Barré, two French neurologists. Little was known of the cause of GBS or the mechanism for its symptoms, however, until the 1970s. Since then, symposia sponsored by the National Institute of Neurological and Communicative Disorders and Stroke have shed more light on this condition.

Most individuals with GBS have a rapidly progressing muscular weakness in more than one limb and also experience paresthesia (tingling) and numbness in the hands and feet. These sensations have the effect of reducing fine muscle control, balance, and one's awareness of limb location. The prevailing scientific opinion regarding GBS is that it is an autoimmune disorder involving white blood cells, which for some unknown reason attack nerves and/or produce antibodies against myelin, the insulating covering of nerves. The weakness is usually ascending in nature, beginning with numbness in the toes and fingers and progressing to total limb weakness. The demyelination is more prominent in the nerves of the trunk and occurs to a lesser extent in the more distal nerves. The brain and spinal cord are protected from GBS by the blood-brain barrier, although antibodies to myelin have been found in the cerebrospinal fluid of some patients.

With GBS, there is often a precipitating event such as surgery, pregnancy, upper respiratory infection, viral infection (such as cytomegalovirus), or vaccination. Preexisting debilitating illnesses such as systemic lupus erythematosus (SLE)

Information on Guillain-Barré Syndrome

Causes: Autoimmune disorder; often with precipitating event such as surgery, pregnancy, upper respiratory infection, viral infection (such as cytomegalovirus), vaccination

Symptoms: Weakness; loss of reflex; difficulty maintaining balance; eye muscle paralysis; tingling and numbness in hands and feet; reduced fine motor control, balance, and awareness of limb location; paralysis of vocal cords

Duration: Chronic with acute episodes

Treatments: Plasmapheresis, administration of cyclosporine or corticosteroids

or Hodgkin's disease also seem to predispose a person to GBS. GBS has been diagnosed in patients having heart transplants in spite of the fact that they are receiving immunosuppressive drugs. The increased risk with such surgery may be attributable to the stress associated with the procedure. Most patients who come down with GBS have had some prior condition that placed stress on the immune system prior to the appearance of GBS.

The patient with GBS is frequently incapable of communicating as a result of paralysis of the vocal cords. Typically, motor paralysis will worsen rapidly and then plateau after four weeks, with the patient bedridden and often in need of respiratory support. Autonomic nerves can also be affected, causing gastrointestinal disturbances, adynamic ileus (loss of function in the ileum of the small intestine), and indigestion. Other, less common symptoms include pupillary disturbances, pooling of blood in limbs, heart rhythm disturbances, and a decrease in the heart muscle's strength. These patients are usually hypermetabolic because considerable caloric energy goes into an immune response that is self-destructive and into mechanisms that are attempting to repair the damage.

In addition to the loss of myelin, cell body damage to nerves may result and may be associated with permanent deficits. If the nerve cell itself is not severely damaged, regrowth and remyelination can occur. Antibodies to myelin proteins and to acidic glycolipids are seen in a majority of patients. Blood serum taken from patients with GBS has been shown to block calcium channels in muscle, and experiments in Germany have found that cerebrospinal fluid from GBS patients blocks sodium channels.

Like most autoimmune conditions, GBS is cyclic in nature; the patient will have good days and bad days because the immune system is sensitive to the levels of steroid hormones in the body, which are known to fluctuate. In addition to paralysis, there is significant pain with GBS. Many of the nerve fibers that register the pain response (nociceptors) are nonmyelinated and therefore are not interrupted in GBS. Pain management can be difficult, requiring the use of such drugs as fentanyl, codeine, morphine, and other narcotics. The course of the disease is variable and is a function of the level of reactivity of the patient's immune system. The autoimmune attack is augmented in those patients experiencing activation of serum complement protein induced by antibodies. Recovery usually takes months, and frequently the patient requires home health care. Complications can lead to death, but most patients recover fully, though some have residual weakness.

The physician must be careful to distinguish GBS from lead poisoning, chemical or toxin exposure, polio, botulism, and hysterical paralysis. Diagnosis can be confirmed using cerebrospinal fluid (CSF) analysis. GBS patients have protein levels greater than 0.55 gram per deciliter of CSF. Macrophages are frequently found in the CSF, as well as some B cells. Nerve conduction velocity will be decreased in these patients to a value that is 50 percent of normal in those nerves that are still functioning. These changes can take several weeks to develop.

With GBS, macrophages and T cells have been shown to be in contact with nerves, as evidenced in electron micrographs. T-cell and macrophage activation in these individuals point to an immune response gone awry, possibly precipitated by a virus or exposure to an antigen that is foreign but similar in appearance to one of the proteins in myelin. T cells, upon encountering an unrecognizable antigen, will produce interleukin II, initiate attack, and recruit macrophages to participate. The use of an anti-T-cell drug theoretically should improve nerve function, but researchers at the University of Western Ontario failed to find any benefit from the infusion of an anti-T-cell monoclonal antibody. Unexpectedly, GBS has been found in patients testing positive for the human immunodeficiency virus (HIV) who are asymptomatic, in spite of the fact that their T cells are under attack from the HIV virus and are diminished in number. Although myelin proteins are thought to be the immunogens, other candidates include gangliosides in the myelin. Antiganglioside antibodies have been seen in a majority of GBS patients. This trait may distinguish GBS from amyotrophic lateral sclerosis (Lou Gehrig's disease) and multiple sclerosis, which seem to involve different myelin proteins as antigens.

In GBS, the white blood cells attack peripheral motor nerves more often than other types of nerves, implying a biochemical difference between motor and sensory nerves that has yet to be discovered. One possible cause of this disease is a similarity between a protein or glycolipid that is present normally in myelin and coincidentally on an infectious agent, such as a virus. The immune system responds to the agent, resulting in a sensitization of the macrophages and T cells to that component of myelin. B cells are then stimulated to produce antibodies against this antigen, and they unfortunately cross-react with components of the myelin protein. The severity of the disease will depend on the number of macrophages and lymphocytes activated and whether serum complement-binding antibodies are being produced. Serum complement proteins are activated by a particular class of antibodies, resulting in the activation of enzymes in the blood that potentiate tissue destruction and neurogenic atrophy. Serum complement levels can be determined by a serum complement fixation test.

In severe cases of GBS, intercostal muscles are more severely compromised and respiratory function needs to be monitored closely. The immune response will subside when T-suppressor cells have reached their peak levels. Halting the autoimmune response will not reverse the symptoms immediately, since it takes time for antibody levels to decrease and for the nerves to regrow and remyelinate, which occurs at the rate of 1 to 2 millimeters per day. Some nerves will undergo retrograde degeneration and be lost from the neuronal pool. Other nerves will have more closely spaced nodes and conduct impulses at a lower velocity. Nerve sprouting will also occur, which will result in one nerve's being responsible for more muscle fibers or serving a larger sensory area and in decreased fine motor control.

Treatment and Therapy

In Guillain-Barré syndrome, the amount of muscle and nerve involvement can be assessed by performing an electromyogram, which can reveal the amount of motor nerve interruption and the conduction velocity of the nerves that continue to function. Based upon the assumption that an autoimmune response was in progress, corticosteroids such as prednisolone and methylprednisolone were once administered in high doses, but such drugs have been shown to have a deleterious effect on the disease and are no longer used.

More recently, a procedure known as plasmapheresis has been tried with better results, especially when performed in the first two weeks. This procedure involves removing 250 milliliters (a little more than a pint) of plasma from the blood every other day and replacing this volume with a solution containing albumin, glucose, and appropriate salts. Six treatments are typical and usually result in a faster recovery of muscle control than for those not receiving plasmapheresis. Because relapses may occur if the patient produces new antibodies to myelin, immunosuppressants are given to the patient after plasmapheresis. Another procedure, intravenous immunoglobulin therapy, is based on the strategy of blocking the binding of antibodies to nerves, which lessens the severity of the immune attack.

Cyclosporine, a T-cell inhibitor, is also being tried, with some promising results. Some researchers note, however, that transplant patients, who routinely take cyclosporine, have a higher-than-normal risk of developing GBS. Others emphasize that no one knows what their risk for GBS would be without the administration of cyclosporine. Because of the variability of the body's immune response, the benefits of this drug will depend on whether, in a given individual, it is an antibody response or T-cell response. Cyclosporine will benefit those who have a strong T-cell response. T-cell reactivity can be tested with the mixed lymphocyte assay, and T-cell counts can be done.

Cerebrospinal fluid filtration is also being tried in order to remove antibodies. Serum so filtered loses its nerve-inhibiting effect, as evidenced by its application to in vitro nerve and muscle cells. GBS has been mimicked in animal models, which show antibody and T-cell reactivity to myelin protein. Guillain-Barré syndrome has many of the characteristics of an autoimmune disease and could serve as a model for an acquired autoimmune condition.

Not related to the neurology of this sudden-onset disease, but equally devastating, is the protracted psychological impact of simultaneously being able to think and have emotions while not being able to move limbs, fingers, toes, and facial and eye muscles. Even though most patients recover, progress is always torturously slow, as the myelin sheath gradually regenerates. Ongoing psychological support is an important element in treating these patients.

Perspective and Prospects

Guillain-Barré syndrome is an example of a delicate physiological balance gone awry. The immune system has the difficult task of distinguishing between self and enemy, and if it detects the latter it must either inactivate or eliminate the intruder. Mistakes in recognition or communication between immune cells can cause either an unintended attack or the failure to attack when appropriate. GBS probably represents an unnecessary self-attack on tissue, in this case myelin, and may be considered a form of hyperimmunity. Many diseases fall into this category. They include rheumatoid arthritis, juvenile diabetes, Crohn's disease, ulcerative colitis, Graves' disease, multiple sclerosis, amyotrophic lateral sclerosis, ankylosing spondylitis (inflammation of the joints between the vertebrae), and systemic lupus erythematosus. The other type of response, hypoimmune, is seen in cancer and immunodeficiency diseases such as acquired immunodeficiency syndrome (AIDS).

Questions that arise with GBS are the same ones that arise in many other diseases. It must be determined why the immune system chose this time to initiate an attack against a self-antigen. The answer could be a mistake in recognition, an error in translating the deoxyribonucleic acid (DNA) code in the bone marrow cells, an alteration of the antigen by some environmental factor, or an alteration of an antigen-detector protein on a white blood cell. Researchers also try to discover if there is a genetic predisposition for GBS. Seeking answers about GBS may shed light on other conditions as well, and treatments beneficial to GBS patients have a high probability of benefiting patients with other immune disorders. GBS is a reminder that physiological stress can translate to immunological stress, and under stress the immune system can make mistakes.

—*William D. Niemi, Ph.D.*

See also Ataxia; Autoimmune disorders; Electromyography; Immune system; Immunology; Motor neuron diseases; Nervous system; Neuralgia, neuritis, and neuropathy; Neurology; Neurology, pediatric; Numbness and tingling; Paralysis; Stress.

For Further Information:

Abbas, Abul K., Andrew H. Lichtman, and Shiv Pillai. *Basic Immunology: Functions and Disorders of the Immune System.* 4th ed. Philadelphia: Saunders/Elsevier, 2012.

Adelman, Daniel C., et al., eds. *Manual of Allergy and Immunology.* 5th ed. Philadelphia: Lippincott Williams & Wilkins, 2012.

Baron-Faust, Rita, and Jill P. Buyon. *The Autoimmune Connection.* Chicago: Contemporary Books, 2003.

"Guillain-Barré Syndrome." *Genetics Home Reference,* May 13, 2013.

"Guillain-Barré Syndrome." *Medline Plus,* May 21, 2012.

"Guillain-Barré Syndrome Fact Sheet." *National Institute of Neurological Disorders and Stroke,* August 19, 2011.

Kierman, John A., and Nagalingam Rajakumar. *Barr's The Human Nervous System: An Anatomical Viewpoint.* 10th ed. Philadelphia: Wolters Kluwer/Lippincott Williams & Wilkins, 2013.

Lechtenberg, Richard. *Synopsis of Neurology.* Philadelphia: Lea & Febiger, 1991.

Nicholls, John G., et al. *From Neuron to Brain.* 5th ed. Sunderland, Mass.: Sinauer, 2011.

Noback, Charles R., et al. *The Human Nervous System: Structure and Function.* 6th ed. Totowa, N.J.: Humana Press, 2005.

Parker, James N., and Philip M. Parker, eds. *The Official Patient's Sourcebook on Guillain-Barré Syndrome.* San Diego, Calif.: Icon Health, 2002.

Pearlman, Alan L., and Robert C. Collins. *Neurobiology of Disease.* New York: Oxford University Press, 1990.

Sticherling, Michael, and Enno Christophers, eds. *Treatment of Autoimmune Disorders.* New York: Springer, 2003.

GULF WAR SYNDROME

Disease/Disorder

Anatomy or system affected: Blood, brain, cells, chest, eyes, gastrointestinal system, gums, hair, immune system, joints, muscles, psychic-emotional system, skin

Specialties and related fields: Biochemistry, environmental health, epidemiology, ethics, occupational health, psychology, public health

Definition: A popular term used to describe collectively a variety of symptoms, not a specific disease, suffered by veterans of the Gulf War.

Key terms:

cytokines: proteins which are used by white blood cells to communicate with similar cells

organophosphates: chemical pesticides

pyridostigmine bromide: a chemical that prevents damage from possible nerve gas exposure

sarin: a nerve gas that can cause convulsions and death

Causes and Symptoms

A 2008 report by the US Department of Veterans Affairs, Research Advisory Committee on Gulf War Veterans" Illnesses, concluded that what has been called Gulf War syndrome should be recognized as an illness, characterized by a complex of multiple symptoms, that resulted from service in the 1990–1991 Gulf War. This illness affected more than 25 percent of the 700,000 veterans of this war.

Gulf War syndrome is characterized by flulike symptoms, which sufferers complain of experiencing simultaneously but that do not indicate any specific known disease. Such physical symptoms include chronic fatigue, fever, muscle and joint pain and weakness, and intense headaches. Some patients report episodes of memory loss, insomnia, nightmares, and limited attention spans as well as neuropsychological disorders, such as depression, anxiety attacks, and mood swings. Respiratory problems, diarrhea and gastrointestinal distress, blurred vision, arthritis, bleeding gums, hair loss, and skin

Information on Gulf War Syndrome

Causes: Unclear; possibly exposure to wartime toxins, bacteria, or viruses; psychosomatic factors; post-traumatic stress disorder

Symptoms: Vary widely; can include chronic fatigue, fever, muscle and joint pain and weakness, intense headaches, episodes of memory loss, insomnia, nightmares, anxiety attacks, mood swings, respiratory problems, blurred vision, rashes

Duration: Chronic

Treatments: Self-medication with over-the-counter pain relievers, prescribed drug and physical therapy, counseling

rashes sometimes accompany other symptoms.

When returning veterans first complained about these symptoms, physicians disagreed about the causal factors of Gulf War syndrome. Many of the symptoms could also be signs of other war-related disorders, such as post-traumatic stress disorder (PTSD), or exposure to wartime toxins, bacteria, or viruses. Furthermore, it was difficult for researchers to prove any laboratory abnormality or unique characteristic for this disorder or to isolate any organ system as the primary system affected by this condition. Given this, most medical professionals assumed that Gulf War syndrome was a condition representing factors of several diseases but that is not a separate disease. This diagnostic ambiguity frustrated many Gulf War veterans, who wanted and needed accurate diagnoses and effective treatments.

Gulf War illness is associated with biological alterations primarily in the nervous system and brain. Strong evidence exists that the illness is associated with exposure to two types of neurotoxins: pyridostigmine bromide (PB) pills, which had been intended to protect humans from the effects of nerve agents; and organophosphate pesticides, used during deployment. Early evidence suggested that the illness was related to exposure to substances such as multiple vaccines or fumes from burning oil wells, but these causes have since been ruled out. What is clear, however, is that Gulf War illness is not just PTSD. It is true that some Gulf War veterans have PTSD, but this does not explain the separate problem of Gulf War illness. A 2013 study published in *PLoS ONE* identified a number of characteristic brain changes in veterans with Gulf War syndrome, particularly increased axial diffusivity in the right inferior fronto-occipital fasciculus, a part of the brain involved in fatigue, pain, and emotional regulation. Researchers hope that this discovery will lead to the development of more accurate diagnostic criteria for Gulf War syndrome.

Treatment and Therapy

Because they do not think their concerns are being seriously addressed, many veterans rely on self-diagnosis based on other veterans" accounts exchanged orally, in the press, or on the Internet. Self-medication with over-the-counter pain relievers is a common treatment that many veterans depend on

for the alleviation of symptoms. Physicians prescribe more potent pharmaceuticals and physical therapy to alleviate symptoms and to reinforce patients" immune systems. The American, Canadian, and British governments have established medical programs through publicly funded veterans" administrations and privately endowed medical institutions to research the syndrome's causes, ascertain its etiology, identify derivative presentations of the syndrome, develop effective treatment methods, and offer medical care for veterans exhibiting Gulf War syndrome symptoms.

Physicians recommend that some veterans suffering Gulf War syndrome undergo counseling to address neuropsychological symptoms and to assist in the readjustment to peacetime or civilian life and the frustration with enduring a chronic and unidentified illness. Exercise, a nutritional diet, and support groups are also helpful to many veterans suffering Gulf War syndrome. Genetic testing of veterans and their spouses is also sometimes pursued to determine causation of birth defects in some veterans" children, which are often incorrectly attributed to Gulf War service. Complications associated with treatment of Gulf War syndrome include possible common side effects of pain relievers, such as drowsiness. Patients also risk becoming addicted to pain relievers that they use to numb the ever-present aches associated with chronic illnesses.

Perspective and Prospects

Originally identified when some American, British, and Canadian Gulf War veterans complained of various ailments after returning home in 1991, Gulf War syndrome was sensationalized in the press as a mystery illness. Physicians familiar with military medical history recognized similarities with symptoms documented in soldier populations as early as the American Civil War. This awareness suggested that the syndrome was indicative of a common wartime factor rather than a unique occurrence in the Gulf War.

Gulf War syndrome became politicized as government officials and veterans disagreed regarding the description of and funding for treatment of the syndrome. After clinical investigations of twenty thousand Gulf War veterans, the Institute of Medicine declared that no Gulf War syndrome existed, although some soldiers did suffer nonchronic illnesses, such as malaria. Five independent panels confirmed the conclusion that no unique case of an illness had been proven.

Physicians and scientists representing the Departments of Defense, Veterans Affairs, and Health and Human Services stated that the rates of incidence of Gulf War veterans" symptoms, hospitalization, and mortality are not greater than those reported for the general population and that many veterans may have already been genetically predisposed to certain physiological conditions. They also questioned why veterans from other countries, especially Arab nations, did not report syndrome symptoms, nor were any similar reports issued after World War II soldiers returned from the Persian Gulf.

In 2002, in what veterans called a "stunning reversal," the US Department of Defense admitted that there is increasing evidence that neural damage affects some veterans of the

Gulf War and doubled research funding. The change in stance was partly in response to research emanating from the University of Texas Southwestern Medical Center in Dallas and the US Department of Veterans Affairs. Using a statistical technique called factor analysis, researchers at these facilities identified unusual clusters of symptoms that could be divided into syndromes. Syndrome 1 involved sleep and memory disturbances, syndrome 3 involved joint and muscle pain, while syndrome 2, the most serious, involved confusion and dizziness. Using magnetic resonance spectroscopy (MRS), the research team found that veterans with syndrome 2 had lost nerve cells in the brain structures that are involved with the symptoms of the syndrome. Moreover, syndrome 2 veterans were also approximately eight times more likely as healthy veterans to have had a bad reaction to the PB tablets. Researchers surmise that chemical weapons and the PB tablets that were designed to protect against them affect the same physiological pathway. The increasing scientific evidence of real physiological damage among veterans has helped spur the US government to begin more strenuous investigation into its causes. In 2002, the Department of Veterans Affairs appointed a Research Advisory Committee on Gulf War Veterans" Illnesses.

This committee's 2008 report provided a clearer focus for developing better treatment for Gulf War illness and a focus on how this illness may interact with other conditions. Research in this area continues through federally mandated treatment programs with the Veterans Administration (VA) and through work done independently by universities.

—*Elizabeth D. Schafer, Ph.D.*

See also Biological and chemical weapons; Environmental diseases; Environmental health; Epidemiology; Poisoning; Toxicology.

For Further Information:

Blanck, Ronald R., et al. "Unexplained Illnesses Among Desert Storm Veterans: A Search for Causes, Treatment, and Cooperation." *Archives of Internal Medicine* 155 (February 13, 1995): 262–268.

Bloom, Saul, et al. *Hidden Casualties: Environmental, Health, and Political Consequences of the Persian Gulf War.* Berkeley, Calif.: Arms Control Research Center, North Atlantic Books, 1994.

Eddington, Patrick G. *Gassed in the Gulf: The Inside Story of the Pentagon-CIA Cover-up of Gulf War Syndrome.* Washington, D.C.: Insignia, 1997.

"Gulf War and Health: Treatment for Chronic Multisymptom Illness." *Institute of Medicine of the National Academies*, January 2013.

Hersh, Seymour M. *Against All Enemies: Gulf War Syndrome, the War Between America's Ailing Veterans and Their Government.* New York: Ballantine Books, 1998.

Office of the Secretary of Defense. National Defense Research Institution. *A Review of the Scientific Literature as It Pertains to Gulf War Illnesses.* 8 vols. Santa Monica, Calif.: RAND, 1998–2001.

Rayhan, Rakib U., et al. "Increased Brain White Matter Axial Diffusivity Associated with Fatigue, Pain and Hyperalgesia in Gulf War Illness." *PLoS ONE* 8, no. 3 (March 20, 2013): e58493.

Research Advisory Committee on Gulf War Veterans" Illnesses. *Gulf War Illness and the Health of Gulf War Veterans: Scientific Findings and Recommendations.* Washington, D.C.: Government Printing Office, 2008.

Steele, Lea, Antonio Sastre, Mary M. Gerkovich, and Mary R. Cook. "Complex Factors in the Etiology of Gulf War Illness: Wartime Exposures and Risk Factors in Veteran Subgroups." *Environmental Health Perspectives* 120, no. 1 (January, 2012): 112–118.

Wheelwright, Jeff. *The Irritable Heart: The Medical Mystery of the Gulf War.* New York: W. W. Norton, 2001.

GUM DISEASE

Disease/Disorder
Anatomy or system affected: Gums, mouth, teeth
Specialties and related fields: Dentistry
Definition: Inflammation of the soft tissue that surrounds the teeth; in advanced disease, there is also loss of bone that holds the teeth in place.

Causes and Symptoms

Bacterial infection is the most common cause of gum disease. In the early stages of the disease, only the soft tissues—the gums, or gingiva—are affected, but in later stages bacteria also attack the hard tissues underlying the gums.

The bacteria responsible for gum disease accumulate in plaque, which is a sticky biofilm of bacteria that forms on the teeth above and below the gum line. Plaque that remains on the teeth for more than about seventy-two hours may harden into tartar, which cannot be removed completely except by a professional. Plaque accumulation is usually the result of inadequate tooth brushing and flossing.

Plaque contains many different kinds of bacteria. Bacteria that live below the gum line, where oxygen is low or lacking, are the main culprits in gingivitis, an inflammation of the soft gum tissues. Toxins produced by the bacteria destroy the collagen fibers that make up the connective tissue between the gum and the tooth, causing the gum to loosen and detach from the tooth. The widening and deepening of the space between tooth and gum produces a pocket. Whereas in healthy gums there is a crevice about 1 to 3 millimeters deep between the gum and tooth, in gingivitis there is a pocket up to 4 millimeters deep. The gum becomes movable instead of clinging to the tooth. The gum also swells, is red rather than a healthy pink, and bleeds when brushed or probed. At this early stage, there is little or no pain.

From a gum pocket, bacteria can advance to the bone and to the other hard tissues that support the tooth: the cementum, which covers the roots of the tooth, and the periodontal ligament, which anchors the tooth to the jawbone. Gum disease that has progressed to the bone is referred to as periodontitis. It usually results from a long-term accumulation of plaque

---

Information on Gum Disease

Causes: Bacterial infection
Symptoms: Red, swollen gums that bleed easily; may progress to bone loss. loose teeth, abscesses, and pain
Duration: Chronic and sometimes progressive
Treatments: Removal of plaque and tartar, antibiotics (oral and inserted into gum pockets), surgery

and tartar.

In early periodontitis, the crests or peaks of the bone between the teeth have begun to erode. The patient may as yet be unaware of the problem because there is no pain. As the inflammation destroys the fibers of the periodontal ligament and further dissolves the bone, the pocket often deepens to between 4 and 8 millimeters. In advanced stages, most of the bone surrounding the tooth is destroyed and the tooth loosens. Abscesses and pain are common at this point. Advanced periodontitis can cause teeth to fall out or require extraction and is one of the main causes of tooth loss in adults.

In both gingivitis and periodontitis, the damage may be localized. Furthermore, the disease does not progress at a uniform rate but instead advances episodically, with periods of remission. Most adults have had gingivitis at one time or another, but some individuals are especially susceptible, including those who smoke, have certain medical conditions, or take particular medications.

Treatment and Therapy

Gum disease is treatable. To diagnose the disease, the dentist may use x-rays to determine the extent of bone loss and a dental probe to measure the depth of pockets. The dentist removes plaque and tartar by scaling the surfaces of the teeth and planing the surfaces of the roots. An ultrasonic scaler, which cleans the teeth with high-frequency vibrations, may also be used. Once the bacterial biofilm has been removed, the gums are able to heal and reattach to the teeth, thereby shrinking the pockets.

Oral antibiotics are also useful in fighting periodontitis, though they are not effective for gingivitis. In addition, antibiotics inserted directly into deep gum pockets can deliver high concentrations directly to the infected area.

Surgery is performed on some patients, either by a general dentist or by a periodontist. Under local anesthesia, flaps of gum tissue are cut away from the underlying bone, thus allowing better access for scraping and cleaning the tooth roots and for correcting bone defects caused by the infection. Some of the infected gum tissue is also removed, and the remaining gum is sutured back in place.

An important tool in the fight against gum disease is good oral hygiene. Individuals should brush twice a day and use dental floss daily to remove plaque. In addition to toothpastes, effective cleaning agents include baking soda, peroxide, and some mouth rinses. A regular schedule of teeth cleaning by a dental professional is also essential. Depending on how fast a patient accumulates tartar, professional cleaning may be required every three to six months.

Perspective and Prospects

Humans have attempted to clean their teeth since prehistoric times. Early humans fashioned implements out of twigs and bone splinters to remove bits of food trapped between their teeth. Later, the toothpick became the main tooth-cleaning tool. The Chinese are credited with inventing the toothbrush around 1000 CE. It was not until the late 1930s, however, that

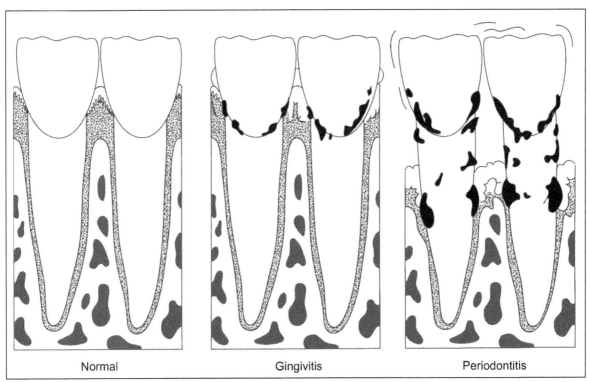

Normal	Gingivitis	Periodontitis

Gum disease begins with poor oral hygiene; if unchecked, it leads to gingivitis (inflammation and infection of the gums) and periodontitis (erosion of supporting bone and tooth loss).

an inexpensive toothbrush became available.

Research on the causes, prevention, and treatment of gum disease is being conducted at dental schools and at the National Institute of Dental and Cranio-Facial Research. Research areas include attempts to regenerate periodontal tissues. Bone grafting can help restore lost bone, and guided tissue regeneration may help re-create periodontal ligament.

—Jane F. Hill, Ph.D.

See also Cavities; Dental diseases; Dentistry; Endodontic disease; Gingivitis; Periodontal surgery; Periodontitis; Plaque, dental; Root canal treatment; Teeth; Tooth extraction; Toothache.

For Further Information:

Amyes, Sebastian G. B. *Bacteria: A Very Short Introduction.* Oxford: Oxford University Press, 2013.

Anand, Vishal, and Minkle Gulati. *Current Trends in Periodontics and Implant Dentistry.* Hauppauge, New York: Nova Science Publishers, 2013.

Blayden, Jessica, and Angie Mott. *Soft-Tissue Lasers in Dental Hygiene.* Oxford: Wiley-Blackwell, 2013.

Christensen, Gordon J. *A Consumer's Guide to Dentistry.* 2d ed. St. Louis, Mo.: Mosby, 2002.

Marsh, P. D. "Dental Plaque." In *Microbial Biofilms,* edited by Hilary Lappin-Scott and J. William Costerton. New York: Cambridge University Press, 1995.

National Institute of Dental and Craniofacial Research. *Periodontal (Gum) Disease: Causes, Symptoms, and Treatments.* Bethesda, Md.: U.S. Department of Health and Human Services, 2012.

Porter, Robert S., et al., eds. *The Merck Manual Home Health Handbook.* Whitehouse Station, N.J.: Merck Research Laboratories, 2009.

Purkait, Swapan Kumar. *Essentials of Oral Pathology.* New Delhi: Jaypee, 2011.

Serio, Francis G. *Understanding Dental Health.* Jackson: University of Mississippi Press, 1998.

Smith, Rebecca W. *The Columbia University School of Dental and Oral Surgery's Guide to Family Dental Care.* New York: W. W. Norton, 1997.

Wood, Debra. "Gingivitis (Gum Disease)." *Health Library,* September 12, 2012.

GYNECOLOGY

Specialty

Anatomy or system affected: Breasts, genitals, reproductive system, uterus

Specialties and related fields: Endocrinology, family medicine, obstetrics, oncology, psychiatry, psychology

Definition: The branch of medicine concerned with the diseases and disorders that are specific to women, particularly those of the genital tract, as well as women's health, endocrinology, reproductive physiology, family planning, and contraceptive use.

Key terms:

menarche: the onset of menstrual cycles in a woman

menopause: the permanent cessation of menstrual cycles, signifying the conclusion of a woman's reproductive life

menstruation: the cyclic bleeding that normally occurs, usually in the absence of pregnancy, during the reproductive period of the human female; typically occurs at twenty-eight-day intervals

Pap test: a screening test for precancer and cancer of the cervix; it is performed by placing a sample of cervical cells on a microscope slide along with a preservative solution or by placing the cells into a small container filled with preservative solution

puberty: the physiological sequence of events by which a child acquires the reproductive capacities of an adult; the growth of secondary sexual characteristics occurs, reproductive functions begin, and the differences between males and females are accentuated

Science and Profession

Gynecology is the branch of medical science that treats the functions and diseases unique to women, particularly in the nonpregnant state. A gynecologist is a licensed medical doctor who has obtained specialty training. Unlike many fields in medicine that are clearly defined by surgical or nonsurgical practice, gynecology involves both. In the early nineteenth century, gynecology was closely tied to general surgery. In fact, one of the first reported cases of abdominal surgery in which the patient survived and was cured of a condition occurred in 1809, with the successful removal of a massive ovarian tumor by Ephraim McDowell (without the benefit of anesthesia or antibiotics).

Gynecology is much more than just a surgical field. With the tremendous progress made in the basic sciences and medical sciences by the twenty-first century, gynecology now involves a broad spectrum of medical fields, including developmental and congenital disorders relating to puberty and adolescence, sexually transmitted infections (STIs) and other infectious diseases, contraception, menstrual disturbances, endocrinology, early pregnancy issues, infertility, preventive health, problems related to menopause, incontinence, and oncology, specifically dealing with cancers of the reproductive system (such as the ovaries, uterus, and breasts). Although much gynecologic care is provided by medical doctors, routine gynecologic care is also often provided by nurse practitioners (especially those with specialty certification in women's health) and certified nurse midwives.

Many of the medical problems dealt with in gynecology have far-reaching social, ethical, and legal consequences. Among the most controversial issues in medicine today involve abortion and STDs (such as human immunodeficiency virus, or HIV), both of which are conditions commonly managed by gynecologists. Another example of a common problem managed by gynecologists with important social implications is contraception. Female steroid hormones were among the first biological substances to be purified in the laboratory in the twentieth century. These hormones were then intentionally fed to animals for their contraceptive effect and eventually given to human beings as well in the form of the birth control pill. The birth control pill is an invention that has been widely credited with providing women with a relatively easy means to control their own fertility. Many social scholars would argue that women's ability to harness their own fertility was key in enabling women to delay childbearing, pursue education and careers, and take roles in society that were formerly occupied almost exclusively by men.

To understand gynecology, it is first necessary to have a working knowledge of relevant female anatomy and physiology. Broadly, the female reproductive organs are divided into two groups, external and internal. Within each group are many specific components, most of which are analogous to structures in the male because they are derived from the same sources during embryological development. The external organs are the vulva (the fleshy "lips" covered with skin), vagina, and clitoris; the internal organs are the uterus (including the cervix), Fallopian tubes, and ovaries. These organs mature during puberty and communicate with regions of the brain, specifically the hypothalamus and pituitary, to coordinate function.

The vagina is a tube of tissue that connects the vulva with the uterus. In adult females, it is nine to ten centimeters in length. When a woman is standing upright, the vagina extends upward and backward from the opening to the uterus. There is a slight cup-like expansion near the uterus. It is here that the actual connection between the vagina and uterus is made through a muscular structure called the cervix. The muscles of the vagina are normally constricted, thus closing the tube. The vagina can stretch to accommodate a penis during intercourse and a fetus during birth.

The cervix is a ring of muscle; the central opening is called the cervical os. Throughout most of the month, the cervical os forms a tight barrier. When the lining of the uterus is sloughed during a menstrual period, the cervix relaxes slightly. During childbirth, the cervix dilates to ten centimeters (about four inches).

The uterus is a hollow, thick-walled, muscular organ. It normally forms a right angle with the vagina, angling upward and anteriorly. The bladder is immediately anterior to the uterus. In a nonpregnant woman, the uterus is pear-shaped. In a woman who has never been pregnant, it is eight centimeters in length, six centimeters wide, and four centimeters thick. It increases in size during pregnancy; after birth, it shrinks but does not quite return to its size prior to pregnancy. The lining of the uterus is shed approximately every twenty-eight days during a normal menstrual period.

The Fallopian tubes are two canals that transport eggs from the ovaries to the uterus. The Fallopian tube is the site where sperm meet the egg and fertilization occurs. The tubes are wide near the ovaries and become narrow toward the uterus. The ovaries are two almond-shaped bodies found in the pelvic cavity, and they brush up against the Fallopian tubes. The ovaries are about 3.5 by 2 by 1.5 centimeters in size, although there can be much variation. The ovaries contain eggs, which are released at monthly intervals between puberty and menopause.

Diagnostic and Treatment Techniques

Many gynecologic visits are done for routine screening of healthy women. When a patient presents with a problem or complaint, a good history from the patient regarding the nature of the problem is crucial for diagnosis. The history is almost always followed by a physical examination. Probably the best known diagnostic technique in gynecology is the pelvic examination. Women should have routine screening examinations beginning at age twenty-one, or three years after onset of sexual activity, whichever age is first. The purpose of the examination is to confirm normal anatomy, rule out pathological conditions, and prevent the development of cancers through early screening tests such as the Pap test.

The pelvic examination is typically performed with the woman on her back, knees apart, with feet and legs supported by stirrups. Visual inspection of the external genitalia is performed; this involves inspecting the pubic region to ensure normal secondary sexual development as well as to look for abnormalities such as unusual lesions on the labia, which may indicate infections (by fungi, bacteria, viruses, or parasites), skin conditions (such as eczema), or cancer. The next portion is a bimanual examination. The examiner places one hand on the patient's abdomen and gently inserts two fingers of the other hand into the patient's vagina; gloves are worn at all times. The examiner proceeds to feel the uterus and ovaries by gently pushing them toward the anterior abdomen. The external hand on the abdomen serves as a counterforce to enable the examiner to feel the contours of the uterus and ovaries and hence to assess their size.

The last portion of the examination is a visual inspection of the interior of the vagina and the surface of the cervix. Because the vagina is normally closed, a device called a speculum is carefully placed in the vaginal canal. The speculum has two "blades"—each blade is analogous to a

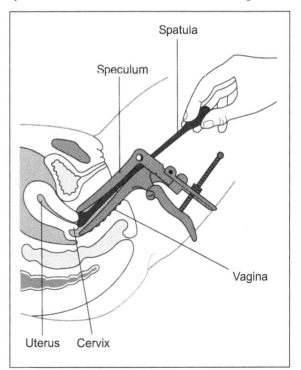

A routine gynecological examination includes a Pap smear, in which a spatula is used to perform a biopsy of the cervix for laboratory analysis.

tongue depressor, which pushes the tongue out of the way to enable inspection of the throat. The blades are then slowly opened to part the vaginal tissues and enable visualization of the vaginal canal and cervix. The vaginal walls and cervix are inspected for abnormalities, and the consistency of vaginal fluid is noted. If any abnormalities are noted, cultures or biopsies may taken to facilitate diagnosis. When indicated, a Pap test is performed by swabbing the exterior of the cervix as well as the cervical canal. The cells that are obtained from the swab can then be sent to the pathology laboratory for analysis to screen for precancer or cancer of the cervix.

Although the bimanual examination is the mainstay of office practice, this examination is but a small fraction of diagnostic modalities commonly employed by gynecologists. A complete physical examination, including breast examination, is often performed for a comprehensive survey to aid in diagnosis. When abnormalities are suspected, imaging techniques and laboratory tests can be invaluable in diagnosis. For instance, when a pelvic mass is felt on bimanual examination, the gynecologist may order an ultrasound to better characterize the mass. Laboratory tests such as CA-125 levels may be indicated to help differentiate the pelvic mass from a benign growth versus a malignancy, such as of the ovary.

Other diagnostic tests commonly employed in gynecological office practices are blood and urine tests for pregnancy, blood or culture tests (for STIs such as HIV, syphilis, gonorrhea, chlamydia, and herpes), and biopsies of the external genitalia, which may assist in diagnosing skin conditions such as lichen sclerosis or precancers. If an endocrinologic abnormality is suspected, then blood tests to check the levels of various hormones (such as thyroid hormone, follicle-stimulating hormone, or prolactin) can help pinpoint the problem. In a patient with urinary incontinence, urodynamic testing, which records the pressures of the bladder and abdomen under different conditions, may help diagnose and characterize the type of incontinence.

A number of diagnostic tests commonly employed by gynecologists require going to an operating room, most often because of the need for patient sedation or anesthesia. One example is hysteroscopy, whereby a small camera mounted on a cannula is introduced through the cervix to visualize the cervical canal and uterine lining. Hysteroscopy can be useful in the diagnosis of polyps or fibroids (benign tumors of the uterus) which may be causing abnormal vaginal bleeding. Another example is diagnostic laparoscopy, whereby a small camera mounted on a cannula is introduced into the abdominal and pelvic cavity to inspect for abnormalities such as pelvic scarring, masses, or endometriosis, a condition in which cells resembling the uterine lining are found in the pelvic or abdominal cavities.

Gynecologic providers have a vast array of treatment options available to them. In the office setting, common treatment modalities include the use of antibiotics for uncomplicated cervical infections, such as chlamydia and gonorrhea, or for vaginal infections, such as trichomoniasis. Another problem commonly treated in the office setting is undesired fertility. A number of contraceptive modalities exist, includ-

ing the prescription of birth control pills, the placement of an intrauterine device (IUD), or the injection of sustained-release hormones. In women experiencing menopausal symptoms such as hot flashes, hormonal pills or other medications may be prescribed. Women with chronic pelvic pain may be treated with medications such as antidepressants. Urinary incontinence may respond to bladder training, pessaries, or medications.

In the operating room, procedures may be carried out in a controlled setting to treat disease. A woman with abnormal vaginal bleeding caused by fibroids who no longer desires childbearing may receive a hysterectomy, with or without removal of the ovaries. If a woman is interested in retaining her uterus, the fibroids can be isolated and removed surgically through a common surgical procedure called a myomectomy. In women who desire permanent sterilization, a common surgical procedure performed by gynecologists is tubal ligation. Another common surgical procedure is the removal of pelvic masses such as ovarian cysts. Endometriosis or pelvic scars can be removed or destroyed through laparotomy (also known as abdominal surgery) or laparoscopy (minimally invasive abdominal surgery). When a Pap test or biopsy indicates noninvasive cancer of the cervix, treatment is possible through excision of the part of the cervix surrounding the cancer. In women with urinary incontinence not helped by medical management, surgery may be indicated to treat the problem. Women who are infertile as a result of blocked Fallopian tubes can be treated with in vitro fertilization. In this procedure, eggs are harvested from the woman in the operating room, and fertilization is performed in the laboratory. When the embryos are sufficiently developed, they are placed in the uterine cavity through an office procedure.

Perspective and Prospects

The formation of a medical field specific to women's diseases largely began in the nineteenth century. At the time, the treatment of women's diseases was inextricably linked with the role of women in society. In the nineteenth century, women were often viewed as frail and limited by their cyclical physiology and childbearing role. Consequently, they were excluded from the male-dominated spheres of politics, professional careers, and education. For instance, influential psychiatrist Henry Maudsley (1835–1918) wrote about the harm that higher education would cause to the physiologic development of postpubescent girls. Edward Clarke (1820–1877), a Harvard Medical School professor, wrote in 1873 that higher education might develop the intellect, but at the expense of the reproductive organs, leading to painful menstrual periods and abnormal uterine function.

The field has evolved dramatically since then, with much of the evolution tied to changes in the role of women in society as well as to technological and scientific advances. Today, one of the major forces changing gynecological practice (as well as many other fields of medicine) is the concept of evidence-based medicine. This movement is based on the idea that medical practice must be guided by scientific evidence as well as good intentions. Without objective evidence that a treatment is effective, even the best of intentions can result in patient harm. Although a physician may practice evidence-based medicine, this does not mean that clinical judgment and the tailoring of treatments to fit individual patients should be ignored. In fact, applying scientific evidence in an automatic way to all patients is not endorsed. Gynecologists today most often practice evidence-based medicine either by examining the available literature themselves, by using evidence-based medical summaries developed by others, or by using evidence-based protocols developed by others.

One example of evidence-based medicine guiding clinical practice involves Pap testing. Although the classical teaching had been that Pap tests were recommended on a yearly basis, this frequency was not based on any direct evidence that this protocol would lead to better outcomes than screening less frequently. Consequently, both the US Preventive Services Task Force and the American Cancer Society have suggested lengthening the period between successive Pap tests in women thirty years of age or older who have had negative results on three or more consecutive Pap tests. In fact, the Preventive Services Task Force recommends Pap tests be performed "at least every three years" rather than every year. The optimum use of limited resources is of concern to patients, physicians, health maintenance organizations (HMOs), and insurance companies alike; the careful application of evidence-based medicine to appropriate situations in medical practice can result in the best overall benefit for all parties involved.

—*Anne Lynn S. Chang, M.D.*

See also Abortion; Amenorrhea; Assisted reproductive technologies; Biopsy; Breast biopsy; Breast cancer; Breast disorders; Breasts, female; Cervical, ovarian, and uterine cancers; Cervical procedures; Chlamydia; Circumcision, female, and genital mutilation; Conception; Contraception; Culdocentesis; Cyst removal; Cystectomy; Cystitis; Cysts; Dysmenorrhea; Electrocauterization; Endocrinology; Endometrial biopsy; Endometriosis; Endoscopy; Episiotomy; Fibrocystic breast condition; Gamete intrafallopian transfer (GIFT); Gender reassignment surgery; Genital disorders, female; Glands; Gonorrhea; Herpes; Hormone therapy; Hot flashes; Human papillomavirus (HPV); Hysterectomy; In vitro fertilization; Incontinence; Infertility, female; Laparoscopy; Mammography; Mastectomy and lumpectomy; Mastitis; Menopause; Menorrhagia; Menstruation; Myomectomy; Nutrition; Obstetrics; Ovarian cysts; Ovaries; Pap test; Pelvic inflammatory disease (PID); Placenta; Postpartum depression; Preeclampsia and eclampsia; Pregnancy and gestation; Premenstrual syndrome (PMS); Rape and sexual assault; Reproductive system; Sexual dysfunction; Sexuality; Sexually transmitted diseases (STDs); Sterilization; Syphilis; Toxic shock syndrome; Tubal ligation; Ultrasonography; Urethritis; Urinary disorders; Urology; Uterus; Warts; Women's health.

For Further Information:

Berek, Jonathan S., and Emil Novak, eds. *Berek and Novak's Gynecology.* 15th ed. Philadelphia: Wolter Kuwer Health/Lippincott Williams & Wilkins, 2012.

Clifford, Annie, et al. *Obstetrics, Gynaecology and Women's Health on the Move.* London: Hodder Arnold, 2012.

Collins, Sally, et al. *Oxford Handbook of Obstetrics and Gynaecology.* [N.p.]: Oxford University Press, 2013.

Doherty, Gerard M., and Lawrence W. Way, eds. *Current Surgical Diagnosis and Treatment.* 12th ed. New York: Lange Medical Books/McGraw-Hill, 2006.

Kasper, Dennis L., et al., eds. *Harrison's Principles of Internal Medicine.* 16th ed. New York: McGraw-Hill, 2005.

Norsigan, Judy, and Boston Women's Health Collective. *Our Bodies, Ourselves: A New Edition for a New Era.* Rev. ed. New York: Touchstone, 2011.

Norwitz, Errol R. *Obstetrics and Gynecology at a Glance.* [N.p.]: Wiley, 2013.

Rushing, Lynda, and Nancy Joste. *Abnormal Pap Smears: What Every Woman Needs to Know.* Rev. ed. Amherst, N.Y.: Prometheus Books, 2008.

Scott, James R., et al., eds. *Danforth's Obstetrics and Gynecology.* 10th ed. Philadelphia: Lippincott Williams & Wilkins, 2008.

Speroff, Leon, and Marc A. Fritz. *Clinical Gynecologic Endocrinology and Infertility.* 8th ed. Philadelphia: Wolters Kluwer Health/ Lippincott Williams & Wilkins, 2011.

Stenchever, Morton A., et al. *Comprehensive Gynecology.* 5th ed. St. Louis, Mo.: Mosby/Elsevier, 2007.

Stewart, Elizabeth Gunther, and Paula Spencer. *The V Book: A Doctor's Guide to Complete Vulvovaginal Health.* New York: Bantam Books, 2002.

Tierney, Lawrence M., Stephen J. McPhee, and Maxine A. Papadakis, eds. *Current Medical Diagnosis and Treatment.* 50th ed. Los Altos, Calif.: Lange Medical Publications, 2011.

Weschler, Toni. *Taking Charge of Your Fertility.* 10th anniversary ed., Rev. ed. New York: Collins, 2006.

GYNECOMASTIA

Disease/Disorder

Anatomy or system affected: Breasts, chest, endocrine system, glands

Specialties and related fields: Endocrinology

Definition: An enlargement of the glandular part of the male breast that may affect one or both breasts and be painless or painful.

Causes and Symptoms

True gynecomastia must be distinguished from malignant or benign breast tumors and from enlargement of the fatty part of the breast due to obesity. Causes of gynecomastia include normal physiological changes with aging, endocrine diseases, other diseases such as chronic liver or kidney disease, tumors, and many drugs.

Some newborn boys may have swollen breasts as a result of the maternal estrogen to which they are exposed during pregnancy. This condition usually lasts for a few weeks following the newborn's birth. This enlargement may be accompanied by the secretion of milk, known as galactorrhea. Also, as boys go through puberty, up to 70 percent will experience gynecomastia, usually between the ages of twelve and fifteen. It is usually one-sided, but it may involve both breasts either at the same time or sequentially. This normally subsides within a year; the only treatment is reassurance that it will resolve on its own.

In athletes who take androgens and anabolic steroids, about half will develop gynecomastia. Other drugs that can cause this problem include alcohol, cimetidine, diazepam, diethylstilbestrol, digitalis, estrogens, some tranquilizers, many of the drugs used to treat schizophrenia, marijuana, methadone, synthetic narcotics, growth hormone, and

Information on Gynecomastia

Causes: Normal physiological changes, endocrine diseases, diseases such as chronic liver or kidney disease, tumors, maternal estrogen during pregnancy, certain drugs (androgens, anabolic steroids, alcohol, cimetidine, diazepam, DES, digitalis, estrogens, some tranquilizers, schizophrenia drugs, marijuana, methadone, synthetic narcotics, growth hormone, tricyclic antidepressants)

Symptoms: Enlargement of breasts in males, sometimes with milk secretion

Duration: For normal causes, less than one year

Treatments: None (self-resolving), cessation of drug use

tricyclic antidepressants.

Elderly men, particularly if they gain weight, may also develop gynecomastia because of the changes in the balance between male and female hormones that come with aging.

Types of cancer treatment leading to gynecomastia include drugs for lung, prostate, and testicular cancers. Likewise, tumors of the adrenal gland may cause this problem. Sometimes the enlargement of the breast tissue is the first sign of some serious underlying disease, but often it occurs for no apparent reason.

Men who develop gynecomastia where the cause is not obvious should have a radiographic study of the chest performed, along with blood studies to measure hormones such as prolactin, testosterone, luteinizing hormone, estradiol, and thyroid hormones. Some men may require genetic testing to determine the cause of their gynecomastia. Finally, a needle biopsy may be necessary.

Treatment and Therapy

The treatment of gynecomastia depends upon the cause. In the case of infant or pubertal boys, nothing is required but time for the problem to resolve on its own. When the condition is the result of a drug, it will usually resolve once the drug is stopped. Weight loss is indicated where the appearance of gynecomastia is attributable to obesity. Treating endocrine disorders, other illnesses, and tumors usually resolves the gynecomastia.

When the problem is painful, it may be treated with an antiestrogen drug. Severe or persistent gynecomastia may be treated by surgical means, although the results are not entirely satisfactory. In some cases, liposuction via the armpit and mastectomy performed under the skin may improve the situation.

—*Rebecca Lovell Scott, Ph.D., PA-C*

See also Breast cancer; Breast disorders; Breasts, female; Endocrine system; Endocrinology; Endocrinology, pediatric; Glands; Hormones; Men's health; Neonatology; Pediatrics; Puberty and adolescence.

For Further Information:

"Gynecomastia." *Medline Plus*, July 26, 2011.

"Gynecomastia (Enlarged Breasts in Men)." *Mayo Clinic*, December 21, 2010.

Komaroff, Anthony, ed. *Harvard Medical School Family Health Guide*. New York: Free Press, 2005.

Masters, William H., Virginia E. Johnson, and Robert C. Kolodny. *Human Sexuality*. 5th ed. New York: HarperCollins College, 1995.

Porter, Robert S., et al., eds. *The Merck Manual of Diagnosis and Therapy*. 19th ed. Whitehouse Station, N.J.: Merck, 2011.

Shannon, Diane W. "Gynecomastia." *Health Library*, September 27, 2012.

Hair

Anatomy

Anatomy or system affected: Hair, skin
Specialties and related fields: Dermatology
Definition: Threadlike outgrowths of nonliving, mostly proteinaceous material that cover much of the body of humans and other mammals.

Key terms:

alopecia: hair loss, especially if noticeable or significant
alopecia areata: loss of hair in patches
follicle: the structure in skin that manufactures hair
hirsutism: excessive hair growth

Structure and Functions

Humans grow three kinds of hair. The downy hair that covers the fetus is lanugo. Soon after birth, it is replaced by vellus (or villus) hair. Vellus hair covers the entire skin surface except for the palms of the hands and the soles of the feet. It is fine, short, nearly colorless, and slow-growing.

The thick, pigmented hair on the head, eyebrows, and eyelids is terminal hair. Somewhere between 65 and 95 percent (by weight) of terminal hair is protein. Other components include water, fats (lipids), trace elements (minerals), and pigment. Because proteins twist into complex three-dimensional shapes held together by chemical bonds, hair is both rigid and flexible. Terminal hair replaces villus hair on the genitals at puberty. Called pubic hair, it is coarse and curly. Also at puberty, terminal hair begins to grow in the armpits and on the faces of males.

The shaft of a single hair has three layers. The outer casing is the cuticle, made of overlapping layers of proteinaceous material. Inside the cuticle lies the cortex, a column of cells containing keratin, the same protein that hardens tooth enamel and fingernails. The central core of the hair is the medulla. Also called the pith, it is made of small, hardened cells snared in a web of fine filaments.

Hair grows from a tiny pouch below the skin's surface called a follicle. At the bottom of the follicle lies the papilla, an upward-growing finger of connective tissue. The papilla forms the root of the hair shaft. The actively growing part of the hair shaft is the hair bulb. The cells that generate the hair lie just above the hair bulb. As soon as hair cells are manufactured, they harden and die, forming the hair shaft.

Tiny blood vessels around each follicle supply nutrients. Sebaceous glands that open into the follicle produce the oily sebum that lubricates hair and skin. In the papilla of the follicle, melanocytes produce melanin, the same pigment that gives skin its color. There are two kinds of melanin: Eumelanin makes hair black or brown, while pheomelanin makes it red or blond. Melanin is deposited in the cortex of the hair shaft of terminal hair, giving it its color.

Hair helps insulate the body. Arrector pili muscles at the base of the follicle elevate hair in response to environmental stimuli, including cold. The high sulfur content of keratin gives it heat-retaining properties. Hair also retards water loss from the body. Body hair augments the sense of touch. Hair's movement facilitates the detection of light touches and slight temperature changes.

Terminal hair cushions the head against blows and protects the scalp from sunburn. Eyelashes keep dirt, insects, and foreign objects out of the eyes. Eyebrows keep sweat from running down into the eyes. The hair inside the ears is coated with the waxy substance cerumen that traps dirt and prevents infections. Hair in the nose filters dust and bacteria from the air.

Hair growth and replacement occur in three stages. Anagen is the active growth stage. It lasts from two to six years. During catagen, lasting about two weeks, the lower segment of the hair follicle breaks down. A "club hair" separates from the papilla and falls out. Then, during telogen, the follicle "rests." Telogen lasts several weeks or months. At any one time, about 80 to 90 percent of the hairs on the head are in anagen, 3 to 4 percent are in catagen, and the remainder are in telogen.

Disorders and Diseases

While a loss of fifty to one hundred scalp hairs per day is normal, alopecia, or noticeable hair loss, occurs in nearly one-third of women and two-thirds of men. Women typically notice a general thinning of the hair, while men usually experience male pattern baldness: loss at the hairline and crown first, followed by loss at top of the head. The cause is neither a loss of follicles nor a cessation of hair growth. Instead, follicles gradually shrink and become less active, producing shorter, finer vellus hairs. Three interacting factors—heredity, hormones, and aging—cause the change in follicles. Genetic programming controls the age when hair loss begins and how fast it progresses. Male hormones (even in women) must be present for balding to occur.

No drug can reverse baldness in its later stages. However, minoxidil (trade name Rogaine) slows the rate of hair loss or promotes regrowth in about 25 percent of men and 20 percent of women. It received the approval of the Food and Drug Administration (FDA) in 1988 and became available without a prescription in 1996. Another drug, finasteride (trade name Propecia), was approved in 1997 for use in men only.

Surgical alternatives are available for those bothered by baldness. To transplant or graft hair, surgeons remove segments of scalp from the sides and back of the head (where follicles are less sensitive to hormones) and transfer them to the top. To perform a scalp reduction, surgeons cut away a portion of hairless scalp, then stitch the remaining scalp together, reducing the total area of baldness. Another alternative is flap surgery. A flap of hair-bearing scalp is turned to cover the spot where bald scalp has been removed.

Alopecia areata is the loss of hair in round patches, usually on the scalp, beard, eyebrows, or pubic area. It is thought to be an autoimmune disease. The immune system "mistakes" the hair follicles for invading disease agents and attacks them, reducing their size and decreasing hair production. The disorder may result from fever, stress, surgery, allergies, crash diets, burns, scalds, and tumors. Other possible causes include radiation exposure, an overactive or underactive thyroid

---

In the News:
Eyelash-Enhancing Drug Latisse

In December, 2008, the Food and Drug Administration (FDA) approved the prostaglandin bimatoprost (Latisse) for a predominantly cosmetic application, eyelash growth. Interest in the drug for eyelash enhancement began when ophthalmologists, who had been prescribing the drug since 2001 under the brand name Lumigen for open-angle glaucoma, began noticing that patients using the drug experienced a beneficial side effect—eyelashes that were darker, thicker, and longer than before.

A three-month proof of concept trial was undertaken to assess the change in subjects' eyelashes from baseline, and 80 percent (thirteen of sixteen) reported "much improved" and 19 percent reporting "improved" eyelash appearance. Growth or darkening of eyelashes was noticed by most subjects by week eight of a subsequent phase 3 clinical trial. The effects continued throughout the treatment period, but returned to baseline following discontinuation of the drug. Researchers think it may be possible to extend the benefits of the drug by tapering use to every few days once an acceptable eyelash length has been reached, but further study is warranted.

Latisse's formulation is identical to Lumigen, a 0.03 percent ophthalmic solution, but the method of application is different. Instead of being instilled into the eye, Latisse is applied to the skin of the upper eyelid just above the eyelashes with sterile disposable applicators.

The drug is not without potential problems; it can lead to itching and red eyes, as well as darkening of the skin in the area of application. There is a small chance that use could lead to a permanent change in eye color, though that is more likely to occur with Lumigen drops due to direct eye contact. A more likely occurrence is that hair growth could happen on unintended areas of the skin, so any excess is recommended to be blotted off. The drug is costly ($120 per month or more) and is unlikely to be covered by insurance. Consumers should beware of over-the-counter products containing unlisted prostaglandins; the FDA has seized some products containing these ingredients.

—*Karen Nagel, R.Ph., Ph.D.*

---

gland, liver or kidney disease, and illnesses ranging from influenza to scarlet fever. A deficiency of iron, zinc, or certain vitamins is the cause in some cases, as is chemotherapy for cancer. Hair loss is also a side effect of many drugs. Alopecia areata is seldom serious or permanent, but it can be disturbing. A doctor may prescribe drugs to combat it, but it generally resolves itself within a year.

Hirsutism, excessive hair growth on the face or body, can cause concern, especially for women. Although it can be triggered by tumors, diseases of the ovaries or adrenal glands, contraceptive pills, hormonal drugs, or anabolic steroids, the most common cause is the menopause. As production of the female hormone estrogen declines, the relative concentration of male hormones (produced naturally by the adrenal glands) rises, causing dark hairs to appear on the upper lip, chin, and cheeks. Shaving, tweezing, waxing, sugaring, or using depilatory creams and lotions removes hair temporarily. Electrolysis, in which a needle inserted into the follicle delivers a current that destroys the follicle, removes hair permanently. In severe cases, doctors may prescribe drugs that block the action of male hormones to treat hirsutism in women.

Perspective and Prospects

Since ancient times, people have sought to prevent or reverse the balding process. The Egyptians of the sixteenth century BCE prescribed a blend of iron, red lead, onions, and alabaster, along with prayers to the sun god. In 420 BCE, the Greek

Hippocrates, often called the founder of modern medicine, recommended a mixture of opium, horseradish, pigeon droppings, beetroot, and spices.

The concept of surgical hair transplantation arose in the early nineteenth century, and in the twentieth century reliable techniques were developed. Japanese physicians pioneered hair transplantation and grafting in the late 1930s and early 1940s, but it was not until the 1980s that procedures yielding cosmetically acceptable results were achieved in the United States. Drug treatments for baldness were discovered by chance as side effects. Minoxidil originally treated hypertension; finasteride ameliorated prostate enlargement.

Attempts to remove unwanted hair have roots in prehistory. Sharpened rocks and shells used for hair removal have been found in archaeological sites dating back twenty thousand years. The ancient Sumerians invented tweezers, and the Egyptians buried razors and arsenic-based depilatories with their dead. Native American men tweezed facial hair with clamshells, and North American colonists in the seventeenth century used caustic lye to burn hair away. In 1903, the American inventor King Gillette marketed the first razor with a disposable blade. Jacob Schick introduced the electric shaver in 1931.

In the 1960s, lasers were first used to heat and disable hair follicles over large areas, and hair removal entered the arena of medical practice. Early lasers emitted a continuous wave that risked overheating and skin damage. The invention of a switching device allowed light energy to enter the follicle in controlled pulses. In 1995, the FDA approved the first laser device for hair removal. Most developed since that time use water or gel to cool the skin and laser light to target the melanin in the hair. Other strategies are being investigated, and studies of such variables as beam width, pulse duration, and delivery rate may result in laser hair removal treatments that are safe, effective, and permanent.

Basic research on the nature and action of the immune system may lead to treatments for autoimmune disorders, including alopecia areata. The cloning of individual, hair follicles may facilitate hair transplantation. Gene therapy could, in theory, be used to alter the genetic control of follicles, preventing inherited baldness entirely.

—*Faith Hickman Brynie, Ph.D.*

See also Dermatology; Gray hair; Hair loss and baldness; Hair transplantation; Laser use in surgery; Pigmentation; Plastic surgery; Skin; Skin disorders.

For Further Information:
Anderson, Richard R. "Lasers in Dermatology: A Critical Update." *Journal of Dermatology* 27, no. 11 (November, 2000): 700–705.

Brynie, Faith Hickman. *101 Questions About Your Skin That Got Under Your Skin . . . Until Now.* Brookfield, Conn.: Twenty-first Century Books, 1999.

Burns, Tony, et al., eds. *Rook's Textbook of Dermatology.* 7th ed. Malden, Mass.: Blackwell Science, 2004.

Dunn, Rob. "Hirsute Pursuits." *New Scientist* 214, no. 2869 (June 16, 2012): 44–47.

Freedberg, Irwin M., et al., eds. *Fitzpatrick's Dermatology in General Medicine.* 7th ed. 2 vols. New York: McGraw-Hill, 2008.

Kuntzman, Gersh. *Hair! Mankind's Historic Quest to End Baldness.* New York: AtRandom, 2001.

Unger, Walter P., Ronald Shapiro, Robin Unger, and Mark A. Unger, eds. *Hair Transplantation.* 5th ed. New York: Informa Healthcare, 2011.

Wood, Debra. "Alopecia." *Health Library*, October 31, 2012.

HAIR TRANSPLANTATION

Procedure

Anatomy or system affected: Hair, head, skin

Specialties and related fields: Dermatology, general surgery, plastic surgery

Definition: The surgical relocation of healthy hair follicles to a part of the scalp where shrunken follicles are producing short, thin hair or no hair.

Key terms:

alopecia reduction: a hair restoration technique that involves surgical removal of a bald portion of scalp followed by stretching of hair-covered scalp to restore hair

donor graft: a segment of hair surgically transplanted as a plug or micrograft from one part of the scalp to another

micrograft: a small filament of donor hair typically containing three or four active hair follicles

Indications and Procedures

Several types of balding may cause a patient to seek out hair transplantation. Perhaps the most common is androgenetic alopecia (common baldness), a condition that can affect both men and women who are genetically predisposed to it. Usually beginning in late adolescence or early adulthood, androgenetic hormones cause hair follicles gradually to grow smaller and eventually to yield hair that can be detected only by a microscope, or no hair at all.

Different patterns of balding have been observed. Frontal recession is a gradual process during which the frontal hairline retreats from the forehead. In vertex thinning, the hair on the crown of the head gradually disappears, exposing the scalp; the denuded area grows slowly in a concentric pattern. With complete balding, progressive frontal recession combines with vertex balding to create a condition in which hair is present only in a rim at the sides and back of the scalp.

Hair replacement via hair transplantation involves surgery, which should be performed by a board-certified physician skilled in this procedure. Hair transplantation has the distinct advantage over all other procedures currently in place for hair restoration because the candidate's own hair is used. Candidates for surgical hair transplantation must have healthy hair growth on the back and sides of the head to serve as donor hair. Choice of location for donor hair will also be influenced by factors such as hair color, hair texture, and growth direction.

All hair transplantation procedures involve the application of anesthesia. It may be administered as local anesthesia applied topically to the donor and recipient areas of the scalp or as general anesthesia if more extensive transplants are undertaken or if the hair transplantation process is more complex.

Following the introduction of anesthesia, the surgeon removes small micrografts of hair typically containing several follicles. They are inserted in narrow slits in the bald areas of scalp or are simply inserted as very small microplugs. Earlier procedures that have largely been discontinued excised plugs containing several dozen hair follicles, which were then inserted into areas of bald scalp, but this left visible and unsightly bumps or plugs from which hair grew in clumps. Some individuals who underwent this earlier plug procedure have since had all or part of their hair restored with modern micrograft or microfollicle procedures.

For many patients, hair transplantation can be accomplished as an outpatient procedure requiring no more than a single day. More extensive and more complicated hair transplantation cases will require additional sessions that may extend over several months. Following the transplant session, the scalp is cleaned, washed, and covered with gauze.

Uses and Complications

All hair restoration procedures require surgery, which may not be suitable for everyone, and patients seeking hair transplantation are cautioned to consult a physician, and perhaps a psychiatrist as well, to determine whether their mental and physical health are optimal for the surgical procedure.

Patients desiring hair transplantation must be cautioned that despite the claims of proponents, there is no certainty that the procedure will be successful. Problems with unsuccessful hair transplantation have led doctors to require patients to sign a form that specifically indicates that the procedure is not guaranteed.

—*Russell Williams, M.S.W.;*
updated by Dwight G. Smith, Ph.D.

See also Dermatology; Grafts and grafting; Hair; Hair loss and baldness; Men's health; Plastic surgery; Skin; Transplantation.

For Further Information:
A.D.A.M. Medical Encyclopedia. "Hair Loss." *MedlinePlus*, May 13, 2011.

A.D.A.M. Medical Encyclopedia. "Hair Transplant." *MedlinePlus*, February 8, 2011.

American Society for Dermatologic Surgery. "Hair Transplants." *American Society for Dermatologic Surgery*, 2013.

Hannapel, Coriene E. "Hair Transplant Advances Add Up to Better Results." *Dermatology Times* 21, no. 6 (June, 2000): 35.

Sams, W. Mitchell, Jr., and Peter J. Lynch, eds. *Principles and Practice of Dermatology.* 2d ed. New York: Churchill Livingstone, 1996.

Scott, Susan Craig, and Karen W. Pressler. *The Hair Bible.* New York: Simon & Schuster, 2003.

Segell, Michael. "The Bald Truth About Hair." *Esquire* 121, no. 5 (May 1, 1994): 111–17.

Thompson, Wendy, and Jerry Shapiro. *Alopecia Areata: Understanding and Coping with Hair Loss.* Rev. ed. Baltimore: Johns Hopkins University Press, 2000.

HAMMERTOE CORRECTION

Procedure

Anatomy or system affected: Blood vessels, bones, feet, musculoskeletal system, nervous system, tendons

Specialties and related fields: General surgery, orthopedics, podiatry

Definition: The surgical removal of ligaments and joining of the middle joints in the toes to correct hammertoe, a deformity in which the toes bend downward abnormally.

Indications and Procedures

A hammertoe is a painful deformity that usually affects the second toe. The clawlike appearance of the toe results from malignancy of the joint surface or shortening and weakening of the foot and toe muscle. People with diabetes mellitus are prone to hammertoe development because of the nerve and muscle damage frequently associated with the disease. In other cases, hammertoe results from the wearing of shoes that are too short and do not fit properly. High-heeled shoes, which place pressure on the front of the foot and compress the smaller toes tightly together, can contribute to hammertoe formation. Painful calluses form on the tops of toes when the deformed toe rubs against the top of the shoe. Special orthotics and pads are often used to redistribute pressure and relieve pain. In severe cases, surgery may be required.

Before the operation, blood and urine studies are conducted and x-rays are taken of both feet. Hammertoe correction surgery begins with the injection of a local anesthetic. To prevent bleeding in the surgical area, a tourniquet is applied above the ankle. An incision is made through the skin above the affected joint. The tendons that attach to the toes are located and cut free of the connective tissue to the foot bone. The tendons are then divided, enabling the toe to straighten. To keep the toe from bending, the middle joints are permanently connected together with fine pins and wires. Fine sutures are used to close the skin, and the tourniquet is removed. After the surgery, additional blood studies are taken. Sutures are usually removed seven to ten days after the procedure.

Uses and Complications

The correction of hammertoe usually arises out of a need to correct severe deformity or relieve persistent pain. During recovery, flat, comfortable shoes should be worn. After recovery, patients should wear shoes that fit well and do not cramp the toes or put undue stress on the front of the foot. Though full recovery from surgery is expected in four weeks, vigorous exercise should be avoided for six weeks after surgery. Once the time for healing has passed, the affected toe will appear in a normal position, and pain will be relieved. Because of the connecting of joints in the toe, however, movement of the toe will be limited.

Possible complications associated with hammertoe correction include excessive bleeding and surgical wound infection.

—Jason Georges

See also Bone disorders; Bones and the skeleton; Feet; Foot disorders; Hammertoes; Lower extremities; Orthopedic surgery; Orthopedics; Podiatry.

For Further Information:

A.D.A.M. Medical Encyclopedia. "Hammer Toe Repair." *MedlinePlus*, July 14, 2012.

Copeland, Glenn, and Stan Solomon. *The Foot Doctor: Lifetime Relief for Your Aching Feet*. Rev. ed. Toronto, Ont.: Macmillan Canada, 1996.

Currey, John D. *Bones: Structures and Mechanics*. Princeton, N.J.: Princeton University Press, 2002.

FootCareMD. "Hammer Toe." *American Orthopaedic Foot and Ankle Society*, 2013.

"Hammer Toe Correction." *Health Library*, May 2, 2013.

Lippert, Frederick G., and Sigvard T. Hansen. *Foot and Ankle Disorders: Tricks of the Trade*. New York: Thieme, 2003.

Lorimer, Donald L., et al., eds. *Neale's Disorders of the Foot*. 7th ed. New York: Churchill Livingstone/Elsevier, 2006.

Van De Graaff, Kent M., and Stuart I. Fox. *Concepts of Human Anatomy and Physiology*. 5th ed. Dubuque, Iowa: Wm. C. Brown, 2000.

HAMMERTOES

Disease/Disorder

Anatomy or system affected: Feet

Specialties and related fields: Orthopedics, podiatry

Definition: Toes that are bent permanently at the joint nearest to the foot; the closely related term "clawtoe" denotes a toe that is bent at both joints.

Causes and Symptoms

Hammertoes and clawtoes can occur in one or more of the four smaller toes on each foot, with the second toe being the most common site for these deformities. Hammertoes and clawtoes are thought to be caused by muscle imbalance, contraction of the tendons, and enlargement of the toe joints. Although anyone can develop these conditions, the majority of cases are caused by wearing high heels or shoes that are too tight. It is common for people to develop painful corns and calluses in association with these conditions, particularly on top or on the tip of the toe where it is most likely to rub against the shoe. Furthermore, people with hammertoes or clawtoes may experience considerable pain if the toe gets inflamed. Skin ulcers may also develop when the bent toe rubs against the shoe. These ulcers can become infected and develop abnormal channels to the skin surface called sinus tracts. These conditions may also cause significant problems with walking for the affected individual.

Information on Hammertoes

Causes: Muscle imbalance, tendon contraction, enlargement of toe joints, improper footwear

Symptoms: Pain, inflammation, corns and calluses, skin ulcers

Duration: Typically short-term

Treatments: Change of footwear, use of corrective inserts or devices, sometimes arthroplasty or cutting of affected tendon

---

Treatment and Therapy

Treatment of hammertoes or clawtoes depends on the severity of the condition and whether there are secondary complications such as corns or ulcers. The simplest treatment is to change to shoes with broad toes and soft soles that cushion the foot and to avoid wearing high heels and shoes that pinch the toes. Accompanied by excellent foot care such as callus and corn removal, this may be all that is required to prevent pain and irritation of the toes. In cases that are more advanced, various inserts can be added to the shoes. These include metatarsal bars, orthotics, and other devices. A metatarsal bar supports the ball of the foot and spreads the pressure over a greater part of the foot. Orthotics are specially molded plastic devices that serve much the same purpose. In some cases, podiatrists (foot doctors) or orthopedists recommend toe caps, which are padded sleeves that help prevent friction between the toe and the shoe. In a few cases, it may be necessary to cut the tendons in the toe or to perform arthroplasty (repair of the joint itself) to provide relief.

—Rebecca Lovell Scott, Ph.D., PA-C

See also Bone disorders; Bones and the skeleton; Corns and calluses; Foot disorders; Hammertoe correction; Lower extremities; Skin; Skin disorders.

For Further Information:

Copeland, Glenn, and Stan Solomon. *The Foot Doctor: Lifetime Relief for Your Aching Feet*. Rev. ed. Toronto, Ont.: Macmillan Canada, 1996.

Currey, John D. *Bones: Structures and Mechanics*. Princeton, N.J.: Princeton University Press, 2006.

Fink, Brett Ryan. *The Whole Foot Book*. New York: Demos Medical Publishers, 2011.

Frowen, Paul, and Donald Neale. *Neale's Disorders of the Foot*. New York: Churchill Livingstone/Elsevier, 2010.

Levy, Leonard A., and Vincent J. Hetherington, eds. *Principles and Practice of Podiatric Medicine*. 2d ed. Brooklandville, Md.: Trace, 2006.

Lippert, Frederick G., and Sigvard T. Hansen. *Foot and Ankle Disorders: Tricks of the Trade*. New York: Thieme, 2003.

Lyons, Sonja. "Hammer Toe." *Health Library*, March 28, 2013.

HAND-FOOT-AND-MOUTH DISEASE

Disease/Disorder

Anatomy or system affected: Gastrointestinal system, mouth, skin

Specialties and related fields: Dermatology, pediatrics, virology

Definition: An enteroviral disease that usually affects children, causing vesicular eruptions on the hands, feet, oral mucosa, and tongue.

Causes and Symptoms

Hand-foot-and-mouth disease is usually caused by coxsackievirus A16, but it may also be associated with a number of other coxsackieviruses and enterovirus 71. Outbreaks of the disease are most common in the summer and early fall. Infants and young children ages one to five years are most commonly infected because they have not had previous exposure to the virus and, therefore, have less immunity

---

Information on Hand-Foot-and-Mouth Disease

Causes: Viral infection
Symptoms: Low-grade fever, sore mouth, oral lesions that rupture into painful ulcers, skin lesions on hands and feet
Duration: Seven to ten days
Treatments: None (self-resolving); topical anesthetic agents for mouth lesions

---

than adults. They often become infected through contact with the nasal and oral secretions of infected children, and nursery school outbreaks may occur. Skin lesions and fecal material may also contribute to the spread of the virus. The incubation period is three to six days.

The illness commences with a low-grade fever (100 to 101 degrees Fahrenheit) and a sore mouth. Oral lesions begin as small, red macules and evolve rapidly into fragile vesicles that rupture, leaving painful ulcers. Any part of the mouth may be involved, but the hard palate buccal mucosa and tongue are mainly affected with an average of five to ten lesions. Similar lesions develop on the skin over the next one to two days; they usually number twenty to thirty, but there may be as many as one hundred. Discrete macular lesions, about 4 millimeters in diameter, appear on the hands and feet and sometimes the buttocks. These lesions often occur along skin lines and progress to become papules and white or gray flaccid vesicles containing infective virus. The lesions may be painful or tender. The fever occurs during the first one to two days of the illness, which resolves in seven to ten days. Rarely, the viral infection is complicated by meningoencephalitis, carditis, or pneumonia.

Treatment and Therapy

There is no specific treatment for hand-foot-and-mouth disease. The infection usually resolves without complications in about one week. Topical anesthetic agents, such as viscous lidocaine, may be used to soothe the discomfort of the mouth lesions. Popsicles and cool sherbets may be given to young children to help soothe a sore mouth. Acetaminophen given at an appropriate dosage for the body weight of the child may also help to relieve the pain of this condition. Some pediatricians recommend a blend of Benadryl and liquid antacid to relieve the stinging sensation of the mouth lesions.

Perspective and Prospects

The first described outbreak of this disease occurred in Toronto, Canada, in 1957. British authors first coined the term "hand-foot-and-mouth disease" when they reported an outbreak in Birmingham, England, in 1959. While there currently are no medications available for treating enteroviral infections, a number of antiviral agents are being studied and might be useful for complicated forms of this disease, such as meningoencephalitis.

—H. Bradford Hawley, M.D.;
updated by Lenela Glass-Godwin, M.W.S.

See also Childhood infectious diseases; Dermatology, pediatric; Encephalitis; Enteroviruses; Fever; Lesions; Meningitis; Rashes; Skin; Skin disorders; Viral infections.

For Further Information:

Barnhill, Raymond, and A. Neil Crowson, eds. *Textbook of Dermatopathology*. 3d ed. New York: McGraw-Hill, 2010.

Belshe, Robert B., ed. *Textbook of Human Virology*. 2d ed. St. Louis, Mo.: Mosby Year Book, 1991.

Goldsmith, Lowell, et al., eds. *Fitzpatrick's Dermatology in General Medicine*. 8th ed. 2 vols. New York: McGraw-Hill, 2012.

"Hand, Foot, and Mouth Disease (HFMD)." *Centers for Disease Control and Prevention*, April 27, 2012.

Mandell, Gerald L., John E. Bennett, and Raphael Dolin, eds. *Mandell, Douglas, and Bennett's Principles and Practice of Infectious Diseases*. 7th ed. New York: Churchill Livingstone/Elsevier, 2010.

McCoy, Krisha. "Hand, Foot, and Mouth Disease." *Health Library*, November 26, 2012.

Vorvick, Linda J., and David Zieve. "Hand-Foot-Mouth Disease." *Medline Plus*, August 10, 2012.

HANTAVIRUS

Disease/Disorder

Anatomy or system affected: Kidneys, lungs, respiratory system

Specialties and related fields: Critical care, environmental health, epidemiology, internal medicine, public health, pulmonary medicine, virology

Definition: An often-fatal viral infection carried by rodents that causes influenza-like symptoms and respiratory failure.

Causes and Symptoms

Hantavirus, which is distantly related to Ebola virus, is transmitted through contact with the urine and droppings of wild rodents, such as the deer mouse and cotton rat. Contact usually involves the inhalation of contaminated particles in dust. Hantavirus is not transmissible between humans.

Infection takes two major forms. In South America, one strain causes hemorrhagic fever with renal syndrome, involving kidney failure, hemorrhaging, and shock. In the United States, another strain results in hantavirus pulmonary syndrome. Early symptoms mimic influenza; they include fever, chills, muscle aches, nausea and vomiting, malaise, and a dry cough. After initial improvement, increasing shortness of breath follows and may progress to pulmonary edema, internal bleeding, respiratory failure, and death.

Treatment and Therapy

Diagnosis of hantavirus pulmonary syndrome involves physical examination for hypoxia, hypotension, and acute respiratory distress syndrome. Laboratory tests show an elevated white blood cell count and a decreasing platelet count, and chest X-rays may reveal edema. The presence of hantavirus is confirmed through serological testing.

There is no cure for hantavirus pulmonary syndrome; treatment is focused on alleviating the symptoms. This condition must be treated in the intensive care unit (ICU) of a hospital, as careful monitoring of respiratory function and blood gases is

---

Information on Hantavirus

Causes: Viral infection spread through contact with urine and droppings of wild rodents

Symptoms: Fever, chills, muscle aches, nausea and vomiting, malaise, dry cough, kidney failure, hemorrhaging, shock

Duration: Acute

Treatments: None; alleviation of symptoms

---

essential. In severe cases, the use of an endotracheal tube and a ventilator becomes necessary. Experiments have been performed with intravenous ribavirin therapy; the efficacy of this treatment is being evaluated. Unfortunately, even with aggressive measures, the death rate ranges from 50 to 80 percent.

Perspective and Prospects

The incidence of hantavirus pulmonary syndrome seemed to rise sharply in the 1990s. Epidemiologists were uncertain whether the number of cases increased or more cases were reported following identification of the virus in the United States in 1993.

Because much remains to be learned about the transmission, development, and treatment of hantavirus infection, public health efforts have been in education and prevention. Hikers and campers are thought to be at a greater risk; they are urged to avoid exposure to rodent droppings and questionable water sources. People entering cabins, sheds, or other buildings that have not been used recently should air out the building first and disinfect all surfaces.

—*Tracy Irons-Georges*

See also Ebola virus; Edema; Environmental diseases; Environmental health; Epidemiology; Hypoxia; Lungs; Pulmonary diseases; Pulmonary medicine; Respiration; Viral hemorrhagic fevers; Viral infections; Zoonoses.

For Further Information:

Cockrum, E. Lendell. *Rabies, Lyme Disease, Hanta Virus, and Other Animal-Borne Human Diseases in the United States and Canada*. Tucson, Ariz.: Fisher Books, 1997.

Dugdale, David C., Jatin M. Vyas, and David Zieve. "Hantavirus." *Medline Plus*, March 11, 2011.

"Hantavirus." *Centers for Disease Control and Prevention*, November 1, 2012.

Kumar, Vinay, et al., eds. *Robbins Basic Pathology*. 9th ed. Philadelphia: Saunders/Elsevier, 2012.

McCoy, Krisha. "Hantavirus Infection." *Health Library*, January 4, 2013.

Meyer, Andrea S., and David R. Harper. *Of Mice, Men, and Microbes: Hantavirus*. San Diego, Calif.: Academic Press, 1999.

Murray, Patrick R., Ken S. Rosenthal, and Michael A. Pfaller. *Medical Microbiology*. 6th ed. Philadelphia: Mosby/Elsevier, 2009.

Pan American Health Organization. *Hantavirus in the Americas: Guidelines for Diagnosis, Treatment, Prevention, and Control*. Washington, D.C.: Author, 1999.

Sompayrac, Lauren. *How Pathogenic Viruses Work*. Boston: Jones and Bartlett, 2002.

Strauss, James, and Ellen Strauss. *Viruses and Human Disease*. 2d ed. Boston: Academic Press/Elsevier, 2008.

HARELIP. *See* **CLEFT LIP AND PALATE.**

HASHIMOTO'S THYROIDITIS
Disease/Disorder

Also known as: Struma lymphomatosa, lymphadenoid goiter, chronic lymphocytic thyroiditis, autoimmune thyroiditis

Anatomy or system affected: Endocrine system, glands, immune system, neck

Specialties and related fields: Endocrinology

Definition: An autoimmune disease that results in inflammation of the thyroid gland caused when abnormal blood antibodies and white blood cells infiltrate and attack thyroidal cells.

Causes and Symptoms

Hashimoto's thyroiditis is a common type of hypothyroidism. The cause and etiology of this disorder is not fully understood; however, it is thought to have an autoimmune origin, in which abnormal blood antibodies and white blood cells, called lymphocytes, infiltrate and attack thyroid cells. The combative interplay between the lymphocytes and the thyroid may lead to a complete absence of thyroid cells. A family history of thyroid disease is commonly traced.

The highest incidence of the disease is observed in young or middle-aged women, but it may occur at any age. The onset is very slow, and the disease may progress for many months or years before it is fully detected. The symptoms may vary, but the condition is usually characterized by a mild pressure on the thyroid gland. In some cases, a firm, slightly irregular, and sometimes tender goiter (enlarged thyroid gland) may develop in the neck region. In more severe cases, the disease may cause symptoms related to low thyroid function (hypothyroidism), such as fatigue, weight gain, intolerance to cold, constipation, and hair loss.

The symptomatology of Hashimoto's thyroiditis may resemble other medical conditions. Therefore, in addition to a full medical examination, the diagnostic procedure must also include blood tests to determine the levels of thyroid hormone and thyroid antibodies. If a patient has developed the classic symptoms that accompany Hashimoto's thyroiditis but has a normal blood test, then a biopsy in which a needle is inserted into the thyroid and some cells are removed may be performed to confirm the diagnosis.

Treatment and Therapy

Though a specific treatment is not yet available, the hypothyroidism resulting from Hashimoto's thyroiditis can be treated with hormones. Medical practitioners opt to commence hormone therapy, in the form of thyroxine, as soon as a diagnosis is made, even if thyroid function is normal at the time. The hormone therapy is expected to shrink any goiter that has developed. If there is no response, then surgery may be required. The prognosis for a full recovery is usually good because the disease remains dormant or stable for many years.

—*Nicholas Lanzieri; updated by Sharon W. Stark, R.N., A.P.R.N., D.N.Sc.*

See also Endocrine disorders; Endocrine glands; Endocrinology;

Information on Hashimoto's Thyroiditis

Causes: Unknown; possibly autoimmune in origin

Symptoms: Mild pressure on thyroid gland, goiter, fatigue, weight gain, cold intolerance, constipation, hair loss

Duration: Chronic

Treatments: Hormonal therapy with thyroxine, surgery if required

---

Glands; Goiter; Hormones; Hyperparathyroidism and hypoparathyroidism; Metabolism; Parathyroidectomy; Thyroid disorders; Thyroid gland; Thyroidectomy.

For Further Information:

Bayliss, R. I. S., and W. M. Tunbridge. *Thyroid Disease: The Facts*. 4th ed. New York: Oxford University Press, 2008.

Burman, Kenneth D., and Derek LeRoith, eds. *Thyroid Function and Disease*. Philadelphia: Saunders/Elsevier, 2007.

"Chronic Thyroiditis (Hashimoto's Disease). *Medline Plus*, June 4, 2012.

"Hashimoto's Disease." *National Endocrine and Metabolic Diseases Information Service*, April 6, 2012.

"Hypothyroidism." *Health Library*, March 15, 2013.

Kronenberg, Henry M., et al., eds. *Williams Textbook of Endocrinology*. 11th ed. Philadelphia: Saunders/Elsevier, 2008.

Shannon, Joyce Brennfleck, ed. *Thyroid Disorders Sourcebook: Basic Consumer Health Information About Disorders of the Thyroid and Parathyroid Glands*. Detroit, Mich.: Omnigraphics, 2005.

Wood, Lawrence C., David S. Cooper, and E. Chester Ridgway. *Your Thyroid: A Home Reference*. 4th rev. ed. New York: Ballantine Books, 2005.

HAVENING TOUCH
Treatment

Also known as: Amygdala depotentiation therapy (ADT)

Anatomy or system affected: Mental health, neurobiologic

Specialties and related fields: Psychiatry, mental health, primary care

Definition: A psychosensory healing modality that helps to overcome the powerful effects of extreme stress and trauma, reducing/eliminating symptoms of posttraumatic stress, anxiety, phobia, and pain by disrupting depotentiation of the amygdala pathway.

Overwhelming Life Experience

Overwhelming life events—such as medical illness, violent incidents, and natural disasters—and the extreme stress associated with them are a common feature of contemporary life. Recent technological advances routinely expose the public, often in grotesque detail, to these myriad adverse circumstances via the Internet and social media, resulting in unprecedented exposure to a range of disasters and life-threatening emergencies.

Through personal survival, witnessing or even hearing about an extreme situation, complex automatic biological responses are stimulated, resulting in long term implications. Primitive brain structures and neurobiological processes, designed to protect an organism's survival by enhancing the ability to perceive and escape danger, encode (record) the event to avoid repetition of future life-threatening situations. This indelible encoding may cause vivid recollections and intrusive thoughts, re-experiencing the event as if it were occurring in the present time. Various healing modalities attempt to change underlying brain structure and chemistry to ameliorate the continuing effects of a prior threatening event.

Neuroscience of Traumatic Experience

Brains are "hardwired" to respond automatically to threats of safety, survival, and well-being. Through a complex, integrated electrochemical signal system in the brain, early warnings are perceived, interpreted, and activated to prepare the organism to fight or flee for its survival. This occurs instantaneously by structures in the brain's limbic system that send electrochemical signals to other structures, which activate α-Amino-3-hydroxy-5-methyl-4-isoxazolepropionic acid (AMPA) receptors that facilitate electrical current to the parts of the brain that must initiate the fight-or-flight response. A cascade of neurochemicals (epinephrine, dopamine, cortisol) rapidly prepare the organism to survive the threat by increasing muscle strength, blood flow, and cardiac and respiratory output.

After the threat is resolved, the brain relaxes and embeds the experience so it can rapidly remember the cues, which can increase awareness of future danger. Trauma activation and encoding occurs in the presence of the following three factors: an overwhelming, inescapable event; the meaning of the event (fear of death, etc.); and the neurobiological landscape of the brain (neurochemical state at the time of the event, which shapes vulnerability or resilience to traumatization).

If the early-warning system remains unremitting after the danger subsides, the lack of a shut-off process leads the encoded trauma response to become a continuous, dysfunctional, dysregulated chronic stressor, on high alert, in a constant state of danger. Triggering by general cues that the brain misinterprets as current danger creates an alteration of the neurochemical landscape of the brain. The altered neurobiology increases vulnerability to further traumatization and the risk for other mental health disorders including phobia, major depression, anxiety, panic, posttraumatic stress, substance abuse, somatoform and, obsessive compulsive disorders, which may actually be passed on to descendants by way of altered genetic patterns.

The heightened sense of vulnerability, exaggerated by the lack of a safe haven, can lead to a chronic emotional state (shame, anger, rage, fear, jealously, revenge, helplessness, sadness), which distorts perceptions of worldview, self and others, leading to myriad additional problems. Avoidance behavior and altered social interaction are common outcomes of encoded phobias and traumas.

Therapeutic Approaches

Many therapeutic approaches have been developed to facilitate coping and reduce adverse consequences. Psychosensory therapies use sensory input to alter the underlying responsiveness to the encoded traumatic event, thus modifying thought, mood, and behavior patterns. Some are nonspecific and work towards a global reduction in stress responsiveness (yoga, massage, aromatherapy), while others stimulate specific healing, enhance resilience, and increase the threshold for further traumatization: eye movement desensitization and reprocessing (EMDR), emotional freedom technique (EFT), and thought field therapy (TFT).

Exposure therapies down regulate stress and its impact on information processing and response. Medications alter the brain's response to the exposure. The psychosensory therapies use the body's innate senses to alter neurochemical concentrations and produce changes in the neurochemical landscape, emphasizing the mind-body connection and the ways this connection is manifested. The basis for HT/ADT is altering the response to a fear stimulus by increasing serotonin in the brain using the extrasensory aspects of touch.

Havening Touch/Amygdala Depotentiation

Havening Touch: Amygdala Depotentiation Therapy is a unique psychosensory therapy that connects sensory input and neurobiological memory to alter the neurochemical landscape of the brain. After seven years of active research, HT/ADT originators describe it as the first and only effective therapy that reduces the impact of overwhelming life experience by changing the brain's encoding and storage of the specific traumatic emotional memory and its negative effects.

The HT/ADT approach involves initiating imaginal exposure, which activates glutamate receptors in the brain. A variety of sensory inputs is applied, particularly HT, which stimulates peripheral receptors in the skin, triggering electrochemical changes, including rising serotonin levels. Distraction, involving visual and auditory tasks, interferes with the consolidated memory, destabilizing and immobilizing storage. The elevated serotonin on recall of the trauma creates safety or a haven for the memory. Decreasing cortisol and the production of a delta wave in the amygdala lead to phosphatase in the postsynaptic neuron that depotentiates the activated glutamate receptors associated with the stimulus input. The receptor becomes internalized, de-linking the traumatic memory and current distress. The depotentiation in the receptors allows for a disconnect between the emotional core and the memory, extinguishing the trauma/phobia. The event is no longer perceived as inescapable, thus no longer encoded as a trauma, and permanently eliminated.

Since the event is no longer immutably encoded in the mind and the body, the memory becomes stored in a more typical, adaptive mechanism, without the emotional disturbance. As the brain is "tricked" into thinking it has escaped, the encoded memory will not be retained as a phobia, only as a simple memory without fear or physiological dimensions, thus allowing for normative behavior. Practitioners of HT/ADT describe a rapid, almost instantaneous relief from the magnitude, intensity, and severity of the memory, usually resulting in a complete reduction of traumatic stress symptoms and negative effects.

As repeated stressors increase and potentiate receptors, additional long-term benefits may result in the decreased number of receptors, thus enhancing the neural landscape.

Facilitated Event Self-Havening (FESH) is a system of self-administered techniques that similarly alter the brain's landscape and produce a normalization of neuromodulators and neurochemicals.

Protocol

After a careful history and assessment, the individual is asked to bring to mind the circumstances of the memory, including the emotional content of the specific traumatic moment and the recollection of as many sensory aspects as possible: sights, sounds, smells, etc. This emotional, cognitive, and sensory memory activates the feeling of fear, anxiety, or trauma, creating the fearful, anxious or traumatic response as if it were current. The practitioner then follows a protocol that includes three components: activation of the event and its emotional core, application of HT (kinesthetic component), and active distraction through prescribed techniques.

The practitioner combines a series of kinesthetic touch stimuli, composed of soothing, gentle strokes to arms, shoulders, forehead, hands, and face that leads to a surge in serotonin and low voltage delta waves. A calcium channel opens, triggering a phosphatase that removes molecules from activated glutamate receptors. AMPA receptors are no longer potentiated, and the receptor is removed from the pathway that disrupts the traumatic encoding. At the same time, distracting thoughts and tasks are introduced, which shift focus and displaces the distressing mind-set. The combination of activation of the memory and its emotional core along with the stimulation of neurochemicals helps to disrupt the linkage that was encoded at the time of traumatization. The distraction displaces the thoughts from working memory and inhibits/prevents further excessive responsiveness. Since the circumstances of the previous traumatizing moment are not replicated (landscape, meaning, and inescapability), the intensity fades and becomes a simple memory without emotional content and is unable to produce a fear response.

The emotional memory and stimulating cues are removed, creating a safe haven in which to recall the event, resulting in a feeling of calm and emotional detachment from the trauma. Typically, the individual reports looking at the issue from a distance rather than from inside the eye of the storm, the view of a postage stamp rather than a large screen, leading to resolution of the problem and disappearance of the phobia, anxiety, or traumatic stress response.

Several forms of HT/ADT have been developed, including Event, Transpirational, Facilitated Event Self-Havening (FESH), and Affirmational HT. In the FESH model, the client is directed by the practitioner to follow a series of steps and at the same time apply Self-Havening Touch (SHT).

Applications and Uses

HT/ADT is indicated in the treatment of amygdala-based disorders and is considered unique in the resolution of the trauma memory. Extinction therapy, exposure therapy, or systematic desensitization involves exposure to a fear-related stimulus, and through nonreinforcement or habituation, the stimulus loses its ability to produce the fear response. A new response is learned; however, the old pathway that produced the fear is still intact; only the response is changed. HT/ADT involves the elimination of the relationship between the event and the emotion.

There are three distinct applications for use within a psychotherapeutic setting provided by a professional mental health clinician that has been fully trained and certified in HT. It can also be used as a self-help technique to diminish emotional disturbances, enhance wellness strategies such as stress management and peak performance, and to promote self-modulated healing.

Summary and Conclusion

HT/ADT is an innovative psychosensory intervention for the treatment of trauma-based disorders and to enhance general well-being. It utilizes the individual's thoughts and emotions coupled with the extrasensory components of touch to modify encoded neural pathways, disrupting and eliminating unwanted responses (symptoms) from previous traumatic experiences. The effect of practitioner-applied tactile stimulation triggers γ-Aminobutyric acid (GABA) release and serotonin, increases low frequency delta wave production, and depotentiates activated glutamate receptors. This de-links encoded traumatic memory from the event, resulting in the emotional detachment from its intensity. This nondrug, short duration, individual-focused modality has been demonstrated in thousands of anecdotal cases worldwide to be safe and effective.

HT is considered alternative or complementary to the healing arts that are licensed in the United States. As a relatively new healing approach, the extent of its effectiveness as well as risks and benefits have not been fully studied. Formal large-scale research endeavors are currently being conducted. While yet to be fully researched by Western academic and medical standards, and therefore may be considered experimental, this approach offers promising opportunities for symptom relief and enhanced quality of life.

—Holly K. Shaw, Ph.D., R.N.

For Further Information:

Ruden, R. "A Neurological Basis for the Observed Peripheral Sensory Modulation of Emotional Responses." *Traumatology* 11, no. 3 (2005): 145-158.

Ruden, R. *When the Past Is Always Present: Emotional Traumatization, Causes, and Cures.* New York: Routledge, 2010.

Ruden, R.A. "Harnessing Synaptic Plasticity to Treat the Consequences of Emotional Traumatization by Amygdala Depotentiation (Havening)." Retrieved from https://havening.org/uploads/Harnessing.pdf.

Ruden, S. ISDAM.com. "Facilitated Self-havening for the Treatment of Dental Phobias and Anxiety: Amygdala Depotentiation Therapy." *ISDAM Magazine* (April, 2013): 45-47. Retrieved from https://havening.org/uploads/Havening_article_ISDAM.pdf.

Weintaub, N.V., M. Zhou, A. Lira, et al. "Cortical 5-HT2A Receptor Singing Modulates Anxiety-like Behaviors in Mice." *Science* (2006): 536-540.

HAY FEVER
Disease/Disorder
Also known as: Seasonal allergic rhinitis
Anatomy or system affected: Eyes, immune system, lungs, lymphatic system, nose, respiratory system, throat
Specialties and related fields: Immunology, otorhinolaryngology
Definition: A damaging immune response to otherwise harmless foreign substances such as pollen grains and mold spores.

Causes and Symptoms

Allergic rhinitis, popularly known as hay fever, represents the most common allergic disorder, affecting approximately 10 percent of the population; the most common source of the allergy is wind-dispersed pollen. These tiny grains are produced in phenomenal numbers to ensure transfer of the pollen (which contains the plant's sperm) to other flowers of the same plant species. Trees, grasses, and certain forbs (especially the ragweeds) are the most common culprits. The first time that a susceptible person is exposed, the pollen acts to sensitize the immune system. On second and subsequent exposures, the pollen triggers an allergic response.

This response is triggered by the formation of a specific class of antibody known as IgE against the proteins on the pollen grains (generally called antigens and in this case called allergens). Immunoglobulin E (IgE) attaches to tissue cells called mast cells by one end and to the pollen grains at the other end. This attachment causes the mast cells to release defensive substances, the best known of which is histamine. These substances cause increased permeability of capillaries and the production and release of mucous and watery substances from the nasal passages and eyes. Itching and sneezing accompany the release. The tendency to produce IgE against pollen allergens is an inherited trait; persons with one or both parents who have allergies to certain substances are more likely to exhibit the same allergies than persons whose parents do not exhibit such responses.

Treatment and Therapy

It is generally agreed that avoidance of the allergen is the most effective therapy for hay fever. Staying inside a building with air conditioning or well-filtered air during the worst allergy season helps. However, avoiding an allergen completely, such as ragweed pollen during ragweed's flowering season, is essentially impossible.

The most common treatments employed are desensitization and drugs. Desensitization involves a series of injections of slowly increasing concentrations of the allergen, in the hope of turning the patient's immune system from the production of IgE to the production of immunoglobulin G (IgG), which does not trigger the mast cells. Drugs such as antihistamines, which block the action or the release of histamine and the other substances released by mast cells, are commonly recommended, either in prescription strength or over the counter. Steroid and decongestant sprays have also been successful in relieving the symptoms of hay fever in some individuals.

Information on Hay Fever

Causes: Allergic reaction to pollen
Symptoms: Itchy eyes and nose, sneezing
Duration: Chronic
Treatments: Avoidance of allergens, desensitization, antihistamines

---

Perspective and Prospects

For many persons, long-term avoidance of allergens such as pollen may be difficult. Current drugs such as antihistamines are directed primarily at relieving symptoms without removing the cause: the binding of IgE to the allergen. Future drugs may address the variety of steps involved in the allergic response while causing fewer side effects such as sleepiness. Other treatments may involve augmentation of IgG production in response to immunization with the allergen, since IgG competes with IgE in binding to the allergen.

—*Carl W. Hoagstrom, Ph.D.;*
updated by Richard Adler, Ph.D.

See also Allergies; Antibodies; Antihistamines; Autoimmune disorders; Decongestants; Immune system; Nasopharyngeal disorders; Otorhinolaryngology; Over-the-counter medications; Rhinitis; Sense organs; Sinusitis; Smell; Sneezing.

For Further Information:

Abbas, Abul K., Andrew H. Lichtman, and Shiv Pillai. *Basic Immunology: Functions and Disorders of the Immune System.* 4th ed. Philadelphia: Saunders/Elsevier, 2012.
Carson-DeWitt, Rosalyn. "Allergic Rhinitis." *Health Library*, October 31, 2012.
Delves, Peter J., et al. *Roitt's Essential Immunology.* 12th ed. Malden, Mass.: Blackwell, 2011.
"Hay Fever." *Mayo Clinic*, July 17, 2012.
Janeway, Charles A., Jr., et al. *Immunobiology: The Immune System in Health and Disease.* 6th ed. New York: Garland Science, 2005.
Owen, Judy, Jenni Punt, and Sharon Stranford. *Kuby Immunology.* 7th ed. New York: W. H. Freeman, 2013.
Rabson, Arthur, et al. *Really Essential Medical Immunology.* 2d ed. Malden, Mass.: Blackwell Science, 2005.

HEAD AND NECK DISORDERS
Disease/Disorder
Anatomy or system affected: Bones, brain, head, muscles, musculoskeletal system, neck, nervous system, respiratory system, spine, throat
Specialties and related fields: Dentistry, emergency medicine, neurology, otolaryngology, sports medicine
Definition: Physical trauma or neurological problems affecting the head and neck, including the spinal cord.

The head and neck region of the human body houses a sophisticated collection of structures including the special sense organs (structures for breathing, speaking, and eating) and the brain, brain stem, and cervical (neck) portion of the spinal cord. A multitude of disorders or injuries can occur in this complex region.

Trauma to the head and neck. Head or neck trauma can result from a harsh blow on the head, as can occur in a fall or with a strike from an object. These injuries are commonly seen in young, basically healthy persons who come to emergency rooms during evenings or weekends as a result of sports accidents, automobile accidents, or domestic or street violence. In the older age group, strokes and aneurysms are more common problems. Some of these accidents or events can cause permanent nerve and brain damage to the injured person.

Concussions and contusions of the head are common results of head trauma, which induces an internal neurological response. A concussion is a loss of consciousness or awareness of one's surroundings that may last a few minutes or days. Sometimes a concussion appears only as a moderately decreased level of awareness and not a total loss of consciousness. There is no evidence of a change in the brain's structure but, oddly, there is a change in the way in which the brain operates so that alertness is altered. Concussion is presumably a temporary change in brain chemistry, and the damage is reversible unless repeated head blows, such as a professional boxer may experience, are endured. Concussions may occur from other trauma, such as loss of blood flow to the brain, but such trauma is more closely associated with the more urgent threat of permanent brain damage. A contusion is popularly referred to as a bruise. The color associated with a fresh bruise is attributable to an aggregation of blood in an area that was damaged, causing many small blood vessels to rupture and release blood into the surrounding tissue. A bruise around the eye, temple, or forehead causes a black eye.

Automobile accidents rank as one of the common causes of head and neck injury. One of the more familiar complaints after a car accident is the condition called whiplash. Whiplash is the layperson's term for hyperextension of the neck, whereby the head is thrust backward (posteriorly) abruptly and beyond the normal range of neck motion. Hyperflexion occurs when the head is abruptly thrust in the forward (anterior) direction—sometimes as a recoil from hyperextension. The pain of whiplash originates from the damage to the anterior longitudinal ligament along the neck region of the spinal cord. This ligament can be overly stretched or even torn as a result of a sudden snap or jerk of the neck. Furthermore, the bony vertebrae may also grind against one another after the trauma, causing additional irritation, swelling, and pain in the neck area.

One of the common troubles of a gun or knife wound to the head and neck region is superficial and deep lacerations (cuts). If left unsutured, a deep scalp wound can cause death by hemorrhage. Superficial lacerations to the face may also cause considerable bleeding; such wounds generally are not life-threatening, but they often require stitches in order to heal.

Trauma to the head and neck area can arise from spontaneous internal events such as a stroke, an embolus, or an aneurysm. Each of these conditions is serious and potentially life-threatening because of the risk of losing blood flow to the brain and other vital tissues of the head and neck region.

Neurological problems of the head and neck. Although the

Information on Head and Neck Disorders
Causes: Injury, neurological problems
Symptoms: Pain, bruising, whiplash, alignment problems, inflammation
Duration: Short-term to chronic
Treatments: Surgery, drug therapy, corrective devices

bony cranium offers some protection to the head, the neck is, in some regards, more vulnerable to intrusion. Breathing can be interrupted by severing the left or right phrenic nerve, each of which innervates its corresponding half of the most important muscle of breathing, the diaphragm.

The left or right vagus nerve may also be severed. The vagus nerves supply the sympathetic system of the thorax and abdomen, and they also innervate the vocal cords. Severance of one of the vagus nerves causes a hoarseness of the voice as a result of the loss of function of one-half of the vocal cords. If both vagus nerves are damaged—a rare event—then the ability to speak is forever lost.

The sympathetic trunk is another nerve at risk in the neck. Severance of this nerve leads to Horner syndrome, which consists of a group of signs including ptosis (drooping eyelids), constricted pupils, a flushed face as a result of vasodilation, and dry skin on the face and neck because of the inability to sweat.

Transection (the complete severance) of the lower cervical spinal cord causes upper and lower limb paralysis and trouble with urination, and damage to the upper cervical cord can cause death because of loss of innervation to the muscles of respiration. Hemisection (partial severance) of the cervical spinal cord can also cause Horner syndrome. Damage to the spinal cord can occur from a knife or gun wound or from crushing or snapping the cord by sudden impact, as with an injury from an earthquake or an automobile accident.

—Mary C. Fields, M.D.

See also Amnesia; Aneurysmectomy; Aneurysms; Ataxia; Botox; Brain; Brain damage; Brain disorders; Carotid arteries; Cluster headaches; Coma; Computed tomography (CT) scanning; Concussion; Craniosynostosis; Craniotomy; Dementias; Dizziness and fainting; Electroencephalography (EEG); Embolism; Encephalitis; Epilepsy; Hallucinations; Headaches; Hemiplegia; Hydrocephalus; Laryngitis; Memory loss; Meningitis; Migraine headaches; Nasal polyp removal; Nasopharyngeal disorders; Neuralgia, neuritis, and neuropathy; Neuroimaging; Neurology; Neurology, pediatric; Neurosurgery; Numbness and tingling; Palsy; Paralysis; Paraplegia; Pharyngitis; Quadriplegia; Seizures; Shunts; Sinusitis; Spinal cord disorders; Sports medicine; Strokes; Subdural hematoma; Thrombosis and thrombus; Torticollis; Transient ischemic attacks (TIAs); Unconsciousness; Voice and vocal cord disorders; Whiplash.

For Further Information:

American Medical Association. *American Medical Association Family Medical Guide.* 4th rev. ed. Hoboken, N.J.: John Wiley & Sons, 2004.

Fehrenbach, Margaret J., and Susan W. Herring. *Illustrated Anatomy of the Head and Neck.* 4th ed. St. Louis, Mo.: Elsevier/Saunders, 2012.

Gorlin, Robert J., et al. *Gorlin's Syndromes of the Head and Neck.* 5th ed. New York: Oxford University Press, 2010.

Lee, Keat J. *Essential Otolaryngology: Head and Neck Surgery.* 10th ed. New York: McGraw-Hill Medical, 2012.

Litin, Scott C., ed. *Mayo Clinic Family Health Book.* 4th ed. New York: HarperResource, 2009.

Marieb, Elaine N. *Essentials of Human Anatomy and Physiology.* 10th ed. San Francisco: Pearson/Benjamin Cummings, 2012.

Moore, Keith L., and Arthur F. Dalley II. *Clinically Oriented Anatomy.* 7th ed. Philadelphia: Kluwer/Lippincott Williams & Wilkins, 2013.

Nicholls, John G., A. Robert Martin, and Bruce G. Wallace. *From Neuron to Brain.* 5th ed. Sunderland, Mass.: Sinauer, 2012.

Noback, Charles R., et al. *The Human Nervous System: Structure and Function.* 6th ed. Totowa, N.J.: Humana Press, 2005.

Scanlon, Valerie, and Tina Sanders. *Essentials of Anatomy and Physiology.* 6th ed. Philadelphia: F. A. Davis, 2012.

HEADACHES

Disease/Disorder

Anatomy or system affected: Brain, head, nervous system, psychic-emotional system

Specialties and related fields: Family medicine, internal medicine, neurology

Definition: A general term referring to pain localized in the head and/or neck, which may signal mere tension or serious disorders.

Key terms:

cluster headache: a severe type of headache, characterized by excruciating pain; attacks occur in groups, or clusters

migraine headache: a type of headache characterized by pain on one side of the head, often accompanied by disordered vision and gastrointestinal disturbances

prophylactic treatment: a treatment focusing on preventing disease, illness, or their symptoms from occurring

symptomatic treatment: a treatment focusing on aborting disease, illness, or their symptoms once they have occurred

tension-type headache: a type of headache characterized by bandlike or caplike pain over the head

Causes and Symptoms

In 1988, an ad hoc committee of the International Headache Society developed the current classification system for headaches. This system includes fourteen exhaustive categories of headache with the purpose of developing comparability in the management and study of headaches. Headaches most commonly seen by health care providers can be classified into four main types: migraine, tension-type, cluster, and "other" acute headaches.

Migraine headaches have been estimated to affect approximately 12 percent of the population. The headaches are more common in women, and they tend to run in families; they are usually first noticed in the teen years or young adulthood. For the diagnosis of migraine without aura (*aura* refers to visual disturbances or hallucinations, numbness and tingling on one side of the face, dizziness, or impairment of speech or hearing—symptoms that occur twenty to thirty minutes prior to the onset of the headache), the person must experience at least ten headache attacks, each lasting between four and seventy-two hours with at least two of the following characteristics: The headache is unilateral (occurs on one side), has a pulsating quality, is moderate to severe in intensity, or is aggravated by routine physical activity. Additionally, one of the following symptoms must accompany the headache: nausea and/or vomiting, or sensitivity to light or sounds. The person's medical history, a physical examination, and (where appropriate) diagnostic tests must exclude other organic causes of the headache, such as brain tumor or infection. Migraine with aura is far less common.

Migraines may be triggered or aggravated by physical activity, by menstruation, by relaxation after emotional stress, by ingestion of alcohol (red wine in particular) or certain foods or food additives (chocolate, hard cheeses, nuts, fatty foods, monosodium glutamate, or nitrates used in processed meats), by prescription medications (including birth control pills and hypertension medications), and by changes in the weather. Yet the precise pathophysiology of migraines is unknown. It had been posited that spasms in the blood vessels of the brain, followed by the dilation of these same blood vessels, cause the aura and head pain; however, studies using sophisticated brain and cerebral blood-flow scanning techniques indicate that this is likely not the case and that some type of inflammatory process may be involved related to the permeability of cerebral blood vessels and the resultant release of certain neurochemicals.

The tension-type headache is the most common type of headache; its prevalence is approximately 79 percent. Tension-type headaches are not hereditary, are found more frequently in females, and are first noticed in the teen years or young adulthood, although they can appear at any time of life. For the diagnosis of tension-type headaches, the person must experience at least ten headache attacks lasting from thirty minutes to seven days each, with at least two of the following characteristics: The headache has a pressing or tightening (nonpulsating) quality, is mild or moderate in intensity (may inhibit but does not prohibit activities), is bilateral or variable in location, and is not aggravated by physical activity. Additionally, nausea, vomiting, and light or sound sensitivity are absent or mild. Furthermore, the patient's medical history and physical or neurological examination exclude other organic causes for the headache apart from the following: oral or jaw dysfunction, muscular stress, or drug overuse. Tension-type headache sufferers describe these headaches as a band-like or cap-like tightness around the head, and/or muscle tension in the back of the head, neck, or shoulders. The pain is described as slow in onset with a dull or steady aching.

Tension-type headaches are believed to be precipitated primarily by emotional factors but can also be stimulated by muscular and spinal disorders, jaw dysfunction, paranasal sinus disease, and traumatic head injuries. The pathophysiology of tension-type headaches is controversial. Historically, tension-type headaches were attributed to sustained muscle contractions of the pericranial muscles. Studies indicate, however, that most patients do not manifest increased pericranial muscle activity and that pericranial muscle blood flow and/or central pain mechanisms might be involved in the pathophysiology of tension-type headaches. It is also believed that muscle contraction and scalp muscle ischemia play some role in tension-type headache pain.

Cluster headaches are the least frequent of the headache types and are thought to be the most severe and painful. Cluster headaches are more common in males, with estimates of 0.4 to 1.0 percent of males being affected. Traditionally, these headaches first appear at about thirty years of age, although they can start later in life. There is no genetic predisposition to these headaches. For the diagnosis of cluster headaches, the person must experience at least ten severely painful headache attacks, typically on one side of the face and lasting from fifteen minutes to three hours. One of the following symptoms must accompany the headache on the painful side of the face: a bloodshot eye, tearing, nasal congestion, nasal discharge, forehead and facial sweating, contraction of the pupils, or drooping eyelids. Physical and neurological examination and imaging must exclude organic causes for the headaches, such as tumor or infection. Cluster headaches often occur once or twice daily, or every other day, but can be as frequent as ten attacks in one day, recurring on the same side of the head during the cluster period. The temporal "clusters" of these headaches give them their descriptive name.

A cluster headache is described as a severe, excruciating, piercing, sharp, and burning pain through the eye. The pain is occasionally throbbing but always unilateral. Radiation of the pain to the teeth has been reported. Duration of a headache can range from ten minutes to three hours, with the next headache in the cluster occurring some time the same day. Cluster headache sufferers are often unable to sit or lie still and are in such pain that they have been known, in desperation, to hit their heads with their fists or to smash their heads against walls or floors.

Cluster headaches can be triggered in susceptible patients by alcohol consumption, subcutaneous injections of histamine, and sublingual use of nitroglycerine. Because these agents all cause the dilation of blood vessels, these attacks are believed to be associated with dilation of the temporal and ophthalmic arteries and other extracranial vessels. There is no evidence that intracranial blood flow is involved. Cluster headaches have been shown to occur more frequently during the weeks before and after the longest and shortest days of the year, lending support for the hypothesis of a link to seasonal changes. Additionally, cluster headaches often occur at about the same time of day in a given sufferer, suggesting a relationship to the circadian rhythms of the body. Vascular changes, hormonal changes, neurochemical excesses or deficits, histamine levels, and autonomic nervous system changes are all being studied for their possible role in the pathophysiology of cluster headaches.

Acute headaches, using the International Headache Society's classification scheme, constitute many of the headaches not mentioned above. Distinct from the other headache types, which are often considered to be chronic in nature, acute headaches often signify underlying disease or a life-threatening medical condition. These headaches can display pain distribution and quality similar to those seen in chronic headaches. The temporal nature of acute headaches, however, often points to their seriousness. Acute headaches of concern are usually the first or worst headache the patient has had or are headaches with recent onset that are persistent or recurrent. Other signs that cause a high index of suspicion include an unremitting headache that steadily increases without relief, accompanying weakness or numbness in the hands or feet, an atypical change in the quality or intensity of the headache, headache upon exertion, recent head trauma, or a family history of cardiovascular problems. Such headaches can point to hemorrhage, meningitis, stroke, tumor, brain abscess, hematoma, and infection, which are all potentially life-threatening conditions. A thorough evaluation is necessary for all patients exhibiting the danger signs of acute headache.

Treatment and Therapy

Because there are several hundred causes of headaches, the evaluation of headache complaints is crucial. Medical science offers myriad evaluation techniques for headaches. The initial evaluation includes a complete history and physical examination to determine the factors involved in the headache complaint, such as the general physical condition of the patient, neurological functioning, cardiovascular condition, metabolic status, and psychiatric condition. Based on this initial evaluation, the health care professional may elect to perform a number of diagnostic tests to confirm or reject a diagnosis. These tests might include blood studies, x-rays, computed tomography (CT) scans, psychological evaluation, electroencephalograms (EEGs), magnetic resonance imaging (MRI), or studies of spinal fluid.

Once a headache diagnosis is made, a treatment plan is developed. In the case of acute headaches, treatment may take varying forms, from surgery to the use of prescription medications. For migraine, tension-type, and cluster headaches, there are several common treatment options. Headache treatment can be categorized into two types: abortive (symptomatic) treatment or prophylactic (preventive) treatment. Treatment is tailored to the type of headache and the type of patient.

A headache is often a highly distressing occurrence for patients, sometimes causing a high level of anxiety, relief-seeking behavior, and a dependency on the health care system. The health care provider must consider not only biological elements of the illness but also possible resultant psychological and sociological elements as well. An open, communicative relationship with the patient is paramount, and treatment routinely begins with soliciting patient collaboration and providing patient education. Patient education takes the form of normalizing the headache experience for patients, thereby reducing their fears concerning the etiology of the headache or about being unable to cope with the pain. Supportiveness, understanding, and collaboration are all necessary components of any headache treatment.

There are a number of abortive pharmacological treatments for migraine headaches. Ergotamine tartrate (an alkaloid or salt) is effective in terminating migraine symptoms by either reducing the dilation of extracranial arteries or in some way stimulating certain parts of the brain. Isomethaptine, another effective treatment for migraine, is a combination of chemicals that stimulates the sympathetic nervous system, provides analgesia, and is mildly tranquilizing. Another class of medications for migraines are nonsteroidal anti-inflammatory drugs (NSAIDs); these drugs, as the name implies, work on the principle that inflammation is involved in migraine. Both narcotic and nonnarcotic pain medications are often used for migraines, primarily for their analgesic properties; the concern in prescribing potent narcotic pain medications is the potential for their overuse. Antiemetic medications prevent or arrest vomiting and have been used in the treatment of migraines. Sumatriptan, a vasoactive agent that increases the amount of the neurochemical serotonin in the brain, shows promise in treating migraines that do not respond to other treatments.

Prophylactic treatments for migraines include beta-blockers, methysergide, and calcium-channel blockers, which are believed to interfere with the dilation or contraction of extracranial arteries by acting on the sympathetic nervous system or on the central nervous system itself. Antidepressants, medications used typically for the treatment of depression, have also been found to prevent migraine attacks; there appears to be an analgesic effect from certain antidepressants that is effective for chronic migraines. Antiseizure medications have been found to be useful for some migraine patients, although the mechanism of action is unknown. NSAIDs have also been used as a preventive measure for migraines.

There are several nonpharmacological treatment options for migraine headaches. These include stress management, relaxation training, biofeedback (a variant of relaxation training), psychotherapy (both individual and family), and the modification of headache-precipitating factors (such as avoiding certain dietary precipitants). Each of these treatments has been found to be effective for certain patients, particularly those with chronic migraine complaints. For some patients, they can be as effective as pharmacological treatments. The exact mechanism of action for their effect on migraines has not been established. Other self-management techniques include lying quietly in a dark room, applying pressure to the side of the head or face on which the pain is experienced, and applying cold compresses to the head.

The abortive treatment options for tension-type headaches include narcotic and nonnarcotic analgesics, because of their pain-reducing properties. More often with tension-type headaches, the milder over-the-counter pain medications (such as aspirin or acetaminophen) are used. NSAIDs, simple muscle relaxants, or antianxiety drugs can also be used. Muscle relaxants and antianxiety drugs are believed to relax smooth muscles, reducing scalp muscle ischemia and therefore head pain.

Prophylactic treatments for tension-type headaches include antidepressants, narcotic and nonnarcotic analgesics, muscle relaxants, and antianxiety drugs. Occasionally, "trigger-point injections" are used to relieve tension-type headaches. Trigger points are areas within muscles, primarily in the upper back and neck, that are hypersensitive; when stimulated, they can cause headaches. These trigger points can be injected with a local anesthetic or steroid to decrease their sensitivity or to eliminate possible inflammation in the area.

Nonpharmacological treatment of tension-type headaches is similar to that for migraines and includes stress management, relaxation training, biofeedback, and psychotherapy. Psychotherapy has been found to be a very important adjunct to any treatment of tension-type headaches because the illness, particularly when chronic, can lead to a pain syndrome characterized by family dysfunction, medication overuse, and vocational disruptions. Other self-management techniques include taking a hot shower or bath, placing a hot water bottle or ice pack on the head or back of the neck, exercising, and sleeping.

For cluster headaches, one of the most excruciating types of headache, the most common abortive treatment is administering pure oxygen to the patient for ten minutes. The exact mechanism of action is unknown, but it might be related to the constriction of dilated cerebral arteries. Ergotamine tartrate or similar alkaloids given orally, intramuscularly, or intravenously can also abort the attack in some patients. Nasal drops of a local anesthetic (lidocaine hydrochloride) or cocaine have been used to interrupt the activity of the trigeminal nerve that is believed to be involved in cluster attacks. The efficacy of these treatments is inconclusive.

Prophylactic treatment of this headache type is crucial. Ergotamine, methysergide, calcium-channel blockers, antiseizure medications, and steroidal anti-inflammatory medications have been used with some success in the prevention of cluster attacks. The mechanism of action for these medications is unknown. Lithium carbonate, a drug commonly prescribed for bipolar disorders, has been found to be effective for some cluster patients. This medication is believed to affect certain regions of the brain, possibly the hypothalamus.

While no nonpharmacological treatment strategies are routinely offered to cluster headache patients, surgery is an option in severe cases, particularly if the headaches are resistant to all other available treatments. Percutaneous radio frequency thermocoagulation of the trigeminal ganglion is a surgical procedure that destroys the trigeminal nerve pathway, the chief nerve pathway to the face. Modest successes have been found with this extreme treatment option.

Perspective and Prospects

Headaches are among the most common complaints to physicians and quite likely have been a problem since the beginning of humankind. Accounts of headaches can be found in the clinical notes of Arateus of Cappadocia, a first century physician. Descriptions of specific headache subtypes can be traced to the second century in the writings of the Greek physician Galen. Headaches are prevalent health problems that affect all ages and sexes and those from various cultural, social, and educational backgrounds.

The prevalence of headaches is greater in women, although the reason is unknown. Age seems to be a mediating factor as well, with significantly fewer people sixty-five years of age or older reporting headache problems. There are no socioeconomic differences in prevalence rates, with persons in high-income and low-income brackets having similar rates. There are data to suggest that people with college educations or higher report headaches more often than those with only some high school education. The only vocational area that has been tied to increased rates of headaches is working at computer terminals.

The total economic costs of headaches are staggering. The expenses associated with advances in assessment techniques and routine health care have risen rapidly. The cost in lost workdays adds to this economic picture. The scientific study of headaches is necessary to understand this prevalent illness. Efforts, such as those by the International Headache Society, to develop accepted definitions of headaches will greatly assist efforts to identify and treat headaches.

—*Oliver Oyama, Ph.D.*

See also Anxiety; Brain; Brain disorders; Caffeine; Cluster headaches; Head and neck disorders; Migraine headaches; Multiple chemical sensitivity syndrome; Neuralgia, neuritis, and neuropathy; Neuroimaging; Neurology; Neurology, pediatric; Sinusitis; Stress; Stress reduction; Tumor removal; Tumors.

For Further Information:

Blanchard, Edward B., and Frank Andrasik. *Management of Chronic Headaches: A Psychological Approach.* New York: Pergamon Press, 1985.

Cohan, Wendy. *What Nurses Know . . . Headaches.* New York: Demos Medical Pub., 2013.

Diamond, Seymour. "Migraine Headaches." *Medical Clinics of North America* 75, no. 3 (May 1, 1991): 545–566.

Diamond, Seymour, and Merle L. Diamond. *A Patient's Guide to Headache and Migraine.* Newtown, Pa.: Handbooks in Health Care Co., 2009.

Eadie, Mervyn J. *Headache: Through the Centuries.* New York: Oxford University Press, 2012.

Giordano, Giovanna M., and Pietro G. Gallo. *Headaches: Causes, Treatment, and Prevention.* New York: Nova Science, 2012.

Ivker, Robert S. *Headache Survival: The Holistic Medical Treatment Program for Migraine, Tension, and Cluster Headaches.* New York: Putnam, 2002.

Lang, Susan, and Lawrence Robbins. *Headache Help: A Complete Guide to Understanding Headaches and the Medications That Relieve Them.* Boston: Houghton Mifflin, 2000.

MedlinePlus. "Headache." *MedlinePlus*, January 7, 2013.

National Headache Foundation. *Headaches.org,* 2013.

National Institute of Neurological Disorders and Stroke. "Headache: Hope through Research." *National Institute of Neurological Disorders and Stroke*, July, 2, 2013.

Paulino, Joel, and Ceabert J. Griffith. *The Headache Sourcebook.* Chicago: Contemporary Books, 2001.

Rapoport, Alan M., and Fred D. Sheftell. *Headache Relief.* Boston: Little, Brown, 1995.

Saper, Joel R., et al. *Handbook of Headache Management: A Practical Guide to Diagnosis and Treatment of Head, Neck, and Facial Pain.* 2d ed. Philadelphia: Lippincott Williams & Wilkins, 1999.

Wood, Debra. "Cluster Headache." *Health Library*, June 24, 2013.

Wood, Debra. "Migraine." *Health Library*, October 24, 2012.

HEALING

Biology

Anatomy or system affected: All

Specialties and related fields: Alternative medicine, cytology, dermatology, family medicine, hematology, histology, immunology, plastic surgery, vascular medicine

Definition: The process of mending damaged tissue by which an organism restores itself to health.

Key terms:

collagen: a white fibrous protein produced by the body to fill in areas destroyed by injury; the healing component more commonly thought of as scar tissue

delayed primary closure: a procedure in which the wound is left open four to six days and then sewn closed; used for infected or contaminated wounds

healing by primary intention: the most desirable healing in the least amount of time, with minimal scar tissue formation; the edges of the wound close together

healing by secondary intention: less desirable healing of a wound, with replacement of damaged area by granulation tissue; delayed healing and excessive scar formation occur

regeneration: the renewal, regrowth, or restoration of destroyed or missing tissue; the production of new tissue

tensile strength: the greatest stress that can be placed on a tissue without tearing it apart; relative to the strength of a tissue

wounds: injuries classified as open or closed depending on whether the skin is broken; types of open wounds include abrasions, lacerations, avulsions, punctures, and incisions

The Healing Process

The human body is not able to reproduce injured parts during the healing process. Most injured tissue in the body is replaced with collagen, a white protein known as scar tissue. Body areas capable of reproducing, or regenerating, include the outer layer of skin and the inner layers of the intestines.

The human body is involved in a continuous process of self-healing. The outer layer of the skin is constantly rubbed off, yet the body is able to replace (regenerate) new skin to take its place. Another body area capable of regeneration is the innermost layer of the intestine. All other types of tissue, however, such as muscle, fat, blood vessels, or even bones, must rely on other ways to heal when injured. How quickly the body heals depends on many factors, but the process is a

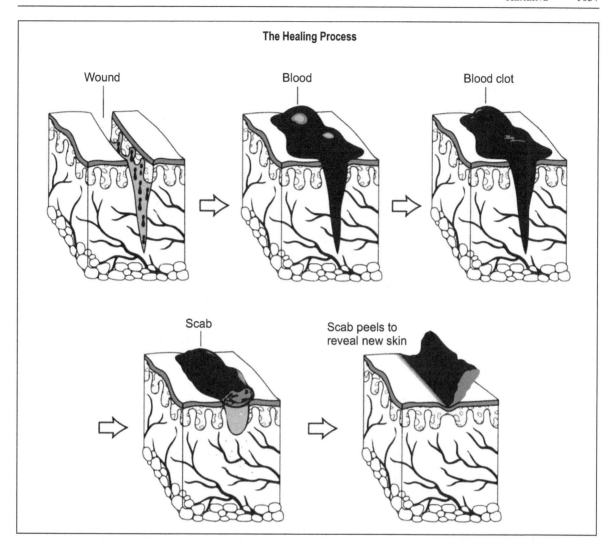

The Healing Process

Wound

Blood

Blood clot

Scab

Scab peels to reveal new skin

predictable one. The healing process includes three phases: the acute inflammatory phase, the repair or regeneration phase, and the remodeling phase.

The first phase of healing, the immediate inflammatory phase, includes the first three or four days after the injury. This process, carried out by vascular, chemical, and cellular events, leads to the repair of tissue, to regeneration, or to scar tissue formation. If the hand is sliced open by a piece of broken glass, the first healing response would be a temporary decrease in blood flow, known as vasoconstriction, or narrowing of the blood vessels at the injury site to prevent the person from bleeding to death. With extensive vessel damage, however, the body is unable to close off enough vessels, and life-threatening hemorrhaging may occur.

The blood begins to seal the broken vessels by coagulation, also known as blood clot formation. The next step is activation of the chemicals needed in the healing process, which is possible only after the blood vessel diameter increases in a process called vasodilation. During vasodilation, the blood

flow is slowed and the blood becomes thicker, resulting in swelling. At this point, a buildup or accumulation of fluid results from the seeping of plasma, the fluid portion of the blood, through the vessel walls. This seeping or leakage results from the difference in pressure within the vessel and outside its walls, as well as in the increased permeability of blood vessel walls during the inflammatory process. The amount of swelling at the injury site depends on the amount of seeping, which in turn depends on how much tissue damage has occurred.

Because the blood flow is slower, the concentration of red blood cells and white blood cells is increased. The white blood cells line up and adhere to the inside walls of small blood vessels, known as venules. These white blood cells then pass through the venule walls and are chemically attracted to the injury site over the next several hours. A specialized connective tissue cell, known as a mast cell, is also sent to the injury site. Mast cells contain heparin and histamine. Heparin prolongs the clotting time of blood by temporarily preventing coagulation, while histamine causes dilation of the capillaries. During this earliest phase, both heparin and histamine are important factors, since their actions allow other specialized cells to move into the injured area. The amount of bleeding and fluid buildup at the injury site depends on the extent of damage and how easily materials can cross the walls of intact vessels. Both of these conditions influence the healing process.

The second phase of healing can be called the repair or regeneration phase. For tissue capable of regeneration, this phase involves the restoration of destroyed or missing tissue. For other types of tissue, this second phase would entail the repair process. The healing of a deep cut in the hand would not be considered regeneration, since the body is not able to remake all the different layers of skin and muscle injured. This healing phase would extend forward from the previously described inflammatory phase. During this phase, the cut is naturally cleaned through the body's ability to remove cellular waste, the help of the red blood cells, and the formation of a blood clot.

Two types of healing can occur. Primary healing, or healing by primary intention, could take place in the hand laceration example, since the edges are even and close together. If this injury resulted in a large piece of tissue being removed, then the body would fill the gap with scar tissue. The replacement of tissue with scar tissue is an example of secondary healing, or healing by secondary intention. A torn muscle would be an example of secondary healing if it is allowed to heal on its own by the formation of scar tissue within the muscle.

No matter which type of healing occurs, several factors regulate how quickly and how completely this process takes place. Because blood vessels and cells are deprived of oxygen and die from the injury, this new cellular waste or debris must be cleaned from the area before repair or regeneration can take place. This tissue death promotes the formation of new capillary buds on the walls of the intact vessels. As these mature, the injury site is newly supplied with oxygenated blood and the healing process continues into the third phase.

The third phase of healing, known as the remodeling phase, includes the laying down of young scar tissue that increases in strength over the next year. Although the healing process has no distinct time frame, it is believed that three to six weeks are needed for the production of scar tissue. There must be a balance between the toughness and the elasticity of the scar. The amount of stress placed on a newly formed scar will determine the tensile strength of the collagen content. If stress or strain is placed on this forming scar tissue too early, the healing process will take longer. A desirable outcome would be a scar of adequate collagen content through the development of sufficient mature collagen fibers of proper tensile strength. Adequate tensile strength is also affected by how long inflammation is present.

If an injury site has inflammation that lasts up to one month, it is considered a subacute inflammation. When it lasts for months or years, it is then called chronic inflammation. Chronic inflammation is a condition in which small trau-

mas happen repeatedly; it is often seen in overuse injuries. Because this type of injury lasts longer, different types of chemicals try to initiate complete healing. The role of some of these special chemicals is not completely understood.

The healing of a broken bone, similar in many ways to the healing of the skin, is somewhat easier to understand. The first phase shows the same acute inflammation that lasts about four days, involving clotting blood, dead bone cells, and soft tissue damage around the injury site. The second phase, the repair and regeneration phase, differs slightly when a bone is broken, since the blood clot (hematoma) becomes granulated and builds between the two bone ends. The bone produces a specialized cell that turns into a soft or hard fibrous callus, matures into cartilage, and finally becomes bone with a firmly woven network of cells.

The beginning soft callus is a network of unorganized bone that forms at the two broken edges and is later absorbed and replaced by a hard callus. With appropriate care, a broken bone will develop a new network in the center and eventually become primary bone. The amount of oxygen available in the area determines this development. It is important to keep in mind that when the injury is severe enough to break a bone, then the blood supply is interrupted, lowering the amount of oxygen that is available. Low oxygen could result in the formation of only fibrous tissue or cartilage. Strong, healthy bone results when oxygen and the correct amount of compression are available. The third phase, the remodeling phase, describes the time when the callus has been reabsorbed and special intersecting bone fibers cover the broken area. It may take many years for this entire process to be completed, until the bone has regained its normal shape and ability to withstand stresses.

Disorders and Treatment

Any of the three stages of healing can be delayed or prevented. The three main causes for failed healing are poor blood supply, poor immobilization, or infection.

The healing process within the body can be seriously hampered if the blood supply is poor, since the delivery of nutrients, chemicals, hormones, and specialized building materials to the injury site is hampered. It is extremely important that oxygen levels are adequate for proper healing. If the blood supply is not sufficient, then the tissue may die, especially in broken bone fragments. Fortunately, most tissues of the body have a good blood supply, as demonstrated by the amount of bleeding that takes place when the skin and underlying tissues are injured.

The second condition that interferes with healing is excessive movement because the body part was not immobilized. For the scar tissue or even new bone to become well organized, the two edges of the injured tissue must be kept close together.

The third reason for poor healing is infection. Although the body has many defenses against infection, foreign material can slow healing. If this infectious material invades the space between the two bone ends of a fracture, the necessary building materials may not reach the site. Infection invading the

---

In the News:
Role of Growth Hormone in Healing

Growth hormone (GH) has been shown to be a stimulating, but not an essential, factor in healing of the colon in dwarf rats. In the September, 2006, issue of the *Scandinavian Journal of Surgery*, researchers investigated the physiological role of growth hormone deficiency on the healing of colonic anastomoses and whether any reduced healing capacity in growth-hormone-deficient rats could be reversed by treatment with growth hormone.

Dwarf rats were treated with recombinant human growth hormone (rhGH) for seven days prior to surgery and for four days postoperatively. The surgery involved cutting out a one-centimeter-wide portion of rat intestine and reconnecting the cut ends in a procedure called end-to-end anastomosis. Researchers measured the strength of the anastomoses of the dwarf rats compared to control groups as an indication of the degree of healing. It was found that treatment with rhGH stimulated healing of the colonic anastomoses in dwarf rats, compared to dwarf rats not treated with rhGH and untreated normal rats that have normal pituitary function. Although healing also occurred in the dwarf rats not treated with rhGH and untreated normal rats, it was not as extensive as the healing that occurred in dwarf rats treated with rhGH.

An interesting finding is that there was no difference in healing between the untreated dwarf rats and the untreated normal rats. This indicates that, although growth hormone plays a role in healing in dwarf rats, growth hormone is not essential to the healing process and other factors may be involved in regulation of healing. Further studies will be needed to examine the possibility of using growth hormone in a clinical setting to stimulate postsurgery healing and to determine the appropriate patient population to treat.

Jason J. Schwartz, Ph.D., J.D.

---

hand tissue cut by the glass could prevent the edges from healing together because of pus, scab formation, or the interference of germs.

There are many different types of injuries, and several steps must be taken in caring for each type. Soft tissues, the first line of defense against injuries, can be used to describe all tissues other than bone. Soft tissue injuries are classified as either closed or open. In a closed wound, the damage lies below the surface of the skin and the skin remains intact. A sprained ankle or a bruised knee are classified as closed wounds. In an open wound, the skin or mucous membranes, such as the lining of the mouth, are broken or torn.

There are four types of open soft tissue injuries; each has specific characteristics and heals differently. The first type is an abrasion, in which part of the outer layer of the skin and some underlying tissue is rubbed or scraped off. A common injury of this type is a scraped knee resulting from a fall on the sidewalk. The second type, a laceration, results from a sharp object cutting the skin, such as the previous example of a piece of glass cutting the skin either superficially or very deeply. The third type, an avulsion, results when a piece of skin or even an entire fingertip is torn off or left loosely hanging by a small flap of skin. It is important that this flap not be removed since a physician can sometimes reattach the part. The last type of soft tissue injury is the puncture wound, which results when a sharp object penetrates the skin and into a body part. Such an injury could be a stab from a knife or an ice pick, a splinter stuck in the foot, or even a bullet shot into the leg. The initial management is the same for all four types of injury.

Management of open wounds must include the control of bleeding, infection prevention, and immobilization. Two of the above injuries, an avulsion and a puncture wound, require additional special care. In the case of an avulsed body part, the amputated part should be saved; wrapped in a dry, sterile piece of gauze; and placed in a plastic bag. If this bag is kept in something cool, such as a bucket of ice, the possibility of reattachment is increased. An impaled object remaining in a puncture wound should never be removed but held in place, all movement restricted until medical care can be given.

Several medical treatments can aid in promoting the healing process, as can commonsense first aid measures taken immediately after an injury occurs. For example, with a glass cut to the hand one should immediately stop the bleeding by placing a sterile piece of gauze, or a very clean cloth, directly over the laceration. By adding direct pressure over the gauze, the circulation is reduced. If the cut is deep, if the bleeding cannot be controlled, or if a piece of glass remains in the wound, then it is advisable to seek medical attention. A physician would then thoroughly clean the injury site and stitch the two edges together. Immobilizing the two flaps of skin together by sewing them will allow the first two phases of healing to progress. By having the wound inspected and cleaned by medical personnel, the risk of infection is reduced. A small injury can be cared for at home, but infection must be prevented through proper cleansing. Even soap and water, along with a bandage or dressing, will help ward off infections.

Perspective and Prospects

Many strategies to improve the healing of human tissue have evolved over time—from ancient times, when healers packed mud on the top of sores to draw out the infection, to modern alternative medicines. Every person, at one time or another, receives a cut, scrape, bump, or bruise. Therefore, there is much interest in speeding up the healing process.

Renewed interests in nontraditional approaches to medicine explore the healing powers locked within the human body. The use of homeopathy, acupuncture, and acupressure are examples of alternatives to antibiotics and standard first aid measures to help an injury heal. Holistic health care, hypnosis, and osteopathic medicine offer other areas of exploration. The practice of Chinese medicine includes the use of herbs, crystals, massage, and meditation to allow healing to proceed quickly but through natural means. Even the use of aromatherapy—treatment through the inhalation of specific smells—has gained a foothold in the medical world. The manipulations done by chiropractic doctors offer other possibilities. Some seek cures in nature, from sources below the sea or deep in the forest. Yet, many untapped resources remain. The continuing research in genetics offers vast possibilities, and the link between mental attitude and the immune system presents a rich area for further exploration. Even innovations as simple as a special glue, used to replace sutures or staples for closing wounds, would have an important influence on the future of the healing process.

—*Maxine M. Urton, Ph.D.*

See also Antibiotics; Aromatherapy; Bleeding; Blood and blood disorders; Chiropractic; Circulation; Dermatology; First aid; Grafts and grafting; Histology; Host-defense mechanisms; Hyperbaric oxygen therapy; Immune system; Immunology; Infection; Inflammation; Laceration repair; Meditation; Skin; Surgery, general; Vascular system; Wounds.

For Further Information:

American Academy of Orthopaedic Surgeons. *Emergency Care and Transportation of the Sick and Injured.* Edited by Benjamin Gulli, Les Chatelain, and Chris Stratford. 10th ed. Sudbury, Mass.: Jones and Bartlett, 2011.

"Bruises." *MedlinePlus,* June 10, 2013.

DiPietro, Luisa A., and Aime L. Burns, eds. *Wound Healing: Methods and Protocols.* Totowa, N.J.: Humana Press, 2003.

Eisenberg, David. *Encounters with Qi.* New York: W. W. Norton, 1995.

"Fractures." *MedlinePlus,* May 15, 2013.

Gach, Michael R. *Acupressure's Potent Points: A Guide to Self-Care for Common Ailments.* New York: Bantam Books, 1990.

Goldberg, Linn, and Diane L. Elliot. *The Healing Power of Exercise: Your Guide to Preventing and Treating Diabetes, Depression, Heart Disease, High Blood Pressure, Arthritis, and More.* New York: Wiley, 2002.

Handal, Kathleen A. *The American Red Cross First Aid and Safety Handbook.* Boston: Little, Brown, 1992.

"Handout on Health: Sports Injuries." *National Institute of Arthritis and Musculoskeletal and Skin Diseases,* April 2009.

Heller, Jacob L, et al. "Cuts and Puncture Wounds." *MedlinePlus,* January 1, 2013.

Kemper, Kathi J. *The Holistic Pediatrician: A Pediatrician's Comprehensive Guide to Safe and Effective Therapies for the Twenty-five Most Common Ailments of Infants, Children, and Adolescents.* 2d ed. New York: HarperCollins, 2007.

Kopec, Tom. "Wound Healing and Care." *TeensHealth.* Nemours Foundation, November 2011.

"Nutrition Guidelines to Improve Wound Healing." *Cleveland Clinic,* November 1, 2007.

Subbarao, Italo, et al., eds. *American Medical Association Handbook of First Aid and Emergency Care.* Rev. ed. New York: Random House Reference, 2009.

Woodham, Anne, and David Peters. *The DK Natural Health Encyclopedia of Natural Healing.* 2d ed. New York: DK, 2000.

HEALTH CARE REFORM

Health care system

Definition: Changes in major governmental policies regarding health care access, services, cost, fairness, and delivery.

Key terms:

health care system: the collection of services in a given country that provide hospital, emergency, preventive, and other outpatient care to citizens

health insurance: the promise by an insurance provider to pay specified costs related to the health care of an individual or group of individuals who pay premium fees

outpatient: evaluation and treatment that does not require overnight stay

reform: a change to improve conditions

Organization and Function

The function of health care is to provide preventive diagnostic treatment and emergency care for the citizens of a country. The physical organization of the health care system in the United States consists of hospitals, outpatient clinics, pharmacies, home health care services, long-term care facilities, public health clinics, and other supportive services such as occupational therapy. There are many layers of staff including physicians, nurses, physician assistants, other medical support staff, office staff, and administrative staff. These organizations are regulated by state and federal agencies. Naturopathic, dental, optometric, and other services are often excluded from insurance or other health care plans.

Health Care in the United States

There are many misconceptions about the existing health care systems in North America and around the world. In the United States, access to services and direct cost to the patient depend on the insurance plan or lack of insurance plan. In Canada, patients are prevented from paying for a service in their own province if it is covered by the provincial health care plan. To reduce costs, a specific number of services are available per quarter or year in some parts of Canada.

To understand health care reform, one has to understand the existing system. In his book *The Healing of America: A Global Quest for Better, Cheaper, and Fairer Health Care* (2009), T. R. Reid outlines four basic health care delivery systems present worldwide today.

The Bismark model is named after the inventor of this German system. It consists of private nonprofit insurance plans that provide universal coverage through public and private hospital services. Cost control is achieved by tight regulation of services and fees.

The Beveridge model is named after a health care reformer in Britain. In this model, the United Kingdom's National Health Care System is financed through taxes. It provides services in public and private hospitals and clinics. The government is responsible for fees and services, and patients do not receive a bill.

The National Health Insurance model involves government insurance with premiums. The most familiar example is the Canadian system, which is credited to Tommy Douglas, the premier in Saskatchewan from 1944 to 1961. The Canadian system is provincially based, so each provincial government decides what services are covered, what fees are paid per service to the provider, and what premiums are charged.

Finally, the out-of-pocket model is a fee-for-service system in which patients pay a fee for each service. This is the prevailing system in developing countries and among the millions of uninsured Americans.

The United States has elements of all four systems. People

with insurance through employers will have coverage for many health care services similar to the Bismark model, with the important difference that many insurance companies in the United States are for-profit. Depending on the insurance plan, copayments may be due and certain services may not be offered. Citizens with Veterans Administration health care, Indian Health Services, or Pentagon's Tri-Star have coverage that is similar to the Beveridge system, in which the government pays for services. For those over sixty-five years old, the national health insurance plan known as Medicare applies. Medicare is similar to the Canadian national health insurance system. For the millions of people who have no insurance, the health care system is a purely fee-for-service system like that found in developing countries. For those who cannot pay, a patchwork of government services such as state-run plans or county hospitals may pay for emergency care.

The number of people in the United States who have no insurance is greater than the entire population of Canada and more than five times the population of Sweden. According to the United States Census Bureau, 48.6 million Americans, or 15.7 percent of the population, had no insurance in 2011. This is a significant health and financial burden. The linkage of affordable insurance to employment also makes many people reluctant to change jobs or to start small businesses, since doing so could require them to give up their health insurance.

When considering health care reform, the government of each country must decide what type or types of health care delivery systems are desired. In a democratic country, this decision will include input from citizens.

Services and Cost

There is a balance between the services provided by any system, the cost per service, and the reimbursement of the provider. The provision of health care varies from simple procedures such as suturing a wound to very complex care such as diagnosing a rare neurologic disorder. Cost will also increase with the time a provider spends with a patient. In systems that have a fixed cost per service, the provider will have a financial incentive to see as many patients as quickly as possible. Malpractice insurance costs and claims also may affect cost and services. In some cases, tests or treatments may be recommended in order to reduce chances of malpractice claims. Some providers will discontinue high-risk procedures because of malpractice insurance costs.

It is a complex equation to determine this balance of service to patients; cost to patients via insurance, taxes, or cash; and reimbursement to providers. Geography and ethnic diversity will also complicate the equation. The population of the United States is more than 300 million, while Canada is about 34 million and Sweden is under 10 million. The United States covers about 3.7 million square miles, Canada about 3.8 million square miles, and Sweden about 170,000 square miles. These factors will influence the feasibility of services in some cases. For example, in the sparsely populated arctic in Canada, it is difficult to provide the same services that may be available in a more densely populated metropolitan area.

Cost is also influenced by insurance company profits, health care provider reimbursement, technology, and preventive care. Some health care systems attempt to limit overall costs by providing preventive education and care. Immunization programs are an example of preventive health care that can reduce illness and therefore reduce cost to the system. Other systems use government control such as rationing to control costs. Rationing may lead to long waiting lists for services.

The balance between services and cost is at the core of any health care reform debate. This balance will be influenced by decisions such as preventive care provisions, what is considered to be elective care versus necessary care, individual needs versus the needs of the population, long-term care provision, and a host of other factors.

Perspective and Prospects

People with steady employment with health care benefits will not necessarily perceive that there is any problem with the existing system. A portion of the 48 million uninsured in the United States may also not perceive a problem if they have not had a need to access services. However, those uninsured with serious health issues, those who become unemployed and lose their insurance, or those who are disqualified from insurance due to preexisting conditions may feel there is a need for reform.

In spite of leading in health care expenditure, the United States places low in many rankings of health indicators. Some use these statistics to point to the need for health care reform in the United States. According to the World Health Organization (WHO), average life expectancy at birth for Americans was 79 years in 2011; the country ranks below numerous industrialized nations, including Japan, France, and Israel. Life expectancy may be affected by other factors such as homicide, so some believe this is not a true indicator of the quality of health care. Other indicators are similarly complex.

Health care reform in the United States is a particularly difficult task due to the large population, the variety of health care delivery systems that exist, and the many diseases and other health concerns that must be treated.. Chronic diseases such as heart disease, depression, asthma, and diabetes account for a large amount of spending. Some politicians and health care professionals believe that early intervention in these cases would ultimately save money. Reform that includes more access to care, preventive care, and early intervention for people with these chronic diseases may improve health quality while decreasing health costs.

There are several things to consider regarding health care reform in the United States. It comes down to the collective philosophy of the citizens, the financial assessment of the benefit of investing in care for the underserved populations, the cost to the citizens through taxation, the cost to citizens for poor health in a segment of the population, and the cost to businesses for employee insurance.

Points under debate include whether providing insurance and preventive care to the currently uninsured might save money, as such individuals might otherwise access costly emergency care when untreated preexisting conditions lead to more serious illness. Lack of affordable insurance may discourage people from becoming self-employed or may cause small businesses to hire only part-time employees to avoid having to pay for expensive employee insurance plans. People with preexisting conditions may be reluctant to change employment due to possible loss of insurance.

Philosophical issues such as whether health care is to be considered a fundamental right are also being discussed. If health care is a fundamental right, then the debate involves what level of services should be considered and whether more wealthy citizens should be allowed to purchase care for faster or more extensive services. The question of whether citizens have a responsibility to have insurance and the role of low-cost insurance as a stimulus to small businesses and self-employed people are other factors to consider. Profit versus nonprofit provision of care, as well as reimbursement for providers, also affects the debate.

The 2009 United States health care bill, the Patient Protection and Affordable Care Act, is more than two thousand pages long and attempts to address a number of these issues. It includes individual and group market reforms such as no lifetime or annual limits and access to insurance for individuals with preexisting conditions. Health insurance market reforms include guaranteed availability and renewability of insurance.

The bill attempts to improve choice through federal assistance in establishment of member-run nonprofit health insurance issuers and state flexibility in the establishment of alternate health care plans for low-income groups. There are also tax credits for individuals and small businesses to encourage individual and employee-sponsored insurance coverage. Individual and employer responsibilities to require minimum insurance for individuals and employees are included in the bill.

There are specific provisions against assisted suicide and to allow for individual choice not to participate in federal health care plans. Additional provisions relate to Medicare and Medicaid reform, rural protections, improvements in payment accuracy, and improvements in Medicare prescription drug coverage. Health care quality and preventive health with the goal of improving public health are also included in this bill, as well as provisions to improve the health care workforce, community health initiatives, and fiscal transparency.

The Patient Protection and Affordable Care Act, passed by Congress and signed into law by President Barack Obama on March 23, 2010, is very complex and not surprisingly has generated strong opinions both for and against many of the provisions within it. As this debate continues to unfold, the philosophical basis for the delivery of health care in the United States will drive the discussion. For those who favor coverage of all citizens, this law offers the hope of providing care to many millions of uninsured. Others are concerned about costs via increased taxation and government involvement. Balancing the complexities of reforming the amalgam that is the United States health system is a challenge that has the goal of improvements in cost, access, and quality of care

for millions of Americans.

—*E. E. Anderson Penno, M.S., M.D., FRCSC*

See also Department of Health and Human Services; Health Canada; Medicare; National Institutes of Health (NIH).

For Further Information:

Armstrong, Pat, and Hugh Armstrong. *About Canada Health Care.* Black Point, N.S.: Fernwood, 2008.

Greer, Scott L., and Paulette Kurzer, eds. *European Union Public Health Policy: Regional and Global Trends.* New York: Routledge, 2013.

Halvorson, George C. *Health Care Reform Now! A Prescription for Change.* San Francisco: John Wiley & Sons, 2007.

Kominski, Gerald F. *Changing the US Health Care System: Key Issues in Health Services Policy and Management.* 4th ed. Malden: Wiley-Blackwell, 2013.

Reid, T. R. *The Healing of America: A Global Quest for Better, Cheaper, and Fairer Health Care.* New York: Penguin Press, 2009.

United States Census Bureau. "Health Insurance." *US Department of Commerce,* 2011.

Weissert, William G. *Governing Health: The Politics of Health Policy.* 4th ed. Baltimore: Johns Hopkins University Press, 2012.

HEALTH MAINTENANCE ORGANIZATIONS (HMOs)

Organizations

Also known as: Competitive medical plans

Definition: A business competitor within a free market economy that provides health care insurance and services to group and individual clients for an established, prepaid monthly premium and that generally attempts to provide care at a lower cost than traditional fee-for-service insurance programs by transferring financial risk to physicians through capitation and other incentives.

Key terms:

disability insurance: a health coverage policy that protects against loss of income resulting from sickness or accident, whereby benefits are structured to pay approximately 40 to 60 percent of earnings up to a maximum total amount

group model HMO: an HMO organized by physicians whereby a private professional corporation is established which then individually contracts with an HMO to provide services exclusively for its subscribers

independent practice association model HMO: a flexible arrangement whereby several office physicians in a community form a networked professional corporation that seeks group contracts among local employers and provides all medical care for a capitated rate per client per month to subscribers, who often choose a personal primary care physician

managed care: the techniques by which an HMO, a health insurance carrier, or a self-insuring employer makes certain that the health care services it is endorsing are cost-effective and of a high quality

point-of-service model HMO: also called an open-ended HMO; a model that includes an option which allows subscribers to seek medical care outside the established network and receive partial reimbursement, with all remaining expenses paid out-of-pocket

preferred providers: physicians and other health care providers and hospitals who choose to provide health care at a reduced cost for subscribers to an HMO

staff model HMO: an HMO that is directly controlled at its headquarters, with all physicians and other health care workers being full-time, salaried employees

Role in the Health Care Industry

A health maintenance organization (HMO) in a free market economy functions in a dual role as both a health insurance company and a provider of health services, roles that were previously separated within the American health care system. HMOs-also known as competitive medical plans, managed care plans, or alternative delivery systems-are generally organized by an employer, physician group, union, consumer group, insurance company, or for-profit health care company. Originally, they were formed from one or more of the following models: point of service, staff, group, and independent practice association (IPA).

The HMO as insurer seeks group contracts with employers and individual patients and negotiates premiums in exchange for covering specified, preagreed-to benefits. It affiliates with or directly hires physicians and other health care providers to treat the expected volume of care that is required for all subscribers (referred to as "covered lives") under contract. An HMO owns or contracts with one or more health centers (e.g., clinics, offices) for ambulatory care and with hospitals and other facilities for inpatient care. Within its private health center or in contracts with freestanding providers, an HMO furnishes services from other providers such as physical and occupational therapy, pharmacy, and behavioral/mental health care, which are rapidly increasing in their level of responsibility.

HMOs are attractive to employers because the annual medical bill for the average subscriber-patient consistently has proved to be approximately 30 percent less than that of conventional commercial insurers. One advantage of HMO membership is that all medical expenses, from routine and emergency care to hospitalization, are covered within a single, fixed monthly premium. In addition, presenting an HMO membership card at time of services with a small co-payment means that paperwork is often reduced. A distinct disadvantage to the HMO model is that that new subscribers often cannot keep a trusted physician they have had for years; also, there is less flexibility in plan design, providers are often too busy, and subscribers often must accept fewer choices in treatment options. Often, subscriber satisfaction with HMO plans is low.

Practices and Procedures

The term "managed care" describes the techniques by which an HMO, a health insurance carrier, or a self-insuring employer investigates that the health care services that it endorses are high quality and cost-effective. This system was once used in many countries. Workers joined a mutual aid

association and paid premiums, and the association was responsible for hiring enough quality full-time or part-time physicians to meet the acute and chronic health needs of its members. These restrictive arrangements could not survive within a country that has a national health insurance law because every covered citizen would then have the right to choose any provider and subsequently bill the system. Managed care has been able to survive in the United States because a compulsory national health insurance law had not been enacted. Since the passage of the Affordable Care Act in 2010, health insurance became compulsory with graduated penalties assessed on individuals who refuse to purchase coverage. The impact of this paradigmatic change in health insurance on individual HMOs and the HMO model itself has yet to evolve, though the impact is expected to be great.

The headquarters of an HMO competitively markets its services to employer groups and individuals and administers the revenue and payments. An HMO generally contracts or directly hires a limited number of physicians in addition to building, staffing, and equipping the necessary number of health centers and hospitals. Its marketing claim is to provide good quality care within the employer's group premium, without seeking further supplements from the employer. Because an HMO and its providers are at personal financial risk, the organization directly imposes financial discipline upon its physicians, hospitals, and other health care providers. The HMO retains a percentage of the premiums paid from employers for its administrative and facility costs and pays a monthly "capitated rate" per client to the providers. HMOs have historically had persistent difficulty in recruiting and retaining physicians, and patients have consistently informed the HMOs that they prefer private offices to health centers.

Managed care procedures generally involve the HMO establishing a network of physicians with superior reputations in each region, with these physicians agreeing to bill the carriers according to limited reimbursement rules. Each client is assigned to a "primary care gatekeeper" who is expected to provide most care in his or her private office for limited fees. When a referral to a specialist, laboratory, or hospital is necessary, authorization is required from the headquarters of the managed care organization. Hospitals contract with these organizations to limit their charges and follow established rules about economical care and prompt discharge. The managed care organization reviews utilization by physicians and hospitals, attempts to correct wasteful practices, and subsequently drops health care providers with expensive and/or poor practice styles.

In contrast to more traditional HMOs, point-of-service (POS) plans have more recently emerged. These enable patients some choice with respect to providers and treatment options but requires them personally to pay the balance for their chosen higher-priced services. If the patient goes to physicians, hospitals, and other providers within the network and follows rules about utilization and authorization, the out-of-pocket financial costs are minimal. The patient retains the option to go to an out-of-plan provider, pay the bill in full, and then be reimbursed for the limited amount established in the individual plan. The employer's group contract with the managed care organization provides for limited and predictable premiums. The considerable costs of out-of-plan services thus are shifted from the group contract to the individual patient.

Managed care plans will continue to monitor closely the treatment patterns of physicians and encourage them to prescribe cheaper medications, to develop standards that physicians are expected to follow in treatment of various diseases, and to hold utilization review panels that review patient records and decide which treatments a patient's health plan will cover and which it will not. Because of the numerous consumer complaints that arose from actions resulting from the decisions of case managers, who often do not have any medical training, nineteen states had passed comprehensive managed care laws by 1997. In that year, states passed a record 182 laws related to managed care, up from 100 in 1996. Legislation during the late 1990s and into the twenty-first century focused on issues such as adopting measures to ban physician gag clauses, establishing consumer grievance procedures, requiring disclosure of financial incentives for physicians to withhold care, holding external reviews of internal decisions to deny care, and ensuring the ability to sue an HMO for malpractice. In 2001, many of these issues were addressed via a legislative "Bill of Rights" for patients. The bill led to a contentious debate over whether and how to regulate managed care plans. The bill was passed, but critics claim its provisions do not apply to all of the more than 160 million people enrolled in health insurance plans and fail to give unhappy patients the right to sue their health plans for punitive damages. Several states have also attempted-with some, like Washington State, succeeding-to implement their own managed care reforms.

Perspective and Prospects

The first HMOs in the United States were established in the 1930s with the pioneering efforts of the Ross-Loos Medical Group in California, but most experienced only minimal growth until the 1970s. Beginning in the early 1970s, HMOs proliferated rapidly, primarily as a result of escalating costs for health care services and increasing competition among a growing number of physicians. The Health Maintenance Organizations Act of 1973 provided federal grants and loans for the establishment of HMOs and required many employers to offer HMO membership to employees as a health insurance alternative. The federal government began to promote the HMO concept as a means by which to control costs by discouraging physicians from performing unnecessary and costly procedures, to meet the increased demand for health insurance particularly in under-served areas, and to foster preventive medicine. Monetary incentives, which are strongly supported by numerous politicians, are in theory the major forces behind personal freedom of choice, containment of costs, and assurance of quality. Innovated by the Kaiser Foundation Health Plan in California, the Health Insurance Plan of Greater New York, and the Group Health Cooperative of Puget Sound, greater numbers of preferred provider

organizations began to appear in the 1980s and 1990s as a more flexible alternative to standard HMOs. Many major health insurers such as Blue Cross and Blue Shield then began exerting control over the daily operations of both HMOs and preferred provider organizations. Managed care was spread rapidly across the United States by the large health insurance companies, largely stimulated by the ongoing difficulties experienced by national policy in containing medical costs. In 1970, there were approximately thirty different managed care plans; by 1997, this number had grown to more than fifteen hundred. In 1997, more than 80 percent of HMOs were for-profit organizations. The significance of this figure is that an increasing amount of money that could be spent on medical care is now being spent on marketing costs and stockholder dividends.

A looming question regarding the future of HMOs is whether physicians and other health care workers, as well as patient subscribers, will continue to enroll and support the system. Managed care necessarily adds substantial administrative overhead, with the ongoing question of whether the final result is greater efficiency for the entire system or simply for subscribing employers. Another controversy involves the responsibility of an HMO to provide disability insurance, which becomes necessary when a client incurs loss of income resulting from sickness or an accident that is not covered by workers' compensation.

An organization that has exerted considerable influence in future HMO developments is the American Association of Retired Persons (AARP), a large, nonprofit advocacy group for Americans over the age of fifty with more than 37 million members. It has begun giving endorsements to HMOs that meet its standards of quality and price.

In other industrialized nations, both the services covered and the extent of coverage equal or exceed the coverage of a standard HMO in the United States. Several countries have universal health care insurance, although in many industrialized nations certain categories of residents may be exempt. Notable examples include Germany, which requires the purchase of private health insurance by law; Canada and Sweden, which have public insurance coverage for essentially any citizen; and Great Britain, which has a majority of medical services located within the public sector. In the United States, the Affordable Care Act is revolutionizing how health care can be purchased by individuals and organizations, what models of health care delivery will be employed, and what metrics and quality measures will be used to evaluate health care quality. Unless repealed by Congress, full implementation of the law will occur by 2020. Under its current provisions coverage is guaranteed regardless of community rating, pre-existing medical conditions, or age, all of which were factors considered in whether individuals could belong to particular HMO plans. The law provides for more coverage options depending upon income, family size, and residing state. All Americans will be required to be covered by health insurance through employers, public programs, or by purchasing coverage from state-based health insurance exchanges, and these exchanges may end up reformulating the

HMO model all together. It is certain, however, that HMOs are in the early stages of transformation that may well result in their extinction as they have been previously known.

—*Daniel G. Graetzer, Ph.D.;*
updated by Althea Williams, M.B.A.

See also Allied health; Ethics; Law and medicine; Malpractice; Managed care

For Further Information:

Birenbaum, Aaron. *Wounded Profession: American Medicine Enters the Age of Managed Care.* Westport, CT: Greenwood Press, 2002. Traces the evolution of health care in the United States during the 1990s and examines the rising costs, consumer backlash, and new legislation.

Brink, Susan, and Nancy Shute. "Are HMOs the Right Prescription?" *U.S. News and World Report* 123, no. 4 (October 13, 1997): 60-65. Covered in this well-researched article is the growing dissatisfaction of subscribers with the quality of health care received, with a rating of the best HMOs in the United States.

Dranove, David. *The Economic Evolution of American Health Care: From Marcus Welby to Managed Care.* Princeton, NJ: Princeton University Press, 2002. Traces the economic, technological, and historical forces that have transformed the health care field.

Freeborn, Donald K., and Clyde R. Pope. *Promise and Performance in Managed Care: The Prepaid Group Practice Model.* Rev. ed. Baltimore: Johns Hopkins University Press, 2000. This excellent text highlights the evolution of several common promises of HMOs that employ the prepaid practice model and evaluates their performance based on relevant criteria.

Johnsson, Julie. "HMOs Dominate, Shape the Market." *American Medical News* 39, no. 4 (1996): 1-3. A well-written article that outlines the competition among HMOs and how t

Kongstvedt, Peter R. *Managed Care: What It Is and How It Works.* 3rd ed. Sudbury, MA: Jones and Bartlett, 2009. Provides a historical overview of managed care and covers organizational structures, concepts, and practices of the managed care industry.

Lairson, D.R., et al. "Managed Care and Community-Oriented Care: Conflict or Complement?" *Journal of Health Care for the Poor and Underserved* 8, no. 1 (1997): 36-55. This informative article evaluates models for community health planning and health care reform designed for the medically indigent, including programs that receive support from the U.S. government and programs that do not.

Ludmerer, Kenneth M. *Time to Heal: American Medical Education from the Turn of the Century to the Managed Care Era.* New York: Oxford University Press, 2005. Ludmerer looks at the future of medicine in America and reveals some very disturbing trends in managed care, education, and research funding. Contains a wealth of factual details and insightful questions.

Zelman, Walter A. *The Changing Health Care Marketplace.* San Francisco: Jossey-Bass, 1996. An excellent evaluation of past trends in HMOs and predictions of what the future might hold.

HEARING

Anatomy

Also known as: Auditory process, audition, auditory sense, sense of hearing

Anatomy or system affected: Bones, brain, cells, ears, nerves

Specialties and related fields: Audiology, neurology

Definition: The series of events in which sound is processed by the sensory system.

Key terms:

cochlea: a structure in the inner ear that receives sound vibrations from the ossicles and transmits them to the auditory nerve

incus: a small bone within the middle ear; also called the anvil because of its shape

malleus: a small bone within the middle ear; also called the hammer because of its shape

nerves: bundles of sensory and motor neurons held together by layers of connective tissue

stapes: a small bone within the middle ear; also called the stirrup because of its shape

tympanic membrane: the eardrum, which separates the external ear canal from the middle ear and ossicles and which transmits sound vibration to the ossicles

Structure and Functions

The human ear can be divided into three distinct regions: the outer ear, the middle ear, and the inner ear. The outer ear consists of two parts, the external pinna (also known as the auricle) and the auditory canal. The external pinna is the external visible part of the ear, made of cartilage. The external pinna and auditory canal channel sound waves into the ear and direct them to the tympanic membrane, or eardrum. The tympanic membrane serves as the division between the outer ear and the middle ear, and vibrates with sound. The vibrations are channeled to three small bones within the middle ear, the malleus (hammer), incus (anvil), and stapes (stirrup). These bones further transmit the vibrations to the membranous oval window, located just below the stapes. The middle ear also opens to the eustachian tube, which is connected to the pharynx and serves as a pressure stabilizer between the middle ear and the atmosphere. This connection allows for the "pop" of ears during a flight or scuba diving.

The oval window serves as the link between the middle and inner ear. The inner ear consists of a long, coiled snail-like structure consisting of fluid-filled chambers. The chambers include the semicircular canals, involved in maintaining balance, and the cochlea, which has a role in hearing. The cochlea consists of two canals, the vestibular canal and the tympanic canal, which are separated by the cochlear duct. The canals are filled with perilymph, and the cochlear duct is filled with endolymph. The perilymph and endolymph are fluids that detect differences in pressure, which correlates with sound. However, the two fluids contain very different concentrations of electrolytes and must stay isolated from each other. The endolymph in the cochlear duct surrounds the sensitive organ of Corti, which contains the cells that respond to sound in the inner ear.

When sound enters the ear, pressure changes in the cochlea travel down the fluid-filled tympanic and vestibular canals. The organ of Corti is situated on the basilar membrane within the cochlear duct. The membrane contains four rows of specialized cells, called hair cells, which protrude from its surface. Above the organ of Corti, just above the hair cells, is the tectoral membrane, which moves in response to pressure variations in the canals. The sound waves cause the basilar membrane to vibrate, which causes excitation of the hair cells. Like other nerve cells, their response to stimuli is to send a voltagepulse called an action potential down the nerve fiber (axon). These impulses travel to the auditory nerve, which carries the sensation of sound to the brain for interpretation.

The volume of the sound is interpreted by the intensity of the vibration of the basilar membrane, also known as the amplitude of the sound wave. The louder the sound, the more vigorous the vibration in the inner ear and the more intensely the hair cells are stimulated to create a stronger sensation to the brain. Differences in pitch are detected by the number of vibrations per second, also known as the frequency of the sound wave. Pitch is measured in hertz (Hz). The higher the frequency of the vibrations, the higher the pitch of the sound, and the lower the frequency of the vibrations, the lower the pitch of the sound. The basilar membrane is not uniform in its width and is sensitive to differing pitches at varying points. Therefore, the most sensitive area on the basilar membrane to the pitch of the particular sound sends a message to the brain that perceives that specific pitch.

The inner ear also contributes to human equilibrium and balance. Located just behind the oval window is a structure containing three components: the utricle, the saccule, and three semicircular canals. The utricle and saccule detect changes in the body's linear movement, such as leaning to one side. The three semicircular canals detect changes in the body's rotational movement, such as shaking or nodding the head. These structures also communicate with hair cells to incorporate special movements with coordination and balance.

Disorders and Diseases

Disturbances in any part of the hearing process can cause varying degrees of hearing loss or deafness. Deafness can be congenital, meaning present from birth, or may occur later in life. Hearing loss can be categorized into many types, including sensorineural hearing loss, conductive hearing loss, central hearing loss, functional hearing loss, or mixed hearing loss. Hearing loss can be bilateral, affecting both ears, or unilateral, affecting only one ear. The identification of the type of hearing loss is imperative for diagnosis and possible treatment. Audiologists and otologists are professionals who work to diagnose and treat hearing loss.

Sensorineural hearing loss is the most common type of congenital hearing loss, accounting for about 90 percent of all hearing loss. This type of hearing loss is caused by a disruption in the inner ear, the acoustic nerve, or a combination of the two. The majority of human sensorineural hearing loss is caused by abnormalities in the hair cells of the organ of Corti in the cochlea. The hair cells may be abnormal at birth or damaged during the lifetime of an individual. There are both external causes of damage, such as trauma or infection, and intrinsic abnormalities, such as mutations in genes that code for the structure of these cells. Sensorineural hearing loss may also present as part of a larger genetic syndrome, where hearing loss is one feature. Sensorineural hearing loss is diffi-

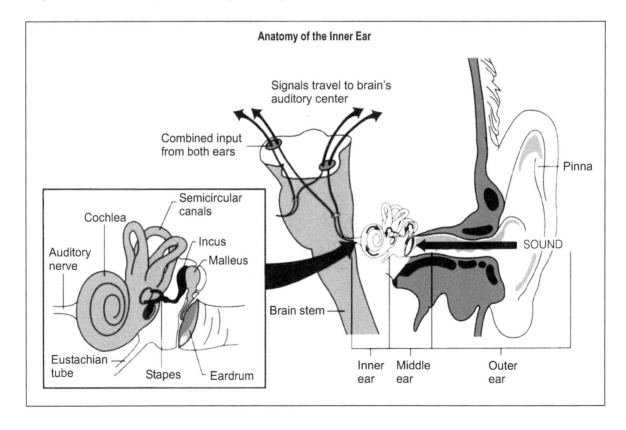

cult to treat. Treatments include the controversial cochlear implant for some qualifying types of sensorineual hearing loss. The cochlear implant is a surgically implanted device that provides sound perception through direct electrical stimulation of the auditory nerve, bypassing the inner ear. For individuals who have sensorineural hearing loss resulting from malformations or damage to the inner ear, the cochlear implant can provide restoration of hearing.

Conductive hearing loss is caused by the disruption of sound waves being transmitted from one part of the ear to the other. The disruption can be caused by physical differences in the external ear canal; the malleus, incus, and stapes; the middle ear cavity; or connections between the outer, middle, or inner ear. Conductive hearing loss can also be caused by a collection of fluid in the eustachian tube, frequent ear infections, or a foreign body in the ear. A loud noise or intense pressure can also rupture the tympanic membrane, which can lead to conductive hearing loss. Conductive hearing loss can often be treated, with surgical interventions, medication, a hearing aid for amplification of sound, or a combination of interventions.

Mixed hearing loss can involve a combination of conductive and sensorineural hearing loss in one individual. Mixed hearing loss can be the most difficult to treat, and it is often is treated with a focus on the conductive hearing loss. Central hearing loss involves damage to the central nervous system, usually the brain, in interpreting sound. Individuals with central hearing loss usually have normal hearing and ear structures, but cannot create meaning of the sound into words or specific noises. Similarly, functional hearing loss results from a psychological condition in which sound cannot be interpreted for emotional or psychological reasons. Treatment for functional hearing loss includes psychotherapy and psychiatric medications rather than surgical interventions or auditory amplification.

Perspective and Prospects

Domenico Cotugno, a physician, was the first individual to describe the anatomy of the inner ear and its relation to hearing. His dissertation in 1761 correctly described the vestibule, semicircular canals, and cochlea of the internal ear and identified the nerve that reaches the semicircular canals as well as the nerve that reaches the cochlea. In disagreement with another published physician, he rightly claimed that the auditory receptive surface is on the membranous lamina of the cochlea, that this lamina changes size with response to identifying different sounds, and that the ear is filled with fluids rather than air as originally hypothesized. Many physicians and researchers have contributed to the understanding of the workings of the ear over time, but none as comprehensively as Cotugno.

Recent interventions to treat hearing loss involve the less invasive hearing aid and the more invasive surgical option of cochlear implants. Hearing aids are small electronic devices that serve to amplify sound and have three basic parts: a microphone, amplifier, and speaker. The hearing aid receives sound through the microphone, which converts the sound waves to electrical signals and sends them to an amplifier. The amplifier increases the power of the signals and then sends them to the ear through a speaker. The hearing aid is worn on the outside of the ear. The hearing aid has become more technologically advanced over time, decreasing in size and increasing in strength.

The cochlear implant is a surgically implanted electrical device. The implant is made up of a microphone, which picks up sound from the environment similar to the hearing aid; a speech processor, which interprets and rearranges sounds picked up by the microphone; a transmitter and receiver/stimulator, which receive signals from the speech processor and convert them into electric impulses; and an electrode array, which is a group of electrodes that collects the impulses from the stimulator and sends them to different regions of the auditory nerve. The cochlear implant can be used to restore hearing to some individuals with sensorineural hearing loss. The implant cannot give normal hearing but can provide some increase in the identification of sounds and speech.

—*Leah M. Betman, M.S., C.G.C.*

See also Aging; Audiology; Deafness; Ear infections and disorders; Ear surgery; Ears; Earwax; Hearing aids; Hearing loss; Hearing tests; Otorhinolaryngology; Sense organs; Tinnitus.

For Further Information:

"Ear Disorders." *MedlinePlus*, June 12, 2013.
"Ears, Nose, and Throat." *MedlinePlus*, January 7, 2013.
Gelfand, Stanley A. *Essentials of Audiology.* 3d ed. New York: Thieme, 2009.
Katz, Jack, ed. *Handbook of Clinical Audiology.* 6th ed. Philadelphia: Wolters Kluwer/Lippincott Williams & Wilkins, 2009.
Lane, Harlan, Robert Hoffmeister, and Ben Bahan. *Journey into the Deaf World.* San Diego, Calif.: DawnSignPress, 1996.
Manni, E., and L. Petrosini. "Domenico Cotugno (1736–1822)." *Journal of Neurology* 257 (October, 2009): 152–153.
Reece, N., and J. Campbell. "Sensory and Motor Mechanisms." In *Biology*, edited by Beth Wilbur. 9th ed. San Francisco: Pearson Education, 2011.
Wilson, B., et al. "Better Speech Recognition with Cochlear Implants." *Nature* 352 (July, 1991): 236–238.

HEARING AIDS

Treatment

Anatomy or system affected: Ears

Specialties and related fields: Audiology, otorhinolaryngology

Definition: Electromechanical devices meant to improve ease of communication and minimize listening fatigue. Patients with profound sensorineural hearing loss receive little or no benefit from conventional hearing aids but may use a cochlear implant, an electronic prosthetic device surgically placed in the inner ear to deliver electrical signals to the brain, where they are interpreted as sounds.

Key terms:

assistive listening devices: earphones or a headset with amplification to supplement or substitute for traditional hearing aids

audiogram: a graph used to display one's hearing ability for average speech sounds, in which decibels have been converted from sound pressure levels to hearing levels

audiologist: a diagnostician who administers hearing tests and dispenses hearing aids

cochlea: an inner ear cavity shaped like a snail surrounded by fluid; when set in motion, this fluid displaces rows of thousands of microscopic hair cells, each of which functions to receive electrical activity and transfer it to the central auditory system

presbycusis: a hearing loss of unknown cause, often attributed to aging

Indications and Procedures

Hearing loss is one of the most common conditions affecting older adults, but it is not limited to that age group. According to the World Health Organization, disabling hearing loss affected more than 350 million people worldwide by 2013, with many more experiencing mild forms of hearing loss. The use of hearing aids is one of the primary strategies for the treatment of hearing loss. These devices were developed to help those people affected by hearing loss ranging from mild to severe and resulting from a number of causes. The most common type of hearing loss, sensorineural, is linked to a variety of physical and psychosocial dysfunctions (isolation, depression, hypertension, and stress) as well as illnesses such as ischemic heart disease and arrhythmias.

Over the years, hearing aids have evolved in several ways. Two major trends have been in signal processing and size. Prior to the 1940s, hearing aids were large and required carrying a battery pack strapped to one's body. In the 1940s, vacuum tubes reduced the size of hearing aids to that of a transistor radio. Hearing aids worn in the ear or on the head were not available until the 1960s. At that time, the best available hearing aids helped in quiet only; in loud situations, they made things worse. Therefore, it was common practice to remove them around noise. Beginning in the 1980s and 1990s, advanced circuitry offered consumers improved quality of hearing in quiet as well as some increased ability to hear in noise; sound distortion was minimal. In the decades since, hearing aids have become more comfortable and less noticeable. Certain hearing aids can be electronically adjusted for individual users; for example, they can be reprogrammed to accommodate increased hearing loss. Some hearing aids have volume controls, while others adjust automatically. Research has shown that consumers report greater satisfaction with sound quality than they did in the past, and people with hearing loss in both ears tend to be more satisfied with two hearing aids, enabling them to determine the direction of sounds.

For patients with bilateral profound sensorineural hearing loss, which does not respond to traditional hearing aids, a cochlear implant is now possible. A cochlear implant is an electronic prosthesis surgically implanted in the inner ear. It has

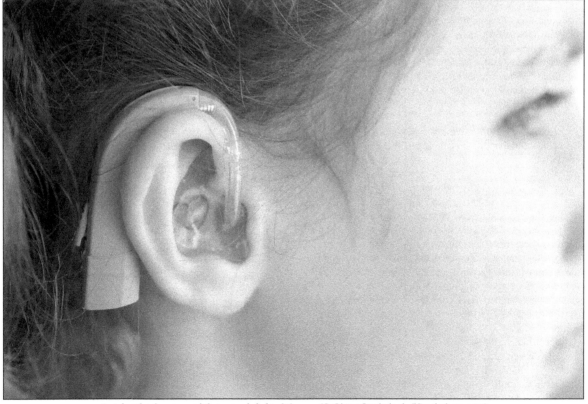

A girl with a hearing aid that extends behind the ear. (© Oktay Ortakcioglu/iStockphoto.com)

In the News: Lyric Hearing Aid

Clinical trials started in 2001 for InSound Medical's Lyric Hearing Aid (LHA), which is located entirely in an ear canal and not externally visible. The device became the sole Food and Drug Administration-approved auditory aid enhancing hearing while hidden from view. Patients began buying LHAs in January, 2007. By April, 2008, *The New York Times* reported the LHA had been inserted in approximately five hundred people.

Through a nonsurgical process, the LHA is placed so its receiver is four millimeters (0.158 inch) near a patient's eardrum. The LHA's microphone is less than four millimeters from where the canal opens into the outer ear. Each aid is adjusted for individuals' auditory requirements. The LHA can remain inside the ear canal for a maximum of four months, at which point it is pulled out with a magnet and replaced. Wearers subscribe to annual LHA services, costing several thousand dollars depending if aids are placed in one or both ears. They receive advanced technology when new devices are inserted because researchers continue to improve design.

InSound Medical reported 90 percent wearer satisfaction with auditory capabilities of the LHA compared to other aids that they had used. Audiologists intend to study possible correlations of LHAs and infections because 2 to 3 percent of users experience that problem. An estimated 50 percent of patients cannot have LHAs inserted due to incompatible ear canal anatomy or severity of deafness.

The LHA received *Medical Device and Diagnostic Industry*'s Medical Design Excellence Award in May, 2009. The December, 2009, issue of *Popular Science* featured LHA's selection for a Best of What's New Award.

—*Elizabeth D. Schafer, Ph.D.*

external parts that are worn outside the ear, including a microphone, speech processor, headpiece antenna, and cable. It is not a hearing aid. A cochlear implant delivers electrical signals to the brain, where they are interpreted as sounds. Potential candidates for these implants include both children and adults in a wide age range. Generally, children should be at least eighteen months old, and many successful implant recipients are in their eighties. Adults who become deaf later in life and who have fully developed speech and language before their hearing loss have better results with the implant than do those who were born deaf or who lost their hearing early in life. It has been shown, however, that children who are born deaf but are given cochlear implants early in life can receive great benefit from them. In adults, the memory of sound appears to be one of the most important factors for success. For children, early implantation and placement in an educational program that emphasizes the development of auditory skills appear to be important factors for success.

Uses and Complications

One of the biggest impediments to hearing aid use is patient reaction to hearing loss. Many people try to cover up the fact that they have hearing difficulties, and when hearing loss is confirmed, they experience a wide range of emotions, from horror, denial, disbelief, and withdrawal to embarrassment, sadness, resentment, and gradual acceptance and coping. People's coping skills and behavior patterns vary, in part because hearing loss generally occurs gradually and may take a long time to be recognized.

For those who embrace hearing aids, a variety of technological and cosmetic choices are available. A number of options exist regarding hearing aid style: behind-the-ear, custom in-the-ear, in-the-canal, and the smallest, the completely

in-canal hearing aid. In addition to aesthetic considerations and sound fidelity, one's anatomy and manual dexterity may dictate the style that is most effective and efficient. The degree of hearing loss and other medical conditions are also important factors when evaluating the best hearing aid.

Perspective and Prospects

Hearing aid technology has improved such that patients with mild to moderate hearing loss will be candidates for hearing aids and those with severe loss will be candidates for hearing aids or cochlear implants, depending upon how well they function with a particular device. Patients with profound hearing loss will benefit best from cochlear implants.

Initially, only those patients who were completely deaf in both ears were considered candidates for cochlear implants. With significant improvements in implant technology, however, the benefits gained by implanted patients, both children and adults, have markedly improved. This, in turn, has led to a broadening of criteria for implant patients. Select patients with severe hearing loss who receive some benefit from hearing aids are considered possible implant candidates.

—*Marcia J. Weiss, M.A., J.D.*

See also Aging; Audiology; Deafness; Ear infections and disorders; Ear surgery; Ears; Earwax; Hearing; Hearing loss; Hearing tests; Otorhinolaryngology; Sense organs.

For Further Information:

A.D.A.M. Medical Encyclopedia. "Devices for Hearing Loss." *MedlinePlus*, July 7, 2011.

Biderman, Beverly. *Wired for Sound: A Journey into Hearing*. Toronto, Ont.: Trifolium Books, 1998.

Carmen, Richard, ed. *The Consumer Handbook on Hearing Loss and Hearing Aids: A Bridge to Healing*. 3d rev. ed. Sedona, Ariz.: Auricle Ink, 2009.

Carson-DeWitt, Rosalyn. "Hearing Loss." *Health Library*, September 10, 2012.

Dillon, Harvey. *Hearing Aids*. New York: Thieme, 2001.

National Institute on Deafness and Other Communication Disorders. "Hearing Aids." *National Institutes of Health*, June 7, 2010.

Romoff, Arlene. *Hear Again: Back to Life with a Cochlear Implant*. New York: League for the Hard of Hearing, 1999.

World Health Organization. "Deafness and Hearing Loss." *World Health Organization*, February 2013.

HEARING LOSS

Disease/Disorder

Anatomy or system affected: Brain, ears

Specialties and related fields: Audiology, speech pathology

Definition: Loss of sensitivity to sound as a result of disease, infection, injury, noise, or aging.

Key terms:

conductive hearing loss: hearing loss resulting from interference with sound vibration; occurs in the external and middle ear

hearing aid: a hearing device that amplifies sounds

sensorineural hearing loss: hearing loss resulting from disease or aging; occurs in the inner ear

Causes and Symptoms

The causes of hearing loss vary, although three major factors enhance the progression of loss as one ages: exposure to noise, previous middle-ear disease, and vascular disease. There are basically two types of hearing loss, conductive hearing loss and sensorineural hearing loss. Conductive hearing loss results from interference with sound vibration through the external and middle ear. In other words, the sound cannot get to the inner ear. In some types of conductive hearing loss, if the sound amplitude is increased enough, then the person may be able to hear. Possible reasons for conductive hearing loss include impacted or large amounts of cerumen (wax) in the ear, foreign bodies (such as soap, food, or insects) in the ear canal, otitis media (middle-ear infection), rheumatoid arthritis, and otosclerosis, in which the stapes becomes fixed to the oval window of the cochlea. Sensorineural hearing loss is caused by damage to the inner ear, the auditory nerve, or the brain.

Earwax buildup is a common and treatable cause of conductive hearing loss. There have been reports that as much as 25 percent of nursing home residents have impacted cerumen. Older adults can be taught how to remove the wax on their own. Cerumenex (by prescription only) and Debrox (sold without a prescription) can be used as directed, followed by lavage to remove the wax and residual medication. Some health care providers recommend the instillation of mineral oil into the ear canal twenty-four hours before removal to help soften the wax, followed by lavage with one part hydrogen peroxide to three parts water at room temperature.

Sensorineural hearing loss means the presence of disease anywhere from the organ of Corti to the brain. The result is loss of hearing high tones, for it is the hair cells in the basal curvature of the organ of Corti that are sensitive to high tones. Presbycusis is sensorineural hearing loss caused by aging of the inner ear. The onset of presbycusis may begin anytime from the third to the sixth decade of life, depending on type. Presbycusis affects more than 50 percent of individuals over age sixty-five. Older adults suffering from these disturbances show distinct and differing audiograms, which are used clinically to diagnose types of impairment. The standard type of presbycusis with hearing loss at high Hertz is often associated with sensory and neural presbycusis. There are four types of presbycusis: sensory, neural, metabolic, and cochlear conductive.

The elderly first start to lose hearing in the high-frequency range. High-frequency consonants and sibilants become more difficult to recognize—for example, *f, g, l, t, s, ch, sh,*

Information on Hearing Loss

Causes: Buildup of earwax, perforated eardrum, disease, congenital malformation, swelling of external ear canal, otitis media, traumatic injury, long-term exposure to loud and continuous noise, tumors

Symptoms: Difficulty understanding speech, difficulty hearing in presence of background noise, social isolation

Duration: Ranges from short-term to chronic

Treatments: Rehabilitation programs, use of hearing aids, surgery

---

and *th.* In presbycusis, high-frequency sounds become unintelligible. Understanding spoken words depends largely on the clear perception of high-frequency consonants rather than low-frequency vowel sounds. This is why words starting with the above letters or combinations become unintelligible. Many times, older adults have both conductive and sensorineural frequency losses. The precise cause of the defect requires help from a specialist and the use of sophisticated audiometric testing.

The sound waves that travel through the ear have two main characteristics, frequency and amplitude. Frequency is related to the pitch of a sound and is measured by the number of vibrations or cycles per second. The higher the vibration frequency, the higher the perceived pitch of the sound. Hertz (Hz) is the unit of measurement to denote cycles per second. Amplitude is related to the loudness of a sound. The greater the intensity with which a sound strikes the eardrum, the louder the tone. The unit of measurement of intensity of sound is decibels (dB).

Among the offenders to hearing are radio headphones, lawn mowers, diesel trucks, heavy machinery, and loud music. A single very loud noise can damage the middle ear. An eardrum can be broken by sounds reaching 160 decibels to 1,000 Hertz. Also, continuous noise of more than 80 to 85 decibels can cause harm to hearing. Normal conversation is measured at 60 decibels. A noisy restaurant, a vacuum cleaner, an electric shaver, and a screaming child can reach decibels between 80 and 85 decibels. Louder everyday noises include a blow-dryer (100 decibels), a subway train (100 decibels), and a car horn (110 decibels). Anyone exposed to noise in the 80 decibel range should wear hearing protection.

Another common hearing problem is tinnitus (ringing in the ears). Medications such as aspirin, aminoglycoside antibiotics, and diuretics can cause toxic effects to the hair cells of the organ of Corti, thereby resulting in sensorineural hearing loss. Tinnitus, an internal noise generated within the hearing system, occurs in many types of hearing disorders at all ages, but it is reported more frequently in the elderly. Tinnitus affects seven million people, of which 10 to 37 percent are elderly, and that number is growing. The ringing sound is generally high pitched with sensorineural loss and low pitched with conductive hearing loss. However, tinnitus may be present with or without hearing loss. Some types of tinnitus do not usually awaken people out of sleep nor do they interfere with

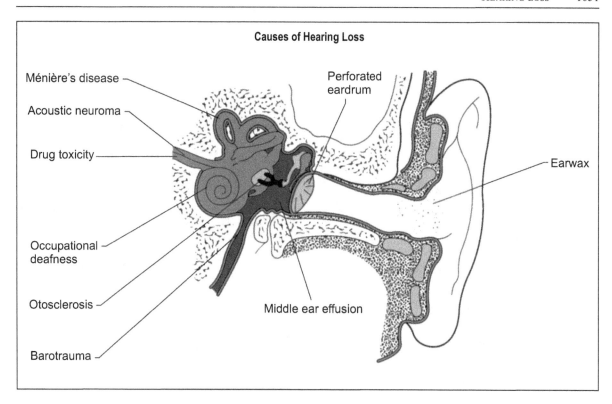

Causes of Hearing Loss

Ménière's disease

Acoustic neuroma

Drug toxicity

Occupational deafness

Otosclerosis

Barotrauma

Perforated eardrum

Earwax

Middle ear effusion

leisure activities. Older adults can attempt to alleviate the condition through biofeedback or by disguising the sound. Soft radio music and other distracting sounds may offer some comfort.

Treatment and Therapy

There are many treatments for hearing loss and, depending on the type of loss, some treatments work better than others. For example, with conductive hearing loss, if the cause is excessive earwax buildup, then the results can be remarkable when the wax is removed. For both types of hearing loss, conductive and sensorineural, simple measures can be used to facilitate better communication.

One technique that can help in communicating with someone with hearing loss is facing the person when speaking, so that he or she can see one's face and lips. Using simple, short sentences or phrases and speaking slowly in a low voice can be helpful. Loudness is not helpful and can be irritating, whereas a low voice enables people to hear lower frequencies, which usually can be heard more easily.

Although hearing aids may help certain types of hearing loss, many people do not like to use them. A person wearing such a device for the first time needs to go through an adjustment period, and some older adults do not give themselves enough time to get used to the hearing aid. Some hearing aids have been known to cause irritation to the external ear. Also, the increased humidity within the external auditory canal may cause infectious otitis externa.

There are basically three kinds of hearing aids: the body type, the behind-the-ear-type, and in-the-ear type. The body type resembles a handheld amplifier with a wire that attaches to an earpiece. The behind-the-ear type is worn behind and in the ear. A person with poor eyesight and rheumatoid arthritis would probably benefit from the body type or behind-the-ear type. These types are easier to see and handle because of their larger size. The in-the-ear devices are small and cosmetically more acceptable, but they are more difficult to manipulate. The selection often depends on the wearer's personal preference, vision capabilities, and manual dexterity.

It takes time to adjust to using a hearing aid. Sounds and voices are made louder, not clearer. The wearer must become accustomed to the background noise. Often, the user must be encouraged to continue using the hearing aid during this adjustment period. The greatest satisfaction is achieved with hearing aids if hearing loss is between 55 and 80 decibels. There is only partial benefit if the loss is greater than 80 decibels.

Perspective and Prospects

Hearing is regarded by some to be the most important of the five senses. It is imperative for people to protect their hearing for as long as they can. In today's world, where excessive noises are bombarding eardrums everyday, people need to protect themselves.

Hearing loss occurs when hair cells in the ear are damaged or destroyed by excessively loud noise or moderately loud noise for prolonged periods of time. Hearing loss usually occurs gradually and without pain. Over time, sounds become muffled and higher frequency sounds become hard to distinguish. Normal conversation occurs around 60 decibels. Anything higher than 60 decibels for extended periods of time may lead to hearing loss. According to the Ear Institute in Los Angeles, about 30 percent of hearing loss is due to exposure to loud sounds.

There are ways to reduce excessive noise levels in the environment. First, the time exposed to loud noises should be limited. This can be accomplished by removing the sound or decreasing the volume. The popular audio products now on the market can pose a risk to hearing. Most people are not aware of the potential dangers of listening to music at high volumes. A person listening to music by wearing earphones should not be heard by the person standing next to them. Similarly, a loud device such as a vacuum cleaner should be operated for no more than ten minutes at a time, with a five-minute break between uses.

It is interesting to note that hearing loss results from both loudness and time exposure. For example, a one-time gunshot noise near the ear can be just as damaging as extended exposure to loud music at 120 decibels for fifteen minutes or more. Anyone working in an environment that reaches noise levels of more than 85 decibels for extended periods of time should wear protective devices. Earplugs and hearing protection devices are needed for construction workers, traffic personnel, musicians, disc jockeys, air traffic personnel, nightclub employees and patrons, or anyone exposed to loud noises.

Scientists are conducting research to discover whether damaged hair cells of the ear are capable of rebuilding their structure over a forty-eight-hour period (the time that it takes for hearing to return after a temporary loss). Researchers speculate that permanent hearing loss may occur when self-repair mechanisms are compromised.

Scientists are studying blood flow in the cochlear section of the ear to evaluate how drugs may affect hair cells. Researchers are also examining blood flow to the cochlea when people are exposed to conversational sound and loud sounds. It seems that when a person is exposed to loud sounds, the blood flow in the cochlea drops. Drugs that are used to treat blood flow problems, such as in peripheral vascular disease, may show a benefit to maintaining blood flow to the cochlea. These and other drug therapies may show promising results in helping people with hearing loss. Finally, with a reduction in harmful noise, hearing loss will decrease.

—*Janet Mahoney, R.N., Ph.D., A.P.R.N.*

See also Aging; Audiology; Deafness; Ear infections and disorders; Ear surgery; Ears; Earwax; Hearing; Hearing aids; Hearing tests; Ménière's disease; Nasopharyngeal disorders; Neuralgia, neuritis, and neuropathy; Otorhinolaryngology; Sense organs; Speech disorders; Tinnitus.

For Further Information:

Carmen, Richard, ed. *The Consumer Handbook on Hearing Loss and Hearing Aids: A Bridge to Healing.* 3d rev. ed. Sedona, Ariz.: Auricle Ink, 2009.

Carson-DeWitt, Rosalyn. "Hearing Loss." *Health Library*, September 10, 2012.

Craine, Michael. *Hear Well Again: A Step by Step Program to Better Hearing.* Chapel Hill, N.C.: Professional Press, 1999.

Gallo, Joseph J., et al., eds. *Handbook of Geriatric Assessment.* 4th ed. Sudbury, Mass.: Jones and Bartlett, 2006.

"Hearing Loss." *Medline Plus*, May 22, 2012.

"Hearing Loss." *National Institute on Aging*, April 30, 2013.

Mahoney, Janet. "Hearing Loss and Assessment: A Concern for All." *Nursing Spectrum* 13, no. 1 (January 10, 2000).

Paterson, J. "What You Need to Know About Hearing Loss." *USA Weekend*, November 21, 1997.

Shelp, Scott G. "Your Patient Is Deaf, Now What?" *RN* 60, no. 2 (February, 1997): 37–41.

Tabloski, Patricia A. *Gerontological Nursing.* 2d ed. Upper Saddle River, N.J.: Pearson, 2010.

HEARING TESTS
Procedure

Anatomy or system affected: Ears, nervous system

Specialties and related fields: Audiology, neurology, occupational health, otorhinolaryngology, pediatrics, speech pathology

Definition: Evaluation techniques for determining the type and severity of hearing loss in children and adults.

Key terms:

auditory brainstem response: measurement of the nervous discharge produced by the central auditory system as a response to sound stimulation; also known as brainstem auditory evoked response (BAER) or auditory brainstem potentials (ABR)

auditory nerve: the nerve that conducts sound stimuli to the brain for interpretation

behavioral audiometry: a technique that the audiologist employs to evaluate hearing in infants, toddlers, or uncooperative patients (both children and adults) with developmental deficits

cochlea: the organ localized in the inner portion of the auditory system that detects sound

mastoid: referring to the bone behind the ear

middle ear: the part of the auditory system, consisting of the ossicular chain and the auditory tube, that serves as a conductor of and transducer of sound

otoacoustic emissions: sound produced in the middle ear as a response to the vibration produced by the cochlea when it is stimulated by external sounds

Indications and Procedures

Hearing tests are done to establish the presence, type, and severity of hearing impairment in children and adults. Such tests are conducted by an audiologist, although screening tests can also be done by a technician under the supervision of an audiologist. The severity of hearing loss is classified as mild, moderate, moderately severe, severe, and profound. It is also classified according to the anatomic region affected: conductive, sensorineural, or mixed hearing loss.

The selection of tests to evaluate hearing will depend on the patient's age and ability to follow directions and the ability of the audiologist to elicit responses from the patient. When a patient cannot follow instructions such as lifting a hand or pressing a button, a test that does not require the patient's cooperation is used. Two tests that do not require the patient's cooperation are the auditory brainstem potential (ABR) test and the evoked otoacoustic emissions (EOAE) test. Both tests require only that the patient be quiet. For this purpose, the patient may need sedation if normal sleep cannot be induced.

The ABR test requires the placement of four electrodes on the patient's head: in both mastoid regions and in the mid forehead and upper center of the head. A stimulus is sent through a small microphone placed in the patient's external ear canal or via headphones. The instrument records the average of the electrical discharges generated by the auditory nerve in response to sound stimuli and produces a tracing of waves that correspond to the different electrical potentials generated in response to the stimuli. Analysis of the waves can determine the presence of hearing loss and measure its severity. The ABR test may be used for screening, to determine whether the subject can hear, or for the clinical evaluation of hearing loss. It can be done at any age. An automated method of ABR testing is available for screening newborn infants for hearing loss; it automatically determines if the patient has passed or failed. The clinical ABR test requires specially trained personnel and takes from forty-five to fifty minutes to perform. The automated method can be applied by a technician.

The EOAE test involves recording the sound produced by hair cells within the cochlea by way of a microphone placed in the outer ear canal. Normally, when sound enters the cochlea, the hair cells produce a sound that bounces backward and can be recorded. This sound correlates with the sound sent to the auditory nerve. If there is damage to the hair cells in the cochlea, then no sound is elicited. The EOAE test can be performed without sedation if the patient cooperates by staying quiet. It can be done by a technician and takes approximately ten minutes or less. The EOAE test is used for universal screening of newborn infants. It can be done at all ages to help determine the integrity of the cochlea and thus whether an observed hearing defect is within the cochlea.

Behavioral techniques are the most practical, cost-effective, and time-efficient methods for the accurate assessment of hearing. They give more complete information on the child's hearing as well as functional information about how the child uses his or her hearing. The simplest test is behavioral observation audiometry, in which the audiologist records the behavioral response to an applied sound stimuli of a known frequency. This test can be done with infants up to six months of age, toddlers, and uncooperative patients, such as children or adults with developmental delays. Visual reinforcement audiometry (VRA) is done with infants and toddlers from six months to twenty-four months of age. It is also used with uncooperative patients. In this test, the patient is submitted to sounds of different intensity and trained to respond to the sound stimuli by means of an attractive stimulus. Every time that the sound appears, the stimulus illuminates. When the patient hears the sound, he or she will look for the reinforcement. Play audiometry is a test that can be used in

children over two years of age. The child is taught to move a block or place a puzzle piece every time he or she hears a sound.

In 2002, Ruth Litovsky, an University of Wisconsin–Madison communicative disorders professor, introduced a binaural hearing test to evaluate how people respond to sounds in a noisy environment resembling public areas and schools. Using computers showing images related to words being broadcasted on loudspeaker, her test assesses which sounds people ignore and which sounds secure their attention.

In 2003, the *Ear, Nose, and Throat Journal* provided information describing the Otogram from Tympany, a Sonic Innovation subsidiary. This device enables patients to test their hearing at sites using automated technology. During the twenty-minute testing period, patients undergo an audiogram that thoroughly evaluates their acoustic capabilities with tympanometry and other standard diagnostic tests, responding to the tests via touchscreens with results recorded by computer.

In 2005, Bio-Logic Systems Corporation and House Ear Institute researchers introduced the hearing in noise test (HINT), which assesses how hearing functions in police and emergency personnel whose hearing is vital to their work. The test involves subjects repeating sentences while exposed to a variation of noise and quiet. The source azimuth identification in noise test (SAINT) evaluates subjects" ability to detect where sounds are located.

Perspective and Prospects

Early detection of hearing loss has become a priority among intervention services because it has devastating effects on language development and consequently on social adaptation. It has been found that the mean age at which deafness is diagnosed is around three, which is after speech development should have occurred. Thus, children with hearing loss are placed at a disadvantage with their peers.

In 1993, the National Institutes of Health (NIH) developed a consensus statement by which all newborn infants in the United States were to be screened for hearing loss. The aim was that by the year 2000, all newborns would have been screened before being discharged from the hospital. By 1999, many US states had passed legislation requiring hearing screening of newborns, but a study described in the July, 1999, issue of *American Journal of Otology* recommended screening only babies with a risk for impaired hearing, stating that pediatricians and child care providers would detect deafness in infants and toddlers.

The October, 2001, the *Journal of the American Medical Association* evaluated nineteen studies, emphasizing that screening newborns was not superior to tests by pediatricians when infants were several months old and stressing that determining the value of newborn screening required additional study. In October, 2005, the *Archives of Pediatrics & Adolescent Medicine* estimated that more than half of children whose hearing test results revealed that they needed additional tests never underwent such testing.

The role of otitis media (middle-ear infections) in producing hearing impairment is an area of great concern and controversy. Special attention to the hearing evaluation of children with recurrent and chronic otitis media is indicated.

—*Gloria Reyes Báez, M.D.,*
and Hilda Velez Rodriguez, M.S.;
updated by Elizabeth D. Schafer, Ph.D.

See also Audiology; Deafness; Ear infections and disorders; Ears; Hearing; Hearing aids; Hearing loss; Neonatology; Otorhinolaryngology; Physical examination; Screening; Sense organs.

For Further Information:

"Audiometry." *MedlinePlus*, August 30, 2012.

Bess, Fred H., and Judith S. Gravel, eds. *Foundations of Pediatric Audiology*. San Diego, Calif.: Plural, 2006.

Dobie, Robert A. and Susan B. Van Hemel, eds. *Hearing Loss: Determining Eligibility for Social Security Benefits*. Washington, D.C.: National Academies Press, 2005

de la Rocha, Kelly. "Audiometry." *Health Library*, November 11, 2012.

Elder, Nina. "Now Hear This—Check Your Baby's Hearing." *Better Homes and Gardens* 78, no. 5 (May, 2000): 264.

Glaser, Gabrielle. "Pediatricians Urge Hearing Tests at Birth." *The New York Times*, April 6, 1999, p. 7.

Hall, James W., III. *New Handbook of Auditory Evoked Responses*. Boston: Pearson Education, 2006.

Hearing Exchange. http://www.hearingexchange.com.

Koike, Kazunari J. *Everyday Audiology: A Practical Guide for Health Care Professionals*. San Diego, Calif.: Plural, 2006.

Montemayor-Quellenberg, Marjorie. "Newborn Hearing Test." *Health Library*, March 15, 2013.

McCormick, Barry, ed. *The Medical Practitioner's Guide to Paediatric Audiology*. New York: Cambridge University Press, 1995.

Martin, Frederick N., and John Greer Clark. *Introduction to Audiology*. 10th ed. Boston: Pearson, 2010.

Northern, Jerry L., and Marion P. Downs. *Hearing in Children*. San Diego, Calif.: Plural, 2011.

Roush, Jackson, ed. *Screening for Hearing Loss and Otitis Media in Children*. San Diego, Calif.: Singular, 2001.

Sataloff, Robert T., and Joseph Sataloff. *Hearing Loss*. 4th ed. New York: Taylor & Francis, 2005.

Heart

Anatomy

Anatomy or system affected: Blood, blood vessels, chest, circulatory system

Specialties and related fields: Cardiology, exercise physiology

Definition: The muscle that pumps blood through the body by means of rhythmic contractions.

Key terms:

arteries: vessels that take blood away from the heart and toward the tissues

atria: the upper receiving chambers of the heart that lie above the ventricles

atrioventricular (A-V) node: a small region of specialized heart muscle cells that receives the electrical impulse from the atria and begins its transmission to the ventricles

coronary arteries: the arteries that supply blood to the heart muscle

diastole: the period of relaxation of the heart between beats

sinoatrial (S-A) node: a small region of specialized heart muscle cells that spontaneously generates and sends an electrical signal that gives the heart an automatic rhythm for contraction

systole: the period of contraction of the heart when blood moves out of the heart chambers and into the arteries

veins: vessels that take blood to the heart and from the tissues

ventricles: the lower pumping chambers of the heart located below the atria; they force blood into the arteries

Structure and Functions

All the cells in the human body are dependent on the blood in the cardiovascular system (the heart and blood vessels) for the transport of gases, nutrients, hormones, and other factors. Likewise, the tissues must have a way to dispose of waste products so that they do not build to harmful levels. All these substances are dissolved in the blood, but something must provide the force to transport the blood to all parts of the body at all times—the heart. This organ must beat continuously from early in development to death. It beats without conscious control and can vary how quickly it moves blood throughout the body depending on the needs and activities of the tissues.

In humans, an individual's heart is about the size of his or her fist and is enclosed in the center of the chest cavity between the lungs. The heart contains specialized muscle cells known as cardiac muscle. These cardiac cells make up most of the thickness of the walls of the heart; they are responsible for moving blood out of the heart and are also involved in maintaining the rhythm of the heartbeat. This heavily muscled layer is referred to as the myocardium. The inner lining of the heart is called the endocardium; it is continuous with the lining of all the blood vessels in the body. The outermost layer of the heart is the epicardium, which covers the myocardium. The heart moves as it beats and is contained within a fluid-filled bag called the pericardial sac. The rhythmically beating heart has the potential to rub against adjacent structures (such as the lungs), harming itself and those structures. Therefore, it is important that the heart be encased in the pericardial sac, with its lubricating fluid.

The human heart has four separate chambers. These internal cavities can be identified by their location and function. The upper pair of smaller chambers are known as atria, and the lower larger chambers are called ventricles. Because the atria and ventricles have a muscular wall which separates them into right and left halves, one can refer to the individual chambers as the right atrium and left atrium, and the right ventricle and left ventricle. The wall that separates the right and left halves of the heart is called the septum. The septum prevents any mixing of blood from the right and left sides of the heart. The atria and ventricles on the same side, however, must allow blood to pass between them in a single direction. This action is accomplished by one-way valves between the atria and ventricles. The valve that allows blood to pass from the right atrium to the right ventricle is called the tricuspid valve because it is made of three flaps. On the left side of the heart is the bicuspid valve (with two flaps), which is also known as the mitral valve. The bicuspid valve allows blood from the left atrium to flow only into the left ventricle. This rather complex anatomy is necessary because the heart must pump blood in one direction and into two separate systems.

The anatomy of the heart often makes more sense if one understands its function or physiology. As an example, one may consider an active cell in the body, perhaps a muscle cell that moves the foot. This cell utilizes oxygen to help metabolize food for energy. During this process, carbon dioxide is produced as a waste product, and high levels of carbon dioxide can be harmful to cells. Therefore, one of the jobs of the cardiovascular system is to deliver oxygen and take away carbon dioxide. Once the carbon dioxide is picked up by the blood, it travels back to the heart via veins and enters the right atrium. From the right atrium, the blood passes the tricuspid valve and enters the right ventricle. The right ventricle then sends the blood past a one-way semilunar valve called the pulmonic valve into blood vessels that transport it to the lungs. At the lungs, the blood loses carbon dioxide and picks up oxygen. This oxygenated blood must now be delivered to the tissues. First, the blood returns to the heart and enters the left atrium. From the left atrium, blood is pushed past the bicuspid mitral valve into the left ventricle. The blood is then pumped from the powerful left ventricle through another semilunar valve (the aortic) into the blood vessels that will carry the blood to all the tissues of the body, including the heart itself. The blood vessels that feed the heart directly are known as coronary vessels.

The orderly pattern by which blood flows through the heart, lungs, and body requires the chambers of the heart to work in a coordinated fashion. The atria contract together to help send blood into the ventricles. The ventricles then contract together so that blood flows through the lungs from the right ventricle and through the tissues of the body from the left ventricle. The tricuspid and bicuspid valves prevent a backflow of blood into the atria when the ventricles contract, and the semilunar valves prevent blood from returning to the ventricles after they have contracted.

Something must coordinate the contraction of the heart so that the atria contract together before the ventricles do so. Highly specialized cells of the myocardium have the ability to conduct electrical impulses rapidly and to discharge spontaneously at a certain rate. These properties allow the heart to be stimulated in a synchronous way and for it to generate its own rate and rhythm. One region of the right atrium is known as the sinoatrial (S-A) node; it functions as the heart's pacemaker. The S-A node has the ability to generate spontaneously an electrical signal with a relatively rapid rhythm. Therefore, it serves to "pace" the heart rate. When the S-A node sends its electrical impulse throughout the atria, the atria contract. There is a slight delay before the impulse reaches the ventricles, which allows the atria to contract fully before the ventricles. The atrioventricular (A-V) node will then pick up the electrical signal and send it through both ventricles via specialized conductive heart muscle fibers known as Purkinje's fibers.

Purkinje's fibers transmit the electrical signal ensuring that all the ventricular muscle cells contract at nearly the same time. The ventricles contract in such a way that the bottom tip of the heart (apex) contracts slightly before the region of the ventricles next to the atria (base). Additionally, the ventricles contract in a somewhat twisting motion that causes the heart to "wring out" the blood.

This rather complex system allows the heart to contract at its own rate and in a highly synchronous fashion. Nevertheless, one's heart rate varies depending on one's physical activity or emotional state. For example, during exercise or when an individual is under stress, the heart rate goes up. When one is relaxed, the heart does not beat as rapidly. Therefore, the body must have a way to regulate the rate at which the S-A node signals the heart to contract.

The autonomic nervous system, which functions without one's conscious control, regulates the heart rate. It is divided into two systems: parasympathetic and sympathetic. The parasympathetic nervous system is active during periods of rest and has the ability to slow the heart. During periods of physical or emotional stress, the sympathetic nervous system stimulates the heart to contract more forcefully and at a more rapid rate. The parasympathetic and sympathetic systems communicate with the heart via chemical messengers known as neurotransmitters. The parasympathetic nervous system uses the neurotransmitter acetylcholine to slow the heart, while norepinephrine and epinephrine are the chemicals used by the sympathetic nervous system to increase the heart rate.

Disorders and Diseases

Even though the heart seems to be adaptable to a variety of situations throughout one's life, it can malfunction. In fact, diseases of the heart and blood vessels are the number-one killer in the United States. One common disease that affects the heart directly is coronary artery disease, which can lead to life-threatening heart attacks. Although medical researchers are still investigating the causes of coronary artery disease, most of the evidence points to hypertension (high blood pressure) and atherosclerosis (a buildup of fatty plaque in the walls of arteries).

Hypertension is usually defined as a blood pressure greater than 140/90 millimeters of mercury (mmHg) at rest. A typical blood pressure for a young, healthy adult is 120/80 mmHg. The top number measures the force of blood against an artery wall during the contraction of the heart; this is referred to as the systolic pressure. The bottom number, the diastolic pressure, is a measurement of force when the heart is relaxed. If either systolic or diastolic pressure exceeds 140/90 mmHg, the patient is considered hypertensive. The cause of hypertension has not been determined, but it is known that with hypertension the heart must work harder to push the blood through the arteries, including the coronary arteries. Physicians treat hypertension by prescribing drugs that block the effect of the sympathetic nervous system on the heart, such as metoprolol (Lopressor). They may also prescribe drugs such as prazosin (Minipress) that prevent the arteries from becoming too narrow.

Hypertension is also seen in patients who have atherosclerosis. This buildup of fatty materials such as cholesterol under the lining of the artery causes the plaque to protrude, narrowing the diameter of the vessel. This can lead to blood clot formation on artery walls that are irregular. This clot, also known as a thrombus, may dislodge and travel in the bloodstream. Eventually, it may block a small artery, thereby preventing the flow of blood to the tissue. If this happens in a coronary artery, a myocardial infarction (heart attack) will result.

A heart attack occurs when a portion of the heart dies because of a lack of oxygen or a buildup of waste products. Heart muscle has no way of repairing itself, and the resulting damage is permanent. If the patient is transported to the hospital immediately, the emergency room physician may give drugs to prevent further blood clot formation (aspirin and heparin) and to help dissolve the already formed clot (reteplase and tenecteplase-tissue plasminogen activator, or TNK-TPA). If the coronary artery is only partially blocked,

the patient may suffer from angina pectoris, a chest pain that radiates down the left arm. These patients usually take drugs such as nitroglycerin, which help dilate (widen) blood vessels, reestablishing adequate flow to the heart.

Another devastating disease of the heart is congestive heart failure, a condition in which the heart fails to pump enough blood to meet the demands of the body's tissues. The heart becomes enlarged because of the resulting excessive increase in blood volume. There are several causes of heart failure, most of which stem from the fact that the heart loses its ability to pump efficiently. For example, a patient who has had a heart attack may have lost significant function as a result of heart damage. Even without a heart attack, some individuals may have malfunctioning heart valves or other problems that cause an inefficient ejection of blood and thus heart failure.

The cardiovascular system attempts to compensate for heart failure in several ways. The sympathetic nervous system increases the heart rate, and the kidneys retain more fluid

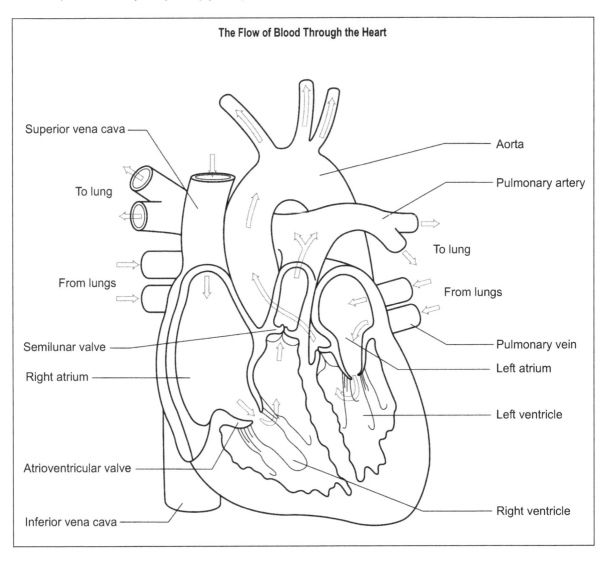

The Flow of Blood Through the Heart

to increase blood volume. These compensatory mechanisms help to reestablish adequate blood flow for a while. Because of the increase in blood volume, however, more blood enters the chambers of the heart and causes them to stretch. At some point, the ventricles can no longer force out the increased amount of blood entering them, and they enlarge. This increase in the size of the heart chamber further enlarges the heart and strains the heart muscle. The heart will continue to weaken, unable to keep up with the body's demands. Compensatory mechanisms attempt to meet the body's need for continuous blood flow but in doing so further overload the heart. This vicious circle may lead to complete heart failure and death.

Congestive heart failure may involve only one side of the heart, perhaps because of a heart attack that affected that side. If the heart failure occurs on the left side, the right ventricle is pumping blood to the lungs in an efficient manner but the left ventricle cannot pump all the blood returning from the lungs. Therefore, blood backs up and pools in the lung tissues. Similarly, if the right ventricle begins to fail and the left ventricle is normal, blood begins to pool throughout the body since the right side of the heart cannot keep up in its pumping.

Physicians are able to slow the progression of congestive heart failure by prescribing drugs such as digoxin that increase the force of heart muscle contraction and thereby the amount of blood ejected with each beat. Therapeutic agents such as captopril (Capoten) help to reduce the fluid retention in the kidneys.

Heart failure is related to the inability of the heart to contract well due to coronary artery disease or other conditions. In addition, the specialized heart muscle cells that provide the heart's rhythm and conduct the electrical signals necessary for a coordinated heartbeat may be affected by disease. In the resting adult, the heart normally beats about seventy to eighty times per minute. Several conditions exist whereby the heart loses control of its normal rate and rhythm, a serious condition.

For example, if the heart begins to beat too rapidly, the ventricles do not have enough time to fill and the movement of blood to the heart muscle and the rest of the body is impaired. The atria or ventricles may contract at a high rate and lose their coordinated sequence of contraction; this is referred to as atrial or ventricular fibrillation. Atrial fibrillation may be tolerated under some circumstances; ventricular fibrillation is a medical emergency. If immediate action is not taken to reestablish the normal rate and conduction sequence, the patient will die. Emergency measures such as electrical defibrillation may shock the heart into reestablishing its normal rhythm and conduction pathways. It is easy to understand how these abnormal patterns of heart activity occur if one imagines more than one pacemaker attempting to control heart function. The cause of these and other, less severe heart rhythms may be heart damage affecting the conductive pathway, drugs, or even psychological distress.

Heart disease is a major cause of death, but most experts agree that many heart problems are preventable. High blood pressure and high blood levels of fat and cholesterol are asso-ciated with an increased incidence of coronary artery disease. Cigarette smoking and excessive weight are also correlated with heart disease. Additionally, exercise seems to be critical in maintaining a healthy heart, as sedentary individuals have a twofold increase in their risk of heart disease when compared to active people.

It is likely that individuals who are at risk can lessen the probability of having heart problems by adopting a more healthful lifestyle, including stopping smoking, reducing excessive weight and mental stress, and engaging in enjoyable physical activities (with their physicians' permission).

Perspective and Prospects

The role of the heart in the functioning of the human body was questioned by the ancient Egyptians, who attributed breathing to the heart. It was the Chinese who first documented that the heart is responsible for the pulse and movement of blood. They also believed that the heart was the seat of happiness. The ancient Greeks had a different idea about the function of the heart, believing that it was the region where thinking originated.

It was not until William Harvey (1578–1657), an English physiologist, published his experiments on the heart and circulation that scientists believed blood was pumped continuously by the heart. He observed that both ventricles of the heart contracted and expanded at the same time. Harvey also noted that when the heart was removed from an animal, it continued to contract and relax; that is, it had an automatic rhythm.

More than one hundred years after Harvey published his work, Stephen Hales made the first blood pressure measurements. He did so by inserting a tube into the neck artery of a horse and watching the blood rise 3 meters above the animal. Then early in the twentieth century Willem Einthoven invented an instrument to measure electrical currents. This instrument was used by Thomas Lewis to measure the electrical activity in the heart, the first electrocardiograph (ECG).

By the mid-twentieth century, heart surgeries were being performed to correct heart defects. These early surgeries had to be done with the heart still beating. In 1953, the heart-lung machine was used to take over the pumping function of the heart during surgery so that the surgeon could stop the heart. In 1967, Christiaan Barnard performed the first heart transplantation in a human. Heart transplants were performed during the next ten years with no long-term survivors, usually because of tissue rejection. In 1982, a completely artificial heart was implanted into a patient. This patient died in the spring of 1983.

Heart transplants have become much more successful, however, mainly because of the use of immunosuppressive drugs that help to prevent rejection of the transplanted heart. In January 2012, the US National Heart, Lung, and Blood Institute reported that heart transplant patients had a one-year survival rate of 88 percent, a five-year survival rate of 75 percent, and a ten-year survival rate of 56 percent. Newer drugs and procedures such as coronary bypass surgery, angioplasty, and atherectomy are becoming more effective in treating heart disease. Nevertheless, perhaps the best approach to maintaining a healthy heart is to practice preventive medicine. Scientists are making comparable strides in finding ways to prevent heart disease as they are in treating already existing conditions.

—*Matthew Berria, Ph.D.*

See also Anatomy; Aneurysmectomy; Aneurysms; Angina; Angiography; Angioplasty; Anxiety; Arrhythmias; Arteriosclerosis; Biofeedback; Blue baby syndrome; Bypass surgery; Cardiac arrest; Cardiac rehabilitation; Cardiac surgery; Cardiology; Cardiology, pediatric; Cardiopulmonary resuscitation (CPR); Catheterization; Circulation; Congenital heart disease; Coronary artery bypass graft; Echocardiography; Electrical shock; Electrocardiography (ECG or EKG); Embolism; Endocarditis; Exercise physiology; Heart attack; Heart disease; Heart failure; Heart transplantation; Heart valve replacement; Hypertension; Internal medicine; Mitral valve prolapse; Pacemaker implantation; Palpitations; Plaque, arterial; Resuscitation; Reye's syndrome; Rheumatic fever; Shock; Sports medicine; Strokes; Systems and organs; Thoracic surgery; Thrombolytic therapy and TPA; Thrombosis and thrombus; Transplantation; Vascular medicine; Vascular system.

For Further Information:

American Heart Association. http://www.americanheart.org.

American Heart Association. "Heart Valves Explained." *American Heart Association*, June 25, 2013.

Gersh, Bernard J. *The Mayo Clinic Heart Book: The Ultimate Guide to Heart Health*. 2d ed. New York: William Morrow, 2000.

Hales, Dianne. *An Invitation to Health Brief*. Updated ed. Belmont, Calif.: Wadsworth/Cengage Learning, 2010.

The Incredible Machine. Washington, D.C.: National Geographic Society, 1994.

Mackenna, B. R., and R. Callander. *Illustrated Physiology*. 6th ed. New York: Churchill Livingstone, 1997.

Marieb, Elaine N., and Katja Hoehn. *Human Anatomy and Physiology*. 9th ed. Boston: Pearson, 2013.

MedlinePlus. "Heart Diseases." *MedlinePlus*, July 8, 2013.

NIH National Heart, Lung, and Blood Institute. "What Is a Heart Transplant?" *NIH National Heart, Lung, and Blood Institute*, January 3, 2012.

NIH National Heart, Lung, and Blood Institute. "What Is a Total Artificial Heart?" *NIH National Heart, Lung, and Blood Institute*, July 6, 2012.

Park, Myung K. *The Pediatric Cardiology Handbook*. 4th ed. St. Louis, Mo.: Mosby/Elsevier, 2010.

Tortora, Gerard J., and Bryan Derrickson. *Principles of Anatomy and Physiology*. 13th ed. Hoboken, N.J.: John Wiley & Sons, 2011.

HEART ATTACK

Disease/Disorder

Also known as: Myocardial infarction

Anatomy or system affected: Circulatory system, heart

Specialties and related fields: Cardiology, critical care, emergency medicine, internal medicine

Definition: Myocardial infarction; the sudden death of heart muscle characterized by intense chest pain, sweating, shortness of breath, or sometimes none of these symptoms.

Key terms:

atherosclerosis: narrowing of the internal passageways of essential arteries caused by the buildup of fatty deposits

atria: the chambers in the right and left top portions of the heart that receive blood from the veins and pump it to the ventricles

fibrillation: wild beating of the heart, which may occur when the regular rate of the heartbeat is interrupted

myocardium: the muscle tissue that forms the walls of the heart, varying in thickness in the upper and lower regions

sinoatrial node: the section of the right atrium that determines the appropriate rate of the heartbeat

ventricles: the chambers in the right and left bottom portions of the heart that receive blood from the atria and pump it to the arteries

Causes and Symptoms

Although varied in origin and effect on the body, heart attacks (or myocardial infarctions) occur when there are interruptions in the delicately synchronized system either supplying blood to the heart or pumping blood from the heart to other vital organs. The heart is a highly specialized muscle whose function is to pump life-sustaining blood to all parts of the body. The heart's action involves the development of pressure to propel blood through arriving and departing channels—veins and arteries—that must maintain that pressure within their walls at critical levels throughout the system.

The highest level of pressure in the total cardiovascular system is to be found closest to the two "pumping" chambers on the right and left lower sections of the heart, called ventricles. Dark, bluish-colored blood, emptied of its oxygen content and laden with carbon dioxide waste instead of the oxygen in fresh blood, flows into the upper portion of the heart via the superior and inferior venae cavae. It then passes from the right atrium chamber into the right ventricle. Once in the ventricle, this blood cannot flow back because of one-way valves separating the "receiving" from the "pumping" sections of the total heart organ.

After this valve closes following a vitally synchronized timing system, constriction of the right ventricle by the myocardium muscle in the surrounding walls of the heart forces the blood from the heart, propelling it toward the oxygen-filled tissue of the lungs. Following reoxygenation, bright red blood that is still under pressure from the thrust of the right ventricle flows into the left atrium. Once channeled into the left ventricle, the pumping process that began in the right ventricle is then repeated on the left by muscular constriction, and oxygenated blood flows out of the aortic valve under pressure throughout the cardiovascular system to nourish the body's cells. Because the force needed to supply blood under pressure from the left ventricle for the entire body is

---

Information on Heart Attack

Causes: Pulmonary problems, atherosclerosis, smoking, high blood pressure, diabetes mellitus

Symptoms: Varies but often includes intense chest pain, sweating, shortness of breath

Duration: Acute

Treatments: Drug therapy, surgery, preventive medication, exercise, dietary change, medical devices

greater than the first-phase pumping force needed to move blood into the lungs, the myocardium surrounding the left ventricle constitutes the thickest muscular layer in the heart's wall.

The efficiency of this process, as well as the origins of problems of fatigue in the heart that can lead to heart attacks and eventual heart failure, is tied to the maintenance of a reasonably constant level of blood pressure. If pulmonary problems (blockage caused by the effects of smoking or environmental pollution, for example) make it harder for the right ventricle to push blood through the lungs, the heart must expend more energy in the first stage of the cardiovascular process. Similarly, and often in addition to the added work for the heart because of pulmonary complications, the efficiency of the left ventricle in handling blood flow may be reduced by the presence of excessive fat in the body, causing this ventricle to expend more energy to propel oxygenated blood into vital tissues.

Although factors such as these may be responsible for overworking the heart and thus contributing to eventual heart failure, other causes of heart attacks are to be found much closer to the working apparatus of the heart, particularly in the coronary arteries. The coronary arteries begin at the top of

the heart and fan out along its sides. They are responsible for providing large quantities of blood to the myocardium muscle, which needs continual nourishment to carry out the pumping that forces blood forward from the ventricles. The passageways inside these and other key arteries are vulnerable to the process known as atherosclerosis, which can affect the blood supply to other organs as well as to the heart. In the heart, atherosclerosis involves the accumulation, inside the coronary arteries, of fatty deposits called atheromas. If these deposits continue to collect, less blood can flow through the arteries. A narrowed artery also increases the possibility of a variant form of heart attack, in which a sudden and total blockage of blood flow follows the lodging of a blood clot in one of these vital passageways.

A symptomatic condition called angina pectoris, characterized by intermittent chest pains, may develop if atherosclerosis reduces blood (and therefore oxygen) supply to the heart. These danger signs can continue over a number of years. If diagnosis reveals a problem that might be resolved by preventive medication, exercise, or recommendations for heart surgery, then this condition, known as myocardial ischemia, may not necessarily end in a full heart attack.

A full heart attack occurs when—for one of several possible reasons, including a vascular spasm suddenly constricting an already clogged artery or a blockage caused by a clot—the heart suddenly ceases to receive the necessary supply of blood. This brings almost immediate deterioration in some of the heart's tissue and causes the organ's consequent inability to perform its vital functions effectively.

Another form of attack and disruption of the heart's ability to deliver blood can come either independently of or in conjunction with an arterially induced heart attack. This form of attack involves a sustained interruption in the rate of heartbeats. The necessary pace or rate of myocardial contractions, which can vary depending on the person's rate of physical exertion or age, is regulated in the sinoatrial node in the right atrium, which generates its own electrical impulses. The ultimate sources for the commands to the sinoatrial node are to be found in the network of nerves coming directly from the brain. There are, however, other so-called local pacemakers located in the atria and ventricles. If these sources of electrical charges begin giving commands to the myocardium that are not in rhythm with those coming from the sinoatrial node, then dysrhythmic or premature beats may confuse the heart muscle, causing it to beat wildly. In fact, the concentrated pattern of muscle contractions will not be coordinated and instead will be dispersed in different areas of the heart. The result is fibrillation, a series of uncoordinated contractions that cannot combine to propel blood out of the ventricles. This condition may occur either as the aftershock of an arterially induced heart attack or suddenly and on its own, caused by the deterioration of the electrical impulse system commanding the heart rate. In patients whose potential vulnerability to this form of heart attack has been diagnosed in advance, a heart physician may decide to surgically implant an electronic pacemaker to ensure coordination of the necessary electrical commands to the myocardium.

Pain Associated with Heart Attack

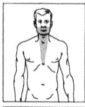

Pain radiating up into jaw and through to back

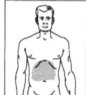

Pain felt in upper abdomen

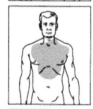

Pressure in the central chest area, from mild to severe

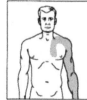

Pain radiating down left arm; may cause sensation of weakness in the arm

Treatment and Therapy

Extraordinary medical advances have helped reduce the high death rates formerly associated with heart attacks. Many of these advances have been in the field of preventive medicine. The most widely recognized medical findings are related to diet, smoking, and exercise. Although controversy remains, there is general agreement that cholesterol absorbed by the body from the ingestion of animal fats plays a key role in the dangerous buildup of platelets inside arterial passageways. It has been accepted that regular, although not necessarily strenuous, exercise is an essential long-term preventive strategy that can reduce the risk of heart attacks. Exercise also plays a role in therapy after a heart attack. In both preventive and postattack contexts, it has been medically proven that the entire cardiovascular system profits from the natural muscle-strengthening process (in the heart's case) and general cleansing effects (in the case of oxygen intake and stimulated blood flow) that result from controlled regular exercise.

The actual application of medical scientific knowledge to assist in the campaign against the deadly effects of heart disease involves multiple fields of specialization. These may range from the sophisticated use of electrocardiograms (ECGs) to monitor the regularity of heartbeats, to specialized drug therapies aimed at preventing heart attacks in people who have been diagnosed as high-risk cases, to coronary bypass surgery or even heart transplants. In the 1980s, highly specialized surgeons at several university and private hospitals began performing operations to implant artificial hearts in human patients.

In the case of ECGs, it has become possible, thanks to the use of portable units that record the heartbeat patterns of persons over an extended period of time, to gain a much more accurate impression of the actual functioning of the heart. Previous dependence on electrocardiographic data gathered during an appointed and limited examination provided only minimal information to doctors.

The domains of preventive surgery and specialized drug treatment to prevent dangerous blood clotting are vast. Statistically, the most important and widely practiced operations that were developed in the later decades of the twentieth century were replacement of the aortic valve, the coronary bypass operation, and, with greater or lesser degrees of success, the actual transplantation of voluntary donors" hearts in the place of those belonging to heart disease patients. Coronary

In the News:
Low-Grade Inflammation as a Trigger

Researchers have suspected for some time that the body's inflammatory response may play a critical role in heart attacks and strokes. It is well known that risk factors for heart attack and stroke include obesity, high cholesterol levels, high blood pressure, and smoking. Blood tests in a 1988 study in Finland, however, showed the presence of a bacterium called *Chlamydia pneumoniae* inside the cells of people with coronary artery disease. It seemed apparent, however, that *C. pneumoniae* alone was not a risk factor or cause of heart disease.

Researchers in the Helsinki Heart Study also looked for the presence of human heat-shock protein 60 (hHsp60), indicating an immune response which could possibly lead to atherosclerosis, and of C-reactive protein (CRP), which sends white blood cells to the site of injury or infection but can cause harm if prolonged or excessive. An eight-year follow-up of this study showed that the risk for heart disease increased when levels of *C. pneumoniae* or hHsp60 antibodies were high. However, the risk was greatest when all three factors were elevated, indicating a possible synergistic effect. It was concluded that chronic infection, autoimmunity, and inflammation in combination contributed to coronary events in the study population.

The research of Paul Ridker of Boston's Brigham and Women's Hospital further showed that levels of CRP over 3 milligrams per liter of blood more than doubled the risk of heart attack and stroke. A test for CRP levels is available, but there are questions of who should be tested and when.

High CRP levels have also been associated with being overweight, a known risk factor for heart disease. Adjusting for age, smoking, and chronic disease, the association was especially strong for obese women, who were six times as likely to have elevated CRP levels, while obese men were twice as likely. One theory to explain this outcome would be that many overweight or obese persons have persistent low-grade inflammation. This may be the result of another protein, interleukin 6, produced by fat tissue, which in turn stimulates the production of CRP by the liver.

Scientific research continues to establish definitive links between heart disease and chronic infections, inflammation, and autoimmune conditions. These links could lead to attacking the basic processes of atherosclerosis, to treatment with anti-inflammatory drugs, and to the prevention of heart attacks and stroke.

—Martha Loustaunau, Ph.D.

bypass operations involve the attachment to the myocardium of healthy arteries to carry the blood that can no longer pass through the patient's clogged arterial passageways; these healthy arteries are taken by the heart surgeon from other areas of the patient's own body.

Another sphere of medical technology, that of balloon angioplasty, held out a major nonsurgical promise of preventing deterioration of the arteries leading to the heart. This sophisticated form of treatment involves the careful, temporary introduction of inflatable devices inside clogged arteries, which are then stretched to increase the space within the arterial passageway for blood to flow. By the 1990s, however, doctors recognized one disadvantage of balloon angioplasty: By stretching the essential blood vessels being treated, this procedure either stretches the plaque with the artery or breaks loose debris that remains behind, creating a danger of renewed clogging. Thus, although angioplasty remains a standard approach to treatment of heart disease, another technique, called atherectomy, was developed to clear certain coronary arteries, as well as arteries elsewhere in the body.

Atherectomy involves a motorized catheter device resembling a miniature drill that is inserted into clogged arteries. As the drill turns, material that is literally shaved off the interior walls of arteries is retrieved through a tiny collection receptacle. Early experimentation, especially to treat the large anterior descending coronary artery on the left side of the heart, showed that atherectomy was 87 percent effective, whereas, on the average, angioplasty removed only 63 percent of the blockage. In addition, similar efforts to provide internal, nonsurgical treatment of clogged arteries using laser beams were being made by the early 1990s.

Perspective and Prospects

The modern conception of cardiology dates from William Harvey's seventeenth-century discovery of the relationship between the heart's function as a pump and the circulatory "restoration" of blood. Harvey's much more scientific views replaced centuries-old conceptions of the heart as a blood-warming device only.

Although substantial anatomical advances were made over the next two centuries that helped explain most of the vital functions of the heart, it was not until the early decades of the twentieth century that science developed therapeutic methods to deal with problems that frequently cause heart attacks. Drugs that affect the liver's production of substances necessary for normal coagulation of blood, for example, were discovered in the 1930s. A large variety of such anticoagulants have since been developed to help thin the blood of patients vulnerable to blood clotting. Other drugs, including certain antibiotics, are used to treat persons whose susceptibility to infection is known to be high. In these cases, the simple action of dislodging bacteria from the teeth when brushing can cause an invasion of the vital parts of the heart by an infection. This bacterialendocarditis, the result of the actual destruction of heart tissue or the sudden release of clots of infectious residue, could lead to a heart attack in such individuals although they have no other symptoms of identifiable heart disease.

The most spectacular advance in the scientific treatment of potential heart attack victims, however, has been in the field of cardiac surgery. Many advances in open heart surgery date from the late 1950s, when the development of heart and lung replacement machines made it safe enough to substitute electronic monitors for some of the organism's normal body functions. Before the 1950s, operations had been limited to surgical treatment of the major blood vessels surrounding the heart.

Various technical methods have also been developed that help identify problems early enough for drug therapy to be attempted before the decision to perform surgery is made. The use of catheters, which are threaded into the coronary organ using the same vessels that transport blood, became the most effective way of locating problematic areas. The process known as angiography, which uses x-rays to trace the course of radiopaque dyes injected through a catheter into local heart areas under study, can actually tell doctors if drug therapy is having the desired effects. In cases where such tests show that preventive drug therapy is not effective, an early decision to perform surgery can be made, preventing the source of coronary trouble from multiplying the patient's chances of suffering a heart attack.

—*Byron D. Cannon, Ph.D.*

See also Angina; Angiography; Angioplasty; Arrhythmias; Arteriosclerosis; Bypass surgery; Cardiac arrest; Cardiac rehabilitation; Cardiac surgery; Cardiology; Cardiopulmonary resuscitation (CPR); Cholesterol; Circulation; Coronary artery bypass graft; Critical care; Defibrillation; Echocardiography; Electrocardiography (ECG or EKG); Embolism; Emergency medicine; Emergency rooms; Heart; Heart disease; Heart failure; Heart transplantation; Heart valve replacement; Hypercholesterolemia; Hyperlipidemia; Hypertension; Ischemia; Mitral valve prolapse; Pacemaker implantation; Palpitations; Phlebitis; Plaque, arterial; Resuscitation; Thrombolytic therapy and TPA; Thrombosis and thrombus.

For Further Information:

American Heart Association. http://www.american heart.org.

Baum, Seth J. *The Total Guide to a Healthy Heart: Integrative Strategies for Preventing and Reversing Heart Disease*. New York: Kensington, 2000.

Berra, Kathleen, et al. *Heart Attack! Advice for Patients by Patients*. New Haven, Conn.: Yale University Press, 2002.

Carson-DeWitt, Rosalyn. "Heart Attack." *Health Library*, September 10, 2012.

Crawford, Michael, ed. *Current Diagnosis and Treatment—Cardiology*. 3d ed. New York: McGraw-Hill Medical, 2009.

Eagle, Kim A., and Ragavendra R. Baliga, eds. *Practical Cardiology: Evaluation and Treatment of Common Cardiovascular Disorders*. 2d ed. Philadelphia: Lippincott Williams & Wilkins, 2008.

Gersh, Bernard J., ed. *The Mayo Clinic Heart Book*. 2d ed. New York: William Morrow, 2000.

Gillis, Jack. *The Heart Attack Prevention and Recovery Handbook*. Point Roberts, Wash.: Hartley & Marks, 1997.

"Heart Attack." *Mayo Clinic*, May 15, 2013.

Kligfield, Paul. *The Cardiac Recovery Handbook: The Complete Guide to Life After Heart Attack or Heart Surgery*. 2d ed. Long New York: Hatherleigh Press, 2006.

"What Is a Heart Attack?" *National Heart, Lung, and Blood Institute*, July 5, 2013.

Yannios, Thomas A. *The Heart Disease Breakthrough: The Ten-Step Program That Can Save Your Life*. Rev. ed. New York: Wiley, 1999.

Zaret, Barry L., Marvin Moser, and Lawrence S. Cohen, eds. *Yale University School of Medicine Heart Book*. New York: William Morrow, 1992.

HEART DISEASE

Disease/Disorder

Anatomy or system affected: Blood vessels, circulatory system, heart

Specialties and related fields: Cardiology, family medicine, internal medicine

Definition: One of the leading causes of death in many industrialized nations; heart diseases include atherosclerotic disease, coronary artery disease, cardiac arrhythmias, and stenosis.

Key terms:

cardiac arrhythmia: a disturbance in the heartbeat

coronary arteries: blood vessels surrounding the heart that provide nourishment and oxygen to heart tissue

nodes: areas of electrochemical transmission within the heart that regulate the heartbeat

plaque: an accumulation of matter within artery walls that can impede blood flow

Causes and Symptoms

The heart is a fist-sized organ located in the lower left quarter of the chest. It consists of four chambers: the right and left atria on top and the right and left ventricles at the bottom. The chambers are enclosed in three layers of tissue: the outer layer (epicardium), the middle layer (myocardium), and the inner layer (endocardium). Surrounding the entire organ is the pericardium, a thin layer of tissue that forms a protective covering for the heart. The heart also contains various nodes that transmit electrochemical signals, causing heart muscle tissue to contract and relax in the pumping action that carries blood to organs and cells throughout the body.

Signals from the brain cause the heart to contract rhythmically in a sequence of motions that move the blood from the right atrium down through the tricuspid valve into the right ventricle. From here, blood is pushed through the pulmonary valve into the lungs, where it fulfills one of its major functions: to pick up oxygen in exchange for carbon dioxide. From the lungs, the blood is pumped back into the heart, entering the left atrium from which it is pumped down through the mitral valve into the left ventricle. Blood is then pushed through the aortic valve into the main artery of the body, the aorta, from which it starts its journey to the organs and cells. As it passes through the arteries of the gastrointestinal system, the blood picks up nutrients which, along with the oxygen that it has taken from the lungs, are brought to the cells and exchanged for waste products and carbon dioxide. The blood then enters the veins, through which it is eventually returned to the heart. The heart nourishes and supplies itself with oxygen through the coronary arteries, so called because they sit on top of the heart like a crown and extend down the sides.

The heart diseases collectively include all the disorders that can befall every part of the heart muscle: the pericardium, epicardium, myocardium, endocardium, atria, ventricles, valves, coronary arteries, and nodes. The most significant sites of heart diseases are the coronary arteries and the nodes; their malfunction can cause coronary artery disease and cardiac arrhythmias, respectively. These two disorders are responsible for the majority of heart disease cases.

Coronary artery disease occurs when matter such as cholesterol and fibrous material collects and stiffens on the inner walls of the coronary arteries. The plaque that forms may narrow the passage through which blood flows, reducing the amount of blood delivered to the heart, or may build up and clog the artery entirely, shutting off the flow of blood to the heart. In the former case, when the coronary artery is narrowed, the condition is called ischemic heart disease. Because the most common cause of ischemia is narrowing of the coronary arteries to the myocardium, another designation of the condition is myocardial ischemia, referring to the fact that blood flow to the myocardium is impeded. Accumulation of plaque within the coronary arteries is referred to as coronary atherosclerosis.

As the coronary arteries become clogged and then narrow, they can fail to deliver the required oxygen to the heart muscle, particularly during stress or physical effort. The heart's

---

Information on Heart Disease

Causes: Pulmonary problems, atherosclerosis, smoking, diabetes, hypertension, infection, high-fat diet and obesity, stress

Symptoms: Varies; can include pain, sweating, shortness of breath, inability to exercise, irregular heartbeat, dizziness, loss of consciousness

Duration: Acute or chronic

Treatments: Drug therapy, surgery, preventive medication, exercise, dietary change, medical devices

---

need for oxygen exceeds the arteries" ability to supply it. The patient usually feels a sharp, choking pain, called angina pectoris. Not all people who have coronary ischemia, however, experience anginal pain; these people are said to have silent ischemia.

The danger in coronary artery disease is that the accumulation of plaque will progress to the point where the coronary artery is clogged completely and no blood is delivered to the part of the heart serviced by that artery. The rough, uneven texture of the plaque instead may cause the formation of a blood clot, or thrombus, which closes the artery in a condition called coronary thrombosis. The result is a myocardial infarction (commonly called a heart attack), in which some myocardial cells die when they fail to receive blood.

Although coronary ischemia is usually thought of as a disease of middle and old age, in fact, it starts much earlier. Autopsies of accident victims in their teens and twenties, as well as young soldiers killed in battle, show that coronary atherosclerosis is often well advanced in young persons. Some reasons for these findings and for why the rates of coronary artery disease and death began to rise in the twentieth century have been proposed. While antibiotics and vaccines reduced the mortality of some bacterial and some viral infections, Western societies underwent significant changes in lifestyle and eating habits that contributed to the rise of coronary heart disease: high-fat diets, obesity, and the stressful pace of life in a modern industrial society. Furthermore, cigarette smoking, once almost a universal habit, has been shown to be highly pathogenic (disease-causing), contributing significantly to the development of heart disease, as well as lung cancer, emphysema, bronchitis, and other disorders. In the early and middle decades of the twentieth century, coronary heart disease was considered primarily an ailment of middle-aged and older men. As women began smoking, however, the incidence shifted so that coronary artery disease became almost equally prevalent, and equally lethal, among men and women.

Other conditions such as hypertension or diabetes mellitus are considered precursors of coronary artery disease. Hypertension, or high blood pressure, is an extremely common condition that, if unchecked, can contribute to both the development and the progression of coronary artery disease. Over the years, high blood pressure subjects arterial walls to constant stress. In response, the walls thicken and stiffen. This "hardening" of the arteries encourages the accumulation of fatty and fibrous plaque on inner artery walls. In patients with diabetes mellitus, blood sugar (glucose) levels rise either because the patient is deficient in insulin or because the insulin that the patient produces is inefficient at removing glucose from the blood. High glucose levels favor high fat levels in the blood, which can cause atherosclerosis.

Cardiac arrhythmias are the next major cause of morbidity and mortality among the heart diseases. Inside the heart, an electrochemical network regulates the contractions and relaxations that form the heartbeat. In the excitation or contraction phase, a chain of electrochemical impulses starts in the upper part of the right atrium in the heart's pacemaker, the sinoatrial or sinus node. The impulses travel through internodal tracts (pathways from one node to another) to an area between the atrium and the right ventricle called the atrioventricular node. The impulses then enter the bundle of His, which carries them to the left atrium and left ventricle. After the series of contractions is complete, the heart relaxes for a brief moment before another cycle is begun. On the average, the process is repeated sixty to eighty times a minute.

This is normal rhythm, the regular, healthy heartbeat. Dysfunction at any point along the electrochemical pathway, however, can cause an arrhythmia. Arrhythmias range greatly in their effects and their potential for bodily damage. They can be completely unnoticeable, merely annoying, debilitating, or frightening. They can cause blood clots to form in the heart, and they can cause sudden death.

The arrhythmic heart can beat too quickly (tachycardia) or too slowly (bradycardia). The contractions of the various chambers can become unsynchronized, or out of step with one another. For example, in atrial flutter or atrial fibrillation, the upper chambers of the heart beat faster, out of synchronization with the ventricles. In ventricular tachycardia, ventricular contractions increase, out of synchronization with the atria. In ventricular fibrillation, ventricular contractions lose all rhythmicity and become uncoordinated to the point at which the heart is no longer able to pump blood. Cardiac death can then occur unless the patient receives immediate treatment.

An arrhythmic disorder called heart block occurs when the impulse from the pacemaker is "blocked." Its progress through the atrioventricular node and the bundle of His may be slow or irregular, or the impulse may fail to reach its target tissues. The disorder is rated in three degrees. First-degree heart block is detectable only on an electrocardiogram (ECG or EKG), in which the movement of the impulse from the atria to the ventricles is seen to be slowed. In second-degree heart block, only some of the impulses generated reach from the atria to the ventricles; the pulse becomes irregular. Third-degree heart block is the most serious manifestation of this disorder: No impulses from the atria reach the ventricles. The heart rate may slow dramatically, and the blood flow to the brain can be reduced, causing dizziness or loss of consciousness.

Disorders that affect the heart valves usually involve stenosis (narrowing), which reduces the size of the valve opening; physical malfunction of the valve; or both. These disorders can be attributable to infection (such as rheumatic fever) or to tissue damage, or they can be congenital. If a valve has narrowed, the passage of blood from one heart chamber to another is impeded. In the case of mitral stenosis, the mitral valve between the left atrium and the left ventricle is narrowed. Blood flow to the left ventricle is reduced, and blood is retained in the left atrium, causing the atrium to enlarge as pressure builds in the chamber. This pressure forces blood back into the lungs, creating a condition called pulmonary edema, in which fluid collects in the air sacs of the lungs. Similarly, malfunctions of the heart valves that cause them to open and close inefficiently can interfere with the flow of blood into the heart, through it, and out of it. This impairment may cause structural changes in the heart that can be life-threatening.

Heart failure may be a consequence of many disease conditions. It occurs primarily in the elderly. In this condition, the heart becomes inefficient at pumping blood. If the failure is on the right side of the heart, blood is forced back into the body, causing edema in the lower legs. If the failure is on the left side of the heart, blood is forced back into the lungs, causing pulmonary edema. There are many manifestations of heart failure, including shortness of breath, fatigue, and weakness.

Numerous diseases afflict the tissues of the heart wall—the epicardium, myocardium, and endocardium, as well as the pericardium. They are often caused by bacterial or viral infection, but they may also result from tissue trauma or a variety of toxic agents.

Treatment and Therapy

The main tools for diagnosing heart disease are the stethoscope, the ECG, and the x ray. With the stethoscope the doctor listens to heart sounds, which provide information about many heart functions such as rhythm and the status of the valves. The doctor can determine whether the heart is functioning normally in pumping blood from one chamber into the other, into the lungs, and into the aorta. The ECG gives the doctor a graph representation of heart function. Twelve to fifteen electrodes are placed on various parts of the body, including the head, chest, legs, and arms. The activities of the heart are printed on a strip of paper as waves or tracings. The doctor analyzes the printout for evidence of heart abnormalities, changes in heart function, signs of a heart attack, or other problems. Generally, the electrocardiographic examination is conducted with the patient at rest. In some situations, however, the doctor wishes to view heart action during physical stress. In this case, the electrodes are attached to the patient and the patient is required to exercise on a treadmill or stationary bicycle. The physician can see what changes in heart function occur when the cardiac workload is increased. The x ray gives the doctor a visual picture of the heart. Any enlargements or abnormalities can be seen, as well as the status of the aorta, pulmonary arteries, and other structures.

Another standard diagnostic tool is the echocardiograph. High-frequency sound waves are pointed at the heart from outside the body. The sound waves bounce against heart tissue and are shown on a monitor. The general configuration of the heart can be seen, as well as the shape and thickness of the chamber walls, the valves, and the large blood vessels leading to and from the heart. Velocity and direction of blood flow through the valves can be determined.

Various procedures can help the doctor assess the degree of ischemia within the heart. In one test, a radioactive isotope is injected into a vein and its dispersion in the heart is read by a scanner. This procedure can show which parts of the heart are being deprived of oxygen. In another test using a radioactive isotope, the reading is made while the patient exercises, in order to detect any changes in expansion and contraction of the heart wall that would indicate impaired circulation. The coronary angiogram gives a picture of the blockage within the coronary arteries. A thin tube called a catheter is threaded into a coronary artery, and a dye that is opaque to x rays is released. The x-ray picture will reveal narrowings in the artery resulting from plaque buildup.

The main goals of therapy in treating heart diseases are to cure the condition, if possible, and otherwise help the patient live a normal life and prevent the condition from becoming worse. In coronary artery disease, the physician seeks to maintain blood flow to the heart and to prevent heart attack. Hundreds of medications are available for this purpose, including vasodilators (agents that relax blood vessel walls and increase their capacity to carry blood). Chief among the coronary vasodilators are nitroglycerin and other drugs in the nitrate family. Also, calcium-channel blockers are often used to dilate blood vessels. Beta-blocking agents are used because they reduce the heart's need for oxygen and alleviate the symptoms of angina. In addition, various support measures are recommended by physicians to stop plaque buildup and halt the progress of the disease. These include losing weight, reducing fats in the diet, and stopping smoking. The physician also treats concomitant illnesses that can contribute to the progress of coronary artery disease, such as hypertension and diabetes.

Sometimes medications and diet are not fully successful, and the ischemia continues. The cardiologist can unblock a clogged artery by a procedure called angioplasty. The physician threads a catheter containing a tiny balloon to the point of the blockage. The balloon is inflated to widen the inner diameter of the artery, and blood flow is increased. This procedure is often successful, although it may have to be repeated. In atherectomy, a miniature drill shaves off the plaque, which is then removed. If neither procedure is successful, coronary bypass surgery may be indicated. In this procedure, clogged coronary arteries are replaced with healthy blood vessels from other parts of the body.

When coronary artery disease progresses to a heart attack, the patient should be treated in the hospital or similar facility. The possibility of sudden death is high during the attack and remains high until the patient is stabilized. Emergency measures are undertaken to minimize the extent of heart damage, reduce heart work, keep oxygen flowing to all parts of the body, and regulate blood pressure and heartbeat.

Cardiac arrhythmias can be managed by a variety of medi-

cations and procedures. Digitalis, guanidine, procainamide, tocanamide, and atropine are widely used to restore normal heart rhythm. In acute situations, the patient's heart rhythm can be restored by electrical cardioversion, in which an electrical stimulus is applied from outside the body to regulate the heartbeat. When a slowed heartbeat cannot be controlled by medication, a pacemaker may be implanted to regulate heart rhythm.

Treatment of heart valve disorders and disorders of the heart wall is directed at alleviating the individual condition. Antibiotics and/or valve replacement surgery may be required. In many cases, valve disorders can be completely corrected. Cardiac transplantation remains a possible treatment for some heart patients. This is an option for comparatively few patients because there are ten times as many candidates for heart transplants as there are available donor hearts.

Perspective and Prospects

Heart disease became a major killer in the United States in the twentieth century. In the early decades, the best that the medical community could do was to treat symptoms. Since then, the emphasis has shifted to prevention. Hundreds of investigative studies have been undertaken to determine the causes of the most prevalent heart dysfunction, coronary artery disease. Many of these studies have involved tens of thousands of subjects, and they point to a general consensus that coronary artery disease is a multifactorial disorder, the primary elements of which are cholesterol and other fatty substances circulating in the bloodstream, smoking, diabetes, high blood pressure, stress, and obesity.

The reasons that mortality from heart disease is declining include improved medications and treatment modalities, and much credit has to be given to the success of preventive measures. Millions of Americans have stopped smoking and have begun watching their diets. Entire industries are devoted to helping Americans eat more intelligently. While fast-food outlets continue to offer high-fat standards, such as hot dogs and hamburgers, they have also added salads and leaner selections.

Perhaps most important, medical and sociological authorities have turned their attention to children. Because advanced atherosclerosis has been detected in young men and women, cholesterol-watching has become a major preoccupation with parents and school dieticians. In addition, national programs have been instituted to discourage smoking among the young. Whether the rates of coronary heart disease will be lower in these individuals than in their parents remains to be seen, but the success of these measures in the older populations indicates that the prognosis is good.

The prognosis is also good for other heart diseases. New drugs continue to be licensed for the treatment of arrhythmias, and more versatile and reliable pacemakers increase the prospects of a normal life for many patients. Improvements in heart surgery have been particularly impressive, especially those for managing congenital heart defects in neonates and infants. Heart transplants have been successfully performed on these patients, and numerous other procedures promise significant improvement in the prospects of young people with heart disease.

Rheumatic fever, however, one of the major causes of heart disease in children, remains a threat. No vaccine is available for immunization against the streptococcus strains that cause rheumatic fever, but fortunately there are effective antibiotics to control infection in these patients. Rheumatic fever usually develops subsequent to a streptococcal throat infection that has not been treated adequately with antibiotics. Careful evaluation of the child with a sore throat and prompt, complete antibiotic treatment of those with streptococcal infection can avoid progression of the infection to rheumatic fever.

—*C. Richard Falcon*

See also Aneurysms; Angina; Arrhythmias; Arteriosclerosis; Blue baby syndrome; Bypass surgery; Cardiac arrest; Cardiac rehabilitation; Cardiac surgery; Cardiology; Cardiology, pediatric; Cholesterol; Circulation; Claudication; Congenital heart disease; Coronary artery bypass graft; Diabetes mellitus; Echocardiography; Electrocardiography (ECG or EKG); Embolism; Endocarditis; Heart; Heart attack; Heart failure; Heart transplantation; Heart valve replacement; Hypercholesterolemia; Hyperlipidemia; Hypertension; Ischemia; Mitral valve prolapse; Obesity; Pacemaker implantation; Palpitations; Phlebitis; Plaque, arterial; Pulmonary hypertension; Thrombolytic therapy and TPA; Thrombosis and thrombus; Varicose veins; Venous insufficiency.

For Further Information:

American Heart Association. http://www.american heart.org.

Baum, Seth J. *The Total Guide to a Healthy Heart: Integrative Strategies for Preventing and Reversing Heart Disease.* New York: Kensington, 2000.

Braunwald, Eugene, et al., eds. *Braunwald's Heart Disease: A Textbook of Cardiovascular Medicine.* 9th ed. Philadelphia: Saunders, 2012.

Gerstenblith, Gary, and Simeon Margolis. *Coronary Heart Disease: Your Annual Guide to Prevention, Diagnosis, and Treatment.* New York: Remedy Health Media, 2013.

Gersh, Bernard J., ed. *The Mayo Clinic Heart Book.* 2d ed. New York: William Morrow, 2000.

Goldberg, Nieca. *Women Are Not Small Men: Life-Saving Strategies for Preventing and Healing Heart Disease in Women.* New York: Random House, 2003.

Kramer, Gerri Freid, and Shari Mauer. *Parent's Guide to Children's Congenital Heart Defects: What They Are, How to Treat Them, How to Cope with Them.* New York: Three Rivers Press, 2001.

Litin, Scott C., ed. *Mayo Clinic Family Health Book.* 4th ed. New York: HarperResource, 2009.

Piscatella, Joseph, and Barry Franklin. *Take a Load Off Your Heart: 109 Things You Can Do to Prevent or Reverse Heart Disease.* New York: Workman, 2003.

Scottish Heart and Arterial Prevention Group. "Cardiovascular Disease: Everyday Management." *British Journal of Cardiology* 19, no. 1 (January–March, 2012).

Taylor, George J., ed. *Primary Care Management of Heart Disease.* St. Louis, Mo.: Mosby, 2000.

Thow, Morag K., Keri Graham, and Choi Lee. *The Healthy Heart Book.* Champaign, Ill.: Human Kinetics, 2013.

Yannios, Thomas A. *The Heart Disease Breakthrough: The Ten-Step Program That Can Save Your Life.* Rev. ed. New York: Wiley, 1999.

Zaret, Barry L., Marvin Moser, and Lawrence S. Cohen, eds. *Yale University School of Medicine Heart Book.* New York: William Morrow, 1992.

HEART FAILURE
Disease/Disorder

Anatomy or system affected: Circulatory system, heart

Specialties and related fields: Cardiology, internal medicine, vascular medicine

Definition: A condition in which the heart cannot pump enough blood to meet the needs of the body because its ability to contract is impaired.

Key terms:

congestive heart failure: the stage of heart failure that occurs when a backup of pressure results in accumulation of fluid in the veins and tissues

coronary arteries: the arteries that supply blood to the heart muscle

diuretic: a drug that stimulates the kidneys to eliminate more salt and water from the body

edema: the accumulation of fluid around the cells in tissue

ejection fraction: the ratio of the stroke volume to the residual volume, expressed as a percentage

hormone: a chemical messenger released by a gland which is carried by the blood to its target

inotropic agent: a drug that improves the ability of the heart muscle to contract

optimal length: the length of a heart muscle cell at which stimulation can elicit the maximum possible force development

residual volume: the blood volume left in the heart chamber at the end of a heartbeat

stroke volume: the blood volume leaving either the right or the left side of the heart with each beat; each side usually ejects the same volume per beat

vasodilator: a drug that relaxes blood vessels

Causes and Symptoms

The circulation of the blood has many functions. It is essential for the delivery of oxygen, nutrients, and elements of the immune system to tissues. It also contributes to regulation and communication between different parts of the body by moving chemical messengers from where they are produced to where they have a biological effect. The delivery of warm blood to the surface of the skin is one essential element in temperature control. The blood pressure determines how much water can move across the exchange surfaces in the kidneys, thus affecting water balance in the body. The movement of blood through the kidneys, the lungs, and all tissues is important for waste removal.

All these functions depend on the ability of the heart to contract and eject blood. Blood is pumped, in two serial circuits, from the right heart through the lungs into the left heart and from the left heart around the body back to the right heart. In each circuit, the blood travels through large arteries, then to smaller arterioles, to capillaries (where exchange takes place), and back via small venules and veins to the heart. Heart failure describes the situation in which heart function is reduced. While still able to beat, the heart is unable to meet the circulatory needs of the body. That is, the heart muscle is unable to contract enough to pump the blood adequately.

The severity of the heart failure can be gauged by the ejection fraction, a measure of the pumping capacity of the heart. It is the percentage calculated from the stroke volume (the volume of blood leaving a heart chamber with each beat) divided by the residual volume (the volume left in the heart chamber at the end of a heartbeat). Thus, the ejection fraction measures how much blood in the heart chamber can actually leave when the heartbeat occurs. In normal, healthy hearts, this value is 100 percent: the amount that stays in the heart is approximately equal to the amount that leaves it. In mild or moderate heart failure, it ranges approximately between 15 and 40 percent: Less blood leaves the heart with each beat, and more blood remains behind.

The pressure inside the heart at the end of a heartbeat is another index of heart performance. If the heart is failing and more blood is left behind in the heart at the end of a beat, the pressure inside the heart at the end of the beat will be increased. In cases of severe failure, the pressure in the arteries outside the heart will fall.

In failure, the heart cannot supply enough blood for all the functions of the circulation. This fact accounts for the variety of symptoms that accompany heart failure: labored breathing; light-headedness; generalized weakness; cold, pale, or even bluish skin tone; and accumulation of fluid in the extremities and/or lungs. Other possible symptoms include distended neck veins, accumulation of fluid in the abdomen, abnormal heart rate and rhythm, and chest pain.

The specific symptoms of the condition depend on the type of failure, its severity, its underlying causes, and the ways in which the body attempts to compensate. There are several ways to categorize types of heart failure: acute or chronic, forward or backward, and right-sided or left-sided.

Acute heart failure refers to a sudden decrease in heart function. It can be caused by toxic quantities of drugs, anesthetics, or metals or by certain disease states, such as infections. Most often, however, it is caused by a sudden blockage of the coronary arteries supplying the heart muscle. A sudden blockage caused by a blood clot can induce a heart attack and subsequent heart failure, causing chest pain and often abnormal heart rate or rhythm. These effects are sometimes so rapid that there is little time for the body to attempt compensation.

Chronic heart failure is a progressive reduction in heart function that develops over time. It can be caused by inherited or acquired diseases, allergic reactions, connective tissue or metabolic abnormalities, high blood pressure, and anatomical defects. The most common cause, however, is coronary artery disease. This disease narrows blood vessels and leads to a reduction in the amount of blood reaching the heart muscle. It causes reduced oxygen availability and, eventually, a reduction in the ability of the heart muscle to contract.

In the early stages of chronic failure, the hormone and nervous systems promote compensation in the heart, blood vessels, and kidneys to help the heart continue to pump enough blood. These systems stimulate the heart muscle directly to make it beat harder. They also take advantage of the fact that

---

Information on Heart Failure

Causes: Varies; can include inherited or acquired diseases, allergic reactions, connective tissue or metabolic abnormalities, high blood pressure, anatomical defects, toxic quantities of drugs, sudden blockage of coronary arteries

Symptoms: Labored breathing; light-headedness; generalized weakness; cold, pale, or even bluish skin tone; accumulation of fluid in extremities and/or lungs; distended neck veins; abnormal heart rate and rhythm; chest pain

Duration: Acute or chronic

Treatments: Drug therapy, surgery, preventive medication, exercise, dietary change, medical devices

---

modest stretching of the heart muscle increases its ability to contract. By stimulating the blood vessels to contract, more blood moves back toward the heart, causing a cold, pale, or even bluish skin tone. Stimulation of the kidney to retain water and sodium results in an increase in blood volume, which also moves more blood back to the heart. In each case, the heart muscle is stretched by these increases and, therefore, can contract harder.

Yet these reactions do not constitute a long-term solution. The heart muscle can become fatigued from overwork and can become overstretched. A resulting accumulation of fluid in the heart reduces its ability to contract. Compensation fails, and the additional fluid in the blood starts to back up in the circulation. This condition is called backward heart failure. At the same time, the heart is unable to pump hard enough to move the blood forward against the higher resistance caused by the contraction of the blood vessels. This condition is termed forward heart failure. Congestive heart failure is the stage that occurs when the backup of pressure is worsened by fluid retention and blood vessel contraction. The congestion, or accumulation of fluid, occurs in the veins and tissues.

Left-sided or right-sided heart failure can occur alone or together. The right side of the heart pumps blood to the lungs to be oxygenated, and the left side of the heart pumps oxygenated blood to the organs of the body. Normally, these two sides are well matched so that the same volume moves through each side. When the right heart cannot contract properly, however, blood accumulates upstream in the veins and somewhat less blood reaches the lungs to pick up oxygen, resulting in distended veins and shortness of breath. It is primarily a backward heart failure. Fluid can back up in the veins and increase pressure in the capillaries so that it starts to leak out of the circulation into the surrounding tissues. This leads to an accumulation of fluid (called edema), especially in the liver and lower extremities. In isolated right-sided heart failure, this pressure rarely backs up to such an extent that it causes problems through the rest of the circulation to the left side of the heart.

In contrast, when the left side of the heart cannot contract properly, it can back up pressure so badly that it creates a pressure overload against which the right side of the heart must pump. This increase in the workload on the right side of the heart frequently leads to two-sided heart failure. This outcome is especially common since the disease conditions that exist in the left side are likely to exist on the right as well. In left-sided heart failure, blood accumulates upstream in the lungs, increasing pressure enough to cause a leakage of fluid into the lungs (pulmonary edema). This leakage interferes with oxygen uptake and therefore causes shortness of breath. It also results in inadequate blood flow to the body's tissues, including the muscles and brain, resulting in generalized weakness and light-headedness. Left-sided heart failure is thus both a backward and a forward failure.

Treatment and Therapy

Treatments for cardiac failure, like its symptoms, depend on a variety of factors. The first goal of treatment is to avoid any obvious precipitating causes of the failure, such as alcohol, drugs, the cessation of nonessential medications, acute stress, a salt-loaded diet, overexercise, infection, illness, or surgery. The next approach is to take the simplest measures to reduce distension of the heart by controlling salt and water retention and to decrease the workload of the heart by altering the circulatory needs of the tissues. The former can be achieved by dietary salt restriction, restriction of fluid consumption, or mechanical removal of fluid accumulating around the lungs or abdomen. The latter can be accomplished with bed rest and weight loss.

Typically, drug therapy is also required in order to treat heart failure. No single agent meets all the requirements for optimal treatment, which includes rapid relief of labored breathing and edema, enhanced heart performance, reduced mortality, reduced progression of the underlying disease, safety, and minimal side effects. Therefore, drugs are used in combination to achieve control over sodium and water retention, improve heart contraction, reduce heart work, and protect against blood clots.

The purpose of therapy with diuretic drugs (drugs that increase salt and water loss through the kidneys) is threefold: to reduce the pooling of fluid that can take place in the lungs, abdomen, and lower extremities; to minimize the buildup of back pressure from the accumulation of blood in the veins; and to reduce the circulating blood volume. All these things will lessen the overstretch of the heart muscle and bring it to a level of stretch that is closer to its optimum. Care must be taken, however, not to reduce severely the water content of the blood, which could reduce the stretch on the heart muscle to below the optimum and consequently impair heart contraction. One way to monitor how much water is lost or retained is for patients to empty their bladders and then weigh themselves each day before breakfast. If weight changes steadily or suddenly, then sodium and water loss may be too great or too little. In either case, an adjustment is in order. Some generic diuretic drugs used to treat heart failure include furosemide, ethacrynic acid, the thiazides, and spironolactone.

The purpose of therapy with inotropic drugs (drugs that increase the contractile ability of heart muscle) is to improve the pumping action of the heart. This effect causes an increase in stroke volume (more blood moves out of the heart per beat) and helps compensate for forward failure. The increased output also reduces the backup of blood returning to the heart and thus also compensates for backward failure.

Digitalis, a derivative of the foxglove plant which originated as a Welsh folk remedy, is still the most frequently used inotropic drug for the treatment of chronic heart failure. Because it improves heart muscle contraction, it reverses to some extent all the symptoms of heart failure. Digitalis exerts its effects by increasing the accumulation of calcium inside the heart muscle cells. Calcium interacts with the structure of the shortening apparatus inside the cell to make more contractile interactions within the cell possible. Its disadvantages are that it becomes toxic in high doses and that it can severely damage performance of an already healthy heart.

Other inotropic agents also act to improve contraction by increasing calcium levels within the heart muscle cells. Some of them mimic the naturally produced hormones and neurotransmitters that are released and depleted in early stages of heart failure. These are called the sympathomimetic drugs. They include drugs such as dopamine, terbutaline, and levodopa. While these drugs improve heart performance, they can have serious side effects: increased heart rate, palpitations, and nervousness. One group of inotropic agents improves cardiac contraction while relaxing blood vessels. These drugs, called phosphodiesterase inhibitors, stop the breakdown of an essential cellular messenger molecule which helps to manage calcium levels and other events inside both heart cells and blood vessel cells. Examples of these drugs include amrinone and milrinone. Their use is not common because they can cause stomach upset and fatigue and because they are not clearly superior to other treatments.

The purpose of therapy with vasodilator drugs (drugs that relax the blood vessels) is to decrease the work of the heart. The resulting expansion of the blood vessels makes it easier for blood to be pumped through them. It also leaves room for pooling some of the blood in the veins, decreasing the amount of blood returning to the heart and so reducing overstretching as well. Some of the vasodilators, such as hydralazine, pinacidil, dipyridamole, and the nitrates, act directly on the blood vessels. Other vasodilators, such as angiotensin-converting enzyme (ACE) inhibitors and adrenergic inhibitors, inhibit the release of naturally produced substances that would make the blood vessels contract. Sometimes it is hard to predict the effects of vasodilators because they may act differently in different blood vessels and the body may attempt to offset the effects of the drug by releasing substances that contract blood vessels. Vasodilator drug therapy is usually added to other treatments when the symptoms of heart failure persist after digitalis and diuretic therapy are used.

The purpose of therapy with antithrombotics (blood clot inhibitors) is to prevent any further obstruction of the circulation with blood clots. Because heart failure changes the mechanics of blood flow and is the result of damaged heart muscle, it can increase the formation of blood clots. When blood clots form an obstruction in the large blood vessels of the

---

In the News:
Homocysteine Levels and Congestive Heart Failure

In the January, 2003, issue of the *Journal of the American Medical Association* (JAMA), a team of researchers from the National Heart, Lung, and Blood Institute's Framingham Heart Study, the U.S. Department of Agriculture Human Nutrition Research Center on Aging, and Boston University reported that elevated levels of total homocysteine in the blood are associated with an increased risk for congestive heart failure, a condition in which the heart is unable to maintain adequate blood circulation to the tissues.

The correlation between elevated homocysteine levels and increased risk of cardiovascular disease in general—and specifically myocardial infarction (heart attack), arteriosclerosis, coronary heart disease, and stroke—has been well established, but this was the first study to pinpoint congestive heart failure.

Homocysteine is an amino acid, but unlike most amino acids, it is not a component of proteins. Its primary role seems to be to act as an intermediate in the formation and breakdown of other molecules. Excess levels of homocysteine probably result from its accumulation when its conversion to the next intermediate occurs too slowly, a process often thought to be caused by folic acid deficiency. This conversion can be accelerated by the administration of folic acid.

The subjects of this eight-year study were 2,491 participants of the Framingham Heart Study, who at the start of the study had no histories of myocardial infarction or congestive heart failure. Their average age was seventy-two years. Patients were examined at various times after the initial measurement of plasma homocysteine, and the examinations included plasma homocysteine measurement, blood pressure measurement, electrocardiogram evaluation, systematic assessment of cardiovascular risk factors, and a review of cardiovascular events in each patient's medical record. There were 156 patients who developed congestive heart failure, and the association between plasma homocysteine levels and the incidence of congestive heart failure was examined. Patients with higher-than-average homocysteine levels were more likely to develop congestive heart failure. Women with higher-than-average homocysteine levels had twice the risk for congestive heart failure when compared to the total female population of the study. Researchers noted, however, that additional studies to evaluate the effect of folic acid supplementation on the risk of congestive heart failure are needed.

—Lorraine Lica, Ph.D.

---

lungs, it is often fatal. Clots can also lodge in the heart, causing further damage to heart muscle, or in the brain, where they could cause a stroke. Both the short-acting clot inhibitor heparin and oral agents such as aspirin are used to prevent these effects.

The combination of all these drug therapies, while unable to reverse the permanent damage of heart failure, makes it possible to treat the condition. Individuals treated for heart failure can lead comfortable, productive lives.

If the heart failure progresses to acutely life-threatening proportions and the patient is in all other ways healthy, the next alternative is surgical replacement of the heart. Artificial hearts are sometimes used as a transition to heart transplant while a donor is sought. Yet transplantation is not a perfect solution. Transplanted hearts do not have the nervous system input of a normal heart and so their control from moment to moment is different. They are also subject to rejection. Nevertheless, they provide an enormous improvement in quality of life for severe heart failure patients.

Perspective and Prospects

The vital significance of the pulse and heartbeat have been part of human knowledge since long before recorded history. Pulse taking and herbal treatments for poor heartbeat have been recorded in ancient Chinese, Egyptian, and Greek histories. Digitalis has been used in treatment for at least two hundred years. It was first formally introduced to the medical community in 1785 by the English botanist and physician William Withering. He learned of it from a female folk healer named Hutton, who used it with other extracts to treat more than one kind of swelling. Withering identified the foxglove plant as the source of its active ingredient and characterized it as having effects on the pulse as well as on fluid retention. The plant is indigenous to both the United Kingdom and Europe and may well have been employed as a folk remedy for far longer.

The developments in physiology and medicine during the nineteenth century set the stage for greater understanding and further treatments of heart failure. It was then that the stethoscope and blood pressure cuff were created for diagnostic purposes. In basic science, cell theory, hormone theory, and kidney physiology led to a better understanding of how heart muscle contraction and fluid balance might be coordinated in the body. The concepts and techniques required to keep organs and tissues alive outside the body with an artificial circulation system were conceived and introduced. Anesthesia and sterile techniques essential for cardiac surgery were developed.

These ideas and accomplishments contributed to important discoveries in the early twentieth century that greatly enhanced the understanding of the early compensatory responses to heart failure. For example, it was found that when heart muscle is stretched, it will contract with greater force on the next beat and that heart muscle usually operates at a muscle length that is less than optimal. Thus, when the amount of blood returning to the heart increases and stretches the muscle in the walls of the heart, the heart will contract with greater force, ejecting a greater volume of blood. This phenomenon, called the Frank-Starling mechanism, was first demonstrated in isolated heart muscle by the German physiologist Otto Frank and in functional hearts by the British physiologist Ernest Henry Starling in 1914.

Subsequent developments in the second half of the twentieth century, such as more specific vasodilator and diuretic drugs as well as the heart-lung machine, have led to the options of more complete drug therapy, artificial hearts (first introduced to replace a human heart by William DeVries in 1982), and heart transplant (first performed by Christiaan Barnard in 1967) as options for the treatment of heart failure.

Researchers have begun clinical trials to assess the viability of using gene therapy for increasing blood flow in patients with advanced heart failure. Though treating heart failure is an ongoing challenge for the medical profession, diagnosing the ailment is becoming easier than before through preventative methods such as annual blood tests and breath tests, findings for the latter of which were published in the *Journal of the American College of Cardiology* in 2013. Furthermore, ongoing stem-cell research may lead to greater advances in the treatment of heart failure.

—*Laura Gray Malloy, Ph.D.*

See also Arrhythmias; Arteriosclerosis; Blood pressure; Cardiac arrest; Cardiology; Cardiology, pediatric; Cholesterol; Circulation; Congenital heart disease; Echocardiography; Edema; Endocarditis; Heart; Heart attack; Heart disease; Heart transplantation; Hypercholesterolemia; Hyperlipidemia; Hypertension; Ischemia; Mitral valve prolapse; Obesity; Palpitations; Vascular medicine; Vascular system.

For Further Information:

American Heart Association. "Costs to Treat Heart Failure Expected to More than Double by 2030." *Circulation*, April 24, 2013.

Campbell, Neil A., et al. *Biology: Concepts and Connections*. 6th ed. San Francisco: Pearson/Benjamin Cummings, 2009.

Crawford, Michael, ed. *Current Diagnosis and Treatment—Cardiology*. 3d ed. New York: McGraw-Hill Medical, 2009.

Deedwania, Prakash C. *Heart Failure*. Philadelphia: Saunders, 2012.

Dox, Ida G., et al. *The HarperCollins Illustrated Medical Dictionary*. 4th ed. New York: HarperCollins, 2001.

Gardner, Roy S., Theresa A. McDonagh, and Nicola L. Walker. *Heart Failure*. New York: Oxford University Press, 2007.

Gersh, Bernard J., ed. *The Mayo Clinic Heart Book*. 2d ed. New York: William Morrow, 2000.

Heidenreich P.A., et al. "Forecasting the Future of Cardiovascular Disease in the United States: A Policy Statement from the American Heart Association." *Circulation* 123, no. 8 (2011): 933–44.

Roger, V. L. et al. "Heart Disease and Stroke Statistics: 2012 Update—A Report from the American Heart Association." *Circulation* 125, no. 1 (2012): 2–220.

Sherwood, Lauralee. *Human Physiology: From Cells to Systems*. 8th ed. Pacific Grove, Calif.: Brooks/Cole/Cengage Learning, 2013.

Silver, Marc A. *Success with Heart Failure: Help and Hope for Those Coping with Congestive Heart Failure*. 3d ed. Cambridge, Mass.: Da Capo, 2007.

HEART TRANSPLANTATION
Procedure

Anatomy or system affected: Chest, circulatory system, heart, lungs, nervous system, respiratory system

Specialties and related fields: Cardiology, critical care, emergency medicine, general surgery

Definition: The removal of a diseased heart and its replacement with a healthy donor heart.

Key terms:

cardiomyopathy: a serious acute or chronic disease in which the heart becomes inflamed; it may result from multiple causes, including viral infection

congenital: present at birth

congestive heart failure: abnormal heart function characterized by circulatory congestion caused by cardiac disorders, especially myocardial infarction of the ventricles

coronary atherosclerosis: the accumulation of cholesterol, lipids, and other cellular debris in the coronary arteries, thereby limiting circulation in the heart

immunity: a defense function of the body that produces antibodies to destroy invading antigens and other disease-causing organisms

leukocytes: white blood cells that are important in the development of immunity

primary cardiomyopathy: cardiomyopathy that cannot be attributed to a specific cause

secondary cardiomyopathy: cardiomyopathy that is attributable to a specific cause (such as hypertension) and that is often associated with diseases involving other organs

Indications and Procedures

Heart transplantation is performed when congestive heart failure or heart injury cannot be treated by other conventional medical or surgical means. It is reserved for patients with a high risk of dying within two years. The procedure involves

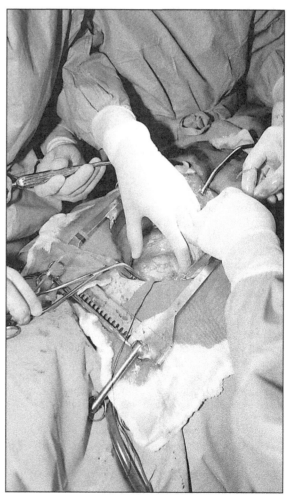

A heart is about to be removed during a transplantation procedure. (PhotoDisc)

In the News:
The AbioCor Artificial Heart

Scientific efforts at developing an artificial heart have been important because only about two thousand human donor hearts are available in the United States per year, despite many thousands of patients requiring a heart transplant. The initial experimental model, the Jarvik-7 in 1982, required a large pump outside the body and tethered the recipient to its 375-pound machine. Technological advances in miniaturization and energy transfer permitted the creation of the AbioCor, the first implantable artificial heart affording full mobility to the patient.

The AbioCor is made of titanium and a unique plastic designed to withstand being flexed forty million times a year. Before receiving Food and Drug Administration (FDA) approval for a clinical trial with fifteen patients, the makers of the AbioCor heart had to demonstrate that it could beat two hundred million times, enough beats to last five years. The device uses a wireless power transfer system. An external battery worn on the waist connects with an external coil on the chest, which transfers energy via radio waves to a coil inside the chest. No wires break the skin or provide a route for infection. A computer chip inside the chest controls the pumping action, and the external battery can operate four or five hours without recharging. An internal battery, kept continually charged by the external battery, provides thirty minutes of emergency power, permitting the user to disconnect the external power when showering.

Only patients likely to die within thirty days and unable to receive a live heart transplant were eligible to take part in the clinical trial. Success was defined as survival for 60 days with clear improvement in quality of life. On July 2, 2001, the first person to receive an implant lived for 151 days. Five more pumps were implanted in 2001, followed by an additional pump in 2002. Two patients died in surgery, but the others lived more than 60 days. The longest surviving recipient lived 512 days and spent several months at home with his family before dying on February 7, 2003. The company temporarily suspended implants in 2002 and modified the AbioCor after two patients died of strokes. Clinical trials resumed in 2003, with three patients receiving artificial hearts in January and March of that year.

The dimensions of the AbioCor heart limit its usability. The human heart is about the size of a fist and weighs about 10 ounces. The AbioCor, the size of a grapefruit, weighs 2 pounds, too large for 50 percent of men and 80 percent of women. The developers hope to overcome this problem in future models.

—*Milton Berman, Ph.D.*

foreign material and attacked it. With an improved understanding of immune system functioning and drug intervention, however, survival rates have gradually improved. Worldwide, approximately 3,500 patients undergo heart transplantation annually, with most occurring in the United States. The one-year survival rate is over 85 percent, the five-year survival rate is over 70 percent, the ten-year survival rate is over 50 percent, and some patients have lived longer than twenty years, according to statistics from the American Heart Association. In the United States, about fifteen thousand Americans aged fifty-five or younger (and forty thousand aged sixty-five or younger) would benefit from heart transplantation. Transplantation has been conducted with newborn babies, and adult patients have run marathons and even played professional sports. The average age at which the procedure is performed is forty-seven years for men and thirty-nine years for women.

The complications immediately following this type of surgery include irreversible damage to the heart, because of coronary atherosclerosis or multiple heart attacks, and primary or secondary cardiomyopathy, because the cardiac muscle cells cannot contract normally. Heart transplant recipients must take immunosuppressive (antirejection) medications for the remainder of their lives to prevent rejection; thus they must also cope with the numerous side effects of these drugs. For at least one year after transplantation, the heart is denervated (cut away from the body's nervous system), causing a resting pulse rate of up to 130 beats per minute, as compared to 60 to 80 beats per minute in a normal heart. The chances for long-term success depend in part on the amount of damage or disease in other organs as a result of stroke, chronic obstructive lung disease, and liver or kidney disease. Transplant recipients must also deal with the psychological and emotional strain of the operation and its aftermath. Patients with a history of alcohol and drug abuse or mental illness, and those who lack a social support network of family and friends, are not considered good candidates for heart transplantation.

removal of a diseased heart and its replacement with a healthy human heart or possibly an animal heart. In special cases, the surgeon may place the donor heart next to the diseased heart without removing it; this is called a piggyback transplant.

Patients who are candidates for heart transplantation include those with valvular disease, congenital heart disease, or rare conditions such as tumors. The selection of recipients is based on which patients are likely to exhibit the most pronounced improvement, functional capacity, and life expectancy after surgery. In the United States, the limited availability of donor hearts has necessitated the creation of a national organ procurement and distribution network called the United Network for Organ Sharing (UNOS), which distributes organs based on severity of illness, waiting time, donor and recipient blood types, and body size match.

Uses and Complications

The first human heart transplantation was performed on December 3, 1967, by Christiaan Barnard in Capetown, South Africa. The heart transplantation procedures that were tried soon afterward usually had a low success rate because the patient's body often rejected the new heart when leukocytes and other cells of the immune system recognized the new heart as

Perspective and Prospects

The rapid increase in the number of heart transplantations performed worldwide is attributable to specialized medical care and to numerous advances in knowledge regarding surgery, tissue preservation, immunology, and infectious

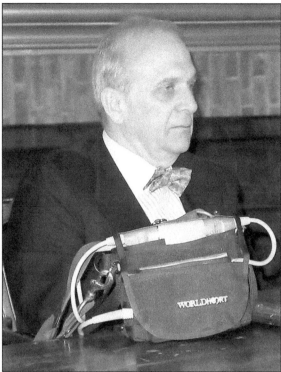

Pete Kenyon survived with an artificial heart for three years until he could receive a donor organ. The pump mechanism is carried in a pouch. (AP/Wide World Photos)

disease. The extraordinary degree of success since the 1970s has enabled many patients who have undergone heart transplantation to live longer and more independent lives. Tremendous strides have been made in diagnosing rejection and developing immunosuppressive medications, and the development of several new antirejection drugs is anticipated soon. New techniques for diagnosing rejection candidates without the performance of a heart biopsy will be a major focus of future research, as will increasing access to donor organs. A better understanding of the immune system may give doctors greater success in transplanting organs from other species (a procedure called a xenograft) instead of human organs. Ongoing research will continue to focus on identifying risk factors for heart disease—such as high blood cholesterol and abnormal lipid subfractions, high blood pressure, diabetes mellitus, family history, and cigarette smoking—as early as possible in order to delay reaching the point at which heart transplantation is necessary.

—*Daniel G. Graetzer, Ph.D.*

See also Cardiac rehabilitation; Cardiac surgery; Cardiology; Cardiology, pediatric; Circulation; Echocardiography; Electrocardiography (ECG or EKG); Grafts and grafting; Heart; Heart disease; Heart failure; Heart valve replacement; Immune system; Immunology; Transplantation; Xenotransplantation.

For Further Information:
American College of Sports Medicine. *ACSM's Guidelines for*

Exercise Testing and Prescription. 8th ed. Philadelphia: Lippincott Williams & Wilkins, 2010.

American Heart Association. *Heart and Stroke Facts.* Dallas, Tex.: Author, 1996.

Baumgartner, William A., et al., eds. *Heart and Lung Transplantation.* 2d ed. Philadelphia: W. B. Saunders, 2002.

Crawford, Michael, ed. *Current Diagnosis and Treatment—Cardiology.* 3d ed. New York: McGraw-Hill Medical, 2009.

Deng, Mario C., et al. "Effect of Receiving a Heart Transplant: Analysis of a National Cohort Entered on to a Waiting List, Stratified by Heart Failure Severity." *British Medical Journal* 321, no. 7260 (September 2, 2000): 540–545.

Eagle, Kim A., and Ragavendra R. Baliga, eds. *Practical Cardiology: Evaluation and Treatment of Common Cardiovascular Disorders.* 2d ed. Philadelphia: Lippincott Williams & Wilkins, 2008.

Ewert, Ralf, et al. "Relationship Between Impaired Pulmonary Diffusion and Cardiopulmonary Exercise Capacity After Heart Transplantation." *Chest* 117, no. 4 (April, 2000): 968.

"Heart Transplant." *Health Library,* September 10, 2012.

"Heart Transplant." *Mayo Clinic,* December 10, 2010.

"Heart Transplant." *MedlinePlus,* May 4, 2011.

HEART VALVE REPLACEMENT
Procedure

Anatomy or system affected: Chest, circulatory system, heart
Specialties and related fields: Cardiology, general surgery
Definition: A surgical procedure that involves removing a defective heart valve and replacing it with another tissue valve or with a mechanical valve.

Key terms:

anticoagulants: a class of drugs that slow the clotting time of blood

bacterial endocarditis: bacterial infection of the heart, which may scar or destroy a valve

murmur: the sound made by blood flowing backward through a heart valve

regurgitation: the leakage of blood backward through a valve

stenosis: a condition in which valve tissue has hardened and thickened, interfering with blood flow through the valve

Indications and Procedures

Valve replacement surgery is a procedure used when a heart valve no longer functions properly. There are several reasons that a heart valve may fail. Sometimes, a major defect present at birth must be repaired immediately. Minor defects present at birth may go undetected for years. When and if these minor defects become worse as a result of aging, valve replacement surgery may be necessary. Another cause of heart valve damage is infection. Rheumatic fever can cause the scarring of a valve. These scars can become more of a problem with age, and surgery may eventually be necessary. Bacterial endocarditis is another type of infection that can damage the heart very quickly. Valve replacement surgery is often needed as a result of this type of infection.

Heart Valve Replacement

When heart valves fail, they can be replaced by mechanical valves, which are made from artificial materials such as plastic, metal, and carbon fibers; by homografts, which are taken

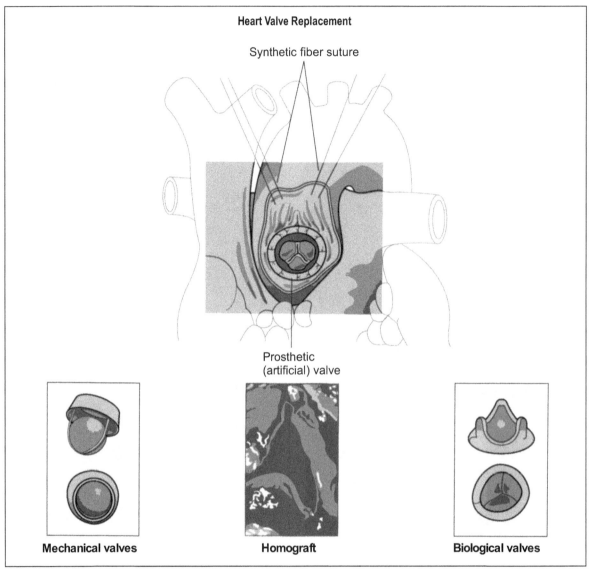

Heart Valve Replacement

Synthetic fiber suture

Prosthetic
(artificial) valve

Mechanical valves   **Homograft**   **Biological valves**

When heart valves fail, they can be replaced by mechanical valves, which are made from artificial materials such as plastic, metal, and carbon fibers; by homografts, which are taken from cadavers; or by biological valves, which are either taken from pigs or constructed from the tissues of the patient or of a cow.

from cadavers; or by biological valves, which are either taken from pigs or constructed from the tissues of the patient or of a cow.

When a heart valve is damaged, the result is usually stenosis or regurgitation. Stenosis occurs when the valve becomes thick and hard. As a result, normal blood flow through the valve is obstructed. A valve that becomes stretched or weak may not close properly, resulting in blood flowing backward through the valve; this is called regurgitation. When the blood flows through an abnormal valve, turbulence occurs and a sound is made. This sound, called a murmur, generally can be heard with a stethoscope.

When a heart valve fails to function properly, the ability of the heart to do work is impaired. In an attempt to maintain normal work levels, the heart begins to enlarge, or experience hypertrophy. When further hypertrophy is no longer possible, the heart fails. This condition will result in permanent damage to the heart muscle and eventually death. Some of the symptoms of valve problems include chest pain or tightness, shortness of breath, temporary blindness, slurred speech, weakness, numbness, lack of coordination, unusually rapid weight gain, fatigue, and loss of consciousness. These symptoms are typically the result of inadequate blood flow, particularly to the brain.

In some cases, surgery can be used to repair the valve. Many times, however, the damage is too extensive for this type of surgery, and the valve must be replaced. The replacement valve may come from a deceased person's heart or from an animal's heart (usually that of a pig), or it may be a mechanical (prosthetic) valve. Prosthetic valves are made from metal, plastic, or carbon ceramic.

During valve replacement surgery, the chest is opened to expose the heart. Blood flow through the heart is diverted through an oxygenator and a pump that maintains the flow of oxygenated blood throughout the body. The surgeon removes the damaged valve and sutures a replacement valve to the heart. Upon completion of the surgery, if the replaced valve functions effectively, normal blood flow is restored through the heart.

Uses and Complications

Heart valve replacement is a very reliable procedure. Although problems with the new valve are possible, the majority of these surgeries are quite effective. Nevertheless, there are two long-term concerns for the patient. Blood thinners or anticoagulants—drugs that slow the clotting process and may prevent blood clots—are usually required with prosthetic valves. These drugs help prevent blood from coagulating in and around the new valve. Some patients must also take antibiotics to prevent additional infections in the heart. Antibiotics are needed especially when patients visit the dentist, when bleeding is likely. If bleeding occurs, bacteria may enter the blood and become lodged in the replacement valve. The ensuing infection can cause further damage to the heart.

When one compares the use of tissue versus mechanical (prosthetic) valves for replacement, some differences emerge. In general, tissue valves work better. In addition, they are less likely to require drugs to increase blood-clotting time. On the other hand, they are harder to obtain. With more people acting as donors and with better preservation techniques becoming available, tissue replacements are preferred.

Perspective and Prospects

Mechanical valves were first used as replacements for damaged valves in the early 1960s. In 1962, the initial clinical use of tissue valves was described. Tissue valve replacements were conducted simultaneously by Donald Ross in England and Sir Brian Barratt-Boyes in New Zealand. The acceptance of tissue valve use was slow because the number of donors was small and the methods for preserving valves for later use were poor. The result was shorter survival times for the replacement valves used in the 1960s and early 1970s.

By the 1980s, better preservation techniques were developed, which allowed surgeons to use living human tissue. These replacements have been found to be superior to nonliving tissues and mechanical valves. In the future, both mechanical and tissue replacements will continue to be used, based on availability and the specific needs of the patient. Newer, less invasive surgical approaches are being investigated in clinical trials.

—*Bradley R. A. Wilson, Ph.D.*

See also Angiography; Angioplasty; Bleeding; Blood and blood dis-

orders; Bypass surgery; Cardiac arrest; Cardiac rehabilitation; Cardiac surgery; Cardiology; Cardiology, pediatric; Circulation; Coronary artery bypass graft; Echocardiography; Electrocardiography (ECG or EKG); Endocarditis; Heart; Heart attack; Heart disease; Heart failure; Heart transplantation; Pacemaker implantation; Rheumatic fever; Thrombolytic therapy and TPA.

For Further Information:

Alpert, Joseph S., James E. Dalen, and Shahbudin H. Rahimtoola, eds. *Valvular Heart Disease*. 3d ed. Philadelphia: Lippincott Williams & Wilkins, 2000.

Altunkaya, Sabri, Sadik Kara, Niyazi GörmüÅŸ, and Saadetdin Herdem. "Comparison of First and Second Heart Sounds after Mechanical Heart Valve Replacement." *Computer Methods in Biomechanics & Biomedical Engineering* 16, no. 4 (April 2013): 368–380.

Bonhoeffer, Philipp, et al. "Percutaneous Replacement of Pulmonary Valve in a Right-Ventricle to Pulmonary-Artery Prosthetic Conduit with Valve Dysfunction." *The Lancet* 356, no. 9239 (October 21, 2000): 1403–1405.

"Choosing the Right Replacement Heart Valve." *Harvard Heart Letter* 21, no. 2 (October 2010): 4–5.

Crawford, Michael, ed. *Current Diagnosis and Treatment—Cardiology*. 3d ed. New York: McGraw-Hill Medical, 2009.

Eagle, Kim A., and Ragavendra R. Baliga, eds. *Practical Cardiology: Evaluation and Treatment of Common Cardiovascular Disorders*. 2d ed. Philadelphia: Lippincott Williams & Wilkins, 2008.

"Heart Valve Replacement." *Health Library*, May 8, 2013.

Kramer, Gerri Freid, and Shari Mauer. *Parent's Guide to Children's Congenital Heart Defects: What They Are, How to Treat Them, How to Cope with Them*. New York: Three Rivers Press, 2001.

Mitka, Mike. "Final Report on Mechanical vs. Bioprosthetic Heart Valves." *Journal of the American Medical Association* 283, no. 15 (April 19, 2000): 1947–1948.

Nauer, Kathleen A., Barbara Schouchoff, and Kathleen Demitras. "Minimally Invasive Aortic Valve Surgery." *Critical Care Nursing Quarterly* 23, no. 1 (May, 2000): 66–71.

Otto, Catherine M. "Timing of Aortic Valve Surgery." *Heart* 84, no. 2 (August, 2000): 211.

HEAT EXHAUSTION AND HEATSTROKE
Disease/Disorder

Anatomy or system affected: Blood vessels, circulatory system, skin

Specialties and related fields: Critical care, emergency medicine, family medicine, internal medicine, sports medicine

Definition: Heat-related illnesses in which the body temperature rises to dangerous levels and cannot be controlled through normal mechanisms, such as sweating.

Causes and Symptoms

The human body is well equipped to maintain a nearly constant internal body temperature. In fact, the body temperature of human beings is usually controlled so closely that it rarely leaves a very narrow range of 36.1 to 37.8 degrees Celsius (97 to 100 degrees Fahrenheit) regardless of how much heat the body is producing or what the environmental temperature may be. Humans maintain a constant temperature so that the millions of biochemical reactions in the body remain at an optimal rate. An increase in body temperature of only one degree Celsius will cause these reactions to move about 10 percent faster. As internal temperatures rise, however, brain function becomes slower because important proteins and enzymes lose their ability to operate effectively. Most adults will go into convulsions when their temperature reaches 41 degrees Celsius (106 degrees Fahrenheit), and 43 degrees Celsius (110 degrees Fahrenheit) is usually fatal.

A special region of the brain known as the hypothalamus regulates body temperature. The hypothalamus detects the temperature of the blood much like a thermostat detects room temperature. When the body (and hence the blood) becomes too warm, the hypothalamus activates heat-loss mechanisms. Most excess heat is lost through the skin by the radiation of heat and the evaporation of sweat. To promote this heat loss, blood vessels in the skin dilate (open up) to carry more blood to the skin. Heat from the warm blood is then lost to the cooler air. If the increase in blood flow to the skin is not enough, then sweat glands are stimulated to produce and secrete large amounts of sweat. The process, called perspiration, is an efficient means of ridding the body of excess heat as long as the humidity is not too high. In fact, at 60 percent humidity, evaporation of sweat from the skin stops. When the body cannot dissipate enough heat, heat exhaustion and heatstroke may occur.

Heat exhaustion is the most prevalent heat-related illness. It commonly occurs in individuals who have exercised or worked in high temperatures for long periods of time. These people have usually not ingested adequate amounts of fluid. Over time, the patient loses fluid through sweating and respiration, which decreases the amount of fluid in the blood. Because the body is trying to reduce its temperature, blood has been shunted to the skin and away from vital internal organs. This reaction, in combination with a reduced blood volume, causes the patient to go into mild shock. Common signs and symptoms of heat exhaustion include cool, moist skin that may appear either red or pale; headache; nausea; dizziness; and exhaustion. If heat exhaustion is not recognized and treated, it can lead to life-threatening heatstroke.

Heatstroke occurs when the body is unable to eradicate the excess heat as rapidly as it develops. Thus, body temperature begins to rise. Sweating stops because the water content of the blood decreases. The loss of evaporative cooling causes the body temperature to continue rising rapidly, soon reaching a level that can cause organ damage. In particular, the brain, heart, and kidneys may begin to fail until the patient experiences convulsions, coma, and even death. Therefore, heatstroke is a serious medical emergency which must be recognized and treated immediately. The signs and symptoms of heatstroke include high body temperature (41 degrees Celsius or 106 degrees Fahrenheit); loss of consciousness; hot, dry skin; rapid pulse; and quick, shallow breathing.

Treatment and Therapy

As with most illnesses, prevention is the best medicine for heat exhaustion and heatstroke. When exercising in hot weather, people should wear loose-fitting, lightweight clothing and drink plenty of fluids. When individuals are not prepared to avoid heat-related illness, however, rapid treatment

---

Information on Heat Exhaustion and Heatstroke

Causes: Dehydration
Symptoms: For heat exhaustion, cool and moist skin that appears either red or pale, headache, nausea, dizziness, exhaustion; for heatstroke, cessation of perspiration, hot and dry skin, rapid pulse, quick and shallow breathing
Duration: Acute
Treatments: Cooling of body, replacement of body fluids, treatment of shock, emergency resuscitation

---

may save their lives. When emergency medical personnel detect signs and symptoms of sudden heat-induced illness, they attempt to do three major things: cool the body, replace body fluids, and minimize shock.

For heat exhaustion, the initial treatment should be to place the patient in a cool place, such as a bathtub filled with cool (not cold) water. The conscious patient is given water or fruit drinks, sometimes containing salt, to replace body fluids. Occasionally, intravenous fluids must be given to return blood volume to normal in a more direct way. Hospitalization of the patient may be necessary to be sure that the body is able to regulate body heat appropriately. Almost all patients treated quickly and effectively will not advance to heatstroke. The activity that placed the patient in danger should be discontinued until one is sure all symptoms have disappeared and steps have been taken to prevent a future episode of heat exhaustion.

Heatstroke requires urgent medical attention, or the high body temperature will cause irreparable damage and often death. Body temperature must be reduced rapidly. With the patient in a cool environment, the clothing is removed and the skin sprinkled with water and cooled by fanning. Contrary to popular belief, rubbing alcohol should not be used, as it can cause closure of the skin's pores. Ice packs are often placed behind the neck and under the armpits and groin. At these sites, large blood vessels come close to the skin and are capable of carrying cooled blood to the internal organs. Body fluid must be replaced quickly by intravenous administration because the patient is usually unable to drink as a result of convulsions or confusion and may even be unconscious. Once the body temperature has been brought back to normal, the patient is usually hospitalized and watched for complications. With early diagnosis and treatment, 80 to 90 percent of previously healthy people will survive.

—*Matthew Berria, Ph.D.*

See also Critical care; Critical care, pediatric; Dehydration; Emergency medicine; Emergency rooms; Fever; First aid; Hyperthermia and hypothermia; Resuscitation; Shock; Sweating; Unconsciousness.

For Further Information:

American Academy of Orthopaedic Surgeons. *Emergency Care and Transportation of the Sick and Injured.* Edited by Benjamin Gulli, Les Chatelain, and Chris Stratford. 9th ed. Sudbury, Mass.: Jones and Bartlett, 2005.
Armstrong, Lawrence E. "Return to Exercise Training After Heat

Exhaustion." *Journal of Sport Rehabilitation* 16, 3 (August 2007): 182–189.

Gilchrist, J., et al. "Heat Illness Among High School Athletes—United States, 2005–2009." *Morbidity & Mortality Weekly Report* 59, 32 (August 2010): 1009–1013.

Hales, Dianne. *An Invitation to Health Brief.* Updated ed. Belmont: Wadsworth/Cengage Learning, 2010.

Leikin, Jerrold B., and Martin S. Lipsky, eds. *American Medical Association Complete Medical Encyclopedia.* New York: Random House Reference, 2003.

McArdle, William, Frank I. Katch, and Victor L. Katch. *Exercise Physiology: Energy, Nutrition, and Human Performance.* 7th ed. Boston: Lippincott Williams & Wilkins, 2010.

Marieb, Elaine N., and Katja Hoehn. *Human Anatomy and Physiology.* 9th ed. San Francisco: Pearson/Benjamin Cummings, 2010.

Nelson, Nicolas G., et al. "Exertional Heat-Related Injuries Treated in Emergency Departments in the U.S., 1997–2006." *American Journal of Preventative Medicine* 40, 1 (January 2011): 54–60.

Subbarao, Italo, et al., eds. *American Medical Association Handbook of First Aid and Emergency Care.* Rev. ed. New York: Random House Reference, 2009.oxy_options track_changes="on"?

HEEL SPUR REMOVAL

Procedure

Anatomy or system affected: Bones, feet, musculoskeletal system

Specialties and related fields: General surgery, orthopedics, podiatry

Definition: The surgical removal of a heel spur, a hard, bony growth on the heel.

Indications and Procedures

Heel spurs, also known as calcaneal spurs, are hard, bony growths on the heel bone. Pain and tenderness in the sole of the foot under the heel bone are common first indicators of this condition. Painful heel spurs can cause difficulty in walking and standing. Running, jogging, and prolonged standing often contribute to their development, especially when unpadded shoes are worn. When efforts to alleviate pain, such as activity modification and the use of shoes with cushioned heels, have been exhausted, it may be necessary for the spur to be surgically removed.

Most heel spur removal operations are performed at outpatient surgical facilities. Before the operation, blood and urine studies are conducted, and x-rays are taken of both feet. Local or spinal anesthetics are administered. The surgeon, orthopedist, or podiatrist conducting the operation will choose a convenient site to make an incision, usually over the spur, and use special instruments to remove the growth. The opening in the skin is closed with sutures. Barring complications, the sutures can be removed ten to fourteen days later. After the surgery, additional blood studies are taken, and laboratory examination of the removed tissue is performed.

Uses and Complications

Heel spurs form as a result of hard pounding or prolonged stress on the heel of the foot. Shock-absorbing soles in shoes and orthopedic inserts that cushion hard blows to the heel during vigorous exercise can help prevent and aid in recovery from heel spur operations. Following a removal operation, vigorous exercise can be resumed in approximately three months.

Clean cloths or tissues can be pressed against the wound for ten minutes if bleeding occurs within the first twenty-four hours after the surgery. The scar from the incision will recede gradually. Although it is important to keep the foot clean, the wound must be kept dry between baths. For the first two or three days after surgery, the wound should be covered with a dry bandage. Complications associated with heel spur removal surgery can include excessive bleeding and surgical wound infection, which should be examined by a doctor.

—*Jason Georges*

See also Bone disorders; Bones and the skeleton; Feet; Foot disorders; Lower extremities; Orthopedic surgery; Orthopedics; Podiatry.

For Further Information:

A.D.A.M. Medical Encyclopedia. "Heel Pain." *MedlinePlus,* February 19, 2012.

American Podiatric Medical Association. "Heel Pain." *American Podiatric Medical Association,* 2012.

Copeland, Glenn, and Stan Solomon. *The Foot Doctor: Lifetime Relief for Your Aching Feet.* Rev. ed. Toronto, Ont.: Macmillan Canada, 1996.

Currey, John D. *Bones: Structures and Mechanics.* Princeton, N.J.: Princeton University Press, 2002.

Levy, Leonard A., and Vincent J. Hetherington, eds. *Principles and Practice of Podiatric Medicine.* 2d ed. Brooklandville, Md.: Trace, 2006.

Lippert, Frederick G., and Sigvard T. Hansen. *Foot and Ankle Disorders: Tricks of the Trade.* New York: Thieme, 2003.

Lorimer, Donald L., et al., eds. *Neale's Disorders of the Foot.* 7th ed. New York: Churchill Livingstone/Elsevier, 2006.

Polsdorfer, Ricker. "Surgical Procedures for Foot Pain." *Health Library,* March 15, 2013.

Van De Graaff, Kent M., and Stuart I. Fox. *Concepts of Human Anatomy and Physiology.* 5th ed. Dubuque, Iowa: Wm. C. Brown, 2000.

HEIMLICH MANEUVER

Procedure

Anatomy or system affected: Chest, lungs, mouth, neck, respiratory system, throat

Specialties and related fields: Emergency medicine

Definition: An emergency technique used to prevent suffocation when the airway becomes blocked.

Indications and Procedures

The Heimlich maneuver is an emergency technique, introduced in 1974 by Henry J. Heimlich, that guides a rescuer through a set of manipulative procedures to prevent suffocation when a victim's airway (windpipe) becomes blocked by food, water, or other foreign material. The maneuver lifts the diaphragm and forces enough air from the lungs to create an artificial cough. This cough intends to move the obstructive foreign body from the windpipe in order to resume normal and functional breathing (ventilation).

The Heimlich maneuver should be performed only if a choking victim cannot speak, cough, or breathe. Several indications may signal such a situation: frantic gestures to the throat, a face that turns blue in color because of lack of oxygen, and the production of loud noises in an attempt to take in breaths of air.

Before attempting the Heimlich maneuver, permission in the form of an affirmative nod or gesture should be given by a conscious victim to the intended administrator of the maneuver. When performing the technique, the rescuer is usually positioned behind the sitting or standing victim, with his or her arms around the victim's waist. The rescuer makes a fist with one hand and places that hand, with the thumb toward the victim, just above the victim's navel or below the rib cage and above the waist. The free hand should clasp the fisted hand tightly. Then, in a series of sharp thrusts upward and inward, the rescuer attempts to develop enough air pressure in the airway to force the lodged foreign object back up the trachea. The procedure may have to be repeated several times before the foreign object is expelled. Once the airway is cleared, the victim should start coughing and/or regain normal breathing. In cases when breathing is not resumed, then cardiopulmonary resuscitation (CPR) may have to be administered. In more serious choking cases in which the airway is not cleared of the obstruction, a small incision to the windpipe called a tracheostomy may have to be completed.

Uses and Complications

In addition to choking victims, the Heimlich maneuver may be administered to asthmatics and drowning victims. While it can be performed on all people, modifications should be adapted when executed upon infants (it is not recommended for infants less than one year old), children, and very obese, pregnant, or unconscious adults. The Heimlich maneuver may also be self-administered.

The Heimlich maneuver is one of the best courses to follow for the prevention of asphyxiation during a choking episode, but it does come with several precautions. In addition to modifications depending on the age and situation of the victim, incorrect administration of the Heimlich maneuver by incorporating techniques such as chest thrusts, back slaps, and abdominal thrusts can cause bruised ribs, broken bones, damage to internal organs, and even death. If all the guidelines are effectively followed by the administrator, however, then the victim should feel little or no bodily discomfort and should recover quickly.

—Nicholas Lanzieri

See also Asphyxiation; Asthma; Cardiopulmonary resuscitation (CPR); Choking; Drowning; Emergency medicine; Emergency medicine, pediatric; First aid; Hypoxia; Lungs; Pulmonary medicine; Pulmonary medicine, pediatric; Respiration; Resuscitation; Trachea.

For Further Information:

Chillag, Shawn, Jake Krieg, and Ranjana Bhargava. "The Heimlich Maneuver: Breaking Down the Complications." *Southern Medical Journal* 103, no. 2 (February 2010): 147–150.

"Choking: First Aid." *Mayo Clinic*, October 13, 2011.

"Heimlich Maneuver." In *Everything You Need to Know About Medical Treatments*. Springhouse, Pa.: Springhouse, 1996.

"Heimlich Maneuver." *MedlinePlus*, July 16, 2011.

Icon Health. *Heimlich Maneuver: A Medical Dictionary, Bibliography, and Annotated Research Guide to Internet References*. San Diego, Calif.: Author, 2004.

Subbarao, Italo, et al., eds. *American Medical Association Handbook of First Aid and Emergency Care*. Rev. ed. New York: Random House Reference, 2009.

Tintinalli, Judith E., ed. *Emergency Medicine: A Comprehensive Study Guide*. 6th ed. New York: McGraw-Hill, 2004.

White, R. D. "Foreign Body Airway Obstruction: Considerations in 1985." *Circulation* 74, no. 6, pt. 2 (1986): IV60–62.

HEMATOLOGY
Specialty

Anatomy or system affected: Blood, circulatory system, immune system, liver, musculoskeletal system, spleen

Specialties and related fields: Cardiology, cytology, forensic medicine, genetics, immunology, oncology, pathology, serology, vascular medicine

Definition: The study of the blood, including its normal constituents, and such blood disorders as anemia, leukemia, and hemophilia.

Key terms:

anemia: a condition characterized by a deficiency of red blood cells or hemoglobin

bone marrow: the soft substance that fills the cavities within bones and that is the site of blood cell production

clotting factors: chemicals circulating in the blood that are necessary for the process of blood clotting

hematologist: one who specializes in the study of blood, its components and disorders

hemoglobin: the iron-containing molecule within red blood cells responsible for oxygen and carbon dioxide transport

leukemia: a condition characterized by the presence of numerous immature white blood cells in the circulating blood

plasma: the fluid portion of blood, containing water, proteins, minerals, nutrients, hormones, and wastes

platelets: specialized cell fragments that initiate blood clotting

red blood cell: a flexible, biconcave blood cell that contains hemoglobin

white blood cell: one of several types of colorless, large blood cells that work together to combat infections

Science and Profession

Most branches of medical science study a particular organ that is made of specific tissues and is located in a definite part of the body. Hematology is unique because its subject, the blood, is a liquid tissue constantly in motion and therefore in constant contact with every other tissue and organ of the body.

It has been estimated that blood travels about sixteen kilometers (ten miles) per hour. It takes six seconds for blood to travel from the heart to the lungs, about eight seconds to travel from the heart to the brain, and only fourteen seconds to travel from the heart all the way to the toes. Hematologists studying these shifting currents of the blood are able to detect patterns that allow the early discovery of many disorders of the blood itself and of the organs that it supplies.

Blood is a complex material composed of approximately 55 percent plasma and 45 percent cells, which are also called formed elements. The plasma, or liquid portion of the blood, is about 90 percent water and 10 percent substances dissolved or suspended in that water. Part of that 10 percent consists of a remarkable array of substances, including nutrients, gases, salts, wastes, and hormones being transported around the body. The other, larger part of the 10 percent is another remarkable array: plasma proteins such as fibrinogen, albumin, and globulins with a great diversity of functions to accomplish. The modern hematologist's ability to measure and monitor all these plasma components precisely has greatly aided physicians in the treatment of innumerable diseases.

Beyond an analysis of the ingredients of the plasma, hematologists focus on the normal and abnormal conditions of the blood's cells. An individual has twenty-five trillion red blood cells; ten million of these cells die or are destroyed each second, and two hundred billion new ones need to be made each day. Hematologists discovered that these tiny, biconcave discs packed with hemoglobin transport the vast majority of the oxygen constantly needed by every cell of every organ for energy production.

Before each red blood cell is released from the bone marrow where it is produced, the bulk of its living nucleus is expelled. A small amount of nuclear material remains as a fine network in these young cells, called reticulocytes. The number of reticulocytes released into the blood is an indication of the activity of the bone marrow. Hematologists use this number both to diagnose conditions such as anemia in its various forms and to assess the patient's response to treatment.

Not only the total number and maturity but also the shape, diameter, and flexibility of red blood cells can give the hematologist important information. For years, such information was gathered by laborious manual methods. Electronic counters can now obtain this information with great speed and even greater accuracy.

Hematologists can also gauge the effectiveness of red blood cells by seeing how much hemoglobin they contain. The amount of this red pigment present, and therefore functioning, was once estimated by being matched against progressively darker-colored glass "standards." Now this figure too is accurately determined using a precise photoelectric technique.

Another useful test is called the packed cell volume (PCV) test. It not only reveals the proportion of the red blood cells to the plasma but also allows the calculation of those cells' average size and hemoglobin content.

An equally common blood investigation is the erythrocyte sedimentation rate (ESR). The erythrocytes, the term that hematologists use to describe red blood cells, normally fall slowly down through the plasma in a standard tube. A very rapid sedimentation rate demonstrates a disturbance in the plasma proteins that may be very dangerous. Usually, the faster the erythrocytes settle out, the sicker the patient, with a

wide variety of inflammations as possible causes.

Beginning in the mid-twentieth century, an increasing number of radioactive tests were developed by which hematologists could more accurately assess total blood volume and the survival time of red blood cells or platelets in circulation. Assessing total volume is important. A loss of more than one liter (two pints) is quite dangerous because it can cause a total collapse of the blood vessels.

This reaction gives a clue about the importance of a second kind of blood cell, the platelet, and its work in stopping bleeding. When a blood vessel is first cut, platelets (or thrombocytes) rush to the site. They swell into irregular shapes, become sticky, and clog the cut, creating a plug. The smallest blood vessels rupture hundreds of times a day, and platelets alone are able to make the necessary repairs. If the cut is too large, then platelets, which are like sponges filled with diverse and biologically active compounds, disintegrate. Their ingredients react with numerous clotting factors in the plasma to initiate clot formation.

Hematologists check blood samples carefully to ascertain whether their patients possess the normal number of platelets—more than a trillion for the average adult. Since platelets live only about ten days, it is necessary to monitor those patients who exhibit significantly low amounts of these cells. If their bone marrow is not constantly replacing these platelets, these patients might bleed to death from a small cut. Doctors must also monitor any tendency toward the formation of too many platelets, as this can lead to thrombophlebitis, the blockage of a vein by a blood clot.

As with red blood cells, the widespread use of electronic counters has made the measurement of the numbers of platelets and of white blood cells (the third type of blood cell) rapid, efficient, and extremely accurate.

White blood cells are hardest to count because they are the least numerous, making up only 0.1 percent of the total blood. Their number also varies dramatically, from four thousand to eleven thousand per cubic centimeter of blood, according to the individual, the time of day, the outside temperature, and many other ordinary factors.

Hematologists can deduce the degree of maturity of circulating white blood cells from the appearance of their nuclei. There are five kinds of white blood cells (or leukocytes), whose normal proportions in the blood are quite specific and change drastically if an infection is present. The number of monocytes, for example, is normally 5 percent of the total number of white blood cells. If typhus, tuberculosis, or Rocky Mountain spotted fever organisms are present, that number will rise to 20 or 30 percent. The normal 60 percentage of neutrophils will increase to 75 percent or more in the presence of pneumonia or appendicitis.

Diagnostic and Treatment Techniques

Blood to be tested by a hematologist is withdrawn from a vein. A thin smear or film of the blood is placed on a glass slide and stained to bring out identifying features more prominently. The microscope then reveals the proportion of different cell types and any variation from the normally expected amount. This examination alone may give an immediate diagnosis of a particular blood disorder. For example, a red blood cell count that is less than four million or more than six million per cubic centimeter of blood is considered unusual and is probably an indication of disease.

It often becomes necessary to study not only the circulating blood cells but also the original cells within the bone marrow that produce the erythrocytes, thrombocytes, and leukocytes. To do so, the hematologist must use a long, thin needle to remove a sample of the marrow from within the tibia (shinbone) of a child or the pelvis (hipbone) or sternum (breastbone) of an adult. This test can provide a reliable diagnosis of a specific blood disorder.

The blood disorders that hematologists are routinely called on to diagnose and treat include diseases of the red blood cells, white blood cells, platelets, and clotting factors and failures of correct blood formation.

Disorders involving a deficiency of red blood cells or their hemoglobin are called anemias. There are many types of anemia, which are named, distinguished, and treated according to their causes. Some anemias exist because of a lack of the materials needed to build red blood cells: iron, vitamin B_{12}, and folic acid. Other anemias are caused by a shortening of the life span of red blood cells or by inherited abnormalities in hemoglobin. Still others are attributable to chronic infections or cancer.

Iron-deficiency anemia is by far the most common; it is particularly prevalent in women of childbearing age and in children. In young children who are growing rapidly, constant increase in muscle mass and blood volume will cause anemia unless a high enough level of iron is present in the diet. All women between puberty and the menopause lose iron with the menstrual flow of blood and, therefore, are always prone to iron-deficiency anemia. A pregnant woman is even more likely to develop this condition, as iron is literally removed from her body and transferred through the placenta to the developing fetus.

The symptoms of iron-deficiency anemia may include a reduced capacity for physical work, paleness, breathlessness, increased pulse, and possibly a sore tongue. The hematologist witnessing small, misshapen red blood cells deficient in hemoglobin will recommend an increase in iron in the diet. The hematologist will also send the patient for various gastrointestinal tests because of the possibility of internal bleeding or failure of the intestine to absorb iron properly.

Another class of anemias involves a lack of vitamin B_{12} or folic acid. Without the help of these two substances, the bone marrow cannot build red blood cells correctly. These anemias are diagnosed when the hematologist finds bizarre cells called megaloblasts in the patient's bone marrow. Both vitamin B_{12} and folic acid can be added to the diet or given by injection. The problem may stem, however, not from an insufficient amount of vitamin B_{12} in the diet but from the inability of the stomach lining to produce a substance called intrinsic factor. In this case, the patient will never be able to absorb the vitamin properly and is said to suffer from pernicious anemia.

Those anemias characterized by the early and too-frequent destruction of red blood cells are grouped together as hemolytic anemias. Some of these disorders are acquired, while others are inherited. In both types, hemoglobin from the destroyed red blood cells can be detected by the hematologist in the plasma, the urine, or the skin, where it causes the yellowing called jaundice.

Because the many types of anemia are so common, hematologists find that the diagnosis and treatment of these diseases form a large part of their everyday practice. All types of leukemia, on the other hand, are quite rare. They are caused by a change in one kind of primitive blood cell in the bone marrow. The result is uncontrolled growth of these cells, which do not mature but rather invade the blood as badly functioning cells. Leukemia is often thought of as cancer of the blood.

Although it is not known what causes leukemia in a particular person, the disease seems to be associated with certain factors, including injury by chemicals or radiation, viruses, and genetic predisposition. Many cases of acute leukemia occur in either children under fourteen or adults between fifty-five and seventy-five years of age. In children, it is almost always a disorder in the bone-marrow cells that produce the white blood cells, called lymphocytes. This disorder is called acute lymphoblastic leukemia, or ALL. Adult leukemia usually occurs in the bone marrow that forms some other type of white blood cell and is called acute nonlymphoblastic leukemia, or ANLL.

Hematologists diagnose both conditions by their shared symptoms: abnormal bone-marrow tissue and a lack of normal white blood cells and platelets in the circulating blood. The patient will often have been referred to the hematologist because of an uncontrollable infection (due to lack of normal white blood cells) or uncontrollable bleeding (due to lack of normal platelets). In both children and adults, anemia usually accompanies acute leukemia because defective bone marrow is not able to produce red blood cells properly either.

Less rare than acute leukemia are the various chronic types. One type, called chronic granulocytic leukemia (CGL), occurs most often after the age of fifty. Unfortunately, its early symptoms are few and vague, so that the disease may have progressed greatly before its presence is even suspected. By such time, an enormous enlargement of the spleen, along with elevations in both white blood cell and platelet counts, can be noted.

Two stages are usually seen in chronic granulocytic leukemia. Early treatment can relieve all symptoms, shrink the spleen, and return all blood cells to normal values. Eventually, however, the leukemic condition recurs, and the patient usually lives an average of only three years. Bone marrow transplantation from a suitable donor and a more recent process in which one's own marrow is removed, irradiated, and returned to the bones have increasingly become the recommended treatments for this condition.

A second type of chronic leukemia is known as chronic lymphatic leukemia (CLL). Unlike most of the other leukemias, CLL has no known cause, but it is most often found in male patients over the age of forty. Often quite symptomless, it is only discovered by chance. The hematologist is able to diagnose CLL by an increased proportion of abnormal white blood cells present in the blood. Surprisingly, this form of leukemia can vary from a case that remains symptomless, with the patient surviving twenty years or more, to a rapidly progressing case with increasing anemia and constant infections.

The third major class of disorders diagnosed and treated by hematologists consists of those involving abnormal bleeding. The diagnosis is quite simple. The hematologist notes whether bleeding from a tiny puncture in the ear lobe stops within three minutes, as it should. If the bleeding does not stop, the determination of the cause may be difficult; it may involve too few platelets or abnormal or missing clotting factors.

Very precise tests of an increasingly sophisticated nature are now used by hematologists to determine whether a bleeding disorder is attributable to inheritance (as with hemophilia), a vitamin K deficiency, or a side effect of medication or is secondary to a type of leukemia.

Perspective and Prospects

That blood and the vessels that carry it are important to life and health was evident even to ancient peoples. Around 500 BCE, Alcmaeon of Croton, a Greek philosopher and medical theorist, was the first to discover that arteries and veins are different types of vessels. A century later, Hippocrates observed that blood, left to stand, settles into three distinct layers. The top layer, the largest, is a clear, straw-colored liquid that is now called plasma. The middle layer is a narrow white band that is now known to contain white blood cells. The bottom, quite large layer contains the cells that are now called red blood cells.

Very little else of value seems to have been learned about the blood until the seventeenth century, which witnessed many discoveries in medical science. In 1628, William Harvey, an English doctor, demonstrated scientific evidence of circulation. He found proof of a circular route and of the purpose of circulation. By 1661, the Italian scientist Marcello Malpighi reported seeing the tiny vessels called capillaries in the lungs of a frog.

Another giant step toward modern hematology occurred in the 1660s due to the efforts of Richard Lower of England and Jean-Baptiste Denis of France. Almost simultaneously, they accomplished blood transfusions from dog to dog and, soon after, from animal to human. Some transfusions were very successful; others were fatal to the patient. Almost 250 years would pass before the reason for success or failure would be learned.

In 1688, the Dutch scientist Antoni van Leeuwenhoek was able to describe and measure red blood cells accurately. He also observed that they changed shape to squeeze through tiny blood vessels. It was almost a hundred years later, in the 1770s, that Englishman Joseph Priestley found that the oxygen in the air changed dark blood from the veins into a bright red color. Only in the 1850s did the German researcher Otto Funke find within those red blood cells the compound hemoglobin, which is affected by the presence or absence of oxygen.

Although the first research on blood clotting was done by William Hewson in 1768, the disease called hemophilia, or the failure of the blood to clot, was not described until 1803, by John Otto.

In the United States in the early twentieth century, Karl Landsteiner discovered why certain blood can be safely transfused: the existence of the ABO blood types. This renowned hematologist was still advancing his science forty years later when he discovered the Rh system of blood types.

Another renowned hematologist, Max Perutz, worked steadily from 1939 to 1978 to understand fully the structure and function of the hemoglobin molecule. The 1940s had seen another breakthrough when Edwin Cohn, another American, discovered how to separate and purify the various plasma proteins. His work gave fellow hematologists the tools to study individual plasma components in order to learn the exact role of each in the blood. Since that time, scores of hematologists have so advanced this medical science that blood seems to have yielded most of its secrets. The ability of hematologists to treat so many types of anemia, leukemia, and other blood disorders successfully is the fruit of their tireless work.

—Grace D. Matzen

See also Acquired immunodeficiency syndrome (AIDS); Anemia; Bleeding; Blood and blood disorders; Blood testing; Blood vessels; Bone marrow transplantation; Cholesterol; Circulation; Cytology; Cytopathology; Dialysis; Disseminated intravascular coagulation (DIC); Ergogenic aids; Fluids and electrolytes; Forensic pathology; Hematology, pediatric; Hemolytic disease of the newborn; Hemophilia; Histiocytosis; Histology; Hodgkin's disease; Host-defense mechanisms; Hypercholesterolemia; Hyperlipidemia; Immune system; Immunology; Infection; Ischemia; Jaundice; Kidney disorders; Kidneys; Laboratory tests; Leukemia; Liver; Lymphadenopathy and lymphoma; Lymphatic system; Nephrology; Nephrology, pediatric; Phlebotomy; Rh factor; Septicemia; Serology; Sickle cell disease; Thalassemia; Thrombocytopenia; Thrombolytic therapy and TPA; Thrombosis and thrombus; Transfusion; Vascular medicine; Vascular system; Von Willebrand's disease; Wiskott-Aldrich syndrome.

For Further Information:

American Society of Hematology. http://www.hematology.org

Avraham, Regina. *The Circulatory System*. Philadelphia: Chelsea House, 1989.

Bick, Roger L. *Disorders of Thrombosis and Hemostasis: Clinical and Laboratory Practice*. 3d ed. Philadelphia: Lippincott Williams & Wilkins, 2002.

Eads, Jennifer R., Neal J. Meropol, and Jerry L. Spivak. "Update in Hematology and Oncology: Evidence Published in 2012." *Annals of Internal Medicine* 158, no. 10 (May 2013): 755–760.

Hoffman, Ronald, et al., eds. *Hematology: Basic Principles and Practice*. 6th ed. Philadelphia: Saunders/Elsevier, 2013.

Kaushansky, Kenneth, et al., eds. *Williams Hematology*. 8th ed. New York: McGraw-Hill, 2010.

Rodak, Bernadette F., George A. Fritsma, and Elaine M. Keohane, eds. *Hematology: Clinical Principles and Applications*. 4th ed. St. Louis, Mo.: Saunders/Elsevier, 2012.

Tortora, Gerard J., and Bryan Derrickson. *Introduction to the Human Body: The Essentials of Anatomy and Physiology*. 9th ed. Hoboken, N.J.: John Wiley & Sons, 2012.

HEMATOMAS

Disease/Disorder

Anatomy or system affected: Blood, blood vessels, musculoskeletal system, skin, vascular system

Specialties and related fields: Neurology, sports medicine

Definition: Localized, semisolid masses of pooled blood in tissue, caused by spontaneous or posttrauma blood leakage through the vessel walls of arteries, capillaries, or veins and subsequent clotting in surrounding tissue; they may occur in skin, soft tissue (muscles, mucosa), and organs or within the skull.

Key terms:

anticoagulant: medication that increases the length of time required for blood to clot

computed tomography (CT): a type of scan that uses X ray waves to produce detailed computerized images

magnetic resonance imaging (MRI): a type of scan that uses radio waves and a powerful magnet to produce detailed computerized images; the equipment is less commonly available and the process is longer in duration than that of CT scan

---

Information on Hematomas

Causes: Spontaneous leakage from fragility of blood vessel wall, posttrauma leakage from events ranging from violent sneeze to bodily injury

Symptoms: Localized edema (swelling), inflammation, pain

Duration: Varies due to individual differences, size and location of hematoma

---

Causes and Symptoms

A hematoma is caused by blood leakage through the wall of an artery, capillary, or vein; subsequent pooling in surrounding tissue; and resultant coagulation in a semisolid mass. This leakage may occur spontaneously due to fragility of a vessel wall or due to an aneurysm. Leakage may also occur posttrauma due to events ranging from a violent sneeze to bodily injury. Symptoms usually consist of localized edema, inflammation, and pain.

A hematoma can occur anywhere along the circulatory system pathway and may be given a descriptive label indicative of its location. Superficial hematomas include aural, intramuscular, scalp, septal, subcutaneous, and subungual hematomas. An aural (ear) hematoma is a blood mass that accumulates between the ear cartilage and the periphondrium (connective tissue) as a result of blunt force trauma to the external ear. Symptoms include ecchymosis (discoloration to the area) and swelling. An intramuscular hematoma is a blood mass that accumulates within a muscle, often in the forearm or lower leg, as a result of blunt force trauma that leaves skin intact but damages muscle fibers and connective tissue. Symptoms include ecchymosis and swelling. A scalp hematoma is a blood mass that accumulates in the skin and muscle layer covering the skull as a result of head injury. Although not usually serious, it nonetheless could be indicative of bleeding within the skull. A septal hematoma is a blood mass that accumulates in the nasal septum, usually in conjunction with a broken nose or injury to nearby soft tissue. Symptoms include nasal congestion, septal swelling, and resultant difficulty breathing. A subcutaneous hematoma is a blood mass that accumulates under the skin as a result of damage to superficial blood vessels. It occurs more frequently to those who take anticoagulants. Symptoms include ecchymosis and swelling. A subungual hematoma is a blood

mass that accumulates under the nail plate of a finger or toe. Symptoms include pain due to pressure buildup in the nail bed.

Internal hematomas include cranial, fracture site, and intraabdominal hematomas. Cranial hematomas can be epidural, subdural, or intracerebral; all are potentially life threatening. An epidural hematoma (also called *extradural hematoma*) is a blood mass that accumulates in the epidural space (inside the skull but outside the dura mater, the membrane that covers the brain), often as a result of damage to the middle meningeal artery, located in the temple area, following skull fracture. Symptoms include asthenia (weakness), confusion, dizziness, drowsiness, nausea and vomiting, severe headache, unmatched pupil size, and often intermittent loss of consciousness.

An acute, subacute, or chronic subdural hematoma (also called *subdural hemorrhage*) is a blood mass that accumulates in the subdural space (inside the dura mater but outside the brain tissue) as a result of damage to cerebral veins, most often due to head injury. Symptoms in adults include asthenia, balance difficulties, confusion or lethargy, headache, nausea and vomiting, seizures, speech difficulties, and visual disturbances. Symptoms in infants include bulging fontanelles, high-pitched crying, increased head circumference, seizures, and vomiting. Symptom onset is more gradual than for epidural hematoma due to a slower leakage rate for venous blood compared to arterial blood and a larger space for blood to fill before pressure buildup is sufficient to affect brain function. For an acute-onset hematoma, which is associated with the highest rate of death or permanent injury, symptoms usually occur immediately after severe head injury. For a subacute-onset hematoma, symptoms may occur days or weeks after injury occurrence. For a chronic-onset hematoma, symptoms may occur weeks after a less severe head injury.

An intracerebral hematoma (also called *intraparenchymal hematoma*) is a blood mass that accumulates in the brain tissue as a result of aneurysm, anticoagulant use, arteriovenous malformation, autoimmune diseases, bleeding disorders, brain tumor, drug abuse (amphetamines, cocaine), encephalitis (central nervous system infection), or uncontrolled chronic hypertension. It may be accompanied by shear injury—tearing of the axon portion of the cranial nerves located in the substantia alba (white matter of the brain)—resulting in severe brain damage due to loss of ability to transmit neural impulses from the brain to the body. A fracture site hematoma is a blood mass that accumulates near a fracture, especially that of the femur (thigh), humerus (upper arm), or pelvis, all of which can result in significant internal hemorrhage. An intraabdominal hematoma is a blood mass that accumulates somewhere within the abdomen—in any of the abdominal organs, in any abdominal component of the gastrointestinal tract, in the peritoneum, or in the retroperitoneal space.

Treatment and Therapy

Initial treatment of superficial hematomas consists of rest-ice-compression-elevation (RICE) of the affected area, if possible, as well as oral administration of nonsteroidal anti-inflammatory drugs (NSAIDs) or other analgesics, if pain management is required.

For an aural hematoma, more aggressive treatment may be necessary due to the potential compromise of blood supply and subsequent cartilage atrophy resulting in a deformity of the pinna (outer ear) that is commonly known as cauliflower ear. Treatment consists of lancing and draining the hematoma followed by application of a compression bandage to enable reperfusion of the cartilage and to prevent hematoma reformation. This bandage is usually removed after three to seven days.

For intramuscular hematoma, more aggressive treatment may be necessary due to the potential compromise of blood supply and subsequent damage to the muscle, connective tissues, and nerves, a condition known as compartment syndrome. It most commonly occurs in muscles of the forearm and lower leg. Treatment consists of surgical intervention to drain the hematoma.

For septal hematoma, more aggressive treatment may be necessary due to the potential compromise of blood supply and subsequent cartilage atrophy resulting in perforation of the septum. Treatment consists of lancing and draining the hematoma followed by application of a gauze sponge or cotton ball in the nasal cavity.

For subungual hematoma, more aggressive treatment may be necessary to relieve pressure between the nail plate and the nail bed. Treatment consists of trephination (hole boring) of the nail plate and drainage of the hematoma.

Cranial hematomas (epidural, subdural, and intracerebral) are potentially life threatening and require immediate medical attention at the onset of signs or symptoms due to the risk of irreversible brain damage and possible death. Administration of anticonvulsant medication may be necessary to control or prevent seizures, and administration of corticosteroid medication may be necessary to reduce cerebral edema (brain swelling).

For epidural hematoma, diagnosis of increased intracranial pressure and location of hematoma are confirmed via computed tomography (CT) scan. Treatment consists of prompt surgical intervention to drain or remove the hematoma. For acute, subacute, and chronic subdural hematoma, diagnosis and location of the hematoma are confirmed via CT scan or magnetic resonance imaging (MRI) scan. Increased risk factors include advanced age, alcohol abuse, and daily use of anticoagulants, anti-inflammatory

medication, or aspirin. Treatment consists of prompt surgical intervention to drain or remove the hematoma.

For intracerebral hematoma, diagnosis of increased intracranial pressure and location of hematoma are confirmed via CT scan or MRI scan. Treatment may consist of surgical intervention to drain or remove the hematoma.

Perspective and Prospects

Although intrinsic factors—such as aneurysm, arteriovenous malformations, autoimmune diseases, bleeding disorders, brain tumor, encephalitis, or uncontrolled chronic hypertension—and extrinsic factors—such as anticoagulant use, alcohol abuse, or drug abuse (amphetamines, cocaine)—may increase the likelihood of hematoma formation, the most common cause is trauma. Minor traumas, ranging from a violent sneeze to a mild sports injury, as well as major traumas, including car accidents and severe falls, all have the potential to cause hematoma formation.

While the size, type, and severity of hematomas vary according to location and causality, a common complication is infection risk as a result of the colonization of bacteria in stagnant blood. Attenuation or avoidance of complications may be achieved by early diagnosis and, if warranted, prompt medical treatment.

As is the case with all undesirable medical conditions, prevention is preferable to treatment. Although trauma prevention may not always be possible, risk may be minimized via lifestyle choices and proper use of safety equipment.

—*Cynthia L. De Vine*

See also Accidents; Bleeding; Blood and blood disorders; Brain damage; Circulation; Emergency medicine; First aid; Hematology; Hematology, pediatric; Hemophilia; Hemorrhage; Intraventricular hemorrhage; Subdural hematoma; Vascular medicine.

For Further Information:

Beers, M. H., ed. *The Merck Manual of Medical Information*. 2d ed. Whitehouse Station, N.J.: Merck, 2003.

Bluestone, C. D., S. E. Stool, and C. M. Alper, et al. *Pediatric Otolaryngology*. 4th ed. Philadelphia: W. B. Saunders: 2002.

DeBerardino, Thomas, and Mark D. Miller. Blunt Trauma Injuries in the Athlete. Philadelphia: Elsevier, 2013.

Hockberger, R. S., R. M. Walls, and J. A. Marx. *Rosen's Emergency Medicine: Concepts and Clinical Practice*. 6th ed. Philadelphia: Mosby/Elsevier, 2006.

Lawton, Michael T. *Seven Aneurysms: Tenets and Techniques for Clipping*. New York: Thieme Medical Publishers, 2011.

Neff, Deanna M. "Subdural Hematoma." *Health Library*, November 26, 2012.

Raimondi, Anthony J., Maurice Choux, and Concezio Di Rocco. *Head Injuries in the Newborn and Infant*. New York: Springer-Verlag, 2013.

Salazar, Misael F. Garza, and Araceli Ruiz Mendoza. *Hematomas: Types, Treatments and Health Risks*. New York: Nova Biomedical Publishers, 2012.

HEMATURIA

Disease/Disorder

Anatomy or system affected: Bladder, blood, kidneys, urinary system

Specialties and related fields: Internal medicine, microbiology, nephrology

Definition: The presence of blood or red blood cells in the urine.

Causes and Symptoms

Hematuria can present as bloody urine that is visible to the naked eye, or it can be subtle, detectable only by microscopic analysis. The source of the blood can be from any part of the urinary system, including the kidneys, bladder, and urethra. Hematuria can be accompanied by a variety of symptoms, or it can be completely asymptomatic.

The presentation, source, and symptoms of hematuria are functions of its broad range of causes. Possibly the most common cause of hematuria is a urinary tract infection (UTI), which includes infections of the kidney (pyelonephritis), bladder (cystitis), and urethra (urethritis). UTIs generally are caused by bacteria such as *Escherichia coli* and are accompanied by symptoms such as fever, pain with urination, and urinary frequency or urgency.

Another common cause of hematuria is kidney stones (nephrolithiasis). Stones are most commonly composed of calcium and can present with severe pain, nausea, and vomiting.

Hematuria can also be the presenting symptom of innocent causes such as benign familial hematuria (a mild inherited condition), benign prostatic hyperplasia (BPH or enlarged prostate, a common condition in middle-aged and elderly men), medication, and exercise. In other situations, it can be the first sign of life-threatening problems such as bladder or kidney cancer and trauma.

Treatment and Therapy

The therapeutic options for treating hematuria depend on its cause. For a UTI, treatment can be a course of oral antibiotics, or it may require hospitalization and intravenous antibiotics in the case of a severe infection. In the case of kidney stones, the stones will usually pass on their own, but in some cases interventions such as surgery or lithotripsy (breaking up the stones) are necessary to clear the obstruction.

If the cause is benign familial hematuria or exercise, then reassurance may be all the treatment that is required. BPH may also be treated with reassurance and lifestyle change, or medication and surgical intervention may be initiated to help reduce the size of the prostate. If medication is the cause of hematuria, the condition may be self-limited, or a patient may be advised to change or stop the medication.

Cancers of the bladder and kidneys are treated with chemotherapy, radiation, surgery, immunotherapy, or a combination of these options, depending on the type and severity of the cancer. Hematuria as a sign of trauma to the kidneys is treated based on careful consideration of various options, and treatment may include surgery.

—*Jennifer Birkhauser, M.S., M.D.*

See also Bladder; Bladder cancer; Bleeding; Cancer; Kidney cancer; Kidneys; Laboratory tests; Noninvasive tests; Prostate enlargement; Proteinuria; Stone removal; Stones; Urethritis; Urinalysis; Urinary disorders; Urinary system; Urology; Urology, pediatric.

For Further Information:

"Blood in Urine (Hematuria)." *Mayo Clinic*, September 1, 2011.

Domino, Frank, ed. *The Five-Minute Clinical Consult*. Philadelphia: Lippincott Williams & Wilkins, 2006.

Kilmartin, Angela, ed. *The Patient's Encyclopaedia of Urinary Tract Infection, Sexual Cystitis, and Interstitial Cystitis*. London: Angela Kilmartin, 2002.

Lopez, Ralph. "The Kidneys." In *The Teen Health Book: A Parents" Guide to Adolescent Health and Well-Being*, edited by Kate Kelly. New York: W. W. Norton, 2003.

Shannon, Diane W. "Blood in Urine (Hematuria—Adult)." *Health Library*, January 10, 2013.

U.S. Department of Health and Human Services. "Hematuria: Blood in the Urine." *National Kidney and Urologic Diseases Information Clearinghouse*, April 16, 2012.

HEMIPLEGIA

Disease/Disorder

Anatomy or system affected: Arms, brain, head, joints, legs, muscles, musculoskeletal system, nervous system, tendons

Specialties and related fields: Exercise physiology, family medicine, neurology, orthopedics, physical therapy

Definition: Paralysis of one side of the body, usually caused by brain damage.

Causes and Symptoms

Hemiplegia is paralysis or partial paralysis of one side of the body, typically involving the leg, arm, and trunk. It is caused by damage to or disease of the part of the brain that controls the motor system. The damage may occur prior to birth, during birth, or after birth as a result of an accident, illness, or stroke. The most common cause is a cerebrovascular disease that leads to clotting of the cerebral arteries or bleeding from the diseased arterial wall, eventually producing a stroke. The site most often affected is the internal capsule, where packed nerve fibers descend from the cortex of the brain into the spinal cord.

Immediately after a stroke, the affected body parts are initially limp. In a few days or weeks, the limbs become stiff and spastic. Symptoms of hemiplegia can include paralysis on one side of the body, muscle weakness and spasticity, poor balance, speech difficulties, epileptic seizures, visual field defects, emotional and behavioral problems, and gait problems, including limping and toe drop. Increased energy ex-

---

Information on Hematuria

Causes: Urinary tract infection, kidney stones, benign familial hematuria, benign prostatic hyperplasia, medication, exercise, cancers, trauma

Symptoms: May be asymptomatic; pain, fever, urinary frequency/urgency

Duration: Days to years, depending on cause and treatment

Treatments: Depends on cause; reassurance, antibiotics, chemotherapy, radiation, surgery

penditure results from compensatory adjustments during walking that produce abnormal movements of the body's center of gravity.

Treatment and Therapy

Treatments for hemiplegia are designed to improve strength and range of motion, increase bodily functions, and reduce or prevent spasticity. Long-term care is very important. Depending on the severity of the disorder, physical therapy, speech therapy, occupational therapy, braces or orthotics, electrical stimulation, drugs, Botox injections, or surgery may be used as corrective procedures. Acupuncture and electroacupuncture procedures may be promising treatments for hemiplegia. Children who suffer from hemiplegia may also receive special educational services to help improve specific learning difficulties caused by the disorder. Affected children should involve the weaker side of the body in everyday activities so that they become as two-sided as possible.

Perspective and Prospects

The side of the body affected by hemiplegia depends on which side of the brain has been damaged. The left side of the brain controls the right side of the body, while the right side of the brain controls the left side of the body. Depending on which side of the body is affected, the disease is often referred to as right hemiplegia or left hemiplegia.

Childhood hemiplegia affects up to one child per one thousand. An associated rare neurological disorder, alternating hemiplegia of childhood (AHC), produces periodic transient attacks of hemiplegia that affect one side of the body or the other. An attack of AHC may last from a few minutes up to days. The attacks may alternate from one side of the body to the other. The symptoms are usually relieved with bed rest and proper sleep.

—*Alvin K. Benson, Ph.D.*

See also Brain; Brain damage; Brain disorders; Nervous system; Neuroimaging; Neurology; Neurology, pediatric; Paralysis; Paraplegia; Physical rehabilitation; Quadriplegia; Strokes.

For Further Information:

Bobath, Berta. *Adult Hemiplegia: Evaluation and Treatment.* 3d ed. London: Butterworth/Heinemann, 1998.
Davies, Patricia M. *Steps to Follow: The Comprehensive Treatment of Patients with Hemiplegia.* 2d ed. New York: Springer, 2004.
"Hemiplegia." *Children's Hemiplegia and Stroke Association,* 2013.
"Hemiplegia." *Christopher and Dana Reeve Foundation,* 2011.
Neville, Brian, and Robert Goodman, eds. *Congenital Hemiplegia.* London: MacKeith, 2001.
"NINDS Alternating Hemiplegia Page." *National Institute of Neurological Disorders and Stroke,* September 16, 2011.
Spivack, Barney S., ed. *Evaluation and Management of Gait Disorders.* New York: Marcel Dekker, 1995.

HEMOCHROMATOSIS
Disease/Disorder
Also known as: Bronze diabetes
Anatomy or system affected: Genitals, heart, liver, pancreas
Specialties and related fields: Cardiology, endocrinology, gastroenterology, internal medicine
Definition: A multisystem disease characterized by increased iron absorption and storage.

Causes and Symptoms

Iron is used by the body for various processes, such as making hemoglobin, the oxygen-carrying molecule in blood. Hemochromatosis is an inherited disorder, usually caused by a mutation of the HFE gene, characterized by the excessive absorption and accumulation of iron from the diet. This excess iron is deposited in various organs. Damage to these organs from years of iron accumulation results in the symptoms of hemochromatosis. The most commonly affected organs are the pancreas (causing diabetes), the skin (causing bronzelike skin pigmentation), the joints (causing arthritis), the testes (causing loss of libido and erectile dysfunction), and the heart (causing abnormal heart rhythms or heart failure). The pituitary gland, which regulates sex hormones and metabolism, can also be affected. Although the liver is commonly involved as well, this usually results in mild abnormalities in blood tests of liver enzymes rather than liver failure. However, cirrhosis of the liver can occur, and these patients are at risk for developing liver cancer. Unfortunately, most of the above warning symptoms occur late in the disease, after decades of iron accumulation and organ damage have already taken place.

Information on Hemochromatosis

Causes: Genetic defect in iron production
Symptoms: Damage to pancreas, skin, testes, and heart, causing diabetes mellitus, bronzelike skin pigmentation, loss of libido and erectile dysfunction, and abnormal heart rhythms or heart failure
Duration: Chronic
Treatments: Phlebotomy (blood removal) to create mild anemia

Treatment and Therapy

Ideally, hemochromatosis should be detected and treated before the onset of symptoms. Screening for patients with a family history of this disease can be performed via blood tests, such as the iron saturation index. More recently, a genetic test for a common mutation that causes hemochromatosis has been developed. Liver biopsy is sometimes needed to confirm the diagnosis. Treatment consists of repeated phlebotomy, or the removal of blood. Typically one unit of blood is removed per week until the patient becomes mildly anemic. Hemochromatosis may require the removal of up to 150 units of blood over several years. Subsequently, phlebotomy is repeated every three to four months, and the patient's iron stores (ferritin) are monitored. If phlebotomy is started before liver cirrhosis develops, then many complications can be avoided. Some patients may benefit from treatment with desferroxamine, a chelating agent that removes iron.

Perspective and Prospects

Hemochromatosis was initially described in 1865 as a triad of glucose in the urine, dark pigmentation of the skin, and liver cirrhosis. Research into the disease has resulted in tremendous advances in the understanding of iron metabolism. The HFE gene, responsible for most diagnoses of hemochromatosis, has been mapped to chromosome 6. Although the genetic defect is present in both men and women, men develop the disease much more often, since menstruation removes excess iron in women. A test to screen for one common mutation in this gene is available, but its usefulness is limited since several other mutations may cause the disease, especially in non-Caucasian ethnic groups.

—*Ahmad Kamal, M.D.*

See also Hematology; Hematology, pediatric; Liver disorders; Metabolic disorders; Metabolism; Nephrology; Nephrology, pediatric.

For Further Information:

Barton, James C., and Corwin Q. Edwards, eds. *Hemochromatosis: Genetics, Pathophysiology, Diagnosis, and Treatment.* New York: Cambridge University Press, 2000.

Everson, Gregory T., and Marilyn Olsen. *Living with Hemochromatosis.* New York: Hatherleigh Press, 2003.

Garrison, Cheryl D., ed. *The Iron Disorders Institute Guide to Hemochromatosis.* 2d ed. Naperville, Ill.: Cumberland House, 2009.

"Hemochromatosis." *Mayo Clinic,* December 13, 2012.

"Hemochromatosis." *National Digestive Diseases Information Clearinghouse,* May 10, 2012.

Parker, James N., and Philip M. Parker, eds. *The Official Patient's Sourcebook on Hemochromatosis.* San Diego, Calif.: Icon Health, 2002.

Weinberg, E. D., and Cheryl D. Garrison. *Exposing the Hidden Dangers of Iron: What Every Medical Professional Should Know About the Impact of Iron on the Disease Process.* Nashville: Cumberland House, 2004.

"What Is Hemochromatosis?" *National Heart, Lung, and Blood Institute,* February 1, 2011.

Hemolytic Disease of the Newborn
Disease/Disorder

Also known as: Erythroblastosis fetalis, Rh incompatibility, ABO incompatibility

Anatomy or system affected: Blood, brain, liver, skin

Specialties and related fields: Hematology, neonatology, neurology

Definition: The destruction of red blood cells in a fetus by antibodies transferred from the mother.

Key terms:

antibodies: proteins produced by the immune system to destroy invading organisms or those perceived as foreign to the body

bilirubin: a pigment derived from the breakdown of red blood cells

Coombs' test: a test used to determine whether sensitization has occurred

exchange transfusion: the exchange of all or most of a patient's blood for donor blood; in a baby with hemolytic disease, usually performed through the umbilical vein

hemolysis: the rapid destruction of red blood cells

jaundice: yellow pigmentation resulting from the deposition of bilirubin in the skin

kernicterus: brain damage produced by the deposition of bilirubin in the brain

Rhogam: a protein that destroys Rh-positive cells

sensitization: the development of antibodies to a substance

Causes and Symptoms

Hemolytic disease of the newborn is a disorder in which maternal antibodies induce hemolysis of the red blood cells of the fetus or newborn, producing jaundice. The most common causes are ABO or Rh incompatibilities. ABO incompatibility occurs when the mother's blood is type O and the baby's blood is either type A or type B. The newborn develops jaundice within the first forty-eight hours of birth as a result of increasing bilirubin levels in the blood. Rh incompatibility can arise when an Rh-negative woman is carrying a second Rh-positive fetus. During the delivery of the first Rh-positive baby, blood from the newborn may pass into the mother's circulation. If no treatment is given, the woman may develop anti-Rh antibodies, which will remain in her circulation. If the fetus in her next pregnancy is also Rh-positive, the anti-Rh antibodies will cross over into the baby's blood, causing hemolysis of the red blood cells. In severe cases, the hemolysis starts in utero and the fetus will develop anemia, progressing to generalized edema with heart failure (hydrops fetalis) and death if the anemia is not corrected.

During the pregnancy, a positive Coombs" test indicates that the woman has been exposed and thus sensitized to Rh factor. A woman who is Rh-negative can become sensitized in three ways: by having delivered an Rh-positive baby following a previous pregnancy and not having received the protein Rhogam; by receiving an erroneous infusion of Rh-positive blood; and by having a spontaneous or induced abortion of an Rh-positive embryo or fetus. A rising concentration of antibodies during the course of the pregnancy indicates that hemolysis is occurring in the fetus. A small amount of amniotic fluid is obtained through a needle inserted through the mother's abdomen to determine the severity of the disease in the fetus. At birth, the baby may have pale skin and an enlarged liver and spleen. Progressive jaundice and anemia develop within the first twenty-four hours. High levels may cause the bilirubin to enter the brain and produce kernicterus. The baby with kernicterus shows little activity (hypoactivity), refuses to suck milk, and experiences seizures that can progress to permanent neurologic damage or to coma and death. Deafness may be a consequence of high bilirubin levels during the newborn period.

Treatment and Therapy

There is no preventive treatment for ABO incompatibility. Phototherapy, or light therapy, is used to decrease the level of bilirubin. Phototherapy acts on the bilirubin deposited in the skin and makes it water soluble, so that the pigment can be excreted through the gastrointestinal tract. An exchange transfusion may be required to decrease the concentration of

---

Information on
Hemolytic Disease of the Newborn

Causes: Blood incompatibilities between mother and fetus

Symptoms: Pale skin, enlarged liver and spleen, progressive jaundice and anemia within twenty-four hours of birth, deafness

Duration: Varies

Treatments: Light therapy, drug therapy, blood transfusions, iron and folic acid supplementation

---

bilirubin if it rises to dangerous levels. These levels will depend on the baby's maturation and clinical condition.

Preventive treatment for Rh incompatibility consists of giving Rhogam to all Rh-negative pregnant women at twenty-eight weeks of gestation and within the first seventy-two hours after the delivery of an Rh-positive baby. All Rh-negative women who have experienced an abortion or who have erroneously received a transfusion of Rh-positive blood should also receive Rhogam.

An Rh-negative pregnant woman with a positive Coombs" test needs to have periodic Coombs titers, or antibody concentration measurements, to determine what type of intervention, if any, is required. This test should first be done between sixteen and eighteen weeks of gestation. Rising Coombs titers indicate that hemolysis is occurring in the fetus. Prenatal interventions may include correcting fetal anemia by giving red blood cells directly to the fetus, either into the abdomen or into the umbilical vein. The fetus must be observed with sonography for the development of fetal edema, an ominous sign. At birth, the baby may have severe anemia requiring immediate correction. Phototherapy and an exchange transfusion may be needed if bilirubin rises above acceptable levels. Other modes of therapy, such as phenobarbital, agar gel, and rectal suppositories, are of limited value in reducing bilirubin in infants with hemolytic disease.

Before discharge from the hospital nursery, a hearing test must be done for all infants who have had jaundice during the neonatal period. Anemia may develop during the first six weeks of life as a result of the persistence of antibodies in the baby's blood. Close follow-up of hemoglobin levels must be done after discharge from the hospital. Blood transfusions may be indicated, as well as iron and folic acid supplementation.

Perspective and Prospects

The incidence of Rh incompatibility has decreased remarkably since the advent of Rhogam. Nevertheless, it still occurs, particularly when unidentified miscarriages have occurred. Rh-negative fetuses can be identified early using special techniques available only in large medical centers. Therapy for hydrops fetalis has improved with the use of cordocentesis. This therapy, which consists of obtaining and transfusing blood directly into the umbilical cord while the fetus is in utero, is available in specialized medical centers and has helped many sensitized babies to survive.

Immunoglobulin has been used to block hemolysis, but it cannot be used for treatment. Agents that can metabolize bilirubin are currently under investigation.

—Gloria Reyes Báez, M.D.

See also Anemia; Antibodies; Blood and blood disorders; Critical care, pediatric; Emergency medicine, pediatric; Hearing loss; Immune system; Jaundice; Neonatology; Pregnancy and gestation; Rh factor; Umbilical cord.

For Further Information:
Behrman, Richard E., Robert M. Kliegman, and Hal B. Jenson, eds. *Nelson Textbook of Pediatrics.* 19th ed. Philadelphia: Saunders/Elsevier, 2011.

"Hemolytic Disease of the Newborn." *MedlinePlus*, November 14, 2011.

"Hemolytic Disease of the Newborn." *University of Iowa Hospitals & Clinics*, November 14, 2011.

Kemper, Kathi J. *The Holistic Pediatrician: A Pediatrician's Comprehensive Guide to Safe and Effective Therapies for the Twenty-five Most Common Ailments of Infants, Children, and Adolescents.* Rev. ed. New York: Quill, 2002.

Levy, Joseph. "Newborn Jaundice." *Parents Magazine* 69, no. 7 (July, 1994): 59–60.

Martin, Richard J., Avroy A. Fanaroff, and Michele C. Walsh, eds. *Fanaroff and Martin's Neonatal-Perinatal Medicine: Diseases of the Fetus and Infant.* 2 vols. 9th ed. Philadelphia: Mosby/Elsevier, 2010.

Nathanson, Laura Walther. *The Portable Pediatrician: A Practicing Pediatrician's Guide to Your Child's Growth, Development, Health, and Behavior from Birth to Age Five.* 2d ed. New York: HarperCollins, 2002.

"Rh Incompatibility." *MedlinePlus*, January 28, 2013.

HEMOLYTIC UREMIC SYNDROME
Disease/Disorder

Also known as: Gasser syndrome

Anatomy or system affected: Blood, circulatory system, gastrointestinal system, kidneys, nervous system, urinary system

Specialties and related fields: Family medicine, gastroenterology, hematology, nephrology, nutrition, pediatrics, urology

Definition: A predominantly childhood disorder produced primarily by a strain of *Escherichia coli* bacteria and characterized by acute kidney failure, hemolytic anemia, and a low platelet count.

Causes and Symptoms

In the majority of cases, hemolytic uremic syndrome develops after the digestive system has been infected by the O157:H7 strain of *Escherichia coli* (*E. coli*). Undercooked meats, contaminated fresh vegetables and fruits, unpasteurized dairy products and juices, and contaminated water are the primary sources of this bacterium. Hemolytic uremic syndrome can be passed from person to person. Less common sources include *Shigella, Salmonella, Yersinia*, and *Campylobacter* bacteria.

Following a siege of gastroenteritis that typically lasts for three to ten days and usually includes vomiting, fever, cramping, and diarrhea, hemolytic uremic syndrome develops

---

Information on Hemolytic Uremic Syndrome

Causes: Infection with *E. coli* or other bacteria that produce toxins which enter the bloodstream

Symptoms: Initially, vomiting, fever, cramping, and diarrhea; progressing to red blood cell destruction, poor kidney function, reduced urine output, paleness, bruises, blood in urine and feces, extreme fatigue, irritability, seizures, increased blood pressure, swollen limbs

Duration: Acute

Treatments: Supportive measures; in severe cases, dialysis or kidney transplantation

---

when the *E. coli* produce toxins that enter the bloodstream and begin destroying red blood cells and platelets. The damaged red blood cells block tiny blood vessels in the kidneys, making it more and more difficult for the kidneys to function. Resulting symptoms can include reduced urine output, paleness, small body bruises, blood in the urine and stool, extreme fatigue, irritability, seizures, increased blood pressure, and swollen limbs.

Treatment and Therapy

Once an individual is diagnosed with hemolytic uremic syndrome, the typical treatment is mostly supportive. Maintaining normal electrolyte and water levels in the body eases the immediate symptoms and helps prevent further complications. Vital signs are monitored frequently, as is the weight of the patient. Blood transfusions are necessary only when there is severe anemia.

Depending on urine output and electrolyte abnormalities, dialysis may be used. On rare occasions, the victim may require a kidney transplant. Administration of antimotility agents, antibiotics, or platelet transfusions seems to worsen the outcome.

Perspective and Prospects

Hemolytic uremic syndrome was first described by Swiss hematologist Conrad von Gasser in 1955. Although it is an uncommon illness, striking examples exist in which many individuals have been infected during a particular time frame. In 2000, more than two thousand people developed hemolytic uremic syndrome symptoms after drinking contaminated water in Walkerton, Ontario, Canada; seven died. Three months later, forty individuals experienced hemolytic uremic syndrome symptoms after eating at a Sizzler restaurant in Milwaukee, Wisconsin; one died. In 2006, more than 180 individuals were identified with hemolytic uremic syndrome symptoms in the United States as a result of contaminated spinach grown in California; three died. In 2011, fenugreek seeds contaminated with *E. coli* O104:H4 caused an epidemic of hemolytic uremic syndrome, affecting 3,800 people, most of whom were adults; thirty-six died.

Research into treating hemolytic uremic syndrome has focused on preventing its onset by using chemical agents that bind the toxins produced by *E. coli* O157:H7 within the intestines. Strategies involving immunization are also being developed.

—*Alvin K. Benson, Ph.D.*

See also Bacterial infections; Bacteriology; Blood and blood disorders; Childhood infectious diseases; Dialysis; *E. coli* infection; Food poisoning; Hematology; Hematology, pediatric; Kidney disorders; Kidney transplantation; Kidneys; Nephrology; Nephrology, pediatric.

For Further Information:

Boyer, Olivia, and Patrick Niaudet. "Hemolytic Uremic Syndrome: New Developments in Pathogenesis and Treatment." *International Journal of Nephrology*, August 2011.

Buchholz, Bernard, et al. "German Outbreak of *Escherichia coli* O104:H4 Associated with Sprouts." *New England Journal of Medicine* 365, no. 19 (2011): 1763–70.

Hoffman, Ronald, et al., eds. *Hematology: Basic Principles and Practice*. 5th ed. Philadelphia: Churchill Livingstone/Elsevier, 2009.

Kaper, James B., and Alison D. O'Brien, eds. *Escherichia coli O157:H7 and Other Shiga Toxin-Producing "E. coli" Strains*. Washington, D.C.: ASM Press, 1998.

Parker, James N., and Philip M. Parker, eds. *The Official Patient's Sourcebook on Hemolytic Uremic Syndrome: A Revised and Updated Directory for the Internet Age*. San Diego, Calif.: Icon Health, 2002.

Tintinalli, Judith E. *Emergency Medicine: A Comprehensive Study Guide*. 7th ed. New York: McGraw-Hill, 2011.

HEMOPHILIA
Disease/Disorder
Anatomy or system affected: Blood

Specialties and related fields: Genetics, hematology, serology

Definition: A genetic disorder characterized by the blood's inability to form clots as a result of the lack or alteration of certain trace plasma proteins.

Key terms:

clotting factors: substances present in plasma that are needed for the coagulation of blood

hemophilia A: a genetic blood disease characterized by a deficiency of clotting factor VIII

hemophilia B: a genetic blood disease characterized by a deficiency of clotting factor IX

hemostasis: the process of stopping the flow of blood at an injury site

von Willebrand's disease: a genetic blood disease characterized by a deficiency of the von Willebrand clotting factor

Causes and Symptoms

The circulatory system must be self-healing; otherwise, continued blood loss from even the smallest injury would be life-threatening. Normally, all except the most catastrophic bleeding is rapidly stopped in a process known as hemostasis. Hemostasis takes place through several sequential steps or processes. First, an injury stimulates platelets (unpigmented blood cells) to adhere to the damaged blood vessels and then to one another, forming a plug that can stop minor bleeding. This association is mediated by what is called the von Willebrand factor, a protein that binds to the platelets. As the

Information on Hemophilia

Causes: Genetic blood defect
Symptoms: Loss of large amounts of blood from even small injuries, hemorrhaging without apparent cause, bruising, pain, swelling, joint lesions, urinary bleeding, pseudotumors
Duration: Chronic
Treatments: Fresh frozen plasma, clotting factor concentrates, drug therapy

platelets aggregate, they release several substances that stimulate vasoconstriction, or a reduction in size of the blood vessels. This reduces the blood flow at the injury site. Finally, the aggregating platelets and damaged tissue initiate blood clotting, or coagulation. Once bleeding has stopped, the firmly adhering clot slowly contracts, drawing the edge of the wounds together so that tough scar tissue can form a permanent repair on the site.

Formation of a blood clot involves the participation of nearly twenty different substances, most of which are proteins synthesized by plasma. All but two of these substances, or factors, are designated by a roman numeral and a common name. A blood clot will be defective if one of the clotting factors is absent or deficient in the blood, and clotting time will be longer. The clotting factors, with some of their alternative names, are factor I (fibrinogen), factor II (prothrombin), factor III (tissue factor or thromboplastin), factor IV (calcium), factor V (proaccelerin), factor VII (proconvertin), factor VIII (antihemophilic factor), factor IX (Christmas factor), factor X (Stuart factor), factor XI (plasma thromboplastin antecedent), factor XII (Hageman factor), and factor XIII (fibrin stabilizing factor).

Several of the clotting factors have been discovered by the diagnosis of their deficiencies in various clotting disorders. The inherited coagulation disorders are uncommon conditions with an overall incidence of probably no more than 10 to 20 per 100,000 of the population. Hemophilia A, the most common or classic type of coagulation disorder, is caused by factor VIII deficiency. Hemophilia B (or Christmas disease) is the result of factor IX deficiency. It is quite common for severe hemophilia to manifest itself during the first year of life. Hazardous bleeding occurs in areas such as the central nervous system, the retropharyngeal area, and the retroperitoneal area. Bleeding in these areas requires admission to the hospital for observation and therapy. Joint lesions are very common in hemophilia because of acute spontaneous hemorrhage in the area, especially in weight-bearing joints such as ankles and knees. Urinary bleeding is often present at some time. The appearance of pseudotumors, caused by swelling involving muscle and bone produced by recurrent bleeding, is also common.

Hemophilia is transmitted entirely by unaffected women (carriers) to their sons in a sex-linked inheritance deficiency. Congenital deficiencies of the other coagulation factors are well recognized, even though bleeding episodes in these cases are uncommon. Deficiency of more than one factor is also possible, although documentation of such cases is rare, perhaps because only patients with milder variations of the disease survive.

Von Willebrand's disease, unlike the hemophilias that mainly involve bleeding in joints and muscles, involves mainly bleeding of mucocutaneous tissues or skin. It affects both men and women. This disease shares clinical characteristics with hemophilia A, or classic hemophilia, including decreased levels of clotting factor VIII. This similarity made the differentiation between the two diseases very difficult for a long time. It has been established that there are two different factors involved in von Willebrand's disease, each with a different function. The von Willebrand factor is involved in the adhesion of platelets to the injured blood vessel wall and to one another and, together with factor VIII, circulates in plasma as a complex held by electrostatic and hydrophobic forces. The von Willebrand factor is a very large molecule, consisting of a series of possible multimeric structures. The bigger and heavier the multimer, the better it works against bleeding. Von Willebrand's disease is one of the least understood clotting disorders. Three types have been identified, with at least twenty-seven variations. With type I, all the multimers needed for successful clotting are present in the blood, but in lesser amounts than in healthy individuals. In type II, the larger multimers, which are more active in hemostasis, are lacking, and type III patients exhibit a severe lack of all multimers.

Treatment and Therapy

The normal body is continually producing clotting factors in order to keep up with natural loss. Sometimes the production is stepped up to cover a real or anticipated increase in the need for these factors, such as in childbirth. Hemophiliacs, lacking some of these clotting factors, may lose large amounts of blood from even the smallest injury and sometimes hemorrhage without any apparent cause. The symptoms of their diseases may be alleviated by the intravenous administration of the deficient clotting factor. How this is done depends on the specific factor deficiency and the magnitude of the bleeding episode, the age and size of the patient, convenience, acceptability, cost of product, and method and place of delivery of care.

There are many sources for clotting factors. Fresh frozen plasma contains all the clotting factors, but since the concentration of the factors in plasma is relatively low, a large volume is required for treatment. Therefore, it can be used only when small amounts of clotting factor must be delivered. Its use is the only therapy for deficiencies of factors V, XI, and XII. Plasma is commonly harvested from single donor units to minimize the risk of infection by the hepatitis virus or human immunodeficiency virus (HIV), thus eliminating the risk involved in using pooled concentrates from many donors. Cryoprecipitates are the proteins that precipitate in fresh frozen plasma thawed at 4 degrees Celsius. The precipitate is rich in factors VIII and XIII and in fibrinogen, and carries less chance of infection with hepatitis. Its standardization is difficult, however, and is not required by the Food and Drug Administration. As a result, dosage calculation can be a problem. In addition, there is no method for the control of viral contamination. Therefore, cryoprecipitates are not commonly used unless harvested from a special known and tested donor pool. Clotting factor concentrates present many advantages. They are made from pooled plasma obtained from plasmapheresis or a program of total donor unit fractionation and are widely available. Factors VIII and IX can also be produced from plasma using monoclonal methods. Porcine factor VIII presents an alternative to patients with a naturally occurring antibody to human factor VIII.

Other substances can replace missing clotting factors as well. The synthetic hormone desmopressin acetate (also known by the letters DDAVP) has been used to stimulate the release of factor VIII and von Willebrand factor from the endothelial cells lining blood vessels. It is commonly used for patients with mild hemophilia and von Willebrand's disease. DDAVP has no effect on the concentration of the other factors, and aside from the common side effect of water retention, it is a safe drug. Antifibrinolytic drugs prevent the natural breakdown of blood clots that have already been formed. Although such drugs are not useful for the primary care of hemophiliacs, they are useful for use after dental extractions and in the treatment of other open wounds, after a clot has formed.

Between 10 and 15 percent of the patients affected with severe hemophilia develop factor VIII inhibitors (antibodies), which prevents their treatment with the usual methods. Newer therapeutic approaches have provided additional options for the management and control of bleeding episodes. The use of prothrombin complex concentrates or porcine factor VIII concentrates is indicated for low responders (those with a low amount of antibodies present in their system). An option for high responders is to try to eradicate the inhibitor present in their systems. One way to do this is with a regimen of immunosuppressive drugs. These are very limited in value, however, and cannot be used with HIV-positive hemophiliacs. The drugs used in this approach include substances such as cyclophosphamide, vincristine, azathioprine, and corticosteroids. Another approach utilizes intravenous doses of gamma globulin to suppress, but not eradicate, the inhibitors. Yet another strategy is an immune tolerance regimen, in which factor VIII is administered daily in small amounts. This method causes the inhibitors to decrease and, in some cases, disappear. The regimen can also involve the prophylactic use of factor VIII (or factor VIII in combination with immunosuppressive drugs).

The introduction of plasma clotting factor concentrates has changed the treatment of patients with clotting factor deficiencies. It has brought about a remarkable change in the longevity of these patients and their quality of life. The availability of cryoprecipitates and concentrates of factors II, VII, VIII, IX, X, and XIII has made outpatient treatment for bleeding episodes routine and home infusion or self-infusion a possibility for many patients. Hospitalization for inpatient treatment is rare, and early outpatient therapy of bleeding episodes has decreased the severity of joint deformities.

Nevertheless, other problems are apparent in hemophiliac patients. Viral contamination of the factor concentrates has allowed the development of chronic illnesses, infection with HIV, immunologic diseases, liver and renal diseases, joint disorders, and cardiovascular diseases. While the use of heat for virus inactivation, beginning in 1983, resulted in a reduction in HIV infections, the majority of patients exposed to the virus had already been infected. The strategies to prevent contraction of hepatitis from these concentrates include vaccination against the contaminating viruses and the elimination of viruses from the factor replacement product. The non-A, non-B hepatitis virus is difficult to remove, however, and the use of monoclonal factors seems to be the only solution to this problem. In general, difficulties associated with treatment have been largely eliminated through the production of the required clotting factors using recombinant DNA techniques, a process performed independent of human blood.

Treatment of von Willebrand's disease also includes pressure dressing, suturing, and oral contraceptives. A pasteurized antihemophiliac concentrate that contains substantial amounts of von Willebrand factor is used in severe cases.

Hematomas, or hemorrhages under the skin and within muscles, can frequently be controlled by application of elastic bandage pressure and ice. The ones that cannot be controlled easily within a few hours may cause muscle contraction and require factor replacement therapy. Exercise is recommended for joints after bleeding, as it helps protect joints by increasing muscle bulk and power and can also help relieve stress. Devices to protect joints, such as elastic bandages and splints, are commonly used. In extreme cases, orthopedic surgical procedures are readily available.

Analgesics, or painkillers, play an important part in the alleviation of chronic pain. Because patients cannot use products with aspirin and/or antihistamines, which inhibit platelet aggregation and prolong bleeding time, substances such as acetaminophen, codeine, and morphine are used. Chronic joint inflammation is reduced by the use of anti-inflammatory agents such as ibuprofen and drugs used with rheumatoid arthritis patients.

The need for so many specialties and disciplines in the management of hemophilia has led to the development of multidisciplinary hemophilia centers. Genetic education (information on how the disease is transmitted), genetic counseling (the discussion of an individual's genetic risks and reproductive options), and genetic testing have provided great help to patients and affected families. Early and prenatal diagnosis and carrier detection have provided options for family planning.

Perspective and Prospects

Descriptions of hemophilia are among the oldest known accounts of genetic disease. References to a bleeding condition highly suggestive of hemophilia go back to the fifth century, in the Babylonian Talmud. The first significant report in medical literature appeared in 1803 when John C. Otto, a

Philadelphia physician, described several bleeder families with only males affected and with transmission through the mothers. The literature of the nineteenth century contains many descriptions of the disease, particularly the clinical characteristics of the hemorrhages and family histories. The disease was originally called haemorrhaphilia, or "tendency toward hemorrhages," but the name was later contracted through usage to hemophilia ("tendency toward blood"), the accepted name since around 1828.

Transfusion therapy was proposed as early as 1832, and the first successful transfusion for the treatment of a hemophiliac patient was reported in 1840 by Samuel Armstrong Lane. The use of blood from cows and pigs in the transfusions was explored but abandoned because of the numerous side effects. It was not until the beginning of the twentieth century that serious studies on clotting in hemophilia were started. Attention was directed to the use of normal human serum for treatment of bleeding episodes. Some of the patients responded well, while others did not. This result is probably attributable to the fact that some had hemophilia A—these patients did not respond because factor VIII, in which they are deficient, is not present in serum—while some others had hemophilia B, for which the therapy worked. In 1923, harvested blood plasma was used in transfusion, and it was shown to work as well as whole blood. With blood banking becoming a reality in the 1930s, transfusions were performed more frequently as a treatment for hemophilia.

The history of the fractionation of plasma began around 1911 with a Dr. Addis, who prepared a very crude fraction by acidification of plasma. In 1937, Drs. Patek and Taylor produced a crude fraction which, on injection, lowered the blood-clotting time in hemophiliacs. In the period from 1945 to 1960, a number of plasma fractions with antihemophiliac activity were developed. The use of fresh frozen plasma increased as a result of advances in the purification of the fractions. Some milestones can be identified in the production of the plasma fractions: the development of quantitative assays for antihemophiliac factors, the discovery of cryoprecipitation, and the development of glycine and polyethylene precipitation.

In 1952, four significant and independent publications indicated that there is a plasma-clotting activity separate from that concerned with classic hemophilia—in other words, that there are two types of hemophilia. One (hemophilia A) is characterized by a deficiency in factor VIII, while the other (hemophilia B) is characterized by deficiency in factor IX. Carriers of hemophilia A can have a mean factor VIII level that is 50 percent lower than that of normal females, while carriers of hemophilia B show levels of factor IX that are 60 percent below normal. The two diseases have the same pattern of inheritance, are similar in clinical appearance, and can be distinguished only by laboratory tests.

Hemophilias are caused by a disordered and complex biological mechanism that continues to be explored. Recombinant DNA techniques have now revealed the molecular defect in factor VIII or factor IX deficiencies in some families, demonstrating that a variety of gene defects can produce the classic phenotype of hemophilia. These techniques have also provided new tools for carrier detection and prenatal diagnosis.

Current treatment of hemophilia has converted the hemophiliac from an in-hospital patient to an individual with more independent status. Crucial in this development has been the creation of comprehensive care centers and of the National Hemophilia Foundation, which provide comprehensive treatment for the hemophilia patient. Home treatment with replacement therapy has become common. With the advancement of recombinant DNA technology, the future looks brighter for the sufferers of this disease.

—Maria Pacheco, Ph.D.

See also Acquired immunodeficiency syndrome (AIDS); Bleeding; Blood and blood disorders; Genetic diseases; Genetics and inheritance; Transfusion; Von Willebrand's disease.

For Further Information:
Bloom, Arthur L., ed. *The Hemophilias*. New York: Churchill Livingstone, 1982.
Hilgartner, Margaret W., and Carl Pochedly, eds. *Hemophilia in the Child and Adult*. 3d ed. New York: Raven Press, 1989.
Hoffman, Ronald, et al. *Hematology: Basic Principles and Practice*. Philadelphia: Saunders/Elsevier, 2013.
Jones, Peter. *Living with Haemophilia*. 5th ed. New York: Oxford University Press, 2002.
Judd, Sandra J., ed. *Genetic Disorders Sourcebook: Basic Consumer Information About Hereditary Diseases and Disorders*. 4th ed. Detroit, Mich.: Omnigraphics, 2010.
King, Richard A., Jerome I. Rotter, and Arno G. Motulsky, eds. *The Genetic Basis of Common Diseases*. 2d ed. New York: Oxford University Press, 2002.
Leenhardt, Christine, Erik E. Berntorp, and Keith W. Hoots. *Textbook of Hemophilia*. 2d ed. Hoboken, N.J.: Wiley-Blackwell, 2010.
Ma, Alice D., Harold Ross Roberts, and Miguel A. Escobar. *Hemophilia and Hemostasis: A Case-Based Approach to Management*. Hoboken, N.J.: John Wiley & Sons, 2013.
Makris, M., and C. Kasper. "The World Federation of Hemophilia Guideline on Management of Haemophilia." *Haemophilia* 19, no. 1 (December, 2012): 1ff.
National Hemophilia Foundation. http://www.hemo philia.org.
Parker, James N., and Philip M. Parker, eds. *The Official Patient's Sourcebook on Hemophilia: A Revised and Updated Directory for the Internet Age*. San Diego, Calif.: Icon Health, 2005.
Rodak, Bernadette, ed. *Hematology: Clinical Principles and Applications*. 4th ed. St. Louis, Mo.: Saunders/Elsevier, 2012.
Voet, Donald, and Judith G. Voet. *Biochemistry*. 4th ed. Hoboken, N.J.: John Wiley & Sons, 2011.

HEMORRHAGE. *See* BLEEDING.

HEMORRHOID BANDING AND REMOVAL
Procedure

Anatomy or system affected: Anus, blood vessels, circulatory system, gastrointestinal system, intestines

Specialties and related fields: Family medicine, gastroenterology, general surgery, proctology

Definition: The surgical ligation and removal of protruding veins from the lower rectum.

Indications and Procedures

Hemorrhoids, or piles, result from the protrusion or varicosity of veins found within the mucous membranes of the rectum. Hemorrhoids may develop inside or outside the rectum, and they are among the more common of human afflictions.

Hemorrhoids generally develop as a result of increased pressure placed on veins within the rectum. The pressure may be attributable to straining as a result of constipation or to prolonged sitting. In women, they often develop during pregnancy and following childbirth. Treatment depends on the severity of discomfort and location of the hemorrhoid.

External hemorrhoids are often not painful, and they may respond to the application of cool compresses or over-the-counter astringent creams. Creams and suppositories containing steroids may be prescribed by a physician. Internal hemorrhoids may not be noticeable unless a vein ruptures, causing some bleeding, pain, and itching. Since bacteria regularly pass through the rectal area, infection may increase the itching and pain, eventually requiring treatment. If discomfort continues and is not relieved through simple medication, the hemorrhoids may require surgical removal. Several methods exist for removal. Often, the vein is stretched and cut off at its base. Local anesthetics may be necessary, and there may be bleeding and discomfort. Internal hemorrhoids may also be eliminated through cryosurgery, the application of subfreezing temperatures to eliminate tissue. The complete surgical removal of the hemorrhoid, hemorrhoidectomy, may be warranted under certain circumstances.

Hemorrhoid banding, also referred to as rubber band ligation and Barron ligation, involves the placement of a tight rubber band at the base of the hemorrhoid. Over the next few days, the vein will degenerate and slough off. The procedure is relatively simple and can be performed on an outpatient basis. Aside from some discomfort for several days, there are few side effects associated with the banding procedure. Warm sitz baths and local astringents may be helpful in reducing any swelling or pain, and the patient should eat a diet conducive to a soft stool.

—Richard Adler, Ph.D.

See also Blood vessels; Colonoscopy and sigmoidoscopy; Colorectal surgery; Constipation; Cryosurgery; Hemorrhoids; Pregnancy and gestation; Proctology; Rectum; Varicose veins; Vascular medicine; Vascular system.

For Further Information:

A.D.A.M. Medical Encyclopedia. "Hemmorrhoid Surgery." *MedlinePlus*, January 24, 2011.

Becker, Barbara. *Relief from Chronic Hemorrhoids*. New York: Dell, 1992.

"Hemorrhoid Banding." *Health Library*, October 11, 2012.

The Hemorrhoid Book: A Look at Hemorrhoids—How They're Treated and How You Can Prevent Them from Coming Back. San Bruno, Calif.: Krames Communications, 1991.

Mahnke, Daus. "Hemorrhoidectomy." *Health Library*, May 23, 2013.

Parker, James N., and Philip M. Parker, eds. *The Official Patient's Sourcebook on Hemorrhoids*. San Diego, Calif.: Icon Health, 2002.

Peikin, Steven R. *Gastrointestinal Health*. Rev. ed. New York: Quill, 2001.

Sachar, David B., Jerome D. Waye, and Blair S. Lewis, eds. *Pocket Guide to Gastroenterology*. Rev. ed. Baltimore: Williams & Wilkins, 1991.

Wanderman, Sidney E., with Betty Rothbart. *Hemorrhoids*. Yonkers, N.Y.: Consumer Reports Books, 1991.

The Removal of Hemorrhoids

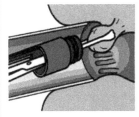 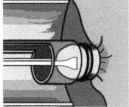

A proctoscope applying
a band to a hemorrhoid

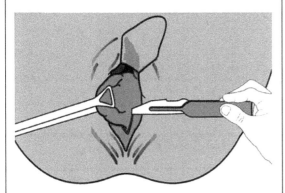

A hemorrhoid being withdrawn
by a clamp and cut off with a scalpel

Severe and distended hemorrhoids may be removed in one of two ways: through the placement of a rubber band around the base of the hemorrhoid, which constricts its blood supply and causes it to wither and drop off; or through surgical excision.

HEMORRHOIDS

Disease/Disorder

Anatomy or system affected: Anus, blood vessels, circulatory system, gastrointestinal system, intestines

Specialties and related fields: Family medicine, gastroenterology, proctology

Definition: Blood-swollen enlargements of specialized tissues that help close the anus, as a result of intravenous pressure in the hemorrhoidal plexus; sometimes called piles.

Key terms:

anus: the valve at the end of the rectum that prevents waste matter from leaking out until a person is ready to defecate

cauterize: to sear tissue with heat or a corrosive substance

dentate line: the junction in the anus where the external skin meets the internal mucosa

gastroenterologist: a physician who specializes in the gastro-intestinal tract and related organs

mucosa: the mucus-secreting membrane that lines the surface of internal organs directly exposed to elements from out-side the body, such as the lungs and intestines

proctologist: a physician who specializes in diseases of the rectum

rectum: the storage compartment at the end of the colon where wastes collect before defecation

stool: the excreted waste products of digestion

thrombosis: the condition of having a clot in a blood vessel

Information on Hemorrhoids

Causes: Increased pressure in lower abdomen result-ing from constipation, diarrhea, long periods of sit-ting, pregnancy and childbirth

Symptoms: Burning, itching, bleeding around anus

Duration: Often short-term but can be chronic

Treatments: Change in dietary and/or lifestyle habits; use of ointments, creams, medicated pads, and sup-positories; surgery if needed

---

Causes and Symptoms

Hemorrhoids, some physiologists suggest, are one of the prices that humans pay for walking upright. The vascular sys-tem—the veins and arteries that circulate blood—evolved in an animal that walked on all fours. Now that humans spend most of their time standing, gravity puts awkward pressure on the system, and at the bottom of major parts of the system, as in the tissue around the anus, the column of blood above weighs heavily on the network of small blood vessels there. It does not take much additional pressure to cause a vessel's wall to balloon out. When it does, the result is a hemorrhoid, a little pouch protruding on the surface of the anus, similar to a hernia or varicose vein. Most people have hemorrhoids, even if they do not realize it, and the major symptoms are rarely dangerous, although they can be annoying and often painful. Sometimes, however, hemorrhoids develop into or mask life-threatening diseases.

The term "hemorrhoid" derives from Greek words mean-ing "blood flowing," an apt description of the circulatory ac-tivity in the anal walls and an inadvertently apt warning of what most alarms people—hemorrhoids occasionally bleed. (The alternative, and now obsolescent, term "piles" comes from Latin *pila*, a ball, apparently a metaphor for the appear-ance of hemorrhoids.) Specifically, the "blood flowing" re-fers to the supple blood vessels of the internal rectal plexus, a series of pouches that act as cushions to help seal the anus shut. When these pouches become enlarged, they turn into hemorrhoids, which jut from the anus wall and swell up to 3 centimeters in length.

Because of the sphincter that controls defecation, not all hemorrhoids are visible without the aid of special instru-ments. The anus, an oval opening about 3 centimeters in front of the spine, is the valve ending the digestive tract. Like the mouth's lips, which begin the tract, the anus can purse shut, a state made possible by two concentric, circular sphincter muscles which act like drawstrings on a cloth bag. When sen-sors in the rectum signal the time to defecate, these muscles relax to pass stool and then immediately contract to close the anus again. As in the mouth, external skin meets the internal mucosal membrane in the anus; the meeting place is a corru-gated joint called the dentate line (or, alternatively, the anorectal juncture or pectinase line). It is in this area—be-tween the skin covering the external (or lower) sphincter and the mucosa over the internal (or upper) sphincter—that hem-orrhoids form. Those that bulge out from the dentate line or above are hidden from sight by the closed anus and are called internal hemorrhoids; those that protrude below the closed anus, and so can be seen or felt, are called external hemorrhoids.

External hemorrhoids are the ones famed for vexing peo-ple. When the skin is stretched over swelled hemorrhoids, its sense receptors are activated, making the hemorrhoids burn and itch, sometimes so intolerably that the urge to scratch them is uncontrollable. Scratching, especially with abrasive materials such as toilet paper, often scrapes and tears the tis-sue. The bright red blood from these lesions is easily notice-able on the toilet paper and may even drip into the toilet bowl or onto underclothes. Likewise, the passage of a hard, dry stool often abrades hemorrhoids to the point of bleeding.

Internal hemorrhoids do not itch or burn and rarely cause pain because the mucosal tissue over them has no nerve end-ings, but they can also bleed when a passing stool damages them. (Pain may be "referred," however, from a damaged in-ternal hemorrhoid to the sciatic nerve, bladder, lower back, or genitals; that is, a person feels little or no pain in the anorectal area, but suddenly pain flares in one of these other areas.) An especially elongated internal hemorrhoid at times can pro-trude through the anus, a condition called prolapse. Usually, it spontaneously recedes or can be pushed back inside with a finger, but upon rare occasion a group of internal hemor-rhoids prolapse, swelling and sending the internal sphincter into painful spasms. A doctor's help may then be required to reduce the pain and fit the hemorrhoids inside.

The blood vessels in the internal rectal plexus swell so eas-ily because they lack valves. Without valves to regulate the local flow of blood, the walls are vulnerable to any sudden in-crease in pressure. Even a small, transient increase above the normal pressure of blood circulation can cause the vessels to bulge. Often, these bulges disappear when the excess pres-sure disappears or remain swollen only briefly afterward. If the increased pressure is high enough, however, a permanent protrusion results, drooping from the anal wall. Even then, if the hemorrhoid is internal, the patient may feel no discomfort and may not realize that a hemorrhoid has formed.

Some people are more susceptible to chronic hemorrhoids than others because of a hereditary lack of elasticity in the blood vessels. In such people, standing for long periods of time can add enough pressure to make hemorrhoids swell.

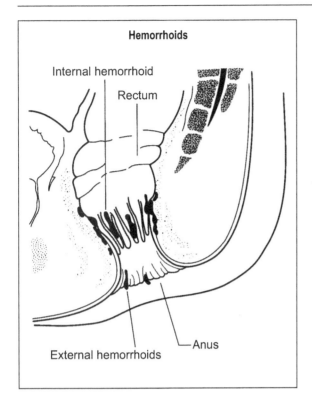

Hemorrhoids

Internal hemorrhoid

Rectum

External hemorrhoids

Anus

from a burst or swollen vessel under the skin—and grow as large as a grape. A doctor can relieve the pain by slicing open the hemorrhoid and squeezing out the clot. Left alone, a thrombosed hemorrhoid may rupture, causing a painful and bloody mess that is ripe for infection. Yet the greatest threat of hemorrhoids lies not in the symptoms themselves but in how they might be confused with those of other, deadly diseases. Colorectal cancer, inflammatory bowel disease, and sexually transmitted diseases such as syphilis, gonorrhea, and herpes can lead to discharges of blood, as can anal fissures (cracks in the anal canal), fistulas (tunnel-like passages between an infected gland and mucosa or skin), and abscesses (pus-filled sacs under the mucosa). A person who dismisses the bloody discharge as simply a flare-up of hemorrhoids may be delaying treatment for the real cause. In the case of colorectal cancer, one of the most common cancers in the United States, such a delay can be fatal. Only a doctor has the tools and vantage point to distinguish between the relatively benign hemorrhoids and a dangerous disorder.

Treatment and Therapy

Since hemorrhoid-like symptoms can be produced by deadly diseases, a thorough checkup at the doctor's office includes an examination of the anus and rectum, especially if the patient has noticed bleeding. In addition to the visual inspection and "digital" examination, during which the doctor inserts a finger and feels around for enlarged hemorrhoids or other masses, patients provide clues by describing the color, amount, and time of bleeding. If the blood is bright red and occurs in small quantities during or just after defecation, hemorrhoids are most likely to blame. If dark red blood or clots appear in the stool or seep out randomly, however, the doctor will look for other causes, inspecting the anus, rectum, and colon with various types of endoscopes, fiber-optic-filled flexible tubes that can also collect tissue samples. Once the doctor rules out other diseases, the patient has three basic choices: change habits, rely on therapy, or have the hemorrhoids removed.

If a person's hemorrhoids do not cause severe discomfort, the doctor will likely recommend a diet with high fiber and water intake. Fiber and water together make stools bulky and soft. They pass more easily during defecation than small, hard, dry stools. The patient does not have to strain, and so no further pressure is put on existing hemorrhoids. Furthermore, soft stools do not scrape hemorrhoids and cause them to bleed. The doctor will also suggest regular exercise, since this helps the bowels work more efficiently and reduces the chance of constipation. Finally, the patient may receive instructions on the proper way to breathe during heavy exertion so as to lessen the stress on the hemorrhoids. With a better diet, more exercise, and less physical straining, patients may find that hemorrhoids have disappeared completely.

Until hemorrhoids shrink, they plague the patient, and to reduce the itching and burning a number of therapies prove effective, if only temporarily. An ice compress eases the discomfort, as does a sitz bath (sitting for at least fifteen minutes in shallow warm water), which also cleanses the site of poten-

Nevertheless, anyone can get hemorrhoids—all that is needed is enough pressure in the lower abdomen. Straining on the toilet to pass stool is the most common cause. People strain when they are constipated or have diarrhea, and since a poor diet can lead to these conditions, hemorrhoids can be a secondary effect of poor eating habits. Those who like to sit on the toilet a long time, reading or watching television while waiting for a bowel movement, also increase pressure on the anus because of the posture and the compressing effect of the toilet ring, and they are likely to develop hemorrhoids. People who regularly lift heavy weights as part of their jobs or for recreation are especially susceptible if they hold their breath while lifting: This action pushes the diaphragm downward on organs below it, including the anus, putting pressure on them. Similarly, during pregnancy women can develop hemorrhoids as the expanding womb crowds and increases pressure on nearby organs; these hemorrhoids are exacerbated by delivery, but they usually go away afterward. Psychologists add to these causes the guilt that some people feel about eating and excreting, guilt spawned by overindulgence in food or bad toilet training; they bear down on their bowels to defecate as quickly as possible and by doing so stress the hemorrhoidal vessels. Finally, hemorrhoids occasionally develop because of some serious diseases, such as heart failure and cirrhosis of the liver, which elevate pressure in the veins, and rectal cancer, which can create a false sense of fullness so that the person strains to pass a stool that is not really there.

Although they seldom do more than itch, external hemorrhoids can thrombose—develop clots of coagulated blood

tially infecting wastes and promotes healing in damaged tissue. Should these relatively simple and cheap measures be impracticable, a variety of ointments, creams, medicated pads, and suppositories, either prescription or nonprescription, may provide relief. Some are inert, such as petroleum jelly, and coat and lubricate the hemorrhoids, protecting them from irritation. Some have an astringent effect, tightening and sealing tissue and thereby protecting it. Others have anesthetic ingredients, numbing the tissue, or anti-inflammatory effects, decreasing swelling. None of these medications has a proven capacity to make swelling go away entirely, and those with active ingredients may cause an allergic response. For patients with

constipation, doctors may prescribe stool softeners to eliminate straining during defecation. Laxatives are usually to be avoided because the chemicals in them irritate hemorrhoids, and the resulting diarrhea often causes urgency and pressure in the rectal area.

When hemorrhoids become chronically and unusually swollen or the patient can no longer endure the discomfort, removing them is the last resort. This cure is certain, although not necessarily permanent, but it has its cost in pain and recovery time. There are seven basic methods, six that cause the target hemorrhoid to shrivel, to drop off on its own, or both, and one, surgery, that removes it directly.

The surgical removal of hemorrhoids, called hemorrhoidectomy, is a relatively simple operation; nevertheless, it is usually reserved for those patients who cannot undergo one of the other methods. The patient is given a local anesthetic to deaden the sensation in the anus, although some patients are rendered unconscious with a general anesthetic. The surgeon cuts off the hemorrhoid at its base and then sews the wound closed with absorbable sutures. The recovery period may require hospitalization for up to a week, during which pain medication, stool softeners, and anal pads are necessary until the tissues heal. Bed rest after hospitalization and sitz baths may also be necessary. Because of this recovery time—as much as a month all together—hemorrhoidectomies are not widely popular among patients or physicians. Moreover, urine retention, infection, and hemorrhaging after the operation are possible complications.

The remaining methods avoid the trauma of cutting, and the first of them, ligation, is one of the oldest of all the methods. Ancient Greek physicians tied a thread around a hemorrhoid to strangle its blood supply; modern gastroenterologists or proctologists use special rubber bands. The effect is the same: The hemorrhoid dries up, shrivels, and falls off. Little pain accompanies the procedure, which is done in the doctor's office.

Likewise, sclerotherapy, cryosurgery, and infrared coagulation are only for internal hemorrhoids because the pain would be too intense on external hemorrhoids. In sclerotherapy, the doctor injects a liquid—usually phenol in oil or quinine in urea—that seals closed the blood vessels at the base of the hemorrhoid. With no blood in them, the vessels eventually shrink to normal dimensions, and, if stressing pressure on them is not resumed, the hemorrhoid disappears.

In cryosurgery, super cold liquid nitrogen or nitrous oxide is applied to the hemorrhoid, freezing it and killing the tissue. The hemorrhoid slowly melts and, as it does, shrinks and finally sloughs off. Popular in the 1970s and early 1980s, cryosurgery lost favor because of the messy and extended recovery time. Useful for mild, small hemorrhoids, infrared coagulation involves a beam of infrared light that, aimed at the hemorrhoid, shrinks it by cauterizing the tissue. The heat of the beam can cause pain in other parts of the anus during the procedure.

The remaining methods, laser surgery and electric current coagulation, can be used on external hemorrhoids. Like infrared coagulation, laser surgery trains a beam of light—in this case intense visible light—that burns and shrinks the hemorrhoid to a stub. Since the laser cauterizes as it destroys tissue and therefore seals off blood vessels, its main advantage over regular surgery lies in reduced bleeding. Recovery time is shorter, about a week, and hospitalization is usually not necessary. This procedure is much more expensive than a hemorrhoidectomy or ligation, however, because of the cost of laser technology. In electric current coagulation, electrodes pass either direct or alternating current through the hemorrhoids. Because tissue is a poor conductor, the resistance to the current creates heat, which cooks the hemorrhoid, coagulating and shrinking it.

Which method the surgeon, gastroenterologist, or proctologist uses depends partly upon the physician's and patient's preferences and partly upon the size and location of the hemorrhoid. Ligation remains the most frequently used method because it is relatively cheap and fast.

Perspective and Prospects

According to Napoleon's personal physician, piles cost the emperor the Battle of Waterloo, which ended his reign. His hemorrhoids were so inflamed and painful on the morning of the battle that he could not get out of bed, much less sit on his horse. Without his personal direction, the French lost. Popular writers often cite this dramatic example, sometimes with humorous overtones, to demonstrate how seriously hemorrhoids can interfere with the lives of even the great.

Certainly, hemorrhoids are no laughing matter. Yet the long-standing taboo in the United States about excretion and the anus has prompted many Americans either to laugh nervously about their hemorrhoids or to keep silent, preferring to suffer stoically rather than to risk becoming the target of jokes. For this reason, it is nearly impossible to say how many sufferers there are in the United States. Estimates vary from several million people to the entire population over the age of thirty.

Whatever the exact statistic, clearly many people share a problem that embarrasses them too much to discuss openly or that they believe is too trivial for medical attention. If they need relief from the itching and pain, they treat themselves. A large industry in home remedies and over-the-counter medications serves them: Rectal medications alone earned drug companies $178 million in 1999, according to the Consumer Healthcare Products Association. The benefits of such medications are difficult to assess, and some authorities claim that petroleum jelly eases the itching and burning as much as any preparation specifically intended for hemorrhoids. Folk remedies, such as suppositories made of tobacco or compresses soaked in papaya juice, can damage tissue outright, making the problem worse. Moreover, throughout the United States specialized clinics offer surgical cures for hemorrhoids, promising patients quick relief on an outpatient basis and using expensive methods, particularly laser surgery.

Many people, therefore, spend considerable money and time, often wasting both, to tend a chronic discomfort that can as readily be prevented or palliated by a change in habits, doctors claim. Like colon cancer and many other intestinal ailments, hemorrhoids are most common in populations whose diet includes a high number of processed foods, which are low in fiber. While fiber is no panacea, people in cultures whose diet contains significant fiber have larger stools and fewer intestinal complaints in general.

Because hemorrhoids are in most cases preventable or controllable without treatment, they have been cited, along with deadly maladies such as colon cancer and inflammatory bowel disease, in criticisms of both the American diet and Americans" eagerness to rely on medical intervention to save them from their own unhealthy habits. In the case of hemorrhoids—while they are not exclusively a malady of Western civilization—the fast pace and pressures of life, the attitudes about defecation, and the eating habits of industrial cultures help give them a distracting prominence.

—*Roger Smith, Ph.D.*

See also Blood vessels; Colon; Colon therapy; Colonoscopy and sigmoidoscopy; Colorectal cancer; Colorectal polyp removal; Colorectal surgery; Cryosurgery; Endoscopy; Hemorrhoid banding and removal; Intestinal disorders; Intestines; Pregnancy and gestation; Rectum; Thrombosis and thrombus.

For Further Information:

Becker, Barbara. *Relief from Chronic Hemorrhoids.* New York: Dell, 1992.
"Help for Hemorrhoids Includes Fiber, Fluids, and Fitness." *Environmental Nutrition* 23, no. 4 (April, 2000): 7.
Litin, Scott C., ed. *Mayo Clinic Family Health Book.* 4th ed. New York: HarperResource, 2009.
Lohsiriwat, Varut. "Approach to Hemorrhoids." *Current Gastroenterology Reports* 15, no. 7 (2013): 1–4.
Minkin, Mary Jane. "Prevent Hemorrhoids." *Prevention* 50, no. 6 (June, 1998): 76.
Okie, Susan. "Colon Susceptible to Other Woes Besides Cancer: The Basics on Everything from Crohn's Disease to Hemorrhoids." *The Washington Post* (February, 1998): Z19.
Okus, Ahmet. "Local Pain-Reducing Methods after Hemorrhoidectomy." *World Journal of Surgery* 37, no. 8 (2013): 2007–2008.
Peikin, Steven R. *Gastrointestinal Health.* Rev. ed. New York: Quill, 2001.
Raspallo, Benjamin M., and Philip Salinitri D. *Hemorrhoids: Symptoms, Diagnosis and Treatment.* New York: Nova Biomedical, 2010.
Sachar, David B., Jerome D. Waye, and Blair S. Lewis, eds. *Pocket Guide to Gastroenterology.* Rev. ed. Baltimore: Williams & Wilkins, 1991.
Wanderman, Sidney E., with Betty Rothbart. *Hemorrhoids.* Yonkers: Consumer Reports Books, 1991.

HEPATITIS

Disease/Disorder

Anatomy or system affected: Liver

Specialties and related fields: Epidemiology, internal medicine, toxicology, virology

Definition: An inflammatory condition of the liver, characterized by discomfort, jaundice, and enlargement of the organ and bacterial, viral, or immunological in origin; may also result from use of alcohol and other toxic drugs.

Key terms:

alanine aminotransferase: a liver enzyme associated with the metabolism of the amino acid alanine; elevated levels are an indication of liver damage

aspartate aminotransferase: a liver enzyme associated with metabolism of the amino acid aspartate; elevated levels are an indication of liver damage

cirrhosis: chronic degeneration of the liver, in which normal tissue is replaced with fibroid tissue and fat; commonly associated with alcohol abuse but can also result from hepatitis

hepatitis A virus: the virus associated with certain forms of hepatitis; generally contracted through fecal contamination of food and water

hepatitis B virus: the agent associated with severe forms of viral hepatitis; contracted through contaminated blood or hypodermic needles or through contaminated body fluids, and sometimes found in association with hepatitis D virus

hepatitis C virus: formerly referred to as the etiological agent for non-A, non-B viral hepatitis; most often passed in contaminated blood

hepato: a prefix denoting anything associated with the liver for example, a hepatocyte is a liver cell

jaundice: a symptom of a variety of liver disorders which manifests as yellowish discoloration of the skin, the whites of the eyes, and other tissues; hepatocellular jaundice results from hepatitis

Causes and Symptoms

Hepatitis, a pathology referring to inflammation of the liver, may result from any of a variety of causes but commonly follows bacterial or viral infection. Hepatitis may be associated with an autoimmune phenomenon in which the body produces antibodies against liver tissue. Liver inflammation may also be an aftereffect of the use of alcohol or various hepatotoxic chemicals, either through the taking of illegal drugs or as a side effect of the legal use of pharmacological agents. Among the pharmaceuticals that can cause liver damage are antibiotics such as isoniazid and rifampin and the painkiller acetaminophen.

Symptoms associated with hepatitis are a reflection of the function of the liver. The liver is arguably the most complex organ in the body. More than five hundred different functions have been associated with the organ, including the production of bile for emulsification of fats and the secretion of glucose,

Information on Hepatitis

Causes: Bacterial or viral infection, immunological disorder, abuse of alcohol and other toxic drugs
Symptoms: Jaundice, liver enlargement, discomfort, fatigue, low-grade fever, nausea, weight loss
Duration: Ranges from short-term to chronic
Treatments: Antibiotics, hospitalization

proteins, or vitamins for use elsewhere in the body. The liver plays a major role in the detoxification of the blood, removing alcohol, nicotine, and other potentially poisonous substances. The Kupffer cells in the liver function in the removal of infectious agents or foreign material from the blood. More than 10 percent of the blood supply in the body is found within the liver at any time.

Among the functions of the liver is the removal of hemoglobin in the blood, which is released as a result of the lysis (disintegration) of red blood cells. A breakdown product of hemoglobin is the yellowish compound bilirubin. It is the buildup of bilirubin in blood that results in the appearance of jaundice in cases of inadequate liver function, such as during hepatitis.

Although hepatitis may develop from a variety of causes, it most commonly results from infection of the liver. Nearly any infectious agent may potentially damage the liver, but generally these involve one of several types of viruses, bacteria, fungi, or amoebas. Liver disease may also be significantly exacerbated by alcohol abuse, as is seen in patients with cirrhosis. Regardless of the specific cause, symptoms of liver disease remain similar in most cases. The liver is often enlarged and tender to physical examination. The person may feel tired and run a low-grade fever. It is not unusual for the person to feel nauseous and lose weight. Jaundice is common in most patients; the concentrations of the enzymes alanine aminotransferase (ALT) and aspartate aminotransferase (AST) may rise. Levels of these enzymes, however, are not necessarily indications of the severity of liver disease; in any event, their levels often fall over the course of the disease.

Three particular viruses have been associated with most forms of viral hepatitis (types A, B, and C), while a fourth (type D) appears as a passenger during some cases of hepatitis B. Several additional viruses, designated hepatitis E (HEV) through hepatitis G (HGV), have also been linked to forms of the disease. Hepatitis A results from infection with the hepatitis A virus (HAV), a virus classified in the same group as the poliovirus and rhinoviruses (cold viruses). The disease is transmitted through a fecal-to-oral method and is self-limited (running a definite and limited course). Often the disease is subclinical (undetectable), particularly as seen in children. Replication of the virus occurs in hepatocytes (liver cells); the virus then passes into the intestine and is eliminated with the feces. A long incubation period following ingestion may occur, sometimes as long as a month, and during the incubation period, the person is capable of transmitting the disease. In otherwise healthy individuals, recovery is complete and occurs over several weeks. Anti-HAV antibodies are present in the blood of about 30 to 40 percent of the general population, reflecting the widespread nature of the disease.

Hepatitis B (HBV), formerly called serum hepatitis, is a potentially much more severe form of the disease. The disease in young children is frequently asymptomatic, with the appearance of symptoms in older individuals being more common. In general, however, the most frequent result of primary infection with HBV is a mild or subclinical course of infection. The disease is most commonly seen in the fifteen-to-thirty-five age group, in part reflecting its method of transmission (through blood or body fluids).

Persistent infection with HBV, occurring in approximately 1 to 3 percent of patients, can be associated with either an asymptomatic carrier state or chronic hepatitis. The chronic state may be severe, with progression to cirrhosis and cellular degeneration or inflammation. In fact, it is the immune response to the presence of HBV that may contribute to liver degeneration. HBV infection results in the expression of viral antigens, which stimulate an immune response on the surface of liver cells. Among the inflammatory cells present at the sites of infection are a large proportion of lymphocytes. These include cytotoxic T cells, which are lymphocytes associated with the killing of virally infected cells. Because immunologically impaired individuals infected with HBV often suffer a mild form of the disease, the possibility exists that it is the immune response itself that contributes to the ensuing liver damage.

Hepatitis B transmission occurs through blood or bodily fluids, including semen and vaginal secretions. Because HBV is also found in saliva, the disease may be transmitted among family members through nonsexual contact. Maternal-neonatal transmission may occasionally occur while the fetus is in the uterus but more likely during the labor or birth process. There is, however, no evidence for transmission through food or water or by an airborne means.

Clinical features of HBV infections are similar to those associated with other forms of hepatitis. In the asymptomatic form of type B disease, AST or ALT levels may be elevated, but jaundice is absent. Adults with symptomatic hepatitis B may suffer jaundice (referred to as *icteric hepatitis*), or they may not (nonicteric hepatitis). There is generally a mild fever, fatigue, and weakness.

Accompanying an indeterminant number of HBV infections is a second virus, designated the hepatitis D virus (HDV). HDV is a defective virus and is capable of replication only in the presence of HBV. Not surprisingly, its geographic distribution and mode of transmission are similar to those of HBV. The prevalence of HDV has been found to be as high as 70 percent in some outbreaks of HBV and nonexistent in others. In most cases, HDV infection results in subclinical or mild hepatitis. In about 15 percent of cases, the disease may progress to a more severe form. HDV may itself be cytopathic (causing pathological changes) for hepatocytes.

Based on the exclusion of other types of etiologic agents, including HAV, HBV, Epstein-Barr virus, and cytomegalovirus, non-A, non-B (NANB) hepatitis was considered a clinical entity. During the late 1980s, NANB hepatitis was determined to be caused by a newly isolated infectious agent, designated hepatitis C virus (HCV). The study of HCV was hampered by the inability to grow the virus in cell culture. Ironically, the virus was cloned and characterized before it was even physically observed, allowing for the development of a screening assay used for the detection of contaminated serum. Before screening procedures were put into place in 1992, HCV infection was the major complication of blood transfusions or transfusions of blood products. Infection now occurs through sexual intercourse, the sharing of intravenous needles, and accidental needle punctures among health care workers. HCV has been increasingly recognized as a major health threat, and in 2012 it was reported that more deaths occurred in the United States from hepatitis C than from HIV, the AIDS-causing virus. HAC creates serious liver damage and is the leading cause of liver transplants. It is all the more dangerous because patients are often asymptomatic and learn of the infection when their blood is screened for other reasons. As a result, many people are unknowing carriers of the virus.

Outbreaks of an enterically transmitted NANB hepatitis (NANB hepatitis transmitted through the intestines), designated hepatitis E, have also been found in some parts of the world. Although hepatitis E was first documented in 1955, it wasn't until the late 1980s that it was determined to be a unique form of the disease. Transmission occurs through eating or drinking contaminated food or water, though there is evidence that household contact with infected persons may also transmit the disease. Hepatitis E is most common in poor countries of Asia, with sporadic outbreaks elsewhere. The few cases found in the United States have involved travelers to these areas.

Acute hepatitis is less commonly associated with infection by other viruses. These include the herpes family of viruses, such as herpes simplex, cytomegalovirus, and Epstein-Barr virus. Because the prevalence of these viruses is quite high, immunosuppressed or immunodeficient patients may be at particular risk.

Certain forms of hepatitis are associated with an autoimmune response. In these cases, the cause is not an infectious agent but rather a form of rejection by the body of its own liver tissue. Autoimmune hepatitis is suspected in individuals in which the disease persists for at least six months with no evidence of exposure to an infectious agent or hepatotoxin. In nearly one-third of these individuals, other immunological diseases such as lupus or arthritis may be present. The clinical manifestations of autoimmune hepatitis are similar to those of other forms of the disease. Most patients exhibit jaundice, a mild fever, weakness, and weight loss. The liver is often enlarged and tender. Unlike other forms of hepatitis, found equally in men and women, autoimmune hepatitis is most commonly found in women. Prognosis of the disease is unclear, as an unknown percentage of cases are subclinical. Severe forms have a high fatality rate.

Treatment and Therapy

Treatment for the various forms of viral hepatitis is, for the most part, symptomatic and supportive. Hospitalization may be required in severe cases, but, in general, any restriction of activity is left up to the patient. This is particularly convenient, since recovery often involves a long convalescence. As long as a healthy diet is maintained, no special dietary requirements exist, but a high-calorie diet is often preferable. Drugs or chemicals that are potentially damaging to the liver, including alcohol and certain antibiotics or painkillers, should be avoided.

Hepatitis induced by other forms of infectious agents such as bacteria or fungi may be treated using an appropriate course of antibiotic therapy. In cases of drug-induced disease, avoidance of the chemical is a key to recovery. Bacterial infections of the liver are often associated with patients who are malnourished, such as the elderly or alcoholics, or who may be immunosuppressed. These problems must also be addressed during the course of treatment.

Prevention of the disease is preferable, however, and because the means of viral spread has been well established in most cases, appropriate measures can often be taken. For the most part, the viruses associated with hepatitis have little in common with one another aside from their predilection for hepatocytes. Thus, preventing their spread involves different strategies.

HAV is almost always spread through a fecal–oral means of transmission. Often the source is an infected person involved in the preparation of uncooked foods. Common sense dictates that the person should wash after every use of a toilet, but this is often not the case. Not surprisingly, children attending day-care centers frequently become infected. Contaminated groundwater is also a potential source of outbreak in areas in which proper sewage treatment does not take place. Less commonly, HAV is spread directly from person to person through sexual contact. A method called immunoprophylaxis can prevent the development of symptoms in individuals exposed to hepatitis A by utilizing a form of passive immunity. Developed during World War II, the procedure involves the pooling of serum from immune individuals. In most cases, inoculation is effective in prevention of the disease.

In 1994, SmithKline Beecham Pharmaceuticals developed and received Food and Drug Administration (FDA) approval for the first vaccine shown to be safe and effective in preventing HAV infection. Manufactured under the trade name Havrix, the vaccine consists of a formalin-inactivated strain of HAV to be administered in three doses to children. In 1996, a similar vaccine was developed by Merck and Co. to be sold under the trade name Vagta. In 2001, a combined hepatitis A and hepatitis B vaccine was developed and approved in the United States for use in individuals eighteen and older. It is given in three doses over a period of six months. In 2002, the Centers for Disease Control recommended that any individuals at risk for hepatitis A infection or those at risk for becoming seriously ill if infected should receive immunization against the virus.

The transmission of HBV generally involves passage via contaminated blood or body secretions. Before blood screening was standard procedure, blood transfusions were the most common means of spreading the disease—hence the designation "serum hepatitis." Since the 1980s, however, the most common means of documented spread has been through either sexual contact or through the sharing of contaminated hypodermic needles. Semen, vaginal secretions, and saliva from infected individuals all contain the active virus, and limiting exchange of these fluids is key to prevention of transmission. Even so, the means of infection in nearly one-third of symptomatic cases remains unknown.

In 2002, the Centers for Disease Control recommended that certain groups of individuals who are at high risk for exposure to HBV be vaccinated against the virus: children (newborn to eighteen years old), intravenous drug users, sexually active heterosexuals and homosexual men, healthcare workers, and those in contact with hepatitis B-infected individuals. It was also recommended that those who would become seriously ill if they contracted the virus be vaccinated: newborns, hemophiliacs, those with any chronic liver disease, and those waiting for a liver transplant.

Because the hepatitis D virus is defective in replication and requires the presence of HBV, no specific measures of prevention are necessary. Immunization against HBV is sufficient to prevent the spread of HDV.

The deadly HCV is treated with antiviral agents, such as ribavirin and shots of interferon. A longer-acting form called pegylated interferon (Pegasys) is shown to help in the early stages of the virus.

Hepatitis E is also transmitted through a fecal-oral route. Drinking water contaminated by sewage has been the most common source of transmission. Because no active means of prevention has been developed, prevention of exposure requires that the individual avoid any food or water potentially contaminated with sewage. This is particularly true in areas of the world in which hepatitis E is found. Though the precaution may seem obvious, the safety of the water, as well as any object washed in the water, is not always readily apparent.

Autoimmune hepatitis results from an aberrant immune system rather than from an infectious agent. Treatment generally involves the use of immunosuppressive drugs to limit the immune response. Corticosteroids such as prednisone, sometimes in combination with azathioprine, have proven effective in the therapy of many patients. Still, in some cases the disease progresses to cirrhosis and results in death. Treatment generally is carried out over a long period of time, at least a year, and relapses are common. Often, the patient requires lifetime therapy. The immunosuppressive activity of the therapy may also leave the patient more susceptible to infection. In some cases, liver transplantation has proven effective, at least in the short term. Because the liver rejection was caused by an autoimmune response in the first place, the transplant may also be subject to the same phenomenon.

Perspective and Prospects

Inflammation of the liver resulting in hepatitis can develop from a variety of mechanisms. Most often, these mechanisms are associated with either a chemical injury or infection by a microbiological agent.

Infections of the liver generally involve one of several viral agents. The association of liver disease, or at least jaundice, with an infectious agent was suspected as early as the fifth century BCE when Hippocrates described a syndrome that was undoubtedly viral hepatitis. The disease was also described in the Babylonian Talmud about eight hundred years later. Epidemics of the disease, which most likely involved outbreaks of hepatitis A, have been reported since the Middle Ages. The spread of this disease through personal contact was confirmed in the 1930s.

Type B, or serum, hepatitis, was described as a clinical entity by A. Lurman in 1855. Lurman observed that 15 percent of shipyard workers in Bremen, Germany, who received a smallpox vaccine containing human lymph developed jaundice within the following six months. In the early years of the twentieth century, jaundice frequently developed among patients who received vaccines prepared from convalescent serums or who underwent procedures such as venipuncture using instruments that had not been properly sterilized. By 1926, the blood-borne nature of the disease had been confirmed. In 1942, more than twenty-eight thousand American soldiers developed jaundice after being vaccinated against yellow fever with a vaccine prepared from pooled human serums. By then it had become obvious that at least two forms of infectious agents were associated with viral hepatitis.

The isolation of HBV occurred as a result of studies initiated by Baruch Blumberg in 1963. Blumberg was actually attempting to correlate the development of diseases such as cancer with particular patterns of proteins found in the serum of individuals. His approach was to collect blood from persons in various parts of the world and then analyze their serum proteins. Blumberg found an antigen, a protein, in the blood of Australian aborigines that reacted with antibodies in the blood of an American hemophiliac. Blumberg called the protein the Australia (Au) antigen. It later became apparent that the Au antigen could be isolated from the blood of patients with serum hepatitis. By 1970, it was established that what Blumberg had referred to as the Au antigen was in fact the HBV particle.

HBV is associated with more than simply viral hepatitis. Chronic hepatitis associated with HBV can often develop into hepatocellular carcinoma, or cancer of the liver. The precise reason is unclear; the cancer may result from the chronic damage to liver tissue associated with long-term infection by HBV.

Cases of HCV continue to climb because of the high numbers of asymptomatic carriers. In 2012, it was reported that deaths as a result of HCV had outnumbered AIDS-related deaths, making HCV one of the next important threats to global health.

—*Richard Adler, Ph.D.;*
updated by Tracy Irons-Georges

See also Addiction; Alcoholism; Autoimmune disorders; Cirrhosis; Immunization and vaccination; Jaundice; Liver; Liver cancer; Liver disorders; Liver transplantation; Nonalcoholic steatohepatitis (NASH); Viral infections.

For Further Information:

Boyer, Thomas D., Teresa L. Wright, and Michael P. Manns, eds. *Zakim and Boyer's Hepatology: A Textbook of Liver Disease*. 5th ed. Philadelphia: Saunders/Elsevier, 2006.

Chwistek, Marcin. "Hepatitis C." *Health Library*, March 2012.

Everson, Gregory T., and Hedy Weinberg. *Living with Hepatitis C: A Survivor's Guide*. 5th ed. New York: Hatherleigh Press, 2009.

Frank, Steven A. *Immunology and Evolution of Infectious Disease*. Princeton, N.J.: Princeton University Press, 2002.

Gorbach, Sherwood L., John G. Bartlett, and Neil R. Blacklow, eds. *Infectious Diseases*. 3d ed. Philadelphia: W. B. Saunders, 2004.

Hepatitis Foundation International. http://www.hepatitisfoundation.org.

Humes, H. David, et al., eds. *Kelley's Textbook of Internal Medicine*. 4th ed. Philadelphia: Lippincott Williams & Wilkins, 2000.

Levine, Arnold. *Viruses*. New York: W. H. Freeman, 1992.

Loftus, Peter. "Patient Dilemma: Treat Hepatitis C Now or Hold Out?" *The Wall Street Journal*, March 4, 2013.

Palmer, Melissa. *Dr. Melissa Palmer's Guide to Hepatitis and Liver Disease*. Rev. ed. Garden City Park, N.Y.: Avery, 2004.

Porter, Lucinda K. *Hepatitis C Treatment One Step at a Time*. New York: Demos Health Publishing, 2013.

Shaw, Michael, ed. *Everything You Need to Know About Diseases*. Springhouse, Pa.: Springhouse Press, 1996.

Spector, Steven. *Viral Hepatitis: Diagnosis, Therapy, and Prevention*. Totowa, N.J.: Humana Press, 1999.

"Viral Hepatitis Headquarters." *Centers for Disease Control/National Prevention Information Network*. April 12, 2013.

Zieve, David, and George F. Longstreth. "Hepatitis A." *The New York Times Health Guide*, May 21, 2013.

HERBAL MEDICINE

Treatment

Also known as: Plant medicine

Anatomy or system affected: All

Specialties and related fields: All

Definition: The traditional and scientific application of chemicals directly derived from any part of plants for medicinal purposes. The medicinal uses of plants are for both preventive and curative purposes.

Key terms:

alkaloid: a large group of compounds that contain nitrogen and usually have a basic reaction (for example, cocaine, caffeine, nicotine, quinine, and morphine)

antiseptic: a chemical substance that inhibits the growth of bacteria

glycoside: a compound containing a carbohydrate molecule (sugar) that yields glucose on hydrolysis and a nonsugar component called aglycone

hormone: chemical messengers produced by the tissues of an organism to act as signaling compounds for the regulation of functions

hypertension: persistent high blood pressure

hypotension: low blood pressure

leukemia: a cancer of the blood-forming organs, marked by the abnormal multiplication and development of leukocytes

pathogen: any agent or microorganism capable of producing disease

pharmaceutical: a medicinal drug

purgative: referring to substances that promote the rapid elimination of material from the digestive tract

The Chemicals of Plant-Derived Medicines

Plants synthesize a wide array of secondary compounds that play a role in the physiology of plants but do not usually constitute an important part of the basic metabolism of plants. Secondary compounds enable plants to attract animals and also help plants to avoid or overcome their natural enemies of infection, parasitism, and predation. These secondary compounds are the main chemicals in plants that humans use as medicinal herbs. Fatty acids, essential oils, gums, resins, alkaloids, and steroids are the most common secondary compounds in plants.

Humans use oils and gums as purgatives and as carriers or emulsifiers in many drug preparations. Volatile oils and resins are often used to help processes that seek to penetrate tissues of the body and are also used as antiseptics. Alkaloids and steroids are the two major classes of plant-derived compounds used in human medicine today. These chemical compounds can occur in different forms that have one or more sugar molecules attached. Such forms, called "glycosides," are often the medicinally active form of a compound.

All forms of steroids are complex chemical compounds that have the same fundamental structure of four carbon rings, called the "backbone." When different chemical groups are added at different places on the backbone, a variety of steroidal compounds are produced as a result. For example, when sugar molecules are added to the carbon rings, steroidal glycosides are produced. Various cardiac glycosides and steroid hormones are produced by the addition of specific side chains or extra rings to the steroid backbone.

The second major group of medicinally important chemicals synthesized in plants is the alkaloids. They contain nitrogen and usually exhibit an alkaline reaction. Alkaloids were formerly considered secondary products, but unlike steroids, they have recently been shown occasionally to enter into the primary metabolism of plants. Some alkaloids are extremely poisonous to humans, and many have been used as poisons in various cultures around the world. Several of these plant chemicals possess antimicrobial properties and are used to kill harmful microorganisms that are pathogenic. A number of them are used as dietary supplements for balanced human nutrition and good health.

Medicinal Plants of Importance

In the past, some natural chemicals and oils were of tremendous medicinal use in treating diseases. Quinine was used for the treatment of malaria, cocaine was used as a stimulant and a local anesthetic, and chaulmoogra oil was employed for the treatment of leprosy. Although these herbal medicines are rarely used today, many plants are still of great importance as sources of medicinal compounds. Both steroids and glycosides occur in many angiosperms.

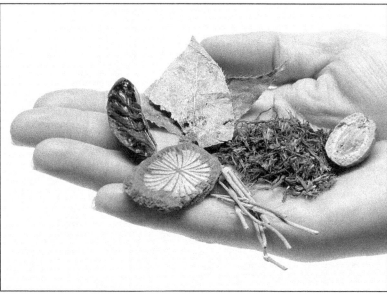

A variety of herbs can be used to prevent and treat illnesses. (PhotoDisc)

To cite a few examples, certain members of the yam genus *Dioscorea* contain particular kinds of steroids in their tubers called "saponins" that are similar to human sex hormones. The chemical diosgenin can be extracted from the tubers, which is a good starting point for the chemical synthesis of saponins. The majority of the hormones synthesized from diosgenin are used in birth control pills, for the production of hormones that regulate the menstrual cycle, or as a component of fertility drugs. Cortisone and hydrocortisone are two other important hormones that are synthesized from diosgenin. They are used for the treatment of severe allergic reactions, arthritis, and Addison disease, which is caused by malfunctioning of the adrenal glands.

Opium poppy, *Papaver somniferum*, is one of the oldest and still predominant sources of analgesics, which relieve pain. More than twenty-six different alkaloids have been isolated from opium, but only three of them—morphine, codeine, and papaverine—are used extensively. Morphine and codeine are used as painkillers, and papaverine is used primarily in drugs for the treatment of internal spasms, particularly those of the intestinal tract.

Another group of alkaloids is obtained from members of the potato family. They are considered analgesics and are used for controlling a variety of muscle spasms and in psychiatry. Alkaloids from *Atropa belladonna* are prescribed for stomach and bladder cramps and to prevent nausea and vomiting caused by motion sickness. They are prescribed for victims of Parkinson's disease to decrease stiffness and tremors and are often given to patients before surgery as a relaxant and to reduce salivation. These alkaloids, especially atropine, may be helpful in cases of nerve gas (organophosphate insecticide) or mushroom poisoning. Alkaloids of the North American lily such as American false hellebore, *Veratrum viride*, have hypotensive properties and are used to treat high blood pressure.

Cinchona, the genus known primarily as a source of quinine, produces about thirty other alkaloids, including the compound quinidine, which is useful in treating heart disease. Quinidine inhibits abnormal rapid contractions of the upper right chamber of the heart and corrects improper heart rhythms.

Rauwolfia serpentina was used in the past for treating snakebites. It was later found to be useful in the treatment of hypertension by relaxing the heart muscle and thus lowering blood pressure; however, it produced the side effects of depression and tremors, and its use was therefore discontinued. In 1952, in Switzerland, the important alkaloid reserpine was isolated from the root where it is concentrated, although it occurs everywhere in the plant. The dramatic effects of reserpine completely altered practices in mental institutions because of its pronounced calming effect on schizophrenics without producing undesirable side effects. A relatively New World species, *R. tetraphylla*, is also a source of the alkaloid.

The few known substances that are able to arrest cancer cells are plant alkaloids. The common periwinkle, *Catharanthus reseus*, has been used in its native range in Europe for hundreds of years as a folk treatment for diabetes. It is now used effectively to treat some cancers and leukemias, especially those that commonly afflict children. The two active alkaloids are vinblastine and vincristine. Mayapple, *Podophylum peltatum*, contains antitumor alkaloids. Today, mayapple alkaloids are used as the basis of VM-26 (teniposide), a drug used to treat testicular tumors and, with other agents, breast and lung cancer. The alkaloid colchicine is extracted from the corms of the autumn crocus, *Colchicum autumnale*. Colchicine is primarily used for the reduction of inflammation and pain caused by gout but is also used in the treatment of cancer. Taxol, a compound most abundant in the bark of the Pacific yew, *Taxus brevifolia*, has been a major success in the treatment of breast and uterine cancer.

Several mucilaginous compounds of plant origin are used in soothing ointments and as carriers for other medicines. Species of *Aloe*, primarily *A. barbadensis*, have been used for their soothing gels. Chymopapain, an enzyme that exhibits specificity in its dissolution of proteins, is obtained from papaya, *Carica papaya*. It is injected by doctors into the soft central area of a deformed spinal disk in humans to dissolve a large part of it and relieve the pressure on adjacent nerves.

Perspective and Prospects

The medicinal uses of plants by humans have been known since ancient times and can be said to predate written history. Every culture on earth has used plants to cure disease, ease pain, and heal the ills and discomforts of the human body. People first started to keep records of herbal medicine about five thousand to seven thousand years ago in China and Mesopotamia. Sumerian drawings of opium poppy capsules from 2500 BCE suggest that considerable knowledge of medicinal plants was in place. A substantial record of the use of herbs in medicine comes from the Code of Hammurabi, a series of tablets carved under the direction of the king of Babylon in about 1770 BCE. These tablets mention plants, such as henbane, licorice, and mint, that are still used in medicines. The Egyptians later recorded their knowledge of illnesses and cures on temple walls and in the Ebers papyrus (1550 BCE), which contains more than seven hundred medicinal formulas.

In Greece, Hippocrates (ca. 460–ca. 370 BCE) prescribed sound nutrition, purgatives, and botanical drugs for humans. He consequently earned the reputation as the founder of medicine by being the first person to document illnesses and their treatments in a rational and orderly fashion. The most significant contribution made by the Greeks toward the documentation of plants with healing properties was made by Dioscorides in his five-volume work entitled *De Materia Medica*. His encyclopedia described the preparation of about one thousand simple drugs. For several centuries afterward, it was the foundation text for practitioners of herbal medicine throughout Europe.

A stronger link was established between the studies of botany and medicine during the Middle Ages, and printed herbals became more available with the invention of the printing press in 1439. More herbs were added to the list from the New World when Europeans arrived in North America and learned American Indian herbal uses. In the fourteenth century, the Renaissance led Europe into the determination of the medicinal uses of plants.

In the seventeenth and eighteenth centuries, science and philosophy advanced to the stage of experiments and hypothesis testing. It was not until the early nineteenth century, however, that scientists first began to isolate and extract healing compounds from plants. This experimental approach to medicine led to an improved understanding of physiology and provided a framework for the careful testing of medical treatments, including medicinal herbs.

The first half of the twentieth century saw tremendous advancements in medicine as more causes of diseases were discovered and new effective drugs were produced. Several modern medicines were produced as isolated and purified products of traditional plant-derived extracts, including morphine, quinine, and ephedrine. Medical chemists then began to determine the structures of these compounds and the possibility of their synthesis. In addition, they explored the chances of using the knowledge of the active ingredients of a natural healing herb to synthesize chemically related compounds that were potentially better medicines than the original one.

In the latter part of the twentieth century and the beginning of the twenty-first century, the prevalence of some diseases in some parts of the world and the emergence of diseases such as acquired immunodeficiency syndrome (AIDS) and severe acute respiratory syndrome (SARS) have challenged scientists, botanists, and doctors to explore plant sources for drugs that will offer possible or better cures.

Medicinal herbs are central to alternative therapies, which are gaining popularity in the twenty-first century. This trend is partly attributable to modern research into plant medicine and the remarkable healing results of herbal application to some diseases. For example, years of studies have shown that garlic can help control blood pressure and cholesterol. Yet few mainstream doctors recommend it, even though garlic is cheaper than pharmaceuticals and causes fewer side effects. This situation is beginning to change, however, because of a growing interest in natural sources of medicine. An estimated 80 percent of the world's population still rely on traditional medicine, and particularly herbs, for treating and preventing disease. Native American herbs are still used by North American doctors in the twenty-first century. Many people do not realize that medical herbs are a key link between alternative therapies and mainstream medicine. Scientists around the world depend on herbs to develop new, more potent medications, and the search continues for plants with healing properties.

According to the World Health Organization, herbal medicines were regulated in over 100 countries in 2008. However, in the United States, herbal remedies do not require testing before use by the public, and the 1994 Dietary Supplement Health and Education Act (DSHEA) does not require proof of safety or efficacy. Since the Federal Food and Drug Administration (FDA) issued good manufacturing practices for the industry in 2007, US herbal supplement manufacturers have been required to ensure the "identity, purity, strength, and composition" of their ingredients.

—Samuel V. A. Kisseadoo, Ph.D.;
updated by LeAnna DeAngelo, Ph.D.

See also Alternative medicine; Antioxidants; Food biochemistry; Homeopathy; Marijuana; Nutrition; Over-the-counter medications; Pharmacology; Pharmacy; Self-medication; Supplements; Toxicology.

For Further Information:

"Botanical Dietary Supplements." *Office of Dietary Supplements, National Institutes of Health*, June 24, 2011.

Castleman, Michael. *Blended Medicine: How to Integrate the Best Mainstream and Alternative Remedies for Maximum Health and Healing*. Emmaus, Pa.: Rodale Press, 2002.

"Herbal Medicine." *Health Library*, July 25, 2012.

"Herbal Products and Supplements." *American Academy of Family Physicians*, February, 2012.

Maleskey, Gale, and the editors of Prevention Health Books. *Nature's Medicines: From Asthma to Weight Gain, from Colds to High Cholesterol—The Most Powerful All-Natural Cures*. Emmaus, Pa.: Rodale Press, 1999.

National Center for Complementary and Alternative Medicine. *Herbs at a Glance: A Quick Guide to Herbal Supplements*. Bethesda, Md.: U.S. Department of Health and Human Services, 2010.

Simpson, Beryl Brintnall, and Molly Conner Ogorzaly. *Economic Botany: Plants in Our World*. 3d ed. Boston: McGraw-Hill, 2001.

"Traditional and Complementary Medicine." *World Health Organization*, 2013.

White, B. Linda, and Steven Foster. *The Herbal Drugstore*. Emmaus, Pa.: Rodale Press, 2003.

Yeager, Selene. *The Doctor's Book of Food Remedies*. Emmaus, Pa.: Rodale Press, 2008.

HERMAPHRODITISM AND PSEUDOHERMAPHRODITISM

Disease/Disorder

Anatomy or system affected: Genitals, reproductive system, urinary system

Specialties and related fields: Embryology, endocrinology, genetics, gynecology, urology

Definition: Abnormal primary sexual characteristics caused by developmental defects.

Information on Hermaphroditism and Pseudohermaphroditism

Causes: Genetic defect of sex organs
Symptoms: Abnormal appearance of primary sexual characteristics
Duration: Chronic unless corrected
Treatments: Hormone therapy, surgery

Causes and Symptoms

Ambiguous genitalia is usually caused by a variation in the number of sex chromosomes or in prenatal exposure to key hormones. Males normally possess one X and one Y chromosome, while females normally have two X chromosomes. When an embryo has a different number or configuration of these chromosomes, normal urogenital development is disrupted and, in some cases, the resulting internal and external sex organs do not match. Inappropriate levels of male and female hormones during fetal development are also responsible for ambiguous genitalia. The main categories of ambiguous genitalia conditions are true gonadal intersex (formerly called "hermaphroditism"), 46, XY intersex ("male pseudohermaphroditism"), and 46, XX intersex ("female pseudohermaphroditism").

True gonadal intersex is a condition in which testicular and ovarian tissues are found in the same person and their urogenital development is ambiguous. A baby with an enlarged clitoris resembling a penis (clithoromegaly) and fused labial-scrotal folds may be assigned to the male sex at birth, whereas a baby with a normal clitoris and open labial-scrotal folds might be considered a female at birth. Hypospadias, a condition in which urethra opens somewhere around or along the clitoris, penis, or vaginal canal, often occurs and lends further ambiguity to the appearance of the external genitalia. Similarly, testicles may be or believed to be undescended. The exact cause of this condition is generally unknown.

Persons with 46, XY intersex may develop internal testes, but their external genitals at birth appear female, incompletely male, or indeterminate. The undervirilization responsible for 46, XY intersex results from a lack of testosterone during fetal development. Among the causes are testicular malfunction; inadequate testosterone production; 5-alpha-reductase enzyme deficiency (sometimes called "guevedoces syndrome"), in which testosterone cannot be converted to 5-alpha-dihydrotestosterone (DHT), the inducer needed for the early development of male tissues; or malfunction in testosterone receptors, known as androgen insensitivity syndrome (AIS) or testicular feminization syndrome (TFS).

Individuals with AIS may lack ovaries, Fallopian tubes, and a uterus, but have a "blind" (dead-end) vagina and breasts; testes may or may not be present. As they enter puberty, they begin to grow genital hair and breasts and have the appearance of normal girls because they are unable to respond to testosterone. Menstruation will not occur, however. When individuals with 5-alpha-reductase enzyme deficiency begin puberty, the clitoris enlarges into a penis-like structure without a urethra. The urethral opening is at the base of the enlarged clitoris. One or both of the internal testes descend into scrotal sacs, and the teenager begins to develop masculine body and facial hair, but there is no breast development. In some cases, the voice deepens, and muscle mass and body shape become more masculine. At puberty, the testes produce very large amounts of testosterone, which is able to make up for the lack of DHT and to stimulate some tissues to develop further.

Persons with 46, XX intersex often have clithoromegaly and fused labia, while the female internal organs develop normally. Female hormones produced at puberty lead to the development of female secondary sex characteristics, unless testosterone is administered. The virilization that causes 46, XX intersex may result from congenital adrenal hyperplasia, a kidney disorder that produces excess androgen in the fetus; ovarian tumors in the mother; aromatase enzyme deficiency, in which male hormones cannot be converted to female hormones; or other sources of prenatal testosterone exposure.

Treatment and Therapy

The most common forms of treatment are hormone therapy and surgery. Hormone therapy might be of value in helping to establish the gender roles affected individuals desire in their culture. Surgery may be required at birth to correct hypospadias or other conditions that impair proper urinary function. Concerned parents should consult with their physicians about the child's specific condition, the possible underlying causes, and the risks and benefits of various treatment options. Psychological counseling is recommended for parents and individuals with ambiguous genitalia, particularly with respective to making treatment decisions.

Perspective and Prospects

In the past, parents and physicians were quick to assign a sex to an infant with ambiguous genitalia and pursue surgery to make the genitalia more recognizably male or female. Immediate surgery is now recommended only to improve or restore function, and families are encouraged to involve the intersex person in making decisions about gender and sexual identity and treatments that support those decisions.

In general, persons with ambiguous genitalia are content with their sexual assignments and are no more likely to seek sex reassignment or to change gender later in life than are persons born with normal genitalia; however, gender-atypical behavior may be associated with some intersex conditions. Intersex individuals also appear just as likely to be heterosexual as the general population. Normal puberty may be absent in affected individuals, and fertility can be an issue in adulthood.

—*Jaime S. Colomé, Ph.D.*

See also Gender reassignment surgery; Genetic diseases; Genetics and inheritance; Hormone therapy; Hormones; Puberty and adolescence; Reproductive system; Sexual differentiation.

For Further Information:

"46, XXX Testicular Disorder of Sex Development." *Genetics Home Reference*, May 20, 2013.

"Ambiguous Genitalia." *MedlinePlus*, May 7, 2012.

"Ambiguous Genitalia." *Mayo Foundation for Medical Education and Research*, March 16, 2012.

"Androgen Insensitivity Syndrome." *MedlinePlus*, July 19, 2012.

"Answers to Your Questions about Individuals with Intersex Conditions." *American Psychological Association*, 2013.

Dreger, Alice Domurat. *Hermaphrodites and the Medical Invention of Sex*. Cambridge, Mass.: Harvard University Press, 2003.

Fausto-Sterling, Anne. *Sexing the Body: Gender Politics and the Construction of Sexuality*. New York: Basic Books, 2000.

Hellinga, Gerhardus. *Clinical Andrology: A Systematic Approach, with a Chapter on Intersexuality*. London: Heinemann, 1976.

Hunter, R. H. F. *Sex Determination, Differentiation, and Intersexuality in Placental Mammals*. New York: Cambridge University Press, 1995.

"Intersex." *MedlinePlus*, August 2, 2011.

Karkazis, Katrina Alicia. *Fixing Sex: Intersex, Medical Authority, and Lived Experience*. Durham, N.C.: Duke University Press, 2008.

Kessler, Suzanne J. *Lessons from the Intersexed*. New Brunswick, N.J.: Rutgers University Press, 2002.

Moore, Keith L., and T. V. N. Persaud. *The Developing Human*. 8th ed. Philadelphia: Saunders/Elsevier, 2008.

Morland, Iain, ed. *Intersex and After*. Durham, N.C.: Duke University Press, 2009.

Hernia
Disease/Disorder

Anatomy or system affected: Abdomen, gastrointestinal system, intestines, reproductive system, stomach

Specialties and related fields: Gastroenterology, internal medicine

Definition: A pouchlike mass consisting of visceral material encased in properitoneal tissue (the hernial sac) protruding through an aperture in the abdomen-a result of a weakening in the abdominal wall.

Key terms:

Bassini technique: the most widely accepted surgical method for treating hernias; named after the Italian surgeon Edoardo Bassini

hernioplasty: the surgery performed to treat hernia patients

incarceration: an advanced and dangerous hernial stage which occurs when the hernial sac protrudes well beyond the abdominal aperture and is constricted at the neck

inguinal hernia: the most common form of hernia, in which the hernial sac protrudes into the lower groin area

reducible hernia: a hernia that has not advanced significantly beyond the weakened aperture in the abdomen; such hernias were formerly treated by means of the externally applied pressure of a truss

Causes and Symptoms

A hernia condition exists when either tissues from, or actual portions of, vital internal organs protrude beyond the enclosure of the abdomen as a result of an abnormal opening in several possible areas of the abdominal wall. In most hernias, the protruding material remains encased in the tissue of the peritoneum. This saclike extension forces itself into whatever space can be ceded by neighboring tissues outside the abdomen. Because of the swelling effect produced, the hernia is usually visible as a lump on the surface of the body. As there are several types of hernias that may occur in different areas of the abdomen, the place of noticeable swelling and the internal organs affected may vary. With the single exception of the pancreas, hernia cases have been recorded involving all other organs contained in the abdomen. The most common hernial protrusions, however, involve the small intestine and/or the omenta, folds of the peritoneum. Another category of hernia, referred to as hernia adipose, consists of a protrusion of peritoneal fat beyond the abdominal wall.

Generally speaking, the cause of hernial conditions involves not only an internal pressure pushing portions of the viscera against the abdominal wall (hence the danger of bringing on a hernia through heavy physical exertion in work or athletics) but also a point of weakness in the abdominal wall itself. Two such points of potential weakness exist in all normal, healthy individuals: the original umbilical ring, which should normally "heal" over after the umbilical cord is severed; and the groin tissues in the lower portion of the abdomen—the region where the most common hernia, the inguinal hernia, occurs. Another possible source of vulnerability to hernia protrusions is connected to the individual's prior surgical history: Scar tissue may prove to be the weakest point of resistance to pressures originating anywhere in the abdominal region.

It should be noted that, because the abdominal tissues of infants and young children are particularly delicate, there is a proportionately higher occurrence of hernial conditions among babies and toddlers. If the hernia is diagnosed and treated early enough, complete healing is almost certain in such cases, most of which do not develop beyond the preliminary, or reducible, stage.

The several stages, or degrees, of hernial development usually begin with what doctors call a reducible hernia condition. At this stage, a patient suffering from hernia, sensing the onset of the disorder, may be able to obtain temporary relief from a developing protrusion by changing posture angle when upright or by lying down. Until the late twentieth century, some physicians preferred to treat reducible hernias by means of an externally attached pressure device, or truss, rather than resorting to surgical intervention. This form of treatment was gradually dropped in favor of increasingly

Information on Hernia

Causes: Presence of scar tissue, heavy physical exertion in work or athletics, obesity, aging, congenital abnormality

Symptoms: Heartburn, swallowing difficulty, chest pain, belching

Duration: Acute or chronic

Treatments: Surgery

effective hernioplasty operations.

When a hernial condition enters what is called the stage of incarceration, the advanced protrusion of the sac containing portions of viscera through the opening, or ring, in the abdominal wall can cause very severe complications. If, as is frequently the case, the protruding hernia sac passes through the ring as a fingerlike tube and then assumes a globular form outside the abdominal wall, a state of incarceration exists. As this state advances, the patient runs the risk of hernial strangulation. The constricting pressure of the ring's edges on the hernial sac interferes with circulatory functions in the herniated organ, causing destruction of tissues and, unless surgical intervention occurs, rapid spread of gangrene throughout the affected organ. The sixteenth-century French surgeon Pierre Franco carried out the first operation to release a strangulated hernia by inserting a thin instrument between the incarcerated bowel and the herniated sac, then incising the latter without touching the extruded vital organ.

A surprisingly wide range of hernial conditions have been noted and studied. These include hernias in the umbilical, epigastric (upper abdominal), spigelian (transversus abdominal muscle), interparietal, and groin regions. Hernias in the groin can be either femoral or inguinal. Inguinal hernias affecting the groin area have always been by far the most common, accounting for more than three-quarters of hernial cases, particularly among males.

Inguinal hernias share a number of common characteristics with one another and with the other closely associated form of groin hernia, the femoral hernia. Inguinal hernias are all caused by the abnormal introduction of a hernial sac into one of the four-centimeter-long inguinal canals located on the sides of the abdomen. These canals originate in the lower portion of the abdomen at an aperture called the inguinal ring. They have an external exit point in the rectus abdominal tissue. Located inside each inguinal canal are the ilioinguinal nerve, the genital branch of the genitofemoral nerve, and the spermatic cord. A comparable passageway from the abdomen into the groin area is found at the femoral ring, through which both the femoral artery and the femoral vein pass.

It may take a long period, sometimes years, for the sac to engage itself fully in the inguinal or femoral ring. Once the ring is passed, however, pressures from inside the abdomen help it descend through the canal rather quickly. If the external inguinal ring is firm in structure, and particularly if the narrow passageway is largely filled with the thickness of the spermatic cord, the inguinal hernia may be partially arrested

at this point. In men, once it passes beyond the external inguinal ring, however, it quickly descends into the scrotum. In women, the inguinal canal contains the round ligament, which may also temporarily impede the further descent of the hernial sac beyond the external inguinal opening.

Treatment and Therapy

Given the widespread occurrence of hernia conditions, especially inguinal hernias, at all age levels in most societies, physicians receive extensive training in the diagnosis and, among those with surgical training, the treatment of hernia patients. Though not always necessary, surgery to repair inguinal hernias is common (external trusses having been largely abandoned), but different schools support different surgical methods. Options include open surgery or laparoscopic surgery, and sutures versus surgical mesh. With the exception of operations involving the insertion of prosthetic devices to block the extension of hernia damage, most modern inguinal hernioplasty methods derive from the model finalized by the Italian Edoardo Bassini in the late nineteenth century.

Bassini believed that the surgical methods of his time fell short of the goal of complete hernial repair, since most postoperational patients were required to wear a truss to guard against recurring problems. In the simplest of surgical terms, his solution involved the physiological reconstruction of the inguinal canal. The operation provided for a new internal passageway to an external opening, as well as strengthened anterior and posterior inguinal walls. After initial incisions and ligation of the hernial sac, Bassini's method involved a separation of tissues between the internal inguinal ring and the pubis. A tissue section referred to as the "triple layer" (containing the internal oblique, the transversus abdominal, and the transversalis fascia tissue layers) was then attached by a line of sutures to the Poupart ligament, with a lowermost suture at the edge of the rectus abdominal muscle. Such local reconstruction of the inguinal canal proved to strengthen the entire zone against the recurrence of ruptures.

Physicians operating on indirect, as opposed to direct, inguinal hernias confront a relatively uncomplicated set of procedures. In the former case, a high ligation of the peritoneal sac (a circular incision of the peritoneum at a point well inside the abdominal inguinal ring) usually makes it possible to remove the sac entirely. Complications can occur if the patient is obese, since a large mass of peritoneal fatty material may be joined to the sac, obstructing access to the inguinal ring. For normal indirect inguinal hernias, the next basic step, after ensuring that no damage has occurred to the viscera either during formation of the hernia or in the process of relocating the contents of the hernial sac inside the abdomen, is to use one of several surgical methods to reduce the opening of the inguinal ring to its normal size. The physician must also ensure that no damage to the posterior inguinal wall has occurred and that its essential attachment to Cooper's ligament does not require additional surgical attention.

One must contrast the relative simplicity of indirect inguinal hernia surgery to treatment of direct inguinal hernias. In these cases, the hernia does not protrude through the existing

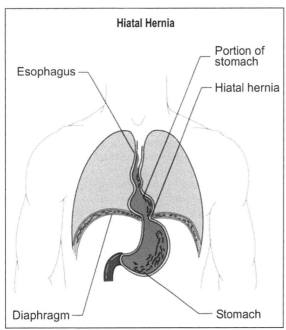

Hiatal Hernia

Esophagus

Portion of stomach

Hiatal hernia

Diaphragm

Stomach

A portion of the stomach has pushed through the weakened abdominal wall.

inguinal aperture, but, as a result of a weakening of local tissues, passes directly through the posterior inguinal wall. The direct inguinal hernia is usually characterized by a broad base at the point of protrusion and a relatively short hernial sac. When a physician recommends surgical treatment of such hernias, the surgeon must be prepared for the extensive task of surgical reconstruction of the posterior inguinal wall as part of the operation.

Two additional reasons tend to discourage an immediate decision to operate on direct inguinal hernias. First, this form of hernia rarely strangulates the affected viscera, since the aperture stretches to allow protrusion of the hernial sac. Second, once physicians find obvious symptoms of a direct inguinal hernia (a ceding of the weakened posterior inguinal wall to pressures originating in the abdomen), they may decide to examine the patient more thoroughly to determine whether the cause behind the symptoms demands treatment as well. Such causes of abdominal pressures may range from the effects of a chronic cough to much more serious problems, including inflammation of the prostate gland or other forms of obstruction in the colon itself.

Perspective and Prospects

Because the phenomenon of hernias has been the subject of scientific observation since the onset of formal medical writing itself, a stage-by-stage development of procedures has been associated with this condition. A main dividing line appears between the mid-eighteenth and mid-nineteenth centuries, however, between the extremely rudimentary surgical treatments of the late Middle Ages and Renaissance and what can be called modern procedures.

The surgical contribution of the sixteenth-century Frenchman Pierre Franco, who performed the first operation to release an incarcerated hernia, must be considered a landmark. The major general cause for advancement in knowledge of hernias, however, is tied to the birth of a new era in medical science, characterized by the use, from about 1750 onward, of anatomical dissection to investigate the essential characteristics of a number of common diseases.

Before the relatively long line of contributions that led to general adoption of the Bassini technique of operating on hernias, surgeons tended to follow the so-called Langenbeck method, named after the German physician who pioneered modern hernioplasty. This method held that simple removal of a hernial sac at the point of its protrusion from the abdomen and closing the external aperture would lead to a closing of the sac by "adhesive inflammation." Such spontaneous closing occurs when a severed artery "recedes" to the first branching-off point.

It took contributions by at least two lesser-known late nineteenth-century forerunners to Edoardo Bassini to convince the surgical world that hernia operations must involve a high incision of the hernial sac. Both the American H. O. Marcy (1837–1924) and the Frenchman Just Marie Marcellin Lucas-Championnière (1843–1913) have been recognized for their insistence on the necessity of high-incision operations. Their hernia operations, by incising the external oblique fascia, were the first to penetrate well beyond the external ring to expose the entire hernial sac. Following removal of the sac, it was then possible for surgeons to close the transversalis fascia and to repair the higher interior tissues that might have been damaged by the swollen hernia.

Following initial acceptance of the technique of high-incision hernial operations, a number of physicians recommended a variety of methods that might be used to repair internal tissue damage. These methods ranged from simple ligation of the sac at the internal ring, without more extensive surgery involving either the abdominal wall or the spermatic cord, to the much more extensive method practiced by Bassini. Even after the Bassini method succeeded in gaining almost universal recognition, other adaptations (but nothing that represented a full innovation) would be added during the middle decades of the twentieth century. One such method, which borrowed from the German physician Georg Lotheissen's use of Cooper's ligament to serve as a foundation for suturing damaged layers of lower abdominal tissues, came to be called the McVay method, after its chief proponent, the American Chester McVay.

Perhaps the most common approach to uncomplicated inguinal hernia repair in the early twenty-first century is the emplacement of synthetic mesh via a laparoscopic procedure, which, like all laparoscopy, has the advantage of greatly reducing recovery times. The most recent developments in this area include the use of biologic mesh, or biomesh, made of human or animal tissue that is fully absorbable by the human body. Studies of this procedure are ongoing, but show promise for reducing the incidence of postsurgical complications.

—*Byron D. Cannon, Ph.D.*

See also Abdomen; Abdominal disorders; Gastroenterology; Gastroenterology, pediatric; Gastrointestinal disorders; Gastrointestinal system; Hemorrhoids; Hernia repair; Intestinal disorders; Intestines; Small intestines.

For Further Information:
Bendavid, Robert, et al., eds. *Abdominal Wall Hernias: Principles and Management.* New York: Springer, 2001.

Fitzgibbons, Robert J., Jr., and A. Gerson Greenburg, eds. *Nyhus and Condon's Hernia.* 5th ed. Philadelphia: Lippincott Williams & Wilkins, 2002.

"Hernia." *MedlinePlus*, December 10, 2012.

Hernia Resource Center. http://www.herniainfo.com.

Kurzer, Martin, Allan E. Kark, and George W. Wantz, eds. *Surgical Management of Abdominal Wall Hernias.* Malden, Mass.: Blackwell Science, 1999.

Ponka, Joseph L. *Hernias of the Abdominal Wall.* Philadelphia: W. B. Saunders, 1980.

Scholten, Amy. "Groin Hernia—Adult." *Health Library*, June 24, 2013.

Scholten, Amy. "Hiatal Hernia." *Health Library*, June 24, 2013.

Stahl, Rebecca J. "Groin Hernia—Child." *Health Library*, June 3, 2013.

HERNIA REPAIR
Procedure
Anatomy or system affected: Abdomen, gastrointestinal system, intestines, stomach

Specialties and related fields: Gastroenterology, general surgery

Definition: Surgery to correct organ or tissue protrusions.

Key terms:

congenital: referring to a disorder which is present at birth

diaphragm: the muscular partition that separates the abdominal and thoracic cavities

esophagus: the muscular tube through which food passes from the throat to the stomach

gangrene: death and decay of a body part as a result of injury, disease, or inadequate blood supply

peritonitis: potentially fatal abdominal inflammation and infection

Indications and Procedures
A hernia is an abnormal protrusion of an organ or organ part from its normal body cavity, most often tissue protruding through the abdominal wall. Abdominal hernias may occur in the groin (inguinal hernia), upper thigh (femoral hernia), navel (umbilical hernia), and diaphragm (hiatal hernia). They may be congenital or acquired in later life. Herniated tissue is most often part of the small or large intestine. It can also be part of the bladder or the stomach in femoral and hiatal hernias, respectively. Most hernias occur as a result of strain to the abdominal wall or its injury. For example, they are often caused by athletic overexertion or hard labor. Consequently, men are more subject to acquired hernias than women.

Hernia Repair
A hernia is the protrusion of a tissue or organ (usually a loop of intestine) into another area of the body. With abdominal wall hernias, which include inguinal and umbilical hernias, the intestine protrudes through a weakness in the abdomen; with femoral hernias, the intestine passes down the canal containing the major blood vessels to the thigh and appears as a bulge in the groin area. When a hernia presents a danger to the patient, the intestine must be surgically returned to its proper position.

Congenital inguinal hernias in male infants can occur when the testicles of a developing fetus work their way down the inguinal canal to the scrotum. If the tissue sac accompanying them does not close off correctly, congenital hernia occurs. In men, acquired inguinal hernias occur when excess abdominal strain ruptures the intestinal wall and releases a loop of intestine. Inguinal hernias are less common in women and are associated with the canal that holds the round ligament of the uterus. Femoral hernias in both sexes lie on the inner sides of the blood vessels of the thighs and are always acquired, often by overexertion. Umbilical hernias, which may be congenital or acquired, protrude from the navel.

Incisional hernia is caused by the incomplete healing of surgical wounds of the abdomen. A fifth hernia type is hiatal hernia, which occurs at the opening where the esophagus passes through the diaphragm (the hiatus). Such hernias, in which part or all of the stomach passes through the diaphragm, may cause no external symptoms and be diagnosed only when chest X rays are taken for other reasons. If symptoms do occur, they usually include heartburn and chest pain.

Hernias are classified according to severity. Reducible hernias are those which can be resolved by pushing herniated tissue back into its proper position. Irreducible hernias are more serious. They cannot be pushed back manually because of their position, or because of the presence of adhesions that bind them in place. Such hernias can only be corrected with surgery. Strangulated hernias are those whose size and location pinch herniated tissue, cutting off blood flow. They require immediate surgical treatment to prevent the development of gangrene or peritonitis, both of which can be fatal.

Surgical repair is the suggested treatment for most hernias. If the patient is temporarily too ill for surgery, a truss may be used to diminish pain and swelling for inguinal, femoral, umbilical, and incisional hernias. Trusses, however, provide only temporary, symptomatic relief, except perhaps in umbilical hernias of very young children. Extreme caution is necessary: Reducible hernias treated with trusses can become irreducible or strangulated.

Standard hernia surgery can be accomplished in several ways. For the correction of inguinal or umbilical hernias, first the muscle wall is opened. Then, after the herniated loop is moved into an appropriate position, the muscle wall is closed as normally as possible. In more severe types of hernia repair involving visible protrusions, the abdominal wall is opened, adhesions are cut away, and the tissue is returned to a normal position. Then, the muscle wall is closed to restore normal muscle layers. When strangulation occurs, damaged tissue is cut away, normal sections are joined together, and viable tissue is returned to the abdomen, followed by abdominal closure. Incisional hernias are treated similarly, in a fashion dependent on the extent of the external damage and the degree of herniation.

Hiatal hernias are treated medically, whenever possible, because they tend to recur after surgery. Medical treatment includes restriction of activity, weight loss, and diet modification. Surgery is carried out when these efforts fail or if severe adhesions and/or strangulation occurs. The goal of this surgery is to strengthen the closure at the junction between the diaphragm and the esophagus.

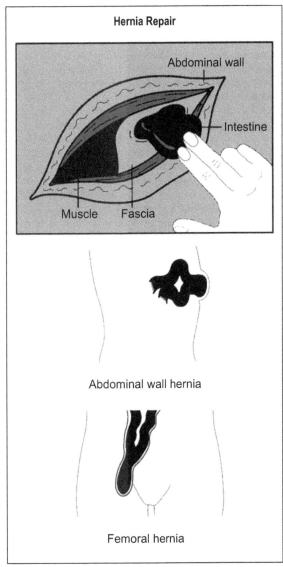

Hernia Repair

Abdominal wall

Intestine

Muscle   Fascia

Abdominal wall hernia

Femoral hernia

A hernia is the protrusion of a tissue or organ (usually a loop of intestine) into another area of the body. With abdominal wall hernias, which include inguinal and umbilical hernias, the intestine protrudes through a weakness in the abdomen; with femoral hernias, the intestine passes down the canal containing the major blood vessels to the thigh and appears as a bulge in the groin area. When a hernia presents a danger to the patient, the intestine must be surgically returned to its proper position.

Uses and Complications

The surgeries to correct inguinal, femoral, umbilical, and incisional hernias are straightforward. In all cases, but especially in strangulation, patients are checked before release to ensure that normal bowel movement occurs, that incisions have not become infected, and that fever has not developed. At this time, patients are also shown how to protect their incisions before coughing, are advised to maintain a high fluid intake to engender normal bowel function, are warned against overexertion, and are made aware of signs of incision infection. Furthermore, they are advised to resume work or physical activity only after consulting the physician involved.

Patients who have undergone surgery to correct a hiatal hernia are given much the same advice. Their surgery, however, is more extensive and prone to more complications. Therefore, they are provided with recommendations concerning which foods and activities to avoid. Furthermore, they are advised of the extended time period required before they can return to normal function and are told that without careful compliance, the problem will recur.

Perspective and Prospects

Major advances in the treatment of hernias have included better diagnosis of their extent and the necessary means of their correction. computed tomography (CT) scanning and other imaging techniques can make possible very accurate diagnoses. Progress in the surgical techniques used in hernia repair includes laparoscopy, in which a fiber-optic tube is used to visualize the chest cavity and thus to minimize incision size in the correction of hiatal hernias. All these methodologies are expected to improve in the future.

—*Sanford S. Singer, Ph.D.*

See also Abdomen; Abdominal disorders; Gangrene; Gastroenterology; Gastroenterology, pediatric; Gastrointestinal disorders; Gastrointestinal system; Hernia; Internal medicine; Intestinal disorders; Intestines; Pediatrics; Peritonitis; Small intestine.

For Further Information:
Beers, Mark H., et al., eds. *The Merck Manual of Diagnosis and Therapy.* 18th ed. Whitehouse Station, N.J.: Merck Research Laboratories, 2006.
"Femoral Hernia Repair." *MedlinePlus*, January 29, 2013.
Fitzgibbons, Robert J., Jr., and A. Gerson Greenburg, eds. *Nyhus and Condon's Hernia.* 5th ed. Philadelphia: Lippincott Williams & Wilkins, 2002.
"Inguinal Hernia Repair." *MedlinePlus*, January 29, 2013.
McCoy, Krishna. "Hernia Repair." *Health Library*, October 11, 2012.
Mulholland, Michael W., et al., eds. *Greenfield's Surgery: Scientific Principles and Practice.* 4th ed. Philadelphia: Lippincott Williams & Wilkins, 2006.
Tierney, Lawrence M., Stephen J. McPhee, and Maxine A. Papadakis, eds. *Current Medical Diagnosis and Treatment 2007.* New York: McGraw-Hill Medical, 2006.
Zinner, Michael J., et al., eds. *Maingot's Abdominal Operations.* 11th ed. New York: McGraw-Hill, 2007.

HERNIATED DISK. *See* **SLIPPED DISK.**

HERPES

Disease/Disorder

Anatomy or system affected: Genitals, mouth, nerves, reproductive system, skin

Specialties and related fields: Dermatology, family medicine, gynecology, urology, virology

Definition: A family of viruses that cause such diseases as cold sores, genital herpes, chickenpox, shingles, and mononucleosis. The term "herpes" is also used to refer to an infection with herpes simplex, either type 1 or type 2.

Key terms:

antiviral agent: a drug that acts against a virus, usually by preventing it from reproducing itself; may be used at the first evidence of symptoms to reduce the severity and length of an episode or continually to prevent episodes from occurring

cold sore: also known as a fever blister; a sore, frequently on the lips but sometimes on the chin, cheeks, nostrils, and occasionally the gums or palate, that causes itching, burning, or tenderness, followed by crusting over

ganglia: clusters of nerves

genitalia: the internal and external reproductive organs

gingivostomatitis: inflammation of the gums and mouth

Kaposi's sarcoma: a rare cancer of connective tissue, found primarily in persons with acquired immunodeficiency syndrome (AIDS)

latent: inactive

lymphoma: one of a number of cancers of the lymphatic system

recurrent: repeated

vesicle: also called a blister; a collection of fluid under the epidermis, or topmost layer of the skin

virus: a tiny disease-causing organism that invades living cells and uses their processes in order to reproduce itself

whitlow: a herpes infection on the finger; it is found commonly in health care workers who must put their fingers into others' mouths and can occur even with the use of protective gloves

Causes and Symptoms

Eight different herpesviruses cause infection in humans. Herpes simplex types 1 and 2 (HHV1 and HHV2) cause cold sores and genital herpes, while herpes zoster, or varicella-zoster virus, (HHV3) causes chickenpox (varicella) and shingles. HHV4, also known as Epstein-Barr virus, causes infectious mononucleosis. A variant of this virus has also been implicated in a rare type of lymphoma. Cytomegalovirus (HHV5) causes a wide variety of health problems, including serious illness in newborn babies, an illness that strongly resembles infectious mononucleosis, and, in persons with AIDS and other immune deficiencies, disease of the retina, stomach, bowels, liver, lungs, and nervous system. Roseola, one of the many rash-and-fever diseases of childhood, is caused by HHV6. HHV7 is associated with seizures and encephalitis, while HHV8 is associated with Kaposi's sarcoma and some lymphomas.

Most commonly, however, the term "herpes" refers to infection with HHV1 and HHV2. A characteristic of both HHV1 and HHV2 infection is blisters clustered on reddened skin or mucous membranes. These blisters then either dry up or break, forming a shallow ulcer, and then crust over and gradually resolve. Another important characteristic is the tendency of infections to recur. This happens because the virus never truly goes away. Rather, it settles in ganglia under the skin and remains latent until some trigger causes it to become active again, resulting in a less severe outbreak at the same site of the body as the primary (first) infection. The trigger may be something physical such as sunburn or a fever, a change in the immune system as with aging, or psychological stress. Recurrences tend to be heralded by itching, tingling, or burning at the site of the original outbreak for hours or days before the blisters occur. Recurrences may be rare or frequent.

Some people are infected with the virus but never have any symptoms. On the other hand, the first infection may cause a person to become very ill. The oral form, called herpetic gingivostomatitis, usually occurs in childhood. Symptoms include painful sores in the mouth, swollen and bleeding gums, swollen glands, and fever. The sores in the mouth may be so severe that it is difficult to eat or drink, and dehydration may become a problem. The genital form of herpes causes painful blisters in the genital area, swollen glands in the groin, fever, and other flulike symptoms. The blisters may make urination extremely painful. Regardless of the site, the first infection usually lasts about two weeks. The blisters themselves may last longer, but they typically scab over without leaving a scar.

Recurrent infections tend to be milder, with a single or small cluster of blisters erupting very close to the original site of infection. Recurrences typically last a shorter time than did the primary infection.

The diagnosis of herpes infection is usually made by observing the characteristic rash. During the first three days of an outbreak, it is possible to culture the virus from the base of one of the ulcers. Blood tests in a person with no current symptoms are not helpful because they do not distinguish between recent infection and one that occurred years before.

Treatment and Therapy

The best treatment for herpes infections is prevention. HHV1 is spread in air droplets, so covering coughs and sneezes is essential. Direct contact with the fluid from the blisters or ulcers can also pass HHV1 or HHV2 from one person to another.

Information on Herpes

Causes: Viral infection

Symptoms: Painful or itchy blisterlike lesions, fever, headache, tiredness, nerve pain, sore throat, swollen lymph nodes, sometimes enlarged liver and spleen

Duration: Varies from short-term to recurrent

Treatments: Antiviral drugs, supportive care

Once the blisters have dried up or crusted over, they are much less contagious. Some people with herpes shed low levels of the virus even when they have no blisters. They may not even know they have the infection.

No treatment eliminates the virus from the body, but antiviral drugs will help shorten the length and severity of an outbreak. Continuous antiviral treatment will suppress the virus and prevent recurrences in most cases. Effective antiviral medications are available by prescription. Of these, oral medications are generally more effective than ointments applied directly to the blister. The common antiviral drugs include acyclovir, famciclovir, valaciclovir, and penciclovir. Over-the-counter lysine supplements seem to be helpful for some people, although scientific studies have not proven their effectiveness.

Perspective and Prospects

A wide variety of vaccines, antibodies, and drugs that stimulate the immune system have been tested in the treatment of herpes, but they have either been ineffective or have caused unacceptable side effects. Researchers in the early twenty-first century, however, have found a new type of drug that works to suppress enzymes produced by the virus that seems to be effective in animal models.

—Rebecca Lovell Scott, Ph.D., PA-C

See also Canker sores; Cervical, ovarian, and uterine cancers; Chickenpox; Chronic fatigue syndrome; Cold sores; Epstein-Barr virus; Genital disorders, female; Genital disorders, male; Gynecology; Mononucleosis; Reye's syndrome; Sexually transmitted diseases (STDs); Shingles; Skin disorders; Viral infections; Warts.

For Further Information:

American Medical Association. *American Medical Association Family Medical Guide.* 4th rev. ed. Hoboken, N.J.: John Wiley & Sons, 2004.

Cozic, Charles P. *Herpes.* San Diego, Calif.: ReferencePoint Press, 2011.

Herpes Resource Center. http://www.herpesresourcecenter.com.

Komaroff, Anthony, ed. *Harvard Medical School Family Health Guide.* New York: Free Press, 2005.

Parker, James N., and Philip M. Parker, eds. *The Official Patient's Sourcebook on Genital Herpes.* San Diego, Calif.: Icon Health, 2002.

Stoppard, Miriam. *Family Health Guide.* London: Dorling Kindersley, 2006.

Sutton, Amy L. *Sexually Transmitted Diseases Sourcebook.* Detroit, Mich.: Omnigraphics, 2013.

HICCUPS

Disease/Disorder

Also known as: Hiccoughs

Anatomy or system affected: Chest, lungs, muscles, respiratory system, throat

Specialties and related fields: Family medicine, gastroenterology, neurology

Definition: Involuntary, spasmodic contractions of the diaphragm and the simultaneous closure of the glottis.

Information on Hiccups

Causes: Overdistension of stomach, gastric irritation from spicy or rich foods, nerve spasms

Symptoms: Involuntary, spasmodic contractions of diaphragm and simultaneous closure of glottis; stomach upset

Duration: Ranges from short-term to chronic

Treatments: Varies; can include holding one's breath, drinking a glass of water, breathing deeply or into a paper bag

---

Causes and Symptoms

A hiccup is caused by an involuntary, spasmodic contraction of the diaphragm, the large partition of muscles and tendons that separates the chest from the abdomen. The diaphragm draws air into the lungs through rhythmic contractions. When it contracts suddenly, an opening located toward the top of the trachea (windpipe) between the vocal cords in the larynx (voice box) called the glottis snaps shut abruptly. The combination of air being forced through the vocal cords in the larynx and the abrupt closure of the glottis causes the sound associated with hiccups.

There are a number of causes of hiccups, the most common being overdistension of the stomach. Other causes include gastric irritation from spicy or rich foods and nerve spasms. There is some indication that hiccups are controlled by the central nervous system.

Hiccups generally last for a very short time, usually stopping within minutes. People who suffer from hiccups for more than twenty-four hours or who have repetitive attacks are said to suffer from chronic hiccups. This condition is very rare.

People of all ages can suffer from hiccups. Pregnant women report that fetuses sometimes have hiccups in the womb.

Treatment and Therapy

An attack of hiccups is not serious and is generally self-limiting. A number of techniques to stop are practiced, including holding one's breath, drinking a glass of water, breathing deeply, or breathing into a paper bag.

Babies often suffer from hiccups, particularly during nursing. Some mothers report that feeding the baby a quarter of a teaspoon of sugar mixed in 4 ounces of water calms the hiccups. Doctors suggest that hiccup-prone babies be fed before they are overly hungry and when they are calm.

—Diane Andrews Henningfeld, Ph.D.

See also Abdomen; Breast-feeding; Coughing; Respiration.

For Further Information:

Gluck, Michael, and Charles E. Pope II. "Hiccups and Gastrointestinal Reflux Disease: The Acid Perfusion Test as a Provocative Maneuver." *Annals of Internal Medicine* 105 (1996): 219–220.

Heuman, Douglas M., A. Scott Mills, and Hunter H. McGuire, Jr. *Gastroenterology.* Philadelphia: W. B. Saunders, 1997.

Howes, Daniel. "Hiccups: A New Explanation for the Mysterious Reflex." *BioEssays* 34, 6 (June, 2012): 451–453.

Hurst, Duane, Catherine Purdom, and Michael Hogan. "Use of Paced Respiration to Alleviate Intractable Hiccups (Singultus): A Case

Report." *Applied Psychophysiology & Biofeedback* 38, 2 (June, 2013): 157–160.

Kaneishi, Keisuke, and Masahiro Kawabata. "Continuous Subcutaneous Infusion of Lidocaine for Persistent Hiccup in Advanced Cancer." *Palliative Medicine* 27, 3 (March, 2013): 284–285.

Launois, J. L., W. A. Bizec, J. C. Whitelaw et al. "Hiccup in Adults: An Overview." *European Respiratory Journal* 6 (1993): 563–575.

Shay, Steven D. S., Robert L. Myers, and Lawrence F. Johnson. "Hiccups Associated with Reflux Esophagitis." *Gastroenterology* 87 (1984): 204–207.oxy_options track_changes="on"?

HIP FRACTURE REPAIR
Procedure

Anatomy or system affected: Bones, hips, joints, legs, musculoskeletal system

Specialties and related fields: Geriatrics and gerontology, orthopedics

Definition: The repair or replacement of a broken hip joint.

Key terms:

arthroplasty: joint replacement

osteoporosis: a loss of bone mass accompanied by increasing fragility and brittleness

Indications and Procedures

Hip fracture repair constitutes one of the most common procedures performed by orthopedic surgeons. The human hip consists of two bones, the hipbone and the thighbone (femur), and their point of intersection, a cup-shaped cavity called the acetabulum. This hip joint forms a ball-and-socket mechanism that allows the leg to move in different directions. As a major weight-bearing joint, the hip is vulnerable both to sudden trauma, such as sports injuries, and to degenerative disorders of aging, such as osteoporosis. If the loss of bone mass associated with osteoporosis is sufficiently advanced, a simple fall from a standing position can shatter the hip joint. The most common fracture involves the femur snapping or cracking just below the rounded end that fits into the acetabulum.

Perspective and Prospects

The repair of hip fractures involves the realignment of the bone fragments and the insertion of a long nail into the bone to hold them together. A plate is attached to the nail and to the healthy bone surrounding the fracture in order to give support.

Because broken bones heal slowly in the elderly, in the past a broken hip almost inevitably resulted in these patients becoming permanent invalids restricted to wheelchairs or, at best, forced to rely on walkers and enjoying only limited mobility. This bleak prognosis changed in the 1960s, when orthopedic specialists working with biomedical engineers developed artificial hip joints. The combination of prosthetic devices and surgical techniques known as total hip arthroplasty (THA) allows physicians to return patients to active, independent lives. In THA, the weakened end of the femur is removed and an artificial replacement installed. The replacement can consist of any of a variety of materials, but typically it is constructed of a chromium steel alloy coated with a ceramic polymer that helps resist corrosion and pro-

vides a surface with which the patient's bone can bond. The end of the prosthesis and the surface of the acetabulum are coated with plastic polymers to reduce friction. Research indicates that artificial hip joints last fifteen years or longer before wear and tear on the lining of the ball-and-socket joint creates problems.

—*Nancy Farm Mannikko, Ph.D.*

See also Aging: Extended care; Arthroplasty; Arthroscopy; Bone disorders; Bone grafting; Bones and the skeleton; Emergency medicine; Fracture and dislocation; Fracture repair; Geriatrics and gerontology; Hip replacement; Orthopedic surgery; Orthopedics; Osteoporosis; Physical rehabilitation.

For Further Information:

A.D.A.M. Medical Encyclopedia. "Hip Fracture Surgery." *MedlinePlus*, November 15, 2012.

Brunicardi, F. Charles, et al., eds. *Schwartz's Principles of Surgery.* 9th ed. New York: McGraw-Hill, 2010.

Currey, John D. *Bones: Structures and Mechanics.* Princeton, N.J.: Princeton University Press, 2002.

Doherty, Gerard M., and Lawrence W. Way, eds. *Current Surgical Diagnosis and Treatment.* 12th ed. New York: Lange Medical Books/McGraw-Hill, 2006.

Mayo Clinic. "Hip Fracture." *Mayo Foundation for Medical Education and Research*, March 22, 2012.

Morrey, Bernard, ed. *Joint Replacement Arthroplasty.* 3d ed. Philadelphia: Churchill Livingstone/Elsevier, 2003.

Nelson, Miriam E., and Sarah Wernick. *Strong Women, Strong Bones: Everything You Need to Know to Prevent, Treat, and Beat Osteoporosis.* Rev. ed. New York: Berkley Books, 2006.

Smoots, Elizabeth. "Hip Fracture." *Health Library*, May 7, 2013.

Townsend, Courtney M., Jr., et al., eds. *Sabiston Textbook of Surgery.* 18th ed. Philadelphia: Saunders/Elsevier, 2008.

Wilmore, Douglas W., et al., eds. *Scientific American Surgery 2006.* New York: Scientific American, 2007.

HIP REPLACEMENT
Procedure

Anatomy or system affected: Bones, hips

Specialties and related fields: Orthopedics, rheumatology

Definition: The removal of diseased bone tissue in the hip and its replacement with an artificial device.

Indications and Procedures

The most common reason for hip replacement surgery is the decline in efficiency of the hip joint that often results from osteoarthritis. Osteoarthritis is a common form of arthritis that causes joint and bone deterioration, which may lead to the wearing down of cartilage and cause the underlying bones to rub against each other. This may result in severe pain and stiffness in the affected areas. Other conditions that may lead to the need for hip replacement include rheumatoid arthritis (a chronic inflammation of the joints), avascular necrosis (loss of bone caused by insufficient blood supply), and injury.

Generally, physicians may be more inclined to choose less invasive techniques such as physical therapy, medication, or walking aids before resorting to surgery. In some cases, exercise programs may help reduce hip pain. In addition, if preliminary treatment does not improve the patient's condition, doctors may use corrective surgery that is not as invasive as hip replacement.

Typically, a candidate for total hip replacement surgery (THR) possesses a hip that has worn out from arthritis, falls, or other conditions. The hip consists of a ball-and-socket joint wherein the head of the femur (thigh bone) fits into the hip socket, or acetabulum. In a normal hip, this arrangement provides for a relatively wide range of motion. For some older adults, however, deterioration caused by arthritis and other conditions reduces the effectiveness of this arrangement, compromising the integrity of the hip socket or the femoral head. This state can lead to extreme discomfort.

Total hip replacement may provide the best long-term relief for these symptoms. Total hip replacement involves the removal of diseased bone tissue and the replacement of that tissue with prostheses (artificial devices used to replace missing body parts). Usually, both the femoral head and the hip socket are replaced. The femoral head is replaced with a metal ball that is attached to a metal stem and placed into the hollow marrow space of the femur. The hip socket is lined with a plastic socket. Other materials have also been used effectively as hip replacements.

In some cases, the surgeon will use cement to bond the artificial parts of the new hip to the bone tissue. This approach has been the traditional method of ensuring that the artificial parts hold. One problem with this method is that over time, cemented hip replacements may lose their bond with the bone tissue. This may result in the need for an additional surgery. However, a cementless hip replacement has been developed. This approach includes a prosthesis that is porous so that bone tissue may grow into the metal pores and keep the prosthesis in place.

Both procedures have strengths and weaknesses. In general, recovery time may be shorter with cemented prostheses, since one does not have to wait for bone growth to attach to the artificial prostheses. However, the potential for long-term deterioration of the replaced hip must be considered. A cemented hip generally lasts about fifteen years. With this in mind, physicians may be more likely to use a cemented prosthesis for patients over the age of seventy. Cementless hip replacement may be more advisable for younger and more active patients. Some physicians have used a combination of approaches, known as a "hybrid" or "mixed" hip. This combination relies on an uncemented socket and a cemented femoral head.

Uses and Complications

Total hip replacements are generally quite successful, with about 98 percent of surgeries proceeding without serious complications. In rare instances, however, complications occur, including blood clots and infections during surgery and hip dislocation or bone fracture after surgery. In addition, in some cases, bone grafts may be used to assist in the restoration of bone defects. In these instances, bone may be obtained from the pelvis or the discarded head of the femur. Other postoperative complications may include some pain and stiffness.

Patients recovering from total hip replacement usually remain in the hospital up to ten days if there are no complications. However, physical therapists may initiate therapy as soon as the day after surgery. Physical therapy involves the use of exercises that will improve recovery. Many patients are able to sit on the edge of their bed, stand, and even walk with assistance as early as two days after surgery. Patients must remember that their artificial hip may not provide the same full range of motion as an undiseased hip. Physical therapists teach patients how to perform daily activities without placing an undue burden on their new hips. This may require learning a new method of sitting, standing, and performing other activities.

While many factors may affect recovery time, full recovery from surgery may take up to six months. At that point, many patients enjoy such activities as walking and swimming. Doctors and physical therapists may discourage patients from participating in such high-impact activities as jogging or playing tennis, which may burden the new hip. Despite these restrictions, many patients are able to perform normal activities without pain and discomfort. Nonetheless, people who have undergone hip replacement surgery are advised to consult with their doctors about proper exercise and activity levels.

Perspective and Prospects

Total hip replacement is one of the most common surgical interventions that older adults face. The American Academy of Orthopedic Surgeons estimates that more than 285,000 hip replacement surgeries are performed in the United States each year. The majority of hip replacements are performed on individuals over the age of sixty-five. One of the reasons for this is that the activity level of older adults is lower than that of younger adults, therefore reducing the concern that the new hip will wear out or fail. However, technological advances have improved the quality of the artificial hip, making hip replacement surgery a more likely intervention for younger adults as well.

—*H. David Smith, Ph.D.*

See also Arthritis; Bone disorders; Bones and the skeleton; Fracture repair; Hip fracture repair; Orthopedics; Osteonecrosis.

For Further Information:

A.D.A.M. Medical Encyclopedia. "Hip Joint Replacement." *MedlinePlus*, June 22, 2012.

Bucholz, Robert, and Joseph A. Buckwalter. "Orthopedic Surgery." *Journal of the American Medical Association* 275, no. 23 (June 19, 1996).

Duffey, Timothy P., Elliott Hershman, Richard A. Sanders, and Lori D. Talarico. "Investigating the Subtle and Obvious Causes of Hip Pain." *Patient Care* 31, no. 18 (November 15, 1997)..

Dunkin, Mary Anne. "Hip Replacement Surgery." *Arthritis Today* 12, no. 2 (March/April, 1998).

Finerman, Gerald A. M., et al., eds. *Total Hip Arthroplasty Outcomes.* New York: Churchill Livingstone, 1998.

Kellicker, Patricia Griffin. "Hip Replacement." *Health Library*, May 6, 2013.

Lane, Nancy E., and Daniel J. Wallace. *All About Osteoarthritis: The Definitive Resource for Arthritis Patients and Their Families.* New York: Oxford University Press, 2002.

MacWilliam, Cynthia H., Marianne U. Yood, James J. Verner, Bruce

D. McCarthy, and Richard E. Ward. "Patient-Related Risk Factors That Predict Poor Outcome After Total Hip Replacement." *Health Services Research* 31, no. 5 (December, 1996).

Morrey, Bernard, ed. *Joint Replacement Arthroplasty.* 3d ed. Philadelphia: Churchill Livingstone/Elsevier, 2003.

National Institute of Arthritis and Musculoskeletal and Skin Diseases. "Hip Replacement." *National Institutes of Health*, April 2012.

OrthoInfo. "Total Hip Replacement." *American Academy of Orthopaedic Surgeons*, December 2011.

Silber, Irwin. *A Patient's Guide to Knee and Hip Replacement: Everything You Need to Know.* New York: Simon & Schuster, 1999.

Trahair, Richard C. S. *All About Hip Replacement: A Patient's Guide.* New York: Oxford University Press, 1999.

Van De Graaff, Kent M., and Stuart Ira Fox. *Concepts of Human Anatomy and Physiology.* 5th ed. Dubuque: Iowa: Wm. C. Brown, 2000.

HIPPOCRATIC OATH

Ethics

Definition: A document, written in the fifth century BCE, to offer guidelines for the emerging medical profession, which continues to be the subject of debate in modern practice because of the ethical issues that it addresses.

Key terms:

euthanasia: the practice (particularly in cases involving patients of advanced age) of withholding medical treatments that might sustain life that would otherwise expire "naturally"; in a more controversial form, it is associated with the administration of drugs by physicians in order to avert prolonged suffering

living will: a legally binding document instructing a physician not to prolong life by externally administered life support systems if the patient is unable to express his or her decision concerning forms of medical treatment recommended by a physician

malpractice insurance: insurance policies held by physicians in order to protect them financially in the event of a patient-initiated lawsuit alleging incidents of improper medical decisions or incompetence

Medical Codes of Ethics

Western civilization has long held the writings of the fifth century BCE Greek physician Hippocrates, and in particular the Hippocratic oath, as a model of ethical values to be followed in the medical profession. As the nature of Western civilization itself has changed over the centuries, interpretations of the ethical values behind the Hippocratic oath have also changed. The circumstances of modern medical practice and ethical values, however, have ironically made certain elements of the classical Hippocratic tradition even more relevant than they may have appeared in previous eras.

In fact, the Hippocratic oath is only the introductory section of the *Corpus Hippocraticum* (Hippocratic Collection) traditionally attributed to Hippocrates. (There is debate about whether he is the author of all the books or only some.) The actual medical observations of Hippocrates were studied and applied for many centuries, until scientific research rendered many of them recognizably obsolete. A number of sections of the corpus, however, reflect the Greek physician's recurring concern for rules to guide the medical profession. Hippocrates" chapters on "The Art," "Decorum," and "The Law" complement the more famous ethical precepts contained in the oath.

The first part of the oath itself covers the physician's lifelong commitment to his or her teachers. This commitment extends not only to the symbolic bonds of respect but also to obligation to share one's medical practice and even to provide financial assistance to one's teachers, if requested. Additionally, the physician is committed to train, free of charge, the families of his or her teachers in the art of medicine.

The second part of the Hippocratic oath contains the more general pledges that would contribute to its value as an ethical guide for the medical profession. The physician is bound, in a very general way, to help the sick according to his or her ability and judgment in a manner that can never be interpreted as involving injury or wrongdoing. The physician is bound both to confidentiality concerning direct experiences in the patient-doctor relationship and to extreme discretion to avoid the circulation of professional knowledge that is not appropriate for publication abroad.

In addition to these general precepts, all of which have an ethical timelessness that would survive the centuries, there were two points in the oath that refer to specific issues that cannot be separated from the modern debate over medical ethics. Addressing the questions of euthanasia ("mercy killing") and abortion, Hippocrates stated: "I will give no deadly drug to any, though it be asked of me, nor will I counsel such, and especially I will not aid a woman to procure abortion."

Anyone searching for wider guidelines can glean many items of timeless wisdom from other sections of Hippocrates" writings. In the pieces titled "The Physician" and "Decorum," for example, the personal behavior of doctors is discussed. In all cases, Hippocrates exhorted physicians to maintain even levels of dignity and patience, to practice exemplary personal hygiene, and to avoid excesses in living habits that could introduce an element of distance between themselves and the patients who depend on them. Many centuries later, as in the eighteenth century English essay by Samuel Bard titled "A Discourse upon the Duties of a Physician," one can see similar concerns for behavioral propriety toward the defenseless: for example, "Never affect to despise a man for the want of a regular education, and treat even harmless ignorance with delicacy and compassion" and protect against the effects of "foolhardiness and presumption." These admonitions are indicative of the defining boundaries of the views of Hippocrates and those of the later, Christian era on the practice of medicine. The main attention of commentators on the Hippocratic corpus in recent generations has been directed to two broad divisions in the main ethical issues that he formulated: the physician's role in abortion and in the decision to end life by either withholding or administering certain treatments. It took many centuries, however, for degrees of emphasis in analyzing the Hippocratic oath to take form. In the interim, and after a delay that separated the classical world from the late medieval world, different interpretations of the Hippocratic oath would appear, each reflecting the cultural environment to which it was meant to apply.

Several factors may explain why centuries passed before systematic attention was given to the rules of medicine first broached in the classical Greek and Roman worlds. The first of these was the general decline of political and economic conditions after the fall of Rome (fifth century CE), which had repercussions in a variety of cultural areas. Medical practices tended to revert to quite crude levels until the rediscovery of early medical texts, including those of Hippocrates, sparked interest in improving conditions of medical treatment in the late Middle Ages.

One can say that, in addition to editing elements of Hippocratic teachings to Christianize the pagan references that they contained, a second important redirection occurred in setting down medieval rules for the practice of medicine. It was Holy Roman Emperor Frederick II, around 1241, who specified for the first time that the higher authority of the state alone should define institutional procedures for certifying physicians. This was to be done through formal training and examinations in the universities of Naples or Salerno, and later in universities throughout the Western world.

In addition to rules leading to physicians" certification, Frederick II stipulated that doctors must take an oath binding them to obligations that, in comparison to the Hippocratic oath or modern codes of medical ethics, covered very specific issues. One of these was an obligation to report any irregularities in an apothecary's preparation of drugs that were to be dispensed to patients. Another enjoined doctors to provide free medical services to the poor.

If one looks at more modern standards for the regulation of relations between physician and patient, it is possible to suggest that—until some very major changes took place in society's views on delicate questions previously reserved for ecclesiastical law—similar operatives continued to govern the guidelines for medical ethics. In the "Code of Medical Ethics" (1846–47) by the American Medical Association (AMA), for example, primary focus is still visibly on the physician's obligation to place the patient's interest before his or her own, particularly in terms of prospects for material or other forms of personal gain. Defense of the public's interest against quackery or the distribution of drugs that are either dangerous or illegally prepared follows, as well as avoidance of "crude hypotheses" or "magnification of the importance of services" sought, merely for the purpose of "temporary effect and popularity." Although there are enormous time spans between the classical Hippocratic model, the medieval variant offered by Frederick II, and the mid-nineteenth century AMA code, all are comparable in their focus on what, in the terminology of the 1847 code, would be called "Duties for Support of Professional Character" (part 1, article 1) or "Duties of the Profession to the Public" (part 2, article 1).

One hundred years later, however, different societal attitudes toward medical ethics would establish themselves in most Western nations, including the United States. Generally stated, the basic changes reflected in ethical debates empha-sized (or questioned the rising emphasis on) the protection of individual rights and privacy in matters relating to human life and the intervention of physicians. On one hand, changing directions in the expression of ethical orientations stemmed from advances made in key areas of medical science in the twentieth century, such as technologies for combating terminal disease, saving the lives of severely preterm infants, and prolonging life in old age. On the other hand, and in an even broader context, extraordinary scientific discoveries concerning the genetic keys behind life itself introduced an entirely different dimension to medical ethics, that of responsibility for monitoring or "engineering" life that has not yet been conceived.

Modern Applications

Although neither the original nor edited versions of the Hippocratic oath are applied today as a condition for becoming a doctor, the medical profession in the United States has definitely formalized publication of what it considers to be a necessary code of medical ethics. Evolving versions of this "Code of Medical Ethics" date from the original (1847) text of the AMA as revised by specific decisions in 1903, 1912, and 1947.

When the AMA adopted a statement under the title "Guide to Responsible Professional Behavior" in 1980, it assigned to a formal body within its organization, the Council on Ethical and Judicial Affairs, the task of publishing, on a yearly basis, updated paragraphs that reflect ethical guidelines for the profession as a whole. These evolving guidelines are organized under such subheadings as "Social Policy Issues," "Interprofessional Relations," "Hospital Relations," "Confidentiality," and "Fees and Charges."

At the turn of the twenty-first century, the public's growing uncertainty about a doctor's role in a market-oriented health care delivery system and increasing mistrust in the face of malpractice suits prompted physicians to question their professional responsibilities and roles within modern medicine. In 2002, a joint effort between the American Board of Internal Medicine (ABIM), the American College of Physicians-American Society of Internal Medicine (ACP-ASIM), and the European Federation of Internal Medicine (EFIM) introduced a new professional code of conduct designed to address these issues and help physicians meet the needs of patients in the twenty-first century. The charter incorporated traditional understanding of professional norms into the unique circumstances of modern medicine by addressing issues such as patient autonomy and choice, working in physician teams and respecting other professionals, managing conflicts of interest, social justice and equality in health care access, and market forces—issues not relevant during the time of Hippocrates. The American-British team noted that they hoped their efforts reaffirmed to a wary public the profession's commitment to putting the needs of the patient first and offered guidelines to physicians for coping with the ethical problems in the modern world.

Along with such modern-day charters, physicians are bound to respect the ethical guidelines provided to them by their professional association. Failure to respect these guidelines is tantamount to breaking one's binding ethical obligations and can lead to expulsion from the medical profession.

Several major changes, both in levels of medical technology and in social attitudes toward issues relating to medical practice, have played key roles in several spheres of an ongoing debate concerning medical ethics. In two cases, those of abortion and euthanasia, debate has focused on the ethics of deciding to end life; in the third, referred to generally as genetic engineering, the central question involves both the living and those yet to be born. In all these spheres, the legal and ethical debates have revolved around potential conflicts between physicians and patients but also in the context of wider social values.

Movement from the historical domain of idealized codes or oaths to the more practical and contemporary realm of changing societal reactions to what constitutes injury or breach of professional ethics in several areas of modern medicine is facilitated by reference to landmark legal decisions that have given a modern and quite different meaning to Hippocratic concepts.

Probably the most widely recognized issue reflecting such ethical conflicts, and one that received specific attention in the Hippocratic oath itself, involves abortion. In the United States, the climate of public opinion toward doctor-assisted pregnancy terminations was altered considerably by the landmark 1973 Supreme Court decision *Roe v. Wade*. In this decision, the Court judged that state laws defining abortion as a criminal offense were unconstitutional. The main thrust of the argument in *Roe v. Wade* was that, although the Constitution does not provide a specific guarantee of a civil right of privacy that could be applied to questions of life and death in medical care, parallels exist in Supreme Court decisions on other matters of individual rights with respect to procreation. These rights tend to fall under the Fourteenth Amendment's concept of personal liberty and restrictions on state action. These rights, in the Court's words, are "broad enough to encompass a woman's decision whether or not to terminate her pregnancy."

Reference to the fundamental right of "personal privacy" in *Roe v. Wade* granted individual women and their physicians recourse against specific state laws criminalizing abortion. It did not, however, consider the right to have an abortion to be unqualified; nor did it extend beyond the domain of pregnancy termination to cover a general assumption that constitutional protection of the right of privacy included the individual's right to "do with one's body as one pleases." In fact, there was an explicit suggestion that the legal definition of protection of an individual's right to privacy where critical medical decisions affecting vital life processes are concerned is "not unqualified and must be considered against important state interests in regulation."

As time passed in the evolving debate over abortion, definitions of what this could mean became colored by the inevitable introduction of religious conceptions of defense of the unborn individual—the fetus—as a possessor of life separate from that of the pregnant woman. This was a precursor to the "right to life" versus "right to choice" debate that would place physicians between two poles of opinion as to where their final obligations should lie.

What seemed most important in the beginnings of the abortion debate (and then, a few years later, the euthanasia debate) was the Supreme Court's inclusion of commentary on Hippocratic ethical precepts as part of its argument justifying recognition of individual rights to final responsibility for the disposition of someone else's "future" life or the disposition of one's own life. The *Roe v. Wade* brief actually argued that the strict Hippocratic injunction against abortion must be recognized as a reflection of only one segment of opinion and values (specifically Pythagorean) at a particular time in history. By underlining the fact that other views and practices were known to be current throughout antiquity, and that later Christian ethics chose to ignore diversity of interpretations of medical ethics in such matters, *Roe v. Wade* implied that diversity of ethical opinion within a social environment must be recognized in order to avoid too narrow a definition of what standards should be followed by physicians in dealing with their patients.

The implications of these two directions in interpreting the ethical bonds between patient and physician—the right to privacy in reaching individual decisions and recognition of a degree of social relativity in defining guidelines for medical ethics—are equally visible in the debate concerning the ultimate source of authority for deciding when to terminate life and the presumed authority of the Hippocratic oath in this process.

Two issues, one involving the ethics of sustaining life by means of advanced medical technology and the other involving the "engineering" of lives according to genetic predictions, fall under the provisions of the Hippocratic oath. As one approaches more contemporary statements of professional obligations of medical doctors, such as the "Principles of Medical Ethics" (1957) of the American Medical Association, one finds that, as certain areas of specificity in classical Hippocratic or Christian medical ethics (the illegality of abortions or the administration of deadly potions) tend to decline in visibility, another area begins to come to the forefront—namely, striving continually to improve medical knowledge and skills to be made available to patients and colleagues.

This more modern concern for the application of advancements in medical knowledge, especially in the technology of medical lifesaving therapy, has introduced a new focus for ethical debate: not "lifesaving" but "life-sustaining" techniques, particularly in cases judged to be otherwise terminal or hopeless. As with the issue of abortion, the question of a doctor's responsibility to use every means within his or her reach to sustain life, even when there is no hope of a meaningful future for the patient, reflects a dilemma regarding Hippocratic injunctions. This debate is more important now than in any earlier era because advanced medical technology has made it possible either to extend the lives of aged patients who would die without life-sustaining machines or—in the case of younger persons afflicted by brain damage, for example—to sustain life although the patient remains in a comatose state.

A prototype in the latter case was a 1976 Supreme Court decision that allowed the parents of New Jersey car accident victim Karen Quinlan to instruct her physician to remove life support systems so that their comatose daughter would die. At issue in this complicated case, which also rested on legal discussions of the constitutional right of privacy, was the question of who should decide that inevitable natural death is preferable to prolongation of life by externally administered means. When the Court took this decision away from an appointed court guardian and gave it to those closest to the patient, the question became whose privacy was being protected. This dilemma is not unlike that inherent in the abortion debate, where the privacy of the pregnant woman is weighed against that of the as-yet-unconscious, unborn child. To whom does the physician's oath to avoid doing injury actually apply?

Legal solutions to subareas of the euthanasia debate were attained in stages, especially in cases of the very aged or patients afflicted with known terminal diseases. A living will, for example, allows individuals to instruct their physicians not to sustain their lives by artificial means if, beyond a certain point, they are unable to express their own will to die. In some cases, this discretion is assigned to the next of kin. In both cases, the objective is to remove ultimate responsibility for inevitable natural death from the physician's shoulders and to place it as closely as possible to within the private sphere of the patient.

A final area of contemporary debate over medical ethics illustrates how far conceptions of ultimate responsibility for the protection of life have gone beyond frames of reference that might have been familiar not only in Hippocrates" time but also as recently as the generation of doctors trained before the 1980s. Impressive advances in the research field of human genetics by the mid-1980s began to make it possible to predict, through analysis of deoxyribonucleic acid (DNA) structures, the likelihood that certain genetic traits (specifically debilitating chronic diseases) might be transmitted to the offspring of couples under study. Inherent in the rising debate over the ethics of such studies, which range from the prediction of reproductive combinations (genetic counseling) through actual attempts to detach and splice DNA chains (genetic engineering), was the delicate question of who, if anyone, should hold the responsibility of determining if individuals have ultimate control over their genes. In the most extreme hypothetical argument, a notion of scientific exclusion of certain gene combinations, or planning of desirable gene pools in future generations, began to appear in the 1980s and 1990s. These notions represent potential problems for medical ethics that, because of exponential changes in technological possibilities, surpass the entire realm of Hippocratic principles.

Perspective and Prospects

Despite the introduction of certain legal precedents that tried to protect both physicians and their patients against dilemmas stemming from the assumed immutable ethical principles of the Hippocratic oath, society continues to witness practical shortcomings in modern understanding of who needs to be protected and how such protection should be institutionalized.

Malpractice insurance offers legal protection to physicians against personal damage claims levied by aggrieved patients or those surviving deceased patients; by the late twentieth century in the United States, these rates had soared. The larger debate regarding whether what physicians have done in individual cases was right or wrong rests on the assumption that his or her judgment can be put to the test by private parties defending their rights against professional incompetence. Therefore, the issue, as well as the institutional and/or legal devices pursued to resolve it, lies beyond the strict realm of a patient's privacy vis-á-vis a physician's responsibilities.

More characteristic examples of the contemporary social-ethical dilemma of whether doctors are fulfilling their appropriate professional responsibilities in recognizing patients" rights to certain types of treatment continue to fall into legally unresolved categories. The most obvious appears to be the ongoing debate concerning the legality of physician-assisted abortions. The considerations that have been introduced clearly go beyond the black-or-white principles that simple comparison with the content of the Hippocratic oath might involve. Courts and legislators involved in the ethics of abortion have had to devote extensive attention to the considerations of how pregnancies were induced (with attention to the anomalies of incest or rape, for example) or to questions of whether tax-appropriated funds gathered from an ethically divided public body can be dispensed to pay for medically approved abortions.

Still other dimensions of contemporary physician-patient relationships reveal that new forms of legislation will be needed before debates over the applicability of Hippocratic principles to modern society will recede from front-page prominence. With living wills having more or less resolved the question of individuals" right to instruct physicians or families to make decisions for them when personal capacities decline to incoherence, signs of new legal dilemmas began to emerge in the 1990s concerning fully coherent, terminally ill patients. Despairing of future suffering that can come well before any question of life support devices arises, some patients contracted their physicians—initially one physician in particular, Jack Kevorkian of Detroit, Michigan—to perform "mercy killing" by the administration of lethal poisons. Thus, one of the specific negative injunctions of the original Hippocratic oath returned the question of individual physicians" ethical and legal obligations to the forefront of public attention and court proceedings more than two millennia after its initial statement.

—Byron D. Cannon, Ph.D.

See also Abortion; American Medical Association (AMA); Cloning; Education, medical; Ethics; Euthanasia; Genetic engineering; Law and medicine; Living will; Malpractice.

For Further Information:
Antoniou, Stavros A. "Reflections of the Hippocratic Oath in Modern Medicine." *World Journal of Surgery* 34, no. 12 (December 2010): 3075–3079.

Campbell, Alistair V., Grant Gillett, and Gareth Jones. *Medical Ethics*. 4th ed. New York: Oxford University Press, 2005.

Casarett, David J., Frona Daskal, and John Lantos. "Experts in Ethics? The Authority of the Clinical Ethicist." *Hastings Center Report* 28, no. 6 (November/December, 1998): 6–11.

Devine, Richard J. *Good Care, Painful Choices: Medical Ethics of Ordinary People*. 3d ed. New York: Paulist Press, 2004.

Fletcher, John C., et al., eds. *Introduction to Clinical Ethics*. 3d ed. Hagerstown, Md.: University Publishing Group, 2005.

Harron, Frank. *Biomedical-Ethical Issues: A Digest of Law and Policy Development*. Binghamton, N.Y.: Vail-Ballou Press, 1983. New Haven, Conn.: Yale University Press, 1983.

Hulkower, Raphael. "The History of the Hippocratic Oath: Outdated, Inauthentic, and Yet Still Relevant." *Einstein Journal of Biology & Medicine* 25 (2010): 41–44.

Jonsen, Albert R., Mark Siegler, and William J. Winslade. *Clinical Ethics: A Practical Approach to Ethical Decisions in Clinical Medicine*. 6th ed. New York: McGraw-Hill, 2006.

Martin, William. "Beyond the Hippocratic Oath: Developing Codes of Conduct in Healthcare Organizations." *OD Practitioner* 45, no. 2 (2013): 26–30.

Munson, Ronald, comp. *Intervention and Reflection: Basic Issues in Medical Ethics*. 7th ed. Belmont, Calif.: Thomson/Wadsworth, 2004.

Pence, Gregory. *Classic Cases in Medical Ethics: Accounts of Cases That Have Shaped Medical Ethics, with Philosophical, Legal, and Historical Backgrounds*. 4th ed. Boston: McGraw-Hill, 2004.

HIRSCHSPRUNG'S DISEASE
Disease/Disorder

Also known as: Congenital megacolon
Anatomy or system affected: Anus, intestines, nerves
Specialties and related fields: Cytology, family medicine, obstetrics, pediatrics, proctology
Definition: A disease of the large intestine that makes bowel movements difficult or impossible.

Causes and Symptoms

Hirschsprung's disease is caused when the lower part of the large intestine (colon), including the rectum, does not have the ganglion nerve cells to control the muscles that produce the contractions necessary for a bowel movement. Occasionally, the whole large intestine and even portions of the small intestine may be missing these nerve cells. The disease develops prior to birth. In the normal development of a fetus, the ganglion nerve cells grow from the top of the intestine down to the anus. For some unknown reason, the nerve cells stop growing at some distance down the intestine in children who are born with Hirschsprung's disease.

The disease manifests itself most often in young children, although it can appear when an individual is a teenager or an adult. In an individual with Hirschsprung's disease, the healthy upper portion of the colon pushes stool down until it reaches the affected part. The stool then stops. New stool backs up behind it. Severe constipation results. In some cases, the victim may not be able to have any bowel movements at

---

Information on Hirschsprung's Disease

Causes: Lack of ganglion nerve cells for muscle control in lower colon
Symptoms: Severe constipation, vomiting of bile, swollen abdomen, enterocolitis
Duration: Acute
Treatments: Surgery to remove affected area of colon

---

all. Babies with Hirschsprung's disease often vomit up bile and experience swollen abdomens after eating. Infections, particularly enterocolitis, may develop in the intestines, which has the potential of bursting the colon.

Treatment and Therapy

Diagnosis of the disorder is confirmed by a barium enema x-ray and a biopsy of the rectum. Barium makes the intestine show up better on an x-ray. Manometry is also often used by the doctor to diagnose the disease. In this procedure, a small balloon is inflated inside the rectum. If the anal muscle does not relax, the patient may have Hirschsprung's disease.

A pull-through operation removes the affected area of the intestine. The remaining ends are joined together. After this surgery, 85 to 90 percent of the patients pass feces normally, although some may experience diarrhea or constipation for a period of time. Eating high-fiber foods can help reduce diarrhea and constipation. Since the intestine is shortened by the surgery, not as much fluid is absorbed by the body. Consequently, the patient will need to drink plenty of fluids.

Perspective and Prospects

Hirschsprung's disease occurs in approximately 1 out of every 5,000 births. About 80 percent of patients are boys. Children with Down syndrome are at a high risk for developing the disorder.

Hirschsprung's disease has been found to be hereditary, with the risk greater if the mother has the condition. Even if the parents have not had the disorder develop in their own lives, they may pass it on to their children. If one child in a family has the disease, other children are at greater risk to be born with it.

—Alvin K. Benson, Ph.D.

See also Colon; Congenital disorders; Constipation; Enterocolitis; Gastroenterology; Gastroenterology, pediatric; Gastrointestinal system; Genetic diseases; Intestinal disorders; Intestines; Neonatology; Peristalsis; Rectum; Surgery, pediatric.

For Further Information:
Eichenwald, Heinz F., Josef Ströder, and Charles M. Ginsburg, eds. *Pediatric Therapy*. 3d ed. St. Louis, Mo.: Mosby Year Book, 1993.

Holschneider, Alexander M., and Prem Puri, eds. *Hirschsprung's Disease and Allied Disorders*. 3d ed. New York: Springer, 2008.

Kaneshiro, Neil K. "Hirschsprung Disease." *MedlinePlus*, November 13, 2011.

Icon Health. *Hirschsprung's Disease: A Medical Dictionary, Bibliography, and Annotated Research Guide to Internet References*. San Diego, Calif.: Author, 2004.

Nuı̈ñı̇fez Nuı̈ñı̇fez, Ramoı̈n. *Hirschsprung's Disease: Diagnosis and Treatment.* New York: Nova Biomedical Books, 2006.

Parisi, MA. "Hirschsprung's Disease Overview." *NCBI*, November 10, 2011.

Wallace, A. S., and R. B. Anderson. "Genetic Interactions and Modifier Genes in Hirschsprung's Disease." *World Journal of Gastroenterology* 17, 45. (December 7, 2011): 4937–4944.

HISTIOCYTOSIS
Disease/Disorder

Also known as: Langerhans cell histiocytosis (LCH), histiocytosis X, eosinophilic granuloma, Hand-Schüller-Christian disease, Letterer-Siwe disease

Anatomy or system affected: Blood, bones, ears, gastrointestinal system, immune system, liver, lungs, nervous system, skin, throat

Specialties and related fields: Hematology, immunology

Definition: A group of relatively rare blood disorders characterized by the abnormal accumulation of white blood cells called histiocytes, leading to a wide range of adverse bodily responses.

Causes and Symptoms

There is no clear understanding of the exact etiology of histiocytoses, blood disorders characterized by an accumulation of white blood cells called histiocytes, including monocytes, and macrophages. Langerhans cell histiocytosis (LCH) is the most common type. At least four or five people per million are affected, with more males affected than females. The disorder affects both children and adults.

LCH may develop in response to underlying immunodeficiency or as a secondary effect from a viral infection. Symptoms vary based on the severity of the disease, and patients may be relatively symptom-free. LCH may be localized to one area or organ, or it may be more diffuse, involving multiple organs. It can cause lesions on bone, especially skull bones, or it may manifest itself as a skin rash. Respiratory symptoms such as cough or shortness of breath may signify that LCH has affected the lungs. Gastrointestinal manifestations of the disease include bleeding within the gastrointestinal tract or elevated liver enzymes. LCH can also affect the lymph nodes or the central nervous system and may contribute to the development of diabetes insipidus, growth hormone deficiency, and hypopituitarism (underactive pituitary gland).

Definitive diagnosis requires a biopsy, and the differential diagnosis (other diseases similar to it) is broad. Making the diagnosis requires a high index of suspicion because it is rare and easily missed. Helpful radiologic tests might include a chest x-ray or a skeletal survey.

Treatment and Therapy

Treatment options vary widely based on the severity of the disease. On one hand, minimal treatment may be needed for symptom-free, single-system involvement, especially as LCH affecting only one system often remits completely. On the other hand, more severe disease affecting many systems

---

Information on Histiocytosis

Causes: Response to underlying immunodeficiency or secondary effect from viral infection

Symptoms: Depends on severity; may include bone lesions (especially skull), rashes, respiratory problems (cough, shortness of breath), gastrointestinal problems (bleeding, elevated liver enzymes)

Duration: Short-term or long-term

Treatments: Depends on the severity; may include chemotherapy

---

may warrant chemotherapy, with characteristic remissions and relapses.

Perspective and Prospects

The histiocytoses are classified into three types: LCH, hemophagocytic lymphohistiocytosis (HLH), and malignant histiocytosis. The impacts of LCH can be many, some with short-term and others with long-term consequences: stunted growth, dental problems, hearing loss, and hepatic fibrosis, to name a few. Though caregivers from a variety of medical specialties are often involved in caring for LCH patients and tremendous strides in diagnosis and treatment have been made, many patients still suffer from problematic, recurrent disease.

—Leonard Berkowitz, D.O.,
and Paul Moglia, Ph.D.

See also Blood and blood disorders; Hematology; Hematology, pediatric; Immune system; Immunology; Immunopathology.

For Further Information:

Arceci, Robert J., B. Jack Longley, and Peter D. Emanuel. "Atypical Cellular Disorders." *Hematology*, 2002, 297–314.

Egeler, R Maarten, and Giulio J. D'Angio, eds. *Langerhans Cell Histiocytosis.* Philadelphia: W. B. Saunders, 1998.

Gersten, Todd. "Histiocytosis." *MedlinePlus*, April 30, 2012.

Histiocytosis Association. http://www.histio.org.

Irvine, Alan, Peter Hoeger, and Albert C. Yan. *Harper's Textbook of Pediatric Dermatology.* Hoboken, N.J.: Wiley-Blackwell, 2011.

Jaffe, Elaine Sarkin. *Hematopathology.* Philadelphia: Saunders/Elsevier, 2011.

James, William D., and Dirk M. Elston. *Andrews' Diseases of the Skin: Clinical Dermatology.* Philadelphia: Saunders Elsevier, 2011.

Lichtman, Marshall A.. *Williams Manual of Hematology.* New York: McGraw-Hill, 2011.

Osband, Micheal E., and Carl Pochedly, eds. *Histiocytosis-X.* Philadelphia: W. B. Saunders, 1987.

HISTOLOGY
Specialty

Anatomy or system affected: All

Specialties and related fields: Biochemistry, cytology, dermatology, hematology, internal medicine, oncology, pathology, vascular medicine

Definition: The study of the body's tissues-epithelial, connective, muscle, and nerve tissues-to find the changes in structure that can be induced by disease.

Key terms:

collagen: a fibrous protein occurring in many types of connective tissue

connective tissues: tissues containing large amounts of matrix outside the cells

epithelia: tissues that originate in broad, flat surfaces

matrix: organic or inorganic material occurring in connective tissues but located outside the cells

muscle tissues: tissues specialized in such a manner that they respond to stimulation by contracting along their long axes

nerve tissues: tissues specialized in such a manner that they respond to stimulation by conducting nerve impulses along their surfaces

tissues: groups of similar cells that are closely interrelated in function and organized together spatially

Types of Tissues

Histology is the study of tissues, which are groups of similar cells that are closely interrelated in their function and are organized together by location and structure. The four major types of tissues are epithelial tissue, connective tissue, muscle tissue, and nervous tissue.

Epithelial tissue (or epithelia) includes those tissues that originate in broad, flat surfaces. Their functions include protection, absorption, and secretion. Epithelia can be one-layered (simple) or multilayered (stratified). Their cells can be flat (squamous), tall and thin (columnar), or equal in height and width (cuboidal). Some simple epithelia have nuclei at two different levels, giving the false appearance of different layers; these tissues are called pseudostratified. Some simple squamous epithelia have special names: The inner lining of most blood vessels is called an endothelium, while the lining of a body cavity is called a mesothelium. Kidney tubules and most small ducts are also lined with simple squamous epithelia. The pigmented layer of the retina and the front surface of the lens of the eye are examples of simple cuboidal epithelia. Simple columnar epithelia form the inner lining of most digestive organs and the linings of the small bronchi and gallbladder. The epithelia lining the Fallopian tube, nasal cavity, and bronchi are ciliated, meaning that the cells have small hairlike extensions called cilia.

The outer layer of skin is a stratified squamous epithelium; other stratified squamous epithelia line the inside of the mouth, esophagus, and vagina. Sweat glands and other glands in the skin are lined with stratified cuboidal epithelia. Most of the urinary tract is lined with a special kind of stratified cuboidal epithelium called a transitional epithelium, which allows a large amount of stretching. Parts of the pharynx, larynx, urethra, and the ducts of the mammary glands are lined with stratified columnar epithelia.

Glands are composed of epithelial tissues that are highly modified for secretion. They may be either exocrine glands (in which the secretions exit by ducts that lead to targets nearby) or endocrine glands (in which the secretions are carried by the bloodstream to targets some distance away). The salivary glands in the mouth, the glandular lining of the stomach, and the sebaceous glands of the skin are exocrine glands.

The thyroid gland, the adrenal gland, and the pituitary gland are endocrine glands. The pancreas has both exocrine and endocrine portions; the exocrine parts secrete digestive enzymes, while the endocrine parts, called the islets of Langerhans, secrete the hormones insulin and glucagon.

Connective tissues are tissues containing large amounts of a material called extracellular matrix, located outside the cells. The matrix may be a liquid (such as blood plasma), a solid containing fibers of collagen and related proteins, or an inorganic solid containing calcium salts (as in bone).

Blood and lymph are connective tissues with a liquid matrix (plasma) that can solidify when the blood clots. In addition to plasma, blood contains red cells (erythrocytes), white cells (leukocytes), and the tiny platelets that help to form clots. The many kinds of leukocytes include the so-called granular types (basophils, neutrophils, and eosinophils, all named according to the staining properties of their granules), the monocytes, and the several types of lymphocytes. Lymph contains lymphocytes and plasma only.

Most connective tissues have a solid matrix that includes fibrous proteins such as collagen and also elastic fibers, in some cases. If all the fibers are arranged in the same direction, as in ligaments and tendons, the tissue is called regular connective tissue. The dermis of the skin, however, is an example of an irregular connective tissue in which the fibers are arranged in all directions. Loose connective tissue and adipose (fat) tissue both have very few fibers. The simplest type of loose connective tissue, with the fewest fibers, is sometimes called areolar connective tissue. Adipose tissue is a connective tissue in which the cells are filled with fat deposits. Hemopoietic (blood-forming) tissue, which occurs in the bone marrow and the thymus, contains the immature cell types that develop into most connective tissue cells, including blood cells. Cartilage tissue matrix contains a shock-resistant complex of protein and sugarlike (polysaccharide) molecules. Cartilage cells usually become trapped in this matrix and eventually die, except for those closest to the surface. Bone tissue gains its supporting ability and strength from a matrix containing calcium salts. Its typical cells, called osteocytes, contain many long strands by means of which they exchange nutrients and waste products with other osteocytes, and ultimately with the bloodstream. Bone also contains osteoclasts, large cells responsible for bone resorption and the release of calcium into the bloodstream.

Mesenchyme is an embryonic connective tissue made of wandering amoebalike cells. During embryological development, the mesenchyme cells develop into many different cell types, including hemocytoblasts, which give rise to most blood cells, and fibroblasts, which secrete protein fibers and then usually differentiate into other cell types.

Muscle tissues are tissues that are specially modified for contraction. When a nerve impulse is received, the overlapping fibers of the proteins actin and myosin slide against one another to produce the contraction. The three types of muscle tissue are smooth muscle, cardiac muscle, and skeletal muscle.

Smooth muscle contains cells that have tapering ends and

centrally located nuclei. Muscular contractions are smooth, rhythmic, and involuntary, and they are usually not subject to fatigue. The cells are not cross-banded. Smooth muscle occurs in many digestive organs, reproductive organs, skin, and many other organs.

The term "striated muscle" is sometimes used to refer to cardiac and skeletal muscle, both of which have cylindrical fibers marked by cross-bands, which are also called cross-striations. The striations are caused by the lining up of the contractile proteins actin and myosin.

Cardiac muscle occurs only in the heart. Its cross-striated fibers branch and come together repeatedly. Contractions of these fibers are involuntary and rhythmic, and they occur without fatigue. Nuclei are located in the center of each cell; the cell boundaries are marked by dark-staining structures called intercalated disks.

Skeletal muscle occurs in the voluntary muscles of the body. Its cylindrical, cross-striated fibers contain many nuclei but no internal cell boundaries; a multinucleated fiber of this type is called a syncytium. Skeletal muscle is capable of producing rapid, forceful contractions, but it fatigues easily. Skeletal muscle tissue always attaches to connective tissue structures.

Nervous tissues contain specialized nerve cells (neurons) that respond rapidly to stimulation by conducting nerve impulses. All neurons contain RNA-rich granules, called Nissl granules, in the cytoplasm. Neurons with a single long extension of the cell body are called unipolar, those with two long extensions are called bipolar, and those with more than two long extensions are called multipolar. There are two types of extensions: Dendrites conduct impulses toward the cell body, while axons generally conduct impulses away from the cell body. Many axons are surrounded by a multilayered fatty substance called the myelin sheath, which is actually made of many layers of cell membrane wrapped around the axon.

Nervous tissues also contain several types of neuroglia, which are cells that hold nervous tissue together. Many neuroglia have processes (projections) that wrap around the neurons and help nourish them. Among the many types of neuroglia are the tiny microglia and the larger protoplasmic astrocytes, fibrous astrocytes, and oligodendroglia.

Two major tissue types make up most of the brain and spinal cord, or central nervous system. The first type, gray matter, contains the cell bodies of many neurons, along with smaller amounts of axons, dendrites, and neuroglia cells. The second type, white matter, contains mostly the axons, and sometimes also the dendrites, of neurons whose cell bodies lie elsewhere, along with the myelin sheaths that surround many of the axons. Clumps of cell bodies are called nuclei within the brain and ganglia elsewhere. Bundles of axons are called tracts within the central nervous system and nerves in the peripheral nervous system.

Histology as a Diagnostic Tool

Many diseases produce changes in one or more body tissues; these changes are so characteristic that the diagnosis of a disease often depends on the microscopic observation of changes in tissues. For such a diagnosis to be made, the tissue must be sliced very thin on a machine called a microtome. Some tissues are sliced while frozen; others must be hardened (or "fixed") in chemical solutions. After being sliced, the tissue is usually stained with chemical dyes that make viewing easier. Some tissues are viewed under a light microscope; others are sliced even thinner for viewing by electron microscopy.

Most hospitals have a pathology department that is responsible for these operations. After the tissues are sliced and examined, the pathologist makes a report that usually includes a diagnosis of the disease shown by the tissue samples.

Many diseases result in marked changes in the tissue at the microscopic level. Adaptively altered changes, which are usually reversible, include an increase in cell size (hypertrophy), increase in cell numbers (hyperplasia), a change from one cell or tissue type to another (metaplasia), and a decrease in size by withering (atrophy). Prolonged or repeated insults to the tissue may result in altered or atypical growth patterns (dysplasia). Overwhelming or sustained injury results in irreversible changes such as tissue degeneration or death. Tissue degeneration often includes the accumulation of abnormal amounts of fatty, fibrous, or pigmented tissue. Tissue death in a body that goes on living is called necrosis, and it may be of several types. If tissue death exceeds a certain limit, then the death of the organism results. Once this occurs, the tissues usually release protein-digesting enzymes that digest their own cell contents, a process known as autolysis.

Changes to cellular organelles can often be seen with an electron microscope before they become apparent at the light microscope level. Disturbances of the cell membrane may alter the flow of fluids (especially water) and cause changes to occur in the fluid composition of the cytoplasm. Too much fluid may result in swelling and eventually in bursting of the cells; too little fluid results either in shrinkage or in the coagulation of proteins. Swelling may also be induced by the lack of oxygen flow to the mitochondria, which can also result in the deposition of fats or calcium. The increase in the water content of the cells can also cause swelling in the endoplasmic reticulum and the detachment of ribosomes from the surfaces of the rough endoplasmic reticulum. Most damaging of all are the disturbances of the lysosomes, which can release their protein-digesting enzymes and cause autolysis.

At the light microscope level, other changes that may result from disease processes include the coalescence of numerous dropletlike vacuoles into a single, large, fluid-filled space. Other changes that may indicate disease are abnormal cell shapes, changes in the proportion of blood cells, and the rupture of cell membranes or other structures. Substances that may accumulate in diseased cells include glycogen (a sugar storage product), fibrous deposits of collagen and other proteins, and mineral deposits such as calcium salts. Abnormalities of the nucleus may include nuclear fragmentation, loss of the staining properties of the nucleus, or pyknosis, a shrinkage of the nucleus that also includes the clumping of its chromosomal material.

Edema, or tissue swelling, is a condition that can easily be confirmed by microscopic examination of histological sections. The swelling is marked by an increase in the amount of extracellular fluid. In the case of pulmonary edema, the fluid stains pink and fills the usually empty lung spaces (alveoli).

A different type of change is seen in Barrett's esophagus, a condition caused by the repeated backflow (or reflux) of gastric fluids into the esophagus. The inner lining of the esophagus is usually a stratified squamous epithelium, but in Barrett's esophagus the surface cells become taller, and the lining is changed into a columnar epithelium resembling that of the stomach.

Most cancers are recognized by abnormalities of the affected tissues, usually including more cells in the process of cell division (mitosis). The most dangerous cancers are marked by large tumors with ill-defined, irregular margins. If the cancer tumor is well-defined, small, and has a smooth, circular margin, the cancer is much less of a threat.

In juvenile diabetes, histological examination of the pancreas reveals a greatly reduced number of pancreatic islets, and those that remain are smaller and more fibrous. Herpes simplex infection causes the epidermal cells of the skin to undergo a buildup of fluid and a consequent balloonlike swelling. Warts of the skin are marked by a thickening of the outermost layer (stratum corneum) of the epidermis. Pernicious anemia, or vitamin B_{12} deficiency, results in a deterioration of the glands in the stomach lining. Crohn's disease produces swelling of the affected parts of the intestine, deposition of fat and lymphoid tissue, and ultimately tissue loss and deposition of fibrous scar tissue; the affected parts typically alternate with healthy regions. Cirrhosis of the liver, which is most commonly the result of chronic alcohol abuse, proceeds through a fatty stage (marked by deposition of fatty tissue), a fibrotic stage (marked by small nodules and scars), and an end stage marked by abnormal shrinkage (atrophy) of liver tissue, scars, and larger nodules up to 1 centimeter in diameter. Emphysema, a lung disease found in many smokers, is recognizable histologically by an enlargement of the air spaces and by the presence of black, tarlike deposits within the lung tissue. Fibrocystic changes of the breast may be marked by the deposition of fibrous tissue, by increasing cell numbers, and by the enlargement of the glandular ducts.

Systemic lupus erythematosus (SLE), a connective tissue disease, often produces red skin lesions marked by degeneration and flattening of the lower layers of the epidermis, drying and flaking of the outermost layer, dilation of the blood vessels under the skin, and the leakage of red blood cells out of these vessels, adding to the red color. (The word "erythematosus" means "red.")

Muscular dystrophy has several forms; the most common form is marked in its advanced stages by enlarged muscles in which the muscle tissue is replaced by a fatty substance. Another muscular disease, myasthenia gravis, is often marked by overall enlargement of the thymus and an increase in the number of thymus cells. Myocardial infarction (heart attack), a form of heart disease marked by damage to the heart muscle, is indicated in histological section by dead, fibrous scar tissue replacing the muscle tissue in the heart wall. In patients with arteriosclerosis, the usually elastic walls of the arteries become thicker and more fibrous and rigid. Many of the same patients also suffer from atherosclerosis, a buildup of deposits on the inside of the blood vessels that partially or completely blocks the flow of blood.

In nervous tissue, damage to peripheral nerves often results in a process called chromatolysis in the cell bodies of the neurons from which these axons arise. The nuclei of these cells enlarge and are displaced to one side, while the Nissl granules disperse and the cell body as a whole undergoes swelling. Increased deposits of fibrous tissue characterize multiple sclerosis and certain other disorders of the nervous system. Some of these diseases are also marked by a degeneration of the myelin sheath around nerve fibers. In the case of a cerebrovascular stroke, impaired blood supply to the brain causes degeneration of the neuroglia, followed by general tissue death and the replacement of the neuroglia by fibrous tissue. Cranial hematoma (abnormal bleeding in any of several possible locations) results in the presence of blood clots (complete with blood cells and connective tissue fibers) in abnormal locations. Alzheimer's disease is marked by granules of a proteinlike substance called amyloid, often containing aluminum, surrounded by additional concentric layers of similar composition. Advanced stages of alcoholism are marked in brain tissue by the destruction of certain neurons and neuroglia. Poliomyelitis, or polio, is marked by the destruction of nervous tissue in the anterior horn of the spinal cord.

Perspective and Prospects

The microscopic study of tissues began historically with Robert Hooke's *Micrographia* (1665) and the studies of Marcello Malpighi (1628–94), but early microscopes were low in quality by today's standards. As microscopes improved, so did their use in studying tissues. During the 1830s, the Scottish botanist Robert Brown (1773–1858) discovered the cell nucleus. Soon, German biologists Matthias Jakob Schleiden (1804–81) and Theodor Schwann (1810–82) developed the so-called cell theory, which proclaimed that all living things are constructed of cells and that all biological processes are rooted in processes occurring at the level of cells and tissues. The greatest advances in microscopic optics were made between 1870 and 1900, mostly in Germany, and the study of histology benefited greatly.

The great pathologist Rudolph Virchow (1821–1902) was the first to emphasize the structural changes in cells caused by the disease process; he showed that many diseases could be detected at the cellular level under the microscope. This claim, coupled with enthusiasm for the cell theory, aroused great interest in the study of cells throughout Europe and later in America. Advances in tissue-staining techniques in microanatomy were made in various countries over a long period; the Czech histologist and physiologist Jan Evangelista Purkinje (1787–1869) was one of the leaders of this early period. Early in the twentieth century, histologists Santiago Ramón y Cajal (1852–1934) of Spain and Camillo Golgi

(1844–1926) of Italy shared the 1906 Nobel Prize in Physiology or Medicine for their detailed work on the tissue structure of the nervous system. In the decades after World War II, the electron microscope became a standard instrument for the ultrafine study of tissue details at and even below the cellular level. Today, pathology laboratories routinely use the microscopic examination of tissues as an important tool in diagnosis.

—*Eli C. Minkoff, Ph.D.*

See also Alzheimer's disease; Arteriosclerosis; Biopsy; Bleeding; Blood and blood disorders; Bones and the skeleton; Cells; Cirrhosis; Crohn's disease; Cytology; Dermatology; Diagnosis; Emphysema; Glands; Herpes; Lymphatic system; Multiple sclerosis; Muscles; Muscular dystrophy; Nervous system; Neurology; Orthopedics; Pathology; Poliomyelitis; Skin; Strokes; Systemic lupus erythematosus (SLE).

For Further Information:

Fawcett, D. W. *A Textbook of Histology*. 12th ed. New York: Chapman & Hall, 1994.

Junqueira, Luiz Carlos, and José Carneiro. *Junqueira's Basic Histology: Text and Atlas*. 13th ed. New York: McGraw-Hill Medical, 2013.

Kerr, Jeffrey B. *Atlas of Functional Histology*. Reprint. St. Louis, Mo.: Mosby/Elsevier, 2006.

Kessel, Richard G. *Basic Medical Histology: The Biology of Cells, Tissues, and Organs*. New York: Oxford University Press, 1998.

Lewin, Benjamin. *Genes*. 9th ed. Sudbury, Mass.: Jones and Bartlett, 2008.

Ross, Michael H., and Wojciech Pawlina. *Histology: A Text and Atlas*. 6th ed. Baltimore: Lippincott Williams & Wilkins, 2011.

"SIU SOM Histology." *Southern Illinois University School of Medicine*, August 2, 2013.

HIV. *See* HUMAN IMMUNODEFICIENCY VIRUS (HIV).

HIVES

Disease/Disorder

Also known as: Urticaria

Anatomy or system affected: Immune system, skin

Specialties and related fields: Dermatology, family medicine, immunology, internal medicine, pediatrics

Definition: Pink swellings called wheals that may occur in groups on any part of the skin.

Causes and Symptoms

Hives are produced by blood plasma leaking through tiny gaps between the cells lining small vessels in the skin. A natural chemical called histamine is released from mast cells, which lie along the blood vessels in the skin. Allergic reactions, foods, drugs, or other chemicals can cause histamine release.

Hives can vary in size from as small as a pencil eraser to as large as a dinner plate, and they may join together to form larger swellings. When hives are forming, they are usually very itchy; they may also burn or sting. Nearly 20 percent of the general population will have at least one episode of hives in their lifetime. Acute hives may last for a few days to weeks.

Information on Hives

Causes: Allergic reactions, foods, drugs, environmental toxins, infections, insect bites, internal diseases, physical stimuli (e.g., heat, cold)

Symptoms: Inflammation, itchiness

Duration: Acute or chronic

Treatments: Antihistamines

If they last for more than six weeks, they are called chronic hives.

The most common causes of acute hives are foods, drugs, infections, insect bites, and internal diseases. Other causes include physical stimuli, such as pressure, cold, and sunlight.

Treatment and Therapy

The best treatment for hives is to find the cause and then eliminate it. Unfortunately, this is not always an easy task. Even if a cause cannot be found, antihistamines are usually prescribed to provide some relief. Antihistamines work best if taken on a regular schedule. It may be necessary to try more than one or use different combinations of antihistamines to find out what works best. In severe cases of hives, an injection of epinephrine (adrenalin) or a cortisone preparation can bring dramatic relief.

Perspective and Prospects

In 1927, Sir Thomas Lewis reported the association between wheals and small blood vessel dilation, which later confirmed the importance of histamine as a cause of hives. Years of research showed that in addition to allergy, nonimmunological stimuli can cause hives as well. A 1993 report in the *New England Journal of Medicine* found that 30 to 40 percent of patients with idiopathic chronic hives have anti-IGE receptor antibodies in their systems, suggesting that the causes of hives could be multifactorial.

—*Shih-Wen Huang, M.D.*

See also Allergies; Antihistamines; Bites and stings; Blood vessels; Dermatology, pediatric; Immune system; Itching; Over-the-counter medications; Rashes; Skin; Skin disorders.

For Further Information:

Adelman, Daniel C., Thomas B. Casale, and Jonathan Corren, eds. *Manual of Allergy and Immunology*. 5th ed. Philadelphia: Lippincott Williams & Wilkins, 2012.

"Chronic Hives." *Mayo Clinic*, September 17, 2011.

Delves, Peter J., et al. *Roitt's Essential Immunology*. 12th ed. Hoboken, N.J.: John Wiley & Sons, 2011.

Hellwig, Jennifer, and Purvee S. Shah. "Hives." *Health Library*, September 10, 2012.

Hide, Michihiro, et al. "Autoantibodies against the High-Affinity IgE Receptor as a Cause of Histamine Release in Chronic Urticaria." *New England Journal of Medicine* 328, no. 22 (June 1993): 1599–1604.

"Hives." *MedlinePlus*, July 10, 2013.

Joneja, Janice M.V., and Leonard Bielory. *Understanding Allergy, Sensitivity, and Immunity: A Comprehensive Guide*. New Brunswick, N.J.: Rutgers University Press, 1990.

Middlemiss, Prisca. *What's That Rash? How to Identify and Treat*

Childhood Rashes. London: Hamlyn, 2002.

Owen, Judith A., Jenni Punt, and Sharon A. Stranford. *Kuby Immunology*. 7th ed. New York: W. H. Freeman, 2013.

Young, Stuart H., Bruce S. Dobozin, and Margaret Miner. *Allergies: The Complete Guide to Diagnosis, Treatment, and Daily Management*. Rev. ed. New York: Plume, 1999.

HODGKIN'S DISEASE

Disease/Disorder

Anatomy or system affected: Lymphatic system

Specialties and related fields: Hematology, internal medicine, oncology, serology

Definition: A neoplastic disorder originating in the tissues of the lymphatic system, recognized by distinctive histologic changes and defined by the presence of Reed-Sternberg cells.

Key terms:

chemotherapy: a modality of cancer treatment consisting of the administration of cytotoxic drugs

combination chemotherapy: the use of multiple chemical agents in the treatment of cancer, each in a lower dosage so that the overall toxicity, but not the effectiveness, is reduced

neoplastic: pertaining to cancerous growths

prognosis: a prediction of the outcome of treatment for a disease on the basis of clinical and pathologic parameters, such as pathology, clinical stage, and presence or absence of symptoms such as fever, night sweats, and unexplained weight loss

radiotherapy: the use of radiation to kill cancer cells or shrink cancerous growth; when high and full doses of radiation (measured in units called rads) are used, the patient is said to be given a "megavoltage"

Causes and Symptoms

Malignant lymphomas are neoplasms of lymphoid tissues and are of two general categories: those related to Hodgkin (also known as Hodgkin's) disease and others that are collectively called non-Hodgkin lymphomas. The lymphoid tissues represent the structural expressions of the immune system, which defends the body against microbes. This system is widely spread throughout the body, is highly complex, and interacts closely with other physiologic systems of the body—especially the mucosa that lines the airways and digestive tract, where there is direct exposure to environmental microbes and other foreign substances. The components of this system are aggregations of lymphocytes in the mucosal linings (such as tonsils and adenoids), lymph nodes, and the spleen. The components of the lymphatic system connect with one another via small lymphatic vessels. The lymph nodes, which are situated in anatomical regions all over the body, interconnect and drain centrally toward the great veins of the body. The cellular components of the immune system are the lymphocytes, also called immunocytes. These account for about 20 percent of blood cells; lymphocytes make up the bulk of the lymphoid tissue that makes up the lymphatic system. The blood cells have a finite life and are

Information on Hodgkin's Disease
Causes: Unknown
Symptoms: Persistent fever and fatigue; chills and night sweats; painless swelling of lymph nodes in neck, armpits, or groin; unexplained weight loss and loss of appetite; eventual tumors
Duration: Possibly recurrent
Treatments: Radiation therapy, chemotherapy, bone marrow transplantation

disposed of in the spleen, which is the largest lymphoid organ in the body.

There are two major functional immunologic classes of lymphocytes and several other subclasses. Nevertheless, all share similar morphologic appearance, being small round cells almost completely occupied by a round nucleus. The B lymphocyte (the B refers to its bone marrow derivation) can, under proper antigenic stimulation, transform and mature into a plasma cell, which is the cell in charge of producing antibodies. Antibodies are the protein products of the immune system that act by capturing and removing foreign substances, called antigens. The other major class of lymphocytes is the T lymphocyte (the T refers to its thymus derivation). T lymphocytes are of at least two major functional subclasses, which either help or suppress the B lymphocytes in their transformation into plasma cells; thus they are termed helper and suppressor T cells, respectively. Other cellular components of the immune system, cellular monocytes and macrophages, play an important role in carrying and transferring specific immunologic information between the various cellular components of the immune-lymphatic system. This, then, is a highly organized and complex system, with positive and negative biofeedback that maintains optimal, balanced proportions of all the cellular components that make up the system.

Hodgkin disease is a neoplasm of the lymphoid tissues that usually arises in lymph nodes, often in the neck, and has a varied histologic appearance characterized by the presence of Reed-Sternberg cells. The Reed-Sternberg cell is a giant cell having two nuclei that are situated in a mirror-image fashion. Treatment and prognosis in Hodgkin disease are determined by two parameters: the histopathologic classification, whereby the morphologic appearance is evaluated by the pathologist, and the clinical staging classification, whereby the extent of spread of the disease and its localization are determined by clinical studies. The pathology is studied by reviewing thinly cut sections of diseased lymph nodes removed from the patient. This study is most important for establishing a diagnosis of Hodgkin disease and ruling out other conditions that may closely simulate its clinical and/or pathologic features. At times, peer consultations are used to confirm the diagnosis.

Reed-Sternberg cells have a characteristic appearance and must be identified to make a diagnosis of Hodgkin disease. The pathologic classification of this disease, based on microscopic study, recognizes four different types, each with its own clinical implications regarding survival and prognosis. The classification is based on the relative dominance of lymphocytes when compared to the number of the neoplastic Reed-Sternberg cells. In the most favorable type, the lymphocytes predominate and Reed-Sternberg cells are sparse; this type is called lymphocyte predominance. In the worst type, the lymphocytes are very sparse and there are many more Reed-Sternberg cells and their variants; this type is called lymphocyte depletion. In between these two extremes are the mixed-cellularity type, in which there is an even mixture of lymphocytes and Reed-Sternberg cells, and nodular sclerosis, which forms nodules of fibrous scar tissue that surround the mixture of lymphocytes and Reed-Sternberg cells.

This classification has important prognostic implications. It correctly presumes that the neoplastic cells are the Reed-Sternberg cells and their variants, and that the lymphocytes are induced by the immune system to multiply and to fight the spread of the neoplastic cells. It follows that the more the process is successful, the better is the prognosis. Hence lymphocyte predominance carries a more favorable outlook than lymphocyte depletion, with mixed-cellularity types somewhere in between. Nodular sclerosis also carries a good prognosis. Other inflammatory cells are invariably mixed with the lymphocytes and Reed-Sternberg cells; these cells are also part of the body's immune response against cancer cells.

The clinical staging classification of Hodgkin disease was formulated by a group of experts who met at a workshop in Ann Arbor, Michigan, in 1971. It is based on the proposition that the disease begins in a single group of lymph nodes (usually in the neck) and then spreads to the next adjacent group of lymph nodes, on the same side, before it crosses over to the other side of the body. The disease then advances farther across the diaphragm muscle, which separates the thorax from the abdominal cavity, and finally disseminates into the blood to involve the bone marrow and other distant sites. In this schema, stage I represents early stage, with involvement of only a single lymph node region, and stage II is the condition in which two or more such regions are involved on the same side of the diaphragm (that is, either above or below the diaphragm).

In the United States, Hodgkin disease is an uncommon neoplasm accounting for an estimated 9,000 cases. As of 2013, the disease accounts for approximately 1,300 deaths annually, according to American Cancer Society statistics. The incidence in the United States is slightly higher in males than females, and in whites than blacks. As of 2010, approximately 94,000 men and 88,000 women were alive who had histories of Hodgkin disease.

Hodgkin disease can occur at any age, although the highest peak incidence occurs in adolescents and young adults, and smaller peaks occur in the fifth and sixth decades of life. Most patients come to clinical attention because of painless, nontender, enlarged lymph nodes in the neck or armpits (above the diaphragm) or, less commonly, in the groin. In the young adult or adolescent, a mass in the chest may press against the airways to produce a dry, hacking cough and shortness of breath, which may be the patient's first symptoms. Some patients may have anemia or severe itching. At times, especially when the disease is aggressive and extensive, the patient may have a fever, which may run for a few days and then disappear, only to recur after a week or two; there can also be night sweats and weight loss. These symptoms—fever, night sweats, and weight loss—indicate a less favorable prognosis. Younger patients and those with lymphocyte predominance and nodular sclerosis histologic types (favorable histologic types) tend to have limited disease—that is, stages I and II—found primarily above the diaphragm. Older patients and those with mixed-cellularity or lymphocyte depletion types are more likely to have extensive disease involving lymph nodes on both sides of the diaphragm (stage III) or even involving the liver, spleen, and bone marrow (stage IV).

When a patient with persistent lymph node enlargement seeks medical attention, a lymph node biopsy is usually made to make sure of the diagnosis. Other cancers that may simulate Hodgkin disease must be excluded, as well as a long list of benign conditions such as infectious mononucleosis and tuberculosis. A series of blood tests, x-ray and other imaging studies, and a bone marrow biopsy are done in order to evaluate the spread of disease and to assign the proper clinical stage. At times, even surgical exploration of the abdomen, with biopsies of abdominal lymph nodes, the liver, and the spleen, is done to assign an accurate stage of Hodgkin disease; this procedure is called staging laparotomy.

Treatment and Therapy

Modern cancer therapy has achieved its greatest triumph in the treatment of Hodgkin disease. The advent of a generally acceptable histopathologic classification, accurate staging, improved radiotherapy, effective chemotherapy, and supportive care, such as antibiotics and the transfusion of platelets, have contributed to the impressive 80 percent overall cure rate. The therapy is enhanced by an effective teamwork of medical experts in oncology, radiation therapy, surgery, pathology, and diagnostic radiology.

Because Hodgkin disease spreads in an orderly fashion through adjacent lymph node groups, effective high-dose radiation can be directed at affected lymph nodes and at their neighboring, uninvolved nodes. Irradiation, with a full dose of 3,500 to 4,000 rads in three to four weeks, can eradicate Hodgkin disease in involved nodes within the treatment field more than 95 percent of the time. In addition, extended-field irradiation of the adjacent uninvolved nodes is a standard practice used to eradicate minimal or early disease in these lymph nodes.

Stages I and II can be treated with radiotherapy alone by an extended field to include all areas above the diaphragm bearing lymph nodes (the axilla, neck, and chest), and in most cases the lymph nodes in the abdomen. Such treatment cures about 90 percent of patients. For patients in which the disease is found extensively in the chest, chemotherapy is added to the radiotherapy and results in prolonged, relapse-free survival in 85 percent of patients.

A variety of cytotoxic drugs (those that kill cells) are available to treat Hodgkin disease. Such drugs are similar to nitrogen mustard (which was once used in war) and are toxic to the body. It has been found that when more than one drug is used, each in a smaller dose, the toxicity can be reduced without diminishing effectiveness. Thus, combination chemotherapy has evolved. There are many effective regimens of combination chemotherapy that are called by the initials of the individual components; the most widely used is MOPP (mechlorethamine, Oncovin, procarbazine, and prednisone). In stage III, chemotherapy with or without radiotherapy is used, depending upon specific variations within the stage, with cure rates achieved in 80 percent of patients. Even in stage IV disease, combination chemotherapy (particularly with MOPP) has produced a complete remission in about 65 percent of patients, with a cure rate of more than 50 percent.

Bone marrow transplantation, which is the intravenous infusion of normal marrow cells into the patient shortly after treatment in order to protect the patient from toxicity, has permitted the use of much higher doses of certain drugs. It allows the therapist to irradiate all the patient's bone marrow, eradicating both "good" and "bad" cells, with the hope that the normal marrow cells that are infused will populate the bone marrow and grow there. Bone marrow transplantation has been successfully used mainly in young patients who were resistant to conventional chemotherapy.

Perspective and Prospects

Thomas Hodgkin of Guy's Hospital in London was the first to recognize the disease that would bear his name. In 1832, he described the autopsy findings and clinical features of seven patients who had simultaneous enlargement of grossly diseased lymph nodes and spleens, and he considered the condition to be a primary affliction of these organs. This condition, he himself records, was vaguely outlined by Marcello Malpighi in 1665. Four years earlier than Hodgkin, David Craige had described the autopsy findings of a similar case. Subsequent histologic examination of tissues from Hodgkin's original cases confirmed the disease in three of them. In 1865, Sir Samuel Wilks elaborated on the autopsy studies of similar cases and published the findings on fifteen patients, calling the condition Hodgkin disease.

Important histopathologic observations were contributed by William Greenfield in 1878 and E. Goldman in 1892. George Sternberg described the giant cells but believed the condition to be a peculiar form of tuberculosis. The recognition that these cells were an integral part of the disease awaited the careful pathologic observation of Dorothy Reed of Johns Hopkins Hospital in Baltimore. These cells, appropriately named Reed-Sternberg cells, are the hallmark of Hodgkin disease.

Controversy as to the nature of this disease led early investigators to study infectious agents as possible etiologic causes, especially the tuberculosis bacillus, but to no avail. More recent studies have examined the roles of other viral infectious agents, especially the agent of infectious mononucleosis, but with no consistent results. At present, the condition is accepted as neoplastic, probably triggered by some unknown environmental agent or agents.

Between 1930 and 1950, major advances included the recognition of meaningful histologic subtypes of Hodgkin disease correlating with prognosis, and the development by Vera Peters of a clinical staging system. Impressive responses to X-ray therapy were reported at the beginning of the twentieth century, and treatment with megavoltage therapy was further developed. By World War II, it became realistic to speak of curing some patients with early Hodgkin disease. The potential for a cure meant that accurate histologic diagnosis and estimation of the extent and localization of disease were imperative in planning treatment; a multidisciplinary approach to diagnosis and treatment was developed. Modern concepts of histologic classification became codified at a conference held in Rye, New York, in 1965, and the clinical staging system was refined into its present form at a workshop held at Ann Arbor, Michigan, in 1971.

Modern effective chemotherapy was developed concurrently with these advances in classification, staging, and radiotherapy. The alkylating agents, created as an outgrowth of studies on nitrogen mustard gas during World War II, provided the first drugs to produce impressive shrinkage of the tumor and significant palliation of the disease. The subsequent developments in modern pharmacology and therapeutics enabled Vince DeVita and his coworkers, in 1970, to design the first effective combination chemotherapy regimen, MOPP.

Today, many more such regimens are being tested; the possibility for cure has become a realistic hope for every patient with Hodgkin disease. This is the case because of the refinement of ancillary therapies with antibiotics (for infections that may occur during the necessary phases of suppression of the immune system by these powerful toxic drugs) and platelet transfusion technology. Bone marrow transplantation technology also offers strong hope of curing patients with advanced cases who are resistant. The bone marrow is harvested and then reintroduced into a patient whose marrow has been effectively disabled. Immunotherapy is also being investigated. It can boost the patient's ability to combat disease by modulating the body's responses. The drawback to aggressive combinations of chemotherapy and radiotherapy, however, is the emergence of therapy-related leukemia and leukemia-like malignancies several years after the completion of successful therapy for Hodgkin disease.

—*Victor H. Nassar, M.D.*

See also Bone marrow transplantation; Cancer; Chemotherapy; Lymph; Lymphadenopathy and lymphoma; Lymphatic system; Malignancy and metastasis; Oncology; Radiation therapy.

For Further Information:

CA: A Cancer Journal for Clinicians 43, no. 1(January/February, 1993).

Dollinger, Malin, et al. *Everyone's Guide to Cancer Therapy.* 5th ed. Kansas City, Mo.: Andrews McMeel, 2008.

Eyre, Harmon J., Dianne Partie Lange, and Lois B. Morris. *Informed Decisions: The Complete Book of Cancer Diagnosis, Treatment, and Recovery.* 2d ed. Atlanta: American Cancer Society, 2002.

Greer, John, et al., eds. *Wintrobe's Clinical Hematology*. 12th ed. Philadelphia: Wolters Kluwer/Lippincott Williams & Wilkins Health, 2009.

Hoppe, Richard. *Hodgkin Lymphoma*. 2d ed. Philadelphia: Lippincott, 2007.

Jacobs, Charlotte. *Henry Kaplan and the Story of Hodgkin's Disease*. Stanford, Calif.: Stanford University Press, 2010.

Lichtman, Marshall A., et al., eds. *Williams Hematology*. 8th ed. New York: McGraw-Hill, 2010.

Lymphoma Information Network. http://www.lym phomainfo.net/hodgkins.

Parker, James N., and Philip M. Parker, eds. *The Official Parent's Sourcebook on Childhood Hodgkin's Disease*. San Diego, Calif.: Icon Health, 2002.

Parker, James N., and Philip M. Parker, eds. *Official Patient's Sourcebook on Adult Hodgkin's Disease*. San Diego, Calif.: Icon Health, 2002.

Specht, Lena, and Joachim Yahalom. *Radiotherapy for Hodgkin Lymphoma*. New York: Springer, 2011.

Williams, Stephanie F., Ramez Farah, and Harvey M. Golomb, eds. *Hodgkin's Disease*. Philadelphia: W. B. Saunders, 1989.

HOME CARE

Health care system

Also known as: In-home care, in-home services, home health care

Specialties and related fields: Medical social work, nursing, occupational therapy, physical therapy, speech therapy

Definition: Skilled health and nonskilled support care services provided in the home.

Key terms:

continuous care: services provided for extended periods of time such as shifts of eight, ten, twelve, or twenty-four hours

home care reimbursement: various payment options for home care services such as private insurance, government-sponsored programs such as Medicare and Medicaid, long-term care insurance, and self-pay

hospice home care: services provided by professionals and support staff to allow a person with a life-threatening diagnosis of six months or less to remain at home with care

intermittent care: services provided one or more times a week with each visit limited in time

nonskilled home care: support care that does not require a professional; also known as custodial in-home care

skilled home care: medically necessary care that requires a service by a professional such as a nurse or physical therapist

Home Care Option

Many health care and support services can be delivered outside the traditional acute care environment, such as a hospital, rehabilitation center, or skilled nursing facility. Home care services allow people to live at home and still receive necessary health and support care. Examples of persons who can benefit from home care include those discharged from a hospital, rehabilitation center, or skilled nursing unit; older adults with limited caregivers or support systems; chronically ill or disabled persons; postsurgical patients; and at-risk newborns or children. Home care makes staying in one's residence while ill or injured a reality. A nurse or medical social worker can help people assess their needs and access appropriate agencies for home care services. Urban areas usually have more home care agencies offering a wider variety of home care services than rural areas.

Skilled and Nonskilled Home Care

Just as people have different care needs, varied types of home care organizations offer diverse services to meet those needs. For example, some people need nonskilled services to remain in their home. Communities and private companies offer continuous care services such as sitters/attendants who can stay with the person for eight- to twelve-hour shifts. These attendants may provide personal care such as bathing or hair washing. Some agencies connect live-in companions that are available twenty-four hours a day with people needing home care help. Homemaker services are offered through community programs for light house cleaning, clothes washing, grocery shopping, and preparing of simple meals. Home care agencies may align with volunteer groups who have visitation programs and assist with light yard work or transportation to the grocery store or doctor's office. These types of services are important, as they provide help with activities of daily living (ADL) necessary for a dependent person to stay in his or her residence. Most nonskilled home care services are self-pay unless covered by a grant, long-term care insurance, or government-sponsored program such as Medicaid.

Many patients are discharged from hospitals earlier than they once were, to recuperate from illness or surgery at home. Home health care is a less costly alternative to institutional care. Medically necessary skilled home care services are often covered by full or partial reimbursement through private insurance or by government-sponsored programs like Medicare or Medicaid; others may access home care services through self-pay. The home care team is usually an interdisciplinary team of professionals and support staff that work together to maintain a person in his or her home and out of the hospital or other institutional care. The interdisciplinary team may include the registered nurse, licensed practical nurse, home health aid/assistant/attendant, physical therapist, occupational therapist, speech therapist, and medical social worker. Chaplains and volunteers may be part of the home care team. The group works under the direction of the agency administrator, providing care with a medical plan and orders from the attending physician.

Services delivered are based on the patient's condition, individual needs, home location, and sources of reimbursement. Home health care services are provided on an intermittent basis, with care delivered several times each week for an average of thirty minutes to an hour per visit. The patient, along with his or her caregiver, remains responsible for daily care. Intermittent care means the nurse or physical therapist will come to the home to teach or provide specific care but will not stay in the home. The skilled provider will teach the caregiver how to perform necessary tasks. Skilled home health care services are not designed to provide home care for extended periods of time but to assist the person to regain independence or optimal functioning.

Skilled nursing services are provided in the home by a registered nurse (RN). Examples of nursing care include monitoring of vital signs such as blood pressure and pulse; teaching the patient and other caregivers medication indications, dosage, and side effects; encouraging medication and treatment compliance; changing dressings; and providing infusion or intravenous (IV) therapy. Patients who need IV antibiotics, chemotherapy, or home parenteral nutritional can receive these safely at home. The RN performs a physical assessment of the patient and a safety assessment of the home, making recommendations to keep the patient safe while recovering at home. The RN is responsible for teaching necessary care to both the patient and the family or significant support person in the home. The RN might teach the patient and family how to manage pain or give medications safely, watching for any untoward side effects. The RN also supervises the licensed practical nurse (LPN) and home health aides (HHA) who may provide home care services.

Physical therapists provide in-home skilled services that strengthen and restore movement of bones, muscles, and joints. Physical therapists set reasonable goals with the patient and family and monitor progress toward those goals. The physical therapist helps the patient regain strength and function to minimize decline and further injury. Sometimes the patient needs special equipment. The physical therapist can recommend what equipment is best for the individual patient and teach the patient how to use the equipment to maintain or increase function and to gain independence.

Another home care team member is the occupational therapist. This professional teaches the critical skills needed to accomplish daily living activities at home. The occupational therapist helps the patient compensate for loss of function. For example, the occupational therapist may assess the layout of the kitchen in the patient's home and reorganize the placement of dishes and cooking pans for patient accessibility. Occupational therapists show patients how to utilize adaptive equipment such as prostheses or eating utensils and garden tools designed for those with arthritis. The goal is to attain and maintain the highest level of patient functioning to live a productive life.

Speech therapists work in-home with patients who have experienced strokes or accidents, have difficulty swallowing or communicating, or have some form of neurological health problem. The goal is to get the patient to the optimal level of receptive and expressive communication possible for normal life at home.

The medical social worker can be one of the most useful members of the home care team. This professional knows the community resources and helps the patient and family access additional care services. The medical social worker serves as a facilitator and liaison, making referrals to community agencies for the patient and family. Trained to provide support and counseling, the medical social worker is an advocate for the patient now living at home.

Home health aides are a vital part of the home care team. In fact, many patients and families consider the home health aide the most valuable care provider in their homes. Supervised by the RN, home health aides provide personal care and hygiene services such as bathing, hair washing, feeding, and dressing. They can assist in ambulation of the patient and provide light housekeeping or a simple meal if covered by the patient's reimbursement source. Home health aides can be critical to positive home care outcomes.

Other professionals may be available for in-home consultation at some home care agencies. Registered dietitians or nutritionists may offer home visits to discuss diet compliance and special cooking considerations. Nutrition and proper diet are important for achieving healthy outcomes at home. When a patient has a prescribed diet that represents a significant lifestyle change, such as a low-salt or low-fat diet, the registered dietitian can support the patient to success.

Hospice is a special type of care often provided within the home. Hospice home care is for patients diagnosed with end-stage or life-threatening disease with a prognosis of six months or less. Like home health care, hospice home care is coordinated by a multidisciplinary team of providers. Many are the same types of professionals and support staff as with home health care, but the purpose of hospice care is different. The goal in hospice home care is quality of life, not restoration of function and wellness. Additional members of the hospice home care team will include spiritual or pastoral counselors or chaplains, bereavement and grief counselors, and volunteers. All hospice home care services are designed to support and maintain the patient and family at home during the illness and death. Hospice home care is usually reimbursed by private insurance, Medicare, and Medicaid. Most hospice programs accept donations and raise funds to cover nonreimbursed care, so that patients are not denied care due to inability to pay.

Perspective and Prospects

The roots of home care in the United States can be traced to the Charleston Ladies Benevolent Society in 1813. These female volunteers are credited with the early efforts that led to public health nursing in South Carolina. After the Civil War, home care evolved into the British visiting nurse or district nursing model. Home care nurses worked six days a week for eight to twelve hours each day providing bedside care for the patient while holistically supporting the family as well. In 1877, trained home care nurses were sent by the New York Mission to care for the sick poor in their homes. By 1890, the United States boasted twenty-one visiting nurse associations. Lillian Wald, a nurse from New York, established and directed the Henry Street Settlement. In 1911, her organization consisted of fifty-five home care nurses, who made over 175,000 home visits. She is credited with defining the term "public health nursing." The year 1919 brought the first reimbursement for home care nursing services through the Metropolitan Life Insurance Company. However, when the economy crashed in the late 1920s, many home care agencies closed. Home care was then provided primarily by charities.

Change came when Medicare laws, established in 1966, included coverage for home care services. By 1988, home care agencies had increased their numbers by 48 percent. Medicare-certified home care agencies expanded their services but became subject to more regulation.

Home care is a significant part of the health care delivery system in the United States. In 2007, more than 7.6 million people in the United States received some form of home care. That same year, the projected expenditures on home care services were $57.6 billion. Home care, along with nurses and other service providers, can boast almost two centuries of history in the United States.

—*Marylane Wade Koch, R.N., M.S.N.*

See also Aging; Aging: Extended care; Geriatrics and gerontology; Hospice; Hospitals; Medicare; Nursing; Palliative medicine; Safety issues for the elderly; Terminally ill: Extended care.

For Further Information:

Buhler-Wilkerson, Karen. *No Place Like Home: A History of Nursing and Home Care in the United States.* Baltimore: Johns Hopkins University Press, 2003.
"Home Health Care." *Eldercare.gov*, April 24, 2013.
"Home Health Care." *MedlinePlus*, May 11, 2012.
Meyer, Maria M., and Paula Derr. *The Comfort of Home: A Complete Guide for Caregivers.* 3d ed. Portland, Oreg.: CareTrust, 2007.
Prieto, Emily. *Home Health Care Provider: A Guide to Essential Skills.* New York: Springer, 2008.
"There's No Place Like Home—For Growing Old." *National Institute on Aging*, June 26, 2013.

HOMEOPATHY

Specialty

Anatomy or system affected: All

Specialties and related fields: Immunology, pathology, pharmacology

Definition: A system of medicine based on the principle that an ill patient can be provided effective and nontoxic treatment through the use of weak or very small doses of a substance that would cause similar symptoms in a healthy individual.

Key terms:

antidote: anything that counteracts the effect of a substance, such as a homeopathic remedy

Materia Medica: the homeopathic pharmacopoeia, a list of remedies with their associated symptoms and uses

potency: the strength of a homeopathic remedy, according to the number of times it has been diluted and succussed

proving: the testing of a substance or remedy on healthy volunteers (provers), who take repeated doses and record in detail any symptoms produced by the substance

Repertory: an index of symptoms, each heading listing the drugs known to cause the symptom

succussion: violent shaking at each stage of dilution in the preparation of a remedy

tincture: a remedy in liquid form, normally with alcohol and water as a solvent; the most concentrated form is called the mother tincture, from which all dilutions are made

Science and Profession

In conventional medicine, diseases—or changes from the normal physiological state—are diagnosed on the basis of symptoms and physical signs. This enables the physician to find a cause for which there is a specific treatment, or to treat the patient's symptoms. There are few treatments, however, that cure the patient as a whole. Sometimes, symptoms are assumed to be the disease, and the method of action is to try to fix the symptoms and not the disease. Suppressing or removing symptoms does not necessarily constitute a cure. Curing patients means restoring them to a sense of well-being that is physical, emotional, and mental. Homeopathic medicine is a form of treatment that studies the person as a whole, with particular interest in the patient as an individual. Homeopathy is a therapeutic method that consists of prescribing for a patient weak or infinitesimal doses of a substance that, when administered to a healthy person, causes symptoms similar to those exhibited by the ill patient. Homeopathic remedies stimulate the defense mechanisms of the body, causing them to work more effectively and making them capable of curing the individual. While controversial and not accepted by most physicians, homeopathy is not intended to substitute for conventional medicine. Rather, it is a system of therapeutics which is meant to enlarge and broaden the physician's outlook, and in some cases, it might bring about a cure not possible with the usual drugs.

Homeopathy

The principle underlying homeopathy is that taking small amounts of a substance that normally produces a certain symptom will stimulate the immune system to counteract that very symptom. For example, a patient suffering from diarrhea may be given an infinitesimally small dose of a laxative which has been ground into a fine powder with a mortar and pestle.

The word "homeopathy" is derived from the Greek words *homoios*, meaning "like" or "similar," and *pathos*, meaning "suffering." A symptom is defined as the changes felt by the patient or observed by another individual that may be associated with a particular disease. When a homeopathic drug or remedy is administered in repeated doses to a group of healthy persons, certain symptoms and signs of toxicity are produced. These symptoms are carefully annotated in what is called the proving of a remedy. In some cases, there are accidental provings—cases in which the symptoms produced by a drug in a healthy person are observed because of an accident, such as being bitten by a snake. Other sources for the proving of a remedy are the cases in which, after a remedy has been successfully prescribed, symptoms cured by it that were not present in the provings are noted. Some of these symptoms are common to many drugs, and a few are characteristic of particular ones. It is then possible to build a symptom-complex picture which is unique to each drug or remedy. In many cases, when the symptom-complex presented by the patient is compared to the symptom-complex produced by a certain remedy, there will be a resemblance—often a close one—between the patient's symptom picture and the effects of a given drug on healthy persons.

The first and fundamental principle of homeopathy is the selection and use of the similar remedy, based on the patient's symptoms and characteristics and the drug's toxicology and provings. A second principle is the use of remedies in extremely small quantities. The most successful remedy for any given occasion will be the one whose symptomatology presents the clearest and closest resemblance to the symptom-complex of the sick person in question. This concept is formally presented as the Law of Similars, which expresses the similarity between the toxicological action of a substance and its therapeutic action; in other words, the same things that cause the disease can cure it. For example, the effects of peeling an onion are very similar to the symptoms of acute coryza (the common cold). The remedy prepared from *Allium cepa* (red onion) is used to treat the type of cold in which the symptoms resemble those caused by peeling onions. In the same way, the herb white hellebore, which toxicologically produces cholera-like diarrhea, is used to treat cholera.

The homeopathic principle is being applied whenever a sick person is treated using a method or drug that can cause similar symptoms in healthy persons. For example, conventional medicine uses radiation therapy, which causes cancer, to treat this disease. Orthodox medicine, however, does not follow other fundamental principles of homeopathy, such as the use of infinitesimal doses.

Homeopathy stimulates the defense mechanism to make it work more effectively and works on the concept of healing instead of simply treating a disease, combating illness, or suppressing symptoms. Individualization plays a crucial role in homeopathic treatment. Even when two individuals have the same ailment, their symptoms can be different. Remedies are therefore selected on an individual basis, depending on the specific, complete symptom picture of the individual. Homeopathic physicians must develop a different approach to their patients, which involves a diagnosis as well as a study of the whole individual. The way in which some homeopathic remedies work is still unknown, but the persistence of homeopathy since the mid-nineteenth century would seem to suggest its effectiveness in helping sick people.

Some conditions do not respond well to homeopathy, such as those requiring surgery, immediately life-threatening situations such as severe asthma attacks, or situations for which an improvement requires a change in diet (such as iron deficiency) or reduced exposure to environmental stress (a change in lifestyle). Nevertheless, homeopathy appears to help in these cases. For example, it can be useful for faster, complete healing after surgery or after the necessary change in lifestyle has been made. In the United States, both the Food and Drug Administration (FDA) and traditional homeopaths have been concerned about the use of homeopathic remedies to treat serious problems, such as cancer, and their use by unlicensed practitioners. In some cases, the ability to prescribe homeopathic remedies has been restricted to osteopaths, naturopaths, and medical doctors. In some cases, homeopathy does not work; the reason is unknown.

Individuals who have benefited from these remedies may

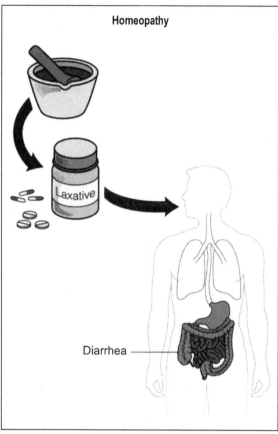

The principle underlying homeopathy is that taking small amounts of a substance that normally produces a certain symptom will stimulate the immune system to counteract that very symptom. For example, a patient suffering from diarrhea may be given an infinitesimally small dose of a laxative which has been ground into a fine powder with a mortar and pestle.

not care whether homeopathy can be scientifically explained or whether research has proven its effectiveness. Nevertheless, some facts suggest that homeopathic medicines are not placebos and that the infinitesimal doses produce true biological action. For example, homeopathic medicines work on animals and are also commonly and successfully used on infants; it is doubtful that psychological suggestion can explain their success in these cases. Moreover, homeopathic microdoses have the capacity to cause symptoms in healthy individuals, and the experience of what is called a healing crisis—temporary exacerbation of symptoms that is sometimes observed during the healing process—cannot be produced by placebos or psychological suggestion. The major drawback to most homeopathic research, however, is that it is rarely published in respected scientific journals, and whatever little has been published has been received with much skepticism from the medical community.

The action of homeopathic medicines supports the theory that each organism expresses symptoms in an effort to heal itself. This homeopathic action can augment, complement, and sometimes replace present medical technologies. For example, abuse of strong medications can lead to resistance to the drugs themselves, allergies, and other unpleasant side effects. In homeopathy, small drug doses have been shown to be more effective than larger ones, which in itself can reduce the undesired side effects associated with the use of common medications.

Diagnostic and Treatment Techniques

The first step in treating an illness using homeopathy is taking the case history or symptom picture (the detailed account of what is wrong with the patient as a whole). This is carried out in a similar way by classical doctors and homeopathic practitioners, since most homeopaths are doctors or have some conventional medical training. The symptoms are divided into three categories: general, mental/emotional, and physical.

The homeopath then consults the *Materia Medica* (the encyclopedia of drug effects) and/or the *Repertory* (an index of symptoms from the *Materia Medica* listed in alphabetical order, used as a cross-reference between symptoms and remedies) to decide on the remedy to be used. The professional homeopath works with a number of *Materia Medica* texts compiled by different homeopaths.

The classical homeopath will give only one remedy at a time in order to gauge its effect more efficiently. The best-known unconventional usage of homeopathic medicines is of combination medicines or complexes, normally a mixture of between three and eight low-potency remedies. This approach is useful when the correct remedy is not available or when the practitioner is unsure as to which one to use. These mixtures are commonly sold in health food stores and are named for the disease or symptom that they are supposed to cure. Another unconventional use is what is called pluralism, which is the application of two or more medicines at a time, each of which is taken at a different time of day. This approach is most commonly used in Europe.

Homeopathy is a natural pharmaceutical system that utilizes microdoses of substances to arouse a healing response by stimulating the patient's immune system. Homeopathic remedies are always nontoxic because of the small concentrations used. They do not act chemically but rather according to a particular physical state linked to the way in which they are prepared. They have the capacity of making the ill subject react to his or her disease, and in this way they are considered specific stimulants.

Homeopathic remedies come from the plant, mineral, and animal kingdoms. Plants are the source of more than half of the remedies. They are harvested in their natural state according to strict norms by qualified specialists and are used fresh after thorough botanical inspection. Mineral remedies include natural salts and metals, always in their purest state. Animal remedies may contain venoms, poisonous insects, hormones, or physiological secretions such as musk or squid ink.

In all cases, the starting remedy is made from a mixture of the substance itself, which has been steeped in alcohol for a period of time and then strained. This starting liquid is called

a tincture or mother tincture. In the decimal scale, a mixture of one-tenth tincture and nine-tenths alcohol is shaken vigorously, a process known as succussion; this first dilution is called a 1X. (The number in the remedy reveals the number of times that it has been diluted and succussed; thus, 6X means diluted and succussed six times.) In the centesimal scale, the remedy is diluted using one part tincture in a hundred, and the letter *C* is used after the number. The number indicates the degree of the dilution, while the letter indicates the technique of preparation (decimal or centesimal). Insoluble substances are diluted by grinding them in a mortar with lactose to the desired dilution. The greater the dilution of a remedy, the greater its potency, the longer it acts, the deeper it heals, and the fewer doses are needed.

A medicine is chosen for its similarity to the person's symptoms, so that the person's bioenergetic processes are hypersensitive to the substance. One theory used to explain the success of homeopathic remedies, even when they are used in such small concentrations, is that they work through some kind of resonance within the individual's system. There are other examples of high sensitivity to small amounts of substances in the animal kingdom, such as in the case of pheromones, sex attractants that affect only animals of the same species in very small amounts and at a very long distance.

Constantine Hering (1800–1880), one of the early pioneers of American homeopathy, was the first to make note of the specific features of the healing process to create a holistic assessment tool that can be used to evaluate a patient's progress. His observations are summarized in Hering's Law of Cure. First, the human body seeks to externalize disease, to dislodge it from more serious, internal levels to more superficial ones. For example, in the healing of asthma the patient may exhibit an external skin rash before complete cure is achieved. Second, the healing progresses from the top of the body to the bottom; someone with arthritis, for example, will feel better in the upper part of the body earlier than in the lower part. Third, the healing proceeds in the reverse order of the appearance of the symptoms; that is, the more recent symptoms will heal first, and old symptoms may reappear before complete healing.

Homeopathic remedies are most commonly available in tablet form, combined with sugar from cow's milk. The tablets can be soft (so that they dissolve easily under the tongue and are easy to crush) or hard (so that they must be chewed and held in the mouth for a few seconds before being swallowed), or they can be prepared as globules (tiny round pills). The liquid remedies are dissolved in alcohol. Also available are powders that are wrapped individually in small squares of paper (convenient if the remedy is needed for only a few doses or is to be sent by mail), wafers, suppositories, and liniments. Homeopathic tablets will keep their strength for years without deteriorating, but they must be stored in a cool, dark, and dry place with their bottle tops screwed on tightly, away from strong-smelling substances.

The prescribed quantities are the same for babies, children, adults, and older people. The size of a dose is immaterial because it is how often it is taken that counts. The strength (po-

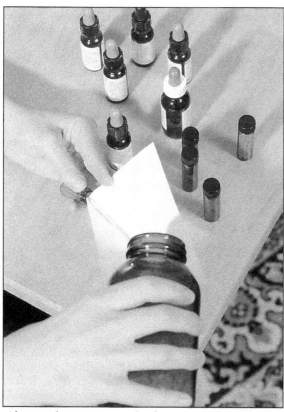

A homeopathist prepares remedies for a patient. (PhotoDisc)

tency) that is needed changes with the circumstances. The greater the similarity between the symptoms and the remedy, the greater the potency to be used (that is, the more dilute the remedy).

The following substances all counteract the effects of a homeopathic remedy to some extent (and as such are considered antidotes): camphor, coffee, menthol/eucalyptus, peppermint, recreational drugs, and any strong-smelling or strong-acting substance.

As with all treatments, there are some dangers associated with homeopathic cures, such as unintentional provings. These take place when, after an initial improvement, the symptoms characteristic of the remedy appear, creating a worse situation for the patient. Sometimes, this reaction takes place because the individual has been taking the remedy for too long, and it can be stopped by discontinuing the remedy or by using an antidote. In other cases, there is a confused symptom picture, the effect being that the remedy is working in a limited way or curing a restricted number of symptoms.

Homeopathy is important in the treatment of bacterial infections (where resistance to antibiotics can develop) and viral conditions. Homeopathic remedies stimulate the person's resistance to infection without the side effects of antibiotics, and they help the body without suppressing the organism's self-protective responses. The remedies used are safer than regular medicines because they exhibit minimal side effects,

and counterreactions between medicines can be prevented.

Homeopathic remedies are exempt from federal review in the United States. In 1938, any drug listed in the *Homeopathic Pharmacopoeia of the United States* was accepted by the FDA. Consequently, prescribed homeopathics do not have to undergo the rigorous safety and effectiveness testing the regulating agency requires of drugs used in orthodox medicine. Nonprescription homeopathics are also exempt and can be purchased in pharmacies, greengroceries, and health food stores throughout the country. The FDA requires that, as with any over-the-counter drug, a remedy be sold only for a self-limiting condition (such as headaches, menstrual cramps, or insomnia) and that the indications be printed on the label. The ingredients and their dilution must also be listed. Nonhomeopathic active ingredients cannot be included in the preparation.

Perspective and Prospects

The Law of Similars was observed twenty-five centuries ago by Hippocrates and was utilized by people of many cultures, including the Mayans, Chinese, Greeks, and American Indians. In the following centuries, other doctors made similar observations, but they did not come to any practical conclusions. It was not until the end of the eighteenth century that a German physician, Christian Friedrich Samuel Hahnemann, studied the matter further, developed it, and gave it a scientific basis.

Hahnemann recruited a group of healthy subjects to take the remedies and report in a diary the symptoms that they caused, a process called proving the substance. He and his subjects proved more than a hundred remedies and produced a very accurate collection for use by other homeopathy practitioners. He also found that the remedies worked better in very small doses. Homeopathy was initially rejected by the medical profession, but its methods became more accepted when Hahnemann obtained astonishing results with his patients. In 1810, he published a book called *Organon der rationellen Heilkunde* (*The Organon of HomÅ"opathic Medicine*, 1836), in which he presented the philosophy of homeopathy. He also published *Materia Medica pura* in six volumes between 1811 and 1821. These volumes contain the compilations of his provings. As new remedies are discovered, they are added to the compilation. By the time of Hahnemann's death in 1843, homeopathy was established around the world.

In the 1820s, homeopathy arrived in the United States at a time when the state of orthodox medicine was worse than in Europe. Many ordinary people consulted herbalists and bonesetters, so homeopathy was easily accepted and soon flourished. In April 1844, the American Institute of Homeopathy was founded. In 1846, however, the American Medical Association (AMA) was founded, and it adopted a code of ethics which forbade its members to consult homeopaths. Nevertheless, public demand continued. The 1860s through the 1880s saw the heyday of homeopathy in the United States, with the institution of training programs, hospitals, and asylums and the training of thousands of homeopaths in the country.

Developments in orthodox medicine around the end of the nineteenth century strengthened this camp, however, while the homeopathic establishment was weakened by internal division. In 1911, the AMA moved to close many homeopathic teaching institutions because they were considered to provide a poor standard of education. By 1950, all the homeopathic colleges in the United States were either closed or no longer teaching homeopathy. By the 1990s, it was roughly estimated that only five hundred to one thousand medical doctors used homeopathics in their practices. Although the AMA has no official statement on homeopathy, it is no longer part of the medical school curriculum.

Homeopathy has exhibited a renaissance, and it is popular throughout the world, especially in France. Perhaps the reasons for this revived popularity include both skepticism surrounding conventional medicine and a need for alternatives in the face of challenging health problems: Homeopathy offers a safe alternative as it seeks to improve the general level of health of the whole person, emotionally as well as physically. It must not be forgotten, however, that this brand of medicine has a long way to go before its curative powers are proven and widely accepted by the medical community.

—*Maria Pacheco, Ph.D.*

See also Alternative medicine; Disease; Herbal medicine; Immune system; Immunology; Pathology; Pharmacology; Toxicology.

For Further Information:

Aubin, Michel, and Philippe Picard. *Homeopathy: A Different Way of Treating Common Ailments*. Translated by Pat Campbell and Robin Campbell. Bath: Ashgrove Press, 1989.

Castro, Miranda. *The Complete Homeopathy Handbook: A Guide to Everyday Health Care*. Rev. ed. New York: Pan Press, 1996.

Josephson, Laura. *A Homeopathic Handbook of Natural Remedies: Safe and Effective Treatment of Common Ailments and Injuries*. New York: Villard Books, 2002.

Matthiessen, Peter F., and Gudrun Bornhoft. *Homeopathy in Healthcare—Effectiveness, Appropriateness, Safety, Costs: AN HTA Report on Homeopathy as Part of the Swiss Contemporary Medicine Evaluation Programme*. Berlin: Springer Verlag, 2011.

McCabe, Vinton. *Practical Homeopathy: A Comprehensive Guide to Homeopathic Remedies and Their Acute Uses*. New York: St. Martin's Press, 2000.

Medhurst, Robert. "Recent Research in Homeopathy." *Journal of the Australian Traditional-Medicine Society* 19, no. 1 (March, 2013): 43–46.

Rutten, Lex, et al. "Plausibility and Evidence: The Case of Homeopathy." *Medicine, Health Care and Philosophy* 16, no. 3 (August, 2013): 525–532.

Ullman, Dana. *Discovering Homeopathy: Medicine for the Twenty-first Century*. 2d rev. ed. Berkeley: North Atlantic Books, 1991.

Ullman, Dana. *Essential Homeopathy: What It Is and What It Can Do for You*. Novato: New World Library, 2002.

H1N1 INFLUENZA

Disease/Disorder

Anatomy or system affected: Lungs, nose, respiratory system, throat

Specialties and related fields: Emergency medicine, epidemiology, family medicine, internal medicine, nursing, pediatrics, public health, virology

Definition: H1N1 influenza is an acute respiratory infection caused by the H1N1 subtype of the influenza A virus.

Key terms:

pandemic: a disease that affects a widespread population

polymerase chain reaction: a technique that multiplies small amounts of genetic material, deoxyribonucleic acid (DNA), into amounts that can be detected by specific genetic probes

reassortment: a process that allows genes to be exchanged between multiple strains of influenza virus infecting a single host

reverse transcriptase: an enzyme that makes complimentary DNA from ribonucleic acid (RNA)

ribonucleic acid: the molecular genetic material of the influenza virus, which is also found in all cells and in some other viruses

Causes and Symptoms

In April 2009, the US Centers for Disease Control and Prevention (CDC) reported two cases of swine influenza A (H1N1) in children residing in Southern California. Neither child had any exposure to pigs or had traveled abroad in the weeks prior to illness. This strain was found to have a unique genetic code that had not previously been identified in either swine or human cases. Specimens collected from an outbreak of influenza in Mexico, beginning in early 2009, proved to be identical to the strains found in California. By May 5, there were 642 confirmed cases of human swine-origin influenza in forty-one states. By May 25, the virus had spread to forty-three countries with 12,515 reported cases and 95 deaths. On June 11, 2009, the World Health Organization (WHO) declared the start of a global pandemic, which lasted until August 2010. Overall, the 2009–2010 H1N1 pandemic caused nearly 15,000 confirmed deaths worldwide. The virus continues to circulate but has not caused widespread infections as it did from 2009 to 2010.

The genetic code of influenza A is sequenced on eight separate segments of single-stranded RNA. When multiple strains of influenza virus infect the same host, such as a pig, these segments of RNA can be exchanged between strains during viral replication, and new strains emerge. Genetic sequence analysis of the H1N1 swine influenza strain which emerged early in 2009 has multiple genetic precursors. Genes from swine H1N2 influenza virus circulating among the North America swine population in the 1990s, genes from H3N2 North American swine influenza, and genes from H1N1 Eurasian swine influenza all have similarity to portions of the 2009 pandemic H1N1 virus genome. The final reassortment of swine (Eurasian and North American), avian, and human influenza A genes may have occurred at a Mexican pig farm with spread of the new quadruple reassortment virus into the human population.

Shifts in the hemagglutinin and neuraminidase surface antigens yielding a novel influenza virus occur every ten to thirty years. In the intervening periods, smaller changes in the hemagglutinin (antigen drift) allow the virus to circulate in the human population, but it does not infect sufficient num-

Information on H1N1 Influenza

Causes: Viral infection
Symptoms: Fever, cough, sore throat, headache, aching muscles, burning eyes, sometimes diarrhea or vomiting;in severe cases, respiratory failure from pneumonia, shock, organ failure
Duration: Incubation period of two to seven days; length of illness dependent on severity
Treatments: Dependent on severity, from home care to admission to intensive care unit with intubation, mechanical ventilation

bers to cause large epidemics or pandemics. These viruses cause severe disease in the very young and elderly individuals who become infected. However, when novel strains emerge after an antigenic shift, children and young adults join those at the extremes of age in having severe disease. This situation is the result of children and young adults having not been exposed to an influenza A subtype similar to the new strain, leaving them without an effective immune response. The 2009 H1N1 swine influenza A followed this pattern, with severe cases and deaths occurring in children and young adults. Infections are worse when there is an underlying illness, such as asthma or diabetes, but nearly half of the severe cases have no underlying medical illness. Obesity emerged as a risk factor for severe and fatal H1N1 disease.

Pregnant women are at high risk for severe influenza caused by any subtype, but the novel H1N1 swine influenza A seems to have struck this group of patients especially hard. Early data from the United States show that pregnant women infected with the H1N1 strain are significantly more likely to be admitted to the hospital or die as a result of their infection than the general population. Pregnancy ratchets down the immune response to allow the developing infant not to be rejected. Further into pregnancy, the enlarging uterus and fetus restrict movement of the diaphragm and facilitate the development of pneumonia. Additionally, these pregnant young adults join their nonpregnant peers in lacking immunity by virtue of having no prior exposure to the H1N1 influenza subtype.

The H1N1 virus's manner of spreading is similar to other strains of influenza. Large droplets from coughing and sneezing by an infected patient are spread to the mucosal surfaces (nose, mouth, and eyes) of uninfected individuals. This droplet spread is most intense when the distances are short, a few feet, but may occur up to ten feet. Direct contact with infected respiratory secretions is also important in the spread of infections and the virus can survive on surfaces and objects for a few hours. Small droplet aerosols may also have a role, but there is less evidence that this is a significant method of transfer. Infected persons can shed the virus and spread disease beginning one day before becoming ill and up to five to seven days after symptoms appear. Infection can result from contact with infected pigs, as probably occurred in the original cases in Mexico, but pork and pork products are not infective.

The incubation period (time between infection and illness) is two to seven days. The most common symptoms have been fever, cough, and sore throat, but 25 percent of patients have had diarrhea or vomiting, which are unusual symptoms for influenza. Headache, aching muscles, burning eyes, and other symptoms accompanying influenza infection may occur. While fever was reported to occur in 94 percent of the first 642 confirmed cases in April and May 2009, subsequent series of cases have reported the absence of fever in 10 to 50 percent of those infected. The severity of illness can vary widely from that of a self-limited mild illness to severe disease requiring admission to a hospital intensive care unit. Individuals that develop severe illness usually show rapid deterioration between day three and five. Respiratory failure from pneumonia, shock, and failure of other organs may follow.

Early diagnosis of H1N1 influenza is important as therapeutic intervention can reduce severity, shorten the course of the illness, and prevent further spread of the infection. A number of rapid influenza diagnostic tests (RIDTs) are available and provide results in thirty minutes or less. A molecular technique called reverse transcriptase polymerase chain reaction (RT-PCR) is able to detect specific influenza RNA in respiratory secretions. This test is highly sensitive and specific and can accurately diagnose infection with H1N1 influenza, but it is performed only in special laboratories and results can take days making them of little use for immediate diagnosis and therapeutic decision making.

Primary viral pneumonia is the most common type of pneumonia in severe cases, but secondary bacteria pneumonia has been found in 30 percent of fatal cases. The most common bacteria are *Streptococcus pneumoniae* and *Staphylococcus aureus*. Overall, it appears that 10 to 20 percent of patients with disease severe enough to require admission to a hospital intensive care unit will die.

Treatment and Therapy

The H1N1 influenza is treated with neuraminidase inhibitors. Oseltamivir, which is available as a capsule and an oral suspension, and zanamivir, which is supplied as an inhaled powder, are oral neuraminidase inhibitors that can be used for both treatment and prophylaxis. A new intravenous neuraminidase inhibitor, peramivir, was approved by the FDA for emergency treatment of H1N1 during the pandemic; however, the emergency-use authorization for peramivir expired in June 2010. Zanamivir is also available for oral use to treat H1N1. Antiviral therapy is most effective when started early in the course of the illness, but viral RNA has been detected in the lower respiratory tract for as long as two weeks, suggesting that antiviral therapy may be beneficial even in the later stages of the illness. Consequently, it is recommended by the CDC that any patient who is not improving receive antiviral therapy even if it is more than forty-eight hours after symptoms have begun.

Complex care in an intensive care unit is necessary for severely ill patients. Respiratory failure must be managed by intubation and mechanical ventilation often involving sophisticated equipment and techniques.

Secondary bacterial pneumonia occurs in some patients

and staphylococci and streptococci have been found to be the most common invading pathogens. Antibacterial agents effective against these bacteria must be given in addition to the antiviral to successfully treat this complicated pneumonia.

Prevention of H1N1 disease can be accomplished by administration of the seasonal flu vaccine, which is available by shot or nasal spray. Vaccines against H1N1 are made from influenza virus that has been grown in chicken eggs and are not recommended for persons allergic to eggs. The nasal mist can be given to healthy individuals between the ages of two and forty-nine, except pregnant women. All others must receive the injectable killed vaccine, including high-risk patients, such as pregnant women and HIV patients who have decreased immunity. Since the protective immune response to H1N1 following vaccination takes two weeks to develop, oral antiviral therapy may be administered during this period to afford protection. In some cases, such as patients allergic to eggs, longer prophylaxis may be warranted and has been shown to be safe and effective for extended duration.

Perspective and Prospects

In 1936, Richard E. Shope first reported antibodies to swine influenza in humans, and shortly thereafter viruses isolated from swine and from humans were linked to the 1918 influenza virus. These viruses are now known to be H1N1 influenza A, and direct descendants of the 1918 virus still persist in pigs and humans. The human H1N1 virus undergoes continual and gradual antigenic drift, causing annual disease and even epidemics. The porcine enzootic H1N1 strain only rarely infects humans. An outbreak of swine H1N1 influenza at Fort Dix, New Jersey, in 1976 caused concern and led to a vaccination campaign, but further spread never occurred. In recent years, analysis of material preserved from fatal cases of 1918 influenza have resulted in complete sequencing of the viral genome. These data have demonstrated that all subsequent pandemic viruses are descendants of the 1918 virus, as are nearly all human influenza A viruses worldwide. Descendants of the 1918 virus resulting from antigenic shifts caused pandemics in 1957 (H2N2) and 1968 (H3N2). Intrasubtype reassortment caused pandemics in 1947 (H1N1), 1957 (H1N1), 1997 (H3N2), and 2003 (H3N2). The origin of the 1918 virus remains unclear, but it is thought to be derived from avian strains with simultaneous adaptation to both humans and swine with possible genetic contributions from an as-yet-to-be-identified different animal host.

Another interesting aspect of the 1918 pandemic is the occurrence of three waves in the Northern Hemisphere. The first wave, beginning in March, lasted six months and had high attack rates, but death rates remained at expected levels. The second wave, from September to November, and a third wave in early 1919 were both characterized by high mortality. Since the autopsy material used for genetic sequencing was from second-wave cases, it has not been possible to determine if any changes in the virus occurred from the less-fatal, first-wave virus.

The 2009 H1N1 virus had a number of similar features to the 1918 virus. The pandemic began in March and spread around the world with continuous activity throughout the summer in the Northern Hemisphere. In September, activity increased and continued to progress. However, there was no increased activity in the winter and into spring 2010, which is unlike the third wave of the 1918 pandemic that occurred in early 1919. While the fatality rate of the 2009 virus was much lower than the 1918 virus, many deaths occurred across all age groups. Vaccines, antivirals, and modern intensive care therapies provided measures to combat influenza that were unavailable in 1918. Demand for vaccines, antivirals, intensive care unit beds, ventilators, and health care providers was high, but resources kept pace. Some H1N1 activity continues worldwide, but the virus has not caused widespread infections since the 2009–2010 pandemic. Successful vaccination, along with handwashing and the use of respirators and masks in health care facilities, significantly slowed the spread of the virus.

—*H. Bradford Hawley, M.D.*

See also Avian influenza; Centers for Disease Control and Prevention (CDC); Emerging infectious diseases; Epidemics and pandemics; Epidemiology; Immunization and vaccination; Influenza; National Institutes of Health (NIH); Viral infections; World Health Organization; Zoonoses.

For Further Information:

Borse, Rebekah H., et al. "Effects of Vaccine Program against Pandemic Influenza A (H1N1) Virus, United States, 2009—2010." *Emerging Infectious Diseases* 19, no. 3 (March, 2013): 439–448.

Jamieson, Denise J., et al. "H1N1 2009 Influenza Virus Infection During Pregnancy in the USA." *The Lancet* 374 (2009): 451–458.

Louie, Janice K., et al. "Factors Associated with Death or Hospitalization Due to Pandemic 2009 Influenza A (H1N1) Infection in California." *Journal of the American Medical Association* 302 (2009): 1896–1902.

Morens, David M., Jeffrey K. Taubenberger, and Anthony S. Fauci. "The Persistent Legacy of the 1918 Influenza Virus." *New England Journal of Medicine* 361 (2009): 225–229.

Myers, Kendall P., Christopher W. Olsen, and Gregory C. Gray. "Cases of Swine Influenza in Humans: A Review of the Literature." *Clinical Infectious Diseases* 44 (2007): 1084–1088.

"Seasonal Influenza (Flu)." *Centers for Disease Control and Prevention*, May 17, 2013.

Stahl, Rebecca J., and Brian S. Alper. "Pandemic (H1N1) Influenza." *Health Library*, October 31, 2012.

Trifonov, Vladimir, Hossein Khiabanian, and Raul Rabadan. "Geographic Dependence, Surveillance, and Origins of the 2009 Influenza A (H1N1) Virus." *New England Journal of Medicine* 361 (2009): 115–119.

HORMONE THERAPY

Treatment

Anatomy or system affected: Blood vessels, bones, brain, breasts, circulatory system, genitals, heart, psychic-emotional system, reproductive system, skin, urinary system, uterus

Specialties and related fields: Cardiology, endocrinology, family medicine, geriatrics and gerontology, gynecology, hematology, internal medicine, oncology, orthopedics, preventive medicine, vascular medicine

Definition: Estrogens, with or without progestins, given to women during perimenopause or menopause, or both, to relieve a variety of symptoms.

Key terms:

hypothalamus: a part of the brain that controls many body functions; its releasing hormones stimulate the pituitary to secrete hormones of its own

incontinence: inability to control the bladder or bowel

menopause: the last menstrual period that a woman experiences

osteoporosis: thinning of the bones, which occurs in all people as they age

perimenopause: a period of years around the menopause, during which changes occur in the balance among the reproductive hormones, leading to the cessation of menses and the end of fertility; this time of transition from reproductive to postreproductive life is also known as the climacteric

pituitary gland: the body's master gland that produces various hormones which in turn stimulate other glands in the body to produce their own hormones; in women, the pituitary produces follicle-stimulating hormone and luteinizing hormone, which stimulate the ovary to produce estrogens and progesterone

progestogen: any of a number of substances (natural or synthetic) that have a progesterone-like effect

prolapse: the slipping out of place of an internal organ, such as the uterus

transdermal: through the skin; transdermal medications are those which are applied as creams, gels, or patches and are then absorbed through the skin

Indications and Procedures

During a woman's reproductive years, a complex feedback loop among the hypothalamus, pituitary gland, and ovaries causes the ovaries to produce various sex hormones, the major ones being estrogens and progesterone. These hormones are responsible for developing the secondary sexual characteristics such as breasts and pubic hair, for governing the menstrual cycle, and for maintaining a pregnancy should one occur. They also have profound effects on a woman's skin, heart, blood vessels, lipids (blood fats such as cholesterol), bones, blood, and other systems.

As women approach menopause, changes begin to occur in the hormone feedback loop. The menstrual cycle typically becomes shorter and more irregular, and then menses cease altogether. As hormone levels decline and the ratio between the estrogens and progesterone changes, the woman's body undergoes other changes such as thinning of the mucous membranes in the reproductive and urinary tract, drying of the skin, thinning of the bones, and alterations in cholesterol levels. Perimenopausal women may also experience hot flashes, night sweats, insomnia, mood swings, and other uncomfortable symptoms. Postmenopausal women do continue to produce sex hormones, although in smaller amounts. The adrenal glands are responsible for much of the postmenopausal hormone production, and some production occurs by conversion of other hormones in the body tissues.

Menopause normally occurs between the ages of forty-five and fifty-five, with an average age of about fifty-one. Menopause before the age of forty is called "premature menopause." A woman who stops menstruating because of a total hysterectomy, in which not only the uterus but also the Fallopian tubes and ovaries are removed, undergoes what is called a "surgical menopause." Women who undergo radiation of the ovaries also experience an artificial menopause. The discomforts associated with menopause may be exaggerated in these women.

Health care providers have used hormone therapy, formerly called "hormone replacement therapy (HRT)," to treat uncomfortable perimenopausal symptoms and to prevent or treat a number of conditions associated with the postmenopausal state. Hormone therapy may include estrogen alone or a combination of estrogen and progesterone. At times, other hormones such as testosterone may be used to treat symptoms, but it is the estrogen-progesterone combination that constitutes what is commonly thought of as hormone therapy. Estrogen therapy is the use of estrogen alone and was formerly known as "estrogen replacement therapy (ERT)."

Hormone therapy may also be prescribed to manage conditions that cause menorrhagia (heavy menstrual bleeding), such as uterine fibroids (noncancerous growths in the uterus), endometriosis (monthly growth of the uterine lining tissue outside the uterus), and ovarian cysts. The long-term risks and contraindications are similar to those for perimenopausal and menopausal women.

Uses and Complications

A variety of estrogens and progestogens are available for the treatment of menopausal symptoms. They include oral estrogens and progestin, transdermal estrogens, injectable estrogens and progestins, and topical estrogens. Oral estrogens for hormone therapy include conjugated estrogens, micronized estradiol, piperazine estrone sulfate, ethinyl estradiol, and quinestrol. Of these, the conjugated equine estrogens have been most extensively studied over a long period of time. They are usually well tolerated by patients. Various estrogens are also available as transdermal patches, inhalable sprays, or vaginal creams or rings. Various combination products are available to administer estrogen with a progestin, including oral and transdermal formulations. Progesterone may be supplied by oral progestins, oral progesterone, topical vaginal preparations, subdermal implants, and levonorgestrel-containing IUDs.

In the 1990s, clinicians provided hormone therapy (then called "hormone replacement therapy") to prevent osteoporosis and heart attacks; the hormone therapy relieved vaginal dryness and hot flashes as well. It was thought that hormone therapy would also provide a number of other benefits for conditions ranging from mood swings to insomnia to prevention of Alzheimer's disease. At various times throughout the twentieth century, health care providers and researchers recommended that all women in perimenopause begin hormone therapy.

In 1998, results from a large clinical trial, the HERS study

(Heart and Estrogen/Progestin Replacement Study), which enrolled women with existing heart disease, demonstrated an unanticipated increase in heart attacks for women in the first year of medication; furthermore, there was no cardiac benefit in the years to follow. In 2002, the Women's Health Initiative (WHI) published groundbreaking results of a large study of women on estrogen and progestin; the trial was ended early because of safety concerns. Findings included blood clots and an increased risk for breast cancer, but a decrease in colon cancer and osteoporotic fractures. Researchers concluded that the risks of taking the medications were not worth the benefits.

A subsequent study of estrogen alone was stopped early because of a small increase in stroke risk. Research has also shown that women using estrogen-only treatments are at higher risk of developing coronary heart disease. Major medical organizations now recommend that hormone therapy should be used only in the smallest effective dose, for the shortest effective period of time, and only for relief of severe symptoms, primarily hot flashes. Hormone therapy should not be used only to prevent osteoporosis.

Women who take estrogen supplementation without a progestogen are at increased risk for developing excessive thickening of the lining of the uterus. This situation can ultimately result in carcinoma (cancer) of the uterus. The development of ovarian cancer is also possible. For this reason, women who have not had a hysterectomy are advised to take only estrogen with concomitant provision of progestogens. If the combination is given on a cyclical basis, however, the woman will most likely experience monthly withdrawal bleeding. This is not always acceptable to postmenopausal women. Most women who take a continuous dose of a lower-dose progestogen will not bleed at all after a year of its continuous use; the remainder will bleed occasionally.

Women who take oral estrogen supplements have an increased tendency to develop blood clots. This risk is greatly decreased with transdermal formulations. Estrogen therapy is also associated with an increased risk of gallbladder disease.

Women who should not take estrogen-containing hormones at all include those with unexplained vaginal bleeding, a history of uterine or breast cancer, liver disease, or a history of blood clots in the veins. Hormone therapy should be used with caution in women with seizure disorders, high blood pressure, diabetes mellitus, migraines, gallbladder disease, and certain other conditions. Minor adverse effects of hormone treatment include swelling, breast tenderness, bloating, headaches, and increased cervical mucus.

As the supply of estrogen decreases, women experience thinning and drying of the vaginal tissues. The cervix, uterus, and ovaries become smaller in size, and the cervix stops producing mucus. In addition, the ligaments that support the reproductive organs become more relaxed. These changes may lead to painful sexual intercourse, bleeding with minor trauma, itching, vaginal discharge, and prolapse of the uterus. Topical vaginal formulations, rather than oral, systemic medications, are recommended if only vaginal thinning and dryness are indicated.

The tissues of the bladder and urethra also become thinner, which may lead to urinary urgency, painful urination, or increased frequency. Some women even become incontinent. The evidence is not entirely clear about the usefulness of estrogen in this setting.

Vasomotor instability refers to the changes that lead to hot flashes and increased sweating. These flashes may be accompanied by heart palpitations, weakness, fatigue, dizziness, or lightheadedness. The episodes may cause nighttime awakening or insomnia, which in turn may lead to memory problems or irritability. The major treatment for vasomotor instability is the administration of estrogen, although progestogens have been used in women who cannot take estrogen. Some women find relief from a different type of drug called clonidine. Other treatments, which have not been studied as thoroughly as estrogen and progesterone, include various vitamin and mineral supplements, tranquilizers, and antidepressants.

All people gradually lose bone mass as they age, but in the years following menopause, this process accelerates in women, particularly in the type of bone known as "trabecular bone." Postmenopausal women's risk for hip fracture becomes two to three times that of men. For this reason, estrogen has been recommended in the past for prevention of osteoporosis, particularly in women who are thin, who smoke cigarettes, who have a strong family history of osteoporosis, who drink large amounts of alcohol, or who have some other risk factor. With concerns about the safety of estrogens, however, other drugs are increasingly used to prevent or treat osteoporosis, including drugs from the classes known as bisphosphonates and selective estrogen receptor modulators (SERMs). Calcitonin and progestogens may also be used, but they do not seem to be as effective as the estrogens, bisphosphonates, or SERMs. All menopausal women should probably take supplemental calcium and vitamin D, exercise regularly, stop smoking if needed, and limit alcohol, caffeine, salt, and animal proteins to minimize their risk of developing osteoporosis.

Before menopause, very few women have heart attacks. This state changes rapidly after menopause, and by age seventy, women have the same risk of heart attack as men. However, major medical organizations have recommended that combination therapy not be used for the prevention of cardiac disease.

As people age, they experience changes in the skin and hair. The skin becomes thinner and less elastic, particularly in sun-exposed areas. There is some loss of pubic hair and hair in the armpits. Some women experience balding, and some develop coarse facial hair. Body hair may either increase or decrease. The skin has estrogen receptors, so those changes are thought to be caused by decreased estrogen. Hair changes are more likely to result from a change in the ratio of estrogen to testosterone in the body after menopause. Testosterone levels remain nearly the same before and after menopause, while estrogen levels drop drastically. Topical hormones have been used to ameliorate or prevent skin changes, especially vaginal atrophy and dryness; however, use of systemic hormones is not supported for these indications.

Some studies have found that women in early menopause experience more irritability, depression, and feelings of anxiety. It is not clear if these changes are attributable to some change in brain chemistry as a result of decreased estrogen, to societal expectations about aging, or to some other factor. Some researchers have suggested that the lack of sleep caused by hot flashes and night sweats, rather than menopause itself, is the source of mood changes. Furthermore, many perimenopausal women have multiple stressors, such as caring for aging parents, which may contribute to depression and anxiety. In contrast to past practice, current evidence does not support the use of hormone therapy for depression or prevention of Alzheimer's disease and other dementias.

In summary, the only indication for systemic hormone administration is for severe menopausal symptoms at the lowest possible dose for the shortest period of time; those with abnormal bleeding conditions should discuss the long-term risks of hormone therapy with their clinicians. Topical preparations may be used for indications such as vaginal dryness or discomfort.

Perspective and Prospects

Feminist thinkers and researchers have raised important questions about the use of sex hormones in women. They point out that many of the conditions that are treated with hormones are a part of women's normal life experience. By declaring such events as pregnancy and menopause as "problems" and treating them with hormones, normal life events become medicalized—a condition to be treated at great expense and some risk to health and well-being. A second important issue raised by feminists is that hormones have been administered to women for various conditions without adequate testing and with serious consequences. For example, in the mid-twentieth century, physicians encouraged perimenopausal women to take estrogen to remain "forever young." Because these women were given estrogen without the progesterone needed to protect against the development of uterine cancer, cancer rates rose dramatically and estrogen alone was withdrawn as a treatment for menopause.

—Clair Kaplan, A.P.R.N./M.S.N.; additional material by Rebecca Lovell Scott, Ph.D., PA-C

See also Aging; Arteriosclerosis; Breast cancer; Cervical, ovarian, and uterine cancers; Endocrinology; Endometrial cancer; Gynecology; Heart disease; Herbal medicine; Hormones; Hot flashes; Hysterectomy; Infertility, female; Menopause; Menstruation; Midlife crisis; Osteoporosis; Sweating; Women's health.

For Further Information:

A.D.A.M. Medical Encyclopedia. "Hormone Therapy." *MedlinePlus*, September 13, 2011.
American College of Obstetricians and Gynecologists. "Hormone Therapy." *American Congress of Obstetricians and Gynecologists*, 2013.
American Society of Health-System Pharmacists. "Estrogen and Progestin (Hormone Replacement Therapy)." *MedlinePlus*, August 1, 2010.
Love, Susan, and Karen Lindsey. *Dr. Susan Love's Menopause and Hormone Book: Making Informed Choices*. Rev. ed. New York: Random House, 2003.
National Women's Health Network. *The Truth about Hormone Replacement Therapy: How to Break Free from the Medical Myths of Menopause*. Roseville, Calif.: Prima, 2002.
Rull, Gurvinder. "Progestogens." *Patient.co.uk*, April 20, 2011.
Seaman, Barbara. *The Greatest Experiment Ever Performed on Women: Exploding the Estrogen Myth*. New York: Seven Stories Press, 2009.
Scholten, Amy, and Brian Randall. "Hormone Replacement Therapy: A Look at the Options." *Health Library*, August 16, 2012.

HORMONES

Biology

Anatomy or system affected: Circulatory system, endocrine system, glands, psychic-emotional system

Specialties and related fields: Biochemistry, endocrinology, pharmacology

Definition: Chemical substances that are secreted by endocrine glands or specialized secretory cells into the blood or nearby tissues to act on those tissues and affect its function.

Key terms:

adrenal glands: endocrine organs located on top of the kidneys; their function is to produce steroid hormones such as cortisol and sex hormones

deoxyribonucleic acid (DNA): the basic building block of life, which bears encoded genetic information; it is found mainly in chromosomes and can reproduce

messenger ribonucleic acid (mRNA): a single-stranded RNA that arises from and is complementary to double-stranded DNA; it passes from the nucleus to the cytoplasm, where its information is translated into proteins

prohormone: a hormone that must be cut or modified in a specific way in order to achieve full activity

receptor: a molecular structure at the cell surface or inside the cell that is capable of combining with hormones and causing a change in cell metabolism or function

Structure and Functions

The definition of the term "hormone" has continued to change over the years. The classic definition is that of an endocrine hormone—that is, one secreted by ductless glands directly into the blood and acting at a distant site. The definition can be expanded to include any chemical substance secreted by any cell of the body that has a specific effect on another cell. A hormone can affect a nearby cell (paracrine action) or the cell that secretes it (autocrine action). Certain hormones are produced by the brain and kidneys, which are not thought of as classic endocrine glands. In fact, the largest producer of hormones is the gastrointestinal tract, which is not usually thought of as an endocrine gland.

Hormones fall into two major categories: peptide hormones, which are derived from amino acids, and steroid hormones, which are derived from cholesterol. The different classes of hormones have different mechanisms of action. Peptide hormones work by interacting with a specific receptor located in the plasma membrane of the target cell. Receptors have different regions, or domains, that perform specialized functions. One part of the receptor has a specific three-dimensional structure similar to a keyhole into which a certain hormone can fit. This design allows a specific action of a hormone despite the fact that the hormone is often circulating in minute quantities in the bloodstream along with myriad other hormones.

There are different classes of plasma membrane receptors. One class is that of the receptor kinases. The insulin receptor is an example. In this case, the part of the receptor molecule that faces the cytoplasm, or inside of the cell, is able to perform a specific function. When insulin interacts with its receptor, a chemical change occurs on the receptor that allows it to activate proteins within the cell. Many hormones use a similar cascade of chemical reactions to control and amplify signals from outside the cell and effect change within the cell itself.

Another class of membrane receptors includes the G-protein coupled receptor. An example is the beta-2 adrenergic receptor. Epinephrine interacts with this receptor, causing the activation of a signal transducer or G protein. This activated G protein then leads to the modification of a specific protein, which leads to a cascade of biochemical events within the cell. This is another example of an amplification mechanism.

Steroid hormones exert their effects by means of a different mechanism. For example, glucocorticoids exert their effects by entering the cell and binding to specific glucocorticoid receptors in the cell nucleus. The glucocorticoid-receptor complex is able to bind specific regulatory DNA sequences, called glucocorticoid response elements. This binding is able to activate gene transcription, which causes an increase in mRNA and, ultimately, the translation of the mRNA to deliver a newly secreted protein. The protein can then act to change the cell's metabolism in some way. Cortisol, a type of glucocorticoid, is produced by the adrenal glands when a person is under stress. It can lead to changes in blood sugar levels, affect immune system function, and, at high levels, increase fat deposition in characteristic areas of the body.

Most hormones that circulate in the blood are attached to binding proteins. The general binding proteins in the body are albumin and transthyreitin. These two proteins bind many different hormones. There are also specific binding proteins, such as thyroid-binding globulin, which binds thyroid hormone, and insulin-like growth factor-binding proteins, which bind to the family of insulin-like growth factors. The bound hormone is considered the inactive hormone, and the free hormone is the active hormone. Therefore, binding proteins make it possible to control an active hormone precisely, without having to synthesize a new hormone.

Hormones can be secreted in a variety of time frames. Some hormones, such as testosterone, are secreted in a pulsatile fashion that changes over minutes or hours. Other hormones, such as cortisol, are secreted in a diurnal pattern, with levels varying depending on the time of day. Cortisol levels are highest at about 8 a.m. and fall throughout the day, with the lowest levels occurring between midnight and 2 a.m. The menstrual cycle is an example of the weekly to monthly variation of hormone production. For instance, progesterone (a steroid hormone) levels rise throughout the menstrual cycle and fall prior to the onset of menses. The exact control mechanisms that determine the rhythmicity of hormone production are unknown.

The ability to study and utilize hormones in treating human disease has been revolutionized by molecular biology. The first hormone to be synthesized for clinical use was insulin. The need for a secure and steady supply of insulin prompted scientists to look for alternative sources of this hormone in the 1970s. At that time, insulin was isolated and purified from animal pancreas glands, mostly those of cows and pigs. It was suspected, however, that insulin could be made in the laboratory via genetic engineering. Native insulin is produced from a prohormone, proinsulin. Recombinant DNA human insulin is currently made by encoding for the proinsulin molecule and then using enzymes to cut the molecule in the proper places, yielding insulin and a piece of protein called C peptide. This process, which is very similar to the process that the body uses to create insulin, produces high yields of active hormone.

Modern molecular biology techniques were used to identify a hormone and receptor involved in weight regulation. Originally discovered in mice, a gene called *ob* was identified in human beings that produced a hormone called leptin. Leptin and its receptor are believed to play a role in signaling satiety to the brain. If the leptin signal does not reach the brain as the result of a faulty receptor, the brain will not produce the satiety signal. Appetite will remain high. Thus, a defective leptin system may contribute to obesity in human beings. The functioning of leptin may also be responsible for cycles of weight loss and gain in dieters. As obese individuals lose adipose tissue, less leptin is synthesized and the brain may not send out sufficient signals to indicate satiety, thus increasing appetite and food consumption. The leptin-obesity connection is under intensive study.

The Medical Use of Hormones

The biological roles of hormones are numerous and critical to the normal function of important organ systems in human beings, and there are many examples of medical uses for hormones. In general, any derangements in the amount of hormones made, or in the timing of their production, can result in significant human disease or discomfort. For example, in women who reach menopause, declining levels of estrogen and progesterone from the ovaries can lead to undesirable consequences such as hot flashes, vaginal dryness, and bone mineral density loss. Taking exogenous estrogen and progesterone, in the form of hormone therapy, can reduce or stop these consequences. Another example of exogenous hormone use in human disease is thyroid hormone. People with thyroid disease, such as Hashimoto's thyroiditis, do not produce adequate levels of thyroid hormone. This condition can lead to intense fatigue and weight gain. These symptoms may be relieved by taking a synthetic thyroid hormone called levothyroxine.

Another example of the medical use of hormones is the

role of synthetic erythropoietin in treating and preventing anemia. Normally, erythropoietin is made by the kidneys. It is essential for the differentiation and development of stem cells from the bone marrow into red blood cells. Most patients who develop kidney failure also suffer from severe anemia because the ability to synthesize erythropoietin is lost as the kidneys are destroyed by disease. Giving this hormone to a patient with kidney disease can lead to the restoration of that patient's red blood cell mass. Correcting the anemia that accompanies chronic renal disease can improve the exercise tolerance and overall quality of life of kidney disease patients. The hormone must be given by injection several times per week. It has been made available to the almost fifty thousand Americans with chronic renal failure who require dialysis. Erythropoietin can also be given to renal failure patients who do not yet require dialysis but who do have anemia.

Another example of a hormone that has been synthesized for treatment of human disease is calcitonin. Calcitonin is a polypeptide hormone secreted by specialized C cells of the thyroid gland (also called parafollicular cells). The parafollicular cells make up about 0.1 percent of the total mass of the thyroid gland, and the cells are dispersed within the thyroid follicles. Calcitonin has been isolated from several different animal species, including salmon, eel, rat, pig, sheep, and chicken. The main physiologic function of the hormone is to lower the serum calcium level. It does this by inhibiting calcium resorption from bone. Calcitonin has been used to treat patients with Paget's disease, a disorder of abnormal bone remodeling that can lead to deformities, bone pain, fractures, and neurological problems. Calcitonin has also been used in the past to treat patients with osteoporosis, a condition of bone density depletion associated with aging that can lead to bone fractures.

The first and most commonly used form of the hormone in the United States is salmon calcitonin. This form is a more potent inhibitor of bone resorption than the human form. A small number of patients given the drug will develop a resistance to it. The etiology of this resistance may be the development of antibodies to the salmon calcitonin. Subsequently, calcitonin was synthesized via recombinant DNA technology. Although the human form is somewhat less potent, the fact that its amino acid structure is identical to that of the native hormone makes it much less immunogenic than salmon calcitonin, and theoretically less likely to produce resistance. In fact, patients who were resistant to salmon calcitonin may be switched to human calcitonin and achieve a therapeutic effect.

An example of a hormone with multiple medical uses is vasopressin, also known as antidiuretic hormone. Normally, vasopressin is produced in the posterior pituitary gland (located in the brain); it is responsible for water conservation. An increase in plasma osmolality or a decrease in circulating blood volume will normally cause its release. Central diabetes insipidus, a disorder involving an absence or abnormal decrease of vasopressin, is characterized by an inappropriately dilute urine. Central diabetes insipidus can be caused by a variety of factors, including trauma, neurosurgery, brain tumors, brain infections, and autoimmune disorder. The clinical symptoms of the disease are polyuria and polydipsia. The patient may put out up to 18 liters of urine per day. If such large volume deficits are not remedied, more serious symptoms will ensue, including dangerously low blood pressure and coma. The acute treatment of any patient with central diabetes insipidus involves the replacement of body water with intravenous fluids. The chronic therapy involves replacement of the hormone vasopressin.

Several different forms of the hormone may be used, depending on the clinical situation. Aqueous vasopressin is useful for diagnostic testing and for acute management following trauma or neurosurgery. For diagnostic testing, it is often given subcutaneously at the end of the water deprivation test to determine whether the patient will respond to the hormone with a decrease in urine output and an increase in urine osmolality greater than 50 percent. After surgery, vasopressin can be given either intramuscularly, with a duration of action of about four to six hours, or by continuous intravenous infusion to ensure a steady level of the hormone.

In obstetrics, vasopressin is also known as pitocin, a hormone that can cause powerful uterine contractions. It is commonly used to augment labor, as when the mother's own uterine contractions are not adequate to expel the baby. It is given intravenously and titrated up until regular contractions of the uterus occur. Another use of vasopressin is in the acute setting of advanced cardiac life support, also known as a code situation. A patient noted to have a cardiac arrhythmia such as ventricular fibrillation may receive vasopressin as well as shocks from a defibrillator in an attempt to restore a perfusing cardiac rhythm.

One of the most important uses of hormones in medicine is for contraception, specifically in the form of birth control pills. In the early twentieth century, the observation was made that mice that were fed extracts from ovaries could be rendered infertile. In the 1920s, the critical substance responsible for this infertility was discovered to be sex steroid hormones. The production of birth control pills dates to the 1920s and 1930s, when steroid hormones such as progesterone were isolated from animal sources, such as pigs. By the 1940s, progesterone could be isolated in large quantities from Mexican yams, which caused the prices for progesterone to fall dramatically. With the fall in prices, the idea that progesterone could be sold in the mass market as a birth control pill became more feasible. The first clinical trial of the birth control pill in human beings occurred in 1956. Since then, several generations of progesterones have been mass produced for the purposes of birth control. Each successive generation of progesterone has caused fewer undesirable side effects, and the dosage necessary to achieve a contraceptive effect has been found to be much lower than those found in the original birth control pills.

Birth control pills and the progesterone contained within them have other medical uses besides contraception. Birth control pills can be used to regulate menstrual cycles in women who suffer from irregular menstrual cycles or abnormal vaginal bleeding. They can be used to decrease heavy menstrual periods. They can even be useful in decreasing acne, which can lead to permanent scarring when it is severe.

Perspective and Prospects

The study of hormones has been instrumental in understanding how human beings adapt to and live in their environment. Hormones are involved in the regulation of body homeostasis and all critical aspects of the life cycle. The study of hormones has expanded as scientists have produced large amounts of synthetic hormones in the laboratory for use in research.

The history of insulin discovery and production is an example of the rapid scientific progress made in the field of hormone research. In 1889, Joseph von Mering and Oskar Minkowski demonstrated that dogs whose pancreases had been removed exhibited abnormalities in glucose metabolism that were similar to those seen in human diabetes mellitus patients. This fact suggested that some factor made by the pancreas lowered the blood glucose. The search for this factor led to the discovery of insulin in 1921 by Frederick C. Banting and Charles H. Best. They were able to extract the active substance from the pancreas and to demonstrate its therapeutic effects in dogs and humans. The chemistry of insulin progressed with the establishment of the amino acid sequence and three-dimensional structure in the 1960s. In 1960, insulin became the first hormone to be measured by radioimmunoassay. With advances in laboratory techniques in the 1970s, it became the first hormone to be commercially available via recombinant DNA technology, thus ensuring the availability of pure hormone without the need for animal sources.

The ability to synthesize hormones and their receptors has increased greatly. In fact, scientists can clone genes, or parts of genes, and synthesize the associated protein in order to make hormones that are encoded by the body. This method involves amplifying small amounts of DNA isolated from the cell using the technique of polymerase chain reaction (PCR). This allows large amounts of the same piece of DNA to be made in a matter of hours, which can then be transcribed into RNA and translated to yield the hormone. These powerful techniques, developed in the research laboratory, have been applied on a commercial basis and have provided enormous benefits to people. One such example is the production of growth hormone.

—RoseMarie Pasmantier, M.D.;
Karen E. Kalumuck, Ph.D.;
updated by Anne Lynn S. Chang, M.D.

See also Addison's disease; Corticosteroids; Cushing's syndrome; Diabetes mellitus; Dwarfism; Endocrine disorders; Endocrinology; Endocrinology, pediatric; Genetic engineering; Gigantism; Glands; Goiter; Growth; Hormone therapy; Hyperhidrosis; Hyperparathyroidism and hypoparathyroidism; Hypoglycemia; Insulin resistance syndrome; Leptin; Melatonin; Menopause; Metabolism; Obesity; Paget's disease; Pancreas; Pancreatitis; Pregnancy and gestation; Puberty and adolescence; Steroid abuse; Steroids; Sweating; Thyroid disorders; Weight loss and gain.

For Further Information:

Barinaga, Marcia. "Obesity: Leptin Receptor Weighs In." *Science* 271 (January 5, 1996): 29.

Bliss, Michael. *The Discovery of Insulin*. 25th anniversary ed. Chicago: University of Chicago Press, 2007.

Bronson, Phyllis J., and Rebecca Bronson. *Moods, Emotions, and Aging: Hormones and the Mind-Body Connection*. Lanham, Md.: Rowman & Littlefield, 2013.

Griffin, James E., and Sergio R. Ojeda, eds. *Textbook of Endocrine Physiology*. 6th ed. New York: Oxford University Press, 2012.

Kronenberg, Henry M., et al., eds. *Williams Textbook of Endocrinology*. 12th ed. Philadelphia: Saunders/Elsevier, 2011.

Marieb, Elaine N. *Essentials of Human Anatomy and Physiology*. 10th ed. San Francisco: Pearson/Benjamin Cummings, 2012.

McPhee, Stephen J., and Maxine A. Papadakis, eds. *Current Medical Diagnosis and Treatment*. 50th ed. New York: McGraw-Hill Medical, 2011.

Pocock, Gillian, Christopher D. Richards, and Dave A. Richards. *Human Physiology*. New York: Oxford University Press, 2013.

Simonsen, Davis. *Hormones and Behavior*. New York: Nova Science, 2013.

HOSPICE

Health care system

Definition: A holistic approach to caring for the dying and their families by addressing their physical, emotional, and spiritual needs.

Hospice is a philosophy of care directed toward persons who are dying. Hospice care uses a family-oriented holistic approach to assist these individuals in making the transition from life to death in a manner that preserves their dignity and comfort. This approach, as Elisabeth Kübler-Ross would say, allows dying patients "to live until they die." Hospice care encourages patients to participate fully in determining the type of care that is most appropriate for their comfort. By creating a secure and caring community sensitive to the needs of the dying and their families and by providing palliative care that relieves patients of the distressing symptoms of their disease, hospice care can aid the dying in preparing mentally as well as spiritually for their impending death.

Unlike traditional health care, where the patient is viewed as the client, hospice care, with its holistic emphasis, treats the family unit as the client. There are usually specific areas of stress for the families of the dying. In addition to the stress of caring for the physical needs of the dying, family members often feel tremendous pressure maintaining their own roles and responsibilities within the family itself. The conflict of caring for their own nuclear families while caring for dying relatives places a huge strain on everyone involved and can be a source of anxiety and guilt for the patient as well. Another area of stress experienced by family members involves concern for themselves, that is, having to put their own lives on hold, keeping from getting physically run down, dealing with their newly acquired time constraints, and viewing themselves as isolated from friends and family. Compounding this is the guilt that many caregivers feel over not caring for the dying relative as well or as patiently as they might, or secretly wishing for the caregiving experience to reach an end.

Due to the holistic nature of the care provided, the hospice team is actually an interdisciplinary team composed of physicians, nurses, psychological and social workers, pastoral counselors, and trained volunteers. This team helps patients, families and caregivers establish goals of care, navigate medical decision-making, communicate with providers, utilize support networks, and coordinate care across a variety of settings, while providing emotional and spiritual support.

Hospice care can be provided in a variety of settings. The majority of hospice care (66 percent in 2012) is provided in the patient's residence, which can range from a nursing home, a residential facility, or their own private residence. There are also hospice inpatient facilities as well as hospice care provided in hospitals. In 2012, approximately 1.6 million patients received hospice services, compared to 1.2 million in 2008.

In the past, palliative care was primarily directed toward patients where curative treatments and life prolongation efforts were no longer effective. While similar to hospice care in that support and relief from suffering are the underlying goals, hospice care is specific to terminally ill patients and palliative care is for any patient with a serious illness.

Today, palliative care is a subspecialty of internal medicine and can be implemented into the plan of care for any age group, at any point during the course of a serious illness, and can be offered in conjunction with curative or life-prolonging treatments depending on the patients' values and preferences. Serious illnesses are those that are complex in nature and may eventually become terminal, such as Alzheimer's, amyotrophic lateral sclerosis (ALS), cancer, cardiac disease, HIV/AIDS, kidney failure, multiple sclerosis, and respiratory disease.

Principles

Hospice care attempts to enhance the quality of dying patients' final days by providing them with as much comfort as possible. It is predicated on the belief that death is a natural process with which humans should not interfere. The principles of hospice care, therefore, revolve around alleviating the anxieties and physical suffering that can be associated with the dying process, and not prolonging the dying process by using invasive medical techniques. Hospice care is also based on the assertion that dying patients have certain rights that must be respected. These rights include a right to absent themselves from social responsibilities and commitments, a right to be cared for, and the right to continued respect and status. The following seven principles are basic components of hospice care.

The first principle is highly personalized and holistic care of the dying, which includes treating dying patients emotionally and spiritually as well as physically. This interpersonal support, known as bonding, helps patients in their final days to live as fully and as comfortably as possible, while retaining their dignity, autonomy, and individual self-worth in a safe and secure environment. This one-on-one attention involves what can be called therapeutic communication. Knowing that someone has heard, that someone understands and is concerned, can be profoundly healing.

Another principle is treating pain aggressively. To this end, hospice care advocates the use of narcotics at dosages that will alleviate suffering while, at the same time, enabling patients to maintain a desired level of alertness. Efforts are made to employ the least invasive routes to administer these drugs (usually orally, if possible). In addition, pain medication is administered before the pain begins, thus alleviating the anxiety of patients waiting for pain to return. Since it has been shown that fear of pain often increases the pain itself, this type of aggressive pain management gives dying patients more time and energy to respond to family members and friends and to work through the emotional and spiritual stages of dying. This dispensation of pain medication before the pain actually occurs, however, has proven to be perhaps the most controversial element in hospice care, with some critics charging that the dying are being turned into drug addicts.

A third principle is the participation of families in caring for the dying. Family members are trained by hospice nurses to care for the dying patients and even to dispense pain medication. The aim is to prevent the patients from suffering isolation or feeling as if they are surrounded by strangers. Participation in care also helps to sustain the patients' and the

Palliative Care	Hospice Care
Serious illness	Terminal illness
Given at any stage of an illness	Given at advanced stages of an illness
Can be given at any age	Can be given at any age
Can be given along with curative therapies	Not given with curative therapies
Life expectancy: any	Life expectancy: 6 months
Location: any	Location: any
Medicare coverage: Variable • Part A (short-term home and hospital coverage) • Part B (equipment, outpatient services)	Medicare coverage: • Part A (short-term home and hospital coverage) • Part B (equipment, outpatient services)
Medicaid coverage: • State variable "wavier" paying family caregivers • Some supplies and equipment	Medicaid coverage: • State variable "wavier" paying family caregivers • Supplies and equipment • Routine care, respite care, short-term inpatient • Grief support, complementary therapies

families' sense of autonomy.

The fourth principle is familiarity of surroundings. Whenever possible, it is the goal of hospice care to keep dying patients at home. This eliminates the necessity of the dying to spend their final days in an institutionalized setting, isolated from family and friends when they need them the most. It is estimated that close to 90 percent of all hospice care days are spent in patients' own homes. When this is not possible and patients must enter institutional settings, rules are relaxed so that their rooms can be decorated or arranged in such a way as to replicate the patients' home surroundings. Visiting rules are suspended when possible, and visits by family members, children, and sometimes even pets are encouraged.

The fifth principle is emotional and spiritual support for the family caregivers. Hospice volunteers are specially trained to use listening and communicative techniques with family members and to provide them with emotional support both during and after the patient's death. In addition, because the care is holistic, the caregivers' physical needs are attended to (for example, respite is provided for exhausted caregivers), as are their emotional and spiritual needs. This spiritual support applies to people of all faith backgrounds, as impending death tends to put faith into a perspective where particular creeds and denominational structures assume less significance. In attending to this spiritual dimension, the hospice team is respectful of all religious traditions while realizing that death and bereavement have the ability to both strengthen and weaken faith.

The sixth principle is having hospice services available twenty-four hours a day, seven days a week. Because of its reliance on the assistance of trained volunteers, round-the-clock support is available to patients and their families.

The seventh principle is bereavement counseling for the survivors. At the time of death, the hospice team is available to help families take care of tasks such as planning the funeral and probating the will. In the weeks after the death, hospice volunteers offer their support to surviving family members in dealing with their loss and grief and the various phases of the bereavement process, always aware of the fact that not all bereaved need or want formal interventions.

History

The term "hospice" comes from the Latin hospitia, meaning "places of welcome." The earliest documented example of hospice care dates to the fourth century, when a Roman woman named Fabiola apparently used her own wealth to care for the sick and dying. In medieval times, the Catholic Church established inns for poor wayfarers and pilgrims traveling to religious shrines in search of miraculous cures for their illnesses. Such "rest homes," usually run by religious orders, provided both lodging and nursing care, since the medieval view was that the sick, dying, and needy were all travelers on a journey. This attitude also reflects the medieval notion that true hospitality included care of the mind and spirit as well as of the body. During the Protestant Reformation, when monasteries were forcibly closed, the concepts of hospice and hospital became distinct. Care of the sick and

dying was now considered a public duty rather than a religious or private one, and many former hospices were turned into state-run hospitals.

The first in-patient hospice establishment of modern times (specifically called "hospice") was founded by Mary Aitkenhead and the Irish Sisters of Charity under her leadership in the 1870s in Dublin, Ireland. Cicely Saunders, a physician at St. Joseph's Hospice in London, which was founded by the English Sisters of Charity in 1908, began to adapt the ancient concept of hospice to modern palliative techniques. While there, Saunders became extremely close to a Holocaust survivor who was dying of cancer. She found that she shared his dream of establishing a place that would meet the needs of the dying. Using the money he bequeathed her at his death as a starting point, Saunders raised additional funds and opened St. Christopher's Hospice in Sydenham, outside London, in 1967. Originally it housed only cancer patients, but with the financial support of contracts with the National Health Service in England and private donations, it later expanded to meet the needs of all the dying. In fact, no patient has ever been refused because of inability to pay. St. Christopher's has served as a model for the hospices to be built later in other parts of the world.

Even though hospice care did not originate with Saunders, she is usually credited with founding the first modern hospice, since she introduced the concept of dispensing narcotics at regular intervals in order to preempt the pain of the dying. She was also the first to identify the need to address other, nonphysical sources of pain for dying patients.

Two years after St. Christopher's Hospice was opened, Kübler-Ross wrote On Death and Dying, which validated the hospice movement by relating stories of the dying and their wishes as to how they would be treated.

In 1974, the United States opened its first hospice, Hospice, Inc. (later called the Connecticut Hospice), in New Haven, Connecticut. Within the next twenty-five years, over three thousand hospice programs would be implemented in the United States. In Canada, the first "palliative care" unit (as hospices are referred to in Canada) was opened in 1975 by Balfour M. Mount at the Royal Victoria Hospital in Montreal. This is considered to be the first hospital-based hospice in North America. Since this time, much advancement has been made in the field of hospice and palliative care in the United States. In 2009, the Accreditation Council for Graduate Medical Education, added hospice and palliative care medicine to its list of accredited training programs for post-MD candidates in the United States.

Cost

Because of hospice care's reliance on heavily trained volunteers and contributions, and because death is seen as a natural process that should not be prolonged by invasive and expensive medical techniques, hospice care is much less costly than traditional acute care facilities. Because hospice care is a philosophy of care rather than a specific facility, though, legislation to provide monetary support for hospice patients took a great deal of time to be approved. In 1982, the U.S. Congress finally added hospice care as a Medicare benefit. In 1986, it was made a permanent benefit. Medicare requires that there be a prognosis of six months or less for the patient to live. There is not, however, a six-month limit to hospice care services. Medicare covers 100 percent of hospice care services. Hospice care is also reimbursable by many private insurance companies, and covered by Medicaid. In 2012, 83.7 percent of all hospice care was paid for by the Medicare Hospice Benefit, 7.6 percent by private insurance, and 5.5 percent by the Medicaid Hospice Benefit.

The National Hospice and Palliative Care Organization (NHPCO) originated in 1978 in the United States as a resource for the many groups across the country who needed assistance in establishing hospice programs in their own communities. The organization included palliative care its mission and goals in 2000. The purpose of this organization is to provide information about hospice and palliative care to the public, to establish conduits so that information may be exchanged between hospice and palliative care groups, and to maintain agreed-upon standards for developing hospice and palliative care centers around the country.

—Mara Kelly-Zukowski, Ph.D.;
updated by Marisela Fermin-Schon

See also Death and dying; Euthanasia; Grief and guilt; Hospitals; Medicare; Palliative medicine; Terminally ill: Extended care.

For Further Information:

Buckingham, Robert W. *The Handbook of Hospice Care.* New York: Prometheus Books, 1996. Covers the history and philosophy of hospice care while providing practical information as to its cost, how to find hospice programs in your own community, and how to manage grief. Focuses on two target populations for hospice care: children and AIDS victims.

Byock, Ira, ed. *Dying Well: Peace and Possibilities at the End of Life.* New York: Riverhead Books, 1998. President of the American Academy of Hospice and Palliative Medicine at the time he wrote this book, Byock uses the personal stories of his patients to show the best ways to die. Provides information for the families of the dying who wish to make their loved ones' final days as comfortable and meaningful as possible.

Center to Advance Palliative Care. "What is Palliative Care?" Retrieved from http://www.getpalliativecare.org/whatis/.

Chun, Audrey, and R. Sean Morrison. "Chapter 31. Palliative Care." *Hazzard's Geriatric Medicine and Gerontology,* 6th ed., edited by Jeffrey B. Halter, Joseph G. Ouslander, Mary E. Tinetti, Stephanie Studenski, Kevin P. High, and Sanjay Asthana. New York: McGraw-Hill, 2009.

Connor, Stephen R. *Hospice: Practice, Pitfalls, and Promise.* Washington, D.C.: Taylor & Francis, 1998. This book provides a useful outline of the history, structure, and function of hospice programs in the United States, with understandably less emphasis on medical issues. There is clear evidence of wide experience and consideration of the real world of hospice care, not secondhand distillation from the literature.

Corr, Charles A., Clyde M. Nabe, and Donna M. Corr. *Death and Dying, Life and Living.* 6th ed. Belmont, CA: Wadsworth/Cengage Learning, 2009. This book provides perspective on common issues associated with death and dying for family members and others affected by life-threatening circumstances.

"Defining Palliative Care." Retrieved from http://www.capc.org/building-a-hospital-based-palliative-care-program/case/definingpc.

Forman, Walter B., et al., eds. *Hospice and Palliative Care: Concepts and Practice.* 2nd ed. Sudbury, MA: Jones and Bartlett, 2003. A text that examines theoretical perspectives on and practical information about hospice care. Other topics include community medical care, geriatric care, nursing care, pain management, research, counseling, and hospice management.

Lattanzi-Licht, Marcia, John J. Mahoney, and Galen W. Miller. *The Hospice Choice: In Pursuit of a Peaceful Death.* New York: Simon & Schuster, 1998. Definitive resource from the National Hospice Organization. Provides practical information such as range of hospice services, methods of payment, and so on. Intersperses stories of families who have received hospice care with a thorough explanation of its history, principles, and benefits.

"Medicare & Hospice Benefits." Retrieved from http://www.medicare.gov/Pubs/pdf/11361.pdf.

Meyer, Maria M., and Paula Derr. *The Comfort of Home: A Complete Guide for Caregivers.* 3rd ed. Portland, OR: CareTrust, 2008. A very useful guide to caregiving in the home. Provides a chronological structure to define preparation for caregiving and the day-to-day expectations, and gives a listing of numerous research resources.

National Hospice and Palliative Care Organization. http://www.nhpco.org. A group that advocates for the terminally ill and their families, develops public and professional educational programs and materials to enhance understanding and availability of hospice and palliative care, and conducts research, among other activities.

Sendor, Virginia F., and Patrice M. O'Connor. *Hospice and Palliative Care: Questions and Answers.* Lanham, MD: Scarecrow Press, 1998. The user-friendly question-and-answer style of this volume allows for use as a quick reference. The purpose is to address the questions often asked by individuals faced with a terminal illness and those involved in the care of the terminally ill.

HOST-DEFENSE MECHANISMS
Biology

Anatomy or system affected: Blood, cells, gastrointestinal system, immune system, skin, urinary system

Specialties and related fields: Hematology, immunology, preventive medicine, serology

Definition: Immunological methods that the body uses to protect against external infectious agents and to maintain internal homeostasis, such as those rooted in the skin, sweat, urine, tears, phagocytes, and "helpful" bacteria.

Key terms:

antibodies: proteins produced by immune cells called lymphocytes; antibodies bind to targets called antigens in a highly specific manner

antigen: any substance that causes the formation of a specific antibody; generally a protein

complement: a series of serum proteins that, when activated, carry out a variety of immune functions; the most notable complement function is the lysis of a target

granulocyte: a white blood cell characterized by large numbers of cytoplasmic granules, including neutrophils, eosinophils, and basophils

innate immunity: nonspecific immunity in the sense that prior contact with an infectious agent is not required for proper innate immune response

interferons: a family of proteins; some of these proteins induce an antiviral state within a cell, while others serve to regulate aspects of the immune response

lymphocyte: either of two kinds of small white blood cells; B lymphocytes function to secrete antibodies, while T lymphocytes function to destroy virus-infected cells

macrophage: any of several forms of either circulating or fixed phagocytic cells of the immune system

neutrophil: a circulating white blood cell that serves as one of the principal phagocytes for the immune system

phagocyte: any cell capable of surrounding, ingesting, and digesting microbes or cell debris; in a certain sense, phagocytes function as scavengers

Structure and Functions

Humans exist in an environment that contains a wide variety of potentially infectious agents. These agents range in size from microscopic viruses—such as rhinoviruses, which cause the common cold—to a wide variety of bacteria and even macroscopic agents such as parasitic worms. In the absence of a functioning immune system, as is observed in persons with acquired immunodeficiency syndrome (AIDS) or congenital immune deficiencies, a person will eventually succumb to overwhelming infections.

Host-defense mechanisms consist of two major components: an innate system that is not dependent on prior exposure to an infectious agent and an acquired immunity that is stimulated by exposure to an agent. In general, the innate system functions in a nonspecific manner, while the acquired immune responses are highly specific.

The first major lines of host defense are the physical barriers to infection. These include the intact skin and the mechanical or physical barriers that serve to protect body openings. Few infectious agents are capable of penetrating intact skin. Numerous sweat glands and follicles are also associated with skin, and their secretion of fatty acids or lactic acid serves to produce an acid environment that inhibits the growth of bacteria. In addition, the high salt content found on the surface of the body also serves to inhibit growth. Bacteria that can resist the high levels of salt and acid, such as *Staphylococcus* or *Streptococcus*, tend to cause skin-related problems such as acne or boils.

Openings of the body, such as the mouth, anus, and vagina, exhibit both the physical barrier of skin and a variety of other defense strategies. Secreted mucus serves to trap foreign particles, which can then be expelled, depending on the tissue, by the ciliary action of the cells, coughing or sneezing, or the washing action of saliva, urine, or tears. Many of these secretions also contain antibacterial or antiviral agents. Gastric juices contain hydrochloric acid, while the enzyme lysozyme, found in tears and saliva, serves to cause the breakdown of certain bacteria.

The normal flora of organisms found within the body also plays an important role in defense. Bacteria in the mouth and gut serve to suppress any external agents that may find their way to those regions. Removal of the innate flora with antibiotics may result in yeast infections of the mouth or vaginal tract, or ulceration by "opportunistic" organisms of the gut.

Penetration of the host by infectious agents initially brings into action other aspects of the innate immune system. This can take the form of a series of "professional" phagocytes, cells that literally eat foreign particles such as bacteria; also included are chemical agents found in tissue and blood.

Two major forms of phagocytes are found in blood and tissues: neutrophils and monocytes/macrophages. Neutrophils represent the most numerous white cells in blood, approximately 60 to 70 percent of the total. They can be recognized by their multilobed nuclei, which confer the ability to pass between the endothelial cells of capillaries into sites of tissue

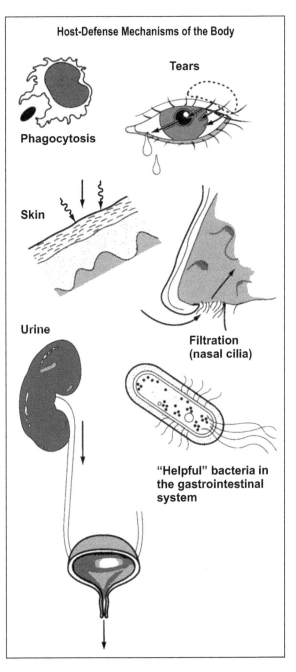

Host-Defense Mechanisms of the Body

Tears

Phagocytosis

Skin

Urine

Filtration (nasal cilia)

"Helpful" bacteria in the gastrointestinal system

infections. When neutrophils locate a target, such as an infectious agent or a dead cell, they surround that target with membranous arms called pseudopods and ingest it. Once the particle is incorporated within this "phagosome," it is ready for killing and digestion.

The killing of ingested organisms such as bacteria involves a series of complicated reactions, the major products of which are highly reactive oxidizing agents such as peroxides or metabolic by-products such as acid. At the same time, digestive organelles within the phagocyte, called lysosomes, fuse with the phagosome. Lysosomes contain numerous digestive enzymes, and these function to digest the engulfed particle. In effect, the particle now ceases to exist.

Monocytes, which are most often observed in their differentiated macrophage stage, function in a similar manner. Unlike circulating cells such as neutrophils, however, macrophages constitute the mononuclear phagocytic system that is associated with many tissues in the body. Examples of tissue-associated macrophages are the Kupffer cells of the liver, the microglia of the brain, and certain alveolar cells of the lungs. In addition to serving a nonspecific phagocytic function, macrophages serve as antigen-presenting cells (APCs) for specific immune responses.

A variety of blood chemicals also can be associated with innate immunity. Complement represents a series of some twenty blood proteins, activated in a cascade fashion, which exhibit a variety of pharmacologic activities. The complement pathway can be initiated upon exposure to certain bacteria. Components of the pathway can serve as chemoattractants for neutrophils. They can increase the efficiency of phagocytosis (opsonization), and they can form a membrane attack complex on the surface of a target, resulting in lysis.

Another type of blood cell may play a role in certain types of parasitic infections: the eosinophil. Granulocytes like the neutrophils, eosinophils contain within their granules digestive enzymes capable of being released against targets such as parasitic worms. The binding of these enzymes on the surface of a target damages the parasite's membrane, resulting ultimately in death of the parasite.

Acquired host defenses, while involving mechanisms similar to those of the innate systems, differ in one important way: they require prior exposure to the antigen. Acquired immunity consists of two major arms: humoral immunity, which represents substances soluble in the blood; and cellular immunity, which utilizes cells targeted against agents in a specific manner.

Humoral immunity centers primarily on proteins called antibodies. Exposure to foreign antigens triggers a series of reactions among three separate types of blood cells: antigen-presenting cells, T lymphocytes, and B lymphocytes. It is the B cell that actually secretes the antibodies.

The process starts when an APC encounters and phagocytizes an antigen. The antigen is digested, and pieces, or determinants, of the antigen are expressed on the surface of the cell. The most common APC is the macrophage, but antigen presentation can also be carried out by dendritic cells found in the dermis of the skin. This portion of the process is analogous to the series of events associated with innate immunity. At this point, however, the determinant is "presented" to appropriate T and B lymphocytes. Only those lymphocytes that possess specific receptors for that antigenic determinant can interact with the APC; it is this aspect that represents the specificity of the reaction. In association with a subclass of T lymphocytes called T helper cells (also known as CD4+ cells), the B cell is stimulated to begin the secretion of large quantities of antibodies. The antibodies recognize and bind only those antigens against which they were produced.

The formation of antigen-antibody complexes is the key to the humoral response. The result of the reaction depends upon the form taken by the antigen. The binding of antibodies to a bacterium or virus results in opsonization, a significantly enhanced ability of phagocytes to engulf the target. Antibody binding to a virus may also inhibit the agent's binding to a target cell, rendering the virus inactive. If the antigen is a toxin, antibody binding will neutralize the molecule.

The other arm of acquired immunity directly utilizes cellular defenses. The key cell here is the T lymphocyte. T lymphocytes mature in an organ called the thymus, which is located in humans near the thyroid in the neck and which provides the basis for the cells" name. One subset of T cells is often referred to as killer cells (or CD8+ cells) because of their function. They possess receptors on their surfaces that bind to specific target cells, which are generally cells infected with viruses, though T cells are also associated with rejection of foreign grafts. Once the T cell binds to the target, pharmacologically active granules are released that bind to and disrupt the membrane of the target. Thus, the humoral response is directed primarily against extracellular agents such as bacteria, while the cellular response is directed primarily against intracellular parasites.

Disorders and Diseases

In their most obvious form, the mechanisms of host defense protect against disease. Humans exist in an environment that is a sea of microorganisms. Most infections, while often uncomfortable, are not life-threatening. It is only when the immune system fails to function properly or is overwhelmed that illness results in the death of the individual. Ironically, the study of these circumstances has provided much knowledge of the functioning of the immune system.

Throughout history, diseases have periodically plagued humanity. Epidemics of viral diseases such as polio and bacterial infections such as bubonic plague or cholera have killed untold millions of persons. Among the most important advances in medicine since the eighteenth century has been the development of vaccination as a means of preventing disease. In the case of passive immunity, host defenses are temporarily augmented, while active immunity, mimicking an actual infection, often provides lifelong protection.

Passive immunity involves the acquisition of preformed antibodies by an individual. Since colostrum, or milk from a nursing mother, contains a form of antibody, this is the most common form of passive immunization. Preformed antibodies may also be given to a person exposed to potentially lethal toxins under circumstances in which there may be insufficient time for a proper immune response. These can include persons exposed to snake venom or tetanus toxin. While temporarily providing protection, passively acquired antibodies survive in the individual only for a short period.

More commonly, vaccines are utilized to provide active immunization by stimulating the acquired host defenses. These vaccines generally utilize inactivated or attenuated parasites that stimulate specific cellular or humoral responses. The prototypes of active immunization are the polio vaccines developed by Jonas Salk and Albert Sabin in the 1950s. Salk's vaccine utilizes a formalin-inactivated poliovirus, while Sabin's consists of attenuated virus. While controversy exists regarding which is superior, both vaccines act in basically the same manner. Exposure to either vaccine results in the production of protective antibodies in the circulation of the individual. In the event of actual infection by poliovirus, the agent would be neutralized before it could reach its target in the central nervous system. Analogous vaccines have been developed against previously common viral diseases such as smallpox, measles, and mumps, and against bacterial diseases such as pertussis (whooping cough) and diphtheria.

The process by which the acquired immune process functions is in part defined by the nature of the antigen. It is also important to remember that the humoral and cellular defense systems are not self-exclusive; each functions in conjunction with the other. If the antigen in question is a bacterium, it is primarily the role of the humoral system to deal with the infection. This can take several forms. The antibody may bind to the surface of the cell, inactivating the cell wall or membrane enzymes, resulting in the death of the cell. The antibody-antigen (bacterium) complex may also activate the complement pathway, resulting in either opsonization or the formation of a membrane attack complex by complement components. Indeed, antibody binding by itself may result in opsonization.

If the antigen is a virus-infected cell, the cellular portion of the response comes into play. Cytotoxic T cells can bind to the target through specific receptors, causing the death of the virus-infected cell. If an antibody binds to viral receptors on the infected cell, cytotoxic cells with receptors for the antibody may show increased affinity for the target in a process called antibody-dependent cell-mediated cytotoxicity (ADCC). The result is the death of the target. The antibody may also serve to neutralize a cell-free virus before the particle can even infect the target cell. Certain bacteria, however, such as the mycobacteria associated with tuberculosis and leprosy, are actually found as intracellular parasites. In such cases, it is the cellular immune system that plays a major role in defense. In this manner, the humoral and cellular defense mechanisms complement each other.

Failure of the immune system to function is clearly illustrated in persons infected with the human immunodeficiency virus (HIV), the virus that causes AIDS. HIV infects the subclass of T lymphocytes called T helper cells. The eventual result is the death and depletion of this subclass of cells. As briefly described earlier, T helper cells are central to the function of both the humoral and the cellular arms of acquired immunity. The interaction of these cells with B lymphocytes is necessary for both antibody production by these cells and their proliferation. The T helper cell is also required for activation and proliferation of the CD8+ cytotoxic T cells.

As AIDS progresses in the individual, the T-helper subclass becomes increasingly depleted. As a result, both the cellular and humoral immune systems become progressively less functional. The person becomes more susceptible to opportunistic organisms in the environment and eventually succumbs to any of a wide variety of diseases.

In rare congenital cases, only certain aspects of the immune system are nonfunctional. These often tragic examples serve to illustrate the role of various cells within the host defense. For example, children with B-cell deficiencies suffer from repeated bacterial infections, while yeast and viral infections rarely result in problems. Children in whom the thymus fails to develop (DiGeorge or Nezelof syndromes), however, suffer from repeated viral infections but rarely from bacterial infections.

Severe combined immunodeficiency syndrome (SCID) affects approximately one of every 150,000 live births. This genetic disorder is the result of a lack of the enzyme adenosine deaminase (ADA), which ultimately causes a lack of functioning T cells. For years, patients with this disorder had been doomed to living in sterile bubble environments and would die at a young age because of their inability to fight even the mildest infection. Bone marrow transplants for patients with compatible donors can sometimes strengthen the immune system; however, this option is not available for everyone.

In 1990, two unrelated girls with SCID, four and nine years old, were the subject of the first clinical trial of gene therapy. T cells in their blood were isolated and cultured, and normal copies of the ADA gene were introduced into the cells. The genetically engineered T cells were then infused back into the patients over a period of approximately two years. Both girls showed remarkable improvement, with near normal levels of ADA and functioning immune systems, and were thereafter able to lead normal lives. These positive results remained several years after cessation of the actual gene therapy, indicating that this first clinical trial of gene therapy was a success. The door is now open for using gene therapy on other disorders, including those of the immune system.

Host defenses are also utilized within the homeostatic process, which can be defined as maintaining the status quo. An example of such a process is the role of the immune system in protecting humans against various forms of cancer. Although immunosuppressed individuals appear to be at no greater risk for most cancers than normal persons, certain types of skin cancers, as well as certain types of B-cell lymphomas, arise more frequently in these persons. Thus, it is likely that the immune system plays at least some role in protecting the individual from certain forms of cancer. Artificial stimulation of the immune system has, however, been utilized in an attempt to treat sundry forms of advanced cancers. The process involves the removal of immune cells from the patient and the incubation of those cells with a form of interferon generally secreted by T helper cells during their regulation of the immune response. The cells are then returned to the patient. The theory is that, by nonspecifically stimulating cytotoxic cells, some of those cells may serve to destroy the cancer. In some instances, patients have shown improvement.

Clearly, the immune system functions by means of a complex process of cellular interactions. The initial encounter with a foreign infectious agent utilizes an innate system that serves as a first line of defense. Then, through a type of learning process, a specific immune response is generated that provides a more rapid, more efficient means of generating protection.

Perspective and Prospects

Manipulating the host's immune system in order to protect against disease dates back more than a thousand years. To protect themselves against smallpox, the Chinese carried out a practice called variolation, in which dried crusts obtained from the pocks of mild cases were inhaled. The practice was copied by early Arabic physicians and eventually made its way to eighteenth century Europe. In the late eighteenth century, an English country physician, Edward Jenner, observed that dairymaids who had recovered from a mild disease called cowpox rarely exhibited the scars associated with smallpox. Jenner reasoned that a person who had been exposed to the cowpox agent would be protected against smallpox. Jenner tested his theory and was proved correct. Smallpox became the first disease that could be prevented by vaccination.

Competition between French and German scientists during the late nineteenth century resulted in much of the existing basic knowledge of host defenses. A Russian, Élie Metchnikoff, working with Louis Pasteur in Paris during the 1880s, developed the views of cellular immunity that are still current. In that same period, the work of Emil von Behring and Paul Ehrlich in Berlin established the role of humoral immunity in protecting against disease.

Active immunization remains the primary method by which an individual may be protected from disease, but the process lends itself to a variety of problems. Not all antigenic determinants of the bacterium or parasite in question are equally important. A response to some antigens may actually hinder the immune response to more important determinants. Furthermore, some individuals react inappropriately to some vaccines, resulting in severe allergic reactions.

For these reasons, much research involves the attempt to isolate only the desired antigen for the vaccine. This has taken several approaches. Purified components, rather than the entire organism, have been used in some vaccines. In some cases, the gene that encodes the desired antigen has been isolated and spliced into the genetic material of a harmless organism. Such an approach has been used to produce a modified hepatitis B vaccine. The gene encoding the surface antigen of the virus has been spliced into the genome of vac-

cinia, long used for vaccination against smallpox. When the individual is vaccinated, the hepatitis gene is expressed (though no virus can be made), and the person becomes immune to the disease. In theory, whole cocktails of vaccines can be prepared in a similar manner.

New illnesses and other environmental hazards that affect host defenses continue to arise. AIDS may be unusually lethal, but as a previously unknown disease, it is by no means unique. Nevertheless, the ability of the host immune system to respond to new infectious agents remains a bulwark for maintaining the health of an individual.

—Richard Adler, Ph.D.;
updated by Karen E. Kalumuck, Ph.D.

See also Antibodies; Bacterial infections; Bacteriology; Blood and blood disorders; Cells; Earwax; Glands; Immune system; Immunization and vaccination; Immunology; Immunopathology; Infection; Skin; Sweating; Tears and tear ducts; Urinary system; Viral infections.

For Further Information:

Adelman, Daniel C., et al., eds. *Manual of Allergy and Immunology.* 5th ed. Philadelphia: Lippincott Williams & Wilkins, 2012.

Bibel, Debra Jan, ed. *Milestones in Immunology.* New York: Springer, 1988.

Delves, Peter J., et al. *Roitt's Essential Immunology.* 12th ed. Malden, Mass.: Blackwell, 2011.

Frank, Steven A. *Immunology and Evolution of Infectious Disease.* Princeton, N.J.: Princeton University Press, 2002.

Hall, Stephen S. *A Commotion in the Blood: Life, Death, and the Immune System.* New York: Henry Holt, 1997.

Hawley, Louise, Richard J. Ziegler, and Benjamin L. Clarke. *Microbiology and Immunology.* Philadelphia: Lippincott Williams & Wilkins, 2013.

Kuby, Janis, et al., eds. *Kuby Immunology.* 7th ed. New York: W. H. Freeman, 2013.

Male, David K., et al., eds. *Immunology.* Philadelphia: Elsevier/ Saunders, 2013.

Murray, Patrick R., Ken S. Rosenthal, and Michael A. Pfaller. *Medical Microbiology.* 7th ed. Philadelphia: Mosby/Elsevier, 2013.

Paul, William E., ed. *Immunology: Recognition and Response.* New York: W. H. Freeman, 1991.

Playfair, J. H. L., and B. M. Chain. *Immunology at a Glance.* 10th ed. Hoboken, N.J.: Wiley-Blackwell, 2013.

HUMAN GENOME PROJECT. *See* GENOMICS.

HUMAN IMMUNODEFICIENCY VIRUS (HIV)
Disease/Disorder

Anatomy or system affected: Immune system

Specialties and related fields: Immunology, microbiology, virology

Definition: A retrovirus that attacks cells of the immune system, leading to a loss of immune function and the development of acquired immunodeficiency syndrome (AIDS).

Causes and Symptoms

HIV is a human retrovirus containing two copies of a 9,749-base ribonucleic acid (RNA) molecule as its genetic material. Among the proteins carried by retrovirus particles is an enzyme called reverse transcriptase, which upon infection of

HIV is transmitted only through the exchange of body fluids, including semen, vaginal fluid, blood, and human milk. Therefore, the primary routes are sexual transmission, the use of dirty needles by intravenous drug users, and HIV-positive mother-to-child transmission during childbirth or from HIV-contaminated breast milk. Transmission through dirty needles used in body piercing or tattooing may occur. Early in the AIDS epidemic, infection was also acquired through the transfusion of contaminated blood or blood products, leading to a very high rate of transmission to hemophiliacs. Today, such transmission is extremely rare, as the blood supply is routinely tested for HIV.

the cell transcribes the RNA genome into a DNA copy. The DNA copy then integrates into a human chromosome and is maintained in a form called a provirus. The provirus acts as a template to produce copies of the HIV RNA genome. Once the provirus has integrated, infection is irreversible.

HIV falls into the subgroup of retroviruses called lentiviruses, "slow viruses" that do not cause a disease state until many years after infection. For example, the period of time between HIV infection and development of disease averages between five and ten years in untreated persons. Despite the absence of symptoms, the person may be infectious during this period.

There are two forms of HIV: HIV-1, which arose in central Africa, is the predominant form throughout most of the world, including the United States; HIV-2, a less common form found in western Africa, is less harmful and reproduces more slowly. These viruses evolved from related agents called simian immunodeficiency viruses (SIV) in apes and monkeys. HIV-1 is believed to have arisen from SIV found in chimpanzees in either the Republic of the Congo or Cameroon, while HIV-2 is believed to have arisen from SIV of the Sootey Mangabey monkey of western Africa.

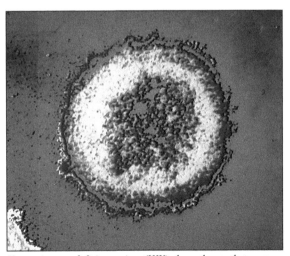

Human immunodeficiency virus (HIV), the pathogen that causes AIDS. (PhotoDisc)

**In the News:
Experimental HIV Vaccine**

Despite more than twenty-five years of intensive research—and a global expenditure of more than $6 billion—a vaccine that prevents HIV infection has remained elusive. One notorious trial was halted early when vaccinated subjects actually suffered an increased risk of infection.

There are a number of complex reasons that candidate vaccines have proven ineffective. One reason is that the molecules on the surface of the virus to which the immune system's antibodies can bind are much more variable than in typical pathogens. The HIV genome, composed of ribonucleic acid (RNA), can accumulate mutations at frequencies up to 100 times higher than genomes composed of deoxyribonucleic acid (DNA) like the human genome. Thus, selection pressure due to an immune response against one set of HIV surface molecules will rapidly lead to the evolution of resistant strains displaying distinct sets of surface molecules. Indeed, multiple highly divergent strains are found in patients in different regions of the globe.

Finally, in September, 2009, a U.S.-Thai team of investigators announced the first demonstration of reduced risk of HIV infection after immunization. The study employed a combination of two vaccines that had individually failed to be effective in previous experiments. Low-to-moderate-risk HIV-negative volunteers aged eighteen to thirty were given injections of vaccine or placebo and subsequently tested for infection every six months for three years. In the control group, 74 of 8,198 subjects were infected by the end of the study; in the vaccinated group, only 51 of 8,197 subjects became infected. Those figures reflect a statistically significant 31.2 percent reduction of probability of infection after vaccination.

Although the observed effect was encouraging, the results include a number of caveats. The vaccine combination targets the HIV strain encountered most frequently in Thailand and therefore would not be expected to provide immunity to the strains responsible for most infections in Africa, Europe, North America, and elsewhere. Vaccination had no apparent effect on the severity of infection in subjects who contracted HIV during the study. Lastly, the vaccine's efficacy is far below the 80 percent threshold required for approval for public distribution.

—*Carina Endres Howell, Ph.D.*

Treatment and Therapy

The lack of fidelity associated with replication of HIV results in a high number of mutations, making it difficult for the immune system of the infected host to respond as it would to infections by other viruses. Consequently, no effective vaccine to prevent infection with HIV has been developed. The Food and Drug Administration (FDA) has approved some two dozen drugs to treat HIV infection; more are in clinical trials. These drugs fall into four categories: nucleoside or nucleotide analogues, which act as direct inhibitors of reverse transcriptase; inhibitors that indirectly inhibit reverse transcriptase by binding to the enzyme; protease inhibitors that interfere with the processing of HIV proteins and assembly of progeny viruses; and inhibitors of entry of

HIV into the cell. Because the virus has a very high rate of mutation, resistance to individual anti-HIV drugs may appear quickly. Present therapy, called highly active antiretroviral therapy (HAART), involves the use of three or four anti-HIV drugs simultaneously. HAART therapy, also termed "cocktail therapy," increases efficacy and reduces the probability of developing simultaneous resistance of HIV to all three or four drugs being used.

—Ralph R. Meyer, Ph.D.;
updated by Richard Adler, Ph.D.

See also Acquired immunodeficiency syndrome (AIDS); Autoimmune disorders; Immune system; Immunodeficiency disorders; Immunology; Immunopathology; Sexually transmitted diseases (STDs); Viral infections.

For Further Information:

Fan, Hung, Ross F. Conner, and Luis P. Villarreal. *The Biology of AIDS.* 4th ed. Sudbury, Mass.: Jones and Bartlett, 2000.

Farnan, Rose, and Maithe Enriquez. *What Nurses Know: HIV/AIDS.* New York: Demos Health, 2012.

Matthews, Dawn D., ed. *AIDS Sourcebook.* 3d ed. Detroit, Mich.: Omnigraphics, 2003.

Sande Merle A., et al. *Sande's HIV/AIDS Medicine: Medical Management of AIDS, 2013.* Philadelphia: Elsevier Saunders, 2012.

Stine, Gerald J. *AIDS Update 2013.* New York: McGraw-Hill Higher Education, 2013.

Strauss, James, and Ellen Strauss. *Viruses and Human Disease.* 2d ed. Boston: Academic Press/Elsevier, 2008.

HUMAN PAPILLOMAVIRUS (HPV)
Disease/Disorder

Also known as: Papovaviruses

Anatomy or system affected: Anus, genitals, reproductive system, skin

Specialties and related fields: Epidemiology, gynecology, oncology, public health, virology

Definition: A group of viruses, some of which are sexually transmitted and associated with genital warts and genital cancer.

Key terms:

Cervarix: a vaccine against the common forms of human papillomavirus that cause cervical cancer

cervical cancer: cancer of the cervix that is associated with human papillomavirus

Gardasil: a vaccine against the common forms of human papillomavirus that cause cervical cancer and genital warts

genital warts: warts occurring in the genital and anal areas and often associated with cancer of the reproductive tract

Pap testing: a screening test to detect precancerous and cancerous cells of the cervix

Causes and Symptoms

Papillomaviruses are deoxyribonucleic acid (DNA) viruses than infect the skin and mucous membranes. Human papillomaviruses belong to a group of papillomaviruses that consists of nearly 120 strains. Most strains are virtually harmless, causing nothing more than benign skin warts (papillomas), while others cause genital warts (condyloma acuminate) and may cause cancer.

Sexual contact is the primary mechanism by which the virus is acquired. About thirty HPV strains are sexually transmitted and can infect the external genitalia, urethra, anus, rectum, and sometimes the mouth and throat. Some low-risk strains cause genital warts, while the ten more virulent, high-risk strains cause abnormal Papanicolaou (Pap) tests and can in some instances cause cancer of the cervix, vagina, vulva, penis, scrotum, anus, and/or the mouth and pharynx. Almost all cases of cervical cancer are the result of persistent HPV infection.

HPV is one of the most common sexually transmitted diseases. It has been estimated that more than 50 percent of sexually active people and up to 75 percent of sexually active women will develop an HPV infection during their lifetimes. Although the active viral infection is usually cleared by the immune system within a few months, it often remains dormant and can later cause a reinfection. Babies of infected women may contract potentially life-threatening HPV infections during delivery.

Women are more susceptible to developing genital warts. Many infected people, however, do not have genital warts. Infected women who are asymptomatic are often diagnosed by an abnormal Pap testing. In 2003, the Food and Drug Administration (FDA) approved the use of testing for high-risk HPV DNA as a routine screening procedure. DNA testing is also used as a confirmatory test for HPV after an abnormal Pap test.

Frequent Pap tests are the best way to diagnose HPV infections in asymptomatic women. About 10 percent of HPV-in-

---

Information on Human Papillomavirus (HPV)

Causes: Viral infection spread through skin (usually sexual) contact

Symptoms: Warts or cancer in genital and anal areas

Duration: Acute in initial infection, then chronic and often recurrent

Treatments: For warts, topical ointments, creams, resins, or gels and electrocautery, cryosurgery, or laser surgery; for cancer, chemotherapy, radiation, surgery; prevention possible with vaccine

fected women will develop precancerous changes in their cervix, and about 8 percent of these women will develop the early stages of cervical cancer. Since persistent HPV infection is a hallmark of developing cervical cancer and since the cancer usually develops slowly over five to ten years, early diagnosis and treatment can be effective in preventing cervical cancer.

Genital warts are highly contagious and are transmitted through skin-to-skin contact from sexual activity. Risk reduction for HPV infection can be achieved by reducing the frequency of sexual contact. Condom use may partially reduce the risk of HPV infection in women. Since condoms do not cover all infected areas, however, their use does not eliminate the risk of infection. Research has suggested that microbicides may prevent infection if they are applied before sexual activity.

Treatment and Therapy

Since there is no cure for an HPV infection, the primary treatments are for warts. Some treatments involve the use of topical ointments, creams, resins, and gels such as imiquimod (Aldara), podophyllin and podofilox (Condylox), and 5-fluorouracil, as well as trichloroacetic acid. Alternatively, warts may be removed by electrocautery, cryosurgery, laser, or conventional surgery.

In 2006, the FDA approved Gardasil, developed by Merck, and in 2009 approved Cervarix, developed by GlaxoSmith Kline, for use as preventive vaccines for the most prevalent HPV strains that cause cervical cancer and genital warts. Gardasil is active against two low-risk HPV strains that are the leading cause of genital warts and, as is Cervarix, active against two high-risk strains that cause up to 70 percent of cervical cancers in the United States. In 2010, the FDA approved the use of Gardasil for the treatment of precancerous lesions in an effort to prevent anal cancer. Gardasil is recommended for women between the ages of nine and twenty-six, and Cervarix is recommended for women between the ages of ten and twenty-five. The Center for Disease Control recommends that all eleven- and twelve-year-old girls receive the HPV vaccine, and that girls and women between thirteen and twenty-six receive "catch up" vaccinations. From 2008 to 2010, the percentage of girls between the ages of thirteen and seventeen who were behind on their vaccinations dropped from 84 to 75 percent. Routine Pap testing is still recommended, because the vaccines do not protect against all strains of HPV.

Perspective and Prospects

HPV was first described as a cause of skin warts in 1907. The relationship between sexual activity and cervical cancer was noted when it was discovered that women who have or who have had multiple sexual partners have a greater risk of developing cervical cancer than do women who have had few or no sexual partners. It was not until the 1980s that HPV was linked to cervical cancer.

The mechanism by which HPV causes cancer has recently been determined. Two proteins encoded by HPV DNA attach to and inactivate cellular proteins that control cell division. With these cellular proteins inactivated, the cell multiplies uncontrollably. Current research is directed toward the development of a vaccine that would inactivate the viral proteins that bind to and inhibit the proteins controlling cell division.

Since sisters of women with cervical cancer have a higher risk of developing cervical cancer, it is thought that genetics may be involved in the progression of the disease.

—Charles L. Vigue, Ph.D.

See also Anal cancer; Anus; Cancer; Carcinogens; Cervical, ovarian, and uterine cancers; Genital disorders, female; Genital disorders, male; Gynecology; Immunization and vaccination; Men's health; Pap test; Reproductive system; Screening; Sexually transmitted diseases (STDs); Skin; Skin cancer; Skin disorders; Viral infections; Warts; Women's health.

For Further Information:

Crum, Christopher P., and Gerard J. Nuovo. *Genital Papillomaviruses and Related Neoplasms*. New York: Raven Press, 1991.

Dizon Don S., and Michael L Krychman. *Questions and Answers About Human Papilloma Virus (HPV)*. Sudbury, Mass.: Jones and Bartlett, 2011.

Eifel, Patricia J., and Charles Levenback, eds. *Cancer of the Female Lower Genital Tract*. Hamilton, Ont.: B. C. Becker, 2001.

Gross, Gerd, and Geo von Krogh, eds. *Human Papillomavirus Infections in Dermatovenereology*. Boca Raton, Fla.: CRC Press, 1997.

McCance, Dennis J., ed. *Human Papilloma Viruses*. New York: Elsevier Science, 2002.

Markowitz, Lauri E., et. al. "Quadrivalent Human Papillomavirus Vaccine: Recommendations of the Advisory Committee on Immunization Practices (ACIP)." *Morbidity and Mortality Weekly Report (MMWR)* 56 (March 23, 2007): 1–24.

Mindel, Adrian, ed. *Genital Warts: Human Papillomavirus Infection*. Boston: Arnold, 1995.

Radosevich, James A. *HPV and Cancer*. New York: Springer, 2012.

Sterling, Jane C., and Stephen K. Tyring, eds. *Human Papillomaviruses: Clinical and Scientific Advances*. New York: Arnold, 2001.

Wailoo, Keith. *Three Shots at Prevention: The HPV Vaccine and the Politics of Medicine's Simple Solutions*. Baltimore, Md.: Johns Hopkins University Press, 2010.

Huntington's disease

Disease/Disorder

Also known as: Huntington's chorea

Anatomy or system affected: Brain, nerves, nervous system

Specialties and related fields: Biotechnology, genetics, neurology, psychiatry, psychology

Definition: In this autosomal dominant genetic neurodegenerative disease, patients have uncoordinated movements as a result of neuron degeneration.

Causes and Symptoms

The mutated gene responsible for Huntington's disease is located on one arm of chromosome 4 and produces the protein huntingtin. The gene contains repeats of the triplet nucleotide sequence CAG. Normal individuals have between nine and thirty-five (on average eighteen or nineteen) CAG repeats in their genes; affected individuals have forty or more repeats,

---

Information on Huntington's Disease

Causes: Genetic protein defect
Symptoms: Uncoordinated movements (chorea), loss of muscle control (dystonias), personality changes, gradual loss of cognition, death
Duration: Progressive, eventually fatal
Treatments: Tricyclic antidepressants for psychological problems and neuroleptics for chorea

---

with an average of forty-six repeats. Individuals with between thirty-six and thirty-nine repeats may or may not develop Huntington's disease. The disease always occurs if the expansion is forty or more repeats. The larger the number of repeats above forty, the earlier the onset of the disease. The disease-causing gene is dominant, so those who inherit the mutated gene develop the disease and have a 50 percent chance of passing the defective gene on to their children.

The triplet CAG codes for the amino acid glutamine. Mutant forms of the huntingtin proteins have forty or more glutamines in the protein. Huntington's disease appears to be caused by a mutation involving a gain of function, in which the expanded polyglutamine region makes the mutant huntingtin protein toxic. Aggregates of mutant huntingtin are observed in the neurons of those who died from Huntington's disease. Normal huntingtin appears to keep neurons alive by stopping programmed cell death.

The neuropathology of Huntington's disease is primarily the degeneration of neurons of the striatum (part of the basal ganglia) and the motor cortex. Clinical manifestations of Huntington's disease typically begin in midlife (thirties and forties), with characteristic motor abnormalities such as uncoordinated movements (chorea) and loss of muscle control (dystonias), personality changes, a gradual loss of cognition, and eventually, death. Huntington's disease primarily affects the central nervous system, but most patients actually die of heart or respiratory complications from long confinement to bed or from head injuries caused by frequent falls.

Treatment and Therapy

The present treatment for Huntington's disease is the use of drugs such as tricyclic antidepressants to control psychological problems and neuroleptics to treat the associated chorea. In 2003, clinical trials were examining the effects of implanting fetal neurons into the brains of Huntington's disease patients.

Perspective and Prospects

In 1872, George Huntington first reported this hereditary disease that he observed in a Long Island, New York, family. Because of the uncoordinated movements of patients, he termed the condition "chorea," from the Greek word for "dance." In 1981, Nancy Wexler began to study a large extended family with Huntington's disease in an isolated village on Lake Maracaibo, Venezuela. Studies of this family aided the work of localizing the gene responsible for this disease. In 1993, that gene was identified by the collaborative work of fifty-

eight scientists, led by James R. Gusella and Francis S. Collins.

—Susan J. Karcher, Ph.D.

See also Brain; Brain disorders; Genetic diseases; Motor neuron diseases; Nervous system; Neuralgia, neuritis, and neuropathy; Neurology; Neurology, pediatric; Tics.

For Further Information:

Alan, Rick. "Huntington's Disease." *Health Library*, September 10 , 2012.

Baréma, Jean. *The Test: Living in the Shadow of Huntington's Disease*. New York: Franklin Square Press, 2005.

Bates, Gillian, Peter S. Harper, and Lesley Jones, eds. *Huntington's Disease*. 3d ed. New York: Oxford University Press, 2007.

Cattaneo, Elena, Dorotea Rigamonti, and Chaiara Zuccato. "The Enigma of Huntington's Disease." *Scientific American* 287 (December, 2002): 92–97.

"Huntington's Disease." *Mayo Clinic*, May 5, 2011.

"Huntington's Disease: Hope Through Research." *National Institute of Neurological Disorders and Stroke*, April 24, 2013.

Lewis, Ricki. *Human Genetics: Concepts and Applications*. 9th ed. Dubuque, Iowa: McGraw-Hill, 2009.

Nussbaum, Robert L., Roderick R. McInnes, and Willard F. Huntington. *Thompson and Thompson Genetics in Medicine*. 7th ed. Philadelphia: Saunders/Elsevier, 2006.

Rubinsztein, David C. "Lessons from Animal Models of Huntington's Disease." *Trends in Genetics* 18 (April 4, 2002): 202–209.

HYDROCELES
Disease/Disorder

Anatomy or system affected: Genitals, reproductive system
Specialties and related fields: General surgery, urology
Definition: A collection of fluid between the lining membranes protecting the testicles in the scrotum.

Causes and Symptoms

Hydroceles occur in 1 percent of adult males. In patients between the ages of eighteen and thirty-five, the presence of an underlying testicular tumor must be ruled out. Accurate diagnosis can be carried out through physical examination. A hydrocele is a smooth, cystlike mass completely surrounding the testicle such that only the mass can be palpated; the testis, inside, cannot be felt. Hydroceles do not involve the spermatic cord. When a light is shined through the cyst, the light is readily transmitted. If the hydrocele is large or tense and the testis cannot be examined, ultrasound examination can eliminate the diagnosis of a testicular abnormality.

Treatment and Therapy

Removal, called hydrocelectomy, is primarily indicated for adult hydroceles that produce discomfort, objectionable scrotal enlargement, or an uncertainty regarding underlying testicular abnormalities upon scrotal ultrasound or physical examination. The presence of a hydrocele does not necessarily require surgical intervention, drainage, or other intervention; it must be accompanied by some significant abnormality to require surgery.

Surgical excision is the most effective method for treatment and can be done on an outpatient basis. A 5.0- to 7.6-centimeter

---

Information on Hydroceles

Causes: Collection of fluid between lining membranes protecting the testicle
Symptoms: Sometimes discomfort, objectionable scrotal enlargement
Duration: Chronic
Treatments: Surgical removal, if desired

(2.0- to 3.0-inch) incision is made in the scrotum, and the wall of the hydrocele is identified and dissected free. The hydrocele sac is removed and its edges sewn or cauterized to eliminate bleeding. The testis is then returned to the scrotum, and the incision is closed. For large hydroceles, a small drainage tube is introduced into the scrotum to limit swelling.

The most frequent complication of hydrocele surgery is scrotal swelling, which may continue for eight weeks. Most patients return to full activity within seven to ten days of surgery, however, and recurrences are rare.

In addition to surgical removal, other treatment options include needle aspiration and aspiration with the injection of sclerosing agents. Needle aspiration is rarely effective and increases infection risk. Fluid usually reaccumulates within three months of aspiration. Aspiration with the injection of sclerosing agents such as tetracycline is successful in fewer than 50 percent of patients and usually requires multiple treatments.

—*Culley C. Carson III, M.D.*

See also Abscess drainage; Cyst removal; Cysts; Genital disorders, male; Men's health; Reproductive system; Testicular surgery.

For Further Information:

Francis, John J., and Laurence A. Levine. "Aspiration and Sclerotherapy: A Nonsurgical Treatment Option for Hydroceles." *Journal of Urology* 189, 5 (May 2013): 1725–1729.

Graham, Sam D., Jr., et al., eds. *Glenn's Urologic Surgery.* 7th ed. Philadelphia: Lippincott Williams & Wilkins, 2010.

"Hydrocele." *Mayo Clinic*, November 3, 2011.

Kay, K. W., R. V. Clayman, and P. H. Lange. "Outpatient Hydrocele and Spermatocele Repair Under Local Anesthesia." *Journal of Urology* 130, no. 2 (August, 1983): 269-271.

Lyons, Sonja. "Hydrocele/Varicocele." *HealthLibrary*, September 26, 2011.

Sherwood, Lauralee. *Human Physiology: From Cells to Systems.* 7th ed. Pacific Grove, Calif.: Brooks/Cole/Cengage Learning, 2010.

Wampler, Stephen M., and Mikel Lianes. "Primary Care Urology: Common Scrotal and Testicular Problems." *Primary Care: Clinics in Office Practice* 37, 3 (September 2010): 613–626.

HYDROCEPHALUS
Disease/Disorder
Also known as: "Water on the brain"
Anatomy or system affected: Brain, head, nervous system, psychic-emotional system
Specialties and related fields: Critical care, general surgery, neonatology, neurology, perinatology
Definition: A collection of excessive amounts of cerebrospinal fluid (CSF) within the cranial cavity, which

can cause increased pressure within the brain and skull, leading to brain tissue damage and, in infants, enlargement of the skull.

Key terms:
cerebrospinal fluid (CSF): the fluid that bathes and nourishes the inner and outer surfaces of the brain and spinal cord
shunt: a tube that is surgically inserted to drain excess fluid away from an area such as the brain
"water on the brain": a common term for hydrocephalus

Causes and Symptoms

Frequently referred to as "water on the brain," hydrocephalus is a disorder most commonly seen in newborns and infants but it sometimes occurs in older children and adults. The fluid is actually a relatively small amount (about 10 cubic centimeters for every kilogram of body weight) of cerebrospinal fluid (CSF), which surrounds and cushions the brain and spinal cord on both the inside and the outside. Within the brain are four CSF-filled spaces called ventricles. The CSF is continuously formed here and then moves down through the central canal, a tube that runs the length of the spinal cord. From the base of the spine, the fluid moves upward on the outside of the spinal cord and returns to the skull where it covers the outer surfaces of the brain. Here it is absorbed by the brain's outer lining. If interference occurs in any part of this process, CSF continues to accumulate in the brain. This usually causes increased pressure to develop within the skull, and abnormally high pressure can lead to permanent brain damage and even death. In the infant, this accumulation also causes the skull to enlarge, since the growth regions of the skull have not yet become firm.

Excessive CSF may develop due to overproduction of fluid in the brain, a blockage of the fluid's circulation, or a blockage of fluid reabsorption on the brain's surface. Hydrocephalus can be congenital or may develop as a result of a head injury, infection, brain hemorrhage, or tumor. Congenital hydrocephalus and most cases of hydrocephalus that begin in infancy are characterized by an enlarged head, which continues to grow at an abnormally rapid pace.

Symptoms and signs that accompany congenital hydrocephalus include lethargy, vomiting, irritability, epilepsy, rigidity of the legs, and the loss of normal reflexes. If left untreated, the condition causes drowsiness, seizures, and severe brain damage and can lead to death possibly within days or weeks. Hydrocephalus is also often associated with other anomalies of the brain and nervous system, such as spina bifida.

Information on Hydrocephalus

Causes: Congenital defect, head injury, infection, brain hemorrhage, tumor
Symptoms: Enlarged head, lethargy, vomiting, irritability, epilepsy, rigidity of legs, loss of normal reflexes
Duration: Typically chronic
Treatments: Surgery

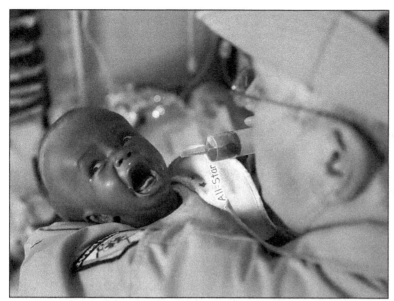

A disaster aid worker feeds a Haitian child suffering from hydrocephalus following the 2010 earthquake. (AP/Wide World Photos)

When hydrocephalus develops in older children and adults, the head size will not increase since the growth lines in the bones of the skull have hardened. If the CSF pressure increases, resulting symptoms include headaches, vomiting, vision problems, problems with muscle coordination, and a progressive decrease in mental activity.

Treatment and Therapy

Diagnosis of hydrocephalus and related nervous system defects sometimes can be made before birth, either by fetal ultrasound or by testing for the presence of an abnormal amount of a brain-associated protein, alpha-fetoprotein, in the pregnant woman's blood. However, even with early diagnosis and surgical intervention promptly after birth, the prognosis is guarded.

Older children and adults suspected of having hydrocephalus should be examined by a neurologist. A computed tomography (CT) scan or magnetic resonance imaging (MRI) of the brain can visualize the structure of the brain and the extent of the hydrocephalus.

Surgical correction is the primary treatment for hydrocephalus. The excess pressure must be drained from within the brain, or a balance between the production and elimination of CSF must be established. In some cases, a combination of surgery and medication is successful. For example, the drugs furosemide (Lasix) and acetazolamide (Diamox), when used for increased CSF pressure from brain hemorrhage, may reduce the amount of CSF fluid produced and thereby decrease the amount of swelling.

Relieving the CSF pressure within the brain is commonly achieved by the surgical insertion of a tube, called a shunt, through brain tissue into one of the cerebral ventricles. A one-way valve is attached to the tube; this allows CSF to escape from the skull cavity when the pressure exceeds a certain level. The tubing is then passed beneath the skin into either the right side of the heart or the abdominal cavity where the excessive CSF can be absorbed safely. Complications of this procedure are fairly common and include repeated infections, septicemia, peritonitis, or meningitis.

A second procedure that is becoming increasingly common in treating hydrocephalus is called an endoscopic third ventriculostomy and involves a surgeon creating a small hold in the bottom of the third ventricle of the brain. There, a thin membrane separates the inside from the outside of the brain, and the tiny hold allows excess CSF to drain normally into the spaces outside the brain in order to be absorbed into the bloodstream. It has become the procedure of choice for children older than six months, but it is also showing promise in younger children.

Perspective and Prospects

The outcome of treated patients with hydrocephalus has improved over the years, but the condition is still associated with long-term problems. A modest percentage of newborns with congenital hydrocephalus will survive and achieve normal intelligence.

—*Cynthia Breslin Beres*

See also Birth defects; Brain; Brain damage; Brain disorders; Childbirth complications; Congenital disorders; Critical care, pediatric; Fetal surgery; Meningitis; Mental retardation; Neonatology; Nervous system; Neuroimaging; Neurology, pediatric; Pediatrics; Shunts; Spina bifida; Spinal cord disorders; Surgery, pediatric.

For Further Information:

Cinalli, G., W. J. Maixner, and C. Sainte-Rose, eds. *Pediatric Hydrocephalus*. New York: Springer, 2004.

Hähnel, Stefan. *Inflammatory Diseases of the Brain*. 2d ed. New York: Springer, 2013.

"Hydrocephalus." *MedlinePlus*, May 7, 2013.

Hydrocephalus Association. http://www.hydroassoc.org.

Kliegman, Robert, and Waldo E. Nelson, eds. *Nelson Textbook of Pediatrics*. 19th ed. Philadelphia: Elsevier/Saunders, 2011.

Leikin, Jerrold B., and Martin S. Lipsky, eds. *American Medical Association Complete Medical Encyclopedia*. New York: Random House Reference, 2003.

Mednick, Adam. *Normal Pressure Hydrocephalus: From Diagnosis to Treatment*. Omaha, Nebr.: Addicus Books, 2013.

Merenstein, Gerald B., and Sandra L. Gardner, eds. *Merenstein and Gardner's Handbook of Neonatal Intensive Care*. 7th ed. Maryland Heights, Mo.: Mosby/Elsevier, 2011.

Mohanty, Aaron. *100 Questions & Answers About Hydrocephalus*. Sudbury, Mass.: Jones & Bartlett Learning, 2012.

Toporek, Chuck, and Kellie Robinson. *Hydrocephalus: A Guide for Patients, Families, and Friends*. Sebastopol, Calif.: O'Reilly, 1999.

HYDROTHERAPY

Treatment

Anatomy or system affected: All

Specialties and related fields: Alternative medicine, physical therapy, rheumatology, sports medicine

Definition: Exercise in warm water, which can aid in the treatments of several disorders.

Indications and Procedures

Hydrotherapy, or water treatment, is one of the oldest therapies still in use. A procedure with origins in ancient Greece has today found a place in alternative medicine.

One use of hydrotherapy is as an alternative method of exercising for patients with chronic heart failure, since the buoyancy effect reduces loading. Exercises to improve mobility, strength, and cardiovascular fitness can be provided easily in water. Immersion in warm water has been used in bathing resorts in Europe since the beginning of the twentieth century to reduce heart failure symptoms as well as to enhance heart function.

Systemic diseases such as diabetes mellitus, peripheral heart disease, neuropathy, steroid dependence, and venous stasis are major contributing factors to forming chronic wounds. The consequence is a nonhealing wound with

A patient receives a therapeutic bath. (Digital Stock)

hypoxia, infection, edema, and metabolic abnormalities. Patients with such wounds, in need of extensive debridement, have traditionally been advised to be immersed in a full-body whirlpool. The reason behind whirlpool therapy is that whirling and agitation of the water, with injected air, removes contaminants and toxic debris and dilutes bacterial contents. The common therapeutic protocol is a five- to twenty-minute session, once daily. Typically, this regimen is continued for a brief period. Other debridement techniques have been gaining in popularity in recent years due to concerns about whirlpool therapy including high water pressure, oversaturation of the skin, and cross-contamination.

Physical therapists have always recommended hydrotherapy to relieve extreme pain. Therefore, it is not surprising that it has found a place in providing relief for patients with fibromyalgia.

Another area where hydrotherapy has found popularity is in labor and childbirth. Studies indicate using hydrotherapy for relief of rapid pain and anxiety in labor. Subjective maternal responses to bathing in labor have been favorable. No maternal or infant infections have been attributed to bathing with intact or ruptured membranes. Maternal bathing in labor does not appear to affect Apgar scores at five minutes or stress hormones at birth.

A 2003 case study indicated that hydrotherapy may be beneficial in treating Rett syndrome. An eleven-year-old girl with stage III Rett syndrome was treated with hydrotherapy in a swimming pool twice a week for eight weeks. After the application of hydrotherapy, stereotypical hand movements had decreased and purposeful hand functions and feeding skills had increased. Research into the effectiveness of hydrotherapy in treating this and other neuromuscular conditions is ongoing.

Perspective and Prospects

Ancient Greek literature contains a considerably large volume of published articles concerning different types of baths and hydrotherapy. These topics were addressed for preventive, hygienic, or therapeutic purposes. These Greek baths were classified in two categories: cold water baths and hot water baths. Cold water baths were said to slow blood circulation; decrease the amount of sweat produced; increase muscular strength, the ability to work, and a sense of well-being; and improve physical, mental, and moral balance. The hot water baths were reported to be relaxing, antispasmodic, and beneficial for treating nervous disturbances.

—*Giri Sulur, Ph.D.*

See also Alternative medicine; Cardiac rehabilitation; Childbirth; Colon therapy; Exercise physiology; Fibromyalgia; Healing; Heart failure; Pain management; Physical rehabilitation; Sports medicine; Wounds.

For Further Information:

Buchman, Dian Dincin. *The Complete Book of Water Healing*. 2d ed. Chicago: Contemporary Books, 2002.

Cole, Andrew J., and Bruce E. Becker, eds. *Comprehensive Aquatic Therapy*. 3d ed. Pullman, Wa.: Washington State University Publishing, 2011.

"Hydrotherapy." *American Cancer Society*, March 7, 2011.

Johnson, Filip. "Hydrotherapy." *North American Spine Society*, March 21, 2011.

Kloth, Luther, and Joseph M. McCulloch. "Wound Bed Preparation/Debridement: Hydrotherapy." In *Wound Healing: Evidence-Based Management*. Philadelphia: F.A. Davis, 2010.

Ruoti, Richard G., David M. Morris, and Andrew J. Cole, eds. *Aquatic Rehabilitation*. Philadelphia: Lippincott, 1997.

Ryrie, Charlie. *The Healing Energies of Water*. North Clarendon, Vt.: Charles Tuttle, 1999.

Tharpe, Nell, Robin G. Jordan, and Cindy L. Farley. "Care of the Woman Using Hydrotherapy in Labor." In *Clinical Practice Guidelines for Midwifery and Women's Health*. 4th ed. Burlington, Mass: Jones & Bartlett Learning, 2013.

HYPERADIPOSIS

Disease/Disorder

Also known as: Severe obesity, extreme obesity

Anatomy or system affected: All

Specialties and related fields: Biochemistry, endocrinology, family medicine, genetics, nutrition

Definition: Having excess body fat; exceeding 200 percent of standard body weight as defined on a height-weight table.

Causes and Symptoms

Obesity results from consuming more calories than the body uses. Severe obesity accounts for less than 1 percent of all obesity in the United States but is linked to a large number of deaths each year, many of them due to heart disease or diabetes. Genetics, socioeconomic status, and emotional disturbances may all contribute to severe obesity.

One leading theory proposes that body weight is regulated by a set point in the hypothalamus (a section of the brain), similar to a home's thermostat setting. A higher-than-normal set point would explain why some people are obese and why losing weight and maintaining weight loss are difficult for them. It is also well established that an increase in the size and/or number of fat cells adds to the amount of fat stored by the body. Those who become obese during early childhood may have up to five times as many fat cells as people of normal weight. Because the number of cells cannot be reduced, weight loss can come about only by decreasing the amount of fat stored in each cell.

Accumulation of excess fat below the diaphragm and in the chest wall places pressure on the lungs, leading to shortness of breath and difficulty in breathing, even with minimal exertion. This may also seriously interfere with sleep. Low back pain and osteoarthritis, especially in the hips, knees, and ankles, may be seen, and skin disorders are common, owing to moisture retention in the folds of the fatty skin. Because of a low ratio of surface area to body weight in severe obesity, the body has a hard time getting rid of excess body heat, leading to excessive sweating and fluid accumulation in the

---

Information on Hyperadiposis

Causes: Sedentary lifestyle, genetic predisposition, diet, emotional disorders

Symptoms: Shortness of breath, difficulty breathing, sleep disruption, low back pain, osteoarthritis, skin disorders, excessive sweating, fluid accumulation in the ankles and feet

Duration: Often chronic

---

ankles and feet.

Fat tends to accumulate in the abdomen in males, and in the thighs and buttocks in females. Abdominal obesity in particular is linked with a high incidence of coronary artery disease, high blood pressure, adult onset diabetes, hyperlipidemia, and gallbladder disease. In addition, an increase in menstrual disorders and in breast, uterine, and ovarian cancer is seen in women. Men have higher rates of colorectal and prostate cancer.

Treatment and Therapy

Self-help and nonclinical weight loss programs rarely work in individuals with severe obesity. Clinical programs that combine supervised weight loss, behavior modification, and exercise have shown good results. Drugs such as amphetamines (ephedrine) have questionable value in cases of severe obesity. Total fasting produces a risk of ketonemia and electrolyte imbalances, leading to cardiac arrhythmias.

Surgery has become an increasingly popular form of treatment. Vertical banded gastroplasty (stomach stapling) and gastric bypass are the most common procedures. Both produce satiety with small food intake and, if coupled with exercise, can result in weight losses approximating one-half of the excess weight (80 to 160 pounds). Jejunoileal bypass is also effective but produces a permanent malabsorption syndrome that may lead to other metabolic problems. Liposuction, where a small incision is made and fatty deposits are suctioned out, produces only moderate results in the severely obese. Because of potential risks to blood vessels and nerves, only a small amount of fat can be removed from each location.

Leptin, the protein hormone product of the *ob* gene, has been suggested as a useful new treatment for severe obesity. However, only about 5 percent of obese individuals fail to produce leptin on their own, and in those individuals either daily injections of leptin or gene therapy to correct the chromosomal defect would be required. Neither is currently considered a practical solution.

Perspective and Prospects

Since 1900, the incidence of severe obesity in the United States has more than doubled, despite the fact that the average number of calories consumed per day has decreased by 10 percent. The most likely explanation is a decrease in physical activity among the population at large. While everyone needs to be conscious of dietary intake and exercise needs, parents of young children in particular need to be careful not to use food as either reward or punishment, as the early years of development appear to be most crucial in setting the stage for later obesity.

—*Kerry L. Cheesman, Ph.D.*

See also Bariatric surgery; Eating disorders; Glands; Leptin; Malnutrition; Nutrition; Obesity; Obesity, childhood; Weight loss and gain; Weight loss medications.

For Further Information:

Bjorntorp, Per, ed. *International Textbook of Obesity*. New York: Wiley, 2001.

Brownell, Kelly D., and Katherine Battle Horgen. *Food Fight: The Inside Story of America's Obesity Crisis, and What We Can Do About It*. New York: McGraw-Hill, 2004.

Goldman, Lee, and Dennis Ausiello, eds. *Cecil Textbook of Medicine*. 23d ed. Philadelphia: Saunders/Elsevier, 2007.

Kushner, Robert, Victor Lawrence, and Sudhesh Kumar. *Practical Manual of Clinical Obesity*. Hoboken, N.J.: Wiley-Blackwell, 2013.

Obesity Society. http://www.obesity.org.

Randall, Brian. "Conditions inDepth: Obesity. *HealthLibrary*, March 20, 2013.

Segel, Carol M. Childhood Obesity: Risk Factors, Health Effects, and Prevention. Hauppauge, N.Y., 2011.

Waddon, Thomas A., and Albert J. Stunkard, eds. *Handbook of Obesity Treatment*. Rev. ed. New York: Guilford Press, 2004.

Widhalm, Kurt. *Morbid Obesity in Adolescents: Conservative Treatment and Surgical Approaches*. London: Springer, 2013.

HYPERBARIC OXYGEN THERAPY

Treatment

Anatomy or system affected: Blood, circulatory system, lungs, respiratory system

Specialties and related fields: Anesthesiology, biotechnology, critical care, emergency medicine, pulmonary medicine, serology

Definition: In hyperbaric oxygen therapy, patients are placed in a chamber where pure oxygen is circulated in an environment whose air pressure is two or three times higher than that at sea level.

Key terms:

decompression sickness: also called the bends; a condition in which bubbles of nitrogen are introduced into the bloodstream

hypoxia: low oxygen in the tissues

ischemia: loss of blood flow

osteomyelitis: bone infection

Indications and Procedures

Hyperbaric oxygen therapy is used in cases that compromise the ability of a person's red blood cells to distribute oxygen throughout the body. This situation usually results in hypoxia, a condition in which the tissues are starved of the life-giving oxygen that they require.

Adult humans consume about three pounds of food and three pounds of water every day. Through respiration, however, they routinely consume twice that amount of oxygen daily. At least one-third of this oxygen enters the bloodstream for distribution to tissues. If these tissues are deprived of oxygen, a condition called ischemia, then they may be destroyed, making people with lowered oxygen levels vulnerable to diseases and infections.

When the oxygen content of the tissues becomes dangerously low, as in cases of hypoxia, immediate treatment is essential. If such treatment is not given, then the results can be fatal. The most effective treatment, often provided in emergency situations, is to place the patient in a hyperbaric chamber, a sealed container in which the pressure is gradually increased to two or three times greater than that at sea level. Pure (100 percent) oxygen is pumped into the chamber. Patients are typically confined to such chambers from one hour to an hour and a half.

The air that humans usually breathe contains about 21 percent oxygen and 78 percent nitrogen. The air pressure within the hyperbaric chamber can increase the number of oxygen molecules in the bloodstream by up to 2,000 percent. With this dramatic increase, oxygen begins to enter oxygen-starved tissue and bone cells.

The hyperbaric chamber was initially used to save the lives of deep-sea and scuba divers who ascended too fast from the ocean's depths, causing them to suffer from decompression sickness (the bends), a potentially fatal condition caused by the formation of nitrogen gas bubbles in the bloodstream. Those suffering from the bends are deprived of the life-sustaining oxygen that the body requires to function effectively. It was found that immersing sufferers in a pressurized environment enabled their red blood cells to absorb sufficient oxygen to nourish their tissues and bones.

Most hospitals set aside rooms into which pure (100 percent) oxygen is piped. Patients in need of hyperbaric oxygen therapy are placed in such rooms and may, through tubes in their noses, be fed the oxygen that they need directly. Such treatment is intermediate. When it proves insufficient, placing patients in pressurized atmospheres for specific lengths of time can result in dramatic increases in the amount of oxygen that they can absorb and in subsequent improvement in their conditions.

Uses and Complications

Besides its use in treating people suffering from the bends, the hyperbaric chamber is employed to treat several other life-threatening conditions. Such therapy is routinely used to treat injuries incurred in automobile or motorcycle accidents in which parts of the body are crushed. Treatment in a hyperbaric chamber heightens the delivery of oxygen to damaged tissues and bones. It can control swelling and limit infection.

Some people have wounds that refuse to heal, such as foot ulcers in diabetic patients whose circulatory systems are compromised, resulting in low oxygen levels. Hyperbaric treatment can increase the amount of oxygen in their bloodstreams and promote healing.

Similarly, such bone infections as osteomyelitis that do not respond to conventional treatment are sometimes controlled by hyperbaric oxygen therapy. The oxygen that such treatment delivers to the bloodstream can control bacterial infec-

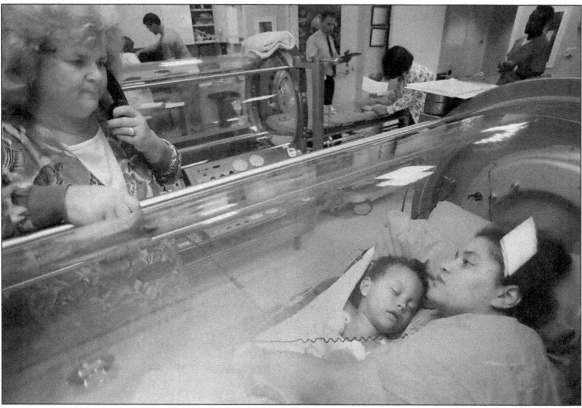

A mother and child receive treatment in a hyperbaric oxygen chamber following exposure to carbon monoxide. (AP/Wide World Photos)

tions and increase the effectiveness of the body's defensive white blood cells.

Cancer patients undergoing radiation may suffer from scarring and compression of important blood vessels, thereby inhibiting the circulation of oxygen throughout the body. Hyperbaric oxygen therapy aids in increasing such circulation, permitting oxygen to reach damaged cells and keep them from dying. This treatment is often used in treating patients with head and neck cancers.

Carbon monoxide poisoning is a pernicious and potentially fatal form of poisoning. Because carbon monoxide is colorless and odorless, it can affect whole families confined in closed houses with defective heating systems. When victims of such poisoning are rescued, immediate hyperbaric oxygen treatment is essential. Such treatment pumps essential oxygen into the bloodstream and aids the body in expelling carbon monoxide. If treatment is given without delay, then damage to the central nervous system and red blood vessels can be circumvented.

This therapy is being used increasingly in the treatment of burn victims, in whom it may reduce swelling, limit infection, and decrease the effects of lung damage resulting from inhaling smoke and overheated air. Because hyperbaric oxygen therapy is often a choice of last resort for people who are dangerously ill, the risks are high and the rate of fatalities is considerable.

Perspective and Prospects

With the remarkable growth of new procedures in medicine, the outlook for hyperbaric oxygen therapy is bright. Once used almost exclusively to treat the bends, such therapy currently is being found effective in dealing with any health problem in which the circulation of oxygen throughout the body is compromised.

—*R. Baird Shuman, Ph.D.*

See also Altitude sickness; Burns and scalds; Cancer; Circulation; Embolism; Healing; Hypoxia; Ischemia; Lungs; Osteomyelitis; Oxygen therapy; Poisoning; Pulmonary medicine; Radiation therapy; Respiration; Ulcers; Vascular medicine; Vascular system; Wounds.

For Further Information:

A.D.A.M. Medical Encyclopedia. "Hyperbaric Oxygen Therapy." *MedlinePlus*, August 30, 2012.

Jain, K. K. *Textbook of Hyperbaric Medicine*. 5th ed. Cambridge, Mass.: Hogrefe, 2009.

Mayo Clinic. "Hyperbaric Oxygen Therapy." *Mayo Foundation for Medical Education and Research*, October 27, 2011.

Oregon Health and Science University Evidence-Based Practice Center. *Hyperbaric Oxygen Therapy for Brain Injury, Cerebral Palsy, and Stroke*. Rockville, Md.: Department of Health and Human Services, Public Health Service, Agency for Healthcare Research and Quality, 2003.

Sheldon, Lisa Kennedy. *Oxygenation*. 2d ed. Sudbury, Mass.: Jones and Bartlett, 2008.

Stuart, Annie. "Hyperbaric Oxygen Therapy." *Health Library*, 11/26/12.

HYPERCHOLESTEROLEMIA
Disease/Disorder

Anatomy or system affected: Blood, blood vessels, circulatory system, heart, liver

Specialties and related fields: Cardiology, hematology, nutrition, pharmacology, vascular medicine

Definition: A high level of cholesterol in the bloodstream, which is considered a major risk factor for heart attack or stroke.

Causes and Symptoms

In the recent past, it has been difficult for medical professionals to establish a clear, causal connection between high cholesterol in the blood and heart disease. After numerous studies involving large numbers of patients over extended periods of time was it possible to establish the now widely accepted statistical correlation between high cholesterol and cardiovascular problems. Cholesterol is a fatty material similar to animal fats, which are called lipids. In the bloodstream, cholesterol lipids combine with proteins to form either a low-density lipoprotein (LDL) or high-density lipoprotein (HDL). LDL transports cholesterol from the liver and intestines to other parts of the body where it is needed. HDL transports excess cholesterol back to the liver where it is metabolized and excreted. HDL prevents excess fat from being deposited on the walls of arteries and therefore is commonly called the "good" cholesterol. Research has established that LDL in blood should be less than 200 milligrams per deciliter, whereas HDL should be greater than 50 milligrams per deciliter, with a ratio of LDL to HDL of preferably four or less. A person is not aware of having high cholesterol. If the condition is not treated, however, then the likelihood of plaque buildup on artery walls and a possible blockage, which could then cause a stroke or heart attack, is increased.

Treatment and Therapy

The first step to reduce excess cholesterol in the bloodstream is a change in diet. As a general guideline, the consumption of vegetables, fruits, and grains should be increased, while red meat, egg yolks, and high-fat dairy products should be decreased. Vegetable oils made from corn, olives, or soybeans, which are low in saturated fats, are preferable to butter and animal fats. The next step is to increase physical exercise, which generally raises HDL, the good cholesterol. Several prescription medications, such as the statins Zocor or Lipitor and nicotinic acid medication such as nicolar and niaspan have been shown to be effective in lowering LDL. A physician needs to monitor a patient's liver function to verify that no harmful side effects are occurring.

Perspective and Prospects

The 1985 Nobel Prize in Physiology or Medicine was awarded to Michael S. Brown and Joseph L. Goldstein for their study of cell-surface receptors that control the entry of LDL into cells. They showed that some people have a deficiency of these receptors. As a result, LDL does not enter cells at the normal rate but continues to circulate in the bloodstream, where it then can adhere to artery walls. In the future, it may be possible to produce drugs that stimulate the body to make more LDL receptors, which would remove excess LDL from the bloodstream.

—*Hans G. Graetzer, Ph.D.*

See also Arteriosclerosis; Blood and blood disorders; Cholesterol; Dietary reference intakes (DRIs); Heart disease; Hyperlipidemia; Lipids; Plaque, arterial; Steroids.

For Further Information:

American Medical Association. *American Medical Association Family Medical Guide.* 4th rev. ed. Hoboken, N.J.: John Wiley & Sons, 2004.

Antman, Elliott M., and Marc S. Sabatine, eds. *Cardiovascular Therapeutics: A Companion to Braunwald's Heart Disease.* Philadelphia: Elsevier/Saunders, 2013.

Cooper, Kenneth H. *Controlling Cholesterol the Natural Way.* New York: Bantam Books, 1999.

Estren, Mark James. *Statins: Miracle or Mistake?* Berkeley, Calif.: Ronin Publishing, 2013.

Kowalski, Robert E. *The New Eight-Week Cholesterol Cure.* New York: Harper & Row, 2006.

Randall, Brian. "High Cholesterol." *Health Library*, March 22, 2013.

Information on Hypercholesterolemia

Causes: Diet, high levels of low-density lipoproteins (LDLs) and low levels of high-density lipoproteins (HDLs)

Symptoms: Plaque buildup on artery walls and possible blockage, causing stroke or heart attack

Duration: Chronic

Treatments: Dietary changes (increase in vegetables, fruits, and grains and decrease in red meat, egg yolks, and high-fat dairy products); increased physical exercise; medications (Zocor, Lipitor)

HYPERHIDROSIS
Disease/Disorder

Also known as: Excessive sweating, excessive perspiration

Anatomy or system affected: Glands, skin

Specialties and related fields: Dermatology, internal medicine, neurology

Definition: Excessive sweating, which may be generalized or limited to certain areas of the body, particularly the hands and feet. The paroxysmal form of this disorder affects approximately 1 percent of the population of the United States.

Causes and Symptoms

The purpose of perspiration is to keep the body at an ideal temperature. The sweat glands are affected by the sympathetic branch of the autonomic nervous system. Two types of sympathetic nerve fibers affect sweat glands: the noradrenergic, which respond to emotional stimuli, and the cholinergic, which respond to temperature. Hyperhidrosis refers to sweating that is greater than is needed to keep the body at a normal temperature.

Hyperhidrosis may be due to a secondary cause, such as hyperthyroidism, hormonal treatments, obesity, menopause, or severe psychiatric disorders. The immediate cause of primary hyperhidrosis (not attributable to another disorder or condition) is dysfunction of the sympathetic branch of the autonomic nervous system; however, the underlying cause of the dysfunction is not clear.

Hyperhidrosis may affect the entire body (general), or it may affect only specific areas, such as the armpits (axillary), palms of the hands (palmar), soles of the feet (plantar), or face (facial). General hyperhidrosis may be a variation on normal sweating. Paroxysmal localized hyperhidrosis, periodic excessive perspiration in a particular area of the body, may also occur. A genetic predisposition may be present. Persons who are obese are more likely to be affected, as are people with certain forms of eczema. Hyperhidrosis can also occur following frostbite.

Hyperhidrosis can vary in severity from being merely embarrassing to quite disabling. It tends to begin in adolescence and gradually increase with age.

Treatment and Therapy

Topical prescription antiperspirants applied to the affected areas may control the symptoms. Drugs that block the sympathetic portion of the autonomic nervous system may also be used. Some people with localized sweating respond to iontophoresis, a technique in which the affected area is placed in an electrolyte solution and stimulated with low-level electrical current. Some success has been shown with injections of botulinum toxin (Botox) into the affected areas. This technique has considerable disadvantages, however. Repeated injections are needed, and they are both painful and costly. Furthermore, the injections may cause temporary weakness of the hand muscles. Surgery to the affected areas of the nervous system has a 90 percent success rate for excessive sweating of the palms but is accompanied by numerous complications, including wound infection, sweating with eating (gustatory sweating), and recurrent hyperhidrosis. Little evidence exists for the effectiveness of psychotherapy, hypnosis, acupuncture, and herbal or homeopathic remedies.
—*Rebecca Lovell Scott, Ph.D., PA-C*

See also Botox; Dermatology; Glands; Hormones; Host-defense mechanisms; Nervous system; Neurology; Obesity; Skin; Sweating; Thyroid disorders.

For Further Information:
American Medical Association. *American Medical Association Family Medical Guide*. 4th rev. ed. Hoboken, N.J.: John Wiley & Sons, 2004.

Carruthers, Jean, and Alastair Carruthers, eds. *Botulinum Toxin: Procedures in Cosmetic Dermatology*. 3d ed. London: Saunders/ Elsevier, 2013.

Carson-DeWitt, Rosalyn. "Hyperhidrosis." *Health Library*, September 30, 2012.

Haider, Aamir. "Hyperhidrosis: An Approach to Diagnosis and Management." *Dermatology Nursing* 16, 6 (December 1, 2004): 515–518.

"Hyperhidrosis (Excessive Sweating)." *Mayo Clinic*, September 21, 2012.

Komaroff, Anthony, ed. *Harvard Medical School Family Health Guide*. New York: Free Press, 2005.

Kreyden, O. P., R. Böni, and G. Burg, eds. *Hyperhidrosis and Botulinum Toxin in Dermatology*. New York: S. Karger, 2002.

Stoppard, Miriam. *Family Health Guide*. London: DK, 2006.

HYPERLIPIDEMIA
Disease/Disorder
Anatomy or system affected: Blood
Specialties and related fields: Family medicine, hematology, internal medicine, serology, vascular medicine
Definition: The presence of abnormally large quantities of lipids (fats) in the blood.

Causes and Symptoms

Although elevated triglyceride levels have been implicated in clinical ischemic diseases, most investigators believe that cholesterol-rich lipids are a more significant risk factor. Although measurements of both cholesterol and triglyceride levels have been used to predict coronary disease, studies suggest that the determination of the alpha-lipoprotein/beta-lipoprotein ratio is a more reliable predictor. Because the alpha-lipoprotein has a higher density than the beta-lipoprotein, they are more often designated as high-density lipoprotein (HDL) and low-density lipoprotein (LDL), respectively. HDL is often referred to as "good cholesterol," and LDL is referred to as "bad cholesterol." The latter is implicated in the development of atherosclerosis.

Atherosclerosis is a disease that begins in the innermost lining of the arterial wall. Its lesions occur predominantly at arterial forks and branch openings, but they can also occur at sites where there is injury to the arterial lining. The initial lesion usually appears as fatty streaks or spots, which have been detected even at birth. With passing years, more of these lesions appear, and they may develop into elevated plaques that obstruct the flow of blood in the artery. The lesions are rich in cholesterol derived from beta-lipoproteins in the plasma. In addition to elevated blood lipids, other risk factors associated with atherosclerosis include hypertension, faulty arterial structure, obesity, smoking, and stress.

Treatment and Therapy

The treatment of hyperlipidemia involves both dietary and drug therapies. Although studies in nonhuman primates indicate that the reduction of hyperlipidemia results in decreased morbidity and mortality rates from arterial vascular disease, studies in humans are less conclusive. Initial treatment involves restricting the dietary intake of cholesterol and saturated fat. Drug therapy is instituted when further lowering of the serum lipids is desired. Among the drugs that have been used as antihyperlipidemic agents are lovastatin and its analogues, clofibrate and its analogues (particularly gemfibrozil), nicotinic acid, D-thyroxine, cholestyramine, probucol, and heparin. A simplified diagram of the endogenous biosynthesis and biotransformation of cholesterol is given below.

acetate → C acetyl SCoA → HMGCoA → MVA → squalene → desmosterol → cholesterol → bile acids

Lovastatin blocks the synthesis of cholesterol by inhibiting the enzyme (HMGCoA reductase) that catalyzes the conversion of beta-hydroxy-beta-methyl glutaryl coenzyme A (HMGCoA) to mevalonic acid (MVA), the regulatory step in the biosynthesis of cholesterol. Both lovastatin and MVA are beta, delta-dihydroxy acids, but lovastatin has a much more lipophilic (fat-soluble) group attached to it. Clofibrate and gemfibrozil block the synthesis of cholesterol prior to the HMGCoA stage. For this reason, they are likely to inhibit triglyceride formation as well. Nicotinic acid inhibits the synthesis of acetyl coenzyme A (acetyl SCoA) and thus would be expected to block the synthesis of both cholesterol and the triglycerides. To be effective in lowering the serum level of lipids, nicotinic acid must be taken in large amounts, which often produces an unpleasant flushing sensation in the patient. A way to inhibit the synthesis of cholesterol at the post-MVA stages has also been sought. Agents such as triparanol, which inhibit biosynthesis near the end of the synthetic sequence, have been developed. Although they are effective in lowering serum cholesterol, they had to be withdrawn from clinical use because of their adverse side effects on the muscles and eyes. Moreover, the penultimate product in the biosynthesis of cholesterol proved to be atherogenic.

D-thyroxine promotes the metabolism of cholesterol in the liver, transforming it into the more hydrophilic (water-soluble) bile acids, thereby facilitating its elimination from the body. An approach to reducing the serum level of cholesterol by a process involving the sequestering of the bile acids utilizes the resin cholestyramine as the sequestrant. The sequestered bile acids cannot be reabsorbed into the enterohepatic system and are eliminated in the feces. Consequently, more cholesterol is oxidized to the bile acids, resulting in the reduction of the serum level of cholesterol. Unfortunately, a large quantity of cholestyramine is required. Sequestration of cholesterol with beta-sitosterol prevents both the absorption of dietary cholesterol and the reabsorption of endogenous cholesterol in the intestines. Here, too, a large quantity of the sequestrant needs to be administered.

Probucol is an antioxidant. Because, structurally, it is a sulfur analogue of a hindered hydroquinone, it acts as a free radical scavenger. Evidence suggests that the antihyperlipidemic effect of probucol is attributable to its ability to inhibit the oxygenation of LDL. The oxygenated LDL is believed to be the atherogenic form of LDL. Heparin promotes the hydrolysis of triglycerides as it activates lipoprotein lipase, thereby reducing lipidemia. Because of its potent anticoagulant properties, however, its use in therapy must be closely monitored. Cholesterol that is present in atherosclerotic plaques is acylated, generally by the more saturated fatty acids. The enzyme catalyzing the acylation process is acyl-CoA cholesterol acyl transferase (ACAT). The development of regulators of ACAT and the desirability of reducing the dietary intake of saturated fatty acids are based on this rationale.

Cholesterol within the cell is able to inhibit further synthesis of cholesterol by a feedback mechanism. Cholesterol that is associated with LDL is transported into the hepatic cell by means of the LDL receptor on the surface of the cell. In individuals who are afflicted with familial hypercholesterolemia, an inherited disorder that causes death at an early age, the gene that is responsible for the production of the LDL receptor is either absent or defective. Studies in gene therapy have shown that transplant of the normal LDL receptor gene to such an individual results in a dramatic decrease in the level of the "bad cholesterol" in the serum. Cholesterol derivatives that are oxygenated at various positions have also been found to regulate the serum level of cholesterol by either inhibiting its synthesis or promoting its catabolism.

—Leland J. Chinn, Ph.D.

See also Arteriosclerosis; Blood and blood disorders; Cholesterol; Heart disease; Hypercholesterolemia; Hypertension; Insulin resistance syndrome; Lipids; Metabolic syndrome; Metabolism; Obesity; Plaque, arterial.

For Further Information:

Alan, Rick. "Hyperlipidemia." *Health Library*, September 1, 2011.

Anderson, J. W. "Diet First, Then Medication for Hypercholesterolemia." *Journal of the American Medical Association* 290, 4. (July 23, 2003): 531–533.

Ball, Madeleine, and Jim Mann. *Lipids and Heart Disease: A Guide for the Primary Care Team*. 2d ed. New York: Oxford University Press, 1994.

Farnier, Michel, and Jean Davignon. "Current and Future Treatment of Hyperlipidemia: The Role of Statins." *American Journal of Cardiology* 82, 4B. (August 27, 1998): 3J–10J.

Haffner, Steven M. "Diabetes, Hyperlipidemia, and Coronary Artery Disease." *American Journal of Cardiology* 83, 9B. (May 13, 1999): 17F–21F.

Hirsch, Anita. *Good Cholesterol, Bad Cholesterol: An Indispensable Guide to the Facts About Cholesterol*. New York: Avalon, 2002.

McGowan, Mary P., and Jo McGowan Chopra. *Fifty Ways to Lower Cholesterol*. New York: McGraw-Hill, 2002.

Rifkind, Basil M., ed. *Drug Treatment of Hyperlipidemia*. New York: Marcel Dekker, 1991.

Safeer, Richard S., and Cynthia L. Lacivita. "Choosing Drug

Therapy for Patients with Hyperlipidemia." *American Family Physician* 61, 11. (June 1, 2000): 3371–3382.

Sorrentino, Matthew J., ed. *Hyperlipidemia in Primary Care: A Practical Guide to Risk Reduction.* New York: Springer, 2011.

Sniderman, Allan, and Paul Durrington. *Fast Facts: Hyperlipidemia.* 5th ed. Oxford: Health Press Limited, 2010.

Witiak, D. T., H. A. I. Newman, and D. R. Feller, eds. *Antilipidemic Drugs: Medicinal, Chemical, and Biochemical Aspects.* New York: Elsevier, 1991.

HYPERPARATHYROIDISM AND HYPOPARATHYROIDISM

Disease/Disorder

Anatomy or system affected: Endocrine system, glands, musculoskeletal system, neck

Specialties and related fields: Endocrinology

Definition: Excessive, uncontrolled secretion (hyperparathyroidism) or reduced secretion (hypoparathyroidism) of parathyroid hormone.

Causes and Symptoms

The precise regulation of calcium is vital to the survival and well-being of all animals. Approximately 99 percent of the calcium in the body is found in bones and teeth. Of the remaining 1 percent, about 0.9 percent is packaged within specialized organelles inside the cell. This leaves only 0.1 percent of the total body calcium in blood. Approximately half of this calcium is either bound to proteins or complexed with phosphate. The other half of blood calcium is free to be utilized by cells. For this reason, it is critical that calcium inside the cell be rigorously maintained at extremely low concentrations. Even a slight change in calcium outside the cell can have dramatic consequences.

The function and regulation of calcium. Calcium plays a vital role in many different areas of the body. For example, the entry of calcium into secretory cells, such as nerve cells, triggers the release of neurotransmitters into the synapse. A fall in blood calcium results in the overexcitability of nerves, which can be felt as a tingling sensation and numbness in the extremities. Similarly, calcium entry into cells is essential for muscle contraction in both heart and skeletal muscle.

Free calcium is thus one of the most tightly regulated substances in the body. The key player in the moment-to-moment regulation of calcium is parathyroid hormone (PTH). PTH is synthesized in the parathyroid glands, a paired gland located in the neck, and released in response to a fall in blood calcium. PTH serves several functions: to increase blood calcium, to decrease blood phosphate, and to stimulate the conversion of vitamin D into its active form, which can then stimulate the uptake of calcium across the digestive tract. Together these actions result in an increase in free calcium, which returns calcium concentrations in the blood to normal.

PTH binds to specific receptors located primarily in bone and kidney tissue. Since most calcium is stored in bone, it serves as a bank for withdrawal of calcium in times of need. Activation of a PTH receptor on osteoclasts, or bone-cutting cells, results in the production of concentrated acids that dissolve calcium from bone, thereby making more free calcium available to the blood supply. PTH also acts on the kidney, where it stimulates calcium uptake from the urine while promoting phosphate elimination. As a result, more calcium is made available to the blood and less phosphate is available to form complexes with the free calcium.

By exerting these effects on its target organs, PTH can restore low calcium concentrations in the blood to normal. Once calcium has returned to a particular set point, PTH secretion is slowed dramatically. If PTH release is not controlled, however, the imbalance in calcium can lead to life-threatening situations. These conditions are termed hyperparathyroidism and hypoparathyroidism.

Hyperparathyroidism. This disorder is defined as the excessive and uncontrolled secretion of PTH. The release of a closely related substance, PTH-related protein, from cancer cells can also cause this condition. Hyperparathyroidism is found in 0.1 percent of the population and is more common in the elderly, who have an incidence rate of approximately 2 percent.

There are two types of hyperparathyroidism: primary and secondary. Primary hyperparathyroidism is caused by disease or damage to the parathyroid glands. For example, cancer of the parathyroid gland can result in the uncontrolled release of PTH and is characterized by an increase in blood calcium. The symptoms associated with primary hyperparathyroidism include osteoporosis, muscle weakness, nausea, and increased incidence of kidney stones and peptic ulcers. These symptoms can all be linked to the presence of excess calcium, which is a result of the oversecretion of PTH.

Secondary hyperparathyroidism often results when PTH cannot function normally, such as in kidney failure or insensitivity of target tissues to PTH. Secondary hyperparathyroidism is usually characterized by an overall decrease in blood calcium levels, even though there is a marked increase in the amount of PTH being released. Its symptoms may include muscle cramps, seizures, paranoia, depression, and, in severe cases, tetany (the tonic spasm of muscles). These symptoms are a direct result of the decline in available calcium.

Hypoparathyroidism. Less common than hyperparathyroidism, hypoparathyroidism is defined by a reduction in

> ## Information on Hyperparathyroidism and Hypoparathyroidism
>
> **Causes:** Endocrine disorder, aging, disease, accidental removal of parathyroid gland or damage to its blood supply
>
> **Symptoms:** Osteoporosis, muscle weakness, nausea, kidney stones, peptic ulcers, muscle cramps, seizures, paranoia, depression
>
> **Duration:** Often chronic
>
> **Treatments:** Drug therapy, hormonal therapy (e.g., estrogen), surgery, vitamin D supplements, calcium restriction or supplements

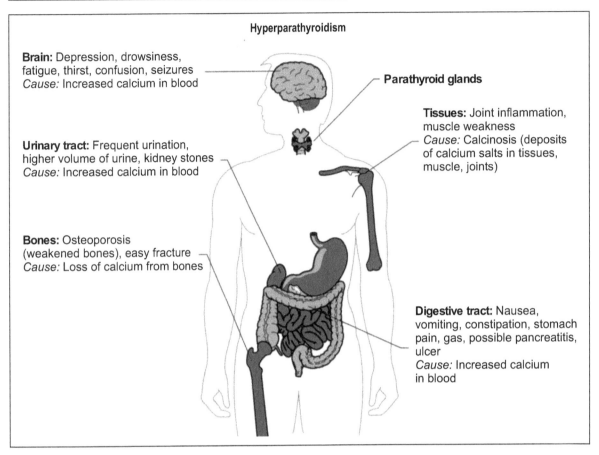

Hyperparathyroidism

Brain: Depression, drowsiness, fatigue, thirst, confusion, seizures
Cause: Increased calcium in blood

Parathyroid glands

Tissues: Joint inflammation, muscle weakness
Cause: Calcinosis (deposits of calcium salts in tissues, muscle, joints)

Urinary tract: Frequent urination, higher volume of urine, kidney stones
Cause: Increased calcium in blood

Bones: Osteoporosis (weakened bones), easy fracture
Cause: Loss of calcium from bones

Digestive tract: Nausea, vomiting, constipation, stomach pain, gas, possible pancreatitis, ulcer
Cause: Increased calcium in blood

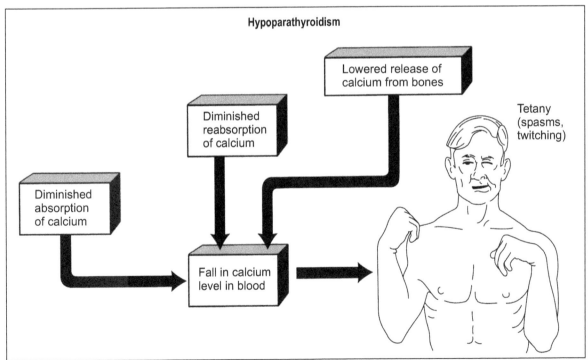

Hypoparathyroidism

Lowered release of calcium from bones

Diminished reabsorption of calcium

Diminished absorption of calcium

Fall in calcium level in blood

Tetany (spasms, twitching)

the secretion of PTH. This condition is normally character-ized by low calcium levels and elevated phosphate levels in response to the lack of PTH. Not only are calcium levels un-usually low, but phosphate levels are unusually high as well, which complicates this condition because phosphate ties up some of the free calcium.

Hypoparathyroidism can also have primary and secondary causes. Primary hypoparathyroidism is known to have two separate origins. The most common is a decrease in PTH re-lease caused by accidental removal of the parathyroid gland. The other is damage of the blood supply around the parathyroid glands. Both occur after there has been some type of surgery or other medical procedure in the neck area. Con-sequently, the decline in PTH results in low calcium and ele-vated phosphate concentrations.

Secondary hypoparathyroidism is a frequent complication of cirrhosis and is characterized by a decrease in both calcium and magnesium concentration. Because magnesium is essen-tial for the release of PTH, this condition can be corrected with magnesium replacement.

Complications associated with all types of hypoparathyroidism include hyperventilation, convulsions, and in some cases tetany of the muscle cells.

Treatment and Therapy

The treatments for primary hyperparathyroidism vary and are dependent on the severity of the condition. Specific drugs can be prescribed that lower elevated blood calcium. Hormone therapy, which includes the administration of estrogen, also acts to restore calcium to normal. Other treatments include di-etary calcium restriction and/or surgery to remove the abnormal parathyroid tissue.

Treatment of secondary hyperparathyroidism often in-volves correcting the problems associated with kidney fail-ure. This can be done by administration of a dietary calcium supplement to restore plasma calcium levels or, in more se-vere cases, by kidney transplantation. Vitamin D therapy has also been attempted for those patients diagnosed in the early stages of renal failure.

Hypoparathyroidism is usually treated with dietary cal-cium and vitamin D supplementation. Both of these treat-ments promote calcium absorption and decrease calcium loss. The duration of the treatment depends on the severity of the condition and may last a lifetime.

—*Jeffrey A. McGowan and Hillar Klandorf, Ph.D.*

See also Endocrine disorders; Endocrine glands; Endocrinology; En-docrinology, pediatric; Glands; Hashimoto's thyroiditis; Hormones; Osteoporosis; Stones; Vitamins and minerals.

For Further Information:

Al Zarani, Ali, and Michael A. Levine. "Primary Hyperparathyroidism." *The Lancet* 349, no. 9060 (April 26, 1997): 1233–38.

Bar, Robert S., ed. *Early Diagnosis and Treatment of Endocrine Dis-orders.* Totowa, N.J.: Humana Press, 2003.

Gardner, David G., and Dolores Shoback, eds. *Greenspan's Basic and Clinical Endocrinology.* 9th ed. New York: McGraw-Hill, 2011.

Kronenberg, Henry M., et al., eds. *Williams Textbook of*

Endocrinology. 12th ed. Philadelphia: Saunders/Elsevier, 2011.

Licata, Angelo A., and Edgar V. Lerma. *Diseases of the Parathyroid Glands.* New York: Springer, 2012.

Neal, J. Matthew. *Basic Endocrinology: An Interactive Approach.* Malden, Mass.: Blackwell Science, 2000.

Ruggieri, Paul, and Scott Isaacs. *A Simple Guide to Thyroid Disor-ders: From Diagnosis to Treatment.* Rev. ed. Omaha, Nebr.: Addicus Books, 2010.

HYPERPLASIA

Disease/Disorder
Also known as: Hypergenesis
Anatomy or system affected: Cells, genitals, urinary system, uterus
Specialties and related fields: Cytology, endocrinology, gyne-cology, urology
Definition: A proliferation of cells in response to either normal or abnormal physiological processes.

Causes and Symptoms

Hyperplasia means that extra cells are present in an organ or tissue. The cells themselves are usually normal, if sometimes enlarged, although in some cases atypical cells (called atypia) may develop. As cells proliferate, they cause the organ or tis-sue to enlarge while affecting normal spacing and ordering. In some cases, the enlargement is a normal stage in a physiologi-cal process, such as the enlargement of breasts for breast-feed-ing. In others, it may be unsightly but harmless, as in sebaceous hyperplasia: small, soft, yellow growths on the face.

Endometrial hyperplasia is enlargement of the endometrium, the lining of the uterus, probably from elevated levels of estrogens. Most instances are benign and cause no symptoms. Hyperplasia with atypia is cause for concern, be-cause in about a quarter of cases it develops into cancer.

Benign prostatic hyperplasia (BPH) is enlargement of the prostate gland by a proliferation of cells in connective tissue and adjacent epithelial tissue. It is common in men over forty years of age and may cause difficult, frequent, or painful urination.

Congenital adrenal hyperplasia is a genetic malformation of the adrenal glands that prevents them from producing the hormones cortisol and aldosterone. Without them, the body produces too much of the male sex hormone androgen. In fe-males, this may lead to abnormal or absent menstruation, genitals that look both male and female, or excessive hair growth. In males, malformed genitals may develop, and there may be early development of male characteristics. In severe cases, newborn infants may experience heart arrhythmias, dehydration, electrolyte imbalances, and vomiting.

Treatment and Therapy

For the majority of hyperplasia cases, when there are no or mild symptoms, physicians do not recommend treatment. In-stead, the condition is monitored regularly—the "wait and watch" approach. However, for severe cases, surgery is often used. For endometrial hyperplasia, removal of the uterus (hysterectomy) is preferred. For the prostate, several

---

Information on Hyperplasia

Causes: Aging, chronic inflammation, abnormal hormone production

Symptoms: Enlarged tissue or organ with impaired function, tumor

Duration: Variable

Treatments: Hormone therapy, surgery, ultrasound, microwave or radio-frequency thermotherapy

---

methods exist to remove the enlarged portion: open surgery, surgery with a resectoscope through the urethra, and laser procedures to destroy excess tissue. Various methods of thermotherapy—heating tissue to destroy or shrink it—use water, microwaves, ultrasound, or radio-frequency energy.

Medications can also reduce the symptoms of hyperplasia. Progestrones are used for endometrial hyperplasia. Several drugs to inhibit production of hormones likewise treat benign prostatic hyperplasia, and other medications may be given to relax the muscles of the prostate and bladder to make urination easier. Medications containing a form of cortisol control androgen levels in the treatment of congenital adrenal hyperplasia.

—*Roger Smith, Ph.D.*

See also Breast-feeding; Congential adrenal hyperlasia; Hypertrophy; Prostrate enlargement.

For Further Information:

Alan, Rick. "Benign Prostatic Hyperplasia." *Health Library*, September 27, 2012.

"Congenital Adrenal Hyperplasia." *Mayo Clinic*, March 4, 2011.

Endometrial Hyperplasia—A Medical Dictionary, Bibliography, and Annotated Research Guide to Internet Resources. San Diego, Calif.: Icon Health, 2004.

Hsu, C. Y., and Scott A Rivkees. *Congenital Adrenal Hyperplasia: A Parents" Guide*. Bloomington, Ind.: AuthorHouse, 2005.

Roehrborn, Claus G. *Contemporary Diagnosis and Management of Benign Prostatic Hyperplasia*. Newton, Pa.: Handbooks in Health Care, 2007.

Stresing, Diane. "Congenital Adrenal Hyperplasia." *Health Library*, November 26, 2012.

HYPERTENSION

Disease/Disorder

Anatomy or system affected: Blood vessels, brain, circulatory system, heart, kidneys, urinary system

Specialties and related fields: Cardiology, family medicine, internal medicine

Definition: An abnormally high blood pressure, an often silent cardiovascular condition that may lead to heart attack, stroke, and major organ failures.

Key terms:

cardiovascular: of, relating to, or involving the heart and blood vessels

cerebrovascular: of, or involving, the brain and the blood vessels supplying it

diastolic blood pressure: the pressure of the blood within the artery while the heart is at rest

hypertension: abnormally high blood pressure, especially high arterial blood pressure; also the systemic condition accompanying high blood pressure

peripheral vascular: of, relating to, involving, or forming the vasculature in the periphery (the external boundary or surface of a body); usually referring to circulation not involving cardiovascular, cerebrovascular, or major organ systems

side effect: a secondary and usually adverse effect (as of a drug); also known as an adverse effect or reaction

sphygmomanometer: a device that uses a column of mercury to measure blood pressure force; pressure is measured in millimeters of mercury

systolic blood pressure: the pressure of the blood within the artery while the heart is contracting

Causes and Symptoms

Hypertension is a higher-than-normal blood pressure (either systolic or diastolic). Blood pressure is usually measured using a sphygmomanometer and a stethoscope. The stethoscope is used to hear when the air pressure within the cuff of the sphygmomanometer is equal to that in the artery. When taking a blood pressure, the cuff is pumped to inflate an air bladder secured around the arm; the pressure produced will collapse the blood vessels within. As cuff pressure decreases, a slight thump is heard as the artery snaps open to allow blood to flow. At this point, the cuff pressure equals the systolic blood pressure. As the cuff pressure continues to fall, the sound of blood being pumped will continue but become progressively softer. At the point where the last sound is heard, the cuff pressure equals the diastolic blood pressure.

Blood Pressure

Blood pressure is measured in two numbers: systolic pressure (the pressure of the blood as it flows out when the heart contracts) over diastolic pressure (the pressure of the blood within the artery as it flows in when the heart is at rest). Readings greater than 140 systolic over 90 diastolic indicate the presence of hypertension.

In hypertension, both systolic and diastolic blood pressures are usually elevated. Blood pressures are reported as the systolic pressure over the diastolic pressure, such as 130/80 millimeters of mercury. It is important to recognize there are degrees of seriousness for hypertension. The higher the blood pressure, the more rigorous the treatment may be. When systolic pressures are in the high normal range, the individual

---

Information on Hypertension

Causes: Stress, genetic factors, obesity, diabetes mellitus, physiological factors

Symptoms: Often asymptomatic

Duration: Often long-term

Treatments: Drug therapy (diuretics, beta-blockers, calcium-channel blockers, ACE inhibitors); lifestyle changes (weight reduction, alcohol restriction, regular exercise)

---

should be closely monitored with annual blood pressure checks. Persistently high blood pressures (greater than 140–159/90–99 millimeters of mercury) require closer monitoring and may result in a decision to treat the condition with medication or other types of intervention.

The blood pressure in an artery is determined by the relationship among three important controlling factors: the blood volume, the amount of blood pumped by the heart (cardiac output), and the contraction of smooth muscle within blood vessels (arterial tone). To illustrate the first point, if blood volume decreases, the result will be a fall in blood pressure. Conversely, the body cannot itself increase blood pressure by rapidly adding blood volume; fluid must be injected into the circulation to do so.

A second controlling factor of blood pressure is cardiac output (the volume of blood pumped by the heart in a given unit of time, usually reported as liters per minute). This output is determined by two factors: stroke volume (the volume of blood pumped with each heartbeat) and the heart rate (beats per minute). As heart rate increases, output generally increases, and blood pressure may rise as well. If blood volume is low, such as with excessive bleeding, the blood returning to the heart per beat is lower and could lead to decreased output. To compensate, the heart rate increases to prevent a drop in blood pressure. Therefore, as cardiac output changes, blood pressure does not necessarily change.

Last, a major controlling factor of blood pressure is arterial tone. Arteries are largely tubular, smooth muscles that can change their diameter based on the extent of contraction (tone). This contraction is largely under the control of a specialized branch of the nervous system called the sympathetic nervous system. An artery with high arterial tone (contracted) will squeeze the blood within and increase the pressure inside. There is also a relaxation phase that will allow expansion and a decrease in blood pressure. Along with relaxation, arteries are elastic to allow some stretching, which may further help reduce pressure or, more important, help prevent blood pressure from rising.

There are two general types of hypertension: essential and secondary. Secondary hypertension is attributable to some underlying identifiable cause, such as a tumor or kidney disease, while essential hypertension has no identifiable cause. Therefore, essential hypertension is a defect that results in excessive arterial pressure secondary to poor regulation by any one of the three controlling factors discussed above. Each factor can serve as a focal point for treatment with medications.

The negative consequences of hypertension are mainly manifested in the deteriorating effect that this condition has on coronary heart disease (CHD). Cardiovascular risk factors for CHD are described as two types, unmodifiable and modifiable. Unmodifiable risk factors cannot be changed. This group includes gender, race, advanced age, and a family history of heart disease (hypertensive traits can be inherited). The modifiable risk factors are cigarette smoking (or other forms of tobacco abuse), high blood cholesterol levels, control over diabetes, and perhaps other factors not yet discov-

ered. For example, additional factors are now recognized for their adverse effects on hypertension, including obesity, a lack of physical activity, and psychological factors.

There is no definitive blood pressure level at which a person is no longer at risk for CHD. While any elevation above the normal range places the person at increased risk for CHD, what are considered high normal blood pressures were previously defined as normal. (Looking back at older data, researchers noted that persons able to maintain pressures at or below 139/89 millimeters of mercury had less severe CHD.) The definition of normal blood pressure may change again in the future as new information is discovered. There is a practical limit as to how low pressure can be while maintaining day-to-day function.

In coronary heart disease, the blood supply to the heart is reduced, and the heart cannot function well. The common term for arteriosclerosis, "hardening of the arteries," indicates the symptom of reduced blood flow, which is a major component of CHD. When the heart cannot supply itself with the necessary amount of blood (a condition known as ischemia), a characteristic chest pain called angina may be produced. The hardening aspect of this disease is the result of cholesterol deposits in the vessel, which decrease elasticity and make the vessel wall stiff. This stiffness will force pressures in the vessel to increase if cardiac output rises. As pressures advance, the vessel may develop weak spots. These areas may rupture or lead to the development of small blood clots that may clog the vessel; either problem will disrupt blood flow, making the underlying CHD worse. Eventually, if the blood supply is significantly reduced, a myocardial infarction (heart attack) may occur. Where the blood supply to the heart muscle itself is functionally blocked, that part of the heart will die.

Besides contributing to an increased risk of heart attack and coronary heart disease, hypertension is a major risk for

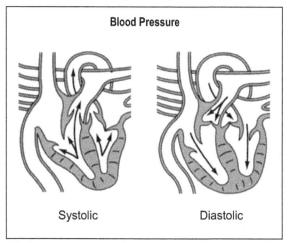

Blood Pressure

Systolic   Diastolic

Blood pressure is measured in two numbers: systolic pressure (the pressure of the blood as it flows out when the heart contracts) over diastolic pressure (the pressure of the blood within the artery as it flows in when the heart is at rest). Readings greater than 140 systolic over 90 diastolic indicate the presence of hypertension.

Blood Pressure and Hypertension

Status	Systolic/Diastolic
Normal	>120/>80
Prehypertension	120-139/80-89
Stage I hypertension	140-159/90-99
Stage II hypertension	<160/100

other vascular problems, such as stroke, kidney failure, heart failure, and visual disturbances secondary to the effects on the blood vessels within the eye. Hypertension is a major source of premature death in the United States and by all estimates affects more than sixty million Americans. Forty percent of all African Americans and more than half of those over the age of sixty are affected. Public awareness of hypertension is increasing, yet less than half of all patients diagnosed are treated. More important, only one in five identified hypertensives have the condition under control. This lack of control is particularly important when one considers the organs influenced by hypertension, most notably the brain, eyes, kidneys, and heart.

Although causative factors of hypertension cannot be identified, many physiological factors contribute to hypertension. They include increased sympathetic nervous activity (part of the autonomic nervous system), which promotes arterial contraction; overproduction of an unidentified sodium-retaining hormone or chronic high sodium intake; inadequate dietary intake of potassium or calcium; an increased or inappropriate secretion of renin, a chemical made by the kidney; deficiencies of arterial dilators, such as prostaglandins; congenital abnormalities (birth defects) of resistance vessels; diabetes mellitus or resistance to the effects of insulin; obesity; increased activity of vascular growth factors; and altered cellular ion transport of electrolytes, such as potassium, sodium, chloride, and bicarbonate.

The kidneys are greatly responsible for blood pressure control. They have a key role in maintaining both blood volume and blood pressure. When kidney function declines, secondary to problems such as a decrease in renal blood flow, the kidney will release renin. High renin levels result in activation of the renin-angiotensin-aldosterone system. The resulting chemical cascade produces angiotensin II, a potent arterial constrictor. Another chemical released is aldosterone, an adrenal hormone which causes the kidney to retain water and sodium. These two actions add to blood volume and increase arterial tone, resulting in higher blood pressure. Normally, the renin-angiotensin-aldosterone system protects kidney function by raising blood pressure when it is low. In hypertensives, the controlling forces seem to be out of balance, so that the system does not respond appropriately. The renin-angiotensin-aldosterone system has a negative effect on bradykinin, a chemical that protects renal function by producing vasodilating prostaglandins that help maintain adequate renal blood flow. This protection is especially impor-

tant in elderly individuals, who may depend on this system to maintain renal function. The system can be inhibited by medications such as aspirin or ibuprofen, resulting in a recurrence of hypertension or less control over the existing disease.

Arteries are largely smooth muscles under the control of the autonomic nervous system, which is responsible for organ function. Yet there is often no conscious control of organs; for example, one can tell the lungs to take a breath, but one cannot tell the heart to beat. The autonomic nervous system has two branches, sympathetic and parasympathetic, that essentially work against each other. The sympathetic system exerts much control over blood pressure. Many chemicals and medicines, such as caffeine, decongestants, and amphetamines, affect blood pressure by mimicking the effects of increased sympathetic stimulation of arteries.

Numerous factors associated with blood pressure elevations will affect one or more of the key determinants of blood pressure; they affect one another as well. An example will show the extent of their relationship. Sodium and water retention will increase blood volume returning to the heart. As this return increases, the heart will increase output (to a point) to prevent heart failure. This higher cardiac output may also raise blood pressure. If arterial vessels are constricted, pressures may be even higher. This elevated pressure (resistance) will force the heart to try to increase output to maintain blood flow to vital organs. Thus, a vicious cycle is started; hypertension can be perceived as a merry-go-round ride with no exit.

Treatment and Therapy

Blood pressure reduction has a protective effect against cardiovascular disease. Generally, as blood pressure decreases, arteries are less contracted and are able to deliver more blood to the tissues, maintaining their function. Furthermore, this decreased blood pressure will help reduce the risk of heart attack in the patient with heart disease. With lower pressures, the heart does not need to work as hard supplying blood to itself or the rest of the body. Therefore, the demand for cardiac output to supply blood flow is less. This reduced workload lowers the incidence of angina.

Treatment of hypertensive patients may involve using one to four different medications to achieve the goal of blood pressure reduction. There are many types of medications from which to choose: diuretics, sympatholytic agents (also known as antiadrenergic drugs), beta-blockers (along with one combined-action alpha-beta blocker), calcium-channel blockers, peripheral vasodilators, angiotensin-converting enzyme inhibitors, and the newest class, angiotension receptor inhibitors. The list of available drugs is extensive; for example, there are fourteen different thiazide-type diuretics and another six diuretics with different mechanisms of action.

Patients prone to sodium and water retention are treated with diuretics, agents that prevent the kidney from reabsorbing sodium and water from the urine. Diuretics are usually added to other medications to enhance those medications" activity. Research into thiazide-type diuretics has shown that these agents possess mild calcium-channel blocking activity,

---

In the News: ACE Inhibitor and Calcium-Channel Blocker Combo

The Seventh Report of the Joint National Committee on Prevention, Detection, Evaluation, and Treatment of High Blood Pressure (JNC 7), which was published in 2003, offers guidelines for treating hypertension, suggests initiating treatment with a thiazide-type diuretic. Due to several large-scale clinical trials, as well as small single-center studies, these guidelines have been challenged as combination therapy with an angiotensin-converting enzyme (ACE) inhibitor and a calcium-channel blocker (CCB) has gained attention as an effective treatment for hypertension and reduced the risk of fatal and nonfatal cardiovascular events. Both ACE inhibitors and CCBs are safe and effective as single agents for hypertension, but the additive effects of these drugs may be greater than the effects of either drug alone on reducing blood pressure and protecting target organs from damage owing to hypertension.

The Avoiding Cardiovascular Events in Combination Therapy in Patients Living with Systolic Hypertension (ACCOMPLISH) trial compared two treatment combinations—the ACE inhibitor benazepril plus the CCB amlodipine, and benazepril plus a diuretic—on cardiovascular events, including death from a cardiovascular event, nonfatal myocardial infarction, nonfatal stroke, hospitalization for angina, resuscitation after sudden cardiac arrest, and coronary revascularization. The study enrolled more than eleven thousand men and women, aged fifty-five years or older, who had hypertension and evidence of cardiovascular, renal, or other organ damage. After thirty-six months of treatment, 75 percent of the patients in both treatment groups achieved the recommended blood pressure goals. However, ACE inhibitor-CCB combination therapy reduced cardiovascular events by 20 percent compared with the ACE inhibitor-diuretic therapy. The results of the ACCOMPLISH trial were presented and published in 2008 and challenged the traditional hypertension treatment guidelines of starting with one-drug therapy and including a diuretic for all hypertensive patients.

Similarly, the Gauging Albuminuria Reduction with Lotrel in Diabetic Patients with Hypertension (GUARD) trial revealed that combination antihypertensive therapy with amlodipine and benazepril resulted in a greater reduction in blood pressure compared to treatment with benazepril and a diuretic. Also, ACE inhibitor-CCB treatment slowed the decline in renal function often associated with hypertension and diabetes.

Further research is needed to extend the results of the ACCOMPLISH and GUARD trials to other agents in the ACE inhibitor or CCB classes or to lower-risk patients. JNC 8 will be published in 2010 and will recommend new guidelines for treating hypertension.

—*Jennifer L. Gibson, Pharm.D.*

---

aiding their ability to reduce hypertension.

Beta-blocking agents are used less often than when they were first developed. They work by decreasing cardiac output through reducing the heart rate. Although they are highly effective, the heart rate reduction tends to produce side effects. Most commonly, patients complain of fatigue, sleepiness, and reduced exercise tolerance (the heart rate cannot increase to adapt to the increasing demand for blood in tissues and the heart itself). These agents are still a good choice for hypertensive patients who have suffered a heart attack. Their benefit is that they reduce the risk of a second heart attack by preventing the heart from overworking.

Calcium-channel blockers were originally intended to treat angina. These agents act primarily by decreasing arterial smooth muscle contraction. Relaxed coronary blood vessels can carry more blood, helping prevent the pain of angina. When calcium ions enter the smooth muscle, a more sustained contraction is produced; therefore, blocking this effect will produce relaxation. Physicians noted that this relaxation also produced lower blood pressures. The distinct advantage to these agents is that they are well tolerated; however, some patients may require increasing their fiber intake to prevent some constipating effects.

Peripheral vasodilators have been a disappointment. Theoretically, they should be ideal since they work directly to cause arterial dilation. Unfortunately, blood pressure has many determinants, and patients seem to become immune to direct vasodilator effects. Peripheral vasodilators are useful, however, when added to other treatments such as beta-blockers or sympatholytic medications.

The sympatholytic agents are divided into two broad categories. The first group works within the brain to decrease the effects of nerves that would send signals to blood vessels to constrict (so-called constrict messages). They do this by increasing the relax signals coming out of the brain to offset the constrict messages. The net effect is that blood vessels dilate, reducing blood pressure. Many of these agents have fallen into disfavor because of adverse effects similar to those of beta-blockers. The second group of sympatholytics works directly at the nerve-muscle connection. These agents block the constrict messages of the nerve that would increase arterial smooth muscle tone. Overall, these agents are well tolerated. Some patients, especially the elderly, may be very susceptible to their effect and have problems with low blood pressure; this issue usually resolves itself shortly after the first dose.

The renin-angiotensin-aldosterone system is a key determinant of blood pressure. Angiotensin-converting enzyme inhibitors (ACE inhibitors) work by blocking angiotensin II and aldosterone and by preserving bradykinin. They have been found quite effective for reducing blood pressure and are usually well tolerated. Some patients will experience a first-dose effect, while others may develop a dry cough that can be corrected by dose reductions or discontinuation of the medication. The angiotensin receptor inhibitors work, instead, by blocking the effects of this substance on the target cells of the arteries themselves. They are proving to be excellent substitutes for people who cannot tolerate the related class of ACE inhibitors.

Unfortunately, and contrary to popular belief, no one can reliably tell when his or her own blood pressure is elevated. Consequently, hypertension is called a "silent killer." It is extremely important to have regular blood pressure evaluations and, if diagnosed with hypertension, to receive treatment.

From 1950 through 1987, as advances in understanding

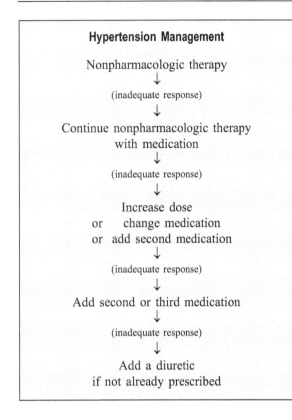

Hypertension Management

Nonpharmacologic therapy
↓
(inadequate response)
↓
Continue nonpharmacologic therapy
with medication
↓
(inadequate response)
↓
Increase dose
or   change medication
or   add second medication
↓
(inadequate response)
↓
Add second or third medication
↓
(inadequate response)
↓
Add a diuretic
if not already prescribed

and treating hypertension were made, the United States population enjoyed a 40 percent reduction in coronary heart disease and a more than 65 percent reduction in stroke deaths. (By comparison, noncardiovascular deaths during the same period were reduced little more than 20 percent.)

It is evident that blood pressure can be reduced without medications. Research in the 1980s led to a nonpharmacologic approach in the initial management of hypertension. This strategy includes weight reduction, alcohol restriction, regular exercise, dietary sodium restriction, dietary potassium and calcium supplementation, stopping of tobacco use (in any form), and caffeine restriction. Often, these methods can produce benefits without medication being prescribed. Stress is another common contributor to hypertension; therefore, stress reduction and management is another strategy to reduce blood pressure. This may be achieved through lifestyle changes, meditation, relaxation techniques, and exercise. Using this approach, medication is added to the therapy if blood pressure remains elevated despite good efforts at nonpharmacologic control.

Other aspects of hypertension and hypertensive patients have been identified to help guide the clinician to the proper choice of medication. With this approach, the clinician can focus therapy at the most likely cause of the hypertension: sodium and water retention, high cardiac output, or high vascular resistance. This pathophysiological approach led to the abandonment of the rigid step-care approach described in many texts covering hypertension. The pathophysiological approach to hypertension management is based on a series of steps that are taken if inadequate responses are seen.

The best strategy for controlling hypertension is to be informed. Each person needs to be aware of his or her personal risk for developing hypertension. One should have regular blood pressure evaluations, avoid eating excessive salt and sodium, increase exercise, and reduce fats in the diet. Maintaining ideal body weight may be a key control factor. Studies have shown that patients who have been successful at losing weight will require less stringent treatment. The benefits could be a need for fewer medications, reduced doses of medications, or both.

—*Charles C. Marsh, Pharm.D.;*
updated by Connie Rizzo, M.D., Ph.D.

See also Angina; Arteriosclerosis; Blood pressure; Cardiology; Cholesterol; Circulation; Claudication; Embolism; Heart; Heart attack; Heart disease; Hyperadiposis; Hypercholesterolemia; Hyperlipidemia; Hypotension; Insulin resistance syndrome; Kidney disorders; Kidneys; Metabolic syndrome; Phlebitis; Physical examination; Preeclampsia and eclampsia; Pulmonary hypertension; Strokes; Thrombolytic therapy and TPA; Thrombosis and thrombus; Vascular medicine; Vascular system.

For Further Information:

Elliott, William J., and Henry black R. *Hypertension: A Companion to Braunwald's Heart Disease.* Philadelphia: Elsevier Saunders, 2013.

McGowan, Mary P., and Jo McGowan-Chopra. *The Hypertension Sourcebook.* Chicago: Contemporary Books, 2001.

Messerli, Franz H., ed. *Cardiovascular Disease in the Elderly.* 3d ed. Boston: Kluwer Academic Publishers, 1993.

Mancia, Giuseppe, and Adel E. Berbari. *Special Issues in Hypertension.* Milano: Springer-Verlag, 2012.

Messerli, Franz H. *The Heart and Hypertension.* New York: Yorke Medical Books, 1987.

Piscatella, Joseph, and Barry Franklin. *Take a Load Off Your Heart: 109 Things You Can Do to Prevent or Reverse Heart Disease.* New York: Workman Publishers, 2003.

Portman, Ronald J., Julie R. Ingelfinger, Joseph T. Flynn. "Pediatric Hypertension." *Clinical Hypertension and Vascular Disease.* 3d ed. New York: Humana Press, 2013.

Rowan, Robert L. *Control High Blood Pressure Without Drugs: A Complete Hypertension Handbook.* Rev. ed. New York: Fireside Books, 2001.

Seeley, Rod R., Trent D. Stephens, and Philip Tate. *Anatomy and Physiology.* 7th ed. New York: McGraw-Hill, 2006.

Tierney, Lawrence M., Stephen J. McPhee, and Maxine A. Papadakis, eds. *Current Medical Diagnosis and Treatment 2007.* New York: McGraw-Hill, 2006.

HYPERTHERMIA AND HYPOTHERMIA
Disease/Disorder

Anatomy or system affected: All

Specialties and related fields: Anesthesiology, critical care, emergency medicine, environmental health, internal medicine

Definition: Hyperthermia is the elevation of the body core temperature of an organism, while hypothermia is a decrease in that temperature; an extreme in either condition is a medical emergency. They both can be induced therapeutically in certain medical and surgical conditions.

Key terms:

ambient temperature: the temperature of the surrounding environment

body temperature: the temperature that reflects the level of heat energy in an animal's body; a consequence of the balance between the heat produced by metabolism and the body's exchange of heat with the surrounding environment

frostbite: injury that results from exposure of skin to extreme cold, most commonly affecting the ears, nose, hands, and feet

hibernation: a condition of dormancy and torpor that occurs in poikilotherm vertebrates and invertebrates; as the environmental temperatures drop, the inner core temperature of such animals also drops to decrease the metabolic rate and physiological functions

homeotherms: animals, such as birds and mammals, that have the ability to maintain a high body core temperature despite large variations in environmental temperatures

Causes and Symptoms

Body temperature reflects the level of heat energy in the body of an animal or human being. It is the consequence of the balance between the heat generated by metabolism and the body's heat exchange with the surrounding environment (ambient temperature). Generally, animal life can be sustained in the temperature range of 0 degrees Celsius (32 degrees Fahrenheit) to 45 degrees Celsius (113 degrees Fahrenheit), but appropriate processes can store animal tissues at much lower temperature. Homeotherms, such as birds and most mammals, have the ability to maintain their high body core temperatures despite large variations in environmental temperatures. Poikilotherms have slow metabolic rates at rest and, as a result, have difficulty maintaining their inner core temperatures. This form of thermal regulation is called ectothermic (outer heated) and is directly affected by the uptake of heat from the environment; such organisms are often termed *cold-blooded*. Homeotherms are endothermic (inner heated) and depend largely on their fast and controlled rates of heat production; such organisms are termed *warm-blooded*. Thus, the lizard, an example of an ectotherm, maintains its body temperature by staying in or out of shade and by assuming a posture toward the sun that will maximize the adjustment for its body heat. At night, the lizard burrows, but its body temperature still drops considerably until the next morning, when it increases with the rising sun.

Body core temperatures vary considerably among mammals and birds. For example, a sparrow's inner core temperature is about 43.5 degrees Celsius (110.3 degrees Fahrenheit), a turkey's is 41.2 degrees Celsius (106.2 degrees Fahrenheit), a cat's is 36.4 degrees Celsius (97.5 degrees Fahrenheit), and an opossum's is 34.7 degrees Celsius (94.5 degrees Fahrenheit). In humans, although the temperature of the inner organs varies by only 1 to 2 degrees Celsius (1.8 to 3.6 degrees Fahrenheit), the skin temperature may vary 10 to 20 degrees Celsius (18 to 36 degrees Fahrenheit) below the core temperature of 37 degrees Celsius (98.6 degrees Fahrenheit), depending on the ambient temperature. This is possible because the cells

---

Information on Hyperthermia and Hypothermia

Causes: Extended exposure to heat or cold

Symptoms: For hyperthermia, headache, nausea, dizziness, heat exhaustion or heatstroke, cessation of perspiration, hot and dry skin, rapid pulse, quick and shallow breathing; for hypothermia, tingling, pain, numbness, sometimes frostbite on nose, ears, hands, and feet

Duration: Acute

Treatments: For hyperthermia, cooling of body, replacement of body fluids, treatment of shock, emergency resuscitation; for hypothermia, warm water on affected body part, hospitalization in intensive care unit

---

of the skin, muscles, and blood vessels are not as sensitive as are those of the vital organs.

An elevation in core temperature of homeotherms above the normal range is called hyperthermia, while a corresponding decrease is called hypothermia. Both can be brought about by extremes in the environment, and an extreme in either condition is a medical emergency. Although the human body can withstand a lack of food for a number of weeks and the absence of water for several days, it cannot survive without thermoregulation, which is the maintaining of the inner core temperature. The core temperature has to be kept within strict limits; otherwise, the brain and heart will be compromised, and death will result. Clinically, the body's core temperature can be monitored by recording the temperature of the rectum, the eardrum, the mouth, the temporal artery, or the esophagus. In elderly people, the body's ability to cope with extreme temperatures may be impaired, so that exposure to even mildly cold temperatures may lead to accidental hypothermia that can be fatal if not detected and treated properly.

All animals produce heat by oxidation of substrates to carbon dioxide. On the average, about 75 percent of food energy is converted to heat during adenosine triphosphate (ATP) formation and its transfer to the functional systems of the cells. In defense against heat, sweating is the primary physiological mechanism in mammals. Dogs, cats, and other furred carnivores increase evaporative heat loss by panting, while small rodents spread saliva. Human beings have two to three million glands that can produce a high volume of sweat for a short period of time.

Fever may occur for at least four main reasons. Infection by microorganisms is the most familiar because of its large variety of causes. An infection may be bacterial (as with septicemia and abscesses), viral (such as measles, mumps, and influenza), protozoal (such as malaria), or spirochetal (such as syphilis). Fever can also occur because of immunological conditions, such as a response to drug allergies or a reaction to a blood transfusion. Other causes are malignancy, such as Hodgkin's disease and leukemia, and noninfectious inflammation, as seen in gout or thrombophlebitis.

Antipyretics are medicines whose consumption results in

the lowering of fever. Aspirin, acetaminophen, and ibuprofen are common, over-the-counter fever-reducing medications. The mechanism of action of the nonnarcotic antipyretics remains a subject of research. Two hypotheses are considered as possible reasons for the suppression of fever. One hypothesis suggests that the drugs reset the temperature in the hypothalamus of the brain by potentially blocking certain brain chemical activity. The other postulates that a modification of the physiological membrane properties takes place, with subsequent incorporation of drug molecules into the tertiary structure of proteins.

Temperature regulation involves the hypothalamus of the brain and the spinal cord, which monitor the difference between the internal and peripheral (core and skin) temperature, with physiological and psychological adjustments to maintain a constant internal temperature. The brain records the various body temperatures via specialized nerve endings called thermoreceptors. Heat transfer occurs between the skin surface and the environment via radiation (which takes place when environmental temperature is lower than body temperature; 60 to 70 percent of body heat is lost through this method), conduction (which takes place by means of physical contact), convection (which occurs through the movement of air), or evaporation (perspiration or sweating).

During cold weather, hikers and climbers are particularly at risk for hypothermia; in extreme cases, body functions are depressed to the extent that victims may be mistaken for dead. Injuries that result from skin exposure to extreme cold are described as frostbite. Frostbite most commonly affects peripheral tissue such as the nose, ears, hands (especially the fingertips), and feet, which first turn unusually red and then unnaturally white. Early symptoms include feelings of coldness, tingling, pain, and numbness. Frostbite takes place when ice crystals form in the skin and (in the most serious cases) in the tissue beneath the skin. If not treated, frostbite may lead to gangrene, the medical term for tissue death. The freezing-thawing process causes mechanical disruption (from ice), intracellular and extracellular biochemical changes, and the disruption of the blood corpuscles. Frostbite treatment includes the removal of wet or restrictive clothing or jewelry. Warm water can be used on the affected body part to restore blood circulation, which will be painful for the victim. Extreme care should be taken when moving the body part with frostbite. The area should never be massaged, as the skin and tissues are very fragile and may be further damaged.

There are several types of hypothermia. Immersion hypothermia occurs when a person falls into cold water. Any movement of the body leads to loss of heat, and the drastic temperature change may trigger a heart attack. Divers are equipped with wet suits to minimize heat loss, but they cool themselves rapidly when they move in cold water and breathe dry air mixtures at the same time.

Submersion hypothermia is actual drowning in cold water. Often during drowning, the person experiences a spasm of the larynx or is able to hold his or her breath. However, the lack of oxygen forces the relaxation of these responses, and water is swallowed. The majority of this water goes into the stomach, but it only takes a very small amount of water in the lungs to cause enough oxygen deprivation to slow or even stop the heart. In cold water, the human body responds by lowering its metabolism, which can allow an individual (especially a child) to survive for a prolonged period without adequate oxygen before death occurs. The exact amount of time that a person can survive in cold-water conditions is unknown. Reports have demonstrated survival in cases of submersion for more than an hour. Unless the person shows evidence of decay, attempts should be made to rescue the individual and involve emergency medical personnel. When removing a victim from the water, care should be taken to remove the individual in a prone (facedown) position to avoid circulatory collapse from the sudden decrease in water pressure. This is a common cause of sudden death for a conscious individual who is rescued from the water.

Clinical reports also indicate hypothermia in alcohol-intoxicated individuals. Shivering is the brain's hypothalamic response to hypothermia. The hypothalamus stimulates reflexes in the spinal cord that trigger a sequence of skeletal muscle contractions, which lead to an increase in body temperature. Other conditions that promote heat loss in an already-hypothermic person include tight and wet clothing, injury causing hemorrhage, fatigue, and even psychosis.

Treatment and Therapy

Nature protects poikilotherm vertebrates and invertebrates in winter by means of hibernation. Hibernation, which is a condition of dormancy and torpor, occurs when the body temperatures of such animals drop in response to a decrease in environmental temperatures. Animals such as bears, raccoons, badgers, and some birds become drowsy in winter because ambient temperature drops of a few degrees considerably decrease their metabolic rates and physiological functions. For example, the body temperature of a bear is 35.5 degrees Celsius (95.9 degrees Fahrenheit) at an air temperature of 4.4 degrees Celsius (39.9 degrees Fahrenheit) and only 31.2 degrees Celsius (88.1 degrees Fahrenheit) at an air temperature of -4 degrees Celsius (24.8 degrees Fahrenheit).

In humans, however, a significant decrease in body temperature is always a medical emergency requiring immediate attention. The treatment for mild cases of hypothermia may consist only of removing wet clothing before providing additional clothing or blankets. Movement of the victim must be minimized to avoid causing abnormal heart rhythms. Providing warm fluids and attempts at rewarming beyond those mentioned are not recommended for laypersons. Severe hypothermia requires hospitalization in an intensive care unit (ICU), where the body temperature is returned to normal by placing the patient under special heat-reflecting blankets; infusing warm intravenous (IV) fluids; irrigating the stomach, abdominal cavity, and bladder with warm fluids; or circulating the victim's blood through a machine to warm it.

Hyperthermia can be in response to illness (fever) or environmental conditions (heat exhaustion or heatstroke). Heatstroke, defined as a core temperature above 40 degrees Celsius (104 degrees Fahrenheit), is a medical emergency that

First Aid for Hypothermia

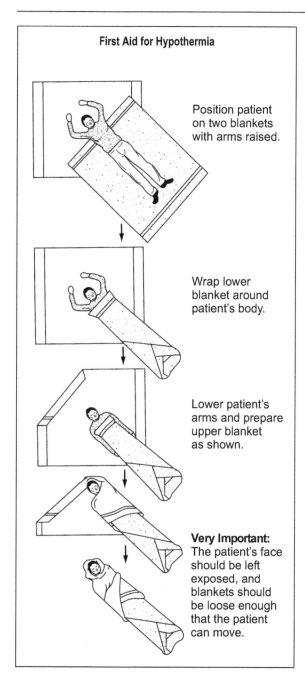

Position patient on two blankets with arms raised.

Wrap lower blanket around patient's body.

Lower patient's arms and prepare upper blanket as shown.

Very Important: The patient's face should be left exposed, and blankets should be loose enough that the patient can move.

occurs when the thermoregulatory system fails. The victim is unable to cool the body's elevated temperature through normal mechanisms of sweating. A sustained elevated temperature can cause seizures in young children and infants. Adults, especially the elderly, are prone to experience confusion. Treatment while waiting for the arrival of emergency medical services includes placing the victim in a cool environment, removing the victim's clothing, and placing ice packs on the groin, neck, and underarm regions. Shivering should be avoided. Salt tablets or solutions should not be given by laypersons because of the risk of elevated sodium levels and the possibility of stomach upset.

Both hyperthermia and hypothermia have been used in medical treatments. Cancer treatment traditionally consists primarily of radiation therapy, surgery, and chemotherapy, but more recent experimental approaches for cancer treatment include immunotherapy and hyperthermia. Hyperthermia has been used with chemotherapy or radiation therapy to improve blood flow to the targeted cancer cells, increase the drug concentration inside those cells, and damage or kill them while preserving the healthy cells nearby. This preservation is attributed to the differences in the structure of cancer cells, which are effectively damaged by heat. Further studies are needed to determine the temperature that is needed to damage or kill the cancer cells without harming other cells. Most body tissues can withstand temperature up to 44 degrees Celsius for up to one hour, with the exception of the brain, spinal cord, and nerves. These structures have been found to have irreversible damage at lower temperatures and shorter exposure time than other tissues.

Ultrasonic irradiation, which uses a thin, stainless-steel tube to induce hyperthermia, is regarded as a promising technique. The heat generated by the energy produced improves the local blood supply by dilating the blood vessels. This dilation, together with an acceleration of enzyme activity, helps cells obtain fresh nutrients and, at the same time, rid themselves of waste products. The other advantage of ultrasonic irradiation is the vibrations that it creates. In the case of a hardened and calcified brain tumor, for example, these vibrations can crush the tumor, which can then be removed via vacuum.

Induced hypothermia is selectively used in various heart and brain surgeries. The patient's body temperature is lowered by the use of cooling blankets and other devices. The core temperature is monitored by bladder and rectal electronic devices. The hypothermia is considered neuroprotective. It is uncertain if the brain protection is from lowered oxygen metabolism or prevention of harmful chemical reactions. The goal of the majority of surgical procedures is to keep the patient's temperature within the normal range. Hypothermia has been associated with increased blood loss, higher infection rates, and other poor outcomes in many surgical situations. Therapeutic hypothermia has also been used after cardiac arrest to preserve heart tissue by decreasing its oxygen demand.

Perspective and Prospects

Both hypothermia and hyperthermia have long had a commanding role in medicine. An Egyptian papyrus roll that can be dated back to 3000 BCE describes the treatment of a breast tumor with hyperthermia. Heat has been used as a therapeutic agent since the days of Hippocrates (c. 460–c. 370 BCE), who stated that a patient who could not be cured by heat was incurable. In the seventeenth century, the Japanese used hyperthermia to treat syphilis, arthritis, and gout, using hot water to increase the body temperature to about 39 degrees Celsius.

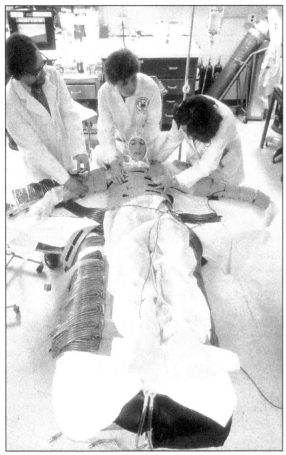

Hyperthermia may be induced in the treatment of cancer. (Mike Mitchell/National Cancer Institute)

The medical use of hyperthermia owes much of its modern-era development to Georges Lakhovsky (1880–1942), a Russian Jew with a brilliant physics background who did most of his work in Paris, France. Although he is not generally given the credit for it, he was the first person to design and build a short-wave diathermy machine, which created artificial fever for the first time in 1923. His work was done primarily on patients with malignant tumors at the Hospital de la Salpetriere and the Hospital Saint-Louis. The first machine that he developed used frequencies from 0.75 megahertz to 3,000 megahertz, a range very much in use in today's clinical hyperthermia. In 1931, he started using a new machine that emitted radio waves of multiple wavelengths. He had partial success with his treatment, as reported to the Pasteur Institute and the French Academy of Sciences. Other scientists in this field include the German physicians W. Busch and P. Bruns, who applied it to erysipelas infection in 1886, and the Swedish gynecologist N. Westermark, who applied it with partial success to nonoperable carcinomas of the cervix uteri in 1898. The combination of hyperthermia and immunotherapy was first applied by William B. Coley, a New York surgeon who managed to cause complete regression of malignant melanoma in patients by inducing artificial fever created by inoculation of infected erysipelas cells.

The practice of hyperthermia in conjunction with chemotherapy, radiation, and surgery for the treatment of cancers is still in its infancy. Research has produced mixed results. Studies have shown that heat is able to kill cancer cells left behind following surgery, and it can kill those cells that tend to be radiation resistant. Unlike radiation, hyperthermia has no known cumulative toxicity. The challenge is to determine the effectiveness of hyperthermia alone compared to with other treatments, the amount of heat needed to kill cancer cells and preserve normal cells, and the proper hyperthermia techniques, such as ultrasound-induced hyperthermia.

The application of hyperthermia in cases of acquired immunodeficiency syndrome (AIDS) has not yet provided decisively positive results. The process involves circulating the patient's blood through a chamber heated to approximately 10 degrees Fahrenheit higher than the body temperature. Although the AIDS virus is killed, many of the patients" other enzymes are found to lose their activity. Consequently, United States health officials have opposed and criticized blood-heating therapy for this disease until more convincing results are produced.

The role of hyperthermia in treating metastatic cancer, in combination with radiation and drugs that sensitize cells to heat and radiation, is increasing. This technique has been made feasible by the technological advancements in deep-heating machines, such as the Magnetrode and the BSD annular phased array, which allow the sequential regional hyperthermia of large body regions such as the thorax and the abdomen. The challenge is to prevent heatstroke during the procedure.

Induced-hypothermia brain surgery protects brain tissue. In stroke patients, a temperature elevation of 1 degree Celsius (1.8 degrees Fahrenheit) can increase the size of the damaged tissue by as much as 50 percent.

—Soraya Ghayourmanesh, Ph.D.;
updated by Amy Webb Bull, D.S.N., A.P.N.

See also Anesthesia; Anesthesiology; Critical care; Critical care, pediatric; Emergency medicine; Fever; Frostbite; Gangrene; Heat exhaustion and heatstroke; Hyperhidrosis; Surgery, general; Sweating.

For Further Information:

Bloomfield, Molly M., and Lawrence J. Stephens. *Chemistry and the Living Organism.* 6th ed. New York: John Wiley & Sons, 1996.

Bucher, Linda. "Emergency Care Situations." In *Medical-Surgical Nursing*, edited by Sharon Lewis, Margaret Heitkemper, and Shannon Dirksen. 6th ed. St. Louis, Mo.: Mosby, 2004.

Calvagna, Mary, and Igor Puzanov. "Radiation Therapy for Cancer Treatment." *Health Library*, September 26, 2012.

"Fever." *MedlinePlus*, July 10, 2013.

Foltz, Patricia, Cheryl Wavrin, and Robert Sticca. "Heated Intraoperative Intraperitoneal Chemotherapy: The Challenges of Bringing Chemotherapy into Surgery." *Association of Operating Room Nurses Journal* 80, no. 6 (December 2004): 1055–1063.

Futterman, Laurie G., and Louis Lemberg. "The Significance of Hypothermia in Preserving Ischemic Myocardium." *American Journal of Critical Care* 13, no. 1 (January 2004): 79–84.

Harries, Mark. "Near Drowning: ABC of Resuscitation." *British*

Medical Journal 327 (December 6, 2003): 1336–1338.

"Hypothermia." *MedlinePlus*, July 4, 2013.

"Inflammation, the Inflammatory Response, and Fever." In *Essentials of Pathophysiology: Concepts of Altered Health States*, edited by Carol Mattson Porth. 3d ed. Philadelphia: Lippincott Williams & Wilkins, 2011.

Martin, Julie J., and Brian Randall. "Hypothermia." *Health Library*, September 27, 2012.

Morcom, Fiona. "Chill Out: Therapeutic Hypothermia Improves Survival." *Emergency Nurse* 11, no. 4 (August 2003): 24–28.

Olson, DaiWai, and Carmelo Graffagnino. "Extremes of Hot or Cold Can Lead to Secondary Injuries." *Nursing* 35, no. 7 (July 2005): 32cc1–32cc2.

Ross, Jennifer Lea. "Near Drowning: Swimming and Other Water Activities Are a Big Part of Summertime Fun, but They're Not without Risk." *RN* 68, no. 7 (July 2005): 36–41.

Van der Zee, J. "Heating the Patient: A Promising Approach?" *Annals of Oncology* 13, no. 8 (August 2002): 1173–1184.

HYPERTROPHY

Biology

Anatomy or system affected: All

Specialties and related fields: Endocrinology, family medicine, internal medicine

Definition: The growth of a tissue or organ as the result of an increase in the size of the existing cells within that tissue or organ; this process is responsible for the growth of the body as well as for increases in organ size caused by increased workloads on particular organs.

Key terms:

atrophy: the wasting of tissue, an organ, or an entire body as the result of a decrease in the size and/or number of the cells within that tissue, organ, or body

compensatory hypertrophy: an increase in the size of a tissue or an organ in response to an increased workload placed upon it

growth: the increase in size of an organism or any of its parts during the developmental process; caused by increases in both cell numbers and cell size

hyperplasia: the increase in size or growth of a tissue or an organ as a result of an increase in cell numbers, with the size of the cells remaining constant

Process and Effects

The growth and development of the human body and all its parts requires not only an increase in the number of body cells as the body grows, a process known as hyperplasia, but also an increase in the size of the existing cells, a process known as hypertrophy. It is true that as humans grow, they increase the number of cells in their bodies, resulting in an increase in the size of tissues, organs, systems, and the body. For some tissues, organs, and systems, however, the number of cells is genetically set; therefore, the number of cells will increase minimally if at all after birth. Thus, if growth is to occur in those tissues, organs, and systems, it must take place by means of an increase in the size of the existing cells.

The process of hypertrophy occurs in nearly all tissues in the body but is most common in those tissues in which the number of cells is set at the time of birth. Among such tissues are adipose tissue, which is composed of fat cells, and nervous tissue, which is found in the brain, in the spinal cord, and in skeletal muscle tissue. Other tissues, such as cardiac tissue and smooth muscle tissue, also show the ability to undergo hypertrophy.

It is generally true that the number of fat cells within the human body is set at birth. Therefore, an increase in body fat is thought to result primarily from an increase in the amount of fat stored within the fat cells. An increase in the amount of fat consumed in the diet increases the amount of fat that is placed inside a fat cell, resulting in an increase in the fat cell's size.

The number of nerve cells within the brain and spinal cord also is set at birth. The cerebellum of the human brain, however, increases in size about twentyfold from birth to adulthood. This increase is brought about by an increase in the size of the existing nerve cells, and particularly by an increase in the number of extensions protruding from each nerve cell and the length to which the extensions grow. Furthermore, there is an increase in the number of the components within the cell. Specifically, there is an increase in the number of mitochondria within the cell, which provide a usable form of energy so that the cell can grow.

The number of skeletal muscle cells is also, in general, preset at the time of birth. The skeletal muscle mass of the human body increases dramatically from birth to adulthood. This increase is accomplished primarily by means of individual skeletal muscle cell hypertrophy. This increase in the diameter of the individual muscle cells is brought about by increases in the amounts of the contractile proteins, myosin and actin, as well as increases in the amount of glycogen and the number of mitochondria within individual cells. As each muscle cell increases in size, it causes an increase in the size of the entire muscle of which it is a part.

Each of the above-mentioned examples occurs naturally as part of the growth process of the human body. Some tissues, however, are capable of increasing in size as the result of an increased load or demand being placed upon them. This increased load or demand is usually brought about by an increased use of the muscle. This increase in the size of cells in response to an increased demand or use is called compensatory hypertrophy. The most common tissues that show the phenomenon of compensatory hypertrophy are the skeletal, cardiac, and smooth muscles.

Skeletal muscle is particularly responsive to being utilized. This response, however, is dependent upon the way in which the skeletal muscle is used. It is well known that an increase in the size of skeletal muscle can be brought about by such exercises as weight lifting. Lifting heavy weights or objects requires strong contractions of the skeletal muscle that is doing the lifting. If this lifting continues over a long period of time, it eventually results in an increase in the size of the existing muscle fibers, leading to an increase in the size of the exercised muscle. Because the strength of a muscle is dependent upon its size, the increase in the muscle's size results in an increase in its strength. The extent to which the size of the muscle increases is dependent upon the amount of time spent lifting the objects and the weight of the objects. The size that a muscle can reach is, however, limited.

Unlike exercises such as weight lifting, endurance types of exercise, such as walking, jogging, and aerobics, do not result in larger skeletal muscles. These types of exercise do not force the skeletal muscles to contract forcibly enough to produce muscle hypertrophy.

In the same way that an increased load or use will cause compensatory hypertrophy in skeletal muscle, a decreased use of skeletal muscle will result in its shrinking or wasting away. This process is referred to as muscle atrophy. This type of atrophy commonly occurs when limbs are broken or injured and must be immobilized. After six weeks of the limb being immobilized, there is a marked decrease in muscle size. A similar type of atrophy occurs in the limb muscles of astronauts, since there is no gravity present in space to provide resistance against which the muscles must work. If the muscles remain unused for more than a few months, there can be a loss of about one-half of the muscle mass of the unused muscle.

Cardiac muscle, like skeletal muscle, can also be caused to hypertrophy by increasing the resistance against which it works. Although endurance exercise does not cause hypertrophy in skeletal muscle, it does result in an increased size of the heart because of the hypertrophy of the existing cardiac muscle cells in this organ. In fact, the heart mass of marathon runners enlarges by about 40 percent as a result of the increase in endurance training. This increase occurs because the heart must work harder to pump more blood to the rest of the body when the body is endurance exercising. Only endurance forms of exercise result in the hypertrophy of the cardiac muscle. Weight lifting, which causes hypertrophy of skeletal muscle, has no effect on the cardiac muscle.

Smooth muscle also is capable of compensatory hypertrophy. Increased pressure or loads on the smooth muscle within arteries can result in the hypertrophy of the muscle cells. This in turn causes a thickening of the arterial wall. Smooth muscle, however, unlike skeletal and cardiac muscle, is capable of hyperplasia as well as hypertrophy.

Complications and Disorders

Hypertrophy also occurs as a result of some pathological and abnormal conditions. The most common pathological hypertrophy is enlargement of the heart as a result of cardiovascular disease. Most cardiovascular diseases put an increased workload on the heart, making it work harder to pump the blood throughout the body. In response to the increased workload, the heart increases its size, a form of compensatory hypertrophy.

The left ventricle of the heart is capable of hypertrophying to such an extent that its muscle mass may increase four- or fivefold. This increase is the result of improper functioning of the valves of the left heart. The valves of the heart work to prevent the backflow of blood from one chamber to another or from the arteries back to the heart. If the valves in the left heart are not working properly, the left ventricle contracts, and blood that should leave the ventricle to go out to the body instead returns to the left ventricle. The enlargement of the left ventricle increases the force with which it can pump the blood out to the body, thus reducing the amount of blood that comes back to the left ventricle despite the damaged heart valves. There is, however, a point at which the enlargement of the left ventricle can no longer help in keeping the needed amount of blood flowing through the body. At that point, the left ventricle finally tires out, and left heart failure occurs.

The same type of hypertrophy can and does occur in the right side of the heart as well. Again, this is the result of damaged valves that are supposed to prevent the backflow of blood into the heart. Should the valves of both sides of the heart be damaged, hypertrophy can occur on both sides of the heart.

High blood pressure, also known as hypertension, may also lead to hypertrophy of the ventricles of the heart. With high blood pressure, the heart must work harder to deliver blood throughout the body because it must pump blood against an increased pressure. As a result of the increased demand upon the heart, the heart muscle hypertrophies in order to pump more blood.

The hypertrophy of the heart muscle is beneficial in the pumping of blood to the body in individuals who have valvular disease and hypertension; however, an extreme hypertrophy sometimes leads to heart failure. One of the reasons this may occur is the inability of the blood supply of the heart to keep up with the growth of the cardiac muscle. As a result, the cardiac cells outgrow their blood supply, resulting in the loss of blood and thus a loss of oxygen and nutrients needed for the cardiac cells to survive.

Smooth muscle, like cardiac muscle, may also hypertrophy under the condition of high blood pressure. Smooth muscle makes up the bulk of many of the arteries and smaller arterioles found in the body. The increased pressure on the arterial walls as a result of high blood pressure may cause the hypertrophy of the smooth muscles within the walls of the arteries and arterioles. This increases the thickness of the walls of the arteries and arterioles but also decreases the size of the hollow spaces within those vessels, which are known as the lumina. In the kidneys, the narrowing of the lumina of the arterioles may result in a decreased blood supply to these organs. The reduced blood flow to the kidneys may eventually cause the kidneys to shut down, leading to renal failure.

Smooth muscle may also hypertrophy under some unique conditions. During pregnancy, the uterus will undergo a dramatic hypertrophy. The uterus is a smooth muscle organ that is involved in the housing and nurturing of the developing fetus during pregnancy. Immediately prior to the birth of the fetus, there is marked hypertrophy of the smooth muscle within this organ. This increase in the size of the uterus is beneficial in providing the strong contractions of this organ that are needed for childbirth.

Skeletal muscle also may be caused to hypertrophy in some diseases in which there is an increase in the secretion of male sex hormones, particularly testosterone. Men's higher levels of testosterone, a potent stimulator of muscle growth, are responsible for the fact that males have a larger muscle mass than do females. Furthermore, synthetic testosterone-like hormones have been used by some athletes to increase muscle size. These synthetic hormones are called anabolic steroids. The use of these steroids does result in the hypertrophy of skeletal muscle, but these steroids have been shown to have harmful side effects.

Obesity is another condition that results largely from the hypertrophy of existing fat cells. In children, however, obesity is thought to result not only from an increase in the size of fat cells but also from an increase in their number. In adults, when weight is lost, it is the result of a decrease in the size of the existing fat cells; the number of fat cells remains constant. Thus, it is important to prevent further weight increases in overweight children to prevent the creation of fat cells that will never be lost.

In the onset of diseases that result in muscle degeneration, such as muscular dystrophy, there is a hypertrophy of the affected muscles. This hypertrophy differs from other forms of muscle hypertrophy in that the muscle cells do not increase in size because of an increase in the contractile protein, mitochondria, or glycogen, but because the muscle cells are being filled with fat. As a result of the contractile protein being replaced with fat, the affected muscles are no longer useful.

Perspective and Prospects

The exact mechanisms that bring about and control the hypertrophy of cells and tissues are not well understood. During the growth and developmental periods, however, the hypertrophy of many tissues is thought to be under the control of blood-borne chemicals known as hormones. Among these hormones is one that promotes growth and is thus called growth hormone. Growth hormone brings about an increase in the number and size of cells. Growth hormone causes the hypertrophy of existing cells by increasing the protein-making capability of these cells. Thus, there is an increase in the number of organelles, such as mitochondria, within the cell, which leads to an increase in cell size.

Growth hormone also causes the release of chemicals known as growth factors. There are several different growth factors, but one of particular importance is nerve growth factor. Nerve growth factor is involved with the increase in number of cell processes of single nerve cells. Such chemicals have been shown to enhance the growth of damaged nerve cells in the brains of animals. As a result, it is possible that nerve growth factor could be used in the treatment of nerve damage in humans by causing the nerves to grow new cell processes and form new connections to replace those that were damaged. This may be of great importance for the treatment of those suffering from brain or spinal cord damage.

Other hormones may have similar effects on tissues other than nervous tissue. For example, the hypertrophy of the smooth muscle in the uterus is thought to be brought about hormonally. Immediately prior to birth, when the hypertrophy of the uterus is occurring, there is an increased amount of estrogen, the primary female hormone, in the blood. It is this increase in estrogen that is thought to lead to the great enlargement of the uterus during this time. Some hormones have the effect of preventing or inhibiting the hypertrophy of body tissues. The enlargement of the uterus prior to birth is brought about not only by an increase in estrogen but also as a result of a decrease in another hormone known as progesterone. Progesterone levels are high in the blood throughout pregnancy. Immediately prior to birth, however, there is a dramatic decrease in the level of progesterone in the blood. Thus, it is believed that the high level of progesterone prevents or inhibits the hypertrophy of the smooth muscle cells in the uterus, since the hypertrophy of this organ will not occur until estrogen levels are high and progesterone levels are low.

It has been suggested that compensatory hypertrophy, such as that which occurs in skeletal, smooth, and cardiac muscle, occurs as a result of the stretching of muscle. Some studies have shown that the stretching of skeletal, cardiac, and smooth muscle does lead to hypertrophy. American astronauts and Russian cosmonauts, however, showed a loss in muscle mass even though they exercised and stretched their muscles as much as three hours per day, seven days per week. This suggests that mechanisms other than the stretching of muscles may be involved in compensatory muscle hypertrophy.

Through an understanding of the mechanisms involved in muscle hypertrophy, it may one day be possible to prevent the atrophy that occurs during space flights, prolonged bed rest, and immobilization necessitated by the injury of limbs. Furthermore, the understanding of the mechanisms that control hypertrophy may help to alleviate the effects of disabling diseases such as muscular dystrophy by reversing the effects of muscle atrophy.

—David K. Saunders, Ph.D.

See also Endocrinology; Endocrinology, pediatric; Ergogenic aids; Exercise physiology; Growth; Hormones; Muscles; Muscular dystrophy; Obesity; Obesity, childhood; Pregnancy and gestation; Steroid abuse; Steroids.

For Further Information:

Alan, Rick. "Muscular Dystrophy." *MedlinePlus*, September 20, 2011.

Guyton, Arthur C., and John E. Hall. *Guyton and Hall Textbook of Medical Physiology.* 12th ed. Philadelphia: Saunders/Elsevier, 2011.

"Is Cardiac Hypertrophy Compensatory or Harmful?" *Medical Roundtable: Cardiovascular Edition* 2, no. 3 (2011): 149–156.

Kronenberg, Henry M., et al., eds. *Williams Textbook of Endocrinology.* 11th ed. Philadelphia: Saunders/Elsevier, 2008.

Marieb, Elaine N., and Katja Hoehn. *Human Anatomy and Physiology.* 9th ed. San Francisco: Pearson/Benjamin Cummings, 2010.

"Muscle Atrophy." *Health Library*, February 5, 2012.

Shier, David N., Jackie L. Butler, and Ricki Lewis. *Hole's Essentials of Human Anatomy and Physiology.* 10th ed. Boston: McGraw-Hill, 2009.

Shostak, Stanley. *Embryology: An Introduction to Developmental Biology.* New York: HarperCollins, 1991.

Tortora, Gerard J., and Bryan Derrickson. *Principles of Anatomy and Physiology.* 12th ed. Hoboken, N.J.: John Wiley & Sons, 2009.

HYPERVENTILATION

Disease/Disorder
Anatomy or system affected: Lungs, respiratory system
Specialties and related fields: Emergency medicine, pulmonary medicine
Definition: Breathing at a faster rate than what is needed for metabolism, resulting in the exhalation of carbon dioxide faster than it is produced.

Causes and Symptoms

Hyperventilation is rapid deep or quick shallow breathing, both of which can result in a dramatic decrease in carbon dioxide levels and an increase in the pH of the blood. While its purpose is an attempt to get more oxygen, hyperventilation can actually result in feeling breathless or dizzy and, in extreme cases, fainting.

There are several possible causes or reasons for hyperventilation, including anxiety, panic attacks, agoraphobia (fear of open spaces), depression, anger, and overconsumption of caffeine. Hyperventilation can also be a symptom of an underlying disease process such as an infection, bleeding, or heart and lung disorder, as well as a response to altitude exposure. Hyperventilation syndrome (HVS) can be manifested either acutely or chronically.

Chronic HVS can cause a variety of physical problems involving respiratory, cardiac, neurologic, or gastrointestinal (GI) systems. Aerophobia, a fear of fresh air, brings on the GI problems such as flatulence, bloating, and belching. Besides rapid breathing, hyperventilation can cause a fast pulse, shortness of breath, chest pain or tightening, dry mouth (from mouth breathing), numbness around the lips and hands, and, in more severe cases, blurred vision, seizures, and loss of consciousness. The chest pain resembles typical angina but does not usually respond to nitroglycerine. Changes in the patient's electrocardiogram (ECG) are common, including ST segment elevation or depression, T-wave inversion, or a prolonged QT interval. Patients with mitral valve prolapse are particularly susceptible to HVS. On occasion, hyperventilation can also be manifested with extreme agitation, tingling in the extremities, or painful hand and finger spasms. The chief characteristic of chronic HVS is multiple complaints without supporting physical evidence. Hence, classic hyperventilation is not readily apparent, but frequent sighing may be evidenced, along with chest wall tenderness, numbness, and tingling sensations. To rule out more serious conditions, arterial blood gases, toxicology screens, and chest X rays are suggested.

Hyperventilation is a technique purposefully used by swimmers and deep-sea divers to enable prolonged breath-holding. Many drownings have been related to this practice, however, because it can cause delayed unconsciousness underwater and subsequent death.

Treatment and Therapy

Contrary to popular belief, breathing into a paper bag to slow down respiration and retain carbon dioxide is not recommended as a treatment for hyperventilation because of the

---

Information on Hyperventilation

Causes: Anxiety, panic attacks, fear, depression, anger, caffeine overconsumption
Symptoms: Rapid deep or quick shallow breathing causing shortness of breath, fast pulse, chest pain or tightening, dry mouth, numbness around lips and hands, blurred vision, seizures, loss of consciousness
Duration: Acute or chronic
Treatments: Reassurance, removal of cause of anxiety; for severe, recurrent cases, antidepressants, beta-blockers, stress management classes, breathing retraining

---

potential life-threatening aggravation of a more serious medical problem such as hypoxia, a myocardial infarction (heart attack), pneumothorax, or pulmonary embolism.

After life-threatening causes of hyperventilation are eliminated, the most successful treatment for hyperventilation is reassurance, discussion of how hyperventilation is causing the patient's symptoms, and removal of the cause of the anxiety, if possible. Instructions from a respiratory therapist on proper abdominal diaphragmatic breathing are also helpful. A patient who faints should be placed flat on the floor with legs elevated. For more severe recurrent cases, antidepressants, beta-blockers, stress management classes, or breathing retraining have all been proven effective in reducing hyperventilation episodes.

—*Bonita L. Marks, Ph.D.*

See also Altitude sickness; Anxiety; Asphyxiation; Caffeine; Choking; Dizziness and fainting; Hypoxia; Lungs; Numbness and tingling; Panic attacks; Pulmonary medicine; Pulmonary medicine, pediatric; Respiration; Resuscitation; Unconsciousness; Wheezing.

For Further Information:

Bradley, Dinah. *Hyperventilation Syndrome: Breathing Pattern Disorders and How to Overcome Them.* Auckland: Random House NZ, 2012.
Callaham, M. "Hypoxic Hazards of Traditional Paper Bag Rebreathing in Hyperventilating Patients." *Annals of Emergency Medicine* 18, no. 6 (1989): 622–628.
Cowley, D. S., and P. P. Roy-Byrne. "Hyperventilation and Panic Disorder." *American Journal of Medicine* 83, no. 5 (1987): 929–937.
Fried, Robert Z. *Hyperventilation Syndrome Research And Clinical Treatment.* Baltimore: Johns Hopkins University Press, 1986.
Gardner, W. N. "The Pathophysiology of Hyperventilation Disorders." *Chest* 109, no. 2 (1996): 516–534.
Hearne, C. R. "Acupuncture in the Treatment of Anxiety in Hyperventilation Syndrome." *Journal of the Acupuncture Association of Chartered Physiotherpaists* (2011): 83–89.
McArdle, William, Frank I. Katch, and Victor L. Katch. *Exercise Physiology: Energy, Nutrition, and Human Performance.* 7th ed. Boston: Lippincott Williams & Wilkins, 2010.
Decuyper, Mieke. "The Relevance of Personality Assessment in Patients with Hyperventilation Symptoms." *Health Psychology* 31, no. 3 (2012): 316–322.

HYPNOSIS
Procedure

Anatomy or system affected: Brain, nervous system, psychic-emotional system

Specialties and related fields: Alternative medicine, anesthesiology, immunology, psychiatry, psychology

Definition: The induction of an altered state of consciousness.

Key terms:

hypnotherapy: a therapeutic method in which hypnosis works in conjunction with the psychotherapeutic process

hypnotic depth: a state frequently measured by the degree of suggestibility possessed by a presumably hypnotized individual

hypnotic induction: the production of hypnosis by means of precise rules and patterns (formal) or rules and patterns that permit limited flexibility (informal)

operator: the person who induces a hypnotic state; synonymous with "hypnotist" and "suggestor"

suggestion: a communication that evokes a nonvoluntary response reflecting the ideational content of the communication

Indications and Procedures

The term "hypnosis" comes from the Greek word *hypnos*, meaning sleep. While scientists and researchers do not understand the exact nature of hypnosis, theorists agree that it is an altered state of consciousness occurring on a continuum of awareness. Hypnosis may occur naturally and spontaneously, as in the case of a daydream. The daydreamer is alert and awake but focuses attention inward rather than outward.

The trance state, often synonymous with the hypnotic state, is characterized by an altered psychological state and minimal motor functioning. A trance can be recognized by the individual's glassy-eyed stare, lack of mobility, and unresponsiveness to external stimuli. A person in a trance state has a heightened receptivity to suggestion. Hypnosis, then, is a natural state that can be induced by another or by oneself (self-hypnosis) for a specific purpose. As a method of treatment, hypnosis, which is often used in conjunction with other approaches to alter psychophysiological states, promotes an understanding that allows for creative problem solving.

In the hypnotic state, the subject is not necessarily docile or submissive and may, because of unconscious processes, reject a suggestion given by even the most expert hypnotist. Four basic types of suggestion have been described: verbal, which includes words and any kind of sound; nonverbal, which applies to body language and gestures; intraverbal, which relates to the intonation of words; and extraverbal, which utilizes the implications of words and gestures that facilitate the acceptance of ideas. Suggestions are also described as being direct or indirect. Suggestibility is a behavior that is not hindered by the individual's logical processes but is enhanced by the subject's motivation, expectation, and trust in the operator as well as by the frequency and manner in which a suggestion is given.

Typically, prior to hypnosis, a subject is seated comfortably opposite or alongside the operator. The operator and subject generally have already discussed what will occur during the hypnotic process. The subject is encouraged to talk about his or her attitudes regarding hypnosis and the operator, as well as any previous experience with hypnosis. If the situation is a clinical one, a full psychiatric history and evaluation will already have been completed. For a positive hypnotic experience to emerge, a comfortable and trusting relationship between subject and operator must exist. There must be a willingness to undergo the experience on the part of the subject and a sensitive, observant, and supportive attitude on the part of the operator. Not all subjects are hypnotizable, but it is believed that most individuals, under appropriate circumstances, can respond to simple suggestions.

The induction process can be one of many types, ranging from directing the subject to close his or her eyes and think of a peaceful scene to having the subject gaze at a particular spot, shiny object, or swinging pendulum until the subject's eyes become heavy and close. Focusing on an object or scene leads the subject to redistribute his or her attention so as to withdraw it from the general surroundings and focus it on a circumscribed area. In the meantime, the subject is encouraged to relax and to allow events to unfold naturally. This induction procedure is sometimes followed, or even replaced, by what are described as "deepening techniques." The direction is given to imagine gradually descending a staircase or elevator or drifting on a boat past a slowly disappearing landscape. Counting forward or backward is another deepening or induction technique. Throughout this procedure, the operator offers comments or suggestions in a slow, repetitive, monotonous voice, exhorting the subject to feel relaxed and calm or to float and drift.

After a period generally lasting from one to several minutes, the operator gives the subject motor and sensory suggestions. For example, the operator may ask the subject to concentrate on the feelings in his or her fingers and hand, to feel the small muscles in the fingers begin to twitch and the arm and forearm begin to feel light. The operator states that these muscles will eventually feel so light that they will lift up off the armrest of the chair and, continually floating upward, ultimately reach the side of the subject's face. The operator might add that the higher the hand floats, the deeper the hypnosis will become, and the deeper the hypnosis becomes, the higher the hand will float. The operator then adds that when the hand reaches the side of the face, the subject will be deeply hypnotized.

When this point is reached, and the hand and arm have "levitated," the operator assumes that the subject is well hypnotized and then adds suggestions that are appropriate to the situation. Not all subjects, however, respond to hypnosis to the same extent or at the same rate.

There is no evidence to support the view that the operator in hypnosis is able to control the experience and behavior of the subject against the latter's wishes. It is the subject's motivation to behave in accordance with the wishes and directions of the operator that creates that erroneous impression. Moreover, there is no evidence to support the idea that a hypnotized subject can transcend his or her normal volitional capacity because of the hypnosis; despite persuasive clinical reports of altered somatic structures in hypnosis, no physiological changes uniquely associated with hypnosis have been demonstrated. Hypnosis is not so much a way of manipulating behavior as of creating increased perception and memory.

Uses and Complications

Because the mind, body, and emotions are interdependent, factors that influence one influence the others as well. The roles of the mind and emotions in functional or psychophysiological (psychosomatic) illness are widely recognized, but in cases of organic illness, their importance is often underestimated.

Regardless of etiology (causes), there are physical and psychological components to all illness. Emotional states that continue over extended periods can produce physiological changes. The fear, resentment, or depression that often accompanies illness may prolong or exacerbate it and interfere with a patient's willingness or ability to participate in treatment. Addressing such issues through hypnosis can greatly improve the overall medical management of a patient, from the initial diagnosis through all forms of treatment, including the treatment of unconscious and critically ill patients.

One advantage of modern clinical hypnosis is that it requires the practitioner to approach the patient as a whole person rather than as a collection of parts, one or more of which may be diseased. For the physician using hypnosis, a medical history goes beyond a list of past illnesses, allergies, and hospitalizations. A more comprehensive picture is developed that includes an understanding of a patient's personality, present state of mind, and life history and the positive aspects as well as the stresses and strains of the patient's present environment.

The use of hypnosis in most, if not all, medical specialties has been well documented. Hypnosis can be used alone or in combination with other approaches to overcome a variety of habit disorders. While some problems, such as thumb-sucking, can be resolved relatively quickly, others, such as overeating, sometimes require extended treatment or a multidimensional approach. Smoking and bed-wetting are examples of habit disorders that may be managed through hypnosis.

There is much evidence that children as a group are more responsive to hypnosis than adults and that infants and young children frequently experience hypnosis as a natural part of their lives. Children can often be helped in a remarkably short period of time. Hypnosis has been used with children in the treatment of such diverse ailments as bed-wetting, soiling, asthma, epilepsy, learning difficulties, some behavioral and delinquency problems, stuttering, and nail-biting.

Hypnosis has been used effectively as an adjunct to the treatment of numerous problems with autonomic (internal) nervous system components. For example, there have been many controlled studies and successful case reports on the use of hypnosis in the treatment of asthma, which is the most common of the psychophysiological respiratory disorders.

Through hypnosis, a patient may be helped to break the vicious cycle in which anxiety and emotional upsets can trigger an acute asthma attack, which in turn can produce anxiety and fear of other attacks.

Hypnosis has also been used effectively in the control and relief of pain. Because pain is experienced psychologically as well as physiologically, hypnosis can help people alter the perception of pain. A patient can learn to block pain to specific areas of the body, lessen the sensation of pain, or move pain from one area of the body to another. This ability is useful in the management of many types of pain, including chronic back pain, postoperative pain, and the pain associated with illness, migraine headache, burns, childbirth, and medical procedures.

In addition to being used to treat chronic conditions such as hypertension, hypnosis has been used to provide symptomatic relief of other chronic conditions, including hemophilia and musculoskeletal disorders such as rheumatoid arthritis, osteoarthritis, fractures, and bursitis.

Hypnosis has been used in dentistry for the relief of anxiety and pain and has been found to be helpful in teeth grinding (bruxism) and gagging. Modern hypnodontics is not primarily concerned with producing a surgical hypoanalgesia except in rare instances in which chemical anesthesia cannot be tolerated. The dentist is concerned with making visits to his or her office more tolerable and less threatening.

In obstetrics and surgery, hypnosis has been used to induce relaxation and relieve anxiety and to reduce the amount of anesthetic necessary. Occasionally, no anesthetic is required. This is sometimes desirable in childbirth, when the mother prefers to be aware of the birth process, or in surgical procedures in which a minimum of anesthetic is desirable.

Hypnosis has also been utilized by the police in what has been termed "investigative hypnosis." Witnesses to crimes are interrogated in an effort to improve their memory retrieval.

Hypnosis has also been helpful in increasing athletic effectiveness. It has been utilized by both team and individual athletes to increase self-confidence and other factors such as self-image and the ability to assess the competition. Hypnosis thus applied to maximize performance in sports has been very effective, but the principles involved are essentially no different from those applied to other areas of living, such as increasing the efficiency of performance in the home, school, or workplace.

Since the mid-1970s, there has been much research into immune system functioning. Studies of the effects of stress on immune system functioning are lending scientific support to anecdotal reports that indicate that hypnosis may be effective in altering the disease process in cancer and AIDS patients. Researchers have found that unless treatments for these illnesses are based on the premise that the mind, body, and emotions are all striving to achieve health, physical intervention alone (radiation or chemotherapy, for example) will not be effective.

Perspective and Prospects

Although medical hypnosis is considered to have had its beginnings with the Viennese physician Franz Anton Mesmer (1733–1815) in the latter half of the eighteenth century, hypnosis, or something very similar to it, has been practiced by religious and other healers in various ways for centuries in most cultures. The earliest evidence of its existence was found among shamans, who were also referred to as "witch doctors," "medicine men," or "healers."

In preparation for healing, a shaman adhered to certain practices that allowed his or her powers of concentration to be heightened. Placing himself or herself in isolation, the shaman began a descent into the "lower world." This often meant visualizing an opening in the earth and a journey downward into that opening. The journey was frequently accompanied by rhythmic drumming, chanting, singing, or dancing. The monotonous rhythm and constancy allowed the shaman's subconscious mind to become strongly focused, seek out the sick spirit of the patient, make it whole, and bring it back to the patient. The shaman actually engaged in a powerful process of visualization and suggestion during which the shaman willed the sick person to be healed.

In the eighteenth century, Mesmer recognized this ancient healing phenomenon and incorporated it into a theory of animal magnetism. Mesmer believed that a "cosmic fluid" could be stored in inanimate objects, such as magnets, and transferred to patients to cure them of illness.

Mesmer dressed flamboyantly. His consulting rooms were dimly lit and hung with mirrors, and he kept soft music playing in the background. The doctor's patients sat in a circle around a vat that contained such elements as powdered glass or iron filings. Then the patients grasped iron rods that were immersed in the vat and were believed to transmit a curing force.

Mesmer's first success was with a twenty-nine-year-old woman who suffered from a convulsive malady, a condition commonly called a "nervous disorder." Her symptoms consisted of blood rushing to her head and a tremendous pain in her ears and head. This state was followed by delirium, rage, vomiting, and fainting. During one of the woman's attacks, Mesmer applied three magnets to the patient's stomach and legs while she concentrated on the positive effects of the "cosmic fluid." In a short time, her symptoms subsided. When her symptoms resurfaced the next day, Mesmer gave her another treatment and achieved similar results. Mesmer believed that the "cosmic fluid," stimulated by the magnets, was directed through his patient's body. Her energy flow was restored, and as a result, she regained her health.

Eventually, Mesmer discarded the magnets. He began to regard himself as a magnet through which a fluid life force could be conducted and then transmitted to others as a healing force. This is what Mesmer described as "animal magnetism."

Despite the fact that no scientific evidence supported the existence of Mesmer's "cosmic fluids" or the concept of "animal magnetism," he had a tremendous rate of success. Thousands flocked to him for treatment. The only explanation for his success is that his patients were literally "mesmerized" into the belief and expectation that they would be cured. "Mesmerism" was a forerunner of the concept of hypnotic suggestion.

During this same period, a new slant on Mesmer's theories was introduced by one of his disciples, the marquis de Puységur. He believed that the "cosmic fluid" was not magnetic but electric. This electric fluid was generated in all living things—in plants as well as animals. Puységur used the natural environment to fill his patients with the healing electric fluid that was expected to end their suffering. His clinic was held outdoors, where the sick were received under an elm tree in the center of the village green. Puységur believed that the tree had an innate healing power and that the force would travel through the trunk and branches to cords that he hung from the tree. At the foot of the tree, patients sat in a circle on stone benches with the cords wrapped around the diseased parts of their bodies. They were "connected" to one another when they touched their thumbs together, which made it possible for the "fluid" to circulate from person to person and to heal.

During this activity, Puységur noticed a strange phenomenon. Some of the patients entered a state of deep sleep as a result of being mesmerized. In this state, the patient could still communicate and be lucid and responsive to the suggestions of the mesmerist. The marquis had discovered the hypnotic trance but had not identified it as such.

In the mid-nineteenth century, the hypnotic trance was used to relieve pain. An eminent London physician, John Elliotson (1791–1868), reported 1,834 surgical operations performed painlessly. In India, a Scottish surgeon named James Esdaile (1808–59) performed many major operations, such as amputation of limbs, using mesmerism (or, as he called it, "magnetic sleep") as the sole anesthetic. One procedure involved conditioning the patient weeks prior to surgery. This was accomplished by inducing a trance state in the patient and offering posthypnotic suggestions to numb the part of the body on which the surgery was to be performed. In a second method, the hypnotist attended to the patient in the operating room, inducing a trance state and suggesting disassociation from any pain. It was possible for the patient to be completely lucid during this state and also to be oblivious to pain, as though completely anesthetized.

Mesmerism continued to provoke new theories and uses. During the late nineteenth century, an English physician, James Braid (1795–1860), gave mesmerism a scientific explanation. He believed mesmerism to be a "nervous sleep" and coined the word "hypnosis," which was derived from the Greek word *hypnos*, meaning sleep. Braid showed that hypnotized subjects are often abnormally susceptible to impressions on the senses and that much of the subjects" behavior was caused by suggestions made verbally.

Soon, other theories began to emerge. Jean Martin Charcot (1825–93), a neurologist who taught in Paris, explained hypnosis as a state of hysteria and categorized it as an abnormal neurological activity.

In France, Auguste Ambroise Leibeault (1823–1904) and

Hippolyte Bernheim (1837–1919) were the first to regard hypnosis as a normal phenomenon. They asserted that expectation is the most important factor in the induction of hypnosis, that increased suggestibility is its essential symptom, and that the hypnotist works on the patient by means of mental influences.

As hypnosis began to receive serious study and be explained rationally, it began to gain acceptance in the scientific community. It was no longer relegated to the realm of the bizarre.

Sigmund Freud became interested in hypnosis at this same time and visited Leibeault and Bernheim's clinic to learn their induction techniques. As Freud observed patients enter a hypnotic state, he began to recognize the existence of the unconscious. Although he was not the first to make this observation, he was the first to recognize the unconscious as a major source of psychopathology. Early in his research, however, Freud rejected hypnosis as the tool to unlock repressed memories, favoring instead his technique of free association and dream interpretation. With the rise of psychoanalysis in the first half of the twentieth century, hypnosis declined in popularity.

Then, a reversal occurred. During World War II, interest in hypnosis was regenerated by the need for short-term therapy (often applied in cases of "battle fatigue") and by the combination of hypnosis and more traditional analytic approaches. Mind-control and "brainwashing" techniques that surfaced during the Korean War again sparked interest in the power of suggestion, especially when the subject was under duress. In the late 1960s and early 1970s, with the rise of public interest in alternative forms of mental health (such as Transcendental Meditation, biofeedback, and yoga) and ways of coping with the stress of the modern world, hypnosis experienced a rebirth. Researchers found new and potent uses for it in therapy, and the trance state began to be recognized as a highly effective tool for modifying behavior and for healing.

—*Genevieve Slomski, Ph.D.*

See also Alternative medicine; Anesthesia; Anesthesiology; Anxiety; Asthma; Bed-wetting; Brain; Meditation; Pain management; Psychiatry; Psychosomatic disorders; Stress; Stress reduction.

For Further Information:

Brown, Peter. *The Hypnotic Brain: Hypnotherapy and Social Communication*. New Haven, Conn.: Yale University Press, 1994.

Burrows, Graham D., Robb O. Stanley, and Peter B. Bloom, eds. *International Handbook of Clinical Hypnosis*. New York: Wiley, 2001.

Forrest, Derek. *Hypnotism: A History*. New York: Penguin, 2000.

"Hypnosis." *American Cancer Society*, November 1, 2008.

"Hypnosis." *Mayo Foundation for Medical Education and Research*, November 20, 2012.

"Hypnotherapy." *Health Library*, March 12, 2013.

Hadley, Josie, and Carol Staudacher. *Hypnosis for Change*. 3d ed. New York: Ballantine Books, 2000.

Yapko, Michael D. *Trancework: An Introduction to the Practice of Clinical Hypnosis*. 4th ed. New York: Routledge, 2012.

Zahourek, Rothlyn P., ed. *Clinical Hypnosis and Therapeutic Suggestion in Patient Care*. New York: Brunner/Mazel, 1990.

HYPOCHONDRIASIS
Disease/Disorder

Also known as: Hypochondriacal neurosis or hypochondriacal reaction

Anatomy or system affected: Psychic-emotional system, all bodily systems

Specialties and related fields: Psychiatry, psychology

Definition: Unwarranted belief about or anxiety over having a serious disease that is based on one's subjective interpretation of physical symptoms or sensations; the belief or anxiety is maintained in spite of appropriate medical assurances that there is no serious disease.

Key terms:

defense mechanisms: automatic, unconscious mental processes that become activated in the presence of emotional distress and anxiety; these processes work to maintain inner harmony by preventing mental awareness of that which would be otherwise too emotionally painful to endure

hypochondria: an earlier term for hypochondriasis; from classical Greek, it means the abdominal region of the body below the rib cage, from which black bile was believed to cause melancholy and yellow bile was believed to cause ill-temper

hypochondriacal neurosis: an earlier, but still-used, term for hypochondriasis; because experts have disagreed about what "neurosis" means precisely, the term is considered less descriptive than "hypochondriasis"

hypochondriacal reaction: another earlier term for hypochondriasis; experts who still prefer this term view hypochondriasis as a transient reaction to life stress and tend not to see it as a mental-emotional disorder in its own right

primary hypochondriasis: hypochondriasis as a disorder in its own right, and not accompanied by another psychiatric disorder such as generalized anxiety or panic

secondary hypochondriasis: the experience of hypochondriacal symptoms as part of an underlying, causal condition such as panic disorder, generalized anxiety disorder, schizophrenia, or major depression with psychotic features

somatization disorder: the somatoform disorder most similar to hypochondriasis; in somatization, the preoccupation is primarily with symptoms that one experiences and not with a disease that one is fearful of getting, an important distinction when these conditions are treated

somatoform disorders: the grouping of disorders that includes hypochondriasis; these disorders feature symptoms that suggest physical disease but that are actually caused by psychological upset

Causes and Symptoms

With hypochondriasis, the real problem is the patient's excessive worry and mental preoccupation with having or developing a disease, not the disease about which the patient is so worried. While concern about contracting a serious disease is

Information on Hypochondriasis

Causes: Psychological disorders
Symptoms: Excessive worry, endless rumination, and obsessive interpretation of symptoms and sensations; impaired normal activity; chronic persistance despite appropriate medical reassurances and contrary evidence
Duration: Chronic, although at times temporary
Treatments: Psychotherapy, limited drug therapy

common and normal and may even make one more prudent, excessive worry, endless rumination, and obsessive interpretation of every symptom and sensation can disable and prevent effective functioning. A diagnosis of hypochondriasis is made when the patient's dread about a disease or diseases impairs normal activity and persists despite appropriate medical reassurances and evidence to the contrary. Even though hypochondriacs can acknowledge intellectually the possibility that their fears might be without rational foundation, the acknowledgment itself fails to bring any relief.

Researchers estimate that 3 to 14 percent of all medical (versus psychiatric) patients have hypochondriasis. Just how prevalent it is in the population as a whole is unknown. What is known is that the disorder shows up slightly more in men than in women, starts at any age but most often between twenty and thirty, shows up most often in physicians" offices with patients who are in their forties and fifties, and tends to run in families.

Most clinicians believe that hypochondriasis has a primary psychological cause or causes but that in general, hypochondriacs have only a vague awareness that they are doing something that perpetuates and worsens their hypochondriacal symptoms. Hypochondriacs do not feign illness; they genuinely believe themselves to be sick or about to become so.

Clinicians usually favor one of four hypotheses about how hypochondriasis starts. The hypotheses are based on anecdotal, clinical experience with patients who have gotten better when treated specifically for hypochondriasis. Researchers have rarely studied hypochondriasis using strict experimental methods. Nevertheless, the anecdotal evidence is important because it gives clinicians a way to think about how to treat the condition.

The most popular belief among mental health professionals is that hypochondriacs have a deep-seated anger. Because their life experience is of hurt, disappointment, rejection, and loss, they engage in a two-stage process. Though many believe themselves to be unlovable and unacceptable as they are, they solicit attention and care by presenting themselves either as ill or as dangerously close to becoming ill. Endless worry and rumination soon render ineffective others" concern. No amount of reassurance allays their preoccupation and anxiety. In this way, those moved to show concern tire, grow impatient, and finally give up their efforts to help, proving to the worried hypochondriacs that no one really does care about them after all. Meanwhile, the hypochondriacs

remain sad and angry.

This view often assumes that hypochondriasis is actually a form of defense mechanism that transfers angry, hostile, and critical feelings felt toward others into physical symptoms and signs of disease. Because hypochondriacs find it too difficult to admit that they feel angry, isolated, and unloved, they hide from the emotional energy associated with these powerful feelings and transfer them into bodily symptoms. This process seems to occur most often when hypochondriacal people harbor feelings of reproach because they are bereaved and lonely. In effect, they are angry at being left alone and left uncared for, and they redirect the emotion inwardly as self-reproach manifested in physical complaints.

Others hypothesize that hypochondriasis enables those who either believe themselves to be basically bad and unworthy of happiness or feel guilty for being alive ("existential guilt") to atone for their wrongdoings and, thereby, undo the guilt that they are always fighting not to feel. The mental anguish, emotional sadness, and physical pain so prevalent in hypochondriasis make reparation for the patients" real, exaggerated, or imagined badness.

A third view is sociological in orientation. Health providers who endorse it see hypochondriasis as society's way of letting people who feel frightened and overwhelmed by life's challenges escape from having to face those challenges, even if temporarily. Hypochondriacs take on a "sick role," which removes societal expectations that they will face responsibilities. In presenting themselves to the world as too sick to function, they also present themselves as excused from doing so. A schoolchild's stomachache on the day of a big test provides a relatively common and potentially harmless example of this role at work. Non-physically disabled adults who seek refuge from life stress by staying in bed and who find themselves with true physical paralysis years later provide a more serious and regrettable example.

A fourth view utilizes some experimental data that suggest that hypochondriacal people may have lower thresholds for (and lower tolerances of) emotional and physical pain. The data suggest that hypochondriacs experience physical and/or emotional sensations that are a magnification of what is normal experience. Thus, a sensation that would be sinus pressure for most people would be experienced as severe sinus headache in the hypochondriac. Hypersensitivity (lower threshold) to bodily sensations keeps hypochondriacs ever on watch for these upsetting, intense sensations because of how amplified the physical and emotional experiences are. What seems to most people an exaggerated concern with symptoms is simply prudent, self-protective vigilance to hypochondriacs.

Regardless of why the disorder develops, the majority of hypochondriacs go to their physicians with concerns about stomach and intestinal problems or heart and blood circulation problems. These complaints are usually only part of broader concerns about other organ systems and other anatomical locations. The key clinical feature of the disorder of hypochondriasis, however, is not where and how many bodily complaints there are but the patients" belief that they are seriously sick, or are just about to become so, and that the disease has yet to be detected. Laboratory tests that reveal healthy organs, physician reassurances that they are well, and long periods in which the dreaded disease fails to manifest itself are not reassuring at all. Hypochondriacs seem genuinely unable not to worry.

Hypochondriacs typically present their medical history in great detail and at great length. Often, they have an elaborate, exotic, and complex pathophysiological theory to explain how they acquired the disease and what it is doing, or will soon do, to them. At times, they cite recent research and give great importance to other causes, tests, or treatments that they and their health providers have not yet tried. Because their actual problem is not, strictly speaking, medical (or not only medical) and because they usually frustrate professional caretakers such as physicians, as well as nonprofessional caretakers such as family and friends, breakdown in the helping process is common. Worried patients tax physicians" time and resources, while busy physicians feel increasingly drained for what they believe is no good reason. The hypochondriacal patients sense that their concerns are not respected or taken seriously; they start to sense resentment. Phone calls to physicians" offices go unreturned for longer and longer periods. The perceived lack of access to their health providers serves to increase a hypochondriac's worry and stress. The physicians increasingly believe that these patients are unappreciative—that they are, in fact, healthy and that they are not cooperating with treatment goals. Instead, hypochondriacal patients are seen as excessively demanding. Anger builds on both sides, relationships deteriorate, and the hypochondriac begins to "doctor-shop," while the physicians lose them as patients.

Although hypochondriasis is usually chronic, with periods in which it is more and less severe, temporary hypochondriacal reactions are also commonly seen. Such reactions most often occur when patients have experienced a death or serious illness of someone close to them or some other major life stressor, including their own recovery from a life-threatening illness.

When these reactions persist for less than six months, the technical diagnosis is a condition called "somatoform disorder not otherwise specified." When external stressors cause the reaction, the hypochondriacal symptoms usually remit when the stressors dissipate or are resolved. The important exception to this rule occurs when family, friends, or health professionals inadvertently reinforce the worry and preoccupation through inappropriate amounts of attention. In effect, they reward hypochondriacal behavior and increase the likelihood that it will persist. A mother may never have received more support and help at home than following breast cancer surgery. A father may never have felt his children's affection as much as when he recuperated from having a heart attack. An employee may have never obtained special allowances on the job or received so many calls from coworkers as when recovering from herniated disk surgery. A student may never have gotten as special treatment or as many gifts from teammates as when treated for rheumatic fever. What began as a

transient hypochondriacal reaction can become chronic, primary hypochondriasis.

The life of hypochondriacs is unhappy and unrewarding. Nervous tension, depression, hopelessness, and a general lack of interest in life mark the fabric of the hypochondriacs" daily routines. Actual clinical, depressive disorders can easily coexist with hypochondriasis to the point that even antidepression medications will simultaneously alleviate hypochondriacal symptoms.

Hypochondriasis often accompanies physical illness in the elderly. As a group, the elderly have declining health, experience diminished physical capacities, and are at increased risk for contracting and developing disease. Earlier tendencies toward hypochondriasis sometimes intensify with age with the condition first appearing in old age. Hypochondriasis is not, however, a typical or expected aspect of normal aging; most elderly people are not hypochondriacal. In those who are, however, hypochondriasis is most likely a symptom of depression, abandonment, or loneliness, which are the conditions that should first be treated.

Treatment and Therapy

The most important aspect of treating hypochondriasis is assessing whether true organic disease exists. Many diseases in their early stages are diffuse and affect multiple organ systems. Neurologic diseases (such as multiple sclerosis), hormonal abnormalities (such as Graves' disease), and autoimmune/connective tissue diseases (such as systemic lupus) can all manifest themselves in ways that are difficult to diagnose accurately. The frantic and obsessive reporting of hypochondriacal patients can just as easily be the worried and detailed reporting of patients with early parathyroid disease; both report symptoms that are multiple, vague, and diffuse. The danger of hypochondriasis lies in its being diagnosed in place of true organic disease, which is exactly the kind of event hypochondriacs fear will happen.

Of course, there is nothing to prevent someone with true hypochondriasis from getting or having true physical illness. Worrying about illness neither protects from nor prevents illness. Moreover, barring a sudden, lethal accident or event, every hypochondriac is bound to develop organic illness sooner or later. Physical illness can coexist with hypochondriasis—and does so when attitudes, symptoms, and mental and emotional states are extreme and disproportionate to the medical problem at hand.

The goal in treating hypochondriasis is care, not cure. These patients have an ongoing mental illness or chronic maladaptation and seem to need physical symptoms to justify how they feel. Neither surgical nor medical interventions will ameliorate a psychological need for symptoms. The best treatments when hypochondriasis cannot itself be the target of treatment are long term in orientation and seek to help patients tolerate and accommodate their symptoms while health providers learn to understand and adapt.

Medications have proved useful in treating hypochondriasis only when accompanied by pharmacotherapy-sensitive conditions such as major depression or generalized anxiety. When hypochondriasis coexists with either mental or physical disease, the latter must be treated in its own right. Secondary hypochondriasis means that the primary disorder warrants primary treatment.

The course of hypochondriasis is unclear. Clinicians" anecdotal experience tends to endorse the perception that hypochondriacs are impossible as patients. Outcome studies, however, belie the pessimism. The research suggests that many who are treated get better, especially if also treated for secondary conditions such as coexisting anxiety or depressive disorder.

A fifty-six-year-old married male, for example, recounted his history as never having been in really good health at any time in his life. He made many physician office visits and had, over the years, seen many physicians, though without ever feeling emotionally connected to them. Over the past several months, he felt increasingly concerned that he was having headaches "all over" his head and that they were caused by an undetected tumor in the middle of his brain, "where no X ray could detect it." He had read about magnetic resonance imaging (MRI) in a health letter to which he subscribed and said that he wanted this procedure performed "to catch the tumor early." Various prescribed medications for his headache usually brought no relief.

While productive at work and promoted several times, he had been passed over for his last promotion because, he believed, his superiors did not like him. He also stated that he believed that many on the job saw him as cynical and pessimistic but that no one appreciated the "pain and mental anxiety" he endured "day in and day out."

His spouse of thirty-two years had advanced significantly at a job she had begun ten years earlier, and she seemed to him to be closer to their three children than he was. She was increasingly involved with outside voluntary activities, which kept her quite busy. She reported that she often asked him to join her in at least some of her activities, but he always said no. She said that when she arrived home late, he was often in a state of physical upset for which she could never seem to do the "right thing to help him." In their joint interview, each admitted often feeling angry at and frustrated with the other. She could never determine why he was sick so often and why her efforts to help only seemed to make his situation worse. He could not understand how she could leave him all alone feeling as physically bad as he did. He believed that she never seemed to worry that something might happen to him while she was out being "a community do-gooder." The husband was suffering from a classic case of hypochondriasis.

Perspective and Prospects

The term *hypochondriasis* has ancient origins and reflects a view that all persons are subject to their own humoral ebb and flow. Humors were once thought to be bodily fluids that maintained health, regulated physical functioning, and caused certain personality traits. In classical Greek, *hypochondria*, the plural of *hypochondrion*, referred to both a part of the anatomy and the condition known today as hypochondriasis. *Hypo* means "under," "below," or "

beneath," and *chondrion* means literally "cartilage" but in this case refers specifically to the bottom tip of cartilage at the breastbone (the xiphoid or, more formally, xiphisternum). Here, below the breastbone but above the navel, two humors were thought to flow in excess in the hypochondriacal person. The liver, producing black bile, made people melancholic, depressed, and depressing; the spleen, producing yellow bile, made people bilious, cross, and cynical. This view, or a variant of it, persisted until the late eighteenth century.

Sigmund Freud and other psychiatrists treated hypochondriacal symptoms with some success while approaching the disorder as a defense mechanism rather than as an excess of bodily fluids. Their treatment for the first time cast a psychological role for what had been seen as a physical problem. Mental health professionals whose theoretical orientation is psychoanalytic or psychodynamic continue to deal with hypochondriasis as they deal with other defense mechanisms.

In the 1970s, some researchers began to suggest that hypochondriasis was being incorrectly applied to describe a discrete disorder. They argued that hypochondriasis is not a true diagnosis. Other researchers disagreed and argued for differentiating between primary and secondary hypochondriasis. Their view has proved to have significant pragmatic utility in treating the wide range of patients who exhibit symptoms of hypochondriasis, and it remains the prevailing view.

Given the general unwillingness of patients with hypochondriasis to admit that they have a psychological problem and not some yet-to-be-found organic condition, the interpersonal difficulties that often arise between health providers and these patients and the serious potential of concurrent organic disease, it is not surprising why hypochondriasis continues to challenge both persons afflicted with this disorder and those who treat them.

—Paul Moglia, Ph.D.

See also Antianxiety drugs; Anxiety; Bipolar disorders; Body dysmorphic disorder; Depression; Factitious disorders; Midlife crisis; Neurosis; Obsessive-compulsive disorder; Over-the-counter medications; Panic attacks; Phobias; Psychiatric disorders; Psychiatry; Psychiatry, child and adolescent; Psychiatry, geriatric; Psychosomatic disorders; Signs and symptoms; Stress; Stress reduction.

For Further Information:
Abramowitz, Jonathan S., and Autumn E. Braddock. Hypochondriasis and Health Anxiety. Cambridge, Mass.: Hogrefe, 2011.

Asmundson, Gordon J. G., et al., eds. *Health Anxiety: Clinical and Research Perspectives on Hypochondriasis and Related Conditions*. New York: Wiley, 2001.

Barsky, Arthur J. "Somatoform Disorders." In *Kaplan and Sadock's Comprehensive Textbook of Psychiatry.* Vol. 1, edited by Harold I. Kaplan and Benjamin J. Sadock. 8th ed. Baltimore: Wolters Kluwer/Williams & Wilkins, 2005.

Belling, Catherine. *A Condition of Doubt: The Meanings of Hypochondria.* New York: Oxford University Press, 2012.

Ben-Tovim, David I., and Adrian Esterman. "Zero Progress with Hypochondriasis." *The Lancet* 352 9143. (December 5, 1998): 1798–1799.

De Jong, Peter J., Marie-Anne Haenen, Anton Schmidt, and Birgit Mayer. "Hypochondriasis: The Role of Fear-Confirming Reasoning." *Behaviour Research and Therapy* 36 . 1 (January, 1998): 65–74.

Hill, John. *Hypochondriasis: A Practical Treatise on the Nature and Cure of that Disorder.* 1766. New York: Wildside Press, 2011.

Randall, Brian. "Hypochondria." *Health Library*, November 26, 2011.

Starcevic, Vladen, and Don R. Lipsitt, eds. *Hypochondriasis: Modern Perspectives on an Ancient Malady.* New York: Oxford University Press, 2001.

Vorvick, Linda J. "Hypochondria." *MedlinePlus*, September 19, 2012.

HYPOGLYCEMIA
Disease/Disorder

Anatomy or system affected: Blood, endocrine system, glands

Specialties and related fields: Endocrinology, family medicine, hematology, internal medicine, serology

Definition: The condition in which concentration of glucose in the blood is too low to meet the needs of key organs, especially the brain; this condition limits treatments for diabetes mellitus.

Key terms:

fasting hypoglycemia: hypoglycemia that occurs when no food is available from the intestinal tract; usually caused by failure of the neural, hormonal, and/or enzymatic mechanisms that convert stored fuels (primarily glycogen) into glucose

glucagon: a pancreatic hormone that signals an elevated concentration of glucose in the circulation

gluconeogenesis: the synthesis of molecules of glucose from smaller carbohydrates and amino acids

glucose: a simple sugar, readily converted to metabolic energy by most cells of the body and essential for the welfare of brain cells

glycogen: a storage form of carbohydrate, composed of many molecules of glucose linked together; is found in many tissues of the body and serves as a major source of circulating glucose

glycogenolysis: the cleavage of glycogen into its constituent molecules of glucose

hypoglycemic unawareness: the occurrence of hypoglycemia without the warning symptoms of trembling, palpitations, hunger, or anxiety

hypoglycemic unresponsiveness: inadequate recovery of the circulating glucose concentration after an episode of hypoglycemia

insulin: a pancreatic hormone that signals a reduced concentration of glucose in the circulation

neuroglycopenia: abnormal function of the brain, caused by an inadequate supply of glucose from the circulation

reactive hypoglycemia: hypoglycemia that occurs within a few hours after ingestion of a meal

Causes and Symptoms

The condition known as hypoglycemia exists when the concentration of glucose in the bloodstream is too low to meet

Information on Hypoglycemia

Causes: Endocrine disorder, malnutrition, advanced stages of cancer, inherited metabolic disorders, severe infections (including overwhelming bacterial infection and malaria), certain drugs

Symptoms: Trembling, pallor, palpitations and rapid heartbeat, sweating, abdominal discomfort, feelings of anxiety and/or hunger, disturbed thoughts, confusion, loss of normal control of behavior, headache, lethargy, impaired vision, abnormal speech

Duration: Temporary to long-term

Treatments: Drugs inhibiting secretion of insulin, hormonal therapy

bodily needs for fuel, particularly those of the brain. Ordinarily, physiological compensatory mechanisms are called into play when the circulating concentration of glucose falls below about 3.5 millimoles. Activation of the sympathetic nervous system and the secretion of glucagon are especially important in promoting glycogenolysis and gluconeogenesis. Symptoms of sympathetic nervous activation normally become apparent with glucose concentrations that are less than about 3 millimoles. Brain function is usually demonstrably abnormal at glucose concentrations below about 2 millimoles; sustained hypoglycemia in this range can lead to permanent brain damage.

Some of the symptoms of hypoglycemia occur as by-products of activation of the sympathetic nervous system. These symptoms include trembling, pallor, palpitations and rapid heartbeat, sweating, abdominal discomfort, and feelings of anxiety and/or hunger. These symptoms are not dangerous in themselves; in fact, they may be considered to be beneficial, as they alert the individual of the need to obtain food. Meanwhile, the sympathetic nervous system signals compensatory mechanisms. The manifestations of abnormal brain function during hypoglycemia include blunting of higher cognitive functions, disturbed mentation, confusion, loss of normal control of behavior, headache, lethargy, impaired vision, abnormal speech, paralysis, neurologic deficits, coma, and epileptic seizures. The individual is usually unaware of the appearance of these symptoms, which can present real danger. For example, episodes of hypoglycemia have occurred while individuals were driving motor vehicles, which can lead to serious injury and death. After recovery from hypoglycemia, the patient may have no memory of the episode.

There are two major categories of hypoglycemia: fasting and reactive. The most serious, fasting hypoglycemia, represents impairment of the mechanisms responsible for the production of glucose when food is not available. These mechanisms include the functions of cells in the liver and brain that monitor the availability of circulating glucose. Additionally, there is a coordinated hormonal response involving the secretion of glucagon, growth hormone, and other hormones and the inhibition of the secretion of insulin. The normal consequences of these processes include the addition of glucose to the circulation, primarily from glycogenolysis, as well as a slowing of the rate of utilization of circulating glucose by many tissues of the body, especially the liver, skeletal and cardiac muscle, and fat. Even after days without food, the body normally avoids hypoglycemia through breakdown of stored proteins and activation of gluconeogenesis. There is considerable redundancy in the systems that maintain glucose concentration, so the occurrence of hypoglycemia often reflects the presence of defects in more than one of these mechanisms.

The other category of hypoglycemia, reactive hypoglycemia, includes disorders in which there is disproportionately prolonged and/or great activity of the physiologic systems that normally cause storage of the glucose derived from ingested foods. When a normal person eats a meal, the passage of food through the stomach and intestines elicits a complex and well-orchestrated neural and hormonal response, culminating in the secretion of insulin from the beta cells of the islets of Langerhans in the pancreas. The insulin signals the cells in muscle, adipose tissue, and the liver to stop producing glucose and to derive energy from glucose obtained from the circulation. Glucose in excess of the body's immediate needs for fuel is taken up and stored as glycogen or is utilized for the manufacture of proteins. Normally, the signals for the uptake and storage of glucose reach their peak of activity simultaneously with the entry into the circulation of glucose from the food undergoing digestion. As a result, the concentration of glucose in the circulation fluctuates only slightly. In individuals with reactive hypoglycemia, however, the entry of glucose from the digestive tract and the signals for its uptake and storage are not well synchronized. When signals for the cellular uptake of glucose persist after the intestinally derived glucose has dissipated, hypoglycemia can result. Although the degree of hypoglycemia may be severe and potentially dangerous, recovery can take place without assistance if the individual's general nutritional state is adequate and the systems for activation of glycogenolysis and gluconeogenesis are intact.

Diagnosis and Treatment

The diagnostic evaluation of an individual who is suspected of having hypoglycemia begins with verification of the condition. Evaluation of a patient's symptoms can be confusing. On one hand, the symptoms arising from the sympathetic nervous system and those of neuroglycopenia may occur in a variety of nonhypoglycemic conditions. On the other hand, persons with recurrent hypoglycemia may have few or no obvious symptoms. Therefore, it is most important to document the concentration of glucose in the blood.

To establish the diagnosis of fasting hypoglycemia, the patient is kept without food for periods of time, up to seventy-two hours, with frequent monitoring of the blood glucose. Should hypoglycemia occur, blood is taken for measurements of the key regulatory neurosecretions and hormones, including insulin, glucagon, growth hormone, cortisol, and epinephrine, as well as general indices of the function of the liver and kidneys. If there is suspicion of an abnormality in an enzyme involved in glucose production, the diagnosis can be confirmed by measurement of the relevant enzymatic activity in circulating blood cells or, if necessary, in a biopsy specimen of the liver.

Fasting hypoglycemia may be caused by any condition that inhibits the production of glucose or that causes an inappropriately great utilization of circulating glucose when food is not available. Insulin produces hypoglycemia through both of these mechanisms. Excessive circulating insulin ranks as one of the most important causes of fasting hypoglycemia, most cases of which result from the treatment of diabetes mellitus with insulin or with an oral drug of the sulfonylurea class. If the patient is known to be taking insulin or a sulfonylurea drug for diabetes, the cause of hypoglycemia is obvious; appropriate modification of the treatment should be made. Hypoglycemia caused by oral sulfonylureas is particularly troublesome because of the prolonged retention of these drugs in the body. The passage of several days may be required for recovery, during which time the patient needs continuous intravenous infusion of glucose.

Excessive insulin secretion may also result from increased numbers of pancreatic beta cells; the abnormal beta cells may be so numerous that they form benign or malignant tumors, called insulinomas. The preferred treatment of an insulinoma is surgery, if feasible. When the tumor can be removed surgically, the operation is often curative. Unfortunately, insulinomas are sometimes difficult for the surgeon to find. Magnetic resonance imaging (MRI), computed tomography (CT) scanning, ultrasonography, or angiography may help localize the tumor. Some insulinomas are multiple and/or malignant, rendering total removal impossible. In these circumstances, hypoglycemia can be relieved by drugs that inhibit the secretion of insulin.

Malignant tumors arising from various tissues of the body may produce hormones that act like insulin with respect to their effects on glucose metabolism. In some cases, these hormones are members of the family of insulin-like growth factors, which resemble insulin structurally. Malnutrition probably has an important role in predisposing patients with malignancy to hypoglycemia, which tends to occur when the cancer is far advanced.

Fasting hypoglycemia can be caused by disorders affecting various parts of the endocrine system. One such disorder is adrenal insufficiency; continued secretion of cortisol by the adrenal cortex is required for maintenance of normal glycogen stores and of the enzymes of glycogenolysis and gluconeogenesis. Severe hypothyroidism also may lead to hypoglycemia. Impairment in the function of the anterior pituitary gland predisposes a patient to hypoglycemia through several mechanisms, including reduced function of the thyroid gland and adrenal cortices (which depend on pituitary secretions for normal activity) and reduced secretion of growth hormone. Growth hormone plays an important physiologic role in the prevention of fasting hypoglycemia by signaling metabolic changes that allow heart and skeletal muscles to derive energy from stored fats, thereby sparing glucose for the brain. Specific replacement therapies are available for deficiencies of thyroxine, cortisol, and growth hormone.

Hypoglycemia has occasionally been reported as a side effect of treatment with medications other than those intended for treatment of diabetes. Drugs that have been implicated include sulfonamides, used for treatment of bacterial infections; quinine, used for treatment of falciparum malaria; pentamidine isethionate, given by injection for treatment of pneumocystosis; ritodrine, used for inhibition of premature labor; and propranolol or disopyramide, both of which are used for treatment of cardiac arrhythmias. Malnourished patients seem to be especially susceptible to the hypoglycemic effects of these medications, and management should consist of nutritional repletion in addition to discontinuation of the drug responsible. In children, aspirin or other medicines containing salicylates may produce hypoglycemia.

Alcohol hypoglycemia occurs in persons with low bodily stores of glycogen when there is no food in the intestine. In this circumstance, the only potential source of glucose for the brain is gluconeogenesis. When such an individual drinks alcohol, its metabolism within the liver prevents the precursors of glucose from entering the pathways of gluconeogenesis. This variety of fasting hypoglycemia can occur in persons who are not chronic alcoholics: It requires the ingestion of only a moderate amount of alcohol, on the order of three mixed drinks. Treatment involves the nutritional repletion of glycogen stores and the limitation of alcohol intake.

Severe infections, including overwhelming bacterial infection and malaria, can produce hypoglycemia by mechanisms that are not well understood. Patients with very severe liver damage can develop fasting hypoglycemia, because the pathways of glycogenolysis and gluconeogenesis in the liver are by far the major sources of circulating glucose in the fasted state. In such cases, the occurrence of hypoglycemia usually marks a near-terminal stage of liver disease. Uremia, the syndrome produced by kidney failure, can also lead to fasting hypoglycemia.

Some types of fasting hypoglycemia occur predominantly in infants and children. Babies in the first year of life may have an inappropriately high secretion of insulin. This problem occurs especially in newborn infants whose mothers had increased circulating glucose during pregnancy. Children from two to ten years of age may develop ketotic hypoglycemia, which is probably related to insufficient gluconeogenesis. These disorders tend to improve with time. Fasting hypoglycemia is also an important manifestation of a variety of inherited disorders of metabolism characterized by the abnormality or absence of one of the necessary enzymes or cofactors of glycogenolysis and gluconeogenesis or of fat metabolism (which supplies the energy for gluconeogenesis). Most of these disorders become evident in infancy or childhood. If there is a hereditary or acquired deficiency of an enzyme of glucose production, the problem can be circumvented by provision of a continuous supply of glucose to the affected individual.

There are several other rare causes of fasting hypoglycemia. A few individuals have had circulating antibodies that caused hypoglycemia by interacting with the patient's own insulin or with receptors for insulin on the patient's cells. Although the autonomic (involuntary) nervous system has an important role in signaling recovery from hypoglycemia, diseases affecting this branch of the nervous system do not usually produce hypoglycemia; presumably, hormonal mechanisms can substitute for the missing neural signals.

Reactive hypoglycemia can occur with an unusually rapid passage of foodstuffs through the upper intestinal tract, such as may occur after partial or total removal of the stomach. Persons predisposed to maturity-onset diabetes may also have reactive hypoglycemia, probably because of the delay in the secretion of insulin in response to a meal. Finally, reactive hypoglycemia need not indicate the presence of any identifiable disease and may occur in otherwise normal individuals.

Diagnosis of reactive hypoglycemia is made difficult by the variability of symptoms and of glucose concentrations from day to day. Adding to the diagnostic uncertainty, circulating glucose normally rises and falls after meals, especially those rich in carbohydrates. Consequently, entirely normal and asymptomatic individuals may sometimes have glucose concentrations at or below the levels found in persons with reactive hypoglycemia. Therefore, the glucose tolerance test, in which blood samples are taken at intervals for several hours after the patient drinks a solution containing 50 to 100 grams of glucose, is quite unreliable and should not be employed for the diagnosis of reactive hypoglycemia. Proper diagnosis of reactive hypoglycemia depends on careful correlation of the patient's symptoms with the circulating glucose level, preferably measured on several occasions after ingestion of ordinary meals. Some persons develop symptoms such as weakness, nausea, sweating, and tremulousness after meals, but without a significant reduction of circulating glucose. This symptom complex should not be confused with hypoglycemia.

When rapid passage of food through the stomach and upper intestine causes reactive hypoglycemia, the administration of drugs that slow intestinal transit may be helpful. When reactive hypoglycemia has no evident pathological cause, the patient is usually advised to take multiple small meals throughout the day instead of the usual three meals and to avoid concentrated sweets. These dietary modifications can help avoid hypoglycemia by reducing the stimulus to secrete insulin.

Two rare inherited disorders of metabolism can produce reactive hypoglycemia after the ingestion of certain foods. In hereditary fructose intolerance, the offending nutrient is fructose, a sugar found in fruits as well as ordinary table sugar. In galactosemia, the sugar responsible for hypoglycemia is galactose, a major component of milk products. Management of these conditions, which usually become apparent in infancy or childhood, consists of avoidance of the foods responsible.

Perspective and Prospects

Fasting hypoglycemia is uncommon, except in the context of treatment of diabetes mellitus. The most serious public health problem associated with hypoglycemia is that it limits the therapeutic effectiveness of insulin and sulfonylurea drugs. Evidence suggests that elevation of the circulating glucose concentration (hyperglycemia) is responsible for much of the disability and premature death among patients withdiabetes. In many of these patients, therapeutic regimens consisting of multiple daily injections of insulin or continuous infusion of insulin through a small needle placed under the skin can reduce the average circulating glucose to normal. Frequent serious hypoglycemia is the most important adverse consequence of such regimens. Persons with diabetes seem to be at especially high risk for dangerous hypoglycemia for two reasons. First, there is often a failure of the warning systems that ordinarily cause uncomfortable symptoms when the circulating glucose concentration declines, a situation termed *hypoglycemic unawareness*. As a consequence, when a patient with diabetes attempts to control his or her blood sugar with more frequent injections of insulin, there may occur unheralded episodes of hypoglycemia that can lead to serious alterations in mental activity or even loss of consciousness. Many patients with diabetes also have hypoglycemic unresponsiveness, an impaired ability to recover from episodes of hypoglycemia. Also, diabetes can interfere with the normal physiologic responses that cause the secretion of glucagon in response to a reduction of circulating glucose, thus eliminating one of the most important defenses against hypoglycemia. If both hypoglycemic unawareness and hypoglycemic unresponsiveness could be reversed, intensive treatment of diabetes would become safer and more widely applicable.

Reactive hypoglycemia, although seldom a clue to serious disease, has attracted public attention because of its peculiarly annoying symptoms. These symptoms, which reflect activation of the sympathetic nervous system, resemble those of fear and anxiety. The symptoms are not specific, and many patients with these complaints do not have hypoglycemia.

In summary, hypoglycemia indicates defective regulation of the supply of energy to the body. When severe or persistent, hypoglycemia can lead to serious behavioral disorder, obtunded consciousness, and even brain damage. Fasting hypoglycemia may be a clue to significant endocrine disease. Reactive hypoglycemia, while annoying, usually responds to simple dietary measures. The study of hypoglycemia has led to many important insights into the regulation of energy metabolism.

—Victor R. Lavis, M.D.

See also Blood and blood disorders; Diabetes mellitus; Endocrine disorders; Endocrinology; Endocrinology, pediatric; Hormones; Metabolism; Obesity; Pancreas; Pancreatitis; Vitamins and minerals.

For Further Information:

Alan, Rick. "Hypoglycemia." *Health Library*, September 2012.

Chow, Cheryl, and James Chow. *Hypoglycemia for Dummies*. 2d ed. New York: Wiley, 2007.

Dods, Richard F. *Understanding Diabetes: A Biochemical Perspective*. Hoboken, N.J.: John Wiley & Sons, 2013.

Harmel, Anne Peters, and Ruchi Mathur. *Davidson's Diabetes Mellitus: Diagnosis and Treatment*. 5th ed. Philadelphia: W. B. Saunders, 2004.

Hypoglycemia Support Foundation. http://www.hypoglycemia.org.

Kahn, C. R., et al., eds. *Joslin's Diabetes Mellitus*. 14th ed. Philadelphia: Lippincott Williams & Wilkins, 2007.

Kalyani, Rita Rastogi, and Simeon Margolis. *Diabetes: Your Annual Guide to Prevention, Diagnosis, and Treatment*. Baltimore, Md.: Johns Hopkins Medicine, 2013.

Lincoln, Thomas A., and John A. Eaddy. *Beating the Blood Sugar Blues: Proven Methods and Wisdom for Controlling Hypoglycemia*. New York: McGraw-Hill, 2001.

McDermott, Michael T. *Endocrine Secrets*. 6th ed. Philadelphia: Elsevier/Saunders, 2013.

Melmed, Shlomo., et al., eds. *Williams Textbook of Endocrinology*. 12th ed. Philadelphia: Saunders/Elsevier, 2011.

Parker, James N., and Philip M. Parker, eds. *The 2002 Official Patient's Sourcebook on Hypoglycemia*. San Diego, Calif.: Icon Health, 2002.

HYPOPARATHYROIDISM. *See* HYPERPARATHYROIDISM AND HYPOPARATHYROIDISM.

HYPOSPADIAS REPAIR AND URETHROPLASTY
Procedure

Anatomy or system affected: Genitals, reproductive system

Specialties and related fields: General surgery, urology

Definition: Urethroplasty is any plastic surgery performed on the urethra; one of these procedures is the repair of hypospadias, the presence of an abnormal opening in the male urethra.

Indications and Procedures

Urethroplasty is performed to correct defects of the urethra, the tube leading from the bladder to the outside of the body through which urine exits the body. Hypospadias is a congenital defect of the distal end of the urethra in which it opens on the underside of the penis instead of at the tip. Less commonly, the opening can occur lower down on the underside of the penis or in the scrotum. Hypospadias is also associated with abnormalities in the kidneys.

The correction of hypospadias involves a technique known as a "flip-flap" repair: two incisions on the undersurface of the glans and shaft of the penis are made, and skin from the glans is fashioned into an opening that is anatomically normal. The operation is usually done under general anesthesia.

The lines for both incisions are drawn and incisions carefully made to avoid damaging adjacent structures and erectile tissue. The prepuce is released from the body of the penis. A *V*-shaped flap is cut from the skin immediately below the hypospadias. The flap is rotated, and one side is sutured into one of the incisions made in the glans. The other side is similarly inserted into the other incision and sutured in place, forming a tube that extends the urethra. Excess skin from the prepuce is removed; the prepuce is sutured back into position on the shaft of the penis. The skin from the underside of the penis is brought together over the repaired urethra and sutured together. A catheter is frequently (but not universally) placed in the urethra and kept in place for up to two weeks. Some surgeons believe that the presence of a catheter helps to establish the new urethra. Others think that it only contributes to postoperative holes (fistulas) and do not use it, allowing the patient to urinate immediately through the newly constructed tube. The patient may return to the surgeon's office in a week for a postoperative check and the removal of sutures.

Another type of urethroplasty is the surgical repair of a discontinuity in the male urethra. Most commonly, this defect occurs on the underside of the penis and is attributable to the incomplete closure of the skin portions that normally fuse over the urethra during embryonic development. The technique is similar to that described above. Under general anesthesia, skin is removed from the prepuce of the penis and is sutured in place over the defect, closing the opening. A catheter may or may not be inserted. The patient returns to the surgeon's office in a week for a postoperative check and the removal of sutures.

Uses and Complications

The techniques associated with urethroplasty are used to repair congenital defects. Complications from these procedures are unusual, but they may include infection and stricture. Such problems can be avoided with careful attention to the finer details of the surgery.

The need for urethroplasty and hypospadias repair is unlikely to disappear. From a psychological standpoint, it benefits the patient to repair a hypospadias as early in life as possible, preferably before the age of three.

—*L. Fleming Fallon, Jr., M.D., Ph.D., M.P.H.*

See also Fistula repair; Genital disorders, male; Men's health; Neonatology; Pediatrics; Reproductive system; Surgery, pediatric; Urinary system; Urology; Urology, pediatric.

For Further Information:

A.D.A.M. Medical Encyclopedia. "Hypospadias Repair." *MedlinePlus*, October 9, 2012.

Baskin, Laurence S., ed. *Hypospadias and Genital Development*. New York: Kluwer Academic/Plenum, 2004.

Beers, Mark H., et al., eds. *The Merck Manual of Diagnosis and Therapy*. 18th ed. Whitehouse Station, N.J.: Merck Research Laboratories, 2006.

Ferrari, Mario. *PDxMD Renal and Genitourinary Disorders*. New York: Elsevier, 2002.

Hadidi, Ahmed T., and Amir F. Azmy, eds. *Hypospadias Surgery: An Illustrated Guide*. New York: Springer, 2004.

Icon Health. *Hyperspadias: A Medical Dictionary, Bibliography, and Annotated Research Guide to Internet References*. San Diego, Calif.: Author, 2004.

Montague, Drogo K. *Disorders of Male Sexual Function*. Chicago: Year Book Medical, 1988.

Neff, Deanna M. "Hypospadias Repair." *Health Library*, September 26, 2012.

Swanson, Janice M., and Katherine A. Forrest, eds. *Men's Reproductive Health*. New York: Springer, 1984.

Urology Care Foundation. "Hypospadias." *American Urological Association*, January 2011.

Hypotension

Disease/Disorder

Also known as: Low blood pressure

Anatomy or system affected: Blood vessels, brain, circulatory system, heart, kidneys

Specialties and related fields: Cardiology, critical care, emergency medicine, exercise physiology, geriatrics and general surgery, internal medicine, pharmacology

Definition: Blood pressure that not only is low but also causes symptoms such as dizziness in the affected individual. It has multiple causes, including blood loss, heart attack, trauma, reactions to medications, and overwhelming infection.

Causes and Symptoms

The body has a complex system for regulating blood pressure, which ensures adequate blood flow to each organ and tissue. The sympathetic and parasympathetic branches of the autonomic nervous system, various hormones produced by the adrenal and pituitary glands, the kidneys, the heart, and local mechanisms in all parts of the body control the amount of blood in the vessels, how much blood is squeezed out of the heart with each beat, and how much blood is available to any body system at a given time. A failure in any of these regulatory areas can cause the blood pressure to become too low for the person to function normally.

Normal blood pressure varies depending on the demands put on the body, how fit a person is, and the age of the individual. For most adults, 120/80 is considered normal; however, the top number (systolic pressure) can be as low as 90 and the bottom number (diastolic) as low as 60 and still be considered normal. When the blood pressure is lower than about 90/60 and the individual develops symptoms related to the low pressure, then that individual is diagnosed with hypotension. Low blood pressure by itself is not unhealthy, especially in athletic people, but when the flow of blood to the organs of the body is inadequate, symptoms develop. They include rapid heartbeat, light-headedness or dizziness, weakness, and possibly fainting. Other symptoms vary with the cause of the low blood pressure.

Low blood pressure associated with insufficient blood flow to the body organs can cause kidney failure, strokes, and heart attacks. Orthostatic hypotension is low blood pressure and its associated symptoms that are most pronounced when a person goes from lying or sitting to standing.

Specific causes of hypotension include adverse drug reactions, diseases such as diabetes that damage the autonomic nervous system, hormone-producing tumors, fever, heart disease, dehydration, hemorrhage, excessive heat, alcohol use, heart attack, heart trauma, abnormal heart rhythms, overwhelming infection, anaphylaxis, burns, vomiting, and diarrhea.

Treatment and Therapy

The treatment of hypotension is primarily aimed at removing the underlying cause—for example, discontinuing a drug that causes blood vessels to dilate or wearing elastic stockings to

---

Information on Hypotension

Causes: Blood loss, heart disease, heart attack, trauma, adverse drug reactions, infection, hormone-producing tumors, fever, dehydration, excessive heat, alcohol use, shock, burns

Symptoms: Low blood pressure accompanied by rapid heartbeat, light-headedness or dizziness, weakness, possibly fainting; sometimes kidney failure, strokes, heart attack

Duration: Acute

Treatments: Supportive measures such as fluids and oxygen therapy; treatment for underlying cause

---

improve blood flow back to the heart. If the low blood pressure is severe enough, then supportive treatment with fluids, oxygen, and other modalities may be required.

—*Rebecca Lovell Scott, Ph.D., PA-C*

See also Blood pressure; Cardiology; Circulation; Dizziness and fainting; Heart; Hypertension; Kidneys; Nephrology; Nervous system; Neurology; Vascular medicine; Vascular system.

For Further Information:

American Medical Association. *American Medical Association Family Medical Guide.* 4th rev. ed. Hoboken, N.J.: John Wiley & Sons, 2004.

"Hypotension." *MedlinePlus*, February 20, 2011.

Komaroff, Anthony, ed. *Harvard Medical School Family Health Guide.* New York: Free Press, 2005.

"Low Blood Pressure." *American Heart Association*, April 4, 2012.

"Low Blood Pressure (Hypotension)." *Mayo Clinic*, May 19, 2011.

Stoppard, Miriam. *Family Health Guide.* London: DK, 2006.

Voyatzis, Diane. "Orthostatic Hypotension." *Health Library*, March 25, 2013.

HYPOTHALAMUS
Anatomy

Anatomy or system affected: Brain, endocrine system, glands, nervous system, psychic-emotional system

Specialties and related fields: Biochemistry, endocrinology, neurology, psychiatry, psychology

Definition: A region of the brain that functions as the control center for all autonomic regulatory activities of the body.

Structure and Functions

The hypothalamus is a small, cone-shaped structure located near the center of the brain immediately below the thalamus. The hypothalamus has many nuclei and fiber tracts. It forms part of the walls and floor of the central chamber of the cerebral ventricles, which is known as the third ventricle. Neurons in the hypothalamus extend axons to the pituitary gland that is hanging on a stalk underneath the hypothalamus.

The hypothalamus controls many automatic functions of the body. Its overall function is to maintain normal, healthy conditions in the body by governing the autonomic nervous system and controlling pituitary output. Its specific functions are controlling the release of eight major hormones in the body, regulating body temperature, controlling food and water intake, controlling daily cycles in physiological state and behavior, mediating emotional responses, and regulating sexual behavior and reproduction.

Disorders and Diseases

If the hypothalamus is not functioning properly, the autonomic nervous system can send wrong neurosignals to the body that can make the victim feel stressed and emotionally empty. This can lead to disordered sleep, dysfunction of the immune system, altered body temperature, or multiple hormonal dysfunctions. These conditions often lead to depression, hyperactivity, malfunctioning of normal brain and limbic activities, or abnormal responses to stress. Disturbances in neural pathways that connect the hypothalamus and thalamus and control mood appear to be related to some of the symptoms of schizophrenia.

Obesity and related disorders are directly related to the critical role that the hypothalamus plays in the central regulation of appetite and metabolism. Insufficient production of antidiuretic hormone by the hypothalamus may cause diabetes insipidus. When the thirst center in the anterior hypothalamus is stimulated, polydipsia occurs, which can lead to polyuria.

Treatment of hypothalamic disorders depends on the cause of the dysfunction. If it is due to a tumor, the growth is either surgically removed or treated with radiation. If it is due to hormonal deficiencies, the missing hormones are replaced. Other specific treatments may be applied if the malfunction is due to infection, bleeding, or other causes.

Perspective and Prospects

The homeostatic function of the hypothalamus was suggested by Claude Bernard in the late 1800s. Many initial studies were focused on identifying the boundaries, structural components, nuclei, tracts, and interconnections of the hypothalamus. During the latter half of the twentieth century, interest shifted to the functions of the hypothalamus that were involved in emotional expression, disease, controlling metabolism, and producing neuroendocrine secretions. This emphasis has led to a better understanding and treatment of medical problems and chemical imbalances associated with hypothalamic dysfunctions.

—*Alvin K. Benson, Ph.D.*

See also Brain; Nervous system; Neurology.

For Further Information:

Hadley, Mac E., and Jon E. Levine. *Endocrinology* 6th ed. Upper Saddle River, N.J.: Pearson, 2007.

Jasmin, Luc. "Hypothalamus." *MedlinePlus*, November 2, 2012.

Norwood, Diane Voyatzis. "Diabetes Insipidus." *Health Library*, March 15, 2013.

Rennert, Nancy J. "Hypothalamus." *MedlinePlus*, December 11, 2011.

Stoll, Walt, and Jan DeCourtney. *Recapture Your Health.* Boulder, Colo.: Sunrise Health Coach, 2006.

Swaab, Dick F. *Human Hypothalamus: Basic and Clinical Aspects, Part 2: Handbook of Clinical Neurology.* Amsterdam: Elsevier, 2003.

HYPOTHERMIA. *See* **HYPERTHERMIA AND HYPOTHERMIA.**

HYPOTHYROIDISM. *See* **CONGENITAL HYPOTHYROIDISM.**

HYPOXIA
Disease/Disorder

Also known as: Inadequate oxygen supply and shortness of breath

Anatomy or system affected: Lungs, respiratory system

Specialties and related fields: Anesthesiology, critical care, emergency medicine, exercise physiology, family medicine, general surgery, internal medicine, neurology, nursing, pulmonary medicine

Definition: An inadequate supply of oxygen to tissues caused by either oxygen delivery not being sufficient for tissue requirements or utilization of oxygen being ineffective.

Information on Hypoxia

Causes: Airway obstruction, apnea, collapse of lung, side effects of certain drugs, anemia, heart failure

Symptoms: Headache, anxiety, dizziness, sweating and flushing, extreme difficulty breathing, increasing pulse and respiratory rates, extreme restlessness and fear, gasping respirations, laryngeal stridor, flared nostrils, cyanosis, vigorous abdominal and diaphragmatic movement with little chest wall movement

Duration: Acute

Treatments: Related to cause; includes oxygen administration, cricothyroidotomy, tracheostomy, mechanical ventilation

---

Causes and Symptoms

Various diseases or conditions of the lungs can cause mechanical problems with air exchange. These problems generally cause a diminished supply of oxygen and an excess of carbon dioxide in the blood. Hypoxia is present in any condition that causes inadequate amounts of oxygen to be delivered to body cells. Various types of hypoxia have been identified, including hypoxemic, anemic, and stagnant. Hypoxemic hypoxia is related to inadequate oxygen in inhaled air or respiratory problems that prevent adequate oxygen from reaching lung capillaries. Anemic hypoxia is related to any condition that causes a reduction in hemoglobin. Although adequate oxygen may reach the blood, it is not adequately transported to tissues. Stagnant hypoxia is related to reduced blood flow to capillaries and may be caused by conditions such as heart failure or obstruction of a blood vessel.

Treatment and Therapy

The treatment of hypoxia depends on its cause. Although oxygen therapy (administration of inhaled oxygen) seems a logical therapeutic measure, it may be helpful in some types of hypoxia but of little value in others. Oxygen therapy is clearly indicated when hypoxia is due to lack of oxygen in environmental air, to hypoventilation, or to problems that interfere with pulmonary diffusion. Oxygen therapy is moderately helpful in hypoxia from anemia and carbon monoxide poisoning. When hypoxia is caused by failure of the circulatory system, oxygen therapy may be slightly beneficial. It is of almost no value when hypoxia is caused by the inability of cells to use oxygen. In addition to oxygen delivered by face mask or cannula, in emergency situations a cricothyroidotomy and tracheostomy may be performed. Mechanical ventilation may also be necessary.

Adequate tissue oxygenation is evaluated by the following: Does the atmospheric air contain enough oxygen and humidification? Is the airway clear, or does it seem to contain excess secretions? Is the client able to ventilate without pain or discomfort? Do both sides of the thorax rise and fall equally with inhalation? Does breathing sound noisy? Are the rate, rhythm, and depth of respiration within normal limitations? Is cough and sputum production present? Is chronic lung disease present? Are blood gases within normal limits? Is the complete blood count within normal limits? Is the radial/apical pulse rate, rhythm, and volume within normal limits? Is blood pressure within normal limits? Is mental confusion, disorientation, or memory loss present?

—*Jane C. Norman, Ph.D., R.N., C.N.E.*

See also Asphyxiation; Choking; Coughing; Hyperbaric oxygen therapy; Hyperventilation; Lungs; Oxygen therapy; Pulmonary diseases; Pulmonary hypertension; Pulmonary medicine; Pulmonary medicine, pediatric; Respiration.

For Further Information:

Des Jardins, Terry. *Clinical Manifestations and Assessment of Respiratory Disease.* New York: Elsevier Science, 2005.

Lei Xi, and Tatiana V. Serebrovskaya, eds. *Intermittent Hypoxia: From Molecular Mechanisms to Clinical Applications.* Hauppauge, N.Y.: Nova Science, 2013.

"NINDS Cerebral Hypoxia Information Page." *National Institute of Neurological Disorders and Stroke.* October 2010.

Roach, Robert C., Peter D. Wagner, eds. *Hypoxia Into the Next Millennium.* New York: Springer Science + Business, 2013.

Vordermark, Dirk. *Hypoxia: Causes, Types and Treatment.* Hauppauge, N.Y.: Nova Science, 2012.

Wilkins, Robert L. *Egan's Fundamentals of Respiratory Care.* New York: Elsevier Health Sciences, 2008.

Wilkins, Robert L. *Respiratory Disease: Case Study Approach to Patient Care.* New York: F. A. Davis, 2006.

HYSTERECTOMY
Procedure

Anatomy or system affected: Reproductive system, uterus

Specialties and related fields: Endocrinology, general surgery, gynecology, oncology

Definition: The removal of the uterus and sometimes the ovaries and surrounding tissues, which is performed for a variety of indications, including uterine cancer and fibroids that cause symptoms.

Key terms:

adenomyosis: a noncancerous disorder in which cells resembling the lining of the uterus are found within the muscle layer of the uterus, leading to abnormal vaginal bleeding and pain

estrogen: the female sex hormone produced by the ovaries and the adrenal gland that is responsible for the development of female secondary sex characteristics; the three types naturally produced by the body are estradiol, estrone, and estriol

Fallopian tubes: the structures located between the uterus and ovaries that are responsible for the transport of the egg; also called the oviducts

fibroid: a noncancerous tumor of the uterus, also known as leiomyoma; when large, these tumors can cause heavy menstrual bleeding leading to anemia or cause pressure symptoms in the pelvis

laparoscopy: a minimally invasive surgical procedure in which an instrument equipped with a small camera, called a laparoscope, is inserted through a small incision in the abdomen to visualize the pelvis or abdomen; surgical manipulation may be carried out during this procedure

menorrhagia: unusually heavy menstrual bleeding; when severe, it can lead to anemia

progesterone/progestin: a hormone produced in the ovaries that sustains pregnancy; birth control pills are composed primarily of progesterone, which works by suppressing ovulation

Indications and Procedures

The term "hysterectomy" comes from the Greek *hystera,* meaning "uterus," and *ektome,* meaning "to cut out." While hysterectomy refers to the removal of the uterus and, most commonly, the attached Fallopian tubes, there are several types of hysterectomies. Total hysterectomy, contrary to popular belief, does not mean that the ovaries are removed with the uterus. Rather, the term indicates the removal of the uterus and cervix. Subtotal, or partial, hysterectomy is the excision of the uterus above the cervix; the cervix is left in place. Either one or both ovaries may be removed with the uterus (unilateral oophorectomy or bilateral oophorectomy). Salpingo-oophorectomy refers to the removal of one of the Fallopian tubes along with the accompanying ovary, while bilateral salpingo-oophorectomy refers to the removal of both Fallopian tubes and ovaries.

Indications for hysterectomy can be divided into noncancerous and cancerous conditions. Within the noncancerous category, the most common indication for hysterectomy is symptomatic fibroids. Many women have fibroids, and the majority of fibroids do not cause symptoms and can be left alone. Symptomatic fibroids are those which are large enough to cause pressure symptoms in the pelvis, compress the bladder or rectum, or cause pain or discomfort during intercourse. Another type of symptomatic fibroids are those which cause excessively heavy menstrual bleeding and, when severe, anemia.

A hysterectomy is indicated in these situations if the pa-

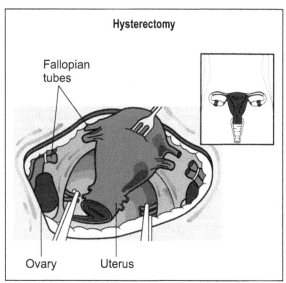

Hysterectomy

Fallopian tubes

Ovary   Uterus

The uterus, and sometimes such accompanying organs as the ovaries and Fallopian tubes, may be removed to treat disease conditions or as a contraceptive measure; the inset shows the location of the uterus.

tient fails to respond to less conservative therapy for symptomatic fibroids. Examples of conservative therapy for heavy bleeding include high-dose estrogen or birth control pills. A hysterectomy is usually performed only when childbearing is no longer desired, since removal of the uterus precludes pregnancy. Prior to hysterectomy, large fibroids may be shrunk with a course of a hormone called gonadotropin-releasing hormone. Unfortunately, this treatment results in menopausal symptoms, including hot flushes and bone density depletion, and therefore cannot be used for prolonged periods of time. More recently, treatments such as uterine artery embolization, in which the arteries feeding the uterus are blocked off using foreign particles such as gel foam, have been tried as an alternative to hysterectomy, in an attempt to preserve the uterus and avoid major surgery.

Another indication for hysterectomy is in patients who have had recurrent fibroids after myomectomy. A myomectomy is the surgical removal of isolated fibroids, rather than removal of the uterus itself. The benefit is that the uterus can be preserved, although the downside is that fibroids may regrow. Hysterectomy is the definitive treatment for uterine fibroids.

Another noncancerous indication for hysterectomy is adenomyosis, a painful condition whereby the cells of the uterine lining are abnormally embedded in the uterine muscle. No good treatments exist for this condition besides hysterectomy. Another indication for hysterectomy occurs in cases of abnormal uterine bleeding in which the bleeding is refractory to management with nonsurgical treatments, such as birth control pills or procedures that ablate the uterine lining. Other less common indications for hysterectomy are uterine prolapse (in which the uterus descends into the vaginal canal, causing discomfort or urinary incontinence), chronic pelvic pain (refractory to more conservative management), and large infections of the uterus and pelvis that are unresponsive to antibiotics. Hysterectomy may also be performed as part of a cesarean section if the surgeon encounters uncontrollable bleeding after delivery of the infant.

Uterine cancer is a clear indication for hysterectomy. Often, the cancer causes abnormal uterine bleeding. Prior to hysterectomy, the cancer has usually been confirmed on biopsy of the uterine lining. If the cancer is small and localized to a small area of the uterus, then removal of the uterus alone may be curative. More often, however, uterine cancer may have spread more deeply into the uterine wall or even grown beyond the uterus. In these cases, hysterectomy may be accompanied by more extensive surgery that includes removing lymph nodes or other pelvic structures.

Most frequently, hysterectomy is accomplished through a 6- to 8-inch midline incision running either down from the navel or across the lower abdomen near or below the hairline (known as a "bikini incision"). This procedure is referred to as an abdominal hysterectomy. Vaginal hysterectomy is the removal of the uterus through the vaginal canal, rather than through a surgical opening in the abdomen. This procedure is most often performed to resolve prolapse (because the uterus has already descended into the vaginal canal) or when the uterus is not massively enlarged and can be pulled down and out through the vagina. If the hysterectomy is performed because of large fibroid tumors, then the abdominal approach is usually used. On rare occasions, a vaginal hysterectomy may be facilitated using laparoscopy. In these cases, laparoscopy enables visualization and manipulation of the uterus via small incisions in the abdomen to assist in removal of the uterus through the vaginal canal.

During the hysterectomy, the patient is almost always under general anesthesia. The patient lies on her back for abdominal hysterectomies. In vaginal hysterectomies, the patient's legs are placed in stirrups and the knees are spread apart to enable the gynecologist to gain access to the vaginal canal. The actual removal of the uterus involves clamping, transecting, and suture ligating the blood vessels that feed the uterus and the tissues that anchor the uterus in the pelvic cavity. Care is taken by the surgeon to avoid the ureters, the tubes carrying urine from the kidney to the bladder. The ureters are very close to the lower part of the uterus and can be damaged easily. If the entire uterus is removed, then the top end of the vagina, called the cuff, is sutured closed. If the cervix is left in place, then the top of the cervix is sutured closed.

After the surgery, the patient receives narcotic pain medication and antibiotics to prevent infection and is monitored carefully to confirm that vital signs are stable and recovery is appropriate. Laboratory tests may be performed to ensure that the patient is not unusually anemic and that important organs such as the kidneys are functioning properly. Until a patient is able to walk, a catheter (a rubber tube attached to a collecting bag) will be used to pass urine. Patients may initially take liquids by mouth. When they can tolerate liquids, indicating no apparent injury to the bowels, patients may begin to take solid food. A patient may be hospitalized for two to four days after the hysterectomy, although hospital stays in general have been shortening in length. On the whole, patients who receive vaginal hysterectomies have shorter hospital stays than patients receiving abdominal hysterectomies, assuming that no complications arise. Patients can usually resume normal sexual functioning six weeks after the surgery.

Uses and Complications

Hysterectomy can be used to provide relief from pressure, pain, and bleeding from the uterus. It may also be curative in the early stages of uterine cancer and can increase survival in later stages. For women who are finished with childbearing and whose lifestyles or responsibilities do not allow them to try more conservative treatments, many of which require several months to take effect, hysterectomy can provide definitive relief from symptoms within the defined time period needed to undergo scheduled surgery. In cases of life-threatening uterine hemorrhage, hysterectomy can save a woman's life.

The common complications of hysterectomy are those which are common to many major surgeries. One complication is excessive blood loss. The average blood loss during a hysterectomy is estimated at between 400 and 500 cubic centimeters (about a pint). When removal of the uterus is difficult, for instance because of the position of large fibroids, increased blood loss is likely to occur. When excessive blood loss is of concern, the patient's blood levels may be checked during the procedure. A patient who is significantly anemic may receive blood transfusions to avoid poor oxygenation of the major organs and to increase blood volume, and hence avoid shock. The number of transfusions depends on the amount of blood estimated to be lost. If a blood vessel continues to bleed after the patient leaves the operating room, then the patient may need to return to the operating room to have the bleeding vessel identified and sutured.

Another common complication of hysterectomy is infection. Even when aseptic techniques are followed, an infection may develop several days after the surgery. This is particularly true in vaginal hysterectomies, where the surgeon works through the vaginal canal, considered a clean but contaminated field. For this reason, patients are given antibiotics immediately prior to surgery in order to prevent infection. A patient who shows signs of infection after the surgery may be placed on an extended course of antibiotics. The source of these infections can range from the vaginal cuff site to the peritoneum (the lining of the pelvic and abdominal cavity) and the urinary tract.

The third major complication that can occur with hysterectomy is inadvertent damage to internal organs. The urinary tract and the bowels are particularly at risk during hysterectomy because of their proximity to the uterus. The ureters can be occluded inadvertently by the misplacement of a suture. If discovered early, this damage can be repaired. If the problem is not recognized, however, then a damaged ureter can result in kidney malfunction. For this reason, kidney function is carefully followed after the hysterectomy through blood tests. Since the bladder sits on the bottom half of the uterus, it is a common organ that can be damaged during a hysterectomy. If the bladder is accidentally entered using the scalpel during surgery, then it can usually be repaired during the procedure. Postsurgery, the patient may need prolonged catheterization of the bladder to enhance bladder recovery. The large and small intestines are another common site of surgical injury. They can be accidentally cut or sutured. Sometimes, this problem is not detected until after the patient has left the operating room, and the problem becomes apparent when normal bowel function does not return in a timely fashion postoperatively. The patient may experience nausea, vomiting, and abdominal distension and discomfort and may not be able to pass gas from the rectum.

Another complication that can occur after surgery is the formation of blood clots, particularly in the leg veins, as a result of the patient's immobility during and after surgery. These clots can be dangerous when they break off from their source and move into the lungs, a condition called pulmonary embolism. Large pulmonary emboli can be life-threatening. Pulmonary emboli can be prevented using warm compression stockings during and after surgery to promote blood flow. Early ambulation (walking) after surgery can also decrease the chances of developing leg vein clots and pulmonary emboli.

Long-term complications of hysterectomy also include scar formation in the pelvis, called adhesions, which can interfere with bowel function or cause pelvic pain. Some patients may experience the prolapse of the remaining pelvic organs (such as the bowels and bladder) into the space formerly occupied by the uterus. Procedures may be employed during the hysterectomy to anchor the vaginal cuff and close any spaces where prolapse might occur.

In rare cases, removal of the uterus can inadvertently decrease blood supply to any remaining ovaries, leading to ischemia and loss of ovarian function. In these cases, the patient may experience the symptoms of estrogen deficiency, also known as menopausal symptoms. They include hot flashes, vaginal dryness, and, when estrogen deficiency is prolonged, bone density loss. In women whose hysterectomies included removal of the ovaries, the hot flashes may become apparent a few days after surgery. In these cases, estrogen therapy or other medications may be of benefit.

The impact of a hysterectomy on a woman's psychological state varies from woman to woman. In women who have been suffering a great deal from their symptoms, be it pressure and pain or abnormal bleeding, a hysterectomy can be a relief and enable them to return to their activities of daily living. Hysterectomy can improve sexual function in many cases. In other women, a hysterectomy can trigger a sense of loss and represent the end of the woman's fertility, which is often associated with youth and vitality.

Perspective and Prospects

In ancient times, the complaints of women and the illnesses of the female organs were viewed as coming from an "unhappy uterus." It was believed that the uterus had the primary purpose of childbearing and that, when the uterus was not occupied with this function, it might show its wrath by abnormal bleeding and pain. These beliefs prevailed for centuries; early medical history indicates that women's gynecologic complaints were largely ignored. Moreover, no safe surgical procedures had been developed.

A noteworthy event in early American medical history was the operation attempted and documented by a frontier physician and surgeon, Ephraim McDowell. In 1809 in Danville, Kentucky, this daring young doctor carried out experimental surgery on a middle-aged woman to remove a huge ovarian tumor. Without the benefit of anesthesia and a sterile technique, he performed successful abdominal surgery on four out of five other patients.

Myomectomy, or removal of a fibroid tumor of the uterus, was the next procedure to be performed—first in France and later (about 1850) in Massachusetts by Washington Atlee. The first hysterectomy was successfully performed by Walter Burnham in the same decade, but he lost twelve of his next fifteen hysterectomy patients. In the text *Operative Gynecology* (1898), Howard A. Kelly of Baltimore describes one hundred hysterectomies that he performed in the late nineteenth century, all done because of pelvic infection. He lost only four patients, though convalescence for some survivors was prolonged.

Remarkable medical progress occurred in the nineteenth century in abdominal and vaginal surgical techniques. In the 1850s, Marion Sims of South Carolina was the first to perform vaginal surgery in the United States. He successfully repaired a vesicovaginal fistula, an abnormal opening between the bladder and the vagina through which urine escapes into the vagina. In the late nineteenth century, the "Manchester" operation for uterine prolapse was performed by A. Donald in Manchester, England. Prior to this procedure, uterine prolapse was treated with a pessary, a device inserted into the vagina to hold the uterus in place.

In the 1930s, N. Sproat Heany of Chicago devised the present-day technique of vaginal hysterectomy. Vaginal (as opposed to abdominal) hysterectomy, it was believed, resulted in a less complicated procedure with shorter convalescence and more cosmetically pleasing results for most patients. For some time, vaginal hysterectomy was viewed as superior to abdominal hysterectomy. In the 1970s, between 25 and 40 percent of all hysterectomies were accomplished vaginally, depending on the age of the woman at the time of surgery. In 1981, however, a landmark study published by the US Congress, weighing the costs, risks, and benefits of hysterectomy, stated that women undergoing vaginal hysterectomy are more likely to have postoperative fever and to receive antibiotic treatment. Moreover, vaginal hysterectomy patients may undergo further surgery at a rate as high as 5 to 10 percent.

By the late 1980s and early 1990s, the trend among many gynecologists had shifted away from hysterectomy to more conservative treatments, when possible. Physicians began to question whether hysterectomies were, in some or even in most cases, medically necessary. As more information became available to women regarding alternatives to hysterectomy (a major revenue-producing surgical procedure in the United States), many women became more apt to question their physicians when told that hysterectomy was the only possible solution to their gynecological problems.

—*Genevieve Slomski, Ph.D.;*
updated by Anne Lynn S. Chang, M.D.

See also Cancer; Cervical, ovarian, and uterine cancers; Contraception; Dysmenorrhea; Ectopic pregnancy; Endometriosis; Ethics; Gender reassignment surgery; Genital disorders, female; Gynecology; Hormone therapy; Hormones; Menorrhagia; Oncology; Ovaries; Reproductive system; Sterilization; Tubal ligation; Uterus; Women's health.

For Further Information:

Clark, Jan. *Hysterectomy and the Alternatives: How to Ask the Right Questions and Explore Other Options.* Rev. ed. London: Vermilion, 2000.

Dennerstein, Lorraine, Carl Wood, and Ann Westmore. *Hysterectomy: New Options and Advances.* 2d ed. New York: Oxford University Press, 1999.

Doherty, Gerard M., and Lawrence W. Way, eds. *Current Surgical Diagnosis and Treatment.* 12th ed. New York: Lange Medical Books/McGraw-Hill, 2006.

"Hysterectomy." *MedlinePlus*, February 26, 2012.

"Hysterectomy—Laparoscopic Surgery." *Health Library*, March 15, 2013.

"Hysterectomy—Open Surgery." *Health Library*, September 27, 2012.

Ikram, M., M. Saeed, and Shazia Jabeen. "Hysterectomy Comparison of Laparoscopic Assisted Vaginal Versus Total Abdominal Hysterectomy." *Professional Medical Journal* 19, no. 2 (March/April, 2012): 214–220.

Moore, Michele C., and Caroline M. de Costa. *Do You Really Need Surgery? A Sensible Guide to Hysterectomy and Other Procedures for Women.* New Brunswick, N.J.: Rutgers University Press, 2004.

Stenchever, Morton A., et al. *Comprehensive Gynecology.* 5th ed. St. Louis, Mo.: Mosby/Elsevier, 2007.

IATROGENIC DISORDERS
Disease/Disorder
Anatomy or system affected: All
Specialties and related fields: All
Definition: Health problems caused by medical treatments.

Causes and Symptoms

Iatrogenic disorders may be attributable to inefficient or uncaring physicians or to the risks inherent in medical procedures that are necessary to prevent death or crippling disease. Such disorders are usually divided into those caused by medications, surgery, and medical misdiagnosis.

The average patient of any age expects physicians and the medical infrastructure to deliver perfect cures for all diseases. This is not possible because some diseases have no cure and because medical treatment always involves some potential risk to the persons being treated. In fact, a percentage—usually a small one—of the patients treated for any disease develop unexpected health problems (adverse reactions) which can be diseases themselves.

The term "iatrogenic disorder" is a catchall used to encompass the many different adverse reactions that accompany the practice of modern medicine. The number of such problems has grown as medical science has become more sophisticated. They are often blamed entirely on physicians and other medical staff involved in cases producing iatrogenic disorders.

This blame is correctly directed in instances where a physician and other staff involved are uncaring, inattentive, careless, or incompletely educated. However, iatrogenic disorders often result from the nature of modern medicine. Doctors frequently attempt therapeutic methods (such as surgery) that are innovative efforts that cure serious diseases but have some inherent risk of failure. They may also use therapeutic drugs that are powerful agents for cure of specific disease processes but that have side effects causing other health problems in some people who take them. In addition, doctors will often utilize complicated overall therapy having adverse consequences that patients may not acknowledge despite physicians" attempts to explain them orally and with consent forms.

Treatment and Therapy

Despite careful efforts of most physicians—who are informed, caring, and efficient—iatrogenic disorders accompany many medical procedures. Public attention is, however, focused most on the effects of therapeutic agents, drugs and vaccines, because patients are often unaware that no therapeutic agent in use is ever perfectly safe. Even a clear physician description of the dos and don'ts associated with such therapy may be flawed by biological variation among patients, causing problems in one individual but not others. Furthermore, the explosion of new diseases and new versions of old diseases since the late 1980s has led to much more complex treatment regimens. Consequently, iatrogenic disorders occur much more often.

The increase in iatrogenic disorders has become particularly germane in treatment of the aged, acquired immunodeficiency syndrome (AIDS) patients, and the very young.

Information on Iatrogenic Disorders

Causes: Inherent medical risk, misdiagnosis, physician malpractice, medication error, surgical error
Symptoms: Wide ranging
Duration: Varies from acute to fatal
Treatments: Depends on circumstances

Hence, several rules must be followed concerning therapeutic agents. First, wherever possible, these medications should be used only after other means fail and the benefits to be gained clearly outweigh the risks entailed. Second, therapy should begin with the lowest possible effective dose, and all dose increases should be accompanied by frequent symptom relief and toxicity monitoring. Third, patients and responsible family members must be made aware of all possible adverse symptoms, how to best counter them, and the foods or other medications to be avoided to diminish iatrogenic potential. Such problems, in the aged, are due to biochemical changes that alter their tolerance for many medications.

Many iatrogenic disorders are caused by the presence of bacterial contamination in wounds and the fact that surgical maintenance of sterility is not absolutely perfect. For example, iatrogenesis occurs after 30 percent of surgical procedures carried out at heavily contaminated surgical sites (such as emergency surgery of abdominal wounds). In addition, the use of antibiotics can be problematic. In many cases, the large doses of these therapeutic agents required to fight primary bacterial infection will cause superinfection by other microbes, such as fungi. Furthermore, wide antibiotic use in hospitals has led to the creation of antibiotic-resistant bacteria.

For these reasons, treatment of surgical sites requires individualized attention. Clean wounds can be closed up immediately without high risk of infection, but deep wounds known to be contaminated prior to surgery are often best handled by closing up interior tissues and leaving skin and subcutaneous tissues open until it is clear that infection is under control. Many patients are frightened by such procedures and the pain involved, not understanding that it is in their best interest. Hence, they may resist treatment and accuse conscientious physicians of causing iatrogenic disorders. Such treatment is most crucial in the aged and in young children. In elderly patients the cause is diminution of body defenses against infection (for example, the immune system). It has been reported that the elderly experience a doubled or tripled chance of experiencing postoperative complications that may be seen as iatrogenic by their families. Young children are also more at risk than postpubertal individuals and "younger" adults, for reasons related to their incompletely developed immune systems.

Iatrogenesis resulting from misdiagnosis is too complicated an issue to be considered in depth here. In some cases, it is caused by physician inadequacy, but more often such problems are attributable to the great difficulty in diagnosing any disease absolutely.

It is essential for patients and physicians to communicate

effectively. Such interaction lowers the occurrence of iatrogenic disorders because patients can decide to forgo treatment or to learn how to comply exactly with complex treatment protocols. Patients who do not receive adequate answers to questions posed to physicians should seek treatment elsewhere. Physicians should completely explain potential problems associated with therapeutic procedures by oral communication, informative consent forms, and well-educated counselors.

Because of the many iatrogenic disorders associated with medical therapy, physicians often believe that the best course of treatment—where a symptom is unclear and severe danger to patients is not imminent—is to allow nature to take its course so as to do no harm. This approach is often misunderstood by patients. To clarify the issue and to satisfy them, it should be explained—by the physician—that treatment can often be more dangerous than a perceived health problem.

It is hoped that the continued development of medical science, careful and complete therapy explanations by medical staffs, and better medical understanding and better treatment compliance by patients will decrease the incidence of iatrogenic disorders.

—*Sanford S. Singer, Ph.D.*

See also Antibiotics; Bacterial infections; Drug resistance; Ethics; Hospitals; Law and medicine; Malpractice; Nausea and vomiting; Side effects; Surgery, general; Surgical procedures; Wounds.

For Further Information:

Apfel, Roberta J., and Susan M. Fisher. *To Do No Harm: DES and the Dilemmas of Modern Medicine.* New Haven, Conn.: Yale University Press, 1984.

Camus, Philippe, and Edward C. Rosenow. *Drug-Induced and Iatrogenic Respiratory Disease.* London: Hodder Arnold, 2010.

Carroll, Paula. *Life Wish: One Woman's Struggle Against Medical Incompetence.* Alameda, Calif.: Medical Consumers, 1986.

Farmer, Paul. *Infections and Inequalities: The Modern Plagues.* Berkeley: University of California Press, 2001.

Levy, Stuart B. *The Antibiotic Paradox: How the Misuse of Antibiotics Destroys Their Curative Powers.* 2d ed. Cambridge, Mass.: Perseus, 2002.

Morath, Julianne M., and Joanne E. Turnbull. *To Do No Harm: Ensuring Patient Safety in Health Care Organizations.* San Francisco: Jossey-Bass, 2005.

Preger, Leslie, ed. *Iatrogenic Diseases.* 2 vols. Boca Raton, Fla.: CRC Press, 1986.

Sharpe, Virginia F., and Alan I. Faden. *Medical Harm: Historical, Conceptual, and Ethical Dimensions of Iatrogenic Illness.* New York: Cambridge University Press, 1998.

Vincent, Charles, Maeve Ennis, and Robert J. Audley, eds. *Medical Accidents.* New York: Oxford University Press, 1993.

Wilson, Michael, Brian Henderson, and Rod McNab. *Bacterial Disease Mechanisms: An Introduction to Cellular Microbiology.* New York: Cambridge University Press, 2002.

ILEOSTOMY AND COLOSTOMY

Procedures

Anatomy or system affected: Abdomen, gastrointestinal system, intestines

Specialties and related fields: Gastroenterology

Definition: Surgical procedures that reroute the intestines to a hole, or stoma, in the abdomen after the removal of all or part of the colon.

Key terms:

anastomosis: the surgical connection of one tubular organ to another

appliance: any device for collecting or removing stool from a stoma

colon: the last section of the intestines, where most fluids are absorbed, located between the ileum and the rectum; also called the large bowel or intestine

ileum: the lower third of the small intestine, which joins with the colon

ostomy: a popular term for any operation that results in a stoma

rectum: the intestinal storage area for feces between the colon and anus

stoma: a surgically created passage between the intestines and the outer skin

stool: the waste matter of digestion excreted from the body through the anus or stoma

Indications and Procedures

Despite great advances in drugs and nonsurgical procedures, doctors can cure some disabling or life-threatening diseases of the intestines only on the operating table. Common procedures of this type are the colostomy and ileostomy, both of which replace the anus with a stoma on the abdominal wall.

Colostomy and ileostomy are medical terms compounding *stoma* (from the Greek word for "mouth") and a prefix identifying the section of gut that ends in the newly created "mouth." If a portion of the colon is retained and ends in a stoma, the operation constructing it is called a colostomy. If the entire colon is removed and the lower section of the small bowel, or ileum, ends in a stoma, the operation constructing it is called an ileostomy. Nonmedical support groups for patients commonly use the back-formation "ostomy" to refer to any operation that creates a stoma (including a urostomy, in which a stoma is created for the excretion of urine) and to such patients as "ostomates," although neither term belongs to medical technical vocabulary.

Physicians determine that an ileostomy or a colostomy is necessary after inspecting the damaged intestinal segments by endoscopy, by imaging, or during surgery. In consultation with a surgeon, the patient agrees to undergo the procedure. The patient fasts before the surgery and receives laxatives and enemas (except in the case of obstructions or severe ulcerative colitis) to clean as much feces from the intestines as possible and thus reduce the chance of infection during surgery. The surgeon, often with the advice of an enterostomal therapist (ET), examines the patient's abdomen carefully, checking where the skin naturally folds and stretches when the patient assumes various common body positions, and a spot for the stoma is selected that is convenient for the patient and free of stress from muscles and skin tension. That place is marked. An area to the right and below the navel is the usual location for an ileostomy. The left side is commonly chosen for a colostomy.

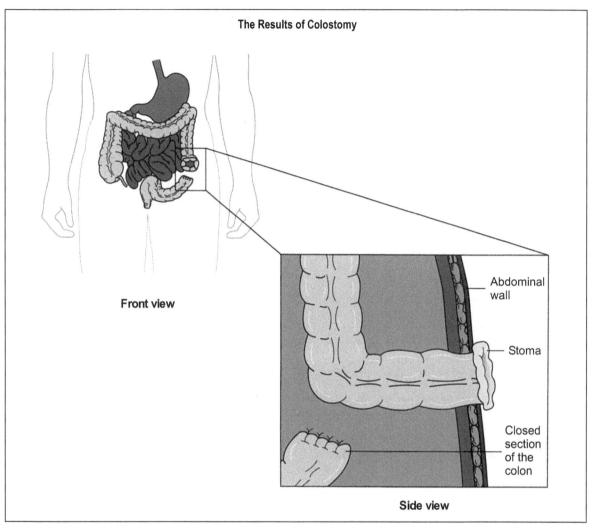

The Results of Colostomy

Front view

Abdominal wall

Stoma

Closed section of the colon

Side view

In colostomy, the colon is severed, the uppermost end of the intestine is extended through the abdominal wall to create a stoma through which fecal matter will be expelled, and the remaining section of the colon is closed off with sutures.

In ileostomy, the surgeon makes the opening incision, starting a few centimeters above the navel and continuing to the pelvic area. After the abdominal cavity is exposed, the tissues connecting the colon to surrounding structures are severed, starting at the cecum; the blood supply is cut and tied off; and clamps are placed over theileum and rectum. Then the colon is cut free of the small intestine and rectum and is removed. If the operation is a subtotal procedure, the rectum is sutured shut and left in place or the open end is pulled through the abdominal wall as a mucous stoma. (Such a second stoma is sometimes fashioned because the surgeon plans to connect the ileum and rectum in a later operation.) If the surgeon performs a proctocolectomy, the rectum is removed after the stoma is made and the anus is sutured shut.

The stoma is built by cutting a small round opening first in the skin and then in the abdominal wall and pulling the end of the ileum through the hole. The end sticks above the skin, is

folded back over itself, and is sutured to the edges of the hole, leaving the stoma protruding two to three centimeters. This basic ileostomy is called a Brooke ileostomy, after the English surgeon Bryan Brooke.

Variations on this basic procedure are employed depending on the wishes and health of the patient. A Kock pouch, named after its inventor, Nils Kock of Sweden, can be fashioned just behind the stoma in the abdominal cavity to act as an artificial rectum, collecting liquid waste until the ostomate wishes to void it; because this arrangement gives the patient control over defecation, it is called a continent ileostomy. The surgeon uses about forty-five centimeters of ileum to form the pouch and adjusts the stoma so that it acts as a valve until a tube is inserted for drainage. In some cases, when the underlying condition necessitating removal of the bowel segment is ultimately determined to be cured, and if there is sufficient remaining bowel, the ostomy can be reversed by closing the stoma and then reconnecting the bowel either to the rectum or to the anus.

If the ileum and rectum are joined, the procedure is called an ileorectal anastomosis. The rectum resumes its old job as a feces reservoir, and the patient defecates normally through the anus. This arrangement is seldom employed for ulcerative colitis patients, however, since the disease usually persists in the rectum. If the ileum is sutured directly to the anus, the procedure is called an ileoanal anastomosis. Because there is no rectum to collect feces, the surgeon must construct one. The pouch is made from loops of ileum that are slit along their length and stitched together. If not enough ileum remains from which to make a pouch, the surgeon pulls the end through the rectum and ties it directly to the anus, a procedure called an endorectal ileal pull-through. The anastomosis procedures require two operations—one for the temporary stoma and construction of the pouch, one to connect the pouch and the rectum, or anus—to give the artificial rectum a chance to heal properly and so prevent leaking.

Colostomies feature somewhat more variety of stoma placement than ileostomies, but since removal of the rectum, sigmoid colon, or both are the most common reasons for the creation of the stoma, it is usually placed on the lower left of the abdomen, near the hipbone. If more of the colon is removed, the stoma may be higher up toward the rib cage. The operation begins much as for an ileostomy, except that only the portion of the colon from the damaged or diseased area to the anus is removed and the initial incision begins near that damaged section. The remaining, healthy colon is pulled through holes in the abdomen and skin, and its end is rolled back and fastened. The stoma protrudes out about two to three centimeters, so that an appliance for storing waste, if needed, can be attached.

There are three varieties of colostomy. The first, a single-barreled end colostomy, is the classical configuration. The rectum and anus are removed, and a single circular stoma, about twenty-five millimeters (one inch) in diameter, is the permanent exit for stool. If, however, the surgeon believes that the colon and rectum can be rejoined, the rectum is left intact and closed. Either of two procedures can be used to give the colon a rest period between the removal of the diseased section and reconnection to the rectum. A double-barreled colostomy involves slicing through the colon and making side-by-side stomas from the ends. In a loop colostomy, the colon is not cut through; instead, a slit is made in one side, which is pulled through the skin and made into an oval stoma, usually larger than other stomas. In both cases, the upper colon discharges stool, and the lower length passes mucus.

Uses and Complications

Both colostomy and ileostomy are last-resort or emergency treatments. When a wound, such as one caused by a knife or gunshot, punctures the intestines, waste matter, full of bacteria, spills into the abdominal cavity. The severe infection that is sure to follow can kill a patient in days; thus, an emergency operation is required. The surgeon pulls healthy bowel through the abdominal wall and forms a temporary stoma (so that no more waste can leak out of the intestines), cleans out the spillage, and repairs the damaged bowel. In many cases, it is possible to reconnect the healthy bowel to the damaged portion after the wound has healed; at the same time, the stoma is closed, and the patient resumes defecation through the anus.

Emergency operations, however, account for only a small percentage of colostomies and ileostomies. About two-thirds of surgeries to form stomas are colostomies, most of which follow operations removing cancer (usually in the lower colon or rectum) or an obstruction. Diverticulitis, the inflammation of little pouches in the colon wall, may also require a colostomy; the diversion of wastes allows the inflammation to subside and the colon wall to heal, after which the stoma may be removed and the colon reconnected. Additionally, repair of some rare birth defects may entail a colostomy.

Ileostomies account for about one-quarter of stoma-creating procedures. Most are performed to eradicate ulcerative colitis, a chronic inflammation of the colon that begins in the rectum and may spread upward until the whole colon is involved. No drug or dietary treatment cures ulcerative colitis; when the condition becomes too unbearable for a patient to endure, the colon is removed and an ileostomy is performed. Long-standing ulcerative colitis is particularly likely to become cancerous, and the colon may be removed for that reason alone. Likewise, familial polyposis, a hereditary disease that dots the colon with toadstool-shaped lumps that are likely to become cancerous, may require removal of the colon and ileostomy.

Wounds, diverticulitis, familial polyposis, and birth defects, while not particularly rare, are the reasons for relatively few stomas. Stoma surgery is more commonly performed to treat colorectal cancer (particularly in the elderly) and ulcerative colitis (commonly disabling patients in their twenties). As the average age of the population increases, so does the incidence of colon cancer and the need for ostomies.

Recovery from stoma surgery is prolonged. Surgery shocks the intestines, and several days pass before the gut resumes the wavelike contractions (called peristalsis) that enable digestion and push wastes toward the stoma. In the meantime, patients live on intravenous fluid nourishment. When bowel motion restarts and wastes begin coming through the stoma, the ileostomate must develop new habits to cope with the flow of wastes (which are always fluid because the ileum does not remove sufficient water to solidify the waste matter) by learning to attach and empty appliances and to keep the stoma clean. Colostomates, especially those who have lost only their sigmoid colon, can look forward to passing firm stools and may eventually be able to live without an appliance, but months of diarrhea occur before the bowel regains full operation.

Many complications can plague the new anatomy, some of which require surgical correction. The most serious include intestinal obstruction, scar adhesions that distort the shape of the bowel, retraction of the stoma, abscesses, prolapse (more of the bowel pushing out of the body), and kidney stones (which form because persistent diarrhea can dehydrate ostomates). Less threatening, but demanding attention, are offensive odors, diarrhea, skin irritation, and bowel inflammation. Steady advances in surgical technique have lowered the complication rates, and few patients die because of the surgery.

Ostomates often must live with the stoma for the rest of their lives. Feces exit through the stoma, rather than the anus, forcing patients to "toilet train" themselves all over again. Some stomas, known as continent stomas, hold back wastes until the patient is ready to defecate by draining them with a tube. Many, however, are not, and stool and gas steadily seep through the opening, where the waste matter is collected in an appliance, usually a plastic bag that seals over the stoma.

Having a plastic bag of stool on the abdomen and needing to empty it periodically to prevent it from leaking, instead of defecating by sitting down on a toilet, proves a difficult adjustment for some patients, both physically and psychologically. Several aid resources help new ostomates adjust. Specially trained registered nurses called enterostomal therapists teach patients how to manage their new stomas and how to attach appliances or insert catheters to drain continent stomas; they also help care for the stomas after the operation and periodically review their patients" progress. Gastroenterologists, physicians who specialize in the intestinal tract, can provide medical guidance and directly inspect the bowel wall behind the stoma through an endoscope, a flexible fiber-optic tube, should trouble develop. Support groups offer various resources to those ostomates who feel isolated and depressed because of the stoma.

Out of the hospital, ostomates face a new and different life. As well as learning to handle appliances or irrigate artificial rectums, they must face the fact that a major organ of their bodies is changed. The need for the stoma may anger or depress them, and this fixation on the change, if unalleviated, can evolve into loss of self-esteem and attendant social withdrawal. Many ostomates experience guilt in the belief that the disease and stoma, as well as the effects of the stoma on their families, are somehow their own fault.

These reactions require social and psychological therapy, extending care well beyond that afforded by the surgeon and the hospital. Support groups and the enterostomal therapist supply the majority of this care, but occasionally professional psychological help is required. The repulsion that patients feel for stomas and the consequent chance of morbid psychological reactions have encouraged surgeons to prefer anastomoses to stomas when possible, even though anastomoses are more difficult, have higher failure rates, and require a longer recovery period.

Fortunately, the great majority of ostomates do adjust to their new lives; they seldom have any other alternative. Providing that the original need for surgery has been eliminated—the cancer has been removed, for example—they can look forward to an undiminished life span and few if any restrictions upon appetite, sexual function, or exercise. The majority of ostomates recover completely and are able to return to their previous occupations after recovery. Without the operations, all of them would have led drastically impaired lives, and many would have died. The high success rate places the ileostomy and colostomy procedures among the ranks of surgical interventions that rescue the seriously ill from otherwise incurable organic diseases.

Perspective and Prospects

Although drastic techniques requiring much skill from surgeons and stamina from patients, ostomies did not originate with modern medicine and its sophisticated technology for sustaining patients during operations. Some colostomies date from the last quarter of the eighteenth century. In the nineteenth century, the number of operations creating a stoma—then called "artificial" or "preternatural" anus—increased, although without antiseptic conditions or anesthesia a patient's chances for survival were not good. Surgeons sometimes placed the stomas on the back instead of the abdomen. In 1908, William Ernest Miles conducted the first operation to remove a cancerous rectum; since the patient's intestines were still moving waste matter, which needed an exit, Miles created a stoma, thereby establishing one of the most common surgeries of the twentieth century.

Still, colostomies and ileostomies did not proliferate until after World War II. Since then, refinements in surgical techniques and postoperative care have steadily reduced the chance of complications and the length of the recovery period. At the same time, several variations of permanent and temporary stomas have been developed.

Like many other extreme surgical interventions, the ileostomy and colostomy testify to the limits of biomedical knowledge: most of these surgeries are performed because other remedies fail. Until researchers discover the mechanisms causing cancer, ulcerative colitis, and other deadly lower bowel diseases and develop nonsurgical cures, ileostomies and colostomies will remain common, especially among the elderly.

—*Roger Smith, Ph.D.*

See also Anal cancer; Anus; Bypass surgery; Cancer; Colitis; Colon; Colorectal cancer; Colorectal surgery; Crohn's disease; Digestion; Diverticulitis and diverticulosis; Gastrectomy; Gastroenterology; Gastroenterology, pediatric; Gastrointestinal disorders; Gastrointestinal system; Intestinal disorders; Intestines; Rectum.

For Further Information:

A.D.A.M. Medical Encyclopedia. "Colostomy." *MedlinePlus*, May 6, 2011.

A.D.A.M. Medical Encyclopedia. "Ileostomy." *MedlinePlus*, December 10, 2012.

Adrouny, Richard. *Understanding Colon Cancer*. Jackson: University Press of Mississippi, 2002.

Brandt, Lawrence J., and Penny Steiner-Grossman, eds. *Treating IBD: A Patient's Guide to the Medical and Surgical Management of Inflammatory Bowel Disease*. Reprint. New York: Raven Press, 1996.

Bub, David S., et al. *One Hundred Questions and Answers About Colorectal Cancer*. Sudbury, Mass.: Jones and Bartlett, 2003.

Doherty, Gerard M., and Lawrence W. Way, eds. *Current Surgical Diagnosis and Treatment*. 12th ed. New York: Lange Medical Books/McGraw-Hill, 2006.

Fries, Colleen Farley. "Managing an Ostomy." *Nursing* 29, no. 8 (August, 1999): 26.

Kalibjian, Cliff. *Straight from the Gut: Living with Crohn's Disease and Ulcerative Colitis*. Cambridge, Mass.: O'Reilly, 2003.

Mullen, Barbara Dorr, and Kerry Anne McGinn. *The Ostomy Book: Living Comfortably with Colostomies, Ileostomies, and Urostomies*. Rev. ed. Palo Alto, Calif.: Bull, 1992.

National Digestive Diseases Information Clearinghouse. "Bowel Diversion Surgeries: Ileostromy, Colostomy, Ileoanal Reservoir, and Continent Ileostomy." *National Institutes of Health*, April 23, 2012.

Parker, James N., and Philip M. Parker, eds. *The 2002 Official Patient's Sourcebook on Ulcerative Colitis*. San Diego, Calif.: Icon Health, 2002.

United Ostomy Associations of America. http://www .uoaa.org.

IMAGING AND RADIOLOGY

Procedure

Anatomy or system affected: All

Specialties and related fields: Nuclear medicine, radiology

Definition: Medical imaging uses radiation that passes through the body to construct images of the insides of the body.

Key terms:

computed tomography (CT): a scanning procedure using X rays

fluoroscope: a machine that uses a fluorescent screen instead of photographic film to display X-ray images

magnetic resonance imaging (MRI): an imaging method using radio waves

positron emission tomography (PET): a scanning procedure using gamma rays from injected radioactive pharmaceuticals

single photon emission computed tomography (SPECT): a scanning procedure using gamma rays from injected radioactive pharmaceuticals

tomography: a method to produce a three-dimensional image of the internal structure of the body by observing and recording radiation transmitted, reflected, or emitted by structures inside the body; observations are made of sections, or slices, of the body that are assembled to form the final image

ultrasound: an imaging method using high-frequency sound

Indications and Procedures

Before the advent of radiology, physicians were forced to rely on visual clues, palpation (examination by touch), and exploratory surgery to discover what lay beneath a patient's skin. X-rays provided the first path around this limitation and allowed physicians to peer beneath the skin without surgery. X-rays are electromagnetic radiation similar to visible light, but they have much higher energies than visible light, which makes them more penetrating.

Circumstances under which a doctor needs to see inside the body and might use x-rays to do so include those in which a patient has fallen and experiences localized pain and swelling in the leg (possible broken bone); a patient with severe pain in the lower back passes blood in the urine (possible kidney stone); a patient experiences intermittent and squeezing chest pain, nausea, and shortness of breath (possible constricted arteries in the heart); and a patient has a history of localized stomach pain and heartburn, also called acid reflux (possible inflamed esophagus, hiatal hernia, or ulcer).

All medical imaging devices require a source of radiation, a detector, and a way to position the patient. For x-rays, the patient stands in front of a film holder or lies on a table over a film holder while x-rays from an x-ray tube pass through the patient and cast the patient's shadow onto the film. The film must be as large as the body part being examined. Dense constituents such as bones show up as white on x-ray negatives, while various other body tissues show up as shades of gray depending upon the fraction of the x-rays that they block.

X-ray film has been developed to have excellent resolution and contrast, and an x-ray is a permanent record. It is not easy to take several x-rays in quick succession, however, as might be done to examine the upper gastrointestinal tract. An alternative is to use fluoroscopy, in which a screen coated with special compounds is used in the place of film. These compounds fluoresce when struck by x-rays. Advantages are that the image is immediate (no film to develop) and moving images can be viewed. The image can be made brighter by an image intensifier—a television-camera-like device that amplifies the image—and a permanent record can be made by photographing this final image.

An ultrasound unit adapts sonar to medical purposes. The unit consists of a probe; electronics to generate, receive, and analyze signals; and a monitor to display the results. Such a device is relatively inexpensive compared with other types of scanners, and at the intensities used, ultrasound waves do not harm the body. The ultrasound probe contains a transducer, a crystal that can change electrical signals into sound waves and can also act as a receiver changing sound waves into electrical signals. During the examination, a gel is spread over the patient's skin in the area of interest. The gel provides good acoustical coupling between the probe and the patient's body tissue. To create an image of structures as small as 1 millimeter, ultrasound frequencies between 3 and 7 megahertz are used. The crystal inside the probe emits sound waves while rapidly rocking back and forth, producing a wedge of sound pulses. The crystal then becomes a receiver and picks up sound echoes that form as the sound passes from one type of tissue into another. Distance can be determined from the time elapsed between sending a pulse and receiving the echo. Combining this distance information with the direction and intensity of the echo allows a computer to build an image of the structures inside the body.

This image is displayed on a monitor screen and can also be printed for a permanent record. The probe is moved around to provide the least obstructed view of the target. Since ultrasound waves pass easily through soft tissues such as the liver and fluid-filled organs such as the gallbladder or the uterus during pregnancy, ultrasound is particularly useful to examine these organs. Ultrasound does not penetrate bone or gas, and the latter property makes it difficult to examine the digestive tract with ultrasound.

Like ultrasound, magnetic resonance imaging (MRI), uses no potentially harmful radiation, but it is the most expensive

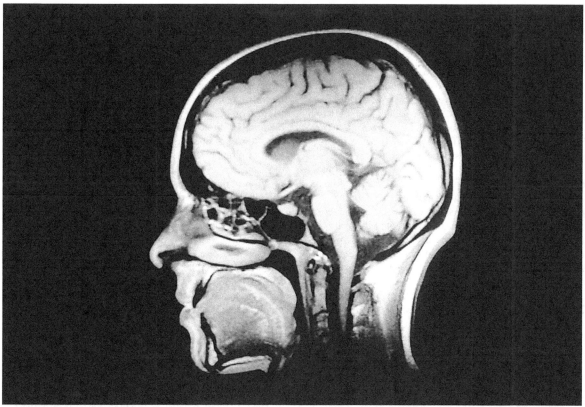

An MRI allows physicians to visualize soft tissues inside the body, such as the brain and nasopharyngeal tissues. (Digital Stock)

of the imaging techniques. MRI uses a very large, superconducting magnet. Once the magnetic field is established, superconducting magnets require very little electrical power. To be superconducting, the magnet is wound with niobium-titanium wire and maintained at liquid helium temperature (about five kelvins above absolute zero). The magnet itself is in the form of a very large, hollow cylinder into which the patient can be inserted. The magnetic field inside the cylinder is uniform and very strong, typically 0.5 to 2.0 tesla; for comparison, the strength of the earth's magnetic field is only about 0.00005 tesla near the surface. There are also three sets of much smaller (.0018 to .0027 of a tesla) "gradient" magnets, which are used to tweak the magnetic field at pinpoint locations during the scan. Hydrogen atoms are among the most abundant atoms in soft tissue. In a strong magnetic field, the spin axis of hydrogen nuclei (protons) precesses about magnetic field lines. The exact frequency with which it precesses depends on the proton's surroundings, or the type of tissue in which it is found.

The patient rests on a table that moves into the tunnel formed by the magnet. The magnetic field causes no noticeable sensation, but claustrophobic patients may become anxious. To combat this effect, newer machines have wider tunnels or have one side open. An insulated wire coil may be placed on the patient over the area to be examined, or coils mounted on the magnet may be used. A brief pulse of radio-

frequency waves is broadcast from the coil at the same time that the gradient magnets adjust the magnetic field to the right value in a narrow slice of the patient. If the radiofrequency is at the precession frequency, then those protons with which it resonates will absorb energy. After the radiofrequency pulse, the protons produce an echo that radiates energy back to the coil. Analysis of this energy allows the identification of the type of tissue, which, along with location information from the gradient magnets, allows a computer to construct an image of the internal tissues of the patient. The image can be either two-dimensional or three-dimensional, as needed. Two-dimensional slices can be vertical, horizontal, or in any plane desired.

A scan of the brain and spinal column can detect areas of damage to the myelin (insulating sheath) surrounding nerve fibers that is the hallmark of multiple sclerosis. MRI scans are also used in diagnosing tumors, infections of the brain, strokes, torn ligaments, and many other conditions. As with x-rays, contrast agents may be injected into the patient to make certain tissues or systems stand out. For example, the blood vessels in the heart may be examined in this fashion. Depending upon the size of the region to be scanned, the procedure takes from twenty to ninety minutes, and the patient must remain as still as possible during this time. Currents in the gradient magnets produce loud thumping sounds. These may be masked by providing the patient with music through earphones during the examination. Physicians now depend heavily on MRI investigations, and the 2003 Nobel Prize in Medicine or Physiology was awarded to Paul C. Lauterbur and Sir Peter Mansfield for their work leading to the development of the MRI technique.

A nuclear medicine scan, also called nuclear radiology or isotope study, uses radioactive pharmaceuticals that have been injected into or ingested by the patient. The radiation dose to the patient is strictly controlled and is the least possible for the procedure to be effective. The radioactive isotopes used emit gamma rays—essentially high-energy x-rays—which easily pass through the body and are observed by an array of gamma detectors. The patient lies on a table while the detector array is positioned near the target organ. In some applications, the array slowly scans a region. A computer receives information on the location and intensity of the detected gamma rays and constructs an image from this information. The image is fuzzy and lacks the fine detail that can be seen with x-rays or ultrasound, but it shows directly how well the target organ functions.

To be useful for this purpose, radioactive isotopes must emit penetrating gamma rays, have a short half-life, and either be taken up by the target organ or be capable of being attached to a molecule that is taken up by the target organ. A short half-life is desirable to ensure that the isotope will cease to be radioactive not too long after it has served its purpose. Technetium-99m is frequently used because it is taken up by the thyroid and salivary glands (if those are the targets), it can be used to tag other biologically active molecules, and its half-life is only 6.01 hours.

For a thyroid study, the patient may be given a drink or a pill containing iodine-123 (13.1 hour half-life). About twenty-four hours later, the gamma emission from the thyroid is measured. This procedure shows how well the thyroid works in general. The patient may then be injected with technetium-99m and several scans made over the next hour. This provides another measure of the thyroid's functioning. It also allows a measure of the thyroid's size and shape. Any area of inactivity suggests a blockage or damage, while an unusual area of activity suggests an abnormally high tissue growth rate such as a tumor. In general, a region of rapidly growing tissue shows up as a hot spot on a nuclear medicine scan, which makes it possible to see a healing bone fracture that an x-ray might miss.

A positron emission tomography (PET) scan is a special type of nuclear medicine scan that capitalizes on a property of the gamma rays emitted during positron annihilation. Positrons are positively charged and are the electron's antiparticle. Since they are oppositely charged, positrons and electrons are strongly attracted to each other, and as soon as they touch, they mutually annihilate, converting their energy into two gamma rays emitted at precisely 180 degrees to each other.

A gantry houses a large ring of gamma ray detectors arranged like a doughnut on its side. The patient rests on a movable table that carries the patient into, and perhaps through, the detector ring. Depending upon the purpose of the exami-

nation, one of several radioactive pharmaceuticals is administered. For example, fluorine-18 (half-life 109.8 minutes) is attached to glucose molecules and used to monitor the brain's metabolism. Since active areas of the brain draw the most glucose, a PET scan can watch the brain at work. When a fluorine nucleus emits a positron, the positron encounters an electron almost at once and is annihilated. The gamma ray detectors continually register hits from natural background radiation, but if two detectors located 180 degrees around the ring from each other record gamma rays of the right energy (0.511 million electron volts) and within a few nanoseconds of each other, it is virtually certain that they originated from a positron annihilation in the patient. A computer then draws a straight line between the two detectors and through the patient. Where two or more lines intersect is the location of the activity.

A single photon emission computed tomography (SPECT) scan is similar to a PET scan, but it detects only one photon at a time instead of a pair. To define the direction of a gamma ray photon, a collimator is placed in front of the detector array. The collimator is a slab of five-centimeter-long lead straws pointing at the patient so that a gamma ray can reach the detector only by traveling up a straw. Such a collimator and detector array is called an Anger camera. A ring of cameras around the patient allows a computer to construct a three-dimensional image of the target organ. SPECT combines the organ function information of nuclear medicine with some of the resolution of a computed tomography (CT) scan.

The CT apparatus consists of a movable table on which the patient rests and a gantry that houses the x-ray equipment. A doughnut hole in the gantry is large enough for the patient and table to pass through. An x-ray tube is mounted in the doughnut, and an array of x-ray detectors are mounted in the doughnut directly opposite from the x-ray source. As the doughnut rotates all the way around, the x-ray beam is sent through a narrow "slice" of the patient. Instead of the normal x-ray silhouette of the patient as illuminated from one direction, silhouettes from all directions are obtained, but only as numbers, not yet as images.

The information available consists of where the detector was when it picked up the signal and how strong the signal was. As the scan continues, the computer uses this information to construct an image of that slice of the patient. While the doughnut carries the x-ray tube and detectors around and around the patient, the table advances slowly and continuously until the whole body (or the desired segment) has been scanned. Blood clots and ruptured vessels in the brain are easily detected, as well as tumors in soft tissues such as the liver.

Uses and Complications

Bones, bone breaks, and some tumors show up well on an x-ray, but soft tissue images may require additional techniques. For examination of the upper gastrointestinal tract, the patient is given a barium solution to drink while standing in front of the x-ray detector. Barium blocks x-rays and coats the esophagus and stomach lining, thereby outlining them in detail on the x-ray. In the "barium swallow," a quick series of x-

Comparison of Radiation Doses for Various Procedures

Procedure	Typical Effective Dose	Natural Background Equivalent
Ultrasound scan	none	none
MRI	none	none
Chest X ray	0.1 mSv	10 days
Thyroid iodine uptake (whole-body dose)	2 mSv	8 months
Thyroid scan Tc-99m (whole-body dose)	5 mSv	1 year, 7 months
Whole-body PET scan with fluorine-tagged glucose	6 mSv	2 years
Chest CT scan	8 mSv	2 years, 8 months
Whole-body CT scan	10 mSv	3 years, 4 months

rays is taken to follow the progress of the barium into the stomach. Constrictions in the esophagus, the action of the stomach valve, and the presence of a hiatal hernia (the upper part of the stomach bulging through a weakened diaphragm) become visible. As the barium proceeds, a stomach ulcer may stand out in outline.

To check for kidney stones and to examine the kidneys, ureters, and urinary bladder, an intravenous pyelogram (IVP) is performed. First, a contrast solution (based on iodine, which blocks x-rays) is injected into the patient's vein. The patient may feel a brief warm flush as the body reacts to the iodine, but this reaction passes quickly. The solution used soon passes through the patient's system: through the kidneys, through the ureters, and to the bladder. A series of x-rays is then taken in which kidney stones may be revealed; any swelling of a kidney or blockage of a ureter will show up, if present.

The angiogram, a similar but more extensive procedure, is used to examine the blood vessels of the heart or other location. In this procedure, a catheter (fine plastic tube) is inserted into the femoral artery at the groin or into a blood vessel in the upper arm. The patient is given medication for pain and anxiety. Using a fluoroscope monitor, the physician maneuvers the catheter to the desired location and then injects the contrast solution through the catheter. Several x-rays are taken from various angles, and any blockages or constrictions are generally apparent. The catheter is then withdrawn, and the patient is required to rest.

CT scanning represents a major step forward in x-ray technology. A patient might suffer a sudden loss of muscle control and feeling in part of the body (possible stroke). The doctor would like to x-ray the brain for signs of a ruptured or blocked blood vessel, but contrast agents are not useful for the brain. Without them, internal organs and tissues appear only as faint ghosts in an x-ray. A CT scan uses computer technology to convert special x-ray images into clear views of the organs.

While prudence dictates that radiation exposure be kept to a minimum, the medical benefits of procedures using radiation generally outweigh the risks. Provided that a radiation dose is not overwhelmingly massive, the body has amazing recuperative properties and is able to repair most radiation damage. Everyone is exposed daily to background radiation from naturally occurring trace amounts of radioactive elements and from cosmic rays. None of the typical imaging procedures generates radiation above allowable limits, but it should be noted that a medical procedure may expose the target organ to many times the average body dose.

A typical x-ray image shows different types of tissue as various shades of gray. Advances in medical imaging include digitizing any image and using powerful computer programs to enhance the subtle differences between different types of tissue, even coloring them so that they are immediately obvious to the physician. Three-dimensional images can be constructed and rotated so that they can be examined from every angle. A physician can see exactly what problems will be encountered in removing a tumor. Computers can scan x-rays used to screen for breast cancer, called mammograms, and draw the radiologist's attention to any questionable regions. Finally, computers can merge images from complementary techniques such as PET (shows functionality of the organ) with MRI (shows high-resolution detail) to give a more complete view.

Perspective and Prospects

On November 8, 1895, Wilhelm Conrad Röntgen made an astounding and disquieting discovery. Many scientists of the day, including Röntgen, were studying cathode rays. The required apparatus was an evacuated glass tube with electrodes sealed inside at either end. When a high voltage was placed across the electrodes, cathode rays (electrons) streamed from the cathode, and where they struck the glass tube, the glass fluoresced.

Röntgen covered the tube with black paper and darkened the room, but still a fluorescent screen some distance away from the tube glowed whenever he operated the tube. Since cathode rays cannot travel far through air, Röntgen deduced that some unknown type of radiation must be coming from the tube. He called it X radiation (X for unknown). Placing bits of wood or metal between the tube and the screen cast shadows on the screen, some darker and some lighter. The key moment came when Röntgen held up a small lead disk. The expected shadow of the lead appeared, but holding the disk, Röntgen saw the shadows of his finger bones. He opened his hand, and the shadowy skeleton hand opened. Röntgen wondered if he could be hallucinating. In those days, some people believed that dreaming about or imagining seeing a skeleton was a premonition of one's impending death. Röntgen was concerned that others might think him insane if he were to describe what he had seen, so he needed proof.

In the ensuing weeks, Röntgen made an intense study of the properties of x-rays. Three days before Christmas, he placed photographic film in a black paper package and had his wife, Bertha, place her hand on it while he exposed it with x-rays for fifteen minutes. The photograph showed the bones of Bertha Röntgen's hand, with a ring on her finger. Röntgen sent a copy of the photograph along with an explanation to a friend, but it soon found its way into newspapers all over the world. Only four months after the public announcement, Thomas Edison's company began marketing "complete outfits for x-ray work." While some considered looking at skeletons while people were still using them revoltingly indecent, the medical usefulness of x-rays was immediately apparent. The first Nobel Prize in Physics ever awarded went to Röntgen in 1901 for his discovery of x-rays.

In spite of the obvious medical advantages, relatively few doctors used x-rays at first, but the public found them a source of entertainment. Edison built a fluoroscope for use at amusement parks. Looking through a hooded visor, spectators placed their hands between an x-ray tube and a fluorescent screen and watched their bones wiggle as they moved their hands. Casual exposure to x-rays continued into the 1950s with the use of fluoroscopes by shoe stores to see how well shoes fit.

The widespread use of medical x-rays was hampered by the lack of trained operators and proper equipment. This situation changed with World War I, when x-ray teams were trained and equipped by the hundreds. Marie Curie was a prime force in establishing such teams for the French and Belgian militaries. From this modest beginning, the various imaging techniques have evolved to provide the physician with "magic eyes" that can peer inside the body.

—*Charles W. Rogers, Ph.D.*

See also Angiography; Angioplasty; Computed tomography (CT) scanning; Diagnosis; Echocardiography; Electromyography; Endoscopic retrograde cholangiopancreatography (ERCP); Magnetic resonance imaging (MRI); Mammography; Neuroimaging; Noninvasive tests; Nuclear medicine; Nuclear radiology; Positron emission tomography (PET) scanning; Radiation sickness; Radiation therapy; Radiopharmaceuticals; Single photon emission computed tomography (SPECT); Ultrasonography.

For Further Information:

A.D.A.M. Medical Encyclopedia. "Imaging and Radiology." *MedlinePlus*, March 22, 2012.

Giger, Maryellen L., and Charles A. Pelizzari. "Advances in Tumor Imaging." *Scientific American* 275, no. 3 (September, 1996): 110–12.

MedlinePlus. "Diagnostic Imaging." *MedlinePlus*, May 24, 2013.

Mould, Richard F. *A Century of X Rays and Radioactivity in Medicine*. Philadelphia: Institute of Physics, 1993.

OrthoInfo. "X-Rays, CT Scans, and MRIs." *American Academy of Orthopaedic Surgeons*, 2013.

Raichle, Marcus E. "Visualizing the Mind." *Scientific American* 270, no. 4 (April, 1994): 58–64.

Ter-Pogossian, Michel M., Marcus E. Raichle, and Burton E. Sobel. "Positron-Emission Tomography." *Scientific American* 243, no. 4 (October, 1980): 170–81.

Weissleder, Ralph, et al. *Primer of Diagnostic Imaging*. 4th ed. Philadelphia: Mosby/Elsevier, 2007.

IMMUNE SYSTEM

Biology

Anatomy or system affected: Blood, cells, circulatory system, glands, liver, lymphatic system, spleen

Specialties and related fields: Cytology, hematology, immunology, microbiology, preventive medicine, serology

Definition: A system-including the spleen, thymus, lymphatic system, and specialized cells-that protects the body from foreign substances.

Key terms:

antibody: any of the proteins produced in the body during an immune response; recognizes and attacks foreign antigen substances

antigen: a substance within the human body recognized as foreign either by antibodies or by special immune cells; the cause behind the stimulation of the immune response

autoimmunity: an abnormal immune reaction against antigens

immunosuppression: a decrease in the effectiveness of the immune system

pathogen: any disease-causing organism, including a virus, bacterium, protozoan, mold or yeast, or other parasite

Structure and Functions

The immune system is capable of recognizing and identifying many different substances foreign to the human body. To function properly, this system must receive, interpret, and transmit large amounts of information about invaders from outside or within the body. These constant and ever-changing threats to the body must be met and destroyed by one complex system—namely, the human immune system. Many organs and parts of the body play a major role in maintaining resistance; some have more important roles than others, but all parts must work in unison. The circulatory and lymphatic systems, along with specific organs, are of primary importance in the overall workings of the immune system.

Blood. Besides the outer protective layer of the skin and mucous membranes, the first line of defense in the immune system includes the blood in the circulatory system. About 50 percent of human blood is made up of a fluid called plasma, which contains water, proteins, carbohydrates, vitamins, hormones, and cellular waste. The other half of blood is composed of white cells, red cells, and platelets. The red blood cells, called erythrocytes, are responsible for moving oxygen from the lungs to the other parts of the body. The special platelet cells, called thrombocytes, enable the blood to form clots, thus preventing severe bleeding. An unborn child produces red and white blood cells in the spleen and liver, while a newborn makes blood in the center of bones, called the marrow. After maturity, all red and most white blood cells are produced in the bone marrow. Although the red cells and platelets are vital, it is the white cells that play a major role in the immune system.

In a broad sense, white blood cells surround and engulf foreign matter and adjacent dying cells in a process called phagocytosis. The function is possible since the white blood cells can move, unlike red corpuscles, by pushing their bodies out and pulling forward. Red corpuscles move because of the flow of the blood within the circulatory system. White blood cells move in the lymph vessels, where they work to defend the body against disease, but are also transported through the blood. Bacteria and other foreign material can remain alive within a white corpuscle, but sometimes the corpuscle dies from the toxins produced by the bacteria. The resulting formation of pus is actually an accumulation of dead white blood cells. At other times, the white corpuscles win and the foreign matter is destroyed.

Three major types of white blood cells, known collectively as leukocytes, are involved in immune responses. All three—granulocytes, monocytes, and lymphocytes—arise from areas in either bone marrow, the spleen, or the liver.

The granulocytes, each of which is about twice the size of a red blood cell, originate from red bone marrow and live only about twelve hours. Under the classification of granulocytes, distinct cells have different structures, sizes, and shapes. These specialized granulocytes include the neutrophils, eosinophils, and basophils. None of these cells has a specific memory for future immune responses. The neutrophil granulocyte eats and digests small foreign matter with the help of special enzymes. Between 40 and 75 percent of the white blood cells in the human body are neutrophils. When these highly mobile neutrophil cells arrive at an injury site, they burst, releasing their enzymes and melting away the surrounding tissues. Eosinophils are similar to neutrophils but seem to be specialized in fighting infection caused by parasites, because of the seven toxic proteins that they use to fight. They are also effective against fungal, bacterial, viral, or protozoan infections. Basophils, which are smaller in size, move from the bone marrow through the body and act as a control

by preventing overreactions during an immune response. Basophils prevent coagulation, but they cannot destroy foreign matter. These cells account for less than 1 percent of the white blood cells found in the blood.

The second group of leukocytes includes the monocytes, the largest cells found in the blood. Monocytes are two to three times as large as red cells, yet they are not very numerous, making up 3 to 9 percent of all the leukocytes in the blood. After only a few days in the blood, they move to areas between tissues. Over the course of months or years, the monocytes enlarge ten times in size in order to specialize in phagocytosis. After this growth, they are called macrophages. They are also referred to as terminal cells since they cannot divide, and thus do not reproduce.

The third type of leukocyte, and the most sophisticated of the white blood cells, are called lymphocytes because they come from the lymph system as well as bone marrow. The T lymphocytes, which are primarily responsible for immunity, can change into helper, killer, and suppressor cells. Besides being able to recognize foreign matter precisely, they can live freely in the blood, grow larger and divide, and then change back to their original form after working against the invader. Lymphocytes circulate throughout the body, moving from the bloodstream through the lymph fluid and back into the blood. The two major types of lymphocytes are T lymphocytes (also called T cells) and B lymphocytes (also called B cells). Both T and B cells can recognize foreign matter and hook onto it. Some of these special "memory" cells remain in the body for life, preventing a specific invader from causing illness when it is encountered again in the future. These specialized cells must have a way to travel through the body; one of these transport systems is the lymphatic system.

The lymphatic system. This system is a closed network of vessels that help in circulating fluids from the body and returning them to the bloodstream. The lymphatic system also defends against disease-causing foreign materials, known as antigens. The smallest components of the lymph system are the lymphatic capillaries that run parallel to the blood capillaries. The fluid inside these capillaries, which has come across the thin wall membrane from tissues all across the body, is called lymph. These capillaries merge into larger lymphatic vessels, which then merge into a type of collecting area called a lymph node. The lymph fluid is drained into trunks that join one of two collecting ducts. The larger left thoracic duct collects lymph from the lower part of the abdomen and the legs, and from the left side of the upper body before emptying into a vein near the neck and shoulder. The right lymphatic duct does the same for the right side of the upper body. After leaving the collecting ducts, the lymph fluid becomes part of the blood plasma in the veins and returns to the right atrium of the heart. Lymph does not flow like blood in veins and arteries; instead, it is controlled by muscular activity.

The spleen. This largest lymphatic organ is located in the upper left part of the abdominal cavity, behind the stomach and under the diaphragm. The hollow spaces within the spleen are filled with blood, making it soft and elastic. The white blood cells in the lining of these hollow cavities engulf and destroy foreign materials, as well as damaged red blood cells that pass through the spleen.

The thymus. This gland is located between the lungs and above the heart, just behind the upper part of the breastbone. It contains large numbers of white cells; some are inactive, but others develop and leave the thymus to become functional in the immune system.

The liver. Located in the upper right part of the abdominal cavity below the diaphragm, the liver is well protected by the ribs. Since it is the largest gland in the body, it plays a major role in metabolism while also aiding the body's ability to clot blood. In addition, various liver cells, called macrophages, help in destroying damaged red blood cells. The liver's connection to the immune system is its ability to also destroy foreign substances through phagocytosis.

Bone marrow. Marrow is located in the center of bones. It can be divided into two types, red or yellow marrow. It is the red marrow that aids in the formation of white and red blood cells. The yellow marrow stores fat and is not involved in producing blood cells. Some white blood cells come from bone marrow cells. They are released into the blood and are carried to the thymus gland, where they undergo special processing that changes them into T lymphocytes (the letter *T* shows that they came from the thymus gland). The other lymphocytes that do not reach the thymus after leaving the bone marrow are named B lymphocytes (*B* because they came from bone marrow). These B lymphocytes are abundant in lymph nodes, the spleen, bone marrow, secretory glands, intestinal lining, and reticuloendothelial tissue.

The Responses of the Immune System

Failures of the immune system can lead to devastating diseases, either because the immune system attacks itself or because it fails to defend against outside foreign antigen matter. An antigen can be any substance that stimulates the body to fight, ranging from a bacterial infection to the virus that causes acquired immunodeficiency syndrome (AIDS).

When the body fights against an antigen, the immune system can produce two types of response, either a cellular immune response or a humoral immune response. The cellular response involves specific types of cells that recognize, attack, and destroy the invading pathogen or antigen. It is the primary response against most viruses, many fungi, parasitic organisms and some bacteria (for example, mycobacteria), and against transplanted tissues. The humoral immune response, which consists of complement and antibodies, is the body's main defense against most other bacteria. The two systems work together, however, communicating by complex chemical mediators.

Another way of looking at how the body fights to keep itself healthy is to separate the immune responses into either primary or secondary responses. The second time that a given antigen enters the body, the immune system attacks with what is called the secondary immune response stored in special immune memories, making it faster and more extensive than the primary response that occurred when the antigen was first en-

countered. This immune memory must be built for each antigen before the body becomes immune to the wide variety of diseases and conditions to which one is exposed on a daily basis.

The body begins to build this memory prior to birth by making an inventory of all the molecules within the body. Foreign substances not in this memory are considered to be antigens, which will activate an immune response. When an antigen is first encountered, the primary response occurs, producing lymphocytes that are sensitized to the invader. Many types of lymphocytes can respond in order to create the appropriate antibody molecules, which are then released into the lymph and transported to the blood. This process may last several weeks. During this primary immune response, the B cells and T cells serve as memory cells. Because a memory for the antigen has been stored, if this antigen is encountered in the future the memory cells can react more quickly and effectively. In this secondary immune response, the antibodies are ready to react by attaching themselves to the surfaces of the antigens. There must be a specific type of antibody produced for every type of antigen. These new antibodies may survive only a few months, but the memory cells live much longer.

There are four main ways that an antibody can bind to an antigen. The antibody can pull together clusters of invading organisms to prevent the antigens from spreading. Another possibility is for this special component of the blood to punch a hole in the invader and destroy it. The antibody can also combine with the antigen, which makes it easier to destroy. In the case of a virus or a toxin, the antibody can neutralize the harmful activity by covering the outside of the antigen. With so many ways for an antibody to attach to an antigen, it is equally important for the antibody memory to be established. It is this special memory that leads to future immunity.

These memory cells are responsible for the four different types of immunity, two of which are acquired actively and two of which are acquired passively. The first type is naturally acquired active immunity, which results after the body is exposed to a live pathogen and develops the disease. The second type is artificially acquired active immunity, such as that gained after a vaccination. The immune response is triggered after an injection of weakened or dead pathogens is received, but the body does not suffer the severe symptoms of the disease. An example would be a smallpox vaccination. The third type of immunity is artificially acquired passive immunity, gained through an injection of prepared antibodies. This method is considered passive since the antibodies, called gamma globulin, were made by another person. This type of immunity usually does not last more than a few weeks, and the person will be susceptible to that pathogen in the future. Naturally acquired passive immunity occurs when the antibodies pass to the fetus from the mother, but it includes only those antibodies available in the blood of the mother. This process gives an infant certain short-term immunities for the first year of life.

These types of immunity are usually desirable, but there are occasions when an immune response is not wanted, such as after an organ transplant. When tissue or organs are transplanted from one person to another, the body may reject the foreign tissue, triggering an immune response and possibly destroying the new organ. Consequently, attempts are made to match the tissue between recipient and donor. In an effort to halt the immune response, immunosuppressive drugs are given to interfere with the recipient's ability to form antibodies, and drugs can be administered to destroy the lymphocytes that produce these antibodies. Unfortunately, the recipient is often left unprotected against infections, since the immune system is not functioning normally.

Perspective and Prospects

In the same way that the discovery of penicillin shocked the world, immunology has created endless possibilities in medicine. When surgeons found that they could transplant an organ from one person to another, the interest in immunology exploded.

This field of medicine has discovered that the immune system's power and effectiveness can be lessened because of several factors. Improper diet, stress, disease, and excessive physical activity levels can depress the immune system. Other factors that can modify immunity include age, genetics, and metabolic and environmental factors. The anatomical, physiological, and microbial factors are shown in the susceptibility of the young and the very old to infections. For the young, the system is immature, while the aged have suffered a lifetime of assaults from pathogens. The impact of psychological stress is difficult to measure, yet it holds the potential for negatively affecting the immune system.

Before immunology can be fully understood, more knowledge must be gained about how antibodies are made and how they develop memories. Lymphocytes must be examined to discover what role they play in the immune response. Studies must look at not only the whole picture of the immune system but also its smaller parts—the organs and how each participates. Such studies could lead to better success in transplanting these organs. Unanswered questions remain about how the immune system relates to other body systems. The relationships among the brain and nervous system, hormones, and the respiratory system leave many areas ripe for further study.

Recent research has identified the significant importance of Class I major histocompatibility proteins (I-MHCPs) in the cellular immune system. When disease-associated proteins occur in a cell, they are broken into pieces by the cell's proteolytic machinery. Cell proteins become attached to antigen fragments and transport them to the surface of the cell, where they are "presented" to the body's defense mechanisms. I-MHCPs are these transport molecules. The I-MHCPs holding an antigen fragment can attach to certain immature T cells. Once such a T cell and I-MHCP-antigen complex hook up, the T cell reproduces many times. This important link between the cellular immune system and I-MHCPs has been shown in recent times by the epidemic of diseases like AIDS, which kills T cells. Class II MHCPs (II-MHCPs) interact similarly in antibody production by the humoral immune system. Understanding of the genes used in production of the I-MHCPs and the II-MHCPs has led to great hope for methods to control their production, possibilities for eventual cure of AIDS, emerging cancer treatments, and better understanding of the production of antibodies.

Additional information is needed on defects in the system, as are explanations for its dysfunctions. With greater knowledge of immunology, it may be possible to conquer AIDS, allergies, and asthma and to develop birth control methods based on the immune response. Doctors may be able to cure cancer, diabetes, herpes, infertility, multiple sclerosis, and rheumatoid arthritis. The possibilities are endless and could also include perfecting transplants of organs and skin grafts and preventing birth defects and even obesity. Through human gene therapy, those at risk for genetic disorders could be diagnosed and those with existing genetic conditions could be treated. Genetically engineered drugs and gene replacement therapy could relieve the stress on the human immune system. Until these methods become feasible, however, individuals must protect the natural immunity supplied by their bodies.

—*Maxine M. Urton, Ph.D.*

See also Acquired immunodeficiency syndrome (AIDS); Allergies; Antibodies; Antioxidants; Autoimmune disorders; Blood and blood disorders; Bone marrow transplantation; Cells; Chemotherapy; Circulation; Cytology; Cytopathology; Dialysis; Endocrinology; Endocrinology, pediatric; Glands; Healing; Hematology; Hematology, pediatric; Histiocytosis; Homeopathy; Hormones; Host-defense mechanisms; Human immunodeficiency virus (HIV); Immunization and vaccination; Immunodeficiency disorders; Immunology; Immunopathology; Infection; Kawasaki disease; Liver; Lymph; Lymphatic system; Multiple chemical sensitivity syndrome; Oncology; Preventive medicine; Serology; Severe combined immunodeficiency syndrome (SCID); Skin; Stress reduction; Systems and organs; Transfusion; Transplantation; Wiskott-Aldrich syndrome.

For Further Information:
Adelman, Daniel C., et al., eds. *Manual of Allergy and Immunology.* 5th ed. Philadelphia: Lippincott Williams & Wilkins, 2012.
Delves, Peter J., et al. *Roitt's Essential Immunology.* 12th ed. Malden, Mass.: Blackwell, 2011.
Frank, Steven A. *Immunology and Evolution of Infectious Disease.* Princeton, N.J.: Princeton University Press, 2002.
Immune Web. http://www.immuneweb.org.
Hawley, Louise, Richard J. Ziegler, and Benjamin L. Clarke. *Microbiology and Immunology.* Philadelphia: Lippincott Williams & Wilkins, 2013.
Janeway, Charles A., Jr., et al. *Immunobiology: The Immune System in Health and Disease.* 7th ed. New York: Garland Science, 2007.
Kuby, Janis, et al., eds. *Kuby Immunology.* 7th ed. New York: W. H. Freeman, 2013.
Life, Death, and the Immune System. New York: W. H. Freeman, 1994.
Male, David K., et al., eds. *Immunology.* Philadelphia: Elsevier/ Saunders, 2013.
Marieb, Elaine N. *Essentials of Human Anatomy and Physiology.* 10th ed. San Francisco: Pearson/Benjamin Cummings, 2012.
Tortora, Gerard J., and Bryan Derrickson. *Principles of Anatomy and Physiology.* 13th ed. Hoboken, N.J.: John Wiley & Sons, 2012.

IMMUNIZATION AND VACCINATION
Procedure

Anatomy or system affected: Blood, cells, immune system

Specialties and related fields: Immunology, microbiology, preventive medicine, public health

Definition: Immunization is the process by which exposure to an infectious agent or chemical confers an organism with resistance to that agent; vaccination involves the injection of a killed or attenuated microorganism, with the intention of inducing immunity.

Key terms:

active immunity: immunity resulting from antibody production following exposure to an antigen

antibody: a protein secreted by lymphocytes in response to antigen stimuli, such as bacteria or viruses; also referred to as immunoglobulin

antigen: any chemical substance that stimulates the production of antibodies

attenuation: the weakening or elimination of the pathogenic properties of a microorganism; ideally, the organism is rendered harmless

passive immunity: immunity resulting from the introduction of preformed antibodies

serotype: a subgroup member within a larger species that is similar, but not identical, to other members of the species

toxoid: a toxin that has been chemically treated to eliminate its toxic properties but that retains the same antigens as the original

vaccinia: a virus that causes a poxlike illness in cattle (cowpox) and serves as smallpox vaccine in humans because of its similarity to the smallpox virus

The Fundamentals of Immunization

The major day-to-day function of the immune response is to protect the body from infection. Exposure to foreign antigens such as infectious agents results in the stimulation of either of two components of the immune system: the humoral (or antibody) immune response or the cellular immune response. Although no clear division exists between these two facets of the immune system, the antibody response deals primarily with organisms such as bacteria that live outside the cell. The cellular response deals primarily with microbes that live within a cell, such as intracellular bacteria or viruses.

A specialized class of white cells called B lymphocytes carries out the production of antibodies. Stimulation of these cells results from a complicated interaction between a variety of cells, including antigen-presenting cells (macrophage and dendritic cells) and both T and B lymphocytes. The response is specific in that each type of T or B cell can interact with only a single antigen. The B cell that produces antibodies against a particular characteristic or shape on the surface of a bacterium reacts only with that particular determinant. In turn, the antibodies secreted by that B cell can interact only with specific determinants.

Antibodies secreted by B cells are themselves inert proteins. A variety of effects can result, however, when an anti-body binds to an antigen. The specific results depend on the nature of the antigen. For example, binding of an antibody to a toxin results in the neutralization of that substance. If the antigen is on the surface of a bacterial cell, then the antibody can act as a flag that attracts other chemicals circulating in the blood. The technical term for an antibody bound to a bacterium is *opsonin*. The antibody-bacterium complex becomes much more likely to be ingested and destroyed by a specialized cell called a phagocyte than if the antibody were not present. Likewise, if the antigen is an extracellular virus particle, binding of the antibody may inhibit the ability of the virus to infect a cell.

The cellular immune system also reacts in a specific manner. A subclass of T lymphocytes called cytotoxic T cells reacts with specific antigenic determinants on the surface of infected cells. When the T cells bind to a target, the result is the local release of toxic chemicals that ultimately kill the target.

The development of vaccines against specific infectious microbial agents resulted in the control or elimination of many diseases caused by these agents. The first formal vaccine developed for the prevention of disease was that used by Edward Jenner against smallpox during the 1790s. Another century passed before the molecular basis for vaccine function began to be understood.

Immunity to an antigen or disease may be induced using either of two methods. If preformed antibodies produced in another human or animal are inoculated into an individual, the result is passive immunity. Passive immunity can be advantageous in that the recipient achieves immunity in a short period of time. For example, if a person has been exposed to a toxin or has come into contact with an infectious agent, passive immunity can provide rapid, short-term protection. However, because the individual does not generate the capacity to produce that antibody, and the preformed antibodies are gradually removed from the body, no long-range protection is achieved.

The stimulation of antibody production through exposure to antigens, such as those found in a vaccine, results in active immunity. Development of effective active immunity requires a time span of several days to several weeks. The immunity is long term, however, often lasting for the life span of the individual. Furthermore, each additional exposure to that same antigen, either through a vaccine booster or through natural exposure, results in a more rapid, greater response than those achieved previously. This increased rate of reaction is referred to as an anamnestic response.

The actual material used in a vaccine is variable, depending on the form of antigen. The earliest vaccine, that used by Jenner against smallpox, consisted of a virus that caused a disease in cattle called cowpox. The word *vaccination* is itself derived from this use; *vacca* is the Latin word for cow. While cowpox is distinct from the disease smallpox, the viruses that cause the two diseases contain similar antigenic determinants. Jenner made this observation and exploited the fact that exposure to the cowpox virus results in active immunization against smallpox.

The use of attenuated strains of bacteria or viruses applies

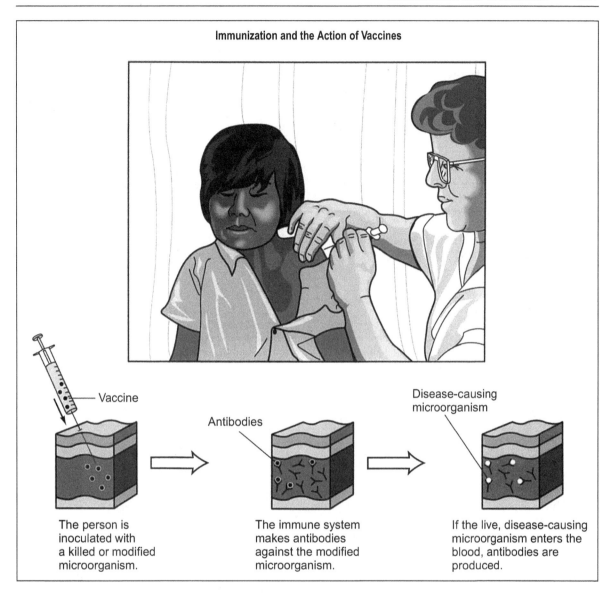

Immunization and the Action of Vaccines

Vaccine

Antibodies

Disease-causing microorganism

The person is inoculated with a killed or modified microorganism.

The immune system makes antibodies against the modified microorganism.

If the live, disease-causing microorganism enters the blood, antibodies are produced.

the same principle of cross-reaction. Attenuated organisms are mutants that have lost the ability to cause disease but that retain the antigenic character of the virulent strain. The most notable application of attenuation is the Sabin oral poliovirus vaccine (OPV). By testing hundreds of virus isolates for the ability to cause polio in monkeys, Albert Sabin was able to isolate certain strains that did not cause disease. These strains formed the basis for his vaccine. Similar testing resulted in the development of attenuated virus vaccines against a wide variety of agents, including measles, mumps, and rubella. Likewise, the Bacillus Calmette-Guérin (BCG) strain of *Mycobacterium tuberculosis* serves as a vaccine against the agent that causes tuberculosis. Unfortunately, the latter vaccine does not always result in immunity for the recipient. It generally is not used in the United States but is widely used in

countries where tuberculosis is common.

In some cases, the isolation of attenuated strains of microorganisms has proved difficult. For this reason, inactivated or killed microorganisms often serve as the basis for vaccine production. The Salk inactivated poliovirus vaccine represents the best-known example. By treating poliovirus with a solution of the chemical formalin, Jonas Salk was able to inactivate the organism. The virus retained its antigenic potential and served as an effective vaccine. A similar process has resulted in vaccines to protect against other bacterial diseases, such as bubonic plague, cholera, and pertussis (whooping cough), and against viral influenza.

In some cases, the vaccine is directed not against the etiological agent itself but against toxic materials produced by the agent. This is the case with diphtheria and tetanus. The vaccines are produced by treating the diphtheria and tetanus toxins secreted by these bacteria with formalin. The toxoids that result are antigenically similar to the actual toxins and so are able to induce immunity. They are incapable, however, of causing the deleterious effects of the respective diseases.

Only those determinants of a virus or bacterium that stimulate neutralizing antibodies are necessary in most vaccines. For this reason, the use of genetically engineered vaccines was begun in the 1980s. The first example put into use was the production of a vaccine against the hepatitis B virus (HBV). The gene that encodes the surface antigen of HBV was isolated and inserted into a piece of genetic material within the yeast *Saccharomyces*. The HBV antigen produced by the yeast was purified and subsequently found to be as effective in a vaccine as the whole virus. Since no live virus is involved, there is no danger of an attenuated strain reverting to its virulent parent. Recently, similar technology has been applied to produce vaccines that protect against chickenpox and hepatitis A virus.

History and Major Successes

Since the first use of vaccination by Jenner in the 1790s for the prevention of smallpox, immunization techniques have been developed for protection against most major infectious illnesses. The term *vaccination* was originally applied to immunization against smallpox, but its definition has long been expanded to include most immunization techniques. The terms *vaccination* and *immunization* are used interchangeably, although there are technical differences in their definitions.

The nineteenth-century improvements in public health measures, combined with the passage of laws for compulsory vaccination, resulted in a steady decrease in the number of smallpox cases in the United States and most countries of Europe. Even as late as 1930, however, approximately 49,000 cases were reported in the United States. In the 1950s, large numbers of cases were still being reported in areas of Africa and Asia. At that time, the World Health Organization (WHO) of the United Nations decided on a plan for the elimination of smallpox based on the fact that humans served as the sole reservoir for the smallpox virus; animals are not naturally infected with smallpox. Through the use of mass immunization techniques, the plan was to isolate areas of infection into smaller and smaller pockets.

The plan for the elimination of smallpox developed by WHO ultimately proved completely successful. There are actually two different forms of smallpox. The last known natural case of variola major was reported in Bangladesh in 1974. The last known case of variola minor was reported in Somalia in 1976. Although an outbreak of smallpox resulting from a laboratory accident was reported in Great Britain, there were no additional naturally caused cases of smallpox. In 1978, WHO declared the world to be free of smallpox.

Ironically, the origins of the vaccine in use during this successful campaign are unknown. The original strain of cowpox used by Jenner was lost sometime during the nineteenth century. The strain used in the vaccine during the twentieth century, called vaccinia virus, may have originated from an isolate obtained during the Franco-Prussian War in the 1870s.

Although vaccination was effective in immunizing most persons against smallpox, use of the vaccine itself had some risk. Serious complications were rare but did occasionally occur. With the disappearance of the disease, the need for routine immunization lessened, and, in 1971, compulsory vaccination of children in the United States was discontinued. In 1976, the routine vaccination of hospital employees was discontinued as well. By the 1990s, the only known sites of existence of smallpox virus were freezers in four laboratories. The September 11, 2001, terrorist attacks at the World Trade Center in New York City and at the Pentagon introduced a new era in which the fear of terrorists" use of biological agents has prompted renewed discussions about the reintroduction of the smallpox vaccine.

The use of vaccines for the elimination of poliomyelitis represents another success story. Although sporadic outbreaks of polio occurred in earlier centuries and probably as long ago as the time of ancient Egypt, the first epidemics appeared in the late nineteenth century. Ironically, this increase in the incidence of polio was caused by improvements in public health. Poliovirus is easily transmitted through a fecal-oral route, but the majority of cases, particularly in young children, are without symptoms, or asymptomatic. With improvements in sanitation, the first exposure to polio was often delayed until later childhood or, as in the case of President Franklin D. Roosevelt, in the adult years. Under these circumstances, the disease is often more severe.

In 1955, the inactivated poliovirus vaccine developed by Salk was introduced for general use; in 1961, Sabin's oral poliovirus vaccine was licensed for use. By the 1990s, polio had been eliminated from the Western Hemisphere and from developed countries elsewhere. In 2003, WHO developed the Global Polio Eradication Initiative, the purpose of which is both to monitor outbreaks of polio and to address the means of preventing its transmission. Despite setbacks in portions of Asia and Africa, the number of reported cases of polio worldwide was reduced to 223 by 2012, according to WHO data. Since eradication of polio is not complete, the American Academy of Pediatrics (AAP) recommends that children receive immunizations at intervals during their first two years of life and again before starting school. Adults who plan to travel to areas of the world in which polio is found should also be immunized.

The most significant advancement in twentieth-century health care in the United States has been the elimination of most major childhood diseases. In addition to poliovirus immunization, children routinely receive a variety of early immunizations. Measles, mumps, and rubella (MMR) vaccines are first administered in a single preparation at twelve to fifteen months of age. All three contain live attenuated viruses. The measles vaccine was first introduced in 1966 and resulted in a decline in reported measles cases of nearly 99 percent by the 1980s. Beginning about 1986, however, increasing numbers of cases of measles were reported among young adults who had been previously immunized. For this reason, the AAP recommends that children receive a second dose of MMR vaccine prior to entering school, at approximately four to six years of age. A series of the diphtheria, pertussis, and tetanus (DTaP) vaccine is administered at two, four, six, and fifteen to eighteen months, with tetanus and diphtheria boosters recommended at ten-year intervals throughout the remainder of a person's life.

With the elimination of most other major childhood illnesses, *Hemophilus influenzae* type B infections moved into the dubious position of being among the most significant causes of illness and death among young children. In 1985, a vaccine developed from the outer coat of the bacterium was licensed for use. The vaccine worked poorly in children under the age of two, the major population at risk. Consequently, an improved vaccine was developed and licensed by 1987. The second vaccine consisted of a portion of the bacterial coat of *H.influenzae* joined to diphtheria toxoid. Immunization with the vaccine is recommended at two, four, six, and twelve to fifteen months.

Understandings of immunity and immunization grew, and vaccine technology continued to evolve. For example, in 1986, a genetically engineered hepatitis B virus vaccine was developed and licensed. The gene that encodes the virus surface antigen was placed in a small piece of deoxyribonucleic acid (DNA), a plasmid, and inserted into the common baker's yeast *Saccharomyces cerevisiae*. The antigen that is produced is used in a three-dose series to immunize individuals at risk for the disease: health care workers, institutional staff, and anyone else who is likely to come into contact with the virus. It is also recommended in all children in an effort to eradicate disease through universal immunization.

Other vaccines developed during the late twentieth century include pneumococcal vaccine, meningococcal vaccine, hepatitis A vaccine, rotavirus vaccine, and varicella (chickenpox) vaccine. All of these have become part of routine immunization in children and adolescents.

Additionally, preparations of some long-standing vaccines have been improved through new technology. For example,

Recommended Childhood Immunization Schedule, Ages 0-6 (2010)

	Birth	1 mo.	2 mos.	4 mos.	6 mos.	12 mos.	15 mos.	18 mos.	19-23 mos.	4-6 yrs.
Hepatitis B	Dose 1	Dose 2			Dose 3					
Rotavirus			Doses 1, 2, 3							
Diphtheria, tetanus, pertussis (DTaP)			Doses 1, 2, 3				Dose 4			Dose 5
***H. influenzae* type B (HiB)**			Doses 1, 2, 3			Dose 4				
Polio			Doses 1, 2		Dose 3					Dose 4
Influenza					Yearly					
Measles, mumps, rubella (MMR)						Dose 1				Dose 2
Chickenpox (Varicella)						Dose 1				Dose 2
Pneumococcal vaccine (PCV)			Doses 1, 2, 3			Dose 4				
Hepatitis A						Doses 1, 2				

Approved by the Advisory Committee on Immunization Practices, the American Academy of Pediatrics, and the American Academy of Family Physicians.

live polio virus vaccine (Sabin) proved more effective than the original injectable vaccine (Salk). However, even the attenuated virus rarely caused disease in some vaccine recipients, and successful efforts were undertaken to improve the effectiveness of vaccine made from killed (inactivated) virus; this enhanced inactivated preparation is now in use in the United States. Likewise, pertussis vaccine, which was poorly tolerated in a significant number of children and adults, has been improved, and the new acellular pertussis vaccine preparation is now recommended for both children and adults.

Although routine vaccination of children has virtually eliminated most health-threatening infectious disease from that population, immunization of adults against preventable diseases has not been as successful. It was estimated that in the late twentieth century, between fifty thousand and seventy thousand adults died yearly from diseases that were preventable through immunization, such as pneumococcal pneumonia, influenza, and hepatitis B.

Historically, pneumococcal pneumonia, caused by the bacterium *Streptococcus pneumonia*, has been a killer of adults. In the 1990s, an estimated forty thousand persons, primarily the elderly, died from this disease. The available vaccine is a polysaccharide vaccine, representing serotypes for twenty-three of the major strains of the bacterium. When administered by the age of fifty, the vaccine provides a significant degree of protection against the organism.

Between 1957 and 2005, seasonal influenza outbreaks averaged between ten thousand to twenty-five thousand deaths per year in the United States alone. Two of the epidemics each resulted in more than forty thousand deaths. Most of these deaths were in elderly adults. Although the usefulness of vaccination among the elderly is limited, immunization against influenza will often lessen the severity of the disease, even if it fails to prevent infection. Furthermore, vaccination of large segments of the population, including health care workers, limits the spread of disease within the population and therefore reduces the exposure to susceptible elderly persons and others at risk for complications from influenza.

Shingles is a blistering skin condition caused by a reactivation of the chickenpox virus (varicella zoster, or herpes zoster) that occurs primarily among the elderly. Although it rarely causes death, it can be extremely painful, and the pain may persist long after the lesions heal. When the condition involves the area around they eye, blindness may result. A vaccine against this disease has been developed.

Some specialized vaccines are recommended only for international travelers. Both killed injectable and live attenuated oral vaccines against typhoid are licensed. The ease of administration of an oral vaccine has made this form the preferred choice. In addition, vaccines against cholera and yellow fever may be used in appropriate circumstances.

Although active immunization in most circumstances remains the preferred method of protection through vaccination, there are situations in which passive immunization may provide temporary protection. Individuals may be immunosuppressed or lack a functional immune system. This condition may result from infection (acquired immunodeficiency syndrome, or AIDS), medical intervention (chemotherapy), or congenital reasons (severe combined immunodeficiency disease, or SCID). Whatever the cause, active immunization does not develop. In addition, there are circumstances in which the necessary time for the development of immunity through active immunization is not available, such as with exposure to tetanus, hepatitis A or B, or rabies. For passive immunization or replacement therapy in immunodeficiency disorders, immunoglobulin is usually prepared from pools of plasma obtained from large numbers of blood donors. Specific immunoglobulins, directed against specific targets such as rabies or tetanus, are prepared from plasma containing high concentrations of these antibodies.

Perspective and Prospects

The elimination of smallpox represents the classic example in which the efficacy of a vaccine resulted in the eradication of disease. Smallpox was an ancient disease, with origins as early as the twelfth century BCE. It appeared in the Middle East in the sixth century CE, with subsequent dissemination into northern Africa and southern Europe as a result of the Arab invasions from the sixth to the eighth centuries. The disease spread throughout Europe during the Crusades of the eleventh and twelfth centuries and reached the Americas early in the colonial period. It has been estimated that at its peak during the eighteenth century, smallpox killed 400,000 persons each year and caused more than one-third of all cases of blindness. It has also been estimated that smallpox or other diseases that traveled to the Americas with settlers killed approximately 85 percent of the American Indians who died during colonial periods.

The principle of immunization in prevention did not originate with Jenner, the English physician credited with development of the smallpox vaccine in the 1790s. A practice called variolation was well known in China and parts of the Middle East for centuries prior to Jenner. Variolation consisted of the inhalation of dried crust prepared from the pocks obtained from individuals suffering from mild cases of smallpox. A variation involved removing small amounts of fluid from an active smallpox pustule and scratching the liquid into the skin of children. Lady Mary Wortley Montagu, wife of the British ambassador to the Ottoman Empire, introduced the practice of variolation into Great Britain during the early eighteenth century. Use of variolation was empirical; the practice was often successful. The possibility remained, however, that immunization might actually introduce the disease.

Born in 1749, Jenner first became aware of the protective effects of cowpox from the story of a local dairymaid who had been exposed to the disease. After years of study and observation, he became convinced of the story's validity. In 1796, he immunized an eight-year-old boy with material from a cowpox lesion. No ill effects were seen. Further immunizations supported the theory that cowpox protected against smallpox. Jenner called this material variolae vaccinae. Richard Dunning, a Plymouth physician, in an 1800 analysis of the proce-

In the News: Combination Vaccine Pediarix for Infants

In December, 2002, the U.S. Food and Drug Administration (FDA) approved a multicomponent vaccine containing diphtheria and tetanus toxoids, acellular pertussis adsorbed (DTaP), hepatitis B (HepB; recombinant), and inactivated poliovirus (IPV) components. This vaccine, manufactured by GlaxoSmithKline Biologicals in Belgium, is called DTaP-HepB-IPV combined vaccine, or Pediarix. It is intended to be given to infants in three injections, one each at two, four, and six months of age. Pediarix provides protection against diphtheria, tetanus, pertussis (whooping cough), hepatitis B, and poliomyelitis in a series of only three injections instead of the nine injections previously given to infants. Thus, for patients and practitioners alike, it provides benefits such as saved office visits and decreased costs. Most important, the shorter injection series makes it much easier for parents, increasing the likelihood that parents will have their children immunized against these serious diseases.

The Pediarix vaccine has been subjected to numerous worldwide clinical trials to evaluate its safety and immunogenicity, or impact on the immune system. Data indicate that the vaccine is both safe and effective, with no significant adverse effects being reported. In these trials, the immunogenicity of each of the components in the combined vaccine was not shown to differ significantly from the immunogenicity of the components administered separately. These studies, involving more than seven thousand infants, reported minor adverse affects, including injection-site soreness (pain, redness, or swelling), fever, and irritability. The Pediarix vaccine has been associated with a greater frequency of fever in comparison to the separately administered vaccine components. Infants who are hypersensitive to any component of the vaccine, including yeast, neomycin, and polymyxin B, should not be given the vaccine. The Advisory Committee on Immunization Practices (ACIP), the Committee on Infectious Diseases of the American Academy of Pediatrics, and the American Academy of Family Physicians all have recommended this vaccine for routine use.

—Steven A. Kuhl, Ph.D.

dure, was the first to use the term *vaccination*.

Wider application of the principle of vaccination followed from Louis Pasteur's studies during the 1870s and 1880s. With his attenuation of the bacterium that caused chicken cholera, Pasteur demonstrated that one could manipulate the virulence of a microorganism. This practice soon led to his development of vaccines against both anthrax and rabies.

The twentieth century saw the development of effective vaccines against most major childhood diseases. Use of the DPT toxoid became routine in the United States about 1945. Development of the oral Sabin vaccine and inactivated Salk vaccines during the 1950s resulted in the complete elimination of poliomyelitis from the Western Hemisphere by the 1990s. The use of genetic engineering, in which only the genes necessary to synthesize specific antigens are used, was first applied to the hepatitis B vaccine. It has also been applied successfully to create vaccines against chickenpox and hepatitis A virus. A vaccine against hepatitis C virus is under development. This technology provides the potential for manufacturing vaccine "cocktails," or combinations of such genes from a variety of infectious agents in a single vaccine.

Some vaccines have more wide-ranging impact than prevention of infection, as some long-standing viral infections have been shown to cause cancer. This is true of both hepatitis B and hepatitis C, which are implicated in the development of primary hepatocellular carcinoma, the most common form of cancer worldwide.

Another such vaccine is directed against infection by cer-

tain strains of the human papillomavirus (HPV). HPV is most commonly associated with genital warts and is usually transmitted sexually, but it may be spread by hand contact as well. Infection by some strains may lead to the development of cervical cancer. According to WHO, more than 500,000 new cases of cervical cancer are diagnosed annually, and more than 250,000 women die of the disease each year. In 2006, a vaccine called Gardasil, directed against the four most common types of HPV, was licensed. A three-dose regimen is recommended for girls and women between nine and twenty-six years old. Some experts recommend that the vaccine be extended to boys and young men as well to interrupt more effectively the most common chain of infection.

Several infections that cause a huge burden of illness and death worldwide have so far eluded efforts to create a successful vaccine. Malaria is one example. Attempts to develop a vaccine against AIDS also have proven largely unsuccessful. The mechanism that has been exploited by other vaccines, namely the stimulation of T cells to produce antibodies that protect a recipient, is nonfunctional in AIDS, and successful development of a vaccine against AIDS will require scientific ingenuity.

New infections also have attracted the attention of vaccine researchers. The appearance of a new outbreak of avian influenza in 2003, usually referred to simply as the bird flu, raised new concerns about particularly virulent strains of influenza. The emergence in 2009 of a new strain of influenza, the novel H1N1 strain, raised fears of a pandemic (a worldwide epidemic) and challenged the capacity of the pharmaceutical industry to develop an effective vaccine and to produce enough of it in a short time to immunize the world's population against an imminent threat. The emergence of new infections, the threat of bioterrorism, and the unique difficulties posed by some microorganisms remain areas of active investigation in the field of vaccine research and development.

—Richard Adler, Ph.D.;
L. Fleming Fallon, Jr., M.D., Ph.D., M.P.H.;
updated by Margaret Trexler Hessen, M.D.

See also Acquired immunodeficiency syndrome (AIDS); Anthrax; Antibiotics; Avian influenza; Bacterial infections; Bacteriology; Biological and chemical weapons; Chickenpox; Childhood infectious diseases; Cholera; Diphtheria; Disease; Emerging infectious diseases; Environmental health; Epidemics and pandemics; Hepatitis; H1N1 influenza; Host-defense mechanisms; Human papillomavirus (HPV); Immune system; Immunology; Influenza; Measles; Microbiology; Mumps; Pathology; Plague; Poliomyelitis; Preventive medicine; Rubella; Smallpox; Tuberculosis; Viral infections; Whooping cough; World Health Organization.

For Further Information:

A.D.A.M. Medical Encyclopedia. "Immunizations." *MedlinePlus*, March 23, 2012.

Behbehani, Abbas. *The Smallpox Story in Words and Pictures*. Kansas City, Mo.: University of Kansas Medical Center, 1988.

Brock, Thomas D., ed. *Microorganisms: From Smallpox to Lyme Disease*. New York: W. H. Freeman, 1990.

Delves, Peter J., et al. *Roitt's Essential Immunology*. 11th ed. Malden, Mass.: Blackwell, 2006.

Glickman-Simon, Richard. "What Are Vaccines?" *Health Library*, February 28, 2013.

Grandi, Guido, ed. *Genomics, Proteomics, and Vaccines*. Hoboken, N.J.: John Wiley & Sons, 2004.

National Institute of Allergy and Infectious Diseases. "How Vaccines Work." *National Institutes of Health*, April 19, 2011.

Playfair, J. H. L., and B. M. Chain. *Immunology at a Glance*. 9th ed. Hoboken, N.J.: Wiley-Blackwell, 2009.

Plotkin, Stanley A., and Walter A. Orenstein, eds. *Vaccines*. 4th ed. Philadelphia: W. B. Saunders, 2004.

Rosario, Diane. *Immunization Resource Guide: Where to Find Answers to All Your Questions About Childhood Vaccinations*. Burlington, Iowa: Patter, 2001.

World Health Organization. *World Health Organization*, 2013.

IMMUNODEFICIENCY DISORDERS
Disease/Disorder

Anatomy or system affected: Immune system

Specialties and related fields: Genetics, immunology

Definition: Genetic or acquired disorders that result from disturbances in the normal functioning of the immune system.

Key terms:

antibody: protein immunoglobulin secreted by B lymphocytes; the production of antibodies is induced by specific foreign invaders, and they combine with and destroy only those invaders

B lymphocytes: also referred to as B cells; white cells of the immune system that produce antibodies; produced within the bone marrow

phagocytes: white cells of the immune system that destroy invading foreign bodies by engulfing and digesting them in a nonspecific immune response; include macrophages and neutrophils

stem cells: multipotential precursor cells within the bone marrow that develop into white cell populations, including lymphocytes and phagocytic cells

T lymphocyte: a type of immune cell that kills host cells infected by bacteria or viruses and secretes chemicals (interleukins) that regulate the immune response

Causes and Symptoms

The defense of the body against foreign invaders is provided by the immune system. In nonspecific immunity, phagocytic cells engulf and destroy invading particles. Specific immunity consists of very specialized cell types that are synthesized in response to a particular type of foreign invader. Self-replicating stem cells within the bone marrow give rise to lymphocytes, which mediate specific immunity. Lymphocytes establish self-replacing colonies within the thymus, spleen, and lymph nodes. The various categories of T lymphocytes are derived from the thymus colonies, while B lymphocytes develop and mature within the bone marrow. B lymphocytes secrete highly specific antibodies that attack bacteria and some viruses.

T lymphocytes do not secrete antibodies. Cytotoxic T cells directly attack body cells that have been infected with a bacterium or virus, while helper T cells regulate the immune response, either by directly interacting with other lymphocytes or by secreting chemicals, called interleukins, that regulate those cells. In immunodeficiency disorders, some or all of these defenses are compromised, which can have life-threatening consequences. Immunodeficiency diseases are generally the result of genetic abnormalities and are present from birth; others may be acquired through infection or exposure to damaging drug or radiation treatments. Depending upon the specific defect, the result may range from limited defects involving a class of cells to an entire shutdown of the immune system; prognosis depends on the severity of the defect. Since these defects generally involve recessive traits, expression of immune deficiencies usually results from mutations on the X chromosome; sex-linked traits are generally observed only in males, since males carry a single X chromosome.

The most severe immunodeficiency disorder is attributable to the absence of stem cells, which results in a total lack of both B and T lymphocytes. This rare genetic condition is referred to as severe combined immunodeficiency syndrome (SCID). Affected infants show a failure to thrive from birth and can easily die from common bacterial or viral infections. The term SCID encompasses a variety of genetic deficiencies. Certain forms are sex-linked, while other types may be autosomal (non-sex-linked). The most common autosomal form is a deficiency in the enzyme adenosine deaminase, resulting in disruption of deoxyribonucleic acid (DNA) synthesis in the stem cells.

Major syndromes that involve defects specific to the T lymphocyte population are characterized by recurrent viral and fungal infections. DiGeorge syndrome results from improper development of the thymus, which in turn results in insufficient production of T lymphocytes, often accompanied by other structural abnormalities in the infant. In severe cases, death results in early childhood from overwhelming viral infections.

The most common disorders affecting B lymphocytes are forms of hypogammaglobulinemia. This condition is characterized by insufficient levels of antibody. The cause is generally associated with increased rates of antibody breakdown or loss in the urine secondary to kidney malfunction. Bruton's agammaglobulinemia is a rare, sex-linked form of the condition, in which B cells fail to mature properly. Severe bacterial infections are the most common symptom. When the disorder is left untreated, infants generally die of severe pneumonia prior to six months of age.

Several immunodeficiency disorders may be the result of partial defects in the production and/or function of B and T lymphocytes. Wiskott-Aldrich syndrome is a genetically inherited disease manifested by recurrent infections and an itchy, scaly inflammation of the skin. Certain classes of antibodies are absent or scarce. Chronic mucocutaneous candidiasis is characterized by chronic fungal infection of the skin and mucous membranes; reduced levels of T cells are responsible for this disfiguring disorder.

Immunodeficiency disorders may also be the result of defects in phagocytic cells; the underlying cause of most of these disorders is ill-defined but often involves deficiencies in hydrolytic enzymes. In chronic granulomatosis, an inherited enzyme deficiency prevents the immune system from destroying bacteria that have been phagocytized. Infants affected by this disorder develop severe infections and chronic inflammations of internal organs and bones. The bacteria responsible for these infections are generally common flora that are not considered pathogens in healthy individuals.

Immune disorders may involve defects in antibody production. However, certain forms of inherited disorders involve another group of proteins called complement. Complement actually represents a group of serum proteins that interact with each other in a series. The pathway may be activated either specifically from antibody-target interactions or nonspecifically by surface components of certain bacteria. Intermediates in the complement pathway attract or stimulate phagocytosis (opsonins), induce inflammation, and play roles in cell destruction. Some of the intermediates are enzymes that regulate the activation of complement components. The most important intermediate in the pathway is the C3 component. C3 is a protein that acts as an opsonin and at the same time is involved in activating later steps in the sequence. Defects in C3 result in increased susceptibility to infection. Similar immune problems may result from defects in other complement intermediates.

Most of the disorders that affect the immune system are not inherited but develop sometime during the person's life. They are either the result of an infection or a consequence of another disease or its treatment. The use of corticosteroids to treat inflammations, or the illicit use of them in muscle-building, can interfere with the proper production and function of T lymphocytes. Other immunosuppressive drugs used to diminish the possibilities of graft or transplant rejection, or in the treatment of autoimmune diseases, can severely depress antibody production. Chemotherapeutic agents used in the treatment of cancer can affect DNA replication and severely compromise the entire immune system. Whole-body radiation can damage or destroy bone marrow stem cells.

Acquired immunodeficiency syndrome (AIDS) is caused by the human immunodeficiency virus (HIV). HIV is transmitted primarily through unprotected sexual contact, sharing of needles for intravenous drug use, transfusion with contaminated blood products, or contact with contaminated body fluids. HIV specifically infects one type of regulatory T lymphocyte, the helper T cell, resulting in severe immune depression. The virus may be harbored in an inapparent form for

---

Information on Immunodeficiency Disorders

Causes: Genetic disorders, infections, damage from drug or radiation treatments, environmental factors

Symptoms: Vary; can include recurrent infections, scaly inflammation of skin, chronic inflammations of internal organs and bones, fever, fatigue

Duration: Often chronic

Treatments: Typically targeted at source of deficiency; can include antibody injections, antifungal medications, bone marrow transplantation, drug cocktails, alternative medicine (acupuncture, herbal medicine, meditation, homeopathy)

---

years. Initial symptoms may be quite mild, but they generally progress so that the affected individual becomes susceptible to a host of opportunistic bacterial and fungal infections. A rare form of cancer called Kaposi's sarcoma is associated with infection by a particular human herpesvirus, HHV8, in persons with AIDS. AIDS also produces neurological damage in about one-third of infected individuals.

Treatment and Therapy

Most treatment of immunodeficient individuals is palliative. Infections are treated with antibiotics whenever possible. Individuals are counseled to avoid situations in which they may be exposed to contagious agents.

Treatment of immunodeficiency disorders may also target the source of the deficiency. For example, in DiGeorge syndrome, characterized by the congenital absence of the thymus, fetal thymus transplants may correct the problem, with improvement in lymphocyte levels seen within hours after the transplants. The use of thymus extracts has also been beneficial. Syndromes such as hypogammaglobulinemia can be managed by injection with mixtures of antibodies. Drug therapy to substitute for some immune components absent in Wiskott-Aldrich syndrome has been shown to have variable effects. The most effective treatment for chronic mucocutaneous candidiasis is aggressive antifungal medication to eradicate the causative organism; treatment must continue for several months because fungal infections are slow to respond to therapy and frequently recur. Chronic granulomatosis is notoriously difficult to treat, and the most effective therapy has been antibiotic and antifungal agents used aggressively during an overt infection.

Because of the magnitude of the defects, many inherited immunodeficiency disorders are difficult to treat successfully and are commonly fatal early in life. Chronic granulomatosis is usually fatal within the first few years of life, and only about 20 percent of patients reach the age of twenty. SCID is a serious disorder in which affected infants can die before a proper diagnosis is made. For individuals with these and other serious immunodeficiency disorders, maintenance in an environment free of bacteria, viruses, and fungi, such as a sterile "bubble," has been the best means to prevent life-threatening infections. Such an approach, however, precludes the possibility of a normal life. The most effective treatment for individuals with severely compromised immune systems is bone marrow transplantation. In this procedure, bone marrow from a compatible individual is introduced into the bone marrow of the patient. If the procedure works—and the success rate is high—in approximately one to six months the transplant recipient's immune system will be reconstituted and functional; full recovery make take up to one year. Bone marrow transplantation is a permanent cure for these disorders, since the transplanted marrow will contain stem cells that produce all the cell types of the immune system. The difficulties in transplantation include finding a compatible donor and preventing infections during the period after the transplant.

Drug therapy for AIDS utilizes treatments that interfere with replication of the virus. The first drug to be approved for use was zidovudine (formerly AZT), a DNA analogue, but its success was somewhat limited, as it was associated with severe side effects and the creation of resistant virus. More recent treatments utilize drug "cocktails," combinations of drugs that act at different stages of viral replication. Vaccines and antibiotic therapy are used to prevent or treat the opportunistic illnesses that accompany AIDS. Various drugs may also help to ease symptoms of AIDS such as appetite disturbances, nausea, pain, insomnia, anxiety, depression, fever, and diarrhea. A combination of therapies has been shown to increase life expectancy in AIDS patients. Many patients choose to participate in clinical trials of experimental drugs not approved for general use in the hope that the new drug will be more effective at alleviating the disease. Others seek out alternative or nontraditional medical treatments that have a long history of use in Western cultures. These treatments include acupuncture, herbology, meditation, and homeopathy. An important aspect of therapy for AIDS patients is maintaining mental health through support groups and supportive caregivers.

Illicit use of corticosteroids can seriously compromise the immune system and may lead to permanent damage. The best therapy for this type of acquired immunodeficiency is prevention—that is, to not misuse the drugs. In their supervised use to control inflammation or other disease symptoms, normal immune function will return after treatment has been completed. A huge risk to cancer patients who are being treated with chemotherapy and/or radiation therapy is the depression of the immune system, which can lead to a host of infections being contracted and not easily fought off by the body's compromised immune system. These individuals should avoid exposure to infectious agents when possible and be attentive to lifestyle modifications that can strengthen the immune system and encourage its speedy recovery, including a nutritious diet, plenty of rest, and avoidance of stress. Close monitoring for any signs of infection facilitates rapid antibiotic therapy, which can prevent serious complications.

Perspective and Prospects

Prior to the gains in scientific knowledge about the mechanics of the immune system, individuals with genetic immunodeficiency disorders would die of serious infections during their first few years of life. Even when it was finally realized that these individuals suffered from defects of the immune system, little could be done for most of the disorders, except to treat infections as they developed and to avoid contact with potential disease-causing organisms—a near impossibility if one is to lead a normal life. Housing persons with SCID in sterile bubbles was uncommon because of the expense and impracticality. During the 1970s, bone marrow transplants were first developed; by the 1990s they had progressed to a greater than 80 percent success rate. As a result of improved transplant-rejection drugs, transplants from donors with less-than-perfect tissue matches are now possible. Bone marrow transplantation has been a source of cure for many individuals with immune disorders.

Bone marrow transplantation is not suitable or possible in every case of immunodeficiency disorder, and scientists have long sought a means to cure the genetic defects themselves. In 1992, French Anderson of the National Institutes of Health conducted the first gene therapy trial on a young girl suffering from SCID. Some of the girl's bone marrow cells were removed from her body and exposed to an inactivated virus containing a normal gene for ADA, the defective enzyme. Some of the stem cells in the marrow incorporated the healthy gene, and the engineered cells were returned to her body. The cells lodged in her bone marrow, where they produced healthy immune cells. The procedure was repeated successfully in three other children shortly afterward.

Among the exciting applications of research into the molecular biology of immunodeficiencies has been the identification of specific genetic defects. Bone marrow stem cells can now be isolated and identified. In the future, such cells may be engineered such that the defective gene associated with the deficiency may be replaced by a normal copy. Since the cells are those from the same individual, transplantation problems can be avoided. However, bone marrow or cord blood transplants remain the only cure for SCID.

—*Karen E. Kalumuck, Ph.D.;*
updated by Richard Adler, Ph.D.

See also Acquired immunodeficiency syndrome (AIDS); Allergies; Arthritis; Asthma; Autoimmune disorders; Blood and blood disorders; Bone marrow transplantation; Cells; Cytology; Cytopathology; DiGeorge syndrome; Gene therapy; Hematology; Hematology, pediatric; Host-defense mechanisms; Human immunodeficiency virus (HIV); Immune system; Immunology; Immunopathology; Serology; Wiskott-Aldrich syndrome.

For Further Information:

Abbas, Abul K., and Andrew H. Lichtman. *Basic Immunology: Functions and Disorders of the Immune System*. 4th ed. Philadelphia: Saunders/Elsevier, 2012.

Bartlett, John G., and Ann K. Finkbeiner. *The Guide to Living with HIV Infection*. 6th ed. Baltimore: Johns Hopkins University Press, 2007.

Canellos George P., and Nancy Berliner. *Immunodeficiency, Infection, and Stem Cell*. Philadelphia: Saunders, 2011.

Delves, Peter J., et al. *Roitt's Essential Immunology*. 12th ed. Malden, Mass.: Blackwell, 2011.

Fehervari, Zoltan, and Shiman Sakaguchi. "Peacekeepers of the Immune System." *Scientific American*, October, 2006, 56–63.

Frank, Steven A. *Immunology and Evolution of Infectious Disease.* Princeton, N.J.: Princeton University Press, 2002.

Geha Raif S., and Luigi Notarangelo. *Case Studies in Immunology: A Clinical Companion.* 6th ed. New York: Garland Science, 2012.

Immune Web. http://immuneweb.org.

Parker, James N., and Philip M. Parker, eds. *The Official Parent's Sourcebook on Primary Immunodeficiency.* San Diego, Calif.: Icon Health, 2002.

Sticherling, Michael, and Enno Christophers, eds. *Treatment of Autoimmune Disorders.* New York: Springer, 2003.

Stine, Gerald J. *AIDS Update 2013.* New York: McGraw-Hill, 2013.

Vickers, Peter S. *Severe Combined Immune Deficiency: Early Hospitalization and Isolation.* Hoboken, N.J.: John Wiley & Sons, 2009.

IMMUNOPATHOLOGY

Specialty

Anatomy or system affected: All

Specialties and related fields: Dermatology, genetics, hematology, immunology, pathology, serology

Definition: The study of disease processes that have an immunological basis or pathogenesis involving either B cells (antibodies) and complement or T cells, including damage to tissues and cells caused by hypersensitivity reactions.

Key terms:

antibody: a molecule of the immune system, produced by B cells and targeted toward eliminating a specific antigen

B cells: also known as B lymphocytes; the antibody-producing cells of the immune system

congenital: something that is present at birth

hypersensitivity: reactions in which the immune system response is exaggerated

immunodeficiency: a state in which the immune system components that are meant to protect an individual are in a weakened state or absent altogether

T cells: also known as T lymphocytes; the immune system cells involved in cellular immunity and regulation of the immune response

Science and Profession

Immunopathology is the subdiscipline of immunology that deals with the four basic types of pathologies caused by the immune system: autoimmune disorders, congenital immunodeficiencies, acquired immunodeficiencies, and hypersensitivity reactions. Physicians who deal with such disorders are trained in immunology and/or pathology.

Autoimmune disorders are those in which the body fails to distinguish between self and nonself, leading to attack by the immune system on the tissues or organs of the body. There are many autoimmune disorders, and the symptoms are extremely varied, depending on the site and extent of the attack. Some disorders are tissue-specific, while others affect tissues and organs throughout the body. Examples of autoimmune disorders are multiple sclerosis (MS), systemic lupus erythematosus (SLE), and myasthenia gravis.

Congenital (primary) immunodeficiencies are those conditions in which there is an absence or a failure of the immune system at birth. Often they are the result of a failure of one or more components of the immune system to develop during the fetal stages. Most congenital deficiencies have a genetic basis. An example of a primary immunodeficiency disorder is DiGeorge syndrome, in which T cells are deficient as a result of a developmental problem of the thymus. The most severe of these disorders is severe combined immunodeficiency disorder (SCID), in which both B and T cells do not develop or function properly. Complement deficiencies fall into this category as well. Complement is a series of proteins that combine to generate an attack on invading cells, such as bacteria.

Acquired (secondary) immunodeficiencies are those that arise later in life, following a change in some environmental condition or exposure, such as accidents or surgery that damages or removes the spleen or lymph nodes, radiation exposure that damages the bone marrow, and cancers that attack or destroy parts of the immune system. Lymphocytic leukemias (malignancies of bone marrow precursors of B and T cells) are an example of acquired immune system diseases. Malnutrition or the use of certain drugs (especially opiates) may also affect the immune system responses in a negative way. Finally, viruses, such as human immunodeficiency virus (HIV), can attack and suppress the human immune system components, leading to a deficient ability to defend the body from daily attack by microorganisms. Some acquired immunodeficiencies occur without identified cause.

In contrast to the immunodeficiency syndromes, hypersensitivity reactions are those in which the immune system overreacts in its attempt to keep the body healthy, and by doing so causes localized or systemic reactions that can range from annoying to life-threatening. Hypersensitivity reactions are classified according to their molecular mechanism of action and may overlap with other categories, such as autoimmune disorders. Type I reactions are those which most people would recognize as allergies. Here, a series of chemicals, including immunoglobulin E (IgE), are released into the bloodstream, triggering the effects commonly associated with allergies: runny nose, itchy eyes, and difficulty breathing. The most severe case is anaphylaxis, sometimes seen in individuals with allergies to bee or wasp venom or to certain food substances. Type II reactions are those in which existing antibodies in the bloodstream bind to antigens that are seen as foreign and begin the process of tissue destruction. Examples include transfusion reactions, in which the wrong blood type is given to an individual, and erythroblastosis fetalis (hemolytic disease of the newborn), in which maternal antibodies attack a developing fetus that has a different set of antigens. Type III disorders are those in which large immune complexes form and are deposited in the bloodstream or kidneys, leading to disorders such as vasculitis and glomerulonephritis. Type IV reactions are those involving T-cell attack; they include contact dermatitis (such as poison ivy reactions) and transplant rejection.

Diagnostic and Treatment Techniques

Specialists who deal with immunopathologies may provide treatments that vary widely, as do the disorders themselves.

The goal of all therapy is to restore the immune system to its normal balance so that it can continue to protect the body from the constant barrage of invading microorganisms. Individuals with immune system deficiencies are told to avoid contact with other individuals as much as possible, since most viruses and bacteria are spread through personal contact. Prophylactic regimens of antibiotics, antivirals, and antifungals are helpful in most of those with immunodeficiencies, but in those with more severe forms, bone marrow transplants are the treatment of choice. The use of passive immunization—transferring antibodies from healthy individuals into those with immunodeficiencies—is helpful in some cases. In acquired immunodeficiency syndrome (AIDS), drug combinations, or "cocktails," are aimed at suppressing replication of HIV, which attacks the T cells and keeps them from functioning.

Because most hypersensitivity reactions are temporary immunopathologies, their treatment involves short-term therapies to restore balance to the system. Antihistamines, for instance, help many allergy sufferers, as do air purifiers and lifestyle changes. Careful tissue and blood typing can eliminate or lower the instances of the other types of hypersensitivities.

Treatment for autoimmune disorders is also quite variable, because of the wide variety of manifestations and underlying causes. Treatments commonly include immunosuppressive drugs and replacement of hormones or other chemicals that the body is lacking.

Perspective and Prospects

Since immunology itself is a field that is still in its infancy, recognition of immune disorders and their treatments is relatively new. Autoimmunity was first described by Paul Ehrlich at the turn of the twentieth century, and he called the phenomenon "horror autotoxicus," a name that struck fear in patients and providers alike. Hypersensitivitiy reactions, especially allergies, were recognized hundreds of years ago, and various chemical prescriptions were used to control the symptoms, but it was not until the mid-twentieth century that the molecular basis of allergies began to be understood. Immunodeficiencies are still being described, and the understanding of their basis is quite incomplete.

Some immunodeficiencies, if detected early enough, may be candidates for future gene therapy. In those cases where a single gene defect can be identified, introduction of the functional gene into the developing tissue may be able to reverse the course of the disease, partially or completely. Other options include transplantation of the thymus or bone marrow in order to allow normal functioning of the immune system components.

One of the most exciting potential treatments for secondary immunodeficiencies is vaccination. The ability to block AIDS through early immunization looks promising, although still many years away from use.

—Kerry L. Cheesman, Ph.D.

See also Acquired immunodeficiency syndrome (AIDS); Allergies; Arthritis; Autoimmune disorders; Blood and blood disorders; Bone

marrow transplantation; Cells; Chemotherapy; Cytology; Cytopathology; Endocrinology; Endocrinology, pediatric; Glands; Hematology; Hematology, pediatric; Hemolytic disease of the newborn; Host-defense mechanisms; Human immunodeficiency virus (HIV); Immune system; Immunization and vaccination; Immunology; Kawasaki disease; Leukemia; Lymphatic system; Multiple chemical sensitivity syndrome; Myasthenia gravis; Oncology; Rh factor; Serology; Severe combined immunodeficiency syndrome (SCID); Skin; Systemic lupus erythematosus (SLE); Transfusion; Transplantation; Wiskott-Aldrich syndrome.

For Further Information:

Abbas, Abul K., Andrew H. Lichtman, and Shiv Pillai. *Basic Immunology: Functions and Disorders of the Immune System*. 4th ed. Philadelphia: Saunders/Elsevier, 2014.

Clark, William R. *In Defense of Self: How the Immune System Really Works*. New York: Oxford University Press, 2007.

Fischer, A. M., et al. "Naturally Occurring Primary Deficiencies of the Immune System." *Annual Review of Immunology* 15 (1997): 93–124.

Janeway, Charles A.. *Immunobiology: The Immune System in Health and Disease*. 7th ed. New York: Garland Science, 2007.

Majno, Guido, and Isabelle Joris. "Part III: Immunopathology." *Cells, Tissues, and Disease: Principles of General Pathology*. 2d ed. New York: Oxford University Press, 2004. 523–610.

MedlinePlus. "Immune System and Disorders." *MedlinePlus*, August 9, 2013.

National Institute of Allergy and Infectious Diseases. "Immune System." *NIH National Institute of Allergy and Infectious Diseases*, July 30, 2013.

IMPETIGO

Disease/Disorder

Anatomy or system affected: Immune system, skin

Specialties and related fields: Bacteriology, dermatology, emergency medicine, family medicine, internal medicine, microbiology, pediatrics, sports medicine

Definition: A superficial bacterial infection of the skin.

Causes and Symptoms

Impetigo is a superficial bacterial skin infection usually caused by group A streptococcus, *Staphylococcus aureus*, or a mixture of both. Group A streptococcus was originally the predominant pathogen, but recently *S. aureus* has become the most common strain. Impetigo caused by either of these bacteria is clinically identical.

Children are most commonly affected by impetigo, and infection is often preceded by minor trauma such as insect bites. Outbreaks predominantly occur during the summer months when the climate is hot and humid. Impetigo is very contagious and easily spread in crowded conditions such as in families, schools, the military, and athletics. Poverty and poor personal hygiene can also predispose individuals to infection.

A typical infection first develops as multiple vesicopustules, which rupture and form a characteristic golden yellow crust. The lesions are painless but commonly pruritic (itchy), and scratching can serve to spread infection. Systemic symptoms are rare, but there can be local lymphadenopathy. The face, particularly the region around the mouth, is a common site of infection.

Information on Impetigo

Causes: Bacterial infection
Symptoms: Skin inflammation, blisters, itchiness, scabbing
Duration: Acute
Treatments: Injection of antibiotics (penicillin, erythromycin)

Treatment and Therapy

Topical and oral antibiotics have been used for the treatment of impetigo. Historically, the treatment of choice was penicillin or ampicillin. This has changed, however, as the most predominant bacteria are now *S. aureus* instead of group A streptococcus, which almost universally produces a beta-lactamase that makes them resistant to penicillin. It is now recommended to use a beta-lactamase-resistant penicillin such as dicloxacillin or a first-generation cephalosporin such as cephalexin. Erythromycin can be used if the patient is allergic to penicillin.

Topical antibiotics such as mupirocin and fusidic acid (not available in the United States) are very effective treatments. Mupirocin has been shown to be as effective as erythromycin. Topical antibiotics are used with mild or moderate cases; and oral antibiotics are reserved for more advanced cases. Topical antibiotics are as effective and have fewer side effects, which make them a better choice in less severe cases. A ten-day course is recommended whether oral or topical antibiotics are used.

Gentle cleansing of the area with soap and water can be helpful. Personal hygiene may be discussed with the patient to help prevent recurrence of infection. Frequent hand washing and not sharing bath linens can help prevent spread of the bacteria. The lesions usually heal without scarring.

—*Jeffrey B. Roberts, M.D.,*
and Jeffrey R. Bytomski, D.O.

See also Antibiotics; Bacterial infections; Blisters; Childhood infectious diseases; Dermatology; Dermatology, pediatric; Rashes; Skin; Skin disorders; Staphylococcal infections; Streptococcal infections.

For Further Information:

Bhumbra, Nasreen A., and Sophia G. McCullough. "Skin and Subcutaneous Infections." In *Update on Infectious Diseases*, edited by Richard I. Haddy and Karen W. Krigger. Philadelphia: W. B. Saunders, 2003.

"Impetigo." *Mayo Clinic*, May 15, 2013.

Larsen, Laura, ed. *Childhood Diseases and Disorders Sourcebook*. Detroit, Mich.: Omnigraphics, 2012.

Plaza, Jose A., and Victor G. Prieto. *Inflammatory Skin Disorders*. New York: Demos Medical Publishing, 2012.

Scholten, Amy. "Impetigo." *Health Library*, September 9, 2012.

Swartz, Morton N., and Mark S. Pasternack. "Cellulitis and Subcutaneous Tissue Infection." In *Mandell, Douglas, and Bennett's Principles and Practice of Infectious Diseases*, edited by Gerald L. Mandell, John E. Bennett, and Raphael Dolin. 7th ed. New York: Churchill Livingstone/Elsevier, 2010.

Taylor, Julie Scott. "Interventions for Impetigo." *American Family Physician* 70, 9. (November 1, 2004).

Van Schoor, Jacky. "Superficial Skin Infections in the Pharmacy."

SAPA 13, 1. (2013): 39–40.

Zappi, Eduardo. *Dermatopathology: Classification of Cutaneous Lesions*. New York: Springer, 2013.

IMPOTENCE. *See* **SEXUAL DYSFUNCTION.**

IN VITRO FERTILIZATION

Procedure

Anatomy or system affected: Cells, reproductive system, uterus

Specialties and related fields: Embryology, genetics, gynecology

Definition: A procedure whereby eggs and sperm are combined in the laboratory to achieve fertilization, usually followed by the introduction of the resulting embryos into the uterus.

Key terms:

chromosome: a structure found in the cell nucleus that is composed of deoxyribonucleic acid (DNA) and associated proteins; chromosomes are responsible for carrying genetic information and can be observed under a microscope

clomiphene: a synthetic estrogenic substance used to induce ovulation in women who do not ovulate regularly; it is taken orally as a medication

endometriosis: a condition whereby cells of the uterine lining are found in abnormal locations, such as the pelvic cavity or ovary; endometriosis can lead to pelvic pain and the development of scars that can block the Fallopian tubes

Fallopian tube: one of two structures that conduct the egg, as it is released from the ovary, into the uterus

follicle: a spherical mass of cells and fluid within the ovary, from which the mature egg is produced

implantation: the process in which an embryo attaches and burrows into the lining of the uterus

in vitro: a Latin term used to indicate a process that has taken place outside an organism, such as in a laboratory test tube or petri dish

ovulation: the process whereby the egg is released from the ovary and can be fertilized by sperm; this event occurs approximately at the middle portion of a woman's menstrual cycle

semen analysis: analysis of a recently ejaculated semen specimen, which includes a sperm count and an estimate of the percentage of motile sperm

zygote: the single cell formed after fertilization that is the result of the fusion of egg and sperm; it can develop into a new individual organism

Indications and Procedures

The purpose of fertilization is to create a new organism or individual that has the same number of chromosomes as the parent individuals but that has a unique mixing of genetic traits from both the mother and the father. In animals, this is accomplished by the fusion of egg and sperm cells. Both egg and sperm contain half the number of chromosomes needed to produce a healthy individual. The fusion of egg and sperm

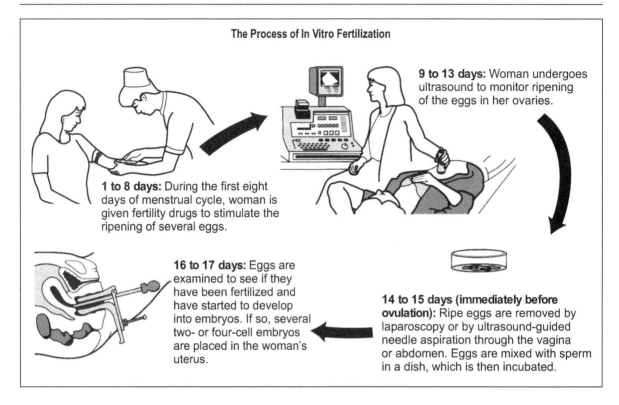

The Process of In Vitro Fertilization

1 to 8 days: During the first eight days of menstrual cycle, woman is given fertility drugs to stimulate the ripening of several eggs.

9 to 13 days: Woman undergoes ultrasound to monitor ripening of the eggs in her ovaries.

14 to 15 days (immediately before ovulation): Ripe eggs are removed by laparoscopy or by ultrasound-guided needle aspiration through the vagina or abdomen. Eggs are mixed with sperm in a dish, which is then incubated.

16 to 17 days: Eggs are examined to see if they have been fertilized and have started to develop into embryos. If so, several two- or four-cell embryos are placed in the woman's uterus.

results in a zygote, or fertilized egg, which can develop into an individual organism.

Eggs and sperm are both gametes, cells that are specialized to carry out reproductive functions. The sperm cells are produced in the testicles of the male. Sperm production is continuous in the male, and millions of sperm are made within the testicles each day. Sperm cells contain genetic material within their head and are equipped with a flagellum, or whiplike tail, to enable them to swim within a liquid medium. The egg, or ovum, is about .01 millimeter in size and hundreds of times larger than the sperm. It is produced in the ovaries of females and contains cytoplasm, the cellular substance and specialized cell structures that are needed for the zygote to form and grow. In women, a single mature egg is usually made with each menstrual cycle and is released from the follicle contained in one of the ovaries. As women age, their ovaries become depleted of follicles, and eventually, at the menopause, ovulation no longer occurs. Therefore, a woman's age can contribute significantly to her ability to conceive. Other causes of ovarian failure that may lead to infertility include the use of chemotherapeutic agents and premature ovarian failure syndrome.

In natural, or in vivo, fertilization, sperm from the male are deposited in the vaginal canal of the female during sexual intercourse. The sperm are contained in nutritive fluid, called semen. The sperm are able to swim up the cervical canal (the lower part of the uterus) only during and around the time of female ovulation, as the cervical mucus becomes permeable to sperm at this time. Once within the uterine cavity, the sperm make their way up into the Fallopian tubes, where they can meet the egg and proceed with fertilization.

Several steps lead to fertilization. The egg is surrounded by a layer of cells called the corona radiata. This layer is loose and easily penetrated by sperm. The next layer is the zona pellucida, which is a critical barrier in fertilization. One of the sugarcoated proteins in the zona pellucida, ZP3, captures a sperm cell by binding to its head. This causes a structure on the head of the sperm, called an acrosome, to release enzymes. This process is called the acrosomal reaction. These enzymes then digest the coat on the head of the sperm cell and digest a path for the sperm through the zona pellucida. After this, the sperm reaches the membrane of the egg, and the sperm and egg cells fuse. The chromosomes of the sperm and egg join, thus completing the process of fertilization. Subsequently, the fertilized egg travels back into the uterus and implants into the lining of the uterus, where it continues to develop as an embryo and then as a fetus.

When the natural anatomy or physiology of the reproductive system is abnormal, infertility can result. For instance, endometriosis in women can cause severe scarring of the pelvic cavity, leading to occluded Fallopian tubes or ovaries that are completely encased in scar tissue. In these cases, the egg may have difficulty reaching the Fallopian tube canal and hence is unable to meet sperm to achieve fertilization. Another cause of pelvic scarring is pelvic inflammatory disease (PID), which can be caused by sexually transmitted diseases (STDs) or ruptures in the gastrointestinal tract.

In vitro fertilization (IVF) may be indicated when a couple

experiences infertility. Infertility is defined as the lack of conception after one to two years of unprotected intercourse. There are many causes of infertility, which may be attributable to either the male or the female partner. Usually when an infertile couple seeks medical attention, they are asked to give a detailed history and receive physical examinations by the physician. Depending on the findings, the couple will be asked to undergo testing to better identify the cause of the infertility. Men will be asked to give a semen sample. The sample will be analyzed in the laboratory to ensure that adequate numbers of sperm are present and that they are able to move appropriately, a procedure called semen analysis. Women may be assessed for anatomic defects, such as whether the Fallopian tubes are blocked or large fibroid tumors in the uterus may prevent sperm from entering the Fallopian tubes. This assessment may be accomplished using a technique called a hysterosalpingogram, in which dye is introduced into the uterine cavity and an X-ray picture is taken. If a woman's Fallopian tubes are blocked, then no dye will spill into the pelvic cavity. If a woman's tubes are open, then dye will be seen spilling into the pelvic cavity. In addition, women may also undergo assessments regarding their ovarian function and ability to produce eggs. Blood tests may be drawn to assess for appropriate hormone levels.

If the cause of infertility is found to be blocked Fallopian tubes, then IVF may be indicated. Sometimes, women with irregular menstrual cycles who do not ovulate at predictable intervals may be treated with a medication called clomiphene, in order to induce ovulation. If a woman fails to achieve spontaneous conception after several months of clomiphene therapy, then the physician may proceed with in vitro fertilization as the next step in the attempt to achieve conception.

Another example of when IVF may be indicated is in cases where the sperm are defective. For instance, some men may have sperm that have difficulty swimming appropriately or penetrating the egg. In such cases, the sperm may need to be injected artificially into the egg to achieve fertilization, a procedure called intracytoplasmic sperm injection (ICSI). To perform this procedure, eggs must be harvested from the woman. The eggs are then placed in a petri dish, where they are injected with the sperm. Because fertilization is occurring outside the body in this situation, this procedure is also a type of in vitro fertilization. After the eggs have matured for a few days in the laboratory, the healthiest-looking zygotes are placed into the woman's uterus, a procedure called embryo transfer.

Another example in which intracytoplasmic sperm injection might be used is when the couple's infertility is caused by the man's inability to ejaculate sperm. This might occur, for instance, with a lack or occlusion of the vas deferens, the tubes that carry sperm from the testicles to the urethra where the sperm can exit the body. To obtain sperm for IVF in these cases, the male partner may undergo testicular sperm extraction, in which sperm are removed from the testicles. The sperm are then injected into the ova to achieve fertilization in vitro.

The procedures for IVF involve the induction of ovulation in the woman using hormones that stimulate the ovaries. These are usually hormones that are similar to endogenous follicle-stimulating hormone (FSH), which is responsible for follicle growth within the ovary. These exogenous hormones lead to the development of multiple follicles within both ovaries. The size and number of these follicles are observed by ultrasound, and when the appropriate number and size are achieved, the ovum harvest is performed. This procedure involves taking the woman to the operating room, where she is given anesthesia and placed on her back with her legs in stirrups and knees apart. A needle attached to a vacuum device is carefully introduced into the vaginal canal with ultrasound guidance. With the ultrasound helping to locate the ovaries and follicles precisely, the needle is inserted into the follicle through the posterior vagina. The fluid within the follicle is aspirated, and the egg usually is suctioned out of the follicle along with the follicular fluid and placed into a test tube. The same procedure is repeated until a sufficient number of eggs have been harvested or the follicles have been depleted. The eggs are then taken to the laboratory, where they are examined under a microscope.

A sperm sample is then collected from the male partner, and the sample is washed and analyzed to ensure that the sperm appear healthy and able to fertilize the eggs. The sperm are then introduced to the eggs within a petri dish containing tissue culture fluid. If intracytoplasmic sperm injection is to be performed, then single sperm are taken up into a glass needle and injected into individual eggs at this time. The petri dish is placed in an incubator for a few days. Once the embryos have developed sufficiently, a few healthy ones are chosen to be introduced into the woman's uterus through embryo transfer. This involves picking up the embryos into a semiflexible tube. The tube is then inserted carefully through the cervical canal into the uterine cavity, where the embryos are released. Embryos that are not transferred into the woman's uterus can be frozen using cryopreservation for future use.

Uses and Complications

IVF enables couples who suffer from infertility to conceive and bear children. Specifically, IVF is most helpful for couples whose infertility is caused by blocked Fallopian tubes or the inability of sperm to reach and penetrate the egg. In couples where the woman is unable to produce her own eggs, donor eggs from another woman may be used in IVF. If a man is unable to produce his own sperm, then sperm donors may be used in IVF.

Recent technology has enabled early prenatal diagnosis for inheritable conditions using cells taken from the early embryo during the six-to-eight-cell stage, called blastomere biopsy. Inheritable diseases caused by single gene defects, such as cystic fibrosis, Duchenne muscular dystrophy, sickle cell disease, hemophilia, and Tay-Sachs disease, have been detected using preimplantation diagnosis. This type of prenatal diagnosis is possible only through the IVF process, as the early embryo would not be accessible to the physician in cases of spontaneous conception. Procedures such as blastomere biopsy are far from common, however, given the technical difficulty and economic costs of such procedures.

The complications associated with the IVF process include a condition called ovarian hyperstimulation syndrome. This situation can occur when a woman receives hormones to stimulate ovulation. In these cases, the follicles within the ovary become excessively stimulated and grossly enlarge the ovary. When this condition is severe, the woman can suffer abdominal pain, fluid imbalances, electrolyte imbalances, abnormal kidney function, and an accumulation of fluid in the abdominal cavity or lungs. Her blood may have an abnormal tendency to form clots, and her blood pressure may become dangerously low. These patients are monitored carefully and require hospitalization, as severe ovarian hyperstimulation syndrome can be fatal.

Other complications of the IVF process can occur during the ovum harvest procedure. These include the risks of anesthesia and infection (because the needle is a foreign body introduced through the vagina, a nonsterile field). Another risk involves bleeding. Although the needle for harvesting the eggs is under ultrasound guidance, the risk of the needle inadvertently puncturing neighboring blood vessels still exists. In addition, the ovaries themselves may bleed when punctured, as they are highly vascular organs. Bleeding that is severe and life-threatening may require abdominal or pelvic surgery to identify the location of the bleeding and to stop the bleeding with sutures. If the patient becomes significantly anemic from the bleeding, she may require a blood transfusion.

Other risks of IVF are incurred during the embryo culture process. During this process, the petri dishes containing the embryos may become contaminated with microorganisms. In addition, problems with the tissue culture medium or with the incubation process may lead to poor embryo development and the lack of any viable embryos to transfer into the woman. Another risk is that embryos transferred into the uterus may not implant themselves in the lining.

The rate of achieving pregnancy after IVF is directly related to the number of embryos transferred into the uterus. When multiple embryos are transferred back into the uterus, however, the woman is at risk for a multiple gestation pregnancy. Multiple gestation pregnancies lead to an increased risk of spontaneous abortion (miscarriage) and preterm birth, as well as other pregnancy complications such as low birth weight, growth restriction in utero, increased risk of congenital anomalies, placental abnormalities, preeclampsia (a hypertensive disease of pregnancy), umbilical cord accidents, and malpresentations (when the fetus is not lying in the uterus with the head down, making vaginal birth difficult). More long-term risks of in vitro fertilization are the increased risk for complications during pregnancy. For instance, women whose pregnancies were a result of assisted reproductive technologies such as IVF are at increased risk for preterm birth, when compared to age-matched women whose pregnancies were a result of spontaneous conception.

In addition, the long-term outcomes of children conceived using IVF is unknown, as the first children born as a result of

this technique are beginning to enter middle age. Whether they will live normal life spans is unknown. Whether they will have normal reproductive outcomes themselves remains unclear. Whether they are more prone to diseases such as cancer later in life is also unknown.

Perspective and Prospects

The first baby conceived through in vitro fertilization was Louise Brown, who was born in 1978. The English team responsible for this important breakthrough consisted of Patrick Steptoe, a surgeon from Oldham Hospital, and Robert Edwards, a reproductive physiologist from Cambridge University. In the 1960s, animal breeding programs had successfully utilized in vitro fertilization. In 1965, Edwards reported that he had successfully induced maturation of a human egg in vitro. Edwards teamed up with Steptoe and another colleague, Jean Purdy. In 1970, they reported that they had achieved in vitro fertilization and cleavage (cell division) in human eggs. The first successful birth of an IVF baby in the United States occurred in 1981 in Norfolk, Virginia. The first successful use of a previously frozen human embryo occurred in Australia in 1984; two years later, a similar procedure was employed successfully in the United States.

A couple can undergo multiple cycles of IVF. A 1996 study reported data from large centers in three countries that showed that the cumulative pregnancy rate after six cycles of IVF is approximately 60 percent. However, if a couple fails to achieve pregnancy after six cycles, then the chances of achieving pregnancy through IVF fall significantly. At that time, the infertile couple may be counseled to seek alternative means of becoming parents, such as adoption.

In vitro fertilization and its related procedures have provided opportunities to conceive for couples who would otherwise be childless. These opportunities have led to many ethical controversies as well. What should be done with frozen embryos that are not used? What are the rights of egg or sperm donors once the child is born? What are the rights of the child to know his or her parentage and family history of medical problems? What are the rights of surrogate mothers? How many embryos should be transferred back into the woman, given that multiple gestations are at increased risk for poor outcomes such as premature delivery? Is there a certain age at which women should not attempt pregnancy? Some countries such as Australia, Norway, Spain, and the United Kingdom have responded to some of these questions by passing legislation regulating IVF. Other countries have been slower to respond, leaving decisions related to IVF to physicians, the patients themselves, and the court system.

As more couples delay childbearing, the prevalence of infertility and the desire for IVF and other assisted reproductive technologies is likely to increase. Human reproduction is not an efficient process, and the older the female partner becomes, the less likely it is that natural conception will occur. For instance, a 1986 survey in the United States reported that the proportion of married women who were infertile between the ages of twenty and twenty-four was only 7 percent. By the ages of forty to forty-four, this proportion became 28 percent.

This statistic is partly attributable to the fact that the total length of time during which conception is possible is less in older women, as older women ovulate less frequently than do younger women.

—Anne Lynn S. Chang, M.D.

See also Assisted reproductive technologies; Conception; Embryology; Ethics; Gamete intrafallopian transfer (GIFT); Genetic engineering; Gynecology; Hormones; Infertility, female; Infertility, male; Multiple births; Obstetrics; Ovaries; Pregnancy and gestation; Reproductive system; Uterus; Women's health.

For Further Information:

Chisholm, Andrea, and Brian Randall. "In Vitro Fertilization." *Health Library*, May 22, 2013.

Gardner, David K., ed. *In Vitro Fertilization: A Practical Approach.* New York: Informa Healthcare, 2007.

"Infertility." *MedlinePlus*, May 20, 2013.

Lentz, Gretchen M., et al. *Comprehensive Gynecology.* 6th ed. Philadephia: Mosby/Elsevier, 2013.

Sher, Geoffrey, Virginia Marriage Davis, and Jean Stoess. *In Vitro Fertilization: The A.R.T. of Making Babies.* 3d ed. New York: Facts On File, 2005.

Speroff, Leon, and Marc A. Fritz. *Clinical Gynecologic Endocrinology and Infertility.* 8th ed. Philadelphia: Lippincott Williams & Wilkins, 2011.

"Treating Infertility: FAQ." *American College of Obstetricians and Gynecologists*, Apr. 2013.

Wisot, Arthur L., and David R. Meldrum. *Conceptions and Misconceptions: The Informed Consumer's Guide Through the Maze of In Vitro Fertilization and Other Assisted Reproduction Techniques.* 2d ed. Point Roberts, Wash.: Hartley & Marks, 2004.

INCONTINENCE

Disease/Disorder

Anatomy or system affected: Abdomen, bladder, gastrointestinal system, urinary system

Specialties and related fields: Family medicine, geriatrics and gerontology, gynecology, internal medicine, obstetrics, pediatrics, psychiatry, urology

Definition: Involuntary loss of urine or feces, primarily a social and hygienic problem that particularly affects the older population.

Key terms:

atonic bladder: a bladder characterized by weak muscles

enuresis: bed-wetting

frequency: urination at short intervals; a common problem accompanying incontinence

micturition: the act of urinating

nocturia: nighttime urination

sphincter: a ring-shaped muscle that surrounds a natural opening in the body and can open or close it by expanding or contracting

urge incontinence: a strong desire to urinate followed by leakage of urine

urgency: a strong desire to void urine immediately

Causes and Symptoms

Continence is a skill acquired in humans by the interaction of two processes: socialization of the infant and maturation of the central nervous system. Without society's expectation of continence, and without broadly accepted definitions of appropriate behavior, the concept of "incontinence" would be meaningless. There are many causes for urinary incontinence. Three broad (interrelated and often overlapping) categories are physiologic voiding dysfunction, factors directly influencing voiding function, and factors affecting the individual's capacity to manage voiding.

The causes of physiologic voiding dysfunction involve an abnormality in bladder or sphincter function, or both. The bladder and sphincter have only two functions: to store urine until the appropriate time for urination and then to empty it completely. Voiding dysfunction involves the failure of one or both of these mechanisms. Four basic types of voiding dysfunction can be distinguished: detrusor instability, genuine stress incontinence, outflow obstruction, and atonic bladder.

Detrusor instability is a condition characterized by involuntary bladder (detrusor muscle) contraction during filling. While all the causes of bladder instability are not fully understood, it can be associated with the following: neurologic disease (brain and spinal cord abnormalities), inflammation of the bladder wall, bladder outlet obstruction, stress urinary incontinence, and idiopathic (spontaneous or primary) dysfunction. Detrusor instability usually causes symptoms of frequency, urgency, and possibly nocturia or enuresis.

Genuine stress incontinence is caused by a failure to hold urine during bladder filling as a result of an incompetent urethral sphincter mechanism. If the closure mechanism of the bladder outlet fails to hold urine, incontinence will occur. This is usually manifested during physical exertion or abdominal stress (such as coughing or sneezing). It can occur in either sex, but it is more common in women because of their shorter urethra and the physical trauma of childbirth. Men can experience stress incontinence following traumatic or surgical damage to the sphincter.

Obstruction of the outflow of urine during voiding can produce various symptoms, including frequency, straining to void, poor urinary stream, preurination and posturination dribbling, and a feeling of urgency with resulting leakage (urge incontinence). In severe cases, the bladder is never completely emptied and a volume of residual urine persists. Overflow incontinence can result. Common causes of bladder outlet obstruction are prostatic enlargement, bladder neck narrowing, or urethral obstruction. Functional obstruction occurs when a neurologic lesion prevents the coordinated relaxation of the sphincter during voiding. This phenomenon is termed detrusor-sphincter dyssynergia.

An atonic bladder—one with weak muscle walls—does not produce a sufficient contraction to empty completely. Emptying can be enhanced by abdominal straining or manual expression, but a large residual volume persists. The sensation of retaining urine might or might not be present. If sensation is present, frequency of urination is common because only a small portion of the bladder volume is emptied each time. Sensation is often diminished, and the residual urine volume can be considerable (100 to 1,000 milliliters). Overflow incontinence often occurs.

Information on Incontinence

Causes: Neurological disease, bladder inflammation, obstruction, prostate gland enlargement, urinary tract infection, diuretics, endocrine disorders (e.g., diabetes mellitus, thyroid disorders), aging, pregnancy and childbirth

Symptoms: Frequent urination, straining to void, poor urinary stream, feeling of urgency with resulting leakage

Duration: Ranges from acute to chronic

Treatments: Drug therapy, surgery, bladder training

An acute urinary tract infection can cause transient incontinence, even in a fit, healthy young person who normally has no voiding dysfunction. Acute frequency and urgency with disturbed sensation and pain can result in the inability to reach a toilet in time or to detect when incontinence is occurring. If an underlying voiding dysfunction is also present, an acute urinary tract infection is likely to cause incontinence.

Many drugs can also disturb the delicate balance of normal functioning. The most obvious category consists of diuretics, those drugs that increase urinary discharge; a large, swift production of urine will give most people frequency and urgency. If the bladder is unstable, it might not be able to handle a sudden influx of urine, and urge incontinence can result. Sedation can affect voiding function directly (for example, diazepam can lower urethral resistance) or can make the individual less responsive to signals from the bladder and thus unable to maintain continence. Other commonly prescribed drugs have secondary actions on voiding function. Not all patients, however, will experience urinary side effects from these drugs.

Various endocrine disorders can upset normal voiding function. Diabetes can cause polydypsia (extreme thirst), requiring the storage of a large volume of urine. Glycosuria (sugar in the urine) might encourage urinary tract infection. Thyroid imbalances can aggravate an overactive or underactive bladder. Pituitary gland disorders can result in the production of excessive urine volumes because of an antidiuretic hormone deficiency. Estrogen deficiency in postmenopausal women causes atrophic changes in the vaginal and urethral tissues and will worsen stress incontinence and an unstable bladder.

Several bladder pathologies can also cause incontinence by disrupting normal functioning. A patient with a neoplasm (abnormal tissue growth), whether benign or malignant, or a stone in the bladder occasionally experiences incontinence as a symptom. These are infrequent causes of incontinence.

Often it takes something else in addition to the underlying problem to tip the balance and produce incontinence. This is especially true for elderly and disabled persons who are delicately balanced between continence and incontinence. For example, immobility—anything that impedes access—is likely to induce incontinence. Immobility can be the result of the gradual worsening of a chronic condition, such as arthritis, multiple sclerosis, or Parkinson's disease, until eventually the individual simply cannot reach a toilet in time. The condition may be acute—an accident or illness that suddenly renders a person immobile might be the start of failure to control the bladder.

In the case of children, most daytime wetting persists until the child reaches school age. It is less common than bed-wetting (enuresis), and the two often go together. One in ten five-year-old children, however, still wets the bed regularly. With no treatment, this figure gradually falls to 5 percent of ten-year-olds and to 2 percent of adults. It is twice as common in boys as in girls, has strong familial tendencies, and is associated with stressful events in the third or fourth year of life. A urinary tract infection is sometimes the cause.

Fecal, as opposed to urinary, incontinence is generally caused by underlying disorders of the colon, rectum, or anus; neurogenic disorders; or fecal impaction. Severe diarrhea increases the likelihood of having fecal incontinence. Some of the more common disorders that can cause diarrhea are ulcerative colitis, carcinoma, infection, radiation therapy, and the effect of drugs (for example, broad-spectrum antibiotics, laxatives, or iron supplements). Fecal incontinence tends to be a common, if seldom reported, accompaniment.

The pelvic floor muscles support the anal sphincter, and any weakness will cause a tendency to fecal stress incontinence. The vital flap valve formed by the anorectal angle can be lost if these muscles are weak. An increase in abdominal pressure would therefore tend to force the rectal contents down and out of the anal canal. This might be the result of congenital abnormalities or of later trauma (for example, childbirth, anal surgery, or direct trauma). A lifelong habit of straining at stool might also cause muscle weakness.

The medulla and higher cortical centers of the brain have a role in coordinating and controlling the defecation reflex. Therefore, any neurologic disorder that impairs the ability to detect or inhibit impending defecation will probably result in incontinence, similar in causation to the uninhibited or unstable bladder. For example, the paraplegic can lose all direct sensation of and voluntary control over bowel activity. Neurologic disorders such as multiple sclerosis, cerebrovascular accident, and diffuse dementia can affect sensation or inhibition, or a combination of both. Incontinence occurs with some people suffering from dementia because of a physical inability to inhibit defecation. With others, it occurs because the awareness that such behavior is inappropriate has been lost.

Severe constipation with impaction of feces is probably the most common cause of fecal incontinence, and it predominates as a cause among the elderly and those living in extended care facilities. Chronic constipation leads to impaction when the fluid content of the feces is progressively absorbed by the colon, leaving hard, rounded rocks in the bowel. This hard matter promotes mucus production and bacterial activity, which causes a foul-smelling brown fluid to accumulate. If the rectum is overdistended for any length of time, the internal and external sphincters become relaxed, allowing passage of this mucus as spurious diarrhea. The patient's symptoms usually include fairly continuous leakage of fluid stool without any awareness of control.

Most children are continent of feces by the age of four years, but 1 percent still have problems at seven years of age. Fecal incontinence or conscious soiling in childhood (sometimes referred to as encopresis) has, like nocturnal enuresis (nighttime urinary incontinence), long been regarded as evidence of a psychiatric or psychologic disorder in the child. The evidence, however, does not support the claim that incontinent children are disturbed.

Such children usually have fastidious, overanxious parents who are intent on toilet training. The child is punished for soiling, so defecation tends to be inhibited, both in the underwear and in the toilet. When toilet training is attempted, the child may be repeatedly seated on the toilet in the absence of a full rectum and be unable to perform. The situation becomes fraught with anxiety, and bowel movements become associated with unpleasantness in the child's mind. The child therefore retains feces and becomes constipated. Defecation then becomes difficult and painful as well.

Treatment and Therapy

The two primary methods of treating urinary incontinence involve medical and surgical intervention (drug therapy and surgery) and bladder training.

Many drugs can be prescribed to help those with urinary incontinence. Often the results are disappointing, although some drugs can be useful for carefully selected and accurately diagnosed patients. Drugs are often used to control detrusor instability and urge incontinence by relaxing the detrusor muscle and inhibiting reflex contractions. This therapy is helpful in some patients. Sometimes when the drug is given in large enough doses to be effective; however, the side effects are often so troublesome that the therapy must be abandoned. Drugs that reduce bladder contractions must be used cautiously in patients who have voiding difficulty, since urinary retention can be precipitated. Careful assessment must be made of residual urine. Drug therapy is also used with caution in patients with a residual volume greater than 100 milliliters. Some drugs are used in an attempt to prevent stress incontinence by increasing urethral tone. Phenylpropanolamine and ephedrine, those most often used, are thought to act on the alpha receptors in the urethra.

Drug therapy can also be used to relieve outflow obstruction. Phenoxybenzamine is commonly used, but this drug can have dangerous side effects, such as tachycardia (an abnormally fast heartbeat) or postural hypotension. If the bladder does not contract sufficiently to ensure complete emptying, drug therapy can be attempted to increase the force of the voiding contractions. Carbachol, bethanechol, and distigmine bromide have all been used with some success. Other drugs might be useful in treating factors affecting incontinence—for example, antibiotics to treat a urinary tract infection or laxatives to treat or prevent constipation.

Many drugs can exacerbate a tendency to incontinence. For those who are prone to incontinence, medications and dosage schedules are chosen that will have a minimal effect on bladder control. For example, a slow-acting diuretic, in a divided dose, can help someone with urgency and weak sphincter tone to avoid incontinence. An analgesic might be preferable to night sedation for those who need pain relief but who wet the bed at night if they are sedated.

Turning to surgical intervention, none of the several surgical approaches that have been used in an attempt to treat an unstable bladder has gained widespread use. Cystodistention (stretching the bladder under general anesthesia) and bladder transection, for example, are presumed to act by disturbing the neurologic pathways that control uninhibited contractions. Many vaginal and suprapubic procedures are available to help correct genuine stress incontinence in women. Surgery can also be used to relieve outflow obstruction—for example, to remove an enlarged prostate gland, divide a stricture, or widen a narrow urethra.

In cases of severe intractable incontinence, major surgery is an option. For those with a damaged urethra, a neourethra can be constructed. For those with a nonfunctioning sphincter, an artificial sphincter can be implanted. In some patients, a urinary diversion with a stoma (outlet) is the only or best alternative for continence. Although a drastic solution, a urostomy might be easier to cope with than an incontinent urethra, because an effective appliance will contain the urine.

Urinary incontinence is occasionally the result of surgery, usually urologic or gynecologic but sometimes a major pelvic or spinal procedure. Such iatrogenic incontinence can be caused by neurologic or sphincter damage, leading to various dysfunctional voiding patterns.

Several different types of bladder training or retraining are distinguishable and can be used in different circumstances. The most important element for success is that the correct regimen be selected for each patient and situation. A thorough assessment identifies those patients who will benefit from bladder training and determines the most appropriate method. Other factors that contribute to the incontinence should also be treated (for example, a urinary tract infection or constipation), because ignoring them will impair the success of a program.

Bladder training is most suitable for people with the symptoms of frequency, urgency, and urge incontinence (with or without an underlying unstable bladder) and for those with nonspecific incontinence. The elderly often have these symptoms. Patients with voiding dysfunction, other than an unstable bladder, are unlikely to benefit from bladder training.

The aim of bladder training is to restore the patient with frequency, urgency, and urge incontinence to a more normal and convenient voiding pattern. Ultimately, voiding should occur at intervals of three to four hours (or even longer) without any urgency or incontinence. Drug therapy is sometimes combined with bladder training for those with detrusor instability.

Bladder training aims to restore an individual's confidence in the bladder's ability to hold urine and to reestablish a more normal pattern. Initially, a patient keeps a baseline chart for three to seven days, recording how often urine is passed and when incontinence occurs. This chart is reviewed with the program supervisor, and an individual regimen is developed. The purpose is to extend the time between voiding gradually, encouraging the patient to practice delaying the need to void, rather than giving in to the feeling of urgency. Initially, the times chosen can be at set intervals throughout the day (for example, every one or two hours) or can be variable, according to the individual's pattern as indicated by the baseline chart. When the baseline chart reveals a definite pattern to the incontinence, it might be possible to set voiding times in accordance with and in anticipation of this pattern.

A pattern of voiding is set for patients throughout the day (timed voiding). Usually no pattern is set at night, even if nocturia or nocturnal enuresis is a problem. Patients are instructed to pass urine as necessary during the night. Sometimes the provision of a suitable pad or appliance helps to increase confidence and means that, if incontinence does occur, the results will not be disastrous. If urgency is experienced, patients are taught to sit or stand still and try to suppress the sensation rather than to rush immediately to the toilet. A normal fluid intake is encouraged because the goal is to have the patient continent and able to drink fluids adequately.

As patients achieve the target intervals without having to urinate prematurely or leaking, the intervals can gradually be lengthened. The speed of progress depends on the individual and on other variables, such as the initial severity of symptoms, motivation, and the amount of professional support. Patients usually remain at one time interval for one to two weeks before it is increased by fifteen to thirty minutes for another two weeks. Once the target of three- to four-hour voiding without urgency has been achieved, it is useful to maintain the chart and set times for at least another month to prevent relapse.

Some people find that practicing pelvic muscle exercises helps to suppress urgency. Any weakness in the pelvic floor muscles will cause a tendency not only to urinary incontinence but also to fecal stress incontinence. Mild weakness can respond to pelvic muscle exercises similar to those used in alleviating the symptoms of stress incontinence, but with a concentration on the posterior rather than the anterior portion of the pelvic muscles. Rectal tone is assessed by digital examination, during which the patient is instructed to squeeze. Regular contractions on the posterior portion of the pelvic muscles are then practiced often for at least two months (usually in sets of twenty-five, three times a day).

In cases of fecal impaction, a course of disposable phosphate enemas—one or two daily for seven to ten days, or until no further return is obtained—is the treatment of choice. A single enema is seldom efficient, even if an apparently good result is obtained, because impaction is often extensive: The first enema merely clears the lowest portion of the bowel. If fecal incontinence persists once the bowel has been totally cleared (a plain abdominal X ray can be helpful in confirming this), the condition is assumed to be neurogenic in origin rather than caused by the impaction.

Perspective and Prospects

Historically, most health professionals have been profoundly ignorant of the causes and management of incontinence. Incontinence was often regarded as a condition over which there was no control, rather than as a symptom of an underlying physiologic disorder or as a symptom of a patient with a unique combination of problems, needs, and potentials. The unfortunate result of such limited understanding was passive acceptance of the symptom of incontinence. Incontinence, often viewed as repulsive, is often a condition that is merely tolerated. As public recognition of the implications of incontinence has increased, however, the stigma associated with it has slowly decreased. It has become common knowledge that millions of Americans suffer from incontinence, and most pharmacies and supermarkets have a section for incontinence products.

At one time, incontinence was primarily regarded as a "nursing" problem, with nurses providing custodial care—keeping the patient as clean and comfortable as possible and preventing pressure ulcers from developing. Gradually, nurses were not alone in acknowledging that incontinence was a symptom requiring investigation and intervention; those in other health professions also began to realize this need. In the 1980s, research funds began to be allocated for the study of incontinence. In 1988, US Surgeon General C. Everett Koop estimated that 8 billion dollars was being spent by the federal government on incontinence in nursing homes in the United States annually.

As incontinence began to be recognized by the public as a health problem rather than as an inevitable part of aging, more people admitted having the symptoms of incontinence and sought medical attention. It has been estimated that, of all cases of incontinence, more than one-third can be cured, another one-third can be dramatically improved, and most of the remainder can be significantly improved.

—*Genevieve Slomski, Ph.D.*

See also Bed-wetting; Constipation; Diarrhea and dysentery; Digestion; Sphincterectomy; Stone removal; Stones; Urinary disorders; Urinary system; Urology; Urology, pediatric.

For Further Information:

Arnold-Long, Mary. "Fecal Incontinence: An Overview of the Causes, Treatments, and Interventions to Address Bowel Incontinence in the Elderly." *Long-Term Living* 59, no. 10 (Octoboer, 2010): 50–53.

Dierich, Mary, and Felecia Froe. *Overcoming Incontinence: A Straightforward Guide to Your Options*. New York: John Wiley & Sons, 2000.

Jeter, Katherine, Nancy Faller, and Christine Norton, eds. *Nursing for Continence*. Philadelphia: W. B. Saunders, 1990.

Khandelwal, C., and C. Kistler. "Diagnosis of Urinary Incontinence." *American Family Physician* 87, no. 8 (April 2013): 543–550.

Nathanson, Laura Walther. *The Portable Pediatrician: A Practicing Pediatrician's Guide to Your Child's Growth, Development, Health, and Behavior from Birth to Age Five.* 2d ed. New York: HarperCollins, 2002.

Newman, Diane Kaschack. *Managing and Treating Urinary Incontinence*. 2d ed. Baltimore: Health Professions Press, 2009.

Parker, William, Amy Rosenman, and Rachel Parker. *The Incontinence Solution: Answers for Women of All Ages*. New York: Fireside, 2007.

Randall, Brain. "Urinary Incontinence—Male." *Health Library*, September, 27, 2012.

Stahl, Rebecca J. "Neurogenic Bladder—Child." *Health Library*, March 1, 2013.

Vasavada, Sandip P., et al., eds. *Female Urology, Urogynecology, and Voiding Dysfunction*. New York: Marcel Dekker, 2005.

INFARCTION

Disease/Disorder

Also known as: Heart attack, stroke, acute abdomen

Anatomy or system affected: Blood vessels, brain, heart, intestine, kidneys, lungs

Specialties and related fields: Cardiology, critical care, emergency medicine, family medicine, gastroenterology, general surgery, internal medicine, neurology, nursing, vascular medicine

Definition: A localized area of tissue damage or necrosis caused by absence of blood supply and oxygen to the part.

Causes and Symptoms

"Infarct" is the term used to indicate a localized area of necrosis resulting when the blood supply to an area falls below the level required for cells to survive. Infarction results from the obstruction of an artery at a point that causes the main blood supply to be blocked. It also occurs when the tissue requirements are raised above the capacity of the diseased vessels to deliver blood. Although an infarction may occur in any tissue, those that require a large supply of blood are particularly vulnerable. Organs in which infarctions are commonly found are the brain, heart, intestine, kidney, and lung. The consequences of an infarction depend on its location and extent. If the infarcted area is extensive enough, then function of the organ is compromised and death or disability may result. A large infarct in a vital organ such as the heart, lung, or brain may be responsible for sudden death.

Symptoms related to infarction include the development of tissue ischemia. The most marked manifestation of acute ischemia is pain. Fear and anxiety are other symptoms that may be exhibited. Myocardial infarction, commonly called a heart attack, is classically associated with a characteristic diagnostic triad. First, there is a clinical picture consisting of severe, prolonged chest pain, frequently associated with sweating, nausea, vomiting, and a sense of impending doom. Second, serum levels of the cardiac enzymes released by the necrotic myocardial cells are elevated. Finally, electrocardiographic changes are evident.

Treatment and Therapy

Acute myocardial infarction requires immediate admission to a hospital with a coronary care unit. Continuous close monitoring of cardiac rhythms and enzymatic changes is especially important. The first twenty-four hours after onset of symptoms is the time of highest risk for sudden death. Myocardial infarction caused by intracoronary thrombi (clots) can be relieved by infusion of thrombolytic agents that dissolve the clots and promote vasodilation. The treatment must be performed within three to four hours after the onset of

---

Information on Infarction

Causes: Lack of blood supply from obstruction, blockage, or spasm of blood vessel supplying organ affected

Symptoms: Pain, ischemia, necrosis

Duration: Acute

Treatments: Bed rest, oxygen, thrombolytic medications, nitroglycerine, morphine, stool softeners, low-sodium diet, surgery

---

infarction and can reestablish blood flow in approximately three minutes. Bed rest followed by a gradual return to activities of daily living reduces the myocardial oxygen demands of the compromised heart.

Pain relief is of utmost importance. If sublingual nitroglycerin is ineffective, then small, carefully titrated doses of morphine sulfate may be given for sedation and vasodilation. Supplementary oxygen is administered to increase arterial oxygen content and deliver more oxygen to the ischemic myocardium. Dietary measures are aimed at preventing nausea and vomiting, and consumption of sodium, saturated fats, sugar, and caffeine is limited. In addition to pain relief, pharmacologic intervention is used to limit infarction size, reduce vasoconstriction, prevent thrombus formation, and augment repair. Treatment for infarction of the brain, kidney, and bowel may require surgery to reestablish circulation and remove necrotic tissue.

—Jane C. Norman, Ph.D., R.N., C.N.E.

See also Angina; Blood vessels; Cardiac arrest; Cardiac rehabilitation; Cardiology; Cardiopulmonary resuscitation (CPR); Circulation; Critical care; Embolism; Emergency medicine; Heart; Heart attack; Ischemia; Necrosis; Stroke; Thrombolytic therapy and TPA; Thrombosis and thrombus.

For Further Information:

Bowman, James P. *Strokes: An Illustrated Guide to Brain Structure, Blood Supply, and Clinical Signs*. New York: Prentice Hall, 2002.

Dracup, Kathleen. *Meltzer's Intensive Coronary Care: A Manual for Nurses*. New York: Prentice Hall, 1995.

Dugdale, David C., Michael A. Chen, and David Zieve. "Heart Attack." *MedlinePlus*, June 22, 2012.

Hankey, Graeme J. *Stroke*. New York: Elsevier Health Sciences, 2002.

Manson, Joann E. *Prevention of Myocardial Infarction*. New York: Oxford University Press, 1996.

Tanner, Dennis C. *Family Guide to Surviving Stroke and Communications Disorders*. New York: Jones and Bartlett, 2008.

INFARCTION, MYOCARDIAL. *See* HEART ATTACK.

INFECTION

Disease/Disorder

Anatomy or system affected: All

Specialties and related fields: Bacteriology, family medicine, hematology, internal medicine, virology

Definition: Invasion of the body by disease-causing organisms such as bacteria, viruses, fungi, and parasites; symptoms of infection may include pain, swelling, fever, and loss of normal function.

Key terms:

antibiotic: a substance that destroys or inhibits the growth of microorganisms, such as bacteria

antibody: a small protein secreted from specialized white blood cells that binds to and aids in the destruction of pathogens

antigen: a substance found on pathogens to which the antibodies bind; also, any substance considered foreign by the body

bacteria: small microorganisms; some bacteria found normally in and on the body have helpful functions, while others that invade the body or disrupt the normal bacteria are harmful and often infectious

edema: an abnormal accumulation of fluid in the body tissues; tissue with edema is swollen in appearance

infectious: referring to a microorganism that is capable of causing disease, often with the ability to spread from one person to another

inflammation: a tissue reaction to injury which may or may not involve infection; pain, heat, redness, and edema are the usual signs of inflammation

pathogen: a microorganism or substance capable of producing a disease, such as a bacterium causing an infection

phagocytosis: the ingestion and destruction of a pathogen or abnormal tissue by specialized white blood cells known as phagocytes

virus: a very small organism that is dependent upon a host cell to meet its metabolic needs and to reproduce

Process and Effects

Healthy people live with potential pathogens; that is, people have on and in their bodies non-disease-causing bacteria. They live in harmony with these organisms and in fact benefit from their presence. For example, some of the bacteria found in the intestinal tract supply vitamin K, which is important in blood-clotting reactions.

The human body has several features that prevent disease-causing organisms from inducing an infection. These features include anatomical barriers, such as unbroken skin, and the mucus in the nose, mouth, and lungs, which can trap pathogens. Another defense is the acid within the stomach, and even bacteria that are normally present in certain areas of the body can force out more harmful bacteria. The immune system is specially developed to ward off intruders.

Immune cells and factors secreted from these cells provide the next line of defense against invading organisms. Antibodies are secreted from specialized white blood cells known as plasma cells. These antibodies are very specific in their recognition of pathogens. For example, an antibody may recognize one particular strain of bacteria but not another. Antibodies attach themselves to the part of the bacterium called the antigen. Once bound to the antigen, they aid in the destruction of the pathogen. In addition to plasma cells, other white blood cells help in combating infections, including two types of

---

Information on Infection

Causes: Exposure to bacteria, viruses, fungi, or parasites

Symptoms: Pain, swelling, fever, fatigue, loss of normal function

Duration: Acute to chronic

Treatments: Drug therapy (antibiotics, antiviral agents, antifungal agents, etc.)

---

phagocytes called macrophages and neutrophils. Both of these types of immune cells have the ability to eat and digest pathogens such as bacteria in a process known as phagocytosis.

In order to cause disease, microorganisms must somehow overwhelm the body's natural defenses and immune system. Bacteria capable of causing infections may even be naturally occurring organisms in the body that have left their normal environment and overcome the elements that usually hold them at bay. For example, some bacteria that typically reside in the mouth may cause pneumonia (inflammation of the lungs) if they gain access to the lungs.

Other infections, such as a cold, the flu, or a sexually transmitted disease, can be caused by pathogens that do not normally reside in the body. These kinds of infections are called communicable or transmissible infections. A physician treating someone who has been bitten by a bat, skunk, or dog will want to know whether the animal has rabies, as rabies is a viral infection that is transmitted via a bite that breaks the skin and contaminates the wound with infectious saliva.

No matter what the route of infection, the body must mount a response to the intruding microorganism. Often the observable signs and symptoms of an infection are not caused by the direct action of the infecting pathogen but rather reflect the immune system's response to the pathogen. The most frequent signs and symptoms include inflammation and pain at the site of infection, as well as fever.

The inflammatory response is a nonspecific defense that is triggered whenever body tissues are injured, as in the case of infection. The goals of this response are to prevent the spread of the infectious agent to nearby tissues, destroy the pathogens, remove the damaged tissues, and begin the healing process. Signs of inflammation include redness, edema (tissue swelling), heat, pain, and loss of normal function. At first glance, these reactions do not appear to be beneficial to the body, but they do help fight the infection and aid in the healing process. The redness is attributable to an increase in blood flow to the area of infection, which helps provide nutrients to the tissue and remove some of the waste products that develop as the immune system fights the infection. With this increase in blood flow comes an increase in the temperature and amount of blood that leaks out of blood vessels into the tissue spaces, causing edema at the site of infection. Some of the blood that leaks into the site of infection contains clotting proteins that help form a clot around the infected area, thereby reducing the chances that the pathogen could escape into the bloodstream or uninfected tissue nearby. Pain is present when the damaged tissue releases waste products and the pathogen releases toxins. The swelling of the injured area and the pain associated with infections keep the patient from using that area of the body and thus aid in healing. While some painkillers such as aspirin reduce the inflammatory reaction by stopping the production of some of the chemicals released during inflammation, these drugs do nothing to harm the pathogen; they only block the body's response to the microorganism.

Some of the same chemicals that are found in inflamed tissues also cause fever, an abnormally high body temperature that represents the body's response to an invading microorganism. The body's thermostat, located in a region of the brain known as the hypothalamus, is set at about 37 degrees Celsius (about 99 degrees Fahrenheit). During an infection, the thermostat is reset to a higher level. Chemicals called pyrogens are released from macrophages. Once again, aspirin-like drugs can be used to reduce the fever by inhibiting the action of some of these chemicals in the hypothalamus.

The body responds to viral infections in a similar way. Virally infected cells secrete interferon, exerting an antiviral action that may provide protection to uninfected neighboring cells. It appears that interferon acts to inhibit the virus from replicating. Cells that are already infected must be destroyed to rid the body of the remaining virus.

In addition to being part of the inflammatory response, certain white blood cells play an important role in attempting to remove the pathogen. Soon after inflammation begins, macrophages already present at the site of infection start to destroy the microorganism. At the same time, chemicals are being released from both the damaged tissue and the macrophages to recruit other white blood cells, such as neutrophils. The neutrophils, like the macrophages, are effective at attacking and destroying bacteria; unlike the macrophages, they often die in the battle against infection. Dead neutrophils are seen as a white exudate called pus.

Other manifestations of infection include systemic (whole-body) effects as well as changes at the site of infection. As noted, fever is a systemic effect mediated by chemicals from the site of infection. Some of these same factors have the ability to act on the bone marrow to increase the production of white blood cells. Physicians look for fever and an increase in the number of white blood cells as signs of infection. If the infection is severe, then the bone marrow may not be able to keep up with the demand, and an overall decrease in white blood cell number will be found.

Complications and Disorders

Physicians and other health-care workers must use patient history, signs and symptoms, and laboratory tests to determine the type of infection and the most appropriate treatment. Patient history can often tell the examiner how and when the infection started. For example, the patient may have cut himself or herself, been exposed to someone with an infectious disease, or had intimate contact with someone carrying a sexually transmitted disease. Signs of infection—edema, pain,

fever—are usually easy to detect, but some symptoms may be rather vague, such as feeling tired and weak. These general signs and symptoms may indicate to a physician that the patient has an infection, but they will not provide information about the type of microorganism causing the infection. Nevertheless, some microorganisms do cause specific symptoms. For example, the varicella-zoster virus that causes chicken pox and the paramyxovirus that causes measles leave characteristic rashes.

When the microorganism does not have a characteristic sign, physicians must use laboratory tests to determine the pathogen involved. Diagnosis of the disease relies on identifying the causative pathogen by microscopic examination of a specimen of infected tissue or body fluid, by growing the microorganism using culture techniques, or by detecting antibodies in the blood that have developed against the pathogen.

Once the physician determines what type of microorganism has caused the infection, he or she will have to determine the best treatment to eradicate the disease. Drug therapy usually consists of antibiotics and other antimicrobial agents. The selection of the appropriate drug is important, as certain pathogens are susceptible only to certain antibiotics. Unfortunately, few effective antiviral drugs are available for many infectious viruses. In these cases, drugs are mainly used to treat symptoms such as fever, pain, diarrhea, and vomiting rather than to destroy the virus.

Anti-infective drugs are commonly used by physicians to treat infections. Agents that kill or inhibit the growth of bacteria are known as antibiotics and can be applied directly to the site of infection (topical), given by mouth (oral), or injected. The latter two modes of administration allow the drug to be carried throughout the body by way of the blood. Some antibiotic drugs are effective against only certain strains of infectious bacteria. Antibiotics that act against several types of bacteria are referred to as broad-spectrum antibiotics. Some bacteria develop resistance to a particular antibiotic, requiring the physician to switch agents or use a combination of antibiotics. Antibiotic therapy for the treatment of infections should be used when the body has been invaded by harmful bacteria, when the bacteria are reproducing at a more rapid rate than the immune system can handle, or to prevent infections in individuals with an impaired immune system.

Some serious common bacterial infections include gonorrhea, which is sexually transmitted and treatable with penicillin; bacterial meningitis, which causes inflammation of the coverings around the brain and is treatable with a variety of antibiotics; pertussis (whooping cough), which is transmitted by water droplets in air and treatable with erythromycin; pneumonia, which causes shortness of breath, is transmitted via the air, and can be treated with antibiotics; tuberculosis, which infects the lungs and is treatable with various antibiotics; and salmonella, which is transmitted in food or water contaminated with fecal material, causes fever, headaches, and digestive problems, and is treatable with antibiotics. It should be noted that antibiotics are not effective in viral infections; only bacterial infections are treated with antibiotics.

Antiviral drugs such as acyclovir, amantadine, and zidovudine (formerly known as azidothymide, or AZT) are used in the treatment of infection by a virus. These drugs have been difficult to develop. Most viruses live within the cells of the patient, and the drug must in some way kill the virus without harming the host cells. In fact, antiviral agents cannot completely cure an illness, and infected patients often experience recurrent disease. Nevertheless, antiviral drugs do reduce the severity of these infections.

There are several common viral infections. Human immunodeficiency virus (HIV) infection, which causes acquired immunodeficiency syndrome (AIDS), is transmitted by sexual contact or contaminated needles or blood products; it is often treated with zidovudine but remains lethal. Chicken pox (varicella-zoster virus), which is transmitted by airborne droplets or direct contact, is treated with acyclovir. The common cold is caused by numerous viruses that are transmitted by direct contact or air droplets and has no effective treatment other than drugs that reduce the symptoms. Hepatitis is transmitted by contaminated food, sexual contact, or blood; it causes flulike symptoms and jaundice (a yellow tinge to the skin caused by liver problems) and may be helped with the drug interferon. Influenza viruses are transmitted by airborne droplets; the only treatment for the flu is of its symptoms. Measles is transmitted by virus-containing water droplets and causes fever and a rash; treatment consists of alleviating the symptoms. Mononucleosis is transmitted via saliva and causes swollen lymph nodes, fever, a sore throat, and generalized tiredness; a patient with mononucleosis can receive treatment only for the symptoms, as no cure is available. Poliomyelitis (polio) is transmitted by fecally contaminated material or airborne droplets and can eventually cause paralysis; no treatment is available. Rabies is caused by a bite from an infected animal, as the virus is present in the saliva; the major symptoms include fever, tiredness, and spasms of the throat. Treatment for rabies must be given before these symptoms have appeared, as after that point, no effective treatment exists, and the virus usually proves fatal. Rubella is transmitted by virus-containing air droplets and is associated with a fever and rash; there is no treatment other than for the symptoms.

A major problem with infectious diseases is that there is almost always a delay between when the microorganism enters the body and the onset of signs and symptoms. This gap may range from a few hours or days to several years. A patient without noticeable symptoms is likely to spread the pathogen, setting up a cycle in which individuals unknowingly infect others who, in turn, pass on the disease-causing agent. Large numbers of people can quickly become infected in this manner.

One way to prevent the spread of infectious agents is to vaccinate patients. Diseases such as diphtheria, measles, mumps, rubella, poliomyelitis, and pertussis are rare in the United States because of an aggressive immunization program. When a patient is vaccinated, the vaccine usually contains a dead or inactive pathogen. After the vaccine is administered, usually by injection, the immune system responds by making antibodies against the antigens on the microorganism. Since the pathogen in the vaccine is unable to cause disease, the patient has no symptoms after immunization. The next time that the person is exposed to the infectious agent, his or her immune system is prepared to fight it before symptoms become evident.

In addition to immunization to prevent infection, individuals can largely avoid serious infectious diseases through good hygiene with respect to food and drink, frequent washing, the avoidance of contact with fecal material and urine, and the avoidance of contact with individuals who are infected and capable of transmitting the disease. When such avoidance is impractical, other protective measures can be taken.

Sexually transmitted diseases are usually preventable by using barrier contraceptives and practicing safer sex. The most common of these diseases include chlamydial infections, trichomoniasis, genital herpes, and HIV infections. Prevention is particularly important in cases of herpes and HIV, as these are viral infections with no known cures.

Some infections can be acquired at birth, including gonorrhea, genital herpes, chlamydial infections, and salmonella. These microorganisms exist in the birth canal, and some infectious agents can even pass from the mother to the fetus via the placenta. The more serious infections transmitted in this manner are rubella, syphilis, toxoplasmosis, HIV, and the cytomegalovirus. The risk of transmitting these infections can be reduced by treating the mother before delivery or performing a cesarean section (surgical delivery from the uterus), thereby avoiding the birth canal.

Perspective and Prospects

The ancient Egyptians were probably the first to recognize infection and the body's response to the introduction of a disease-causing microorganism, as some hieroglyphics appear to represent the inflammatory process. Sometime in the fifth century BCE, the Greeks noted that patients who had acquired an infectious disease and survived did not usually contract the same illness a second time.

More solid scientific evidence about infections was provided in the nineteenth century by Edward Jenner, an English physician and scientist. Jenner was able to document that milkmaids seemed to be protected against smallpox because of their exposure to cowpox. With this knowledge, he vaccinated a boy with material from a cowpox pustule. The boy had a typical inflammatory response, and he showed no symptoms of smallpox after being injected with the disease a few months later. His immune system protected him from the virus. Since that time, scientists have reached a much better understanding of how the body deals with infection.

Many scientists are focusing their attention on how pathogens are transmitted from the source of infection to susceptible individuals. Epidemiology is the study of the distribution and causes of diseases that are prevalent in humans. Since some infectious diseases are communicable (transmittable), epidemiologists gather data when an outbreak occurs in a population. These data include the source of infectious agents (the tissues involved), the microorganisms causing the disease, and the method by which the pathogens are transmitted from one person to another. Physicians and other health-care workers help in the battle against infections by identifying susceptible individuals; developing and evaluating sources, methods, and ways to control the spread of the pathogens; and improving preventive measures, which usually include extensive educational efforts for the general population. With this knowledge, scientists and physicians attempt to eradicate the disease.

While scientists and physicians have made great advances in the understanding of infection, many problems remain. The spread of certain diseases, such as sexually transmitted diseases, is difficult to control except by modifying human behavior. The most difficult to treat are viral illnesses for which the drugs that are used are ineffective in completely eradicating the virus and bacterial diseases for which the bacteria have developed drug resistance. Because these microorganisms evolve rapidly, new strains continually emerge. When a new infectious agent develops, it is often years before scientists can devise an effective drug or vaccine to treat the disease. In the meantime, large numbers of patients may become ill and even die. Perhaps the most effective way to combat infection is to use preventive measures whenever practical.

—Matthew Berria, Ph.D.

See also Bacterial infections; Bites and stings; Childhood infectious diseases; Disease; Ear infections and disorders; Emerging infectious diseases; Epidemics and pandemics; Eye infections and disorders; Fever; Fungal infections; Iatrogenic disorders; Inflammation; Insect-borne diseases; Lice, mites, and ticks; Parasitic diseases; Prion diseases; Staphylococcal infections; Streptococcal infections; Viral infections; Zoonoses; *specific diseases*.

For Further Information:

"Bacterial Infections." *MedlinePlus*, May 13, 2013.

Biddle, Wayne. *A Field Guide to Germs*. 3d ed. New York: Anchor Books, 2010.

Frank, Steven A. *Immunology and Evolution of Infectious Disease*. Princeton, N.J.: Princeton University Press, 2002.

"Fungal Infections." *MedlinePlus*, January 31, 2013.

Gorbach, Sherwood L., John G. Bartlett, and Neil R. Blacklow, eds. *Infectious Diseases*. 3d ed. Philadelphia: W. B. Saunders, 2004.

Infectious Disease: A Scientific American Reader. Chicago: University of Chicago Press, 2008.

Leikin, Jerrold B., and Martin S. Lipsky, eds. *American Medical Association Complete Medical Encyclopedia*. New York: Random House Reference, 2003.

Merrill, Ray M. *Introduction to Epidemiology*. 6th ed. Sudbury, Mass.: Jones and Bartlett, 2012.

"Parasitic Diseases." *MedlinePlus*, April 25, 2013.

Springhouse Corporation. *Everything You Need to Know About Diseases*. Springhouse, Pa.: Author, 1996.

Sompayrac, Lauren. *How Pathogenic Viruses Work*. Boston: Jones and Bartlett, 2002.

"Viral Infections." *MedlinePlus*, September 18, 2012.

Wilson, Michael, Brian Henderson, and Rod McNab. *Bacterial Disease Mechanisms: An Introduction to Cellular Microbiology*. New York: Cambridge University Press, 2002.

INFERTILITY, FEMALE
Disease/Disorder

Anatomy or system affected: Genitals, reproductive system, uterus

Specialties and related fields: Endocrinology, gynecology

Definition: The inability to achieve a desired pregnancy as a result of dysfunction of female reproductive organs.

Key terms:

cervix: the bottom portion of the uterus, protruding into the vagina; the cervical canal, an opening in the cervix, allows sperm to pass from the vagina into the uterus

endometriosis: a disease in which patches of the uterine lining, the endometrium, implant on or in other organs

follicles: spherical structures in the ovary that contain the maturing ova (eggs)

hormone: a chemical signal that serves to coordinate the functions of different body parts; the hormones important in female reproduction are produced by the brain, the pituitary, and the ovaries

implantation: the process in which the early embryo attaches to the uterine lining; a critical event in pregnancy

ovaries: the pair of structures in the female that produce ova (eggs) and hormones

oviducts: the pair of tubes leading from the top of the uterus upward toward the ovaries; also called the Fallopian tubes

ovulation: the process in which an ovum is released from its follicle in the ovary; ovulation must occur for conception to be possible

pelvic inflammatory disease: a general term that refers to a state of inflammation and infection in the pelvic organs; may be caused by a sexually transmitted disease

uterus: the organ in which the embryo implants and grows

vagina: the tube-shaped organ that serves as the site for sperm deposition during intercourse

Causes and Symptoms

Infertility is defined as the failure of a woman to conceive despite regular sexual activity over the course of at least one year. Studies have estimated that in the United States, 10 to 15 percent of couples are infertile. In about half of these couples, it is the woman who is affected.

Female infertility may be caused by hormonal problems, or it may originate in the reproductive organs: the ovaries, oviducts, uterus, cervix, and vagina. The frequency of specific problems among infertile women is as follows: ovarian problems, 20 percent to 30 percent; damage to the Fallopian tubes, 30 percent to 50 percent; uterine problems, 5 percent to 10 percent; and cervical or vaginal abnormalities, 5 percent to 10 percent. Another 10 percent of women have unexplained infertility. Behavioral factors, such as diet and exercise and the use of tobacco, alcohol, or drugs, also play a role in infertility.

The ovaries have two important roles in conception: the production of ova (egg cells), culminating in ovulation, and the production of hormones. Ovulation usually occurs halfway through a woman's four-week menstrual cycle. In the

---

Information on Female Infertility

Causes: Endometriosis, cervical problems, anovulation, hormonal imbalance, abnormally shaped uterus or vagina, pelvic inflammatory disease

Symptoms: Often asymptomatic; can include lack of menstrual periods, blocked Fallopian tubes, abdominal pain with endometriosis

Duration: Short-term to chronic

Treatments: Fertility drugs, surgery, fertility procedures (e.g., in vitro fertilization)

---

two weeks preceding ovulation, follicle-stimulating hormone (FSH) from the pituitary gland causes follicles in the ovaries to grow and the ova within them to mature. As the follicles grow, they produce increasing amounts of estrogen. Near the middle of the cycle, the estrogen causes the pituitary gland to release a surge of luteinizing hormone (LH), which causes ovulation of the largest follicle in the ovary.

Anovulation (lack of ovulation) can result either directly, from an inability to produce LH, FSH, or estrogen, or indirectly, because of the presence of other hormones that interfere with the signaling systems between the pituitary and ovaries. For example, the woman may have an excess production of androgen (testosterone-like) hormones, either in her ovaries or in her adrenal glands, or her pituitary may produce too much prolactin, a hormone that is normally secreted in large amounts only after the birth of a child.

Besides ovulation, the ovaries have another critical role in conception, since they produce hormones that act on the uterus to allow it to support an embryo. In the first two weeks of the menstrual cycle, the uterine lining is prepared for a possible pregnancy by estrogen from the ovaries. Following ovulation, the uterus is maintained in a state that can support an embryo by progesterone, which is produced in the ovary by the follicle that just ovulated, now called a corpus luteum. Because of the effects of hormones from the corpus luteum on the uterus, the corpus luteum is essential to the survival of the embryo. If conception does not occur, the corpus luteum disintegrates and stops producing progesterone. As progesterone levels decline, the uterine lining can no longer be maintained and is shed as the menstrual flow.

Failure of the pregnancy can result from improper function of the corpus luteum, such as an inability to produce enough progesterone to sustain the uterine lining. The corpus luteum may also produce progesterone initially but then disintegrate too early. These problems in corpus luteum function, referred to as luteal phase insufficiency, may be caused by the same types of hormonal abnormalities that cause lack of ovulation.

Some cases of infertility may be associated with an abnormally shaped uterus or vagina. Such malformations of the reproductive organs are common in women whose mothers took diethylstilbestrol (DES) during pregnancy. DES was prescribed to many pregnant women from 1941 to about 1970 as a protection against miscarriage; infertility and other problems have occurred in the offspring of these women.

Conception depends on normal function of the oviducts (or Fallopian tubes), thin tubes with an inner diameter of only a few millimeters; they are attached to the top of the uterus and curve upward toward the ovaries. The inner end of each tube, located near one of the ovaries, waves back and forth at the time of ovulation, drawing the mature ovum into the opening of the oviduct. Once in the oviduct, the ovum is propelled along by movements of the oviduct wall. Meanwhile, if intercourse has occurred recently, the man's sperm will be moving upward in the female system, swimming through the uterus and the oviducts. Fertilization, the union of the sperm and ovum, will occur in the oviduct, and then the fertilized ovum will pass down the oviduct and reach the uterus about three days after ovulation.

Infertility can result from scar tissue formation inside the oviduct, resulting in physical blockage and inability to transport the ovum, sperm, or both. The most common cause of scar tissue formation in the reproductive organs is pelvic inflammatory disease (PID), a condition characterized by inflammation that spreads throughout the female reproductive tract. PID may be initiated by a sexually transmitted disease such as gonorrhea or chlamydia. Physicians in the United States have documented an increase in infertility attributable to tubal damage caused by sexually transmitted diseases.

Damage to the outside of the oviduct can also cause infertility, because such damage can interfere with the mobility of the oviduct, which is necessary to the capture of the ovum at the time of ovulation. External damage to the oviduct may occur as an aftermath of abdominal surgery, when adhesions induced by surgical cutting are likely to form. An adhesion is an abnormal scar tissue connection between adjacent structures.

Another possible cause of damage to the oviduct that can result in infertility is the presence of endometriosis. Endometriosis refers to a condition in which patches of the uterine lining implant outside the uterus, in or on the surface of other organs. These patches are thought to arise during menstruation, when the uterine lining (endometrium) is normally shed from the body through the cervix and vagina; in a woman with endometriosis, for unknown reasons, the endometrium is carried to the interior of the pelvic cavity by passing up the oviducts. The endometrial patches can lodge in the oviduct itself, causing blockage, or can adhere to the outer surface of the oviducts, interfering with mobility.

Endometriosis can cause infertility by interfering with organs other than the oviducts. Endometrial patches on the outside of the uterus can cause distortions in the shape or placement of the uterus, interfering with embryonic implantation. Ovulation may be prevented by the presence of the endometrial tissues on the surface of the ovary. The presence of endometriosis, however, is not always associated with infertility: Thirty percent to forty percent of women with endometriosis cannot conceive, but the remainder appear to be fertile.

Another critical site in conception is the cervix. The cervix, the entryway to the uterus from the vagina, represents the first barrier through which sperm must pass on their way to the ovum. The cervix consists of a ring of strong, elastic tissue with a narrow canal. Glands in the cervix produce the mucus

Common Causes of Female Infertility

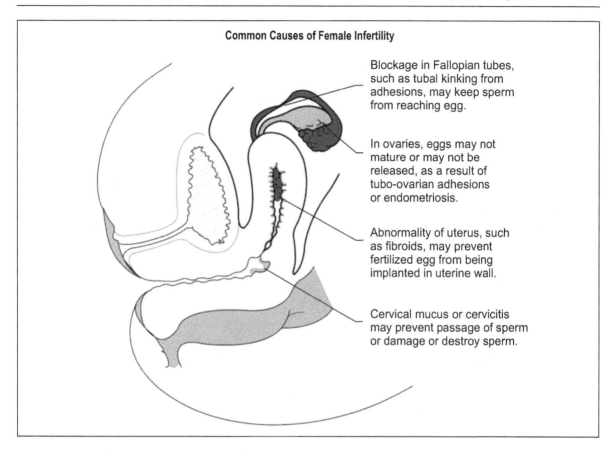

Blockage in Fallopian tubes, such as tubal kinking from adhesions, may keep sperm from reaching egg.

In ovaries, eggs may not mature or may not be released, as a result of tubo-ovarian adhesions or endometriosis.

Abnormality of uterus, such as fibroids, may prevent fertilized egg from being implanted in uterine wall.

Cervical mucus or cervicitis may prevent passage of sperm or damage or destroy sperm.

that fills the cervical canal and through which sperm swim en route to the ovum. The amount and quality of the cervical mucus change throughout the menstrual cycle, under the influence of hormones from the ovary. At ovulation, the mucus is in a state that is most easily penetrated by sperm; after ovulation, the mucus becomes almost impenetrable.

Cervical problems that can lead to infertility include production of a mucus that does not allow sperm passage at the time of ovulation (hostile mucus syndrome) and interference with sperm transport caused by narrowing of the cervical canal. Such narrowing may be the result of a developmental abnormality or the presence of an infection, possibly a sexually transmitted disease.

Treatment and Therapy

The diagnosis of the exact cause of a woman's infertility is crucial to successful treatment. A complete medical history should reveal any obvious problems of previous infection or menstrual cycle irregularity. Adequacy of ovulation and luteal phase function can be determined from records of menstrual cycle length and changes in body temperature (body temperature is higher after ovulation). Hormone levels can be measured with tests of blood or urine samples. If damage to the oviducts or uterus is suspected, a hysterosalpingography will be performed. In this procedure, the injection of a special fluid into the uterus is followed by x-ray analysis of the fluid

movement to reveal the shape of the uterine cavity and the oviducts. Cervical functioning can be assessed with the postcoital test, in which the physician attempts to recover sperm from the woman's uterus some hours after she has had intercourse with her partner. If a uterine problem is suspected, the woman may have an endometrial biopsy, in which a small sample of the uterine lining is removed and examined for abnormalities. Sometimes, exploratory surgery is performed to pinpoint the location of scar tissue or the location of endometrial patches.

Surgery may be used for treatment as well as diagnosis. Damage to the oviducts can sometimes be repaired surgically, and surgical removal of endometrial patches is a standard treatment for endometriosis. Often, however, surgery is a last resort because of the likelihood of the development of postsurgical adhesions, which can further complicate the infertility. Newer forms of surgery using lasers and freezing offer better success because of a reduced risk of adhesions.

Some women with hormonal difficulties can be treated successfully with so-called fertility drugs, which are intended to stimulate ovulation. There are several different drugs and hormones that fall under this heading: Clomiphene citrate (Clomid), human menopausal gonadotropin (hMG), gonadotropin-releasing hormone (GnRH), and bromocriptine mesylate (Parlodel) are among the medications commonly used, with the exact choice depending on the woman's particular problem. One problem with some of the drugs is the risk of multiple pregnancy (more than one fetus in the uterus). Other possible problems include nausea, dizziness, headache, and general malaise.

Aside from fertility drugs, there are a variety of methods in use to try to achieve pregnancy with external assistance, known collectively as assisted reproductive technology (ART). One example of this, artificial insemination, also known as intrauterine insemination (IUI), is an old technique that is still useful in various types of infertility. A previously collected sperm sample is placed in the woman's vagina or uterus using a special tube. Artificial insemination is always performed at the time of ovulation, in order to maximize the chance of conception. The ovulation date can be determined with body temperature records or by hormone measurements. In some cases, this procedure is combined with fertility drug treatment. Since the sperm can be placed directly in the uterus, it is useful in treating hostile mucus syndrome and certain types of male infertility. The sperm sample can be provided either by the woman's partner or by a donor. The pregnancy rate after artificial insemination is highly variable (anywhere from 10 to 70 percent), depending on the particular infertility problem in the couple.

Another assisted reproductive technology is gamete intrafallopian transfer (GIFT), the surgical placement of ova and sperm directly into the woman's oviducts. To be a candidate for this procedure, the woman must have at least one partially undamaged oviduct and a functional uterus. Ova are collected surgically from the ovaries after stimulation with a fertility drug, and a semen sample is collected from the male. The ova and the sperm are introduced into the oviducts through the same abdominal incision used to collect the ova. This procedure is useful in certain types of male infertility, if the woman produces an impenetrable cervical mucus, or if the ovarian ends of the oviducts are damaged. The range of infertility problems that may be resolved with GIFT can be extended by using donated ova or sperm. The pregnancy rate is about 33 percent overall, but the rate varies with the type of infertility present.

The most common assisted reproductive technology is in vitro fertilization (IVF), or the fertilization of the sperm and egg outside the woman's body, followed by implantation of the fertilized egg in the woman's uterus. In this procedure, ova are collected surgically after stimulation with fertility drugs and then placed in a laboratory dish and combined with sperm from the man. The actual fertilization, when a sperm penetrates the ovum, will occur in the dish. The resulting embryo is allowed to remain in the dish for two days, during which time it will have grown to two to four cells. Then, the embryo is placed in the woman's uterine cavity using a flexible tube. In vitro fertilization can be used in women who are infertile because of endometriosis, damaged oviducts, impenetrable cervical mucus, or ovarian failure. As with GIFT, in vitro fertilization may utilize donated ova or donated sperm, or extra embryos that have been produced by one couple may be implanted in a second woman. Embryos created through IVF can either be used immediately or frozen for later implantation. Success rates for in vitro fertilization have improved greatly over time, and in the United States in 2010, the proportion of IVF procedures that resulted in live births was about 56 percent for fresh embryos and 35 percent for frozen embryos, according to the Centers for Disease Control and Prevention.

Some women may benefit from nonsurgical embryo transfer. In this procedure, a fertile woman is artificially inseminated at the time of her ovulation; five days later, her uterus is flushed with a sterile solution, washing out the resulting embryo before it implants in the uterus. The retrieved embryo is then transferred to the uterus of another woman, who will carry it to term. Typically, the sperm provider and the woman who receives the embryo are the infertile couple who wish to rear the child, but the technique can be used in other circumstances as well. Embryo transfer can be used if the woman has damaged oviducts or is unable to ovulate, or if she has a genetic disease that could be passed to her offspring, because in this case the baby is not genetically related to the woman who carries it.

Some infertile women who are unable to achieve a pregnancy themselves turn to the use of a surrogate, a woman who will agree to bear a child and then turn it over to the infertile woman to rear as her own. In the typical situation, the surrogate is artificially inseminated with the sperm of the infertile woman's husband. The surrogate then proceeds with pregnancy and delivery as normal, but relinquishes the child to the infertile couple after its birth.

Perspective and Prospects

One of the biggest problems that infertile couples face is the emotional upheaval that comes with the diagnosis of infertility, as bearing and rearing children is an experience that most people treasure. In addition to the emotional difficulty that may come with the recognition of infertility, more stress may be in store as the couple proceeds through treatment. The various treatments can cause embarrassment and sometimes physical pain, and fertility drugs themselves are known to cause emotional swings. For these reasons, a couple with an infertility problem is often advised to seek help from a private counselor or a support group.

Along with the emotional and physical challenges of infertility treatment, there is a considerable financial burden. Infertility treatments, in general, are expensive, especially for more sophisticated procedures such as in vitro fertilization and GIFT. Since the chances of a single procedure resulting in a pregnancy are often low, the couple may be faced with submitting to multiple procedures repeated many times. The cost over several years of treatment—a realistic possibility—can be very high. Many health insurance companies in the United States refuse to cover the costs of such treatment and are required to do so in only a few states.

Some of the treatments are accompanied by unresolved legal questions. In the case of nonsurgical embryo transfer, is the legal mother of the child the ovum donor or the woman who gives birth to the child? The same question of legal parentage arises in cases of surrogacy. Does a child born using donated ovum or sperm have a legal right to any information about the donor, such as medical history? How extensive should governmental regulation of infertility clinics be? For example, should there be standards for ensuring that donated sperm or ova are free from genetic defects? In the United States, some states have begun to address these issues, but no uniform policies have been set at the federal level.

The legal questions are largely unresolved because American society is still involved in religious and philosophical debates over the propriety of various infertility treatments. Some religions hold that any interference in conception is unacceptable. To these denominations, even artificial insemination is wrong. Other groups approve of treatments confined to a husband and wife, but disapprove of a third party being involved as a donor or surrogate. Many people disapprove of any infertility treatment to help an individual who is not married. Almost all these issues stem from the fact that these reproductive technologies challenge the traditional definitions of parenthood.

—Marcia Watson-Whitmyre, Ph.D.

See also Assisted reproductive technologies; Conception; Contraception; Ectopic pregnancy; Endocrinology; Endometriosis; Gamete intrafallopian transfer (GIFT); Gynecology; Hormones; Hysterectomy; In vitro fertilization; Infertility, male; Menopause; Menstruation; Miscarriage; Obstetrics; Ovarian cysts; Ovaries; Pelvic inflammatory disease (PID); Pregnancy and gestation; Sexual dysfunction; Sperm banks; Sterilization; Stress; Tubal ligation; Uterus; Women's health.

For Further Information:

American Society for Reproductive Medicine. http://www.asrm.org/

"Assisted Reproductive Technology (ART) Report." *Centers for Disease Control and Prevention*, January 6, 2012.

"Female Infertility." *Mayo Clinic*, September 9, 2011.

Harkness, Carla. *The Infertility Book: A Comprehensive Medical and Emotional Guide*. Rev. ed. Berkeley, Calif.: Celestial Arts, 1996.

InterNational Council on Infertility Information Dissemination. http://www.inciid.org.

Phillips, Robert H., and Glenda Motta. *Coping with Endometriosis*. New York: Avery, 2000.

Quilligan, Edward J., and Frederick P. Zuspan, eds. *Current Therapy in Obstetrics and Gynecology*. 5th ed. Philadelphia: W. B. Saunders, 2000.

Riley, Julie. "Infertility in Women." *Health Library*, October 31, 2012.

Speroff, Leon, and Marc A. Fritz. *Clinical Gynecologic Endocrinology and Infertility*. 8th ed. Philadelphia: Lippincott Williams & Wilkins, 2011.

Turkington, Carol, and Michael M. Alper. *Encyclopedia of Fertility and Infertility*. New York: Facts On File, 2001.

Weschler, Toni. *Taking Charge of Your Fertility*. Rev. ed. New York: Collins, 2006.

Wisot, Arthur L., and David R. Meldrum. *Conceptions and Misconceptions: The Informed Consumer's Guide Through the Maze of In Vitro Fertilization and Other Assisted Reproduction Techniques*. 2d ed. Point Roberts, Wash.: Hartley & Marks, 2004.

Zouves, Christo. *Expecting Miracles: On the Path of Hope from Infertility to Parenthood*. New York: Berkley, 2003.

INFERTILITY, MALE

Disease/Disorder

Anatomy or system affected: Genitals, reproductive system

Specialties and related fields: Endocrinology, urology

Definition: The inability to achieve a desired pregnancy as a result of dysfunction of male reproductive organs.

Key terms:

antibody: a chemical produced by lymphocytes (blood cells) that enables these cells to destroy foreign materials, such as bacteria

cryopreservation: a special process utilizing cryoprotectants that enables living cells to survive in a frozen state

cryoprotectant: one of several chemicals that enable living cells to survive in a frozen state; some cryoprotectants are made by animals that survive freezing

epididymis: an organ attached to the testis in which newly formed sperm reach maturity (that is, become capable of fertilizing an egg)

infertility: the inability to produce a normal pregnancy after one to two years of intercourse in the absence of any contraception; it may be caused by male and/or female factors

insemination: the placement of semen in the female reproductive tract, which may occur naturally as a result of sexual intercourse or artificially as a result of a medical procedure

testis: either of two male gonads that are suspended in the scrotum and produce sperm

varicocele: a swollen testicular vein in the scrotum occurring as a result of improper valvular function

Causes and Symptoms

To create a baby requires three things: healthy sperm from a man, a healthy egg from a woman, and a healthy, mature uterus. Anything that blocks the availability of the sperm, egg, or uterus can cause infertility. Infertility can be thought of as an abnormal, unwanted form of contraception.

Many different factors may be responsible for infertility. In general, these factors may be infectious, chemical (from inside or outside the body, such as pharmaceuticals, toxins, or illegal drugs), or anatomical. Genetic factors may be responsible as well, since genes control the formation of body chemicals (such as hormones and antibodies) and body structures (one's anatomy). The way that these factors work is illustrated by male infertility.

Sperm are made in a man's testes (or testicles). Because the creation of sperm is controlled by genes and hormones, abnormalities in these can cause infertility. Sperm are initially formed in the seminiferous tubules, extremely narrow, tightly coiled tubes in the main body of the testes; from there, the sperm are released into another set of tubes to the rear of the testes called the epididymis, where they become mature. Sperm are stored in the epididymis until being released into the vas deferens and then the urethra before leaving the body during intercourse. A blockage of any part of this reproductive tract, or premature release of sperm from the epididymis, can cause infertility.

Information on Male Infertility

Causes: Low sperm count, infection, blockage of sperm ducts (from swollen tissue or tumor), premature release of sperm from epididymis, improper scrotal temperature, varicoceles

Symptoms: Typically asymptomatic

Duration: Short-term to chronic

Treatments: Surgery, hormonal therapy, fertility procedures (e.g., artificial insemination)

A blockage of reproductive ducts can occur as a result of a bodily enlargement, such as swollen tissue, a tumor, or cancer. An infection usually causes tissue swelling and can leave ducts permanently scarred, narrowed, or blocked. Infection can have a direct detrimental effect on the production of normal sperm. Cancer and the drugs or chemicals used to treat cancer can also damage a man's reproductive tract.

Another factor that may be important to male fertility is scrotal temperature. The temperature in the scrotum, the sac that holds the testes, is somewhat lower than body temperature. The normal production of sperm seems to be dependent upon a cool testicular environment.

One cause of male infertility is varicoceles—basically varicose veins of the testes—which occur when one-way valves fail in the veins that take blood away from the testicles. When these venous valves become leaky, blood flow becomes sluggish and causes the veins to swell. Many men with varicoceles are infertile, but the exact reason for this association is unknown. The reasons sometimes given are increased scrotal temperature and improper removal of materials (hormones) from the testis.

Mature sperm capable of fertilizing an egg are normally placed in the female reproductive tract by the ejaculation phase of sexual intercourse. The sperm are accompanied by fluid called seminal plasma; together, they form semen. A blockage of the ducts that transport the semen into the woman or toxic chemicals, including antibodies, in the semen can cause infertility.

For conception to take place—that is, for an egg to be fertilized after sperm enters the female tract—a healthy egg must be present in the portion of the female reproductive tract called the Fallopian tube, and sperm must move through the female tract to that egg. If the egg is absent or is abnormal, or if healthy sperm cannot reach the egg, failure to conceive will result. The female factors that determine whether sperm fertilize an egg are the same as the male factors: anatomy, chemicals, infection, and genes.

For those who seek help with fertility issues, there are many methods available. Female infertility may be treated, depending upon the cause, by surgery, hormone therapy, or in vitro fertilization. Treatment of male infertility may be by surgery, hormone therapy, or artificial insemination. Artificial insemination is often performed when the couple is composed of a fertile woman and an infertile man.

The first step for artificial insemination is for a physician to determine when the woman ovulates or releases an egg into the Fallopian tube. At the time of ovulation, semen is placed with medical instruments in the woman's reproductive tract, either on her cervix or in her uterus.

The semen used by the physician is obtained through masturbation by either the infertile man (the patient) or a fertile man (a donor), depending on the cause of the man's infertility. The freshly produced semen from either source usually undergoes laboratory testing and processing. Tests are used to evaluate the sperm quality. An effort may be made to enhance the sperm from an infertile patient and then to use these sperm for artificial insemination or in vitro fertilization. Other tests evaluate semen for transmissible diseases. During testing, which may require many days, the sperm can be kept alive by cryopreservation, or freezing. Freshly ejaculated sperm remains fertile for only a few hours in the laboratory if it is not cryopreserved.

There are several processes that might enhance sperm from an infertile man. If the semen is infertile because it possesses too few normal sperm, an effort can be made to eliminate the abnormal sperm and to increase the concentration of normal sperm. Sperm may be abnormal in four basic ways: They may have abnormal structure, they may have abnormal movement, they may be incapable of fusing with an egg, or they may contain abnormal genes or chromosomes. Laboratory processes can often eliminate from semen those sperm with abnormal structure or abnormal movement. These processes usually involve replacing the seminal plasma with a culture medium. Removing the seminal plasma gets rid of substances that may be harmful to the sperm. After the plasma is removed, the normal sperm can be collected and concentrated. Pharmacologic agents can be added to the culture medium to increase sperm movement.

Testing for transmissible diseases is especially important if donor semen is used; these diseases may be genetic or infectious. There are many thousand genetic disorders. Most of these disorders are very rare and can be transmitted to offspring only if the sperm and the egg both have the same gene for the disorder. It is impossible, therefore, to test a donor for every possible genetic disorder; he is routinely tested only for a small group of troublesome disorders that are especially likely to occur in offspring. Tests for other disorders that the donor might transmit can be performed at the woman's request, usually based upon knowledge of genetic problems in her own family.

Much of the genetic information about a person is based on family history. Special laboratory procedures allow the genetic code inside individual cells to be interpreted. For this reason, it is important to store a sample of donor cells, not necessarily sperm, for many years after the procedure. These cells provide additional genetic information that might be important to the donor's offspring but not known at the time of insemination.

Semen can also be the source of some infectious diseases. Syphilis, gonorrhea, chlamydia, and acquired immunodeficiency syndrome (AIDS) are examples of sexually transmitted infections (STIs) that can be transmitted by donor semen.

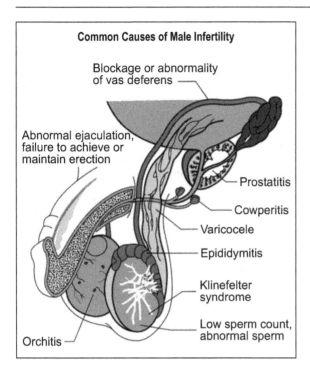

Common Causes of Male Infertility

Blockage or abnormality of vas deferens

Abnormal ejaculation; failure to achieve or maintain erection

Prostatitis

Cowperitis

Varicocele

Epididymitis

Klinefelter syndrome

Low sperm count, abnormal sperm

Orchitis

Screening history and testing are done on donors, but they cannot ensure that there will be no chance of infection. For example, the human immunodeficiency virus (HIV) may be newly present from recently acquired infection, but screening tests depend on the presence of antibodies, which do not show up immediately after someone is infected.

Cryopreservation of sperm is important to artificial insemination for two major reasons. First, it gives time to complete all necessary testing. Second, it allows an inventory of sperm from many different donors to be kept constantly available for selection and use by patients. Sperm have been cryopreserved for over twenty years and then thawed and used successfully.

Cryopreservation involves treating freshly ejaculated sperm with a cryoprotectant pharmaceutical that enables the sperm to survive when frozen; the cryoprotectant for sperm is usually glycerol. Survival of frozen sperm is also dependent upon the rate of cooling, the storage temperature, and the rate of warming at the time of thawing. Sperm treated with a cryoprotectant have the best chance of survival if they are cooled at a rate of about 1 degree Celsius per minute and stored at a temperature of –150 degrees Celsius (about –240 degrees Fahrenheit) or colder. An environment of liquid nitrogen is often used to attain these storage temperatures. The storage temperature must be kept constant to avoid the damaging effects of recrystallization.

Human sperm can be shipped to almost any location for artificial insemination. Sperm is usually cryopreserved before shipment and thawed at the time of insemination.

Treatment and Therapy
The use of artificial insemination to treat two kinds of male

infertility will be considered here. The first example is male infertility that cannot be treated by other means. The second example is a fertile man at high risk for becoming infertile because of his lifestyle or because he is receiving treatment for a life-threatening disease.

The first example might occur when a heterosexual couple, having used no contraception for a year or longer, has been unsuccessful in conceiving a baby. In 40 percent of infertility cases, the woman has the major, but not necessarily the only, problem preventing the pregnancy. In 40 percent of the cases, the man is the major factor. In 20 percent, each person makes a contribution to the problem, or the problem is unidentified. Therefore, both partners must deal with the infertility and be involved in the treatment.

The solution to a couple's infertility involves evaluation and therapy. The couple will be evaluated in regard to their present sexual activity and history, such as whether either one has ever contributed to a pregnancy. The medical evaluation of both partners will include a physical examination, laboratory tests, and even imaging techniques such as x-rays, ultrasonography, or magnetic resonance imaging (MRI). For the man, the physical examination will include a search for the presence of varicoceles, and the laboratory tests will include a semen analysis.

Varicoceles are probably the most readily detected problem that may cause male infertility. They are three times more common in infertile men than in men with proven fertility. This association does not prove that varicoceles cause infertility, however, because surgery that corrects a varicocele does not always correct infertility.

If the medical evaluation determines that the female partner has a normal reproductive tract and is ovulating on a regular basis, and if it determines that the male partner has too few normal sperm to make a pregnancy likely, the couple may be asked to consider adopting a baby or undergoing artificial insemination. With artificial insemination using a sperm donor, if the woman becomes pregnant, half of the baby's genes come from the mother, and the other half of the genes come from the donor, usually a person unknown to the couple. The physician performing artificial insemination may provide the couple with extensive information on several possible donors. Such information might include race, ethnic origin, blood type, physical characteristics, results of medical and genetic tests, and personal information, but the donor usually remains anonymous. The semen from each donor has undergone laboratory testing and cryopreservation. The frozen semen is then thawed at the time of insemination.

Although the idea of artificial insemination is simple, it usually involves some very complicated emotions. Although a couple may be very happy about all other aspects of their lives together, they may be disturbed to learn of the man's infertility. If the couple chooses artificial insemination using a sperm donor, later, they must decide whether to tell the child about the circumstances of his or her birth. Sometimes, a child who originated through artificial insemination may try to learn the identity of the donor.

Although male-factor infertility is the situation that benefits most from insemination and semen cryopreservation procedures, these procedures might be requested by a fertile couple that is at risk for male-factor infertility. Such couples may fear that the man's lifestyle, such as working with hazardous materials (solvents, toxins, radioisotopes, or explosives), may endanger his ability to produce sperm or may harm his genetic information. The man could be facing medical therapy that will cure a malignancy, such as Hodgkin's disease or a testicular tumor, but may render him sterile. A man facing such a situation may benefit from having some of his semen cryopreserved for his own future use, in the event that he does become infertile.

There are ways to compensate for decreased semen quality. The semen may be processed in ways to increase the concentration of normal sperm. The processed semen may be placed directly into the woman's uterus (intrauterine insemination) rather than on her cervix, or in vitro fertilization (IVF) may be used. In this procedure, the sperm and eggs are mixed in a laboratory and the resulting embryo is implanted in the woman. For men with difficulties in sperm production, IVF may be achieved using intracytoplasmic sperm injection (ICSI), which involves the implantation of one sperm directly into an ovum, thus avoiding the need for large numbers of sperm. All these techniques have proved helpful to infertile couples wanting children.

Perspective and Prospects

Studies have shown that about 15 percent of American couples are unable to conceive after one year of unprotected sex, and 10 percent do not conceive after two years. By the early 1990s, artificial insemination produced more than thirty thousand American babies yearly. This procedure advanced in the United States during the latter half of the twentieth century in large measure because of changes in attitudes, more than new medical knowledge.

The medical knowledge to treat male infertility has been available for several centuries, even when the biological basis for pregnancy was not understood. The Bible records stories of patriarchal families that knew the problem of infertility (Abraham and Sarah, Jacob and Rachel) and even indicates, in the story of Onan and Tamar (Genesis 38:9), that semen was understood to be important to reproduction. The possibility of therapeutic insemination was mentioned in the fifth century Talmud. Arabs used insemination in horse breeding as early as the fourteenth century, and Spaniards used it in human medicine during the fifteenth century.

The presence of sperm in semen was first observed by the Dutch scientist Antoni van Leeuwenhoek in the seventeenth century, but their importance and function in the fertilization process was not recognized until the nineteenth century. In 1824, Jean Louis Prévost and J. A. Dumas correctly guessed the role of sperm in fertilization, and in 1876, Oskar Hertwig and Hermann Fol proved that the union of sperm and egg was necessary to create an embryo.

Artificial insemination became an established but clandestine procedure in the late nineteenth century in the United States and England. Compassionate physicians pioneering artificial insemination encouraged secrecy to protect the self-esteem of the infertile man, his spouse, the offspring, and the donor. In an uncertain legal climate, the offspring might have been viewed as the illegitimate product of an adulterous act. Even by the beginning of the twenty-first century, many Americans continued to stigmatize masturbation and artificial insemination. Social attitudes, especially traditional notions of masculinity, have limited the acceptability of artificial insemination to many infertile couples worldwide.

Cryopreservation of sperm became practical with the discovery of chemical cryoprotectants, reported in 1949 by Christopher Polge, Audrey Smith, and Alan Parkes of England. In 1953, American doctors R. G. Bunge and Jerome Sherman were the first to use this procedure to produce a human baby. Cryopreservation made possible the establishment of sperm banks; prior to this development, sperm donors had to provide the physician with semen immediately before insemination was to take place.

Researchers continue to theorize about new fertility-enhancing techniques using sperm. In 2003, scientists discovered that sperm have a type of chemical sensor that causes the sperm to swim vigorously toward concentrations of a chemical attractant. While researchers long have known that chemical signals are an important component of conception, the 2003 findings were the first to demonstrate that sperm will respond in a predictable and controllable way. The findings provided strong evidence that the egg signals its location to the sperm and the sperm respond by swimming toward the egg, a process which could prove promising for future contraception and infertility research. Scientists note that these findings might allow specific tests to be developed to determine if the egg is making the attractant or if the sperm have the receptor, thus helping in identifying those couples who are infertile because of poor signaling between the sperm and egg.

Artificial insemination and other alternative means of reproduction give rise to thorny issues of personal rights of various "parents" (social, birth, and genetic) and their offspring. In the United States, a few states have addressed these issues by enacting laws, usually to grant legitimacy to offspring of donor insemination. In the United Kingdom, Parliament established a central registry of sperm and egg donors. Offspring in the United Kingdom have access to nonidentifying donor information; these children are even able to learn whether they are genetically related to a prospective marriage partner.

—Armand M. Karow, Ph.D.;
updated by Paul Moglia, Ph.D.

See also Assisted reproductive technologies; Conception; Gamete intrafallopian transfer (GIFT); Genital disorders, male; In vitro fertilization; Infertility, female; Men's health; Pregnancy and gestation; Reproductive system; Semen; Sexual dysfunction; Sperm banks; Sterilization; Stress; Testicular surgery; Vas deferens; Vasectomy.

For Further Information:

American Society for Reproductive Medicine. http://www.asrm.org/

Doherty, C. Maud, and Melanie M. Clark. *The Fertility Handbook: A Guide to Getting Pregnant*. Omaha, Nebr.: Addicus Books, 2002.

Fisch, Harry, and Stephen Braun. *The Male Biological Clock: The Startling News About Aging, Sexuality, and Fertility in Men*. New York: Free Press, 2005.

Glover, Timothy D., and C. L. R. Barratt, eds. *Male Fertility and Infertility*. New York: Cambridge University Press, 2003.

InterNational Council on Infertility Information Dissemination. http://www.inciid.org.

"Male Infertility." *Mayo Clinic*, September 15, 2012.

"Male Infertility." *Urology Care Foundation*, March, 2013.

Riley, Julie. "Infertility in Men." *Health Library*, September 26, 2012.

Schover, Leslie R., and Anthony J. Thomas. *Overcoming Male Infertility: Understanding Its Causes and Treatments*. New York: John Wiley & Sons, 2000.

Taguchi, Yosh, and Merrily Weisbord, eds. *Private Parts: An Owner's Guide to the Male Anatomy*. 3d ed. Toronto, Ont.: McClelland & Stewart, 2003.

INFLAMMATION

Disease/Disorder

Anatomy or system affected: All

Specialties and related fields: Family medicine, internal medicine, pathology, rheumatology

Definition: The reaction of blood-filled living tissue to injury.

Causes and Symptoms

In inflammation, the following changes are seen locally: redness, swelling, heat, pain, and loss of function. These changes are chemically mediated. Inflammation may be caused by microbial infection; physical agents such as trauma, radiation, and burns; chemical toxins; caustic substances such as strong acids or bases; decomposing or necrotic tissue; and reactions of the immune system. Acute inflammation is of relatively short duration (from a few minutes to a day), while chronic inflammation lasts longer. The local changes associated with inflammation include the outflow of fluid into the spaces between cells and the inflow or migration of white blood cells (leukocytes) to the area of injury. Chronic inflammation is characterized by the presence of leukocytes and macrophages, as well as by the proliferation of new blood vessels and connective tissue.

Inflammation is a protective mechanism for the body. Redness is attributable to increased blood flow to the injured area. Swelling is caused by the flow of fluid into the spaces between cells. Heat is produced by a combination of increased blood flow and chemical reactions in the local area. Pain results from the presence of two main chemicals found in the bloodstream: prostaglandins and bradykinin. Loss of function is a result of pain (the body limits movement to reduce discomfort) and swelling (interstitial fluid limits movement).

Acute inflammation. Many chemicals are involved in acute inflammation. Mediators of inflammation originate from blood plasma and from both damaged and normal cells. Vasoactive amines are a class of chemicals that increase the permeability of blood vessel and cell walls. The most well studied of these are histamine and serotonin. Histamine is stored in granules in mast cells that are found in both tissue

and basophils, the latter being a type of cell found in the blood. Serotonin is found in mast cells and platelets; it is another type of cell found in the bloodstream. These substances cause vasodilation (expansion of the walls of blood vessels) and increased vascular permeability (leakage through the walls of small vessels, especially veins). Histamine and serotonin can be released by trauma or exposure to cold. Other chemicals that circulate in the blood can release histamine. Two of these are part of the complement system; another is called interleukin-1. The effects of histamine diminish after approximately one hour.

Plasma proteases comprise three interrelated systems that explain much that is known about inflammation: the complement, kinin, and clotting systems. The complement system is composed of twenty different proteins involved in reactions against microbial agents that invade the body. The various chemicals act in a cascade, similar to falling dominoes: Each one sets off another in sequence. The result of these chemical actions is to increase vascular permeability, promote chemotaxis (the attraction of living cells to specific chemicals), engulf invading microorganisms, and destroy pathogens through a process called lysis.

The kinin system is responsible for releasing bradykinin, a chemical substance that causes contraction of smooth muscle tissue, dilation of blood vessels, and pain. The duration of action for bradykinin is brief because it is inactivated by the enzyme kininase. Bradykinin does not promote chemotaxis.

The clotting system is made up of a series of chemicals that result in the formation of a solid mass. The most commonly encountered example is the scab that forms at the site of a cut in the skin. Like the complement system, the clotting system is a cascade of thirteen different chemicals. In addition to producing a solid mass, the clotting system also increases vascular permeability and promotes chemotaxis for white blood cells.

Other substances are involved in acute inflammation. Among the most important of these is a class called prostaglandins. Several different prostaglandin molecules have been isolated; they are derived from the membranes of most cells. Prostaglandins cause pain, vasodilation, and fever. Aspirin counteracts the effects of prostaglandins, which explains the antipyretic (fever-reducing) and analgesic (pain-reducing) properties of the drug.

Another group of substances involved in acute inflammation are leukotrienes. The primary sources for these molecules are leukocytes, and some leukotrienes are found in mast cells. This group promotes vascular leakage but not chemotaxis. They also cause vasoconstriction (a decrease in the diameter of blood vessels) and bronchoconstriction (a decrease in the diameter of air passageways in the lungs). The effect of these leukotrienes is to slow blood flow and restrict air intake and outflow. A different type of leukotriene is found only in leukocytes. This type enhances chemotaxis but does not contribute to vascular leakage. In addition, leukotrienes cause white blood cells to stick to damaged tissues, speeding the removal of bacteria and promoting healing.

Information on Inflammation

Causes: Infection, injury, radiation, burns, chemical toxins, decomposing or necrotic tissue, immune system reactions

Symptoms: Redness, swelling, heat, pain, loss of function

Duration: Acute to chronic

Treatments: Drug therapy (e.g., antibiotics)

Other chemical substances are known to be involved with inflammation: platelet-activating factor, tumor necrosis factor, interleukin-1, cationic (positively charged) proteins, neutral proteases (enzymes that break down proteins), and oxygen metabolites (molecules resulting from reactions with oxygen). The sources of these are generally leukocytes, although some are derived from macrophages. They reinforce the effects of prostaglandins and leukotrienes.

There are four different outcomes for acute inflammation. There may be complete resolution in which the injured site is restored to normal; this outcome usually follows a mild injury or limited trauma where there has been only minor tissue destruction. Healing with scarring may occur, in which injured tissue is replaced with scar tissue that is rich in collagen, giving it strength but at the cost of normal function; this outcome follows more severe injury or extensive destruction of tissue. There may be the formation of an abscess, which is characterized by pus and which follows injuries that become infected with pyogenic (pus-forming) organisms. The fourth outcome is chronic inflammation.

Chronic inflammation. Acute inflammation may be followed by chronic inflammation. This reaction occurs when the organism, factor, or agent responsible for the acute inflammation is not removed or when the normal processes of healing fail to occur. Repeated episodes of acute inflammation may also lead to chronic inflammation, in which the stages of acute inflammation seem to remain for long periods of time. In addition, chronic inflammation may begin insidiously, such as with a low-grade infection or other process that does not display the usual signs of acute inflammation; tuberculosis, rheumatoid arthritis, and chronic lung disease are examples of this third alternative.

Chronic inflammation typically occurs in one of the following conditions: prolonged exposure to potentially toxic substances such as asbestos, coal dust, and silica that are nondegradable; immune reactions against one's own tissue (autoimmune diseases such as lupus and rheumatoid arthritis); and persistent infection by an organism that is either resistant to drug therapy or insufficiently toxic to cause an immune reaction (such as viruses, tuberculosis, and leprosy). The characteristics of chronic inflammation are similar to those of acute inflammation but are less dramatic and more protracted.

—*L. Fleming Fallon, Jr., M.D., Ph.D., M.P.H.*

See also Abscess drainage; Abscesses; Anti-inflammatory drugs; Arthritis; Burns and scalds; Bursitis; Disease; Healing; Immune system; Infection; Wounds; *specific diseases.*

For Further Information:

Challem, Jack. *The Inflammation Syndrome: Your Nutritional Plan for Great Health, Weight Loss, and Pain-Free Living.* Rev. ed. Hoboken: Wiley-Blackwell, 2010.

Dartt, Darlene A. *Immunology, Inflammation and Diseases of the Eye.* Boston: Academic Press, 2011.

Gallin, John I., and Ralph Snyderman, eds. *Inflammation: Basic Principles and Clinical Correlates.* 3d ed. New York: Raven Press, 1999.

Górski, Andrzej, Hubert Krotkiewski, and MichaÅ, Zimecki, eds. *Inflammation.* Boston: Kluwer, 2001.

Guha, Sushovan, Sunil Krishnan, and Bharat B. Aggarwal. *Inflammation, Lifestyle, and Chronic Disease: The Silent Link.* Boca Raton: CRC Press, 2012.

Kumar, Vinay, Abul K. Abbas, and Nelson Fausto, eds. *Robbins and Cotran Pathologic Basis of Disease.* 8th ed. Philadelphia: Saunders/Elsevier, 2010.

McPherson, R. "Inflammation and Coronary Artery Disease: Insights from Genetic Studies." *The Canadian Journal of Cardiology* 28, no. 6 (2012): 662–666.

Meggs, William Joel, and Carol Svec. *The Inflammation Cure.* Chicago: Contemporary Books, 2004.

Preddy, Victor R., and Ronald R. Watson. *Bioactive Food as Interventions and Related Inflammatory Diseases.* Boston: Elsevier/Academic Press, 2013.

Yian, Gu, and Nikolas Scarmeas. "Dietary Inflammation Factor Rating System and Risk of Alzheimer Disease in Elder." *Alzheimer Disease and Associated Disorders* 25, no. 2 (2011): 149–154.

INFLUENZA

Disease/Disorder

Anatomy or system affected: Lungs, nose, respiratory system, throat

Specialties and related fields: Emergency medicine, epidemiology, family medicine, internal medicine, nursing, pediatrics, public health, virology

Definition: An acute respiratory infection caused by an influenza virus.

Key terms:

pandemic: a disease that affects a widespread population

polymerase chain reaction: a technique that multiplies small amounts of genetic material, deoxyribonucleic acid (DNA), into amounts that can be detected by specific genetic probes

ribonucleic acid (RNA): the molecular genetic material of the influenza virus that is also found in all cells and in some other viruses

Causes and Symptoms

Influenza viruses are members of the orthomyxovirus group and are usually spherical or elliptical bodies 80–120 nanometers in size. The core of the virus is a nucleocapsid consisting of matrix or structural proteins, various nonstructural proteins or enzymes, and ribonucleic acid (RNA). The central core is surrounded by an envelope that is studded by two types of surface antigens, rod-shaped trimeric spikes of hemagglutinins and mushroom-shaped tetrameric projections of neuraminidases. Frequent changes in these two antigens produce the waves of influenza, also known as flu or grippe, in people who have no immunity from prior exposure to new strains. When the changes are small, they are referred to as antigenic drift; when they are large, they are called antigenic shift. There are sixteen hemagglutinin and nine neuraminidase subtypes, and all are known to infect birds. Influenza A maintains a reservoir in waterfowl and shorebirds and can infect domestic poultry, horses, pigs, and humans, but influenza B and C viruses principally infect humans. During the past century, H1N1, H2N2, and H3N2 subtypes of influenza A have been the predominant viruses circulating in the human population, and of the 144 possible antigenic combinations these are the only t that have become adapted to human hosts. When antigenic shift occurs, new hemagglutinin and neuraminidase antigens arise to which the population has no immunity. These large changes in the viral surface antigens occur every ten to thirty years, whereas smaller changes (antigenic drift) in the existing circulating subtypes appear every one to three years. Antigenic shift produces epidemics or pandemics, and antigenic drift results in outbreaks or less widespread epidemics.

Influenza epidemics are associated with excess morbidity and mortality. The excess morbidity is calculated by comparing rates of pneumonia- and influenza-associated illness with seasonally expected rates calculated from nonepidemic years. Similarly, excess mortality is determined by comparing pneumonia- and influenza-related deaths to an expected seasonal baseline rate. During epidemics, the attack rate in unvaccinated populations is 10 to 20 percent but may be as high as 40 to 50 percent. These effects were observed in dramatic fashion during the 1918 (H1N1, Spanish), 1957 (H2N2, Asian), and 1968 (H3N2, Hong Kong) influenza A pandemics of the twentieth century. While not associated with pandemics, influenza B virus is capable of causing severe disease, especially in elderly or immunologically impaired individuals. Influenza C is associated with only mild respiratory disease. In temperate climates, influenza is usually a seasonal illness of the winter months. Colder weather and low humidity facilitate transmission, and indoor crowding and school attendance may also contribute to the spread of virus.

The infection is acquired by the transfer of virus in infected respiratory secretions to mucosal surfaces. Aerosols, both large and small droplets from sneezing and coughing, and direct contact are all responsible for viral transfer. The virus attaches to and penetrates the cells lining the respiratory tract and, through a variety of mechanisms, produces cell death. In the hours preceding cellular destruction, however, new viral particles manufactured by the influenza-infected cell are released to infect nearby cells and continue the infection. Viral shedding in respiratory secretions begins about twenty-four hours before the onset of symptoms and continues for five to ten days.

Influenza infection elicits both local (mucosal) and systemic antibodies as well as T-cell lymphocyte responses. Mucosal antibodies of both the IgA and the IgG type have been demonstrated in nasal secretions, and IgA antibodies help protect the cells of the upper respiratory tract from infec-

---

Information on Influenza

Causes: Viral infection
Symptoms: Fever, malaise, headache, muscle pain (particularly in back and legs), coughing, nasal congestion, shivering, sore throat
Duration: Acute
Treatments: Typically alleviation of symptoms; sometimes antiviral drugs (e.g., ribavirin)

---

tion. Systemic antibodies against the hemagglutinin antigen are capable of neutralizing the virus infectivity, while those against the neuraminidase antigen decrease the release of virus from infected cells. If there has been no prior exposure to the particular virus subtype, through either infection or vaccination, then antibody response takes two weeks to develop and peaks at four to seven weeks. Contribution of the T-cell response is less well understood but appears to reduce both the duration of illness and the viral replication.

After an incubation period of one to two days, the illness has an abrupt onset, with chills, fever, myalgia (muscle pain), headache, and anorexia (appetite loss). Ocular symptoms may be prominent, with tearing, burning, and pain with eye movement. Nasal stuffiness and discharge, dry cough, and sore throat are often present. The fever is usually 100 to 104 degrees Fahrenheit on the first day and gradually decreases to normal over the following two to three days, but it may last up to a week. The cough and general feeling of malaise may last for as long as six to eight weeks, even though the acute illness typically resolves in seven to ten days.

Pneumonia is the most important complication of influenza. There may be primary viral pneumonia, secondary bacteria pneumonia, or a combination of both. Autopsies of fatal cases during the 1918 influenza pandemic revealed each of these three varieties of pneumonia in about equal numbers. Primary viral pneumonia more commonly strikes patients with chronic cardiovascular or pulmonary disease; however, new pandemic strains, such as H1N1 influenza, have caused pneumonia in healthy children and young adults. A return of fever during the second week of illness may herald the onset of secondary bacterial pneumonia. This complication is more common in patients with underlying cardiovascular or pulmonary disease and in the elderly. While Richard Pfeiffer originally found *Haemophilus influenzae* as the most common bacterial pathogen, staphylococci and streptococci are the most dominant today. Less common complications include myositis, myocarditis, toxic shock, encephalitis, Guillain-Barré syndrome, and Reye's syndrome.

The influenza virus may be isolated for specific diagnosis and sensitivity testing from nasal swabs or washes, throat swabs, and sputum. Viral cultures usually grow within three days, and special stains combined with specific antibody are then used to identify strains. Susceptibility testing of virus to antivirals is performed in only a few research laboratories. The property of hemagglutination has also been used to identify the virus using a hemagglutination inhibition assay. Currently, the diagnostic "gold standard" is the polymerase chain reaction (PCR), which employs molecular methodology and can discriminate between subtypes. PCR testing is demanding, time-consuming, and expensive. A variety of colorimetric rapid tests to facilitate diagnosis and treatment of influenza A and B are available, and while the results are available in fifteen to twenty minutes, they are able to correctly identify only 40 to 70 percent of influenza patients.

Treatment and Therapy

Four antiviral drugs that are effective against various strains of influenza are currently available for treatment. Amantadine and rimantadine block the ion channel of the matrix protein M2. This ion channel is necessary for acidification of the nucleocapsid, allowing viral RNA to be transported to the nucleus of the invaded cell, which can then be directed to replicate virus. These drugs work to block the ion channels of influenza A and are administered orally. Zanamivir and oseltamivir inhibit neuraminidase, which assists the virus in entering host cells and also enables the newly replicated virus to exit the cell. Neuraminidase cleaves sialic acid from cell wall glycoprotein. Oseltamivir is administered orally, but zanamivir must be given as an aerosol as it is not absorbed from the gastrointestinal tract. These last two medications are effective against both influenza A and B.

All these antivirals must be administered early in the course of illness in order to be effective. They are most efficacious during the first twenty-four hours and lose their efficacy after forty-eight hours. However, therapy after forty-eight hours, while not altering the course of the disease, does reduce viral shedding and infectivity. Furthermore, they have been shown to be useful only in the treatment of uncomplicated influenza.

Widespread usage of these antivirals has resulted in mutations conferring resistance in some influenza A subtypes. For example, the circulating "seasonal" H1N1 virus is resistant to both neuraminidase inhibitors but retains susceptibility to the M2 ion channel blockers, while the reverse was true for the 2009 H1N1 pandemic strain. Specific antiviral treatment must be targeted to the current strain of influenza A or B producing disease in order to be effective.

Antivirals may be used to prevent or ameliorate infection with influenza virus. As with treatment, prophylaxis must be tailored to the specific influenza strain to circumvent resistance. Prophylaxis is often employed during outbreaks to prevent disease during the two weeks following influenza vaccination until the previously susceptible individuals can develop protective antibodies. Antiviral prophylaxis has been shown to be effective for prolonged periods as well.

Influenza vaccines are about 80 percent effective in preventing or reducing illness from the viruses included in the vaccine. The seasonal vaccines for the 2012–2013 season contained two influenza A strains (an H1N1 and an H3N2) plus an influenza B strain. These strains were selected for inclusion by a panel of experts based upon new strains isolated from patients during the later portion of the preceding influenza season to allow sufficient time for the next vaccine to be produced. Virus for inclusion in all these vaccines is grown in chicken eggs and then purified to minimize any contaminating proteins from the chicken egg. Nevertheless, they should not be given to individuals with a prior history of egg allergy. Each of the vaccines is available as a killed injectable preparation or an attenuated live virus nasal preparation. The nasal vaccine is approved only for immunocompetent individuals aged five to forty-nine years. Influenza vaccines are highly recommended for populations at risk for severe or complicated influenza, such as the elderly, patients with underlying cardiopulmonary disease, and pregnant women. Influenza vaccines are also recommended for health care workers to maintain the caregiving workforce and reduce transmission to patients.

Treatment of complicated influenza is mainly supportive by ensuring fluid and electrolyte balance and adequate respiration. In severe cases with pneumonia, me-

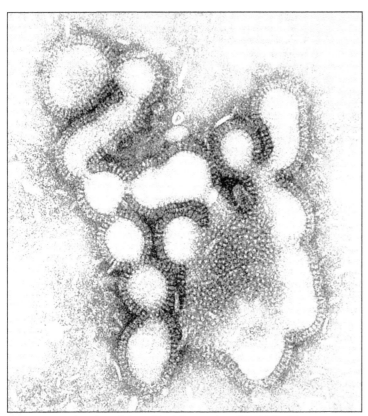

An enlarged view of the influenza virus. (Digital Stock)

chanical ventilation may be necessary. If secondary bacterial pneumonia occurs, then antibacterial therapy with agents directed against likely pathogens, especially *Staphylococcus aureus*, must be administered.

Lastly, because influenza is spread by both aerosols and direct contact, frequent hand washing and the use of masks can prevent or reduce the spread in households and hospitals.

Perspective and Prospects

Epidemics of influenza have been noted to recur every one to three years for at least four hundred years. Such an epidemic prompted Robert Pfeiffer to microscopically identify and cultivate an organism in the purulent sputa of patients with influenza in 1892. This gram-negative bacterium was known as the Pfeiffer influenza bacillus and was thought to be the causative agent of influenza. This organism would later be named *Haemophilus influenzae* in honor of this historic association.

The 1918 influenza pandemic resulted in 21 million deaths worldwide and 549,000 in the United States. Pfeiffer's bacillus could not be consistently isolated from influenza patients during this pandemic, and researchers began to question whether this was the true etiologic agent. In 1932, an American, Richard Shope, was able to transmit swine influenza to other animals using filtered nasal secretions, suggesting a viral, rather than bacterial, etiology. A year later, Wilson Smith and colleagues in England employed similar techniques to transmit human influenza virus from the 1932 epidemic to ferrets. After passage in ferrets, the filtrable agent was injected into mice, producing a pneumonia that resembled that seen during the 1918 pandemic. Smith also demonstrated that sera taken from convalescent influenza patients could neutralize the agent and prevent it from causing disease in ferrets.

While Smith had demonstrated that human influenza was caused by a virus, this association was dependent on transmission to an animal host. An Australian, Sir MacFarlane Burnet, discovered how to cultivate influenza virus in embryonated chicken eggs in 1936. This breakthrough enabled the virus to be grown in quantities that facilitated further study and the development of a protective vaccine in 1944.

The isolation of influenza A by Smith was followed by isolation of another strain of influenza virus from a patient in Puerto Rico by Thomas Francis in 1935. This strain, known as PR-8, served as the prototype for influenza disease worldwide in the 1930s. However, in 1940 a strain of influenza was isolated from a patient during an outbreak that could not be neutralized by antisera from other influenza A strains, and this virus was named influenza B. An influenza outbreak in 1946 led to the discovery that a vaccine made from PR-8 was not protective against this new strain of influenza A; an antigenic shift had occurred. In 1949, a third type, influenza C, was noted.

In 1941, George Hirst observed that influenza virus caused the hemagglutination of red blood cells and, after standing at room temperature, the agglutinated cells would begin to disaggregate, suggesting that the virus was breaking free. Indeed, after about one hour, all the virus could be eluted from the surrounding fluid and the red blood cells were not longer agglutinable. Hirst believed that the virus had altered the red

cell surface to make the cells no longer be able to be agglutinated. It was subsequently shown that a glycoprotein of the red cell membrane contains neuraminic acid which was split off by an enzyme of the influenza virus (neuraminidase).

Molecular techniques have allowed researchers to completely map all eight segments of RNA comprising the influenza A genetic code. Using these techniques on preserved tissue samples from 1918 influenza victims has provided a complete map of this historic strain. It is now known that the genetic legacy of the 1918 virus has been passed on to the subsequent influenza strains causing human disease. Despite these advances, the origin of the 1918 virus remains a mystery, and its ability to cause severe disease with high mortality is still unexplained. These data have shown that the novel H1N1 strain associated with the 2009 pandemic is a fourth-generation descendant of the 1918 virus. It is also known that new pandemic influenza A strains can emerge from two different pathways. The first is for an avian virus to infect a person and become transmissible between human hosts. The second is by reassortment of the eight segments of influenza RNA in hosts, such as pigs, that become infected with multiple strains of influenza A with the emergence of a new pathogenic strain for humans. Such knowledge may help prevent the appearance of a new pandemic strain by altering farming practices and by removing infected domestic poultry or swine when new strains are detected.

In addition to the four specific anti-influenza drugs currently available, several other drug therapies are promising. There are three drugs that inhibit viral RNA. Ribavirin is an antiviral currently available for the treatment of hepatitis C that has activity against influenza, especially at higher dosages. A new experimental drug, viramidine, is a prodrug of ribavirin with activity against influenza and less toxicity than ribavirin. Favipiravir is another RNA inhibitor under investigation. Peramivir is a new neuraminidase inhibitor that can be given intravenously and may soon be available for the treatment of severely ill influenza patients.

Anti-influenza antibody therapies have been tried since 1918, when blood, plasma, and serum from survivors were given to severely ill patients with some successes. Pooled human immunoglobulin from convalescent patients or artificially generated antibodies are both promising therapies.

Vaccine manufacture and development have not progressed significantly in the last fifty years. Perhaps the threat of another pandemic will stimulate new research in ways to produce vaccine strains in large quantities using methods other than chicken egg growth and harvesting. There is also continued hope that a conserved influenza antigen, rather than the ever-changing hemagglutinin and neuraminidase antigens, might yield a protective vaccine.

During the 2012–2013 flu season, a strain of avian influenza A, H7N9, developed in China and infected humans, with 131 cases and 32 deaths reported by the World Health Organization as of May 16, 2013. Very little is known so far about the strain or how it is transmitted, but researchers are studying animal-to-human and human-to-human transmission routes.

—H. Bradford Hawley, M.D.

See also Antibiotics; Avian influenza; Bacterial infections; Centers for Disease Control and Prevention (CDC); Emerging infectious diseases; Epidemics and pandemics; Epidemiology; Fever; H1N1 influenza; Lungs; Microbiology; Nausea and vomiting; Noroviruses; Pneumonia; Pulmonary diseases; Pulmonary medicine; Pulmonary medicine, pediatric; Respiration; Reye's syndrome; Viral infections; World Health Organization; Zoonoses.

For Further Information:

Beigel, John, and Mike Bray. "Current and Future Antiviral Therapy of Severe Seasonal and Avian Influenza." *Antiviral Research* 78 (2008): 91–102.

Carson-DeWitt, Rosalyn. "Influenza (Flu)." *Health Library*, September 30, 2012.

Centers for Disease Control and Prevention (CDC). "Seasonal Influenza (Flu)." *Centers for Disease Control and Prevention*, May 17, 2013.

MedlinePlus. "Flu." *MedlinePlus*, May 17, 2013.

Morens, David M., Gregory K. Folkers, and Anthony S. Fauci. "What Is a Pandemic?" *Journal of Infectious Diseases* 200 (2009): 1018–1021.

Morens, David M., Jeffrey K. Taubenberger, and Anthony S. Fauci. "The Persistent Legacy of the 1918 Influenza Virus." *New England Journal of Medicine* 361 (2009): 225–229.

Preidt, Robert. "HealthDay: Flu Vaccine Safe for Kids with Crohn's, Colitis: Study." *MedlinePlus*, May 6, 2013.

Treanor, John T. "Influenza Viruses, Including Avian Influenza and Swine Influenza." In *Principles and Practice of Infectious Diseases*, edited by Gerald L. Mandell, John F. Bennett, and Raphael Dolin. 7th ed. Philadelphia: Churchill Livingstone/Elsevier, 2009.

World Health Organization/GIP. "Number of Confirmed Human Cases of Avian Influenza A(H7N9), Reported to WHO (Report 6)." *World Health Organization: Influenza*, May 16, 2013.

INFORMED CONSENT
Ethics

Definition: The term used to describe how an individual patient expresses autonomy and self-determination within a medical setting.

Overview

Informed consent is the process in which a clinician provides information on the risks and benefits of a procedure to a patient capable of making informed decisions, who then freely makes a choice on whether to agree to the recommended procedure. A clinician or researcher is legally responsible for obtaining a patient or research participant's informed consent before a medical procedure or participation in clinical research. Laws surrounding informed consent in medical settings are governed by a combination of state common laws and statutes; consequently, they vary by each state and change as judges and legislators pass new legislation.

Informed consent can be either explicit or implied. Express consent is obtained when a patient signs informed consent forms or when they give specific spoken consent to a procedure or medical test. Express consent is most often used before more invasive or risky procedures such as surgery. Implied consent is nonverbal and most often used for low risk and noninvasive procedures. For example, based on a patient's actions and the visit context, a clinician could by implied consent assume a patient's willingness to have the patient's blood pressure or temperature taken as part of health care visits.

Aspects of an Informed Consent

There are several aspects of legally valid informed consent: the consent must be voluntary, informed (the clinician shares information and the patient understands it), and the patient or research participant must be competent to make decisions.

Voluntary. In order for the consent to be voluntary, the patient must be free to choose to accept or reject the medical recommendation without any coercion, fraud, or other constraints.

Informed. The process of making sure consent is informed entails a clinician sharing information and a patient understanding that content. Generally, this disclosure is defined as requiring the clinician to explain the diagnosis, risks, and benefits of the proposed procedure; any available alternative therapies, risks, and benefits of refusing the procedure; any financial costs associated with the procedure; and the level of uncertainty of the information provided. There are two different standards that are often used to determine a clinician's legal responsibility to share information with a patient: the professional and the patient-centered standards. Under the professional standard, a clinician is legally liable for not disclosing information that would be considered the customary practice for clinicians in a similar healthcare role. The patient-centered standard, also known as the "lay standard," is the more stringent standard requiring that the clinician provide all information to the patient that would be "material to the decision making" of a reasonable person.

Competent. Unless they have been formally found to be incompetent, generally patients are assumed to have sufficient cognitive and emotional capacity to understand the proposed medical intervention and make their own medical decisions.

—*Marie Schwartz*

For Further Information:

Goldman, Lee, and Andrew I. Schafer, eds. *Cecil Textbook of Medicine.* 24th ed. Philadelphia: Saunders, 2011.

Halter, J., et. al. *Hazzard's Geriatric Medicine and Gerontology.* 6th ed. New York: McGraw Hill, 2009.

Ryan, Marsha, and Michael S. Sinha. "Informed Consent." *UpToDate,* edited by Hilary Sanfey, Kathryn A. Collins, and Susan B. Yeon. Retrieved from http://www.uptodateonline.com.

Sprung, C.L. J. and B.J.J. Winick. "Informed Consent in Theory and Practice: Legal and Medical Perspectives on the Informed Consent Doctrine and a Proposed Reconceptualization." *Critical Care Medicine* 17 (1989): 1346-1354.

INSECT-BORNE DISEASES
Disease/Disorder

Anatomy or system affected: All

Specialties and related fields: Bacteriology, biochemistry, biotechnology, critical care, environmental health, epidemiology, microbiology, preventive medicine, public health

Definition: Diseases transmitted by insects, which have a significant health and economic impact worldwide, causing illness, disability, and death.

Key terms:

endemic: occurring naturally in a geographic area or population group

epidemic: any disease, injury, or health-related event occurring suddenly in numbers in excess of normal

mucous membranes: the inner lining of the mouth and nasal passages, as well as any membrane or lining containing mucus-secreting glands

parasite: an organism that obtains food and shelter from another organism or host

pathogen: a disease-producing microorganism such as bacteria, viruses, algae, and fungi

vector: an organism that transmits a disease from one host to another

Causes and Symptoms

Insects such as mosquitoes, blackflies, tsetse flies, eye flies, houseflies, fleas, and lice are responsible for transmitting pathogens that inflict disease and illness on hundreds of millions of people each year. Mosquitoes and blackflies are the most medically and economically destructive of the bloodsucking insects. Mosquito-borne diseases kill more than one million people every year and infect hundreds of millions more. These diseases are generally one of three types. The first usually causes fever, rashes, joint pain, and occasional fatal infections. The second type is hemorrhagic,

---

Information on Insect-Borne Diseases

Causes: Transfer of pathogens or parasites via a bite or other contact with mosquitoes, flies, lice, and other insects

Symptoms: Vary; may include fever, nausea, rashes, headache, swollen lymph glands, joint pain, bleeding, shock, blindness, and encephalitis

Duration: Acute and sometimes fatal; may become chronic

Treatments: Sometimes antibiotics, but often none; prevention through vaccines and through biological and chemical control of vectors

---

which causes bleeding from the mucous membranes and occasionally leads to fatal shock. The third type causes symptoms of encephalitis, an inflammation of the brain, and is identified with several epidemics.

The better-known mosquito-transmitted diseases include malaria, yellow fever, dengue fever, and West Nile virus. Malaria, responsible for the deaths of at least one million people in 2002, produces a high fever and chills and does not provide lasting immunity to a relapse. The disease is treated with quinine, but patients can still develop the deadly blackwater fever. Yellow fever is more deadly than malaria and is endemic in Central and South America, the West Indies, and Africa. There is no treatment for yellow fever, although at-risk individuals can be vaccinated to prevent infection. Patients with yellow fever may contract hepatitis and suffer renal (kidney) failure, hemorrhage (blood loss), shock, and death.

Dengue fever, also called breakbone fever, is rarely fatal, but it causes a high fever accompanied by severe pain and stiffness in the joints. The World Health Organization (WHO) estimates that between 50 and 100 million people are infected with Dengue fever annually; in 2010 there were a reported 1.6 million cases in the Americas. The disease is endemic in the tropics, where about 40 percent of the world's population lives. There is no vaccine or cure. Another form, hemorrhagic dengue, produces shock syndrome and follows a previous infection with dengue. The disease may infect people in as many as sixty-one countries.

West Nile virus was first reported in the United States in Queens, New York City, in 1999. In 2012, 5,674 human cases were reported, with 286 deaths. The virus also causes high mortality in many species of birds and results in numerous horse deaths. Most infected people are symptom-free, with mild cases causing flulike symptoms such as fever, coughing, and weakness. Serious infections can progress to more severe headaches, high fevers, tremors, and partial paralysis, as well as encephalitis.

Biting blackflies are a nuisance that can affect tourism, agriculture, forestry, and recreation. For animals, these bites can cause weight loss, stress-related illnesses, and reduced egg, milk, and meat production. One of the most widespread of the blackfly diseases is onchocerciasis, or river blindness, a disease that can be transmitted to humans, cattle, and other large

Mosquito-Borne Diseases

Mosquito	Habits	Features	Diseases
Aedes	Day biter, urban or rural	Head bent, body parallel to surface, black and white in color	Dengue, yellow fever, viral encephalitis
Anopheles	Night biter, mainly rural	Head and body in line, at angle to surface	Malaria, filariasis
Culex	Day biter, urban or rural	Shaped like *Aedes* but brown; whines in flight	Viral encephalitis, filariasis

---

Insect-Borne Viral Diseases

Disease	Principal Vectors
Encephalitis, California	Mosquitoes: Culex tarsalis, Aedes species
Encephalitis, Eastern equine	Mosquitoes: Aedes sollicitans, Culiseta melanura
Encephalitis, St. Louis	Mosquitoes: Culex pipiens pipiens, C. p. quinquefasciatus, C. tarsalis
Encephalitis, Venezuelan	Mosquitoes: Aedes serratus, Ae. scapularis, Ae. taeniorhynchus, Anopheles aquasalis, Culex vomifer, C. taeniopus, Haemogogus species, Mansonia titillans, Psorophora confinnis, P. ferox
Encephalitis, Western equine	Mosquitoes: Culex tarsalis and others
Pappataci or sandfly fever	Sandfly: Phlebotomus papatasii
Rift Valley fever	Mosquitoes: Eretmapodites chrysogaster, Aedes caballus, Ae. deboeri, Ae. circumluteolus, Ae. tarsalis, Culex theileri

---

mammals. The serious effects can occur long after the initial fly bite and are caused by a worm that is transmitted to the host. The worm curls up in lumps on the body, causing coarsening of the skin, depigmentation (loss of color), and intense itching that can drive a person to suicide in severe cases. If the worm enters the eyes, then it can cause reduced peripheral vision, night blindness, and complete loss of vision. Blackfly fever, found in the New England area of the United States, is a severe reaction to bites that causes fever, nausea, headaches, and swollen lymph glands.

Tsetse flies, houseflies, and eye flies are responsible for numerous infections and diseases. The tsetse fly's bite can transmit parasites and cause sleeping sickness, a West African disease in humans. The parasite causes enlarged glands, loss of appetite, and extreme lethargy. The patient eventually lapses into a coma, and the disease is fatal if not treated. A similar fatal disease called nagana occurs in animals, especially imported cattle and horses, cattle, goats, camels, and pigs.

Houseflies are nonbiting insects that can transfer pathogens from infected septic matter (feces) to human foodstuffs, sores, or mucous membranes. These pathogens can transmit cholera germs or cause diarrhea and eye infections. Eye flies drink fluid from eyes or blood from sores, ulcers, and small wounds on humans and animals. These very tiny black flies transmit bacteria, especially to children, and spread eye sores such as conjunctivitis (pinkeye) and other infections.

Biting midges are small flies that can transmit several diseases. Sandfly fever causes a short illness with fever in humans. Bartonellosis, or Carrion's disease, occurs in South America in Peru, Ecuador, and Colombia in higher altitudes. Mild cases usually cause a slight fever, but severe cases can have an 80 percent mortality rate. After five to eight weeks, fever survivors develop large wartlike tumors all over the body, which cause pain and irritation. Leishmaniasis is a parasitic disease and ranges from a mild form with fevers and anemia to a disfiguring type with skin wounds to another form that can cause internal organ damage and death. Most forms infect animals and accidentally transfer to humans. The disease affects approximately twelve million people worldwide, with over one million new cases every year. Other biting midges transmit diseases such as the Oropouche virus, which is found in tropical America. Severe flulike symptoms, with fever and vomiting, can last for up to two weeks but are usually not fatal.

Flea-borne murine (mice) typhus produces a typhuslike fever, eye rash, headache, chills, and general achiness. The most infamous disease transmitted by fleas, however, is the plague, which killed a quarter of the population of Europe in the fourteenth century. People become infected by receiving a flea bite, handling infected animals, or breathing infected respiratory droplets. The plague causes fever, chills, seizures, and severe headaches, followed by swollen lymph glands (or buboes) in the armpit, groin, or neck. Untreated septicemic plague is initially hard to diagnose because it invades the bloodstream directly, eventually spreading to the liver, kidney, spleen, lungs, eyes, and/or lining of the brain. This type of plague has a 40 percent mortality rate with treatment and a 100 percent fatality rate if untreated. Pneumonic plague, which is contracted by inhaling infected drops from another person or animal, causes severe, overwhelming pneumonia, shortness of breath, high fever, and blood in the phlegm. Life-threatening complications include shock, high fever, problems with blood clotting, and convulsions. Untreated pneumonic plague is almost always fatal, but a specific antibiotic treatment must be started fifteen to eighteen hours after symptoms appear in order to be effective.

Insect-Borne Bacterial and Rickettsial Diseases

Disease	Disease Agent	Principal Vectors
Anthrax	Bacillus anthracis	Various horse flies by mechanical transmission
Carrion's disease	Bartonella bacilliformis	Phlebotomus sandflies
Food poisoning	Shigella and Salmonella	Various flies by mechanical transmission
Plague	Yersinia pestis	Xenopsylla cheopis and some other fleas
Trench fever	Rickettsia quintana	Human body louse Pediculus humanus humanus
Tularemia	Francisella tularensis	Deer flies and ticks
Typhus, louse-borne	Rickettsia prowazekii	Human body louse Pediculus humanus humanus
Typhus, murine	Rickettsia mooseri	Rat flea Xenopsylla cheopis; the rat louse Polyplax spinulosa is a zoonotic vector
Yaws	Treponema pertenue	Hippelates gnats

Lice are responsible for several diseases, including louse-borne typhus, which comes from louse feces. Infection occurs through a scratch, contact with mucous membranes, or inhalation. Symptoms include fatigue, muscle aches, headache, coughing, rapid onset of fever, and a blotchy rash on the chest or abdomen. If untreated, the disease can cause delirium, low blood pressure, coma, and possibly death. Treatment with antibiotics usually provides a prompt cure. Brill-Zinsser disease is similar to a mild form of typhus and is a reoccurrence of louse-borne typhus, sometimes waiting as much as thirty years between outbreaks.

Symptoms of louse-borne relapsing fever include head and muscle aches, nausea, appetite loss, dizziness, coughing, vomiting, and the abrupt onset of fever. Severe infections cause the liver and spleen to swell and make breathing painful. Trench fever, or Wolhynian fever, occurred in Central Europe during World War I and World War II and is generally rare and seldom fatal. There may be no symptom or headaches, muscle aches, fever, and nausea.

Chagas" disease is found in South and Central America. Transmission of bacteria occurs through infected feces, and symptoms range from mild and flulike to severe chronic cardiac or digestive system disease. Estimations indicate that eight to eleven million people living in in Mexico, Central America, and South America are infected with Chagas' disease . Between 10 and 30 percent of infected people will develop chronic, life-threatening symptoms or heart failure, and about will fifty thousand die each year from infection. There is no vaccine or cure for Chagas" disease.

Treatment and Therapy

For most insect-borne diseases, treatment includes medical intervention such as antibiotics and vaccines to prevent transmission. As of 2013, vaccines for most of the diseases were still under development, and many of the diseases have no known cure. Educating people on how to avoid infection and treat the symptoms is essential.

Biological control involves reducing a target population by introducing a predator, pathogen, parasite, competitor, or toxin produced by a microorganism. This method of control was used as early as 1889 in California and became popular in the early twentieth century. Insecticides (or pesticides) replaced biological control and proved to be very successful in eliminating the insect vectors. Early pesticides were composed of natural botanicals (plant products) such as nicotine, rotenone, and pyrethrum mixed with chemicals such as lime sulfur, arsenic, mercuric chloride, and soaps. The scientific development of insecticides began as early as 1867, and the structures of botanical insecticides were known in the 1920s. In 1939, the insecticide properties of the first synthetic insecticide, DDT, were discovered. DDT has provided a major benefit in the control of typhus, trench fever, and malaria, and it is still used in indoor insecticides for malaria control.

Pesticides may lose their effectiveness as the parasites become resistant to a specific toxin or insecticide. The focus in the early twenty-first century is on developing pesticides known as third-generation insecticides, mainly aimed at affecting mosquito development. Since these insecticides are developed for mosquitoes, they are less disruptive to the environment and less toxic to humans and other organisms.

Other preventive measures include insect growth regulators (IGRs), which are species-specific and prevent larvae from developing. Genetic control, which involves introducing sterile males to the population or the release of insects with only male-producing properties, results in so few females that the population declines. Genetic control methods also may involve population replacement in which the genetic structure is modified in a particular species of insect to prevent disease transmission. A gene can be inserted that would cause the insect to die after breeding and would be passed to offspring. A different gene insertion would kill the females, which are the bloodsuckers in most species, but not the males.

In addition to pesticides and insecticides, which may be applied over a large area, the elimination of insect breeding and gathering areas is very effective. General measures to prevent infection include using personal repellents on people and livestock, wearing light-colored clothing and long sleeves and pants during feeding times, stabling livestock during peak biting periods, managing sewage and fecal waste, using netting or fine mesh screening, reducing the number of strays and wild animals that can act as hosts, and keeping the air moving with fans.

Perspective and Prospects

Insect-borne diseases have been infecting people throughout history. Malaria was noted in ancient times and written about

prior to the first century CE. Over time, some people speculated about a connection between insects and illness, but the scientific equipment and knowledge were not yet available to prove the existence of the pathogens. Initial observations led to improved hygiene and better housing, which greatly reduced plague and typhus. Malaria and yellow fever, however, did not respond to these developments.

In 1877, Sir Patrick Manson discovered that some mosquitoes can carry a parasite that infects people. This discovery and subsequent work by many others stimulated the research into insect-borne diseases. The insect transmission of plague and typhus took ten to twelve years to understand, and others took decades. There were no specific drugs or vaccines for the diseases until 1925, except for quinine for malaria, which did not always work.

Research continues in an effort to find successful preventive and control measures, including the development of more effective pesticides, insecticides, and genetic controls. Attention must be paid to illnesses in humans and animals and the potential insect connection in order to fight existing diseases and recognize new or mutating ones. For example,

Insect-Borne Protozoan Diseases

Disease	Disease Agent	Principal Vectors
Chagas' disease	Trypanosoma cruzi	Assassin bugs: Panstrongylus megistus and many species of Triatoma
Kala-azar	Leishmania donovani	Sandflies: Phlebotomus chinensis, P. major, P. argentipes, P. perniciosus
Leishmaniasis, American mucocutaneous	Leishmania braziliensis	Sandflies: Phlebotomus intermedius, P. longipalpus, P. pessoai
Leishmaniasis, Mexican	Leishmania mexicana	Sandfly: Phlebotomus flaviscutellatus
Malaria, benign tertian	Plasmodium vivax	Mosquitoes: species of Anopheles
Malaria, malignant tertian	Plasmodium falciparum	Mosquitoes: Anopheles stephensi, A. labranchiae
Malaria, ovale tertian	Plasmodium ovale	Mosquitoes: Anopheles gambiae, A. funestus
Malaria, quartan	Plasmodium malariae	Mosquitoes: many species of Anopheles
Nagana (cattle, etc.)	Trypanosoma brucei	Tsetse fly: Glossina morsitans
Oriental sore	Leishmania tropica	Sandflies: Phlebotomus papatasii and P. sergenti
Sleeping sickness, East African	Trypanosoma rhodesiense	Tsetse flies: Glossina morsitans and G. swynnertoni
Sleeping sickness, West African	Trypanosoma gambiense	Tsetse flies: Glossina tachinoides and G. palpalis
Surra (camels, etc.)	Trypanosoma evansi	Horse flies in the family Tabanidae

Insect-Borne Worm (Helminthic) Diseases

Contracted Through Ingesting Host

Disease	Parasite	Host
Dog tapeworm	Dipylidium caninum	Dog flea Pulex irritans and lice
Rodent tapeworm	Hymenolepis diminuta	Fleas including Xenopsylla cheopis; also roaches, moth and beetle larvae
Spiny-headed worm	Macracanthorhynchus hirudinaceus	Beetle larvae

Contracted from Blood-Sucking Flies

Disease	Parasite	Principal Vectors
Acanthocheilonemasis	Acanthocheilonema perstans	Biting midges: Culicoides austeni and C. grahami
Bancroft's filariasis	Wuchereria bancrofti	Mosquitoes: Culex pipiens quinquefasciatus and other Culex, Aedes, Anopheles, and Mansonia species
Brug's filariasis	Brugia malayi	Mosquitoes: Mansonia, Anopheles, Aedes, and Armigeres species
Dog heartworm	Dirofilaria immitis	Mosquitoes: Culex pipiens, Aedes aegypti, and others
Loiasis or African eyeworm	Loa loa	Mango flies: Chrysops dimidiatus and C. silaceus
Onchocerciasis	Onchocerca volvulus	Black flies: Simulium damnosum, S. neavei, S. ochraceum, and others
Ozzard's filariasis	Mansonella ozzardi	Biting midge: Culicoides furens

some researchers speculate that bloodsucking stable flies may have caused the initial spread of human immunodeficiency virus (HIV) from chimpanzees to humans.

Although many insect-borne diseases were greatly reduced by 1970, they have since made a dramatic recovery in warm areas of the world, perhaps because of the evolution and adaptation of the pathogens. In addition, social problems such as poverty, famine, and war, which often result in overcrowded and unsanitary conditions, offer ideal breeding areas and easy transmission for numerous insect-borne illnesses and diseases.

—Virginia L. Salmon

See also Allergies; Anthrax; Babesiosis; Bites and stings; Chagas' disease; Ehrlichiosis; Elephantiasis; Encephalitis; Epidemiology; Food poisoning; Leishmaniasis; Lice, mites, and ticks; Malaria; Parasitic diseases; Pinworms; Plague; Rocky Mountain spotted fever; Roundworms; Sleeping sickness; Tapeworms; Tropical medicine; Tularemia; Typhus; Worms; Yellow fever; Zoonoses.

For Further Information:

Busvine, James R. *Disease Transmission by Insects: Its Discovery and Ninety Years of Effort to Prevent It.* New York: Springer, 1993.

Carlson, Emily. "Taking the 'Bite' Out of Vector-Borne Diseases." *National Institute of General Medical Sciences*, May 15, 2013.

"Dengue and Severe Dengue." *World Health Organization*, November 2012.

Harder, Ben. "Don't Let the Bugs Bite: Can Genetic Engineering Defeat Disease Spread by Insects?" *Science News* 166, no. 7 (August 14, 2004): 104.

Marquardt, William C., ed. *Biology of Disease Vectors.* 2d ed. New York: Academic Press/Elsevier, 2005.

O'Hanlon, Leslie Harris. "Tinkering with Genes to Fight Insect-Borne Disease: Researchers Create Genetically Modified Bugs to Fight Malaria, Chagas, and Other Diseases." *The Lancet* 363 (April 17, 2004): 1288.

Spielman, Andrew, and Michael D'Antonio. *Mosquito: A Natural History of Our Most Persistent and Deadly Foe.* New York: Hyperion, 2001.

Turkington, Carol A., and Rebecca J. Frey. "Malaria." In *The Gale Encyclopedia of Medicine*, edited by Jacqueline L. Longe. 3d ed. Farmington Hills, Mich.: Thomson Gale, 2006.

"West Nile Virus: What You Need To Know." *Centers for Disease Control and Prevention*, September 12, 2012.

INSOMNIA. *See* **SLEEP DISORDERS.**

THE INSTITUTE OF MEDICINE
Organization
Definition: A nonprofit, nongovernmental organization that provides advice on science, medicine, and well-being to improve health in the United States.

The Institute of Medicine (IOM) was developed in 1970 as a branch of the National Academy of Sciences. The primary goal of the IOM is to provide unbiased, accurate, and authoritative information to aid professionals, government officials, and the general public in making accurate, well informed decisions related to their health, well-being, and healthcare. The information provided by the IOM is evidence-based, meaning that it is rooted in current research.

The Institute of Medicine conducts many research studies every year. These research projects often begin as Congressional mandates or are called for by federal agencies or independent organizations. The IOM's lack of governmental affiliation allows them to report straightforward and sometimes controversial results while remaining unbiased advisors to professionals, political leaders, and government officials.

Study topics are always health-related with focuses on the impact of environment and lifestyle on the health of the general population or specific groups as well as the delivery of healthcare. They include a broad range of subtopics surrounding issues such as vaccination, infectious disease, nutrition and obesity, public health, occupational hazards, and environmental dangers. The goal of these studies is often to provide the hard evidence needed to promote change or improvement in current government policies and practices in order to promote individual, national, and global health. The Institute of Medicine frequently advises Congress on various health topics of immense importance in addition to releasing reports of their findings that are accessible to the general public as well as medical providers and professionals.

The Institute of Medicine holds a yearly meeting where the current president of the IOM gives an address on current, important health issues. This meeting is also published in a formal report with supplemental, pertinent information yearly. In addition, every two years the IOM releases a publication titled Informing the Future, which provides information about the Institute's recent work, how to access it, and the role they play in healthcare delivery and policy.
>   *—Geraldine Marrocco and Carly Stabb*

For Further Information:
Institute of Medicine of the National Academies. "About the IOM." Retrieved from http://www.iom.edu/About-IOM.aspx
Institute of Medicine of the National Academies. "Reports Index." Retrieved from http://www.iom.edu/Reports.aspx

INTENSIVE CARE. *See* **CRITICAL CARE.**

INTENSIVE CARE UNIT (ICU)
Health care system
Definition: A clinical area staffed by a team of highly skilled health care professionals trained to provide total care to patients with severe, life-threatening illnesses or injuries through continuous monitoring of vital signs, supportive care, and intensive medical treatments and therapies.
Key terms:
blood pressure: the amount of force from the blood pushing on artery walls
cardiac: related to the heart
critical care: a multiprofessional health care specialty that cares for patients with severe, life-threatening illness and injury
extubation: removal of a breathing tube
intubation: placement of a breathing tube, most often in the mouth and down the throat
postoperative: referring to the period of time following a surgical procedure
pulmonary: related to the lungs and breathing
sedation: the use of medication to calm patients who are agitated or anxious, to relieve pain, or to relax patients experiencing discomfort from a device being used to support their care (for example, the breathing tube inserted down the throat)

Organization and Types of Units
Critical care is a field of medicine that supports patients with complex and critical medical conditions. This essay provides a description of the structure and staffing of intensive care units (ICUs), and some of the important devices and methods they use to support patients. It is not a comprehensive description of every treatment and therapy used in the ICU.

ICUs are organized in various ways depending on the size, resources, and community needs for a given hospital. Large academic medical centers or teaching hospitals most often have multiple units and cluster specific patient populations on a unit. For example, adult patients undergoing a surgical procedure are admitted to the same unit, while adult patients suffering severe trauma are admitted to a different unit. Large hospitals with multiple ICUs are usually located in densely populated areas, such as an urban or metropolitan area. The other extreme is the small community hospital in a rural area that has multiple beds on a clinical unit that are dedicated for intensive care use.

Intensive care units are organized by clinical specialty and the type of services and treatments needed for that population of patients. The most common type is a combined medical, surgical, and respiratory ICU. Surgical ICUs (SICU) care for postoperative patients, medical ICUs manage patients requiring medical care for one or multiple critical illnesses (for example, pneumonia or a poisoning), and respiratory ICUs manage patients with severe breathing problems. Cardiac ICUs, sometimes called coronary care units (CCUs), provide intensive heart monitoring and treatments for patients with heart problems. Some hospitals will have a cardiac-surgical

ICU that is separate from the CCU and SICU, where patients are admitted following a cardiac operation, such as coronary artery bypass graft surgery. Trauma ICUs manage patients who were severely injured from a gunshot or stabbing wound, a car accident, a fall, or burns. Neurologic ICUs help patients recover from a stroke or spinal cord or brain injury. Most of these ICUs treat adult patients. Children who require critical care are usually admitted to a pediatric ICU or a neonatal ICU (NICU). The pediatric ICU cares for patients from birth until eighteen or nineteen years of age, and neonatal units care for newborns in their first twenty-eight days of life.

Most ICUs have a nurse manager to oversee the nursing staff and a physician director who sets policies, develops protocols, and communicates with patients, their primary care physicians and family members, and other specialists. An ICU either has full-time intensivist physicians who act as the primary care physicians and fully manage each patient (sometimes called a closed ICU) or brings in intensivists to consult on a patient's care (sometimes called an open ICU). The physician in charge (often called the attending) manages the patients and coordinates their medical care with other health care professionals on and off the unit and outside the hospital. Patients are admitted from the emergency room or other inpatient unit in the hospital or from another facility such as a nursing home.

One activity performed to deliver the best care possible is daily patient rounds, in which a critical care team visits each patient. Rounds are usually done early in the morning, and in some units teams may revisit patients in the evening. During rounds, the team discusses each patient's current medical condition and decides what treatments or therapies are needed for the day. The health care professionals performing rounds will vary but always include the attending physician. In teaching hospitals, fellows training to be critical care physicians, residents assigned for a one- or several-month ICU rotation, and medical students from the affiliated medical school will perform rounds with the attending. In some cases, the team is interdisciplinary (multiple clinical disciplines working together), and nurses, pharmacists, respiratory therapists, and others providing medical care to the patients will join rounds.

Staff

Intensive care units are staffed by professionals who are highly trained in a certain clinical discipline (type of job). These individuals work together on the unit as a critical care team to provide total and continuous care to patients. The critical care team on a unit includes intensivists, critical care nurses, a pharmacist, a registered dietitian, a social worker, a respiratory therapist, a physical or occupational therapist, physician assistants, nurse practitioners, a hospital chaplain, and child-life specialists.

Intensivists are board-certified or board-eligible in a medical specialty (for example, surgery or pediatrics). They have additional training, education, and certification to know every organ sys-

An electronic display of a patient's vital signs in an ICU. (©Goran Bogicevic/Dreamstime.com)

tem in the body and how treatments, procedures, and medications may affect critically ill patients.

Critical care nurses are trained to monitor and manage the needs of acutely and critically ill patients. For example, they clean and monitor open wounds and ventilators to prevent patients from developing infections. Moreover, a nurse can receive additional education and training to become certified as a critical care registered nurse (CCRN).

Pharmacists are trained and board-certified or board-eligible in the appropriate and safe use of medications. They also can choose to undertake additional training to understand the specific problems and needs of critical care patients.

Respiratory therapists monitor and manage a patient's breathing using a variety of methods and devices, such as oxygen therapy or mechanical ventilation. Physical therapists work with patients to restore or improve mobility, relieve pain, and limit or prevent physical disability. Occupational therapists assess the impact of the disease or injury on the patients" ability to function at home, at work, and during physical activity after hospital discharge.

Physician assistants and nurse practitioners are licensed with advanced critical care training and work directly under the intensivist. They assist the intensivist, for example, by performing physical exams and procedures, diagnosing and treating illnesses, writing orders, and talking with patients and families. Child-life specialists are licensed professionals who provide play therapy to help children recover from an illness and therapies to distract them during painful procedures. The hospital chaplain offers pastoral support to patients, family members, and staff.

Supportive Care

A wide array of devices, equipment, and medications are used in the ICU to provide supportive care to patients recovering from life-threatening illnesses or injuries. Thus, it is one of the most complex clinical areas in the hospital. In an ICU, lines, tubes, drains, and other devices are attached to or inserted into patients. Any one patient may have as many as fourteen of these different-sized tubes attached in some way to the body. All patients will have heart monitor leads attached to the chest area to monitor the electrical activity of the heart and a pulse oximeter that typically clasps onto a finger to monitor oxygen levels in the blood and pulse rate. Patients may also have a cuff on the arm for periodic blood pressure monitoring and a peripheral IV inserted in a vein on the top of the hand to give fluids or medications. A patient may need a Foley catheter inserted up to the bladder to collect urine or a dialysis catheter inserted in the groin area and attached to a machine to assist the kidneys in cleaning the blood. Other small, tube-like catheters include central line/pulmonary artery (PA) catheters inserted in the neck to monitor blood flow or give medications or life-sustaining nutrition, an arterial line inserted in an artery at the wrist to monitor blood pressure, or an intracranial pressure catheter inserted in the brain to monitor its swelling.

A patient may need assistance breathing. In this case, either an endotracheal tube is inserted in the mouth or a tracheostomy tube is inserted in the neck and attached to a machine (a process called mechanical ventilation) to regulate the patient's breathing and provide the appropriate mix of oxygen and gas. A tracheostomy tube is used only if the patient will need mechanical ventilation for a prolonged period. Chest tubes are inserted under the skin around the rib cage area to remove escaped air or drain blood from the space around the lungs. This type of drainage tube is also used in other areas of the body to remove fluids or blood from a wound. A nasogastric tube inserted through the nose and down into the stomach can remove acid or other unwanted fluids or can supply nutrition. An intra-aortic balloon pump inserted into the groin helps the heart pump blood through the body.

Several emergency procedures can be performed in the ICU to revive a patient who has stopped breathing or is experiencing cardiac arrest. Cardiopulmonary resuscitation (CPR) is a series of things done to open the patient's airway (tilting the chin up, opening the mouth, holding down the tongue), help with breathing (blowing air into the mouth), and help pump blood from the heart into the body (chest compressions). Sometimes manual resuscitation will be done. In this case, a face mask is placed over the patient's mouth or a breathing tube inserted down the throat, and a plastic bag is attached and manually squeezed by the doctor, nurse, or respiratory therapist to fill the lungs with oxygen. Manual resuscitation is a short-term solution for a breathing problem. A patient who continues to require breathing support will be placed on a mechanical ventilator. A patient experiencing cardiac arrest will be defibrillated by placing two paddles attached to a defibrillator on the chest to send an electrical shock through the heart in an attempt to restart the heart's natural rhythm. This procedure may have to be done more than once to convert the heart back to its natural rhythm.

Perspective and Prospects

Intensive care units are relatively new considering the practice of medicine dates to about 4000 BCE, during ancient Egyptian times. The history of intensive care began in the late 1920s when W. E. Dandy opened a three-bed unit for patients following neurosurgery at Johns Hopkins Hospital in Baltimore. About the same time, in 1927, Sarah Morris Hospital in Chicago opened the first center to care for infants born prematurely. The devastation of World War II prompted the creation of wards to resuscitate and care for severely injured soldiers, and afterward, recovery rooms were opened to group postoperative patients together to compensate for a nursing shortage. By 1960, postoperative recovery rooms were in every hospital. Another catastrophic event that contributed to intensive care was the polio epidemic in 1947–48. To compensate for the development of respiratory paralysis and death from polio, doctors in Denmark developed mechanical ventilation therapy to keep patients breathing during this illness. The benefits of this therapy prompted the opening of respiratory ICUs in the 1950s. Then, in 1958, Baltimore City Hospital (now Johns Hopkins Bayview Medical Center) opened the first multidisciplinary ICU in the United States.

By the late 1960s, most US hospitals had at least one ICU, and in the late 1990s there were about six thousand ICUs.

—*Christine G. Holzmueller*

See also Accidents; Blood pressure; Cardiopulmonary resuscitation (CPR); Choking; Coma; Critical care; Critical care, pediatric; Death and dying; Disease; Drowning; Electrocardiography (ECG or EKG); Electroencephalography (EEG); Emergency medicine; Emergency medicine, pediatric; Emergency rooms; First aid; Hospitals; Hyperbaric oxygen therapy; Nursing; Paramedics; Poisoning; Respiration; Resuscitation; Surgery, general; Tracheostomy; Unconsciousness; Wounds.

For Further Information:

American Thoracic Society. "A Primer on Critical Care for Patients and Their Families." *American Thoracic Society*, 2013.

Bongard, Frederick, and Darryl Y. Sue, eds. *Current Critical Care Diagnosis and Treatment*. 3d ed. New York: McGraw-Hill Medical, 2008.

ICU-USA. *ICU-USA*, 1999–2013.

Landrum, Michele Angell. *Fast Facts for the Critical Care Nurse: Critical Care Nursing in a Nutshell*. New York: Springer Pub. Co., 2012.

LeClaire, Sophie E. *Intensive Care Units: Stress, Procedures and Mortality Rates*. New York: Nova Science, 2010.

MedlinePlus. "Critical Care." *MedlinePlus*, August 6, 2013.

Melia, Kath M. *Health Care Ethics: Lessons from Intensive Care*. London: Sage Publications, 2004.

Murray, John F. *Intensive Care: A Doctor's Journal*. Berkeley: University of California Press, 2000.

Occupational Safety & Health Administration. "Intensive Care Unit (ICU)." *Occupational Safety & Health Administration*, n.d.

Page, Karen. *Nursing the Acutely Ill Adult: Case Book*. Buckingham: Open University, 2012.

Singer, Mervyn, and Andrew Webb. *Oxford Handbook of Critical Care*. 3d ed. Oxford: Oxford University Press, 2009.

Society of Critical Care Medicine (SCCM). "About Critical Care." *My ICU Care*, 2001–2013.

Society of Critical Care Medicine (SCCM). "Critical Care Statistics." *Society of Critical Care Medicine*, 2001–2013.

Torpy, Janet M., Lynn Cassio, and Richard M. Glass. "Intensive Care Units." *JAMA The Journal of the American Medical Association*, March 25, 2009.

Vincent, J. L. *Textbook of Critical Care*. 6th ed. Philadelphia: Elsevier/Saunders, 2011.

INTERNAL MEDICINE

Specialty

Anatomy or system affected: Abdomen, bladder, gallbladder, gastrointestinal system, glands, heart, intestines, kidneys, liver, lungs, pancreas, reproductive system, respiratory system, spleen, stomach, urinary system, uterus

Specialties and related fields: Cardiology, endocrinology, gastroenterology, gynecology, nephrology, proctology, pulmonary medicine

Definition: The field of medicine concerned with the diagnosis and treatment of disease of the body's inner organs and structures, usually including surgery on these organs.

Key terms:

acute: referring to a short-term disease process

cellular biology: the study of the processes that take place within a cell

chronic: referring to a long-term disease process

inflammation: redness, pain, and heat resulting from trauma or infection; often the first step in the body's self-healing process

molecular biology: study of the interactions that occur among the molecules that make up living organisms

pathogen: any microorganism that can cause disease, including bacteria, viruses, fungi, yeasts, and parasites

trauma: physical injury to bodily tissue

Science and Profession

Internists, or practitioners of internal medicine, are skilled in the diagnosis and treatment of disease conditions that can occur virtually anywhere within the human body. They must be expert in human biology and anatomy and in pathophysiology (that is, the study of the processes that lead to disease conditions). By its nature, internal medicine embraces many other medical specialties, such as cardiology and gastroenterology. In fact, many internists become certified in related specialties.

The original model for the modern internist was Sir William Osler (1849–1919), a Canadian physician who practiced in the United States for much of his life. Osler was deeply beloved and respected for his compassion and humanity as well as his extraordinary skills in anatomy and diagnosis and in effecting cures for his patients. In his long career as physician and teacher of medicine, Osler formulated many of the guiding principles in the practice of internal medicine.

Knowledge of many scientific disciplines is required of internists. They must understand the physical and biological bases of disease. This involves knowledge of genetics, cellular biology, immunology, and the activities and nature of the various microorganisms that cause disease, such as bacteria, viruses, fungi, yeasts, and parasites.

Internists must understand the components and roles of each type of cell in the human body and know how the cell functions. Human cells are not simple entities, but complex miniature organisms with many activities going on simultaneously, particularly metabolic processes. Just as important, internists must understand what happens within and outside the cell in the disease process. For example, they must know how individual bacteria cause infection and how viruses invade cells, use them for their replication, and then destroy them. Internal medicine involves all the body's organ systems and structures, such as the heart and circulatory system, the gastrointestinal system, the genitourinary system, the respiratory system, the skin, the brain, and the skeletal system.

Internists must also be able to examine patients and diagnose the presence or absence of disease. This process involves a wide variety of techniques and procedures. It usually begins with an introductory interview, followed by physical examination of the patient. Pain is the most common symptom of disease, and manifestation of it is investigated thoroughly.

Diagnostic and Treatment Techniques

Internists understand the intricate pathways of pain throughout the body and know that proper explanation of a pain will often lead directly or indirectly to a correct diagnosis of the underlying disorder. Much of the diagnostic skill of the internist, however, is in the understanding that pain may be ambiguous. Headache can point to the possibility of many disorders, ranging from sinusitis to severe pathologies within the brain. Pain in the chest can be caused by upper respiratory tract infection or heart disease. Pain in the limbs and/or joints may indicate physical trauma as a result of accidents or overexercising, or it may be attributable to arthritic or rheumatic disease or other causes. Abdominal pain can be present in literally dozens of different conditions. Similarly, back and neck pain can be caused simply by physical exertion or may point to a serious underlying disease.

Blood pressure and pulse are checked in the physical examination, and the doctor listens to heart and chest sounds through a stethoscope. The ears, mouth, and nose are examined. Body temperature is an important diagnostic consideration. Excess body heat or fever often accompanies infection and may also be present in other disease conditions. The doctor also checks for enlargement of lymph nodes and other signs that might suggest infection or other disorders.

Blood or urine samples are often taken for laboratory analysis. The internist will specify the tests he or she wants in the laboratory workup. These will include standard assays to give the internist a general picture of the patient's health and may include special tests for individual functions that the doctor may suspect are impaired.

Changes in the function of different body systems can lead the physician through the process of diagnosis. For example, such symptoms as dizziness; fainting; numbness; vision, speech, or hearing disturbances; or coma may be caused by dysfunction of the nervous system or may point to heart disease or other disorder. Abnormalities in respiratory function have specific meaning to the internist and may lead to a diagnosis ranging from a common cold to a more serious respiratory disease or a disease of other organs, such as the heart. Alterations in the skin may indicate a dermatological disorder or may suggest some internal condition.

Sometimes, a diagnosis is easy to make: The presenting symptoms are obvious signs of a specific disease. Sometimes, a group of symptoms, called a syndrome, may be ambiguous and could be related to any of a number of conditions. If the exact nature of a disease or its cause is uncertain, the internist will conduct a differential diagnosis in which possible causes of the disease are investigated in order to eliminate those that are not candidates and to pinpoint the actual cause.

Internists treat a wide variety of disorders. Among the most significant are the infectious diseases. They must study the pathogenesis (from *pathos*, meaning "disease," and *genesis*, meaning "origin" or "source") of infectious diseases in order to know how to diagnose and treat them. Harmful bacteria cause disease in different ways, but all damage and destroy body cells and tissue. Some cause infection at the point where they enter the body, such as at the site of a wound, or in the respiratory tract when they are breathed into the body. Sometimes, bacteria are carried from their site of entry to other parts of the body, where they colonize and cause infection.

The range of bacterial infections is enormous, but one thing that they often have in common is inflammation. Inflammation is the beginning of the immune process by which the body defends itself against invading pathogens. It starts when the body recognizes that the invading organism is a foreign entity by detecting foreign antigens (substances on the surfaces of invading organisms such as bacteria and viruses). The body then releases certain white blood cells, called leukocytes, that are specific for producing antibodies that can destroy the organism. Once the body has identified a foreign organism and created antibodies for it, the immune system will retain a memory of the organism and destroy it whenever it enters the body again.

When confronted with bacterial infection, internists may recognize the organism that causes it from the patient's symptoms, or they may have to take specimens from the site of inflammation and test them in order to identify the organism involved. Sometimes, the organism is identified by microscopic examination, often using a dye that stains certain bacteria. Sometimes, it is necessary to grow the organism in a culture medium in order to identify it. The organism may also be identified by its antigen or by the type of antibody that the immune system produces to fight it.

The signs of viral infection are often exactly the same as those of bacterial infection. The main difference is that the causative organism cannot be isolated and identified as easily. Unlike bacteria, viruses cannot be seen through a microscope or otherwise identified by many of the methods used for bacteria. They can be cultured, however, or antigens or antibodies may be detectable.

In addition to treating infectious diseases, internists are called on to treat dysfunction in all parts of the body. They treat many patients suffering from heart disease, the major killer of Americans. The heart is actually subject to a wide range of disorders, the most common and the most deadly of which is coronary artery disease. Internists have many means of diagnosing heart diseases and, often, predicting them. The patient's presenting symptoms and an analysis of the patient's lifestyle will often suggest the possibility of heart disease. Various in-office and laboratory procedures will inform the internist of the precise status of the patient's heart function and help direct the course of therapy.

Cancer, the second most common cause of mortality in the United States, is often seen by internists. Lung cancer is the leading cause of cancer death, followed by cancer of the colon or rectum, breast, prostate gland, urinary tract, and uterus. The lymph system, blood, mouth, pancreas, skin, stomach, and ovary are also common sites. The term *cancer* describes a large number of disorders. What all cancers have in common is that the cells of an organ multiply uncontrollably. As the cancer cells proliferate, they crowd out other cells and interfere with organ function. Sometimes cancer cells from one organ spread to neighboring organs or are carried to other parts of the body. This process is called metastasis, and it can indicate that the cancer has spread or is spreading throughout the body. Internists may be responsible for treating cancer patients throughout the disease process or may refer them to oncologists, or cancer specialists.

Diseases of the respiratory system are major concerns of the internist. In addition to bacterial and viral infections, there are many acute and chronic respiratory conditions. One major example is asthma. Its cause is unknown, but it is believed to be at least partially attributable to allergy. When an asthma attack occurs, airways in the lungs swell and constrict. Mucus builds up and airflow is restricted, causing the patient to wheeze and gasp for air. Many internists have become skilled in helping asthmatic patients, alleviating symptoms, and preventing attacks.

All parts of the body harbor the potential for disease, infectious and otherwise. They are all, to some degree, the province of internists. The kidneys and the urinary system, the gastrointestinal system, the immune system, the endocrine glands, the brain and the nervous system, and the skeletal system are all within the internist's broad purview. Often disorders in these various organs and systems can be treated fully by internists. When they believe that a patient needs a physician with greater knowledge in a particular area of medicine, however, internists will refer the patient to an appropriate specialist.

In addition to their diagnostic skills, internists must possess a wide knowledge of modern treatment modalities. Surgery is rarely among the procedures mastered by the internist, so surgical procedures are routinely referred to surgeons specializing in the particular techniques involved.

Primary among the internist's tools for fighting infectious diseases are the antibiotics. These are the mainstays of therapy for infections caused by bacteria and other nonviral microorganisms. Since the first antibiotics were developed in the 1930s and 1940s, literally hundreds more have been developed. Scores of these are in use, and new agents are constantly being introduced.

It is vital for internists to keep abreast of new antibiotics because disease-causing organisms are often able to develop resistance against antibiotic agents that have been in use for a long time. For example, many strains of bacteria that were susceptible to penicillin have developed the ability to counteract its antibiotic effect. Other agents had to be found to destroy these resistant strains. This phenomenon occurs across virtually the entire range of the available antibiotics: prolonged use of a given agent often allows the target organism to develop resistance to it. Internists must also be skilled in the proper use of antibiotics. Knowing which agent or combination of agents to prescribe, in what amounts, and for how long are important considerations in developing the patient's treatment plan. Antibiotics are not useful for treating viral infections, but there are a limited number of antiviral agents available for treating certain diseases.

Immunization against infectious diseases can be an important concern of the internist. The most extensive immuniza-tion programs in the United States are directed toward the vaccination of children and thus are generally carried out by pediatricians and family practitioners. Internists are often responsible, however, for the immunization of adult patients. Immunization against influenza is recommended for the elderly, particularly when a new strain of influenza virus arises. It is also recommended that elderly hospitalized patients be vaccinated against pneumococcal pneumonia. Internists are a primary avenue of immunization against hepatitis B, particularly among high-risk target populations, such as medical personnel, intravenous drug abusers, and adult male homosexuals. Internists are also involved in immunizing patients who require special vaccinations because of exposure to disease or for travel to foreign countries.

Patients who require long-term or lifelong therapy for noninfectious diseases include individuals with heart diseases, high blood pressure, diabetes, cancer, respiratory disorders, and a host of other conditions. The challenge to the internist is to develop a regimen that is both efficacious and safe. Drug therapy is prominent in the internist's treatment armamentarium. In either short-term or long-term drug therapy, problems may arise. The patient may develop significant side effects or adverse reactions. The drug may lose its effectiveness after months or years of therapy. The condition may change and require dosage adjustments, additional medications, or a complete change of regimen.

Consistent monitoring of the patient's condition is an important part of therapy. The internist wants to ensure that the prescribed regimen is working and that the therapy is comfortable for the patient. For example, the earliest agents for high blood pressure, or hypertension, often had such disagreeable side effects that patients would stop taking them. Hypertension has virtually no symptoms. After the patient started taking medication, however, he or she could experience loss of energy, listlessness, impotence, dream disturbances, and many other unwelcome effects. Similarly, diabetes patients who are dependent on regular insulin injections sometimes neglect their therapy. They may balk against sticking themselves with needles three or four times a day, and they may not monitor their blood sugar adequately. Preventing the devastating and potentially fatal consequences of diabetes depends on rigorous compliance with all aspects of the diabetes regimen, including diet, insulin, and monitoring.

Thus, patient compliance with therapy becomes one of the major tasks of the internist and virtually any other physician: If the patient does not cooperate with the regimen that the doctor prescribes, the therapy is not likely to be effective. For this reason, many internists now make patient counseling part of their practice. The modern internist recognizes that patients must understand their therapeutic goals, why they are being given certain medicines, and what these drugs can be expected to accomplish. Furthermore, many internists find that it is wise to alert their patients to possible adverse reactions, although they understand the necessity of not frightening the patient. Some internists find the time to discuss their therapeutic regimens thoroughly with their patients. Others use nursing staff or other health care workers to educate patients.

Treatment modalities change constantly, and internists are required to be aware of the latest advances in order to modify their therapy programs to take advantage of improvements in drugs or procedures. Not only are new drugs constantly being approved for use, but modern medical science is continually learning new facts about old diseases as well, and these new insights often radically alter the way a given disease is treated. A good example is a stomach ulcer. For years, it was thought that certain ulcers in the stomach were caused by erosion of the stomach wall by gastric juices. A group of investigators found, however, that a significant number of ulcer patients were also infected with the bacterium *Helicobacter pylori*. It has been suggested that infection may play a role in the development of these ulcers and that, therefore, therapy should be amended to include an antibacterial agent that is effective against *H. pylori*.

Furthermore, the internist's patient load is changing. Most internal medicine practices are treating increasing numbers of elderly patients, who have special needs. Internists must be aware of the constant advances in geriatric medicine in order to modify therapy for older patients.

Perspective and Prospects

In the last decades of the twentieth century, internal medicine became somewhat fragmented as more and more physicians elected to practice in narrower specialties, such as cardiology, gastroenterology, hematology, or oncology, among many others. Specialties are still very much needed, but the practice of medicine seems to be headed back to the broader range of the internist.

As in the past, internists are at the forefront of progress in treatment. Recent generations have seen a far-reaching revolution in an understanding of the basic chemistry of life. As scientists elucidate the activities that occur at the molecular level of physical processes, insights are gained into exactly how the body works, as well as how antagonistic pathogens function. From this knowledge, new treatments have been devised for managing disease states.

A good example is the treatment of hypertension, one of the most common conditions seen by internists. Years ago, the only medications for high blood pressure were sedatives and diuretics. It was not fully understood exactly what occurred at the cellular and molecular level that caused vasoconstriction, which is the main physical characteristic of hypertension. Researchers discovered complex biochemical activities that contributed to vasoconstriction and other aspects of high blood pressure. They were then able to develop agents that could treat the condition more effectively than anything available before. Internists now have a wealth of antihypertensive agents with which to work. Some reduce blood pressure by reducing heart activity, some dilate blood vessels by direct action, and some interfere with the biochemical processes that cause vasoconstriction. In addition, most of the agents that internists and other physicians use for hypertension cause many fewer side effects and adverse reactions than their predecessors.

In the fight against infectious diseases, new research is combining genetics with molecular biology to elucidate the exact biochemical processes by which pathogenic organisms invade and damage body cells and tissues. This research is having an enormous impact on the understanding of bacteria and viruses: how they work, how they mutate, and, perhaps most important, in what ways they are vulnerable. With increased knowledge comes increased capability to design more efficient antibiotics and to find agents that will inhibit the pathogen's ability to develop resistant strains. Internists are among the leaders in the application of these technologies. Because they see such a wide range of disease conditions, internists often function as the main channel by which new medications and treatments reach the patient.

—*C. Richard Falcon*

See also Abdomen; Abdominal disorders; Angina; Arrhythmias; Arteriosclerosis; Bacterial infections; Beriberi; Bladder cancer; Bleeding; Bronchitis; Candidiasis; Cardiac arrest; Cardiology; Cardiology, pediatric; Cholecystitis; Cirrhosis; Colitis; Colon; Colonoscopy and sigmoidoscopy; Constipation; Coughing; Crohn's disease; Diabetes mellitus; Dialysis; Diarrhea and dysentery; Digestion; Diverticulitis and diverticulosis; *E. coli* infection; Emphysema; Endocarditis; Endoscopy; Gallbladder; Gallbladder cancer; Gallbladder diseases; Gangrene; Gastroenterology; Gastroenterology, pediatric; Gastrointestinal disorders; Gastrointestinal system; Glands; Guillain-Barré syndrome; Gynecology; Heart; Heart attack; Heart disease; Heart failure; Heartburn; Hepatitis; Hernia; Incontinence; Indigestion; Influenza; Intestinal disorders; Intestines; Ischemia; Kidney cancer; Kidney disorders; Kidneys; Legionnaires' disease; Leprosy; Liver; Liver disorders; Lungs; Mitral valve prolapse; Multiple sclerosis; Nephritis; Nephrology; Nephrology, pediatric; Nonalcoholic steatohepatitis (NASH); Palpitations; Pancreas; Pancreatitis; Parasitic diseases; Peristalsis; Peritonitis; Pneumonia; Proctology; Pulmonary medicine; Pulmonary medicine, pediatric; Rectum; Renal failure; Reproductive system; Reye's syndrome; Rheumatic fever; Rheumatoid arthritis; Roundworms; Scarlet fever; Schistosomiasis; Small intestine; Staphylococcal infections; Stone removal; Stones; Streptococcal infections; Tapeworms; Tumor removal; Tumors; Ulcer surgery; Ulcers; Urinary system; Urology; Urology, pediatric; Viral infections; Whooping cough; Worms.

For Further Information:

American College of Physicians. "About Internal Medicine." *ACP American College of Physicians*, 2013.

Bureau of Labor Statistics, US Department of Labor. "Physicians and Surgeons." *Occupational Outlook Handbook*, March 29, 2012.

Frank, Steven A. *Immunology and Evolution of Infectious Disease.* Princeton, N.J.: Princeton University Press, 2002.

Hing, Esther, and Susan M. Schappert. "NCHS Data Brief: Generalist and Specialty Physicians: Supply and Access, 2009–2010." *Centers for Disease Control and Prevention*, September 2012.

Kasper, Dennis L., et al., eds. *Harrison's Principles of Internal Medicine.* 18th ed. New York: McGraw-Hill Health Professions Division, 2012.

Kiple, Kenneth F., ed. *The Cambridge World History of Human Disease.* Cambridge: Cambridge University Press, 2008.

Litin, Scott C., ed. *Mayo Clinic Family Health Book.* 4th ed. New York: HarperResource, 2009.

Mullan, Fitzhugh. *Big Doctoring in America: Profiles in Primary Care.* Berkeley: University of California Press, 2002.

Torpy, Janet M., Alison E. Burke, and Richard M. Glass. "Medical Specialties." *JAMA: The Journal of the American Medical Association*, September 5, 2007.

Wagman, Richard J., ed. *The New Complete Medical and Health Encyclopedia.* 4 vols. Chicago: Standard Educational Corp., 2005

INTERNET MEDICINE

Specialty

Also known as: E-medicine

Anatomy or system affected: All

Specialties and related fields: All

Definition: The use of Web-based and other electronic long-distance communication technologies for health information, assessment, service delivery, training, and public health administration.

Key terms:

anonymous: of unknown authorship, unidentified by a singular identity

assessment: a thorough physical and/or psychiatric examination; a process of systematically collecting comprehensive information about health care behavior, physical and psychiatric conditions, and general well-being for the purpose of diagnosis or treatment planning

clinical trials: scientifically based research examinations of new treatment procedures, techniques, devices, or pharmaceuticals that are considered state of the art in the treatment of diseases and other medical disorders

confidential: a situation distinguished by the willing disclosure of intimate information because of assurances that the information will be protected from general distribution or unauthorized disclosure; information which, if disclosed, has the potential to be damaging or dangerous to the patient's reputation, status, or associates

diagnosis: a process of distinguishing knowledge about symptoms and problems that leads to the rendering of conclusions about physical and psychiatric illness; a label used to communicate specific health information among professionals, researchers, health systems, and insurance providers; a label that informs the process of treatment

Internet: a worldwide electronic system connecting individual computer users, computer networks, Web sites, and computer facilities for business, government, organizational, and private purposes

privacy: the state of being free from unwanted or unauthorized observation or other intrusion

professional licensing: state-granted privileges to health care and other professionals allowing them to deliver services or to participate in certain activities; a privilege that is revokable and subject to censure; a privilege usually granted only after thorough examination of the skill and practice of a person seeking licensure

profiling: the collection of data to summarily categorize and track the behavior of individual users or types of users, through electronic or other tracking systems, to learn more about their behavior, usually for the purpose of prediction, done either with or without the knowledge or consent of the user

screening: a triage process; a process of asking a few questions of an individual, as opposed to an assessment, in order to determine whether there is sufficient risk of a problematic condition being present to justify completing a detailed evaluation or, instead, to justify assigning that individual to a category of lesser or no risk

Web site: a location on the Internet that has an individual address and that presents information, usually in the form of individual pages, or Web pages, that the owner of the Web site wishes to make available to Internet users

Science and Profession

The Internet is a computer-based tool that is facilitating communication among vast numbers of individuals, groups, businesses, and governments. In addition to facilitating purely social and business-related ventures, the Internet is proving to be a valuable tool for improving the state of public health. This is because a new type of medical care and medical services has developed. These services, typically called telehealth, telemedicine, and e-medicine, use the Internet as a key tool in their dispensation, organization, and evaluation of health care services. Such services have taken the form of a variety of health care-related websites that provide services once available only through a face-to-face visit with a doctor or other health or social services professional. The websites are valuable in that they provide almost instantaneous information and other communications assistance to patients, their families, treatment professionals, trainers, trainees in the health care and social service professions, and medical researchers.

In terms of assisting patients, Internet-based medical approaches provide a variety of services to individual Internet users. First, they provide a wealth of information on different symptoms and medical conditions. They also allow for screening of such conditions to see if they warrant further attention from medical professionals and advice on how to handle minor health ailments and medical emergencies. They also help consumers to find medical advice, health care providers, self-help or support groups, and therapy over the Internet, all of which may or may not be supervised by medical professionals. Finally, they can give patients and their families information on different treatment options, including common procedures, the latest in alternative medicine, and even current clinical trials information.

Internet medicine can also be very helpful for family members of individuals having medical problems. Often, family members do not know how best to help their significant others in times of medical need. To meet this need, websites may post a wide variety of information that can help people understand the conditions, the requirements of treatment, the limits of treatment, and things they can do to be helpful to the ill family member. Additionally, websites sometimes offer lists of resources for family members.

Health care and social service providers also find the Internet beneficial for their work. For some, it might be as simple as using the Internet to schedule appointments, or to communicate test results, reminder information about treatment procedures, or appointment reminders via e-mail with clients. For others, it might involve using special websites to conduct assessments of clients for the purpose of tracking their treatment success or progress. Professionals may also use telemedicine in order to learn about new treatments and

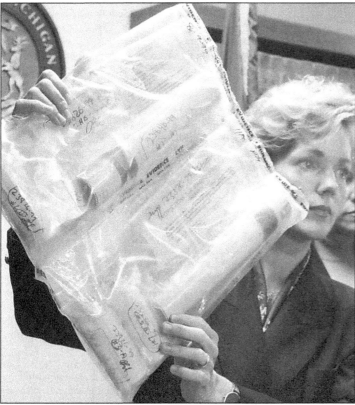

One disadvantage of the Internet is the ease with which illegal or dangerous substances, such as this home manufacturing kit for "date rape" drug gamma hydroxybutrate (GHB), can be distributed. (AP/Wide World Photos)

procedures, or to learn about new drugs and other pharmaceutical products. In addition, health care and social service providers may benefit their general practice by using the Internet to keep abreast of new clinical trials to test state-of-the-art treatments, changes in licensing laws affecting their practice, and the development of new health care databases for tracking, triage, and communication with insurance companies. Finally, some providers are actually using the Internet for health services delivery.

Health care providers in training and their trainers also benefit greatly from telemedicine. To trainees living in remote areas or those who might be highly mobile, such as those in the armed forces, the Internet provides immediate access to large online libraries, knowledgeable online teachers, and databases full of important medical information. Both long-established and new institutions interested in telemedicine increasingly are translating typical face-to-face training approaches into distance-based training programs utilizing the Internet. Encyclopedias, descriptions of techniques, pictures of what different conditions might look like both inside and outside the body, and even video of actual procedures are available online. Similarly, instruction in the use of such material is available online through training programs that lead to certificates of training and actual accred-

ited degrees, ranging from bachelor's to doctoral degrees and postdoctoral training. In addition to helping individuals who are at remote locations, such material also can be used to reach a larger number of trainees than might typically be able to observe or attend such training. The increased ability to teach, show procedures, or give supervision at a distance using pictorial, written, oral, and video information greatly facilitates continuing education and improvement of general health care practice. It also helps to facilitate the evaluation of those practices and training sessions. Since all of the work takes place over the Internet, different aspects of the work can be monitored and evaluated electronically.

Much of the evaluation of this kind of information is done by researchers who are studying client, trainer, provider, or even health care system behavior and organization. This is done by evaluating information, also known as data, in individual sessions or visits to websites, as well as by examining data that are collected over time, across multiple visits. For instance, a person might first go to a website for information on a specific medical condition and then, at a later time or times, come back and look up different treatment approaches, or visit online discussion groups. What they do from time to time would be evaluated by researchers to see how individuals use the site, how long they stay on it, or what things they try searching for that may not yet be on the site. The process of watching behavior over time is called tracking. Tracking allows researchers to profile the users of websites to learn more about their behavior, usually for the purpose of predicting their behavior and response to treatment. The information gathered by creating tracking databases of what happens with Web site users can be used to improve services and to decrease long-term health care service, training, and administration costs on a continuing basis.

Because of all the data being collected on how individuals are using different websites or other Internet-based services, there has been some concern over the individual's right to privacy and the protection of the information collected. For instance, some people have been concerned that if they are searching for information related to the human immunodeficiency virus (HIV) or substance use, they might be identified as being at risk for having that condition whether they do or not. Furthermore, many individuals do not want that information linked to their identities or medical records. On one hand, they may be wishing to avoid solicitation of business from sellers of medical services or products because of their association with the condition; they do not want their personal information sold for that purpose to the providers of such products or services. On the other hand, they may also wish to maintain privacy and keep their information confidential so as to avoid having any threat to their future insurability or their ability to get health care coverage. As an example, if a health care provider such as a health maintenance organization (HMO) tracked users" information on a website and discovered, through the database, that someone who was now applying for coverage had certain medical conditions, that person might have a greater risk of being refused coverage if his or her time on the website was not completely anonymous. In sum, given these concerns, users of Internet medicine need to understand that there are differences between the terms privacy, confidentiality, and anonymity, as well as in the legal issues and protections one can exercise when using this type of medicine. Each website may be operating under different constraints, and so it is always important for users of these services to be sure they understand how the websites handle privacy. Finding out how a website protects or does not protect the privacy of its users is the only way users can determine how safe it is to reveal confidential information when they use a specific website.

Diagnostic and Treatment Techniques

One of the biggest opportunities offered by Internet medicine is that of increasing the ability of individuals to do self-screening for medical conditions to see if they need medical assistance. Likewise, the ability of service providers to do screening and assessment for a larger number of people is increased relative to what can be done in person. This is because the assessments can be administered via the computer, saving valuable provider time. Additionally, assessments can be completed online and sent to providers in advance for immediate evaluation. While it may be some time before conclusive diagnoses can be offered via online technology, such advances are not far off; the differences between online and in-person assessments are being studied.

Intervention via the Internet is also much improved because large quantities of information can be dispensed electronically, printed out by clients or their families, or distributed to large numbers of individuals. Such informational interventions can be important for facilitating proper compliance with medical prescription regimens, helping clients to avoid bad drug interactions, or providing reminders about other things needed to facilitate wellness. Informational interventions can also be used for primary prevention, or preventing problems from happening in the first place. By providing suggestions for problem prevention, much suffering could be spared and many health care dollars can be saved. This is especially true for teenagers and college-age populations, who are often savvy web users.

Treatment also takes place on the Internet via simultaneous online interactions such as in chat rooms, communicating via videoconferencing as in a normal conversation but using video cameras, and simple asynchronous e-mail between the client and the provider. Generally this type of treatment is a complement to face-to-face treatment. For instance, some HMOs use online support groups as additional treatment for

persons already receiving therapy. Others are using programs such as self-guided online courses that clients can work through to benefit their health. In general, practitioners are permitted to do this so long as they are properly licensed. This usually requires being licensed by the state in which they are practicing and/or where the client is receiving the services.

Perspective and Prospects

The Internet continues to grow on a daily basis, with an increasing number of computer owners and websites taking advantage of its capabilities. Communications technologies are also improving constantly, allowing for almost instant individual communication of written, oral, and visual information at distances and speeds that were inconceivable in the past. As a result of these developments, as well as increases in health care costs and the potential economic and health benefits provided by Internet medicine, this specialty area is here to stay. Commitments by governments to examine such developments in health care underscore this likelihood. In 1998, for example, the Health Resources and Service Administration of the United States Department of Health and Human Services established the Office for the Advancement of Telehealth. This office is devoted to advancing the use of telehealth and Internet-based medicine to facilitate improvement in the state of public health and research on public health. The ability of such approaches to provide more services with streamlined administrative procedures and decreased costs holds much promise for improving the state of public health.

—Nancy A. Piotrowski, Ph.D.

See also Allied health; Alternative medicine; Clinical trials; Education, medical; Family medicine; Health maintenance organizations (HMOs); Herbal medicine; Noninvasive tests; Nursing; Pharmacology; Pharmacy; Physical examination; Screening; Self-medication; Telemedicine.

For Further Information:

American Telemedicine Association. *American Telemedicine Association*, 2012.

Armstrong, Myrna L., ed. *Telecommunications for Health Professionals: Providing Successful Distance Education and Telehealth*. New York: Springer, 1998.

Coiera, Enrico. *Guide to Health Informatics*. 2d ed. New York: Oxford University Press, 2003.

Cullen, Rowena. *Health Information on the Internet: A Study of Providers, Quality, and Users*. Westport: Praeger, 2006.

Davis, James B., ed. *Health and Medicine on the Internet: A Comprehensive Guide to Medical Information on the World Wide Web*. 4th ed. Los Angeles: Practice Management Information, 2003.

Goldstein, Douglas E. *E-Healthcare: Harness the Power of the Internet, e-Commerce, and e-Care*. Gaithersburg, Md.: Aspen, 2000.

Hadeed, George, et al. *Telemedicine for Trauma, Emergencies, and Disaster Management*. Boston: Artech House, 2011.

Harding, Anne. "Telemedicine Improves Care for Kids Seen in Rural ERs." *MedlinePlus*, August 19, 2013.

Kinsella, Audrey. *Home Telehealth in the Twenty-first Century: A Resource Book About Improved Care Services That Work*. Kensington, Md.: Information for Tomorrow, 2003.

Maheu, Marlene, Ace Allen, and Pamela Whitten. *E-Health, Telehealth, and Telemedicine: A Guide to Startup and Success*.

San Francisco: Jossey-Bass, 2001.

McKenzie, Bruce C., ed. *Medicine and the Internet.* 3d ed. New York: Oxford University Press, 2002.

MedlinePlus. "Evaluating Internet Health Information: A Tutorial from the National Library of Medicine." *MedlinePlus*, April 19, 2012.

Mayo Clinic. "Telehealth: When Health Care Meets Cyberspace." *Mayo Clinic*, May 13, 2011.

Office for the Advancement of Telehealth. http://www .hrsa.gov/ telehealth.

Price, Joan. *Complete Idiot's Guide to Online Medical Resources.* Indianapolis, Ind.: Que, 2000.

Riva, Giuseppe, and B. K. Wiederhold. *Annual Review of Cybertherapy and Telemedicine 2012: Advanced Technologies in the Behavioral, Social and Neurosciences.* Amsterdam: IOS Press, 2012.

Society of Critical Care Medicine. "What Is Telemedicine?" *My ICU Care*, 2001–2013.

West, Darrell M., Edward Alan Miller, and the Brookings Institution. *Digital Medicine: Health Care in the Internet Era.* Washington, DC: Brookings Institution Press, 2009.

Wootton, Richard, et al. *Telehealth in the Developing World.* Ottawa: International Development Research Centre; London: Royal Society of Medicine Press, 2011.

INTERPARTNER VIOLENCE

Disease/Disorder

Also known as: Intimate partner violence

Anatomy or system affected: Psychic-emotional system, all bodily systems

Specialties and related fields: Emergency medicine, family medicine, geriatrics and gerontology, internal medicine, pediatrics, psychiatry, psychology, public health

Definition: Psychological, physical, or sexual harm from a current or former partner, which can be actual or threatened within heterosexual or homosexual partnerships.

Key terms:

Danger Assessment Tool: An instrument that helps determine the level of danger an abused woman has of being killed by her intimate partner.

mandatory reporting requirements: laws designating groups of professionals that are required to report specific types of violence, abuse, and neglect. In the U.S. these laws vary by state.

Posttraumatic Stress Disorder: A maladaptive condition resulting from exposure to events beyond the realm of normal human experience and characterized by persistent difficulties involving emotional numbing, intense fear, helplessness, horror, reexperiencing of trauma, avoidance, and arousal.

The U.S. Center for Disease Control (CDC) has developed standardized definitions for the four subcategories of interpartner violence:

- Physical is the use of physical force, possibly causing disability, injury, or death.
- Sexual includes the use of physical aggression to force a person to engage in a sex act, when a sex act is attempted or completed with a person who is unable to understand or communicate their unwillingness to be complicit in the act, and abusive sexual contact.

- Threats of physical or sexual violence are when words, gestures, or weapons are used to threaten bodily harm.
- Psychological/emotional abuse describes harm caused by acts, threats of acts, or coercive tactics, and are acts largely defined based on the victim's perception of an act being abusive.

Epidemiology

Interpartner violence affects women at a higher rate than men. It is likely that incidents are underreported, so prevalence data are estimates. In the United States, 35.6 percent of women and 28.5 percent of men report physical violence, stalking, or rape during their lifetimes. Women are more often victims of sexual violence, with 9.4 percent of women in the United States experiencing rape in their lifetimes. Nearly 17 percent of women and 8 percent of men report being victims of sexual violence other than rape during their lifetimes. On the other hand, rates of psychological abuse by an intimate partner are almost equal among genders, with 48.4 percent of men and 48.8 percent of women reporting psychological abuse in their lifetimes.

Worldwide, rates of interpartner sexual and physical violence against women were measured in a World Health Organization (WHO) multicountry study. Among 15 study sites, rates of women reporting they had experienced either sexual or physical violence in their lifetimes ranged from 15 to 71 percent. The rate of participants who reported that they experienced either form of violence in the past year ranged among sites from 4 to 53 percent.

Health Effects of Interpartner Violence

Interpartner violence may lead to direct physical harm. It has also been associated with higher rates of other physical symptoms and comorbid conditions that may persist long after the violent episode has ended. These conditions include headaches, back, musculoskeletal, or chest pain, gynecological disorders, gastrointestinal disorders, sexually transmitted infections, and respiratory infections.

Studies have found a correlation between incidence of interpartner violence and pregnancy. The effects of violence for the year prior to pregnancy have been observed to be far-reaching, and include poor physical outcomes for the mother and fetus, as well as increased risk for postpartum depression in the mother.

Victims of interpartner violence also exhibit increased levels of psychological conditions, especially posttraumatic stress disorder and major depressive disorder. Victims are also more likely to engage in negative health behaviors, such as substance abuse and high-risk sexual behaviors (Roberts, 2003). These comorbidities can equate to long-term health consequences and disability across the lifespan for those who suffer from interpartner violence.

Prevention

The approach to preventing interpartner violence is multifaceted. Prevention efforts must begin by encouraging healthy relationships and emotionally supportive environments.

Services must be readily available for victims, including healthcare, legal assistance, and mental health counseling to enable intervention and prevent reoccurrence. Healthcare providers should be trained to intervene when a victim of interpartner violence is identified. WHO and the Family Violence Prevention Fund have both outlined approaches to addressing patients who are victims of interpartner violence. First and foremost, the patient's immediate risk for danger should be assessed, followed by support and possible referral for counseling. The Danger Assessment Tool is one instrument that can be used to assess how at-risk a female patient is for being murdered by her intimate partner. Some states require clinicians to report acts of violence communicated by patients. Clinicians should be familiar with the mandatory reporting requirements in their state of practice.

—*Beth Williams*

See also: Addiction; Alcoholism; Depression; Domestic Violence; Ethics; Intoxication; Paranoia; Psychiatric disorders; Psychiatry; Psychoanalysis; Psychosis; Rape and sexual assault; Stress

For Further Information:

Bonomi, A.E., M.L. Anderson, R.J. Reid, F.P. Rivara, D. Carrell, and R.S. Thompson. "Medical and Psychosocial Diagnoses in Women with a History of Intimate Partner Violence Diagnoses in Women Abused by Intimate Partners." *Archives of Internal Medicine* 169, no. 18 (2009): 1692-1697.

Campbell, J.Q. "Danger Risk Assessment Tool." Johns Hopkins University, School of Nursing, 2004.

Devries, K.M., J.Y. Mak, L.J. Bacchus, J.C. Child, G. Falder, M. Petzold, and C.H. Watts. "Intimate Partner Violence and Incident Depressive Symptoms and Suicide Attempts: A Systematic Review of Longitudinal Studies." *PLoS Medicine* 10, no. 5 (2013): e1001439.

Garcia-Moreno, C., H.A. Jansen, M. Ellsberg, L. Heise, and C.H. Watts. "Prevalence of Intimate Partner Violence: Findings from the WHO Multi-Country Study on Women's Health and Domestic Violence." *The Lancet* 368, no. 9543 (2006): 1260-1269.

Gazmararian, J.A., S. Lazorick, A.M. Spitz, T.J. Ballard, L.E. Saltzman, and J.S. Marks. "Prevalence of Violence against Pregnant Women." *JAMA: The Journal of the American Medical Association* 275, no. 24 (1996): 1915-1920.

Ludermir, A. B., G. Lewis, S.A. Valongueiro, T.V.B. de Araújo, and R. Araya, R. "Violence against Women by Their Intimate Partner during Pregnancy and Postnatal Depression: A Prospective Cohort Study." *The Lancet* 376, no. 9744 (2010): 903-910.

Roberts, T. A., J.D. Klein, and S. Fisher. "Longitudinal Effect of Intimate Partner Abuse on High-risk Behavior among Adolescents." *Archives of Pediatrics & Adolescent Medicine* 157, no. 9 (2003): 875.

Saltzman, L.E., J.L. Fanslow, P.M. McMahon, and G.A. Shelley. *Intimate Partner Violence Surveillance: Uniform Definitions and Recommended Data Elements: Version 1.0.* Atlanta, GA: Centers for Disease Control and Prevention, National Center for Injury Prevention and Control, 2002.

Weil, Amy. "Intimate Partner Violence: Epidemiology and Health Consequences." *UpToDate,* edited by Suzanne W. Fletcher and H. Nancy Sokol.

INTERSTITIAL PULMONARY FIBROSIS (IPF)
Disease/Disorder

Also known as: Idiopathic pulmonary fibrosis, cryptogenic fibrosing alveolitis

Anatomy or system affected: Heart, lungs

Specialties and related fields: Emergency medicine, internal medicine, pulmonary medicine

Definition: An inflammatory disease that results in the scarring and fibrosis of the lung alveolar tissue (air sacs).

Causes and Symptoms

Interstitial pulmonary fibrosis (IPF) is a chronic lung disease that causes scarring of the tissue between the air sacs (interstitium). It may be the result of a variety of causes, such as occupational exposure to silica or asbestos, drugs, radiation, and diseases such as sarcoidosis or connective tissue diseases (systemic lupus erythematosus, rheumatoid arthritis). When no known cause can be ascertained, the disease is known as idiopathic pulmonary fibrosis. It affects both sexes equally, with the highest incidence between the ages of forty and sixty.

The disease is characterized by an initial inflammation of the alveoli attributable to a known or unknown injury-causing agent, followed by healing by scarring and fibrosis of the interstitium. This results in a decreased transfer of oxygen to the blood, causing symptoms of increasing shortness of breath (dyspnea) and chest pain. The symptoms of the disease appear insidiously, with the patient noticing a dry cough and increasing shortness of breath, initially on exertion and eventually at rest. As the disease progresses, the patient is unable to perform daily activities and may require long-term oxygen therapy. Clubbing of the fingers and blueness of the extremities can be observed in these patients. Death is usually the result of respiratory failure, right-sided heart failure, a blood clot (embolism) in the lungs, stroke, or heart attack.

Diagnosis of IPF is made by correlating a chest x-ray, a computed tomography (CT) chest scan, lung function tests, bronchoscopy, and a measurement of blood oxygen content. Lung biopsy and microscopic examination of the tissue is the only confirmatory test that would also show the extent of damage and help determine the prognosis of the disease.

Treatment and Therapy

Treatment must be initiated as soon as the diagnosis is made. Because of the chronic nature of the disease, most patients require lifelong treatment. Treatment modalities differ with age

---

Information on
Interstitial Pulmonary Fibrosis (IPF)

Causes: Various; may include occupational exposure to silica or asbestos, drugs, radiation, diseases (sarcoidosis, lupus erythematosus, rheumatoid arthritis)

Symptoms: Scarring of lung tissue, shortness of breath, chest pain, dry cough, clubbing of fingers, blue extremities; death may come from respiratory failure, heart failure, blood clot, stroke, heart attack

Duration: Progressive, eventually fatal

Treatments: Drugs (prednisone, cyclophosphamide), oxygen therapy, physical therapy and exercise, lung transplantation

and the stage of the disease, but all aim at reducing the inflammation and stopping the fibrosis. Drugs are the mainstay of treatment, with prednisone (a corticosteroid) and cyclophosphamide being the most commonly used ones. Oxygen therapy improves the blood oxygen level in patients with severe breathlessness, and physical therapy and exercise also help in improving muscle strength and breathing. Patients with severe fibrosis may require lung transplantation.

—*Rashmi Ramasubbaiah, M.D.,*
and Venkat Raghavan Tirumala, M.D., M.H.A.

See also Asbestos exposure; Lungs; Occupational health; Oxygen therapy; Pulmonary diseases; Pulmonary medicine; Respiration; Rheumatoid arthritis; Systemic lupus erythematosus (SLE).

For Further Information:

Kasper, Dennis L., et al., eds. *Harrison's Principles of Internal Medicine.* 18th ed. New York: McGraw-Hill, 2012.

Lynch, Joseph, ed. *Idiopathic Pulmonary Fibrosis.* New York: Marcel Dekker, 2004.

Parker, James N., and Philip M. Parker, eds. *The Official Patient's Sourcebook on Idiopathic Pulmonary Fibrosis.* San Diego, Calif.: Icon Health, 2002.

"Pulmonary Fibrosis." *Mayo Clinic,* March 15, 2011.

Rosenblum, Laurie B. "Idiopathic Pulmonary Fibrosis." *Health Library,* September 1, 2011.

Simpson, John, and Ann Millar. *Advances in Pulmonary Fibrosis.* Boca Raton, Fla.: CRC Press, 2004.

"What Is Pulmonary Fibrosis?" *National Jewish Health,* February, 2010.

Intestinal cancer. *See* Stomach, intestinal, and pancreatic cancers.

Intestinal disorders

Disease/Disorder

Anatomy or system affected: Abdomen, anus, gastrointestinal system, intestines

Specialties and related fields: Family medicine, gastroenterology, internal medicine

Definition: Diseases or disorders of the small intestine, large intestine (or colon), liver, pancreas, and gallbladder.

Key terms:

acute: the stage of a disease or presence of a symptom that begins abruptly, with marked intensity, and subsides after a short time

chronic: the stage of a disease or presence of a symptom that develops slowly and usually lasts for the lifetime of the individual

diarrhea: the passage of approximately six loose stools within a twenty-four-hour period caused by a variety of circumstances, such as infection, malabsorption, or irritable bowel

diverticulitis: inflammation or swelling of one or more diverticula, caused by the penetration of fecal material through thin-walled diverticula and the collection of bacteria or other irritating agents there

diverticulosis: the presence of diverticula in the colon, which may lead to diverticulitis

diverticulum: an outpouching through the muscular wall of a tubular organ, such as the stomach, small intestine, or colon

electrolytes: elements or compounds found in blood, interstitial fluid, and cell fluid that are critical for normal metabolism and function

peristalsis: the involuntary, coordinated, rhythmic contraction of the muscles of the gastrointestinal tract that forces partially digested food along its length

stricture: an abnormal narrowing of an organ because of pressure or inflammation

villi: folds within the small intestine that are important for the absorption of nutrients into the blood

Process and Effects

Intestinal diseases and disorders are sometimes included with those of the digestive system. For the sake of clarity, this article makes the distinction between the structures of the digestive and intestinal tracts. The entire digestive tract, which includes the intestinal tract and is approximately 7.6 to 9.1 meters in length in adults, begins in the mouth and ends with the anus. It includes organs specific to digestion, such as the esophagus and stomach and their substructures. The intestinal tract, which constitutes the major part of the digestive tract, includes the small intestine, the large intestine (also known as the colon), and the organs that branch off these structures (the liver, pancreas, and gallbladder). The function of the small and large intestines is to break down food, absorb its nutrients into the bloodstream, and carry off waste products of digestion as feces.

The small intestine is approximately 6.1 meters long and 3.8 centimeters in diameter and is made up of the duodenum, the jejunum, and the ileum. It is where the process of digestion begins in full. The smaller products broken down by the stomach are received by the small intestine, where they are absorbed into the bloodstream through its lining by villi combined with bile (from the liver) and pancreatic juices.

Almost all food nutrients are absorbed in the small intestine. What passes into the large intestine is a mix of unabsorbed nutrients, water, fiber, and electrolytes. Most of the moisture from this process is removed as the mix passes through the large intestine, leaving solid waste products. Before excretion as feces, approximately 90 percent of the liquid that entered the large intestine has been reabsorbed. This reabsorption is necessary for health because the liquid contains sodium and water.

The large intestine is approximately 1.5 meters long and connected to the small intestine at the ileocecal valve. Waste products from the digestive process pass through this valve into a large holding area of the large intestine called the cecum. The appendix is attached to this structure. The large intestine consists of the ascending colon (which begins on the right side of the abdomen and moves up toward the liver), the transverse colon (which crosses the abdomen), and the descending colon (which moves down the left side of the abdomen). The sigmoid colon is an S-shaped structure that connects to the descending colon and joins the rectum, a tube 12

Information on Intestinal Disorders

Causes: Infection by bacteria or parasites, obstruction, cancer or tumor of rectum and colon, polyps

Symptoms: Vary; can include persistent diarrhea, abdominal cramping or bloating, pain, swelling, fever, fatigue, constipation, nausea and vomiting, loss of appetite

Duration: Acute or chronic

Treatments: Surgery, anti-inflammatory and antidiarrheal medications, antibiotics, chemotherapy and/or radiation therapy

to 20 centimeters long that leads to the anus. Small microorganisms in the large intestine break down waste products not broken down by the stomach and small intestines, resulting in gas (also known as flatus).

Complications and Disorders

Diseases and disorders of the intestinal tract constitute a major health problem affecting many individuals at one point or another in their lives. The common diseases and disorders that affect the intestinal tract include acute inflammatory disorders (such as appendicitis), diverticular disorders (diverticulosis and diverticulitis), chronic inflammatory bowel disease (Crohn's disease and ulcerative colitis), intestinal infections (such as intestinal parasites and bacterial infections with *Salmonella*, *Shigella dysenteriae*, and *Escherichia coli*), intestinal obstructions, cancers or tumors of the rectum and colon, and polyps.

The most common acute inflammatory disorder is appendicitis. Its usually affects individuals between the ages of ten and thirty, and its symptoms include abdominal pain and tenderness, nausea and vomiting, loss of appetite, rapid heart rate, fever, and an elevated white blood cell count. Normally, the appendix, whose function is not clearly understood, fills and empties with food as regularly as does the cecum, of which it is a part. It sometimes becomes inflamed because of either kinking or obstruction, producing pressure and initiating symptoms. The most common major complication associated with appendicitis is perforation, which causes severe pain and an elevation of temperature. In these cases, a physician must be notified immediately. Treatment consists of surgical removal of the appendix.

Diverticular disorders include diverticulosis and diverticulitis. Diverticulosis is the presence of diverticula without any inflammation or symptoms. Diverticulitis is the result of an inflammation or infection of the intestine produced when food or bacteria are retained in a diverticulum. Signs of diverticulosis include cramplike pain in the left lower part of the abdomen, bowel irregularity, diarrhea, constipation, and thin stools. There may be some intermittent rectal bleeding with diverticulitis.

Inflammatory bowel disease (IBD) of unknown cause is most common in whites (usually female) between the ages of fifteen and thirty-five, occurring most frequently in the American Jewish population. The two types of IBD are Crohn's disease, which is also known as regional enteritis, and ulcerative colitis. The disorders are considered to be separate diseases with similar characteristics.

Crohn's disease may affect any part of the intestinal tract but often affects the small intestine. The inflammation usually involves the entire thickness of the intestinal wall. Treatment for Crohn's disease depends on the presence or absence of symptoms. If there are no symptoms, treatment is not necessary. If there is evidence of inflammation, however, anti-inflammatory medication may be prescribed. Vitamin and mineral replacement may be given because of the problems of absorption associated with this disease. Surgery may be required at some point in the disease process because of its associated complications, such as obstruction.

Ulcerative colitis is characterized by tiny ulcers and abscesses in the inner lining of the colon, where it is usually confined. There is a tendency for these ulcerations to bleed, causing bloody diarrhea. The chronic nature of inflammatory bowel disease may cause a stricture, which can result in an obstruction requiring surgical intervention. As with Crohn's disease, the treatment for ulcerative colitis depends on the type of symptoms and may consist of medication, nutrition, or surgery. Anti-inflammatory drugs are used for flare-ups of the disease. Liquid food supplements may be given to compensate for nutrients lost in diarrhea. Intravenous therapy may be prescribed if the colon is considered too diseased to tolerate food.

There are many types of infections that affect the intestinal tract. The most common bacterial infections are caused by microorganisms such as *Salmonella* and *Shigella*. *Salmonella* bacteria are commonly found in meats, fruits (through contaminated fertilizer), poultry, eggs, dairy products, and contaminated marijuana. Pet turtles are also a source of this bacteria. The source of *Shigella* bacterial infection is feces from an infected person, with the route of transmission being oral-fecal—for example, changing the soiled diaper of an infant or having a bowel movement and then eating or preparing food without properly washing one's hands.

Intestinal parasites may also cause infection. The most common of these parasites, *Giardia lamblia*, is present where water supplies are contaminated by raw sewage. The primary treatment for these conditions is replacement of lost fluids and essential electrolytes. Antidiarrheal medications may be prescribed, although they are not normally used because they may interfere with the elimination of the causative agent.

Intestinal obstruction occurs when the normal flow of the intestine is partially or totally impeded due to an accumulation of contents, gas, or fluid. It may also be caused by the intestine's inability to propel contents along the intestinal tract, a process called peristalsis. Peristalsis may be obstructed by scars that bind together two normally separate anatomic surfaces (adhesions), hernias, or tumors. Another cause may be paralytic ileus, a paralysis of the peristaltic movement of the intestinal tract, caused by the effect of trauma or toxins on the nerve endings that regulate intestinal movement. Conservative treatment consists of decompression of the bowel using a nasogastric tube. Surgical treatment may be indicated if the bowel is completely obstructed.

While tumors of the small intestine are rare, those of the colon are common. Cancer of the colon and rectum is the second most common type of cancer in the United States (with lung cancer being the most common). The majority of intestinal tumors are benign (noncancerous) and discovered between the ages of forty and sixty. There are several types of benign tumors, which do not spread. They include lipomas, leiomyomas, angiomas, and adenomas. A small percentage of tumors of the small intestine are malignant (cancerous). The most common are adenocarcinomas, leiomyosarcomas, carcinoid tumors, and lymphomas. The symptoms of these tumors include weight loss, abdominal pain, nausea, vomiting, and bleeding. Treatment is dependent on the stage and location of the tumor. Surgical removal of the tumor may be coupled with chemotherapy or radiation therapy.

Polyps are benign tumors of the large intestine and are common in individuals over the age of sixty. They arise from the lining of the colon and are usually found during tests to diagnose other conditions. Polyps include several different varieties, the most common of which is a hyperplastic polyp. Hyperplastic polyps are less than one-half of a centimeter in diameter and do not pose a health risk. Juvenile polyps can occur in childhood, and inflammatory polyps are believed to result from injury or inflammation, such as after an episode of ulcerative colitis. Neither of these conditions poses a health risk. There is a major category of polyps known as adenomas, however, which have the potential for malignancy. These types of polyps are generally removed to prevent the development of cancer.

Rectal cancer and colon cancer are common among both men and women. Factors that predispose an individual to these types of cancer include family history or a prior history of adenomatous colon polyps, colon cancer, or ulcerative colitis. The precise cause of these cancers is unknown, but diet is believed to play a significant role, specifically diets low in fiber and high in animal fat. One of the key symptoms of these conditions requiring immediate attention (especially for individuals over the age of forty) is rectal bleeding. Treatment consists of surgery to remove the affected part of the colon. The physician may prescribe additional treatment in the form of chemotherapy or radiation therapy.

Perspective and Prospects

Problems associated with the intestinal tract are characterized by a variety of symptoms and treatments. These problems may be temporary in nature or may be manifestations of more serious underlying conditions interfering with the normal functions of absorption, fluid and electrolyte balance, and elimination. Symptoms are signs of malfunction and should not be ignored or go untreated.

Preventing problems associated with the intestinal tract may not always be possible because the causes of some intestinal diseases and disorders are unknown. Nevertheless, there has been substantial research related to intestinal diseases and disorders to support a strong correlation between nutrition and intestinal tract health. For example, there is evidence to support the relationship between the consumption of sugars, high amounts of animal protein and fat, and cholesterol and cancer-causing agents in the intestinal tract. Stress and its resulting influence on stomach acidity also contribute to intestinal ill health. Smoking and lack of regular exercise may also negatively influence normal peristalsis.

The prevention of these and other problems related to intestinal health is important not only to general health but also to work productivity. In the United States, for example, intestinal problems account for a large percentage of lost work time. Education about intestinal health and health issues beginning early in one's life will lower the incidence of some of the more common intestinal diseases and disorders.

—John A. Bavaro, Ed.D., R.N.

See also Abdomen; Abdominal disorders; Anal cancer; Anus; Appendectomy; Appendicitis; Bacterial infections; Bariatric surgery; Bypass surgery; Celiac sprue; Cholecystitis; Colic; Colitis; Colon; Colon therapy; Colonoscopy and sigmoidoscopy; Colorectal cancer;

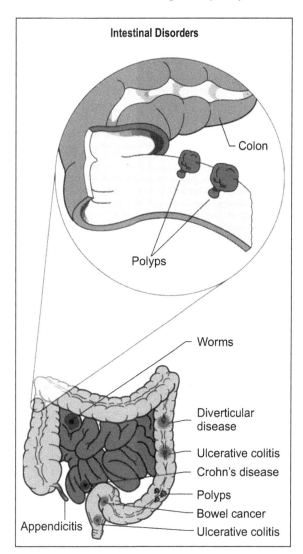

Intestinal Disorders

Colon

Polyps

Worms

Diverticular disease

Ulcerative colitis

Crohn's disease

Polyps

Bowel cancer

Ulcerative colitis

Appendicitis

Colorectal polyp removal; Colorectal surgery; Constipation; Crohn's disease; Diarrhea and dysentery; Digestion; Diverticulitis and diverticulosis; Enemas; Enterocolitis; Fistula repair; Food poisoning; Gastroenteritis; Gastroenterology; Gastroenterology, pediatric; Gastrointestinal disorders; Gastrointestinal system; Gluten intolerance; Hemorrhoid banding and removal; Hemorrhoids; Hernia; Hernia repair; Hirschsprung's disease; Ileostomy and colostomy; Indigestion; Internal medicine; Intestines; Irritable bowel syndrome (IBS); Lactose intolerance; Malabsorption; Malnutrition; Nutrition; Obesity; Obesity, childhood; Obstruction; Parasitic diseases; Peristalsis; Pinworms; Polyps; Proctology; Rectum; Roundworms; Small intestine; Soiling; Stomach, intestinal, and pancreatic cancers; Tapeworms; Tumor removal; Tumors; Worms.

For Further Information:

American Medical Association. *American Medical Association Complete Medical Encyclopedia*. New York: Random House Reference, 2003.

"Colonic Diseases." *MedlinePlus*, September 25, 2012.

Kapadia, Cyrus R., Caroline R. Taylor, and James M. Crawford. *An Atlas of Gastroenterology: A Guide to Diagnosis and Differential Diagnosis*. Boca Raton, Fla.: Parthenon, 2003.

Litin, Scott C., ed. *Mayo Clinic Family Health Book*. 4th ed. New York: HarperResource, 2009.

Payne, Wayne A., Dale B. Hahn, and Ellen Mauer. *Understanding Your Health*. 12th ed. New York: McGraw-Hill, 2013.

Peikin, Steven R. *Gastrointestinal Health: The Proven Nutritional Program to Prevent, Cure, or Alleviate Irritable Bowel Syndrome (IBS), Ulcers, Gas, Constipation, Heartburn, and Many Other Digestive Disorders*. 3d ed. New York: Perennial Currents, 2004.

"Small Intestine Disorders." *MedlinePlus*, February 4, 2013.

Tapley, Donald F., et al., eds. *The Columbia University College of Physicians and Surgeons Complete Home Medical Guide*. Rev. 3d ed. New York: Crown, 1995.

Tortora, Gerard J., and Bryan Derrickson. *Principles of Anatomy and Physiology*. 13th ed. Hoboken, N.J.: John Wiley & Sons, 2012.

INTESTINES

Anatomy

Anatomy or system affected: Abdomen, anus, gastrointestinal system

Specialties and related fields: Gastroenterology, internal medicine

Definition: The portion of the gastrointestinal tract from the lower end of the stomach to the anus, which consists of the small intestine and the colon (large intestine).

Key terms:

amylase: the enzyme responsible for breaking down carbohydrates in the small intestine; amylase enters the intestinal tract from the salivary glands and the pancreas

colon: the large intestine, divided from the small intestine by the cecum (a controlled passageway) and ending at the sigmoid, which leads food waste into the rectum

fiber: food material derived from plant substances that retain the full structure of their cell walls despite the chemical effects of the digestive process

lipases: enzymes secreted by the pancreas into the small intestine; these serve to break down fatty materials (triglycerides) in the first intestinal stage of digestion

peristalsis: the muscular contraction in the walls of the intestines that propels food material forward through the bowels

Structure and Functions

After the initial process of digestion takes place in the stomach, food passes into the intestines, where the chemical action of several gastric juices separates out the nutritive content of fats, carbohydrates, and proteins. This nutritive material is then absorbed into the bloodstream through the walls of the intestines, while waste material is collected for excretion.

In adult humans, thesmall intestine and large intestine together represent a total length of about nine meters (thirty feet). Both small and large intestines are hoselike muscular organs; the former is much longer, but substantially narrower, than the latter. The two intestines are joined at the cecum, which is located in the right-lower abdominal cavity. The appendix, which is sometimes called a "blind pouch" because it is unessential to the main processes performed in the gastrointestinal tract, projects from the cecum.

The physical disposition and function of the large intestine, or colon, are distinct from those of the small intestine. As the large intestinal tube leaves the cecum, it assumes a specific shape, following horizontal and vertical lines within the abdominal cavity. This is not the case with the small intestine, whose extensive length (about seven meters, or twenty-three feet) takes an intertwined "nesting" shape in the limited abdominal space available. By contrast, the colon, which is about 1.5 meters (5 feet) in length, has three easily identifiable sections: the ascending colon on the right side of the abdominal cavity, the transverse colon, and the descending colon on the left side of the abdomen. A final leftward bend in the colon at the sigmoid provides for its attachment to the rectum.

The two parts of the intestines carry out distinct functions in the overall digestive process. As food material passes from the lower end, or pylorus, of the stomach, only a part of the digestive process has occurred. Once partially digested food enters the small intestine, it is propelled through the intestine by means of a process of muscular contraction in the intestinal wall, which is called peristalsis.

As the food moves forward, different substances, some secreted from the lining of the intestine itself, and others—principally, bile and pancreatic fluid, which enter the upper intestine (duodenum) from the liver and pancreas—contribute to a further breaking down of food material.

Very small projections called villi are found along the interior surface of the small intestine. The villi absorb those portions of the food material that have been altered by the digestive process. From the villi, nutritive material is passed into the blood and lymphatic system for distribution to cells throughout the body. This process continues in the middle and end portions (jejunum and ileum, respectively) of the small intestine until, passing through the cecum, the remaining residue enters the large intestine.

The mixture of material contained in the large intestine, or colon, consists of indigestible food, bacteria, and substantial amounts of water. Most of the water is absorbed into the body through the walls of the colon, while the remaining waste material, or feces, is excreted through the rectum.

To understand how food materials are actually absorbed

by the villi inside the small intestine and passed into the bloodstream, one must consider several chemical processes, according to the nature of the material in question.

For example, the triglyceride components of fat, chains of fatty acids attached to glycerol, are chemical compounds that do not dissolve in water (a major part of the main bloodstream). The pancreatic enzymes called lipases split the triglycerides into separate units of fatty acid. Once separated, these fatty acids become coated with bile salts secreted by the liver, a process that allows them to pass into the mucous cells lining the intestine. As this passage occurs, the coated fatty acids (micelles) resume their chainlike form as triglycerides. At this point, however, the triglycerides have assumed an altered chemical state. In this altered form, fats can be absorbed into the blood and carried throughout the body to be used as body "fuel" or, if unused, stored in fatty tissues.

Carbohydrates must be broken down into simple sugars (glucose, galactose, and fructose) before they can be absorbed by the cell linings of the small intestine. This process occurs when the more complex carbohydrates (both starches and sugars) are split by the chemical effects of the enzyme amylase, which enters the small intestine from the salivary glands and the pancreas.

Finally, proteins, which contain the amino acids essential for the process of tissue formation in the body, must be split in several stages, the first of which occurs in the stomach itself. Here, proteins are partially broken down by the action of the gastric juices, mainly pepsin. Once protein material passes into the upper part of the small intestine, or duodenum, the process is accelerated by the influence of two main pancreatic enzymes: trypsin and chymotrypsin. These secretions cause the proteins to release amino acids in three forms: simple, dual, or triplicate bodies. It is not until these three forms are actually inside the cell walls of the small intestine that other enzymes split the dual and triplicate amino acids into their simplest single form, which can be absorbed into the veins that carry nourishment to the various organs of the body.

In the overall chemical process leading to the absorption of various body nutrients by the small and large intestines, there is a certain "absorptive specialization" in different zones of the gastrointestinal tract. Iron and calcium, for example, are absorbed in the duodenum, while proteins, fats, sugars, and all vitamins except vitamin B_{12} are absorbed in the jejunum. Finally, in the ileum, salt, vitamin B_{12}, and bile salts are processed.

Disorders and Diseases

Doctors have always known that the digestive processes of the intestines can be affected in either positive or negative ways by the nature of the food that is consumed. In the simplest terms, negative reactions are manifested by the obvious effects of indigestion and diarrhea. The control of such symptoms of improper or incomplete digestion may appear to the layperson to be a simple matter of using "over-the-counter" tablets such as laxatives or "antigas" pills. Treatment of the symptoms of indigestion, however, may provide only a superficial solution to a problem that is much more serious.

An area of important medical concern that goes beyond the general discomfort caused by imbalanced digestive functioning of the intestines involves peptic ulcers. A peptic ulcer is an open sore on the mucous membrane lining the gastrointestinal tract. The general label "peptic ulcer" was applied to this condition since the discovery, in the mid-1830s, of pepsin, the first clearly identified enzyme known to contribute to the chemical breakdown of ingested foods. Although later stages of research into the digestive process yielded much more extensive knowledge of the component elements of gastric juices, the specific name has remained attached to the general phenomenon of intestinal ulceration. The term "gastric ulcer" refers specifically to ulceration in the stomach lining.

Generally speaking, peptic ulcers occur when there is an imbalance between the task of digestion to be accomplished by the intestines and the amounts and levels of concentration of the gastric juices secreted into the gastrointestinal tract. When the amounts or concentrated strengths of gastric juices in the intestines exceed the level required for digestion (or flow into the intestine when no food has been ingested), these agents actually begin to digest the membranes of the intestine itself.

Various forms of treatment for intestinal ulcers have been developed, including both therapeutic drugs that have the capacity to counteract the corrosive effects of excessive gastric juices and, in the preventive vein, diets that contain natural combatants against intestinal disorders, especially high-fiber, unprocessed, or lightly processed foods.

In recent years, research into the causes of ulcers has extended into the field of gastrointestinal hormonal secretions originating not in the pancreas itself but in the intestine or stomach. These secretions reach the pancreas later through the bloodstream and stimulate its production of digestive juices. Such secretive processes may, if they fail to communicate properly balanced "codes" concerning the task of digestion that needs to take place in the intestines, cause an excessive supply (in volume or strength) of gastric juices, which can cause ulcerations to develop.

The most serious pathological condition that can affect the intestines is cancer of the colon. Thought to develop from a degenerative process originating in benign polyps (stem-based tumors that may develop in areas of the organism lined with mucous membrane, such as the nose, the colon, and, in females, the uterus), cancer of the colon has registered a survival rate that is statistically higher than those of cancers in other vital organs of the abdominal cavity (the liver and stomach, in particular). This is partly because—if the cancer is discovered in time—substantial areas of the colon that have been attacked by cancer can be removed surgically without endangering the continued essential functioning of the intestines.

Almost all questions relating to the pathology of the intestinal tract are somehow connected with the type of food that is eaten. Thus, medical science has turned increasingly to publicizing preventive dietary practices that can have a bearing on all functions of the intestines, from the simplest level of discomfort to the most serious level of chronic diseases.

As stated above, a relatively recent and valuable contribution to the knowledge of natural ways to aid in the absorptive work of both the small intestine and the colon—and to reduce the dangers of ulceration and/or intestinal cancer—involves the role of the fiber content of foods. Fiber is generally described as consisting of polysaccharides and lignin, two plant substances that, more than any other nutritive material, retain their natural forms as plant cell walls and are not broken down by human digestive enzymes. The plant food that is richest in these materials is wheat bran, which contains about 40 percent fiber. As fiber-rich foodstuffs such as bran pass through the gastrointestinal tract, the fiber material they contain is subject to fermentation by anaerobicbacteria in the colon. Two chemical results of this complex process seem to be the removal of deoxycholic acid from the bile and the reduction of the cholesterol saturation level of the bile. Both effects are deemed beneficial, since the reduction of deoxycholic acid and cholesterol in intestinal bile tends, at the very least, to reduce the likelihood of developing gallstones. Fiber-rich diets in combination with the reduction of excess weight became standards of preventive health care by the 1990s.

By the mid-twentieth century, typical personal diets in the Western world contained commercially refined foodstuffs that were rich in sugars and syrups, which are mainly fiber depleted. In addition to the specific disease-related factors mentioned above, medical science has noted that high consumption of fiber-depleted foods results in higher levels of energy intake (absorption of calories) during the digestive process that occurs in the intestines. In simple terms, when calorie intake exceeds the level required by the normally exercised body, the result is weight gain that may continue to the point of obesity.

Perspective and Prospects

Medical science began to become aware of the various digestive functions of hormonal secretions only in the first decades of the twentieth century. Although the early nineteenth century American army surgeon William Beaumont was the first doctor to discover the presence of gastric juices in the intestines, his analysis of digestive fluids remained quite elementary. Beaumont could easily identify hydrochloric acid in stomach secretions. He also took samples of bile from the intestinal tract and performed laboratory experiments that proved the role of bile in breaking down fatty materials. What remained unsolved were the identity and origins of other components of gastric juice and an explanation for their controlled secretion from surrounding organs in the abdominal cavity into the intestines. Beaumont's view that mental concentration (including "negative mental concentration," or anxiety) induced the flow of gastric juices proved eventually to be only partially correct.

It was only in 1902 that the British doctors Ernest Henry Starling and Sir William Maddock Bayliss were able to show that, in addition to nerve "signals," certain chemical factors induced the flow of gastric juices, specifically from the pancreas into the intestinal tract. These doctors found that, in fact, the small intestine released into the bloodstream a "chemical transmitter" that, as it circulated to the other vital organs, stimulated the production and flow of the pancreatic juices necessary for digestion. They called this "chemical transmitter" secretin. To this initial agent would be added a whole category of secretions that are called "hormones," a term taken from the Greek word for "urging on."

A discovery was made in 1928 that helped to clarify the complex relationship of hormones, gastric juice secretion, and the carrying out of the digestive process by the small and large intestines. This was the discovery of pancreozymin, the second main "chemical transmitter" affecting the pancreas, by the American researcher Andrew Ivy. Pancreozymin was found to cause the release by the pancreas of an enzyme-rich fluid made up of three agents: trypsin, lipase, and amylase. Each agent proved to be an activator in the process of breaking down different nutrients (protein, fats, and carbohydrates, respectively).

Although the intestines are the ultimate destination of and seat of activity for the pancreatic juices released by command of this hormone (as well as of the last major digestion-linked hormone, gastrin, which was discovered in 1955), secretin alone has its origin in the intestines themselves. Both pancreozymin and gastrin are secreted from the stomach.

In time, researchers found that most gastrointestinal hormones are secreted by specialized cells that line the interior of the stomach. Such cells react at various levels according to the composition of the food that has been ingested, sending chemical signals, via the hormones they secrete, that determine the relative amounts and strengths of the several gastric juices that enter the intestines from the pancreas. A similar question of varied amounts and strengths of gastric juices was linked to the so-called vagus nerve function, which also activates pancreatic flow to the intestinal tract.

The functional relationship between these two activator agents—the one nervous and the other chemical—has become one of the primary interests of researchers who deal with the most common ailment attacking the intestinal organs: peptic ulceration.

—*Byron D. Cannon, Ph.D.*

See also Abdomen; Abdominal disorders; Anus; Bypass surgery; Colitis; Colon; Colonoscopy and sigmoidoscopy; Colorectal surgery; Digestion; Endoscopy; Enemas; Fiber; Gastroenterology; Gastroenterology, pediatric; Gastrointestinal disorders; Gastrointestinal system; Hemorrhoids; Hernia; Internal medicine; Intestinal disorders; Laparoscopy; Malnutrition; Nutrition; Obstruction; Peristalsis; Polyps; Proctology; Rectum; Small intestine.

For Further Information:

Feldman, Mark, Lawrence S. Friedman, and Lawrence J. Brandt, eds. *Sleisenger and Fordtran's Gastrointestinal and Liver Disease: Pathophysiology, Diagnosis, Management.* New ed. 2 vols. Philadelphia: Saunders/Elsevier, 2010.

Janowitz, Henry D. *Good Food for Bad Stomachs.* New York: Oxford University Press, 1998.

Janowitz, Henry D. *Indigestion: Living Better with Upper Intestinal Problems, from Heartburn to Ulcers and Gallstones.* New York: Oxford University Press, 1994.

LaRusso, Laurie. "Colon Cancer." *Health Library,* February 8, 2013.

Marieb, Elaine N., and Katja Hoehn. *Human Anatomy and*

Physiology. 9th ed. San Francisco: Pearson/Benjamin Cummings, 2010.

Scanlon, Valerie, and Tina Sanders. *Essentials of Anatomy and Physiology.* 5th ed. Philadelphia: F. A. Davis, 2007.

Tortora, Gerard J., and Bryan Derrickson. *Principles of Anatomy and Physiology.* 12th ed. Hoboken, N.J.: John Wiley & Sons, 2009.

Wolfe, M. Michael, et al., eds. *Therapy of Digestive Disorders: A Companion to Sleisenger and Fordtran's Gastrointestinal and Liver Disease.* Philadelphia: W. B. Saunders, 2000.

Tennesen, Michael. "The Ecosystem Inside." *Discover* 32, no. 2 (March, 2011): 35–39.

Wood, Debra. "Peptic Ulcer." *Health Library*, March 18, 2013.

Young, Emma. "Alimentary Thinking." *New Scientist* 2895 (December 15, 2012): 38–42.

INTOXICATION. *See* ALCOHOLISM; POISONING.

INTRAVENOUS (IV) THERAPY
Treatment

Anatomy or system affected: Blood vessels, circulatory system, heart, kidneys, lungs, skin

Specialties and related fields: Anesthesiology, critical care, emergency medicine, general surgery, nursing, obstetrics, oncology, pediatrics

Definition: The infusion of fluids and medications into the general circulation through intravenous tubing and venipuncture.

Key terms:

electrolytes: elements critical for normal metabolism

hemolysis: breakdown of red blood cells and the release of hemoglobin

hyperalimentation: intravenous fluid providing nutrition

hypertonic: a solution that causes cells to decrease their fluid volume

hypocalcemia: low blood levels of calcium

hypotonic: a solution that causes cells to increase in volume

infiltration: movement of fluid into the tissue

isotonic: a solution that causes no change in cell volume

parenteral: administered by injection or infusion

pyrogenic reaction: an increase in body temperature

Indications and Procedures

Because of the dangers inherent in parenteral administration, nutrients and electrolytes should be administered whenever possible by the oral route. However, when a patient must receive fluids, electrolytes, or medications swiftly or over a long period of time, the method of choice is intravenous administration. Intravenous infusions are ordered for patients under the following circumstances: patients in life-threatening situations such as hemorrhage, shock, and severe burns; patients who may have nothing by mouth or who are unable to ingest oral liquids owing to prolonged nausea, vomiting, diarrhea, peritonitis, paralytic ileus, or fistula; patients who require medications that, if given orally, will be destroyed by gastric juices or will not be absorbed by the gastrointestinal tract; or patients who, because of their condition, are unable to digest or absorb a diet administered by mouth or tube.

Uses and Complications

The type of intravenous solution ordered will depend upon the patient's condition and the fluid and electrolyte imbalance present. Parenteral fluids vary in their tonicity: intravenous fluids may be either hypotonic, isotonic, or hypertonic. A hypotonic solution of half-strength saline is an example of a hydrating solution. The primary purpose of hydrating solutions is to provide water. Another common hydrating solution is 5 percent dextrose in water. Hydrating solutions are also used as diluents for intravenous drugs or to deep an intravenous line open at a slow rate in order to be available for medications or other solutions when ordered. Isotonic saline is used in hypovolemic states and corrects mild sodium deficit and metabolic alkalosis. Hypertonic solutions include parenteral nutrition. Because of the grave dangers inherent in parenteral therapy, the physician's orders for intravenous fluids and electrolytes must be as precise, clear, and exact as are prescriptions for any other medication.

Keeping the IV on schedule is a major nursing responsibility. The most accurate way to regulate the intravenous infusion is to calculate the rate of flow mathematically. Intravenous pumps are used to deliver fluids precisely, at a preset drip rate.

To prevent local inflammation of the vein and contamination of solutions, the tubing should be changed every forty-eight hours. No intravenous bag should hang for more than twenty-four hours. Changing the infusion site location should be initiated every seventy-two hours to decrease the potential for phlebitis and infection.

Complications of intravenous therapy include infection as a local reaction as a result of contamination that may spread systemically; mechanical failures, such as solution flow slowing down or stopping because of an obstruction within the venous system or clot in the infusion catheter; pyrogenic reactions caused by contaminated equipment or solutions; and infiltration resulting from dislodging of the needle allowing fluid to infiltrate the nearby tissue. Circulatory overload occurs when a patient receives an excessive amount of solution. Drug overload occurs when a patient receives an excessive amount of fluid containing medications. Superficial thrombophlebitis occurs as a result of overuse of a vein or the infusion of an irritating solution. Air embolism occurs when air enters the circulatory system.

Parenteral hyperalimentation, or total parenteral nutrition, is a method to supply a complete feeding for patients who cannot eat, should not eat, or will not eat as a result of disruption of the integrity of the gastrointestinal tract, neurological injury, severe burns or trauma, or psychiatric pathology. These patients cannot tolerate an oral feeding and may need to allow their gastrointestinal tract to rest from its digestive function until healing occurs. When parenteral hyperalimentation is necessary, the patient is infused with large amounts of essential nutrients required by the body for tissue growth. These solutions contain amino acids for protein and 25 percent dextrose as a carbohydrate source. Vitamins, minerals, trace elements, and electrolytes may be added as necessary. The formulation prescribed can be individualized to meet the nutritional needs of any patient. Parenteral nutrition solutions are administered via the subclavian vein to dilute the highly concentrated glucose solution in the largest quantity of blood available with this route. With these solutions, three thousand calories may be delivered in a twenty-four-hour period. With parenteral nutrition, patients who would have succumbed to illness have a chance to heal and continue to gain weight during what would otherwise be a long, potentially fatal period of starvation.

A major complication of parenteral nutrition therapy is sepsis from the indwelling intravenous catheter caused by either contamination at the time of insertion, later contamination at the insertion site if sterility is not maintained, or contaminated fluids. Another complication is catheter dislocation at the time of insertion, with accidental puncture of an artery. Glucose overload may occur if the infusion rate is too rapid for the patient's ability to handle the glucose load. Finally, hypoglycemic reaction occurs if the infusion is discontinued too suddenly.

Intravenous therapy also includes blood transfusions that are administered to restore blood volume following hemorrhage or severe trauma. Through adverse reactions to blood transfusions are not common, they can be very serious. Complications include circulatory overload, serum hepatitis, and pyrogenic, hemolytic, and allergic reactions.

Perspective and Prospects

The first known intravenous infusion was administered through a goose quill from a pig's bladder that contained the fluid being infused. No record was found related to the success or failure of the treatment. Today, depending upon the severity of the condition, patients with fluid and electrolyte disturbances may have only a few mild symptoms or they may be desperately ill. Consequently, the various medical and nursing interventions used to correct fluid and electrolyte problems range from the simple to the complex. The treatment of patients with fluid, electrolyte, and acid-base disturbances revolves around two concepts: the replacement of fluids, electrolytes, and nutrients or the limitation of the amount of fluids and the correction of electrolyte imbalances.

—*Jane C. Norman, Ph.D., R.N., C.N.E.*

See also Blood vessels; Catheterization; Circulation; Hospitals; Nursing; Nutrition; Pharmacology; Phlebotomy; Respiration; Resuscitation; Surgical procedures; Tracheostomy; Transfusion; Urinary system; Urology; Vascular medicine; Vascular system.

For Further Information:

Booth, Kathryn A. *Intravenous Therapy for Health Care Personnel*. New York: McGraw-Hill, 2007.

Fulcher, Eugenia M. *Intravenous Therapy: A Guide to Basic Principles*. New York: W. B. Saunders, 2006.

Josephson, Dianne L. *Intravenous Infusion Therapy for Nurses*. 2d ed. Clifton Park, New York: Delmar Learning, 2004.

Nentwich, Paul C. *Intravenous Therapy*. New York: Jones and Bartlett, 2007.

"Nutritional Support." *MedlinePlus*, Apr. 18, 2013.

Springhouse, ed. *I.V. Therapy Made Incredibly Easy!* Philadelphia: Lippincott Williams and Wilkins, 2009.

"Total Parenteral Nutrition." *MedlinePlus*, Sept. 1, 2010.

Weinstein, Sharon M. *Plumer's Principles and Practice of Intravenous Therapy*. 8th ed. Philadelphia: Lippincott Williams & Wilkins, 2007.

"What Is Nutrition Support Therapy?" *American Society for Parenteral and Enteral Nutrition*, Mar. 2010.

INTRAVENTRICULAR HEMORRHAGE
Disease/Disorder

Anatomy or system affected: Brain, nervous system
Specialties and related fields: Neonatology, neurology
Definition: Bleeding into or around the normal fluid spaces within the brain.
Key terms:

cerebrospinal fluid (CSF): fluid produced within the ventricles of the brain that flows around the brain and spinal cord

cranial ultrasound: the use of sound waves to obtain a picture of the brain

hydrocephalus: a condition characterized by the abnormal accumulation of fluid within the cranial vault, often accompanied by enlargement of the head and damage to the brain

indomethacin: a nonsteroidal anti-inflammatory drug (NSAID) administered to preterm babies in an attempt to decrease the likelihood of developing intraventricular hemorrhage

ventricles: fluid-filled spaces within the brain

Causes and Symptoms

Intraventricular hemorrhage (IVH) occurs most commonly in premature babies, especially those weighing under 1,500 grams (3 pounds, 5 ounces). IVHs have been seen as well in adults as a secondary complication of hemorrhagic stroke, leaving the individual with a poor prognosis.

IVH in premature babies is thought to occur when there is oxygen deprivation during delivery or complications following delivery. Since the blood vessels in the brain of the baby are fragile, they may rupture easily, resulting in excessive bleeding into (intraventricular) or around (periventricular) the ventricles. Generally, there are no outward symptoms. Some infants with IVH may suddenly develop seizures or anemia. IVH is usually diagnosed by cranial ultrasound routinely done on high-risk infants between three and ten days of life, since most cases occur by day three.

Intraventricular hemorrhages are categorized into four grades based on severity. Grade I involves bleeding confined to the small area where it began. Grade II involves blood extending into the ventricles, with no ventricular enlargement. Grade III involves more blood extending into the ventricles, with ventricular enlargement. Grade IV has blood collecting within the brain tissue (intraparenchymal hemorrhage), reflecting injury to the brain. Hydrocephalus (or too much fluid in the brain wherein the spaces, or ventricles, become enlarged) is a common complication of Grade III or IV bleeds.

Treatment and Therapy

Premature babies are given intravenous indomethacinonce daily for the first three days of life in order to decrease the

---

Information on Intraventricular Hemorrhage

Causes: Unknown; possibly oxygen deprivation during premature delivery or subsequent complications, leading to rupture of blood vessels in brain

Symptoms: Generally none, sometimes seizures or anemia; may result in hydrocephalus

Duration: Acute, with possible long-term consequences if severe (motor problems, developmental delay, seizures, blindness, deafness)

Treatments: Prevention through intravenous indomethacin during first three days of life, steroids given to mother prior to delivery; alleviation of symptoms; insertion of shunt for hydrocephalus

---

likelihood of severe IVH. Steroids (corticosteroids) given to the mother prior to delivery have also decreased the frequency of severe IVH, as have improved monitoring and care of premature babies. No specific treatment exists for IVH, except to treat symptoms and underlying health problems. If hydrocephalus develops, it can be treated with frequent lumbar punctures or ventricular taps. If the condition persists, a shunt may be placed surgically to drain the extra CSF throughout life. In adults who suffer IVH secondary to hemorrhagic stroke, fibrolytic agents (so-called clot busters) are being evaluated as a mode of treatment.

Perspective and Prospects

IVH has been reported in 35 to 50 percent of infants weighing under 1,500 grams (3 pounds, 5 ounces). If IVH is suspected, a doctor may order an ultrasound to diagnose the condition and evaluate the amount of bleeding. As gestational age increases, the likelihood of IVH decreases. The care of sick and premature babies has advanced greatly, but there is still no way to definitively prevent IVH from occurring. Grade I IVHs rarely involve long-term problems. Those classified as Grade IV generally do result in long-term sequelae, including motor problems, developmental delay, seizures, blindness, and deafness.

—*Robin Kamienny Montvilo, R.N., Ph.D.*

See also Bleeding; Brain; Brain damage; Brain disorders; Hydrocephalus; Neonatology; Nervous system; Neurology; Neurology, pediatric; Perinatology; Premature birth; Shunts; Strokes; Subdural hematoma.

For Further Information:

Klaus, Marshall H., and Avroy A. Fanaroff, eds. *Care of the High-Risk Neonate.* 5th ed. Philadelphia: W. B. Saunders, 2001.

Victor, Maurice, and Allan H. Ropper. *Adams and Victor's Principles of Neurology.* 9th ed. New York: McGraw-Hill, 2009.

Volpe, Joseph. *Neurology of the Newborn.* 5th ed. Philadelphia: Saunders/Elsevier, 2008.

INVASIVE TESTS
Procedures
Anatomy or system affected: All
Specialties and related fields: All

Definition: Tests that require the passage of an instrument through the body's protective barriers.

Indications and Procedures

Skin, sphincters, and gag and cough reflex systems are some of the defenses that can be penetrated to gather important diagnostic information. Invasive tests provide medical insights that are unattainable by noninvasive or laboratory tests. Invasive tests are typically performed last in a diagnostic protocol, however, because penetration of the body defenses is not without risk. An anesthetic agent is commonly used to minimize any discomfort or pain that may arise during the tests. Although invasive, these tests often circumvent the trauma of exploratory surgery.

In general, invasive tests may be classified as those that allow the physician to obtain samples of fluid, tissue, or tumors directly from their site of origin (through aspiration, lumbar puncture, and biopsy) or those that allow direct viewing of specific areas of the body through endoscopy. Some test procedures allow both direct viewing and sample collection; bronchoscopy is one such example.

One of the more familiar aspiration tests is amniocentesis. Amniocentesis involves removing 20 to 30 milliliters of fluid from the amniotic sac for analysis. This test is used in prenatal care at weeks fifteen to eighteen in order to assess the genetic makeup of the fetus or to detect developmental abnormalities.

Fluid from effusions can also be aspirated for analysis. Effusions are collections of an abnormally large quantity of fluid within a serous or synovial cavity. While a small amount of fluid is normal in these cavities, a large amount indicates a pathology that should be identified and treated. Once an effusion is tapped, the fluid is grossly examined for color and for clarity or turbidity. Microscopic investigations of the fluids are performed to assess the types of cells present (such as immune cells or malignant cells) and to identify microorganisms that may be present. Paracentesis is the removal of fluid from effusions within the abdominal, or peritoneal, cavity. If the effusion in this region is large, it is called ascites. Removal of fluid from the lung cavity, called thoracentesis, requires penetration of the chest wall between the ribs (intercostal spaces). Common causes of effusions include infections, congestive heart failure, kidney disease, and malignancy.

Synovial fluid is most commonly aspirated from the knee, but other joints can be investigated in this manner. Red blood cells, inflammatory cells, or crystals may be identified by microscopic evaluation of the aspirated fluid. Osteoarthritis, rheumatoid arthritis, and gout are some diseases that can be diagnosed through synovial fluid aspiration.

Cerebrospinal fluid (CSF) is housed within the bony cranium and spinal column. Fluid from this space is collected by lumbar puncture (spinal tap) and is drawn when a viral, bacterial, or fungal meningitis is suspected. Lumbar puncture may also be performed when a tumor or leukemia of the central nervous system is suspected, or to determine whether a subarachnoid hemorrhage is present.

Fine needle aspiration (FNA) is a specific kind of percutaneous (through-the-skin) needle biopsy. FNA can be used to collect a sample of cells from any palpable mass. By directly inserting a needle into the mass and then washing, or flushing, the region, some cells can be eroded from the tissue surface. These cells are set adrift in the fluid, which is sucked back into the flushing syringe. Microscopic evaluation of the cells can then be performed. Breast, neck, abdominal, and lymph nodes are some of the places where FNA is utilized.

Alternative biopsy techniques include gently scraping off a small surface, as in the Papanicolaou (Pap) testing of the cervix, or removing a deeper tissue sample, as in the punch biopsy of the cervix. Biopsy can sometimes require small surgical incisions to reach a certain organ, such as muscle, skin, breast, bone, or renal (kidney) biopsy.

Tissue biopsies may be taken directly from an organ without surgical incisions; one way to do this is with endoscopy. Typically, endoscopes are flexible probing instruments fitted with fiber-optic viewing devices. Often, a tool attachment allows the use of tiny cutting and sampling devices. Small pieces of tissue can be removed from some otherwise inaccessible areas of the body. Different kinds of endoscopes are used to accommodate the unique structural features of body regions, such as the bronchi, stomach, or colon. Sterile techniques are implemented in all cases.

Bronchoscopy is utilized in diagnosing pulmonary infections and lung cancers or in locating and removing foreign objects found in the airways. Esophagealgastroscopy is used to determine the source of upper gastrointestinal problems such as gastric or peptic ulcers, esophageal varices, esophageal reflux, or malignancy. Colonoscopy is similarly used to evaluate the origins of lower gastrointestinal problems. Colon polyps can be identified, and the mucosal lining of the colon can be evaluated for ulcerative colitis, diverticula, or adenocarcinomas.

Finally, arteriography (including angiography) and cardiac catheterization are important and frequently used invasive tests. These tests are used to evaluate the cardiovascular system. Angiography combines radiographic techniques with the injection of dyes into arteries. This combination allows the physician to determine whether an artery is blocked (occluded). Angiography is particularly useful in patients who have heart conditions, such as angina, and can be used to evaluate renal (kidney) arteries, aortic dissection, or cerebral aneurysms. The result of arteriography is a critical component in determining whether surgery or drug intervention is best for a given patient.

As a diagnostic tool, cardiac catheterization provides insight into the health of a heart. Pictures of the heart can be taken as the catheter is advanced into the right side and then the left side of the heart. A dye is injected into the heart so that the flow can be traced as the heart pumps. The heart chambers, valves, and blood vessels can be evaluated. Additionally, pressures within the heart chambers can be recorded.

Uses and Complications

The greatest health risk with any invasive test is infection. For this reason, sterile methods are used to keep infections and mortality caused by infections to a minimum. With proper care, the risks of invasive testing are surpassed by the benefits of the early and proper diagnosis that such tests provide.

—*Mary C. Fields, M.D.*

See also Amniocentesis; Angiography; Arthroscopy; Biopsy; Blood testing; Breast biopsy; Catheterization; Chorionic villus sampling; Colonoscopy and sigmoidoscopy; Cystoscopy; Diagnosis; Endometrial biopsy; Endoscopic retrograde cholangiopancreatography (ERCP); Endoscopy; Laparoscopy; Radiopharmaceuticals.

For Further Information:

Cavanaugh, Bonita Morrow. *Nurse's Manual of Laboratory and Diagnostic Tests.* 4th ed. Philadelphia: F. A. Davis, 2003. Provides information on hundreds of laboratory and diagnostic tests, with each test presented in two distinct, cross-referenced sections: "Background Information" sections provide a complete description of each test and its purposes; "Clinical Application Data" sections focus on the information nurses most commonly need while caring for clients.

Classen, Meinhard, G. N. J. Tytgat, and C. J. Lightdale, eds. *Gastroenterological Endoscopy.* 2d ed. New York: Thieme Medical, 2010. Text that examines such topics as the impact of endoscopy, its history of use, diagnostic procedures and techniques, therapeutic procedures, descriptions of diseases involving the upper and lower intestine, endoscopic features of infectious diseases of the gastrointestinal tract, and pediatric endoscopy.

Dublin, Arthur B., ed. *Outpatient Invasive Radiologic Procedures: Diagnostic and Therapeutic.* Philadelphia: W. B. Saunders, 1989. Discusses such topics as radiography, radiotherapy, and diagnostic imaging. Also covers interventional radiography. Includes bibliographical references and an index.

Griffith, H. Winter. *Complete Guide to Symptoms, Illness, and Surgery.* Revised and updated by Stephen Moore and Kenneth Yoder. 5th ed. New York: Perigee, 2006. Covers more than five hundred diseases and disorders and includes information about causes and risk factors, preventive techniques, and diagnostic tests.

Pagana, Kathleen Deska, and Timothy J. Pagana. *Mosby's Diagnostic and Laboratory Test Reference.* 9th ed. St. Louis, Mo.: Mosby/Elsevier, 2009. A clinical handbook that gives alphabetically organized laboratory and diagnostic tests for easy reference. Each listing includes such things as alternate or abbreviated test names, type of test, normal findings, possible critical values, test explanation and related physiology, and potential complications.

Ravin, Carl E., ed. *Imaging and Invasive Radiology in the Intensive Care Unit.* New York: Churchill Livingstone, 1993. Discusses such topics as critical care medicine, diagnostic imaging, and interventional radiology. Includes bibliographical references and an index.

Sloan, John P. *Biopsy Pathology of the Breast.* 2d ed. New York: Oxford University Press, 2001. A practical guide to diagnosing breast pathology. Second edition examines the ways in which advances in mammographic screening, more treatment options, greater involvement by pathologists in clinical management, and the expansion of molecular pathology have impacted the field.

Zaret, Barry L., Marvin Moser, and Lawrence S. Cohen, eds. *Yale University School of Medicine Patient's Guide to Medical Tests.* Boston: Houghton Mifflin, 1997. Written and edited by Yale University School of Medicine faculty, this resource provides detailed information on types of diagnostic tests, how doctors use them, and what patients can do for themselves.

IRRITABLE BOWEL SYNDROME (IBS)
Disease/Disorder

Also known as: Irritable colon, mucous colitis, nervous colon, spastic colon or bowel

Anatomy or system affected: Abdomen, anus, gastrointestinal system, intestines, nervous system

Specialties and related fields: Alternative medicine, gastroenterology, nutrition

Definition: A common intestinal disorder characterized by abdominal pain or discomfort and by altered bowel habits, consisting of diarrhea or constipation or alternating between diarrhea and constipation.

Key terms:

biofeedback: the technique of making unconscious or involuntary bodily processes perceptible to the senses in order to manipulate them by conscious mental control

biopsychosocial: a model in medicine in which patients are assessed in terms of two important interconnected systems of the mind and the body; in simplest terms, the mind-body connection

cognitive behavioral therapy: a type of psychotherapy that focuses on feelings and actions, especially on replacing negative thoughts with more positive thoughts, thereby resulting in more desirable outcomes

colon: the large intestine

colonoscopy: the use of a small-diameter, flexible tube of optical fibers with an external light source to examine visually the interior of the body, specifically the colon

Crohn's disease: a disease characterized by inflammation of all layers (full thickness) of the intestines or any part of the digestive tract; early symptoms may resemble those of irritable bowel syndrome

defecation: passage of feces through the anus

feces: undigested food and other waste that is eliminated through the anus

gastroenterology: study of the function and diseases associated with the stomach, intestines, and other organs of the digestive tract such as the liver and pancreas

gut: the intestines

ileum: distal part of the small intestine, closest to the starting part of the colon; can be involved in ulcerative colitis

ischemic colitis: inadequate blood supply to the colon

lactose: a sugar found in milk and milk products; some people cannot digest lactose, causing lactose intolerance, which can produce symptoms that resemble those of irritable bowel syndrome

organic: arising from an organ

peristalsis: a series of muscular contractions that move food through the intestines during the process of digestion

physiological: pertaining to functioning; derived from physiology, the study of functions and of the biological, chemical, and physical factors and processes involved in a living organism and its parts

sigmoid: the distal part of the large colon, just before the rectum

sigmoidoscopy: similar to colonoscopy, with the tubular instrument with light instead inspecting only the anus, rectum, and sigmoid colon

somatic: pertaining to the body wall; in contrast to the viscera, which refers to the organs within body cavities

ulcerative colitis: an inflammatory disease that causes superficial ulcers in the ileum, colon, and rectum

Causes and Symptoms

Irritable bowel syndrome (IBS) is a gastrointestinal (GI) disorder characterized by abdominal pain or discomfort associated with diarrhea, constipation, or alternations between these two types of bowel motions. Other GI symptoms are related to this syndrome, including bloating, cramping, gas, heartburn, nausea, passage of mucus, an increased urge to defecate, and a feeling of incomplete defecation. Moreover, non-GI symptoms may accompany IBS, such as discomforts during menstruation, urination, and sexual activities. Although symptoms vary in intensity, they do not grow steadily worse over time but may wax and wane over the years.

IBS is sometimes referred to as a functional disorder. Several causes of IBS have been suggested, but there is no single organic cause that can explain this condition. IBS is understood as a disease with a common set of symptoms that are evaluated based either on the Manning criteria (established in 1978) or the Rome III criteria (updated in 2006) for standardized diagnosis of IBS and for distinguishing organic causes for the syndrome. The Manning criteria include the following: pain relief with defecation, sensation of incomplete defecation, passage of mucus, and frequent and looser stools associated with the onset of pain. The more symptoms are present, the higher the probability of IBS diagnosis. The Rome III criteria include recurrent abdominal pain or discomfort associated with two or more of the following: relief after defecation, change in frequency of stools in association with pain, and change in form or appearance of stools associated with pain. The duration of these symptoms should at least be three days per month for the past three months or the onset of symptoms should at least be six months prior to diagnosis.

Three traditional physiological factors contribute to the symptoms of IBS: changes in GI motility, psychological aspects such as stress, and GI hypersensitivity. The GI motility responds to various stimuli such as food, stress, and gut distension; the resulting changes in activity of the major part of the large intestine or colon can lead to IBS symptoms. Following food digestion by the stomach and the small intestine, the undigested material is propelled toward the rectum by peristalsis. When peristalsis becomes disrupted by IBS, the flow becomes too slow, causing constipation, or too fast, causing diarrhea.

Some foods and drinks appear more likely to trigger IBS attacks by disrupting peristalsis. Fatty foods, fried foods, milk products, chocolate, drinks with caffeine, and alcohol

---

Information on Irritable Bowel Syndrome (IBS)

Causes: Unclear; possibly changes in activity of colon resulting from dietary factors, stress, female reproductive hormones

Symptoms: Abdominal pain and cramps, diarrhea or constipation, bloating, nausea

Duration: Chronic

Treatments: Dietary changes, antispasmodic drugs, psychological counseling, behavioral therapy (e.g., hypnosis and biofeedback, relaxation techniques)

In the News: A Novel Approach to Treating IBS Symptoms

A new target for treatment of the symptoms of irritable bowel syndrome (IBS) is presented by the serotonin (5-HT) receptors that are present in nerves of the gastrointestinal (GI) tract and other organs. Receptors are proteins involved in the response of organs to various signals. Blocking these receptors can modify responses of the nerves in the GI tract. There are several types of 5-HT receptors; they are designated by numbers such as 5-HT3 and 5-HT4.

Alosetron (Lotronex) targets the 5-HT3 receptors in the GI tract. The desired effects of the drug include pain relief, normalization of bowel frequency, and decreased urgency for bowel movements in female patients with diarrhea-predominant IBS. The restrictive guidelines for alosetron were established because of its serious side effects: severe constipation and ischemic colitis that can potentially be fatal. Alosetron was withdrawn from the market but eventually reapproved by the Food and Drug Administration (FDA) with restrictive guidelines for its prescription.

A similar drug called cilansetron also targets the 5-HT3 receptors in the GI tract, and studies have shown that its effects on individuals with IBS are the same as for alosetron. It is the first 5-HT3 blocker specific for both male and female IBS patients suffering from diarrhea. In April, 2005, the FDA did not approve the product registration for cilansetron in the United States, even though the phase III registration trials were complete, and requested additional data from Solvay, the manufacturer. The FDA denial may be related to the challenges under-

gone by alosetron. By the end of 2005, Solvay suspended its product application in the United States, but it continues to discuss the introduction of cilansetron in the United Kingdom through the Medicines and Healthcare Products Regulatory Agency. The United Kingdom is the reference country for the introduction of cilansetron to the member countries of the European Union.

Tegaserod is a drug for treating constipation in IBS patients. It is marketed by Novartis as Zelnorm in the United States and Zelmac outside the United States. Tegaserod was approved by the FDA in 2002 for treatment of female patients suffering from constipation-predominant IBS. Tegaserod targets the 5-HT4 receptors in the GI tract. The desired effects of the drug include decreasing pain perception and reversing constipation through faster food transit in the GI tract. Tegaserod seems to be well tolerated by most patients, with most common side effects including headache, abdominal pain, and diarrhea. Evidence showed a link between the drug and an increased risk of heart attack and stroke, however, and it was withdrawn from the U.S. market in March, 2007.

More treatment options using the novel approach of targeting the serotonin (5-HT) receptors may be on the horizon as researchers learn more about the efficacy and safety of these new drugs in IBS patients.

—*Miriam E. Schwartz, M.D., M.A., Ph.D., and Colm A. Ó'Moráin, M.A., M.D., M.Sc., D.Sc.*

---

can exacerbate the symptoms of IBS, as well as some fruits or vegetables, such as cabbage, broccoli, cauliflower, and brussels sprouts. In some cases, however, no specific foods cause specific symptoms, as any food intake seems to worsen symptoms. Often, IBS-aggravating foods vary from person to person.

The nervous system processing between the brain and the intestines suggest that stress may be the culprit in IBS. Many IBS sufferers report symptoms following a meal when they experience stress. Psychologic stress has been shown to exacerbate GI symptoms in IBS. Stress may also be involved in some people who develop IBS following infection or inflammation of the bowel. In addition, psychiatric diseases are common among IBS patients, especially in those who are hospitalized.

A hypersensitive gut is characterized by enhanced perception of normal motility throughout the digestive tract. Recent studies have shown that specific parts of the brain show greater activation in IBS patients; these activated brain regions are associated with attention and response selection.

IBS is more commonly seen in women than in men, with up to 20 percent of the American population affected. Although it can occur at any time, IBS generally appears in the patient's teens and twenties, and it frequently is found in members of the same family. Americans and Europeans have similar frequencies of IBS.

Treatment and Therapy

Diagnosis of IBS is an involved process that is accomplished through a series of steps. A thorough history should be

provided to the physician. Symptom-based criteria (Manning or Rome III) will be used to identify IBS. Moreover, alarming symptoms such as weight loss, unrelenting diarrhea, family history of colon cancer, and psychiatric aspects such as depression and suicidal thoughts will be ruled out. A physical examination will be performed on the first visit. Laboratory tests and a colonoscopy or sigmoidoscopy may be performed, and a stool sample may be obtained—all of which will rule out serious diseases such as colon cancer, infection, and inflammatory diseases. Traditionally, IBS has been a diagnosis of exclusion.

Treatment options will include dietary and lifestyle changes, medications targeted toward the predominant symptoms, and psychological modalities. Generally, a low-fat, high-fiber diet lessens symptoms, although the tolerance of fiber as well as of all foods varies from person to person. Dietary changes vary according to the severity of the patient's symptoms. In mild cases of IBS, known aggravating foods should be identified and avoided. Symptoms may be eased by eating smaller meals. Since no diet has been found that controls all symptoms, a diary of symptoms and food intake is valuable in determining which foods are offensive. Establishment of fixed times for meals and bathroom visits helps regulate bowel habits as well.

In addition to dietary changes, medications are given to alleviate predominant IBS symptoms. Abdominal pain is treated with antispasmodic drugs such as dicyclomine, especially if the pain is associated with meals; these drugs relax the smooth muscles of the intestines. An antidiarrheal agent such as loperamide is used to reduce loose stools and to relieve abdominal pain. A medication called alosetron (Lotronex) is also used for diarrhea. Because alosetron has serious side effects, such as severe constipation and ischemic colitis, it was withdrawn from the market for a while; it is now available again, but with specific restrictions and only for severe IBS. Physicians must enroll in a special program with the manufacturer in order to prescribe alosetron. For constipation, bulk laxatives that supply increased dietary fiber such as psyllium (Metamucil, Fiberall, Konsyl, Colon Cleanse, and other similar products) are recommended. A medication for constipation called tegaserod (Zelnorm) was made available in 2002 but was withdrawn in 2007 when evidence suggested that it raised the risk of heart attack and stroke. Lubiprostone (Amitiza), which helps promote chloride channel secretions in the bowel and thus aids perstalsis, has been approved for use in women with constipation-predominant IBS and patients with chronic constipation. Linaclotide (Linzess), a guanylate cyclase-C agonist, increases the motility and blocks pain signals in the bowels. It is approved for adults seventeen and older who have IBS with constipation or chronic constipation.

Psychological treatments are imperative for IBS patients whose quality of life is severely impaired. Patients who have concomitant psychiatric conditions such as depression, history of sexual abuse, or any major life stress should be treated for their psychiatric ailments so that they can cope better with IBS.

Psychological counseling, cognitive behavioral therapy, hypnosis, biofeedback, and relaxation techniques are recommended to reduce anxiety and encourage learning to cope better with the pain of IBS. Severe pain from IBS can be treated with antidepressants such as tricyclics. Moderate exercise has also been shown to be beneficial.

In addition to dietary changes prescribed by doctors, alternative practitioners may advise herbal remedies to treat symptoms of IBS, such as Chinese herbal medicines, aloe vera, ginger, evening primrose, fennel, peppermint extract, chamomile, and rosemary. Aromatherapy, hydrotherapy, acupuncture, chiropractic, and osteopathy as alternative treatments may also be useful in some individuals.

Perspective and Prospects

IBS was once believed to be a psychological disorder, but recent studies have shown that it is a true medical disorder with specific physiological characteristics and a significant impact on individuals who are afflicted with it. In addition, IBS has considerable effects on the society's health care burden. It has been reported that IBS is the second most common reason for seeing a physician (the first being the common cold) and accounts for 12 percent of visits to primary care and for the largest group seen by gastroenterologists. In terms of GI diseases, IBS is second only to gastroesophageal reflux disease (GERD) as most prevalent GI disorder in the United States. IBS affects 15.4 million people, and the economic costs (both direct and indirect) are in the billions of dollars. These costs are derived from work absenteeism, doctor visits, medical tests, and procedures, as well as other related expenses.

Although there is no cure for IBS, it is not a life-threatening condition. It has not been shown to cause intestinal bleeding or inflammation, as in Crohn's disease, ulcerative colitis, or cancer. Long-term management, though frustrating, involves commitment to therapy for six months or more to find the best combinations of medicine, diet, counseling, and support for control of IBS symptoms.

—Mary Hurd; updated by
Miriam E. Schwartz, M.D., M.A., Ph.D.,
and Colm A. Ó'Moráin, M.A., M.D., M.Sc., D.Sc.

See also Abdominal disorders; Colitis; Colon; Constipation; Crohn's disease; Diarrhea and dysentery; Gastroenterology; Gastrointestinal disorders; Gastrointestinal system; Intestinal disorders; Intestines; Lactose intolerance; Peristalsis; Small intestine.

For Further Information:

"American Gastroenterological Association Technical Review on Irritable Bowel Syndrome." *Gastroenterology* 123, no. 6 (December, 2002): 2108–2131.
Chey, William D., et al. "Bacterial Overgrowth and IBS: Bridging the Gap." *Gastroenterology and Hepatology* 2, no. 8, supp. (August 9, 2006): 5–13.
Darnley, Simon, and Barbara Millar. *Understanding Irritable Bowel Syndrome*. New York: Wiley, 2003.
Hadley, Susan K., and Stephen M. Gaarder. "Treatment of Irritable Bowel Syndrome." *American Family Physician* 72, no. 12 (December 15, 2005): 2501–2506.
International Foundation for Functional Gastrointestinal Disorders. "Targeted IBS Medications." *AboutIBS*, March 23, 2013.
Irritable Bowel Syndrome Self Help and Support Group. *IBS Group*, April 25, 2013.
MedlinePlus. "Irritable Bowel Syndrome." *MedlinePlus*, May 20, 2013.
Mertz, Howard R. "Irritable Bowel Syndrome." *New England Journal of Medicine* 349, no. 22 (November 27, 2003): 2136–2145.
National Digestive Diseases Information Clearinghouse (NDDIC). "Irritable Bowel Syndrome." *National Digestive Diseases Information Clearing House (NDDIC)*, July 2, 2012.
Wood, Debra. "Irritable Bowel Syndrome." *Health Library*, September 30, 2012.

ISCHEMIA

Disease/Disorder

Anatomy or system affected: Blood vessels, brain, circulatory system

Specialties and related fields: Cardiology, critical care, neurology, vascular medicine

Definition: The interruption or temporary restriction of blood flow to a particular area of the body, such as an organ.

Causes and Symptoms

When a localized area of the brain does not receive enough blood, neurons and supportive tissue such as glia are deprived of the essential oxygen and glucose that keep them alive. If the brain does not receive sufficient blood for even a few minutes, the result is an ischemic stroke.

Although it is possible for ischemia to have no detectable symptoms, when it occurs to the internal carotid, middle cerebral, or vertebral-basilar arteries, symptoms such as confusion, impaired speech, double vision, or numbness on one

Information on Ischemia

Causes: Blood clots, atherosclerosis

Symptoms: Depends on location; may include confusion, impaired speech, double vision, numbness on one side of face, chest pain

Duration: May be temporary or permanent

Treatments: Drug therapy (e.g., aspirin, nitroglycerin), surgery (e.g., angioplasty)

side of the face can be experienced. In some instances, these symptoms are temporary and do not result in permanent damage (these are called transient ischemic attacks, or TIAs), but if the interruption of blood flow lasts long enough, permanent damage (a stroke) occurs. If blood flow is restricted to the coronary artery of the heart (cardiac ischemia), then the heart muscle may suffer permanent damage (myocardial infarction). Symptoms of cardiac ischemia may include chest pain.

Ischemia is commonly caused by the formation of blood clots or by atherosclerosis, in which the walls of the arteries become narrowed as a result of the buildup of fat deposits.

Treatment and Therapy

The risk of ischemia can be assessed with high-resolution ultrasound equipment or magnetic resonance angiography (MRA) to detect blood flow. It is common to use computed tomography (CT) scanning or magnetic resonance imaging (MRI) to visualize damaged brain tissue and determine if the damage is ischemia caused by a blocked blood vessel or by a burst blood vessel (cerebral hemorrhage). Cardiac ischemia can be diagnosed by electrocardiography, echocardiography, or angiography. Drug therapies such as administering aspirin or stronger blood-thinning agents help when ischemia is caused by clotting. Nitroglycerin can quickly open up coronary arteries and reduce the chest pain experienced when the heart is affected. Drugs that lower blood pressure are also helpful treatments.

Surgery might be needed to correct an obstruction that cannot be dissolved. Angioplasty can be used to expand affected arteries, particularly when the cause is atherosclerosis.

Perspective and Prospects

Rudolf Virchow, a nineteenth century German physician, was the first to use the term "ischemia." Since the time that ischemia was originally identified, diagnostics have been improved through the use of echocardiograms that send out sound waves to create an image of the heart's internal structures and through angiograms that can pinpoint the area of arterial narrowing. Treatment improvements for damage to the brain include the administration of unique drugs that can mitigate damage to surrounding nerve cells indirectly affected by the lack of blood.

Much has been learned about the need for a balanced diet, for regular exercise, for controlling hypertension, and for preventing or treating atherosclerosis as means to reduce the likelihood of suffering from an ischemic attack.

—*Bryan C. Auday, Ph.D.*

See also Angioplasty; Arteriosclerosis; Blood vessels; Bypass surgery; Cardiology; Circulation; Claudication; Echocardiography; Heart; Heart attack; Heart disease; Heart failure; Hyperlipidemia; Hypertension; Infarction; Necrosis; Plaque, arterial; Strokes; Thrombosis and thrombus; Transient ischemic attacks (TIAs); Vascular medicine; Vascular system.

For Further Information:

American Heart Association. *Heart Attack Treatment, Prevention, Recovery.* New York: Times Books, 1998.

Anagnostopoulos, Constantinos D., et al., eds. *Noninvasive Imaging of Myocardial Ischemia.* London: Springer, 2006.

Blumenfeld, Hal. *Neuroanatomy Through Clinical Cases.* 2d ed. Sunderland, Mass.: Sinauer, 2011.

Caplan, Louis R. "Patient Information: Ischemic Stroke Treatment (Beyond the Basics)." *UpToDate*, February 1, 2012.

Kalat, James W. *Biological Psychology.* 11th ed. Belmont, Calif.: Wadsworth, 2013.

Kolb, Bryan, and Ian Q. Whishaw. *Fundamentals of Human Neuropsychology.* 6th ed. New York: Worth, 2009.

MedlinePlus. "Transient Ischemic Attack." *MedlinePlus*, April 29, 2013.

Texas Heart Institute at St. Luke's Episcopal Hospital. "Silent Ischemia." *Heart Information Center*, October 2012.

Zillmer, Eric A., and Mary V. Spiers. *Principles of Neuropsychology.* 2d ed. Belmont, Calif.: Thomson/Wadsworth, 2008.

JAUNDICE
Disease/Disorder

Anatomy or system affected: Blood, liver, skin

Specialties and related fields: Gastroenterology, hematology, internal medicine

Definition: Yellow discoloration of skin resulting from increased levels of bilirubin in the blood.

Causes and Symptoms

Jaundice is not a disease, but rather a common sign of various disorders in the liver or the blood. Bilirubin is a pigment formed by the breakdown of hemoglobin, the oxygen-carrying molecule in red blood cells. Bilirubin is then transported to the liver, where it is processed into a water-soluble form. This process is known as conjugation. Conjugated bilirubin is secreted into the bile ducts and eventually excreted in feces. An increase in red blood cell breakdown, impairment in liver function, or blockage of the bile ducts can all result in the buildup of bilirubin. The first visible manifestation of this is often scleral icterus, a yellowing of the white part of the eyes. When levels of conjugated bilirubin are abnormally high, it may be seen in the urine as urobilinogen, which causes a darkening of the urine.

Once the bilirubin level in the blood exceeds 2.5 milligrams per deciliter, the yellow skin discoloration of jaundice can be seen. It is apparent first at the bottom of the tongue and later throughout the skin. Jaundice is sometimes associated with itching, presumably because of the deposition of bilirubin under the skin.

Treatment and Therapy

The treatment of jaundice depends on its cause. The first step is to determine whether there is an excess of conjugated bilirubin or unconjugated bilirubin. High levels of unconjugated bilirubin suggest an increase in red blood cell breakdown, known as hemolysis. This condition can be confirmed by examination of a peripheral blood smear and other laboratory studies. Most cases of hemolysis are the result of another underlying cause, such as infection or drugs. Hemolysis can also result from the body's immune system attacking its own red blood cells. Unconjugated bilirubin is also elevated in inherited disorders such as Gilbert's syndrome and Crigler-Najjar syndrome. These disorders are usually detected in early childhood.

Excess conjugated bilirubin, on the other hand, suggests a blockage in the biliary tree, which can be attributable to gallstones or, less commonly, a tumor. Gallstones can be confirmed with ultrasonography and may require surgery if they cause symptoms. Rarer causes of blockage in the biliary tree include strictures and sclerosing cholangitis. Disease of the liver itself can also result in high levels of conjugated bilirubin, but oftentimes both types of bilirubin are elevated. Such diseases include viral hepatitis (hepatitis A, B, or C), as well as alcohol and drug-induced hepatitis.

—*Ahmad Kamal, M.D.*

See also Cirrhosis; Gallbladder cancer; Gallbladder diseases; Hepa-

---

Information on Jaundice

Causes: Excess of pigment bilirubin resulting from various liver or blood disorders, gallstones, tumors, infection (e.g., hepatitis), or certain drugs

Symptoms: Yellowing of skin and whites of eyes, dark urine, itchy skin

Duration: Acute

Treatments: Depends on cause; may include surgery to remove gallstones or tumors

---

titis; Jaundice, neonatal; Liver; Liver disorders; Signs and symptoms; Stones.

For Further Information:

Arias, Irwin M., and James L. Boyer, eds. *The Liver: Biology and Pathobiology.* Hoboken, N.J.: John Wiley & Sons, 2009.

Casey, Georgina. "Jaundice: An Excess of Bilirubin." *Kai Tiaki Nursing New Zealand* 19, no. 1 (February, 2013): 20–24.

Kasper, Dennis L., et al., eds. *Harrison's Principles of Internal Medicine.* 16th ed. New York: McGraw-Hill, 2005.

Manning, Donal, and Kevin N. Ives. "What's New in Neonatal Jaundice." *Infant* 8, no. 5 (September, 2012): 137–141.

Palmer, Melissa. *Dr. Melissa Palmer's Guide to Hepatitis and Liver Disease.* Rev. ed. Garden City Park, N.Y.: Avery, 2004.

Rosenblum, Laurie. "Jaundice." *Health Library*, June 24, 2013.

Sargent, Suzanne, and Michelle Clayton. "Adult Jaundice—The Pathophysiology, Classification, and Causes." *Gastrointestinal Nursing* 9, no. 4 (May, 2011): 34–40.

JAW WIRING
Procedure

Anatomy or system affected: Bones, gums, mouth, musculoskeletal system, teeth

Specialties and related fields: Dentistry, emergency medicine, nutrition, orthodontics, plastic surgery, speech pathology

Definition: A surgical procedure in which the upper and lower teeth are brought closely together and secured with wire in order to immobilize the jaw.

Key terms:

arch bar: a pliable piece of metal with small hooked attachments; one is fitted along the upper teeth, another is fitted along the lower teeth, the two pieces are connected to the teeth with wires, and other wires are looped around the hooks and brought together to prevent jaw movement

facial edema: swelling of the facial tissue

intermaxillary fixation: the medical term for jaw wiring

mandible: the lower jawbone

maxilla: the upper jawbone

oral hygiene: care of the teeth and mouth

orthognathic surgery: jaw reconstruction

reduction: the restoration of a fractured bone to its normal position

zygoma: the cheekbone

Indications and Procedures

Jaw wiring, also known as maxillomandibular fixation, is often necessary to repair fractures in the jaw. The principles of treatment for facial fractures, in which bones need to be lined up and held in position until healing takes place, are the same as for a fractured arm or leg. Whereas an arm or leg fracture is reduced and casted to hold the bones in proper alignment, however, this method cannot be used for fractures of the face. Instead, once the fractures have been reduced (the bones have been restored to their proper positions), the jaws are wired shut to prevent the displacement of bone or bone fragments until they have healed.

Fractures of the face can involve any of the facial bones. The lower jawbone (mandible) is the most commonly fractured facial bone. Nevertheless, the upper jawbone (maxilla), the cheekbone (zygoma), the nasal bones, or the orbits (formed from bones of the cranium and face around the eyes) may also suffer fractures. A fracture may involve an individual bone or a combination of bones. One of the most common causes of facial fractures is blunt trauma. A blow to the face, the impact from an automobile or motorcycle accident, and a gunshot wound to the face are some examples of such trauma.

When considering fractures of the face, more than simply the bony structures must be evaluated. The skeletal structure encapsulates and protects organs that are vital to the functions of seeing, breathing, eating, talking, and swallowing. Early identification and treatment of fractures of the face are necessary to maintain maximum function of these delicate organs. Therefore, even though facial fractures and related injuries to soft tissue are seldom fatal, they must be treated immediately, since improper care could result in disfigurement, permanent sensory impairment, and lifelong disabilities.

In addition to facial fractures, jaw wiring is sometimes performed to correct malformations of the facial bones, certain birth defects, and acquired disfigurements as a result of trauma or growth-related imperfections. At times, jaw wiring is performed to correct malformations that have caused headaches, chewing disorders, and breathing and speech impairments. This type of surgery is referred to as orthognathic or jaw reconstruction surgery, part of which may involve jaw wiring. This procedure may also be performed as a weight-loss treatment for obese persons.

When a patient is hospitalized for elective facial surgery involving jaw wiring, or intermaxillary fixation, ample time can be given to preparing the patient for the surgical procedure and both preoperative and postoperative care. For the patient who sustains facial trauma, however, the same opportunity for surgical preparation may not be possible.

Facial fractures can often be reduced and immobilized by jaw wiring on the day of the injury. When there is marked facial edema (swelling), when other serious injuries are present, or when the person has eaten within a certain period of time prior to the trauma, however, the surgery will need to be delayed until a general anesthetic can be administered safely and the patient's condition has stabilized to the point that the surgical procedure can be tolerated.

The purpose of jaw wiring is to reduce and stabilize the fracture in such a manner that proper alignment of the bone will be maintained until it has healed. If the surgery is for jaw reconstruction, then the bone is fractured and positioned by the surgeon. These surgical fractures also require stabilization so that they will heal in the intended position. Interosseous wiring (the wiring of one portion of bone to another) using stainless steel wire may be necessary to maintain proper bone alignment. Sometimes, compression plates are used to secure the bones together. At other times, a bite block splint is inserted between the teeth to provide stabilization. This splint resembles a denture plate. An appliance called an external fixation device may be needed to keep the bones in proper alignment until they are healed.

If the patient wears dentures, then the denture plates are wired to the bone, the lower plate to the mandible, and the upper plate to the maxilla, prior to the jaw-wiring procedure. If the patient has no teeth at all, a bite block splint must be wired to the mandible and the maxilla, similar to the way in which dentures would be wired into place.

Jaw wiring is accomplished by first attaching arch bars to the base of the teeth. Arch bars are pliable pieces of metal with small hooked attachments on one side. They come in precut lengths and can also be cut to fit the individual's mouth. One fits along the base of the lower dental arch, and the other fits along the base of the upper dental arch. Thin pieces of stainless-steel wire are passed around the base of each tooth and brought out, then hooked around the arch bar and twisted firmly into place to secure the arch bar itself. The wires are cut, and their edges are tucked down between the teeth to prevent them from poking into gum or cheek tissue. If the patient wears dentures, the arch bar is either wired or glued to the denture plate with a special glue before the plate is wired to the bone structure.

Once the arch bars are positioned and secured, then special rubber bands are drawn around the hooked attachments from the upper to the lower bar. These bands are what actually hold the jaw tightly together. They are usually replaced with thin wires a few days after surgery, when the danger of nausea and vomiting have passed. Wire cutters need to be kept within easy reach at all times, in the event of vomiting. Should this happen, only the wires that hold the teeth together are clipped, and they will need to be reapplied by the physician.

Uses and Complications

Until the 1970s, orthognathic surgery carried a purely cosmetic connotation among the general public. Gradually, with surgical practice, documentation, research, and reports of the results of orthognathic surgery, people have come to understand the importance of such surgery in terms of proper physical functioning, as well as psychological and social functioning. Surgical reconstruction of the face can produce amazing results, but it also comes with a price. The process sometimes takes several years and teamwork by dentists, orthodontists, oral and/or plastic surgeons, and sometimes even psychiatrists to achieve these results. It can also be very costly because some insurance companies still consider orthodontia and corrective surgery cosmetic rather than functional and do not accept claims for these services.

Whatever the reason for jaw wiring, this process involves much more than a simple surgical procedure. Patients are usually hospitalized. Many of them are young, and others have had little hospital experience and may be anxious about the outcome. Lack of family support or financial concerns may increase this anxiety. Other injuries may be present in addition to the facial ones, some of which could be life-threatening and need to be attended to first.

Since jaw wiring usually means that the jaws are tightly wired shut, careful immediate postoperative monitoring by a nurse is needed to ensure that respiratory functioning is adequate, nausea and vomiting are controlled, mouth care is performed, nutritional intake of an all-liquid diet is satisfactory, and facial swelling and pain are reported to the surgeon, if necessary.

Before being discharged from the hospital, patients need to be shown proper mouth care techniques. Primary among them is the use of an electrical appliance that delivers pulsating jets of water, saline, or a mouth care solution to areas between the teeth and under the gum line. It rinses out food debris and harmful bacteria from the mouth. Mouth care is very important during the period of time when the jaws are wired, so that healing is promoted and dental caries (cavities) are prevented.

Good nutritional habits are also important during this time. Since the patient's diet must be liquid in form, concerns about weight loss, adequate food variations, appropriate nutrients for healing, management of food preparation, and possible nutritional supplementation need to be addressed and resolved before a patient is discharged. Patients should have a written diet plan to use at home. Medications needed for pain and nausea, vitamins, and sometimes antibiotics will also need to be obtained in liquid form. Instructions regarding how to administer emergency care, when to call the doctor, and how to cut wires if vomiting occurs must be given.

Follow-up care with the physician will be needed to evaluate progress and to arrange for the clipping of wires and the removal of the arch bars. These procedures are usually done in the physician's office.

Perspective and Prospects

It is likely that attempts were made to treat fractures of the face from the time of the cave dwellers, but no records of such attempts were kept. The earliest known records relating to the treatment of jaw fractures are found in the Smith Papyrus, which is thought to have been written about 25 to 30 centuries BCE. The author advises against the treatment of compound (open) fractures but recommends that the dislocation of the mandible be treated. Definite proof of the art of dentistry was found among the Etruscans, an ancient people living in what is now Tuscany and part of Umbria, in about 600 to 500 BCE: Skeletal remains with the teeth bound with gold wire have been discovered.

In the time of Hippocrates (ca. 460–ca. 370 BCE), the Greek physician known as the founder of medicine, writings bear evidence that facial injuries or fractures were treated with some method of wiring. A section of the Corpus Hippocraticum reads:

If the jaw is broken right across, which rarely happens, one should adjust it in the manner described [one thumb inside the mouth and the fingers outside, for reduction]. After adjustment one should fasten the teeth together as was described above [with gold wire or, lacking that, with linen thread], for this will contribute greatly to immobility, especially if one joins them properly and fastens the ends as they should be.

The use of bandages to treat facial maladies was also practiced by some ancient cultures. Galen of Pergamum (129–ca. 199 CE) and Soranus of Ephesus (98–138 CE) describe such methods. An ancient manuscript by Soranus of Ephesus illustrates the types of bandages used by the ancients to treat head and facial injuries.

Greek writings even suggested dietary practices in cases of jaw injury. When the mandible was fractured, liquid nourishment was recommended, and solid foods were withheld until bone healing was definite. Patients were also advised not to talk for a certain period of time.

In the thirteenth century, the Italian surgeon Guglielmo da Saliceto (ca. 1210–ca. 1277), also known as William of Saliceto, performed one of the first documented cases of jaw wiring, attaching the teeth of the lower jaw to the corresponding teeth of the upper jaw. He used linen and silk thread, twisting them together and then waxing the twist to keep it in place. In the next several centuries, however, the medieval literature lacks any references to the management of facial bone fractures. Whether the work of earlier surgeons was unknown or whether such surgical practices remained standard during these years, without notable progress, remains a mystery. It was toward the end of the nineteenth century that the development of intermaxillary fixation by wiring was developed by an American physician and dentist, Thomas Lewis Gilmer (1849–1931).

Many great names are associated with the twentieth century contributions to improved and refined methods of jaw-wiring techniques and patient care during this process. Much was learned about the nature of facial fractures themselves from the work of French physician Rene LeFort. LeFort conducted a series of experiments in the early twentieth century to study facial fracture combinations. He subjected cadaver skulls to violent blows under many conditions and at various angles and then described the outcomes.

A survey of the progress made in jaw wiring would be incomplete without recognition of the impact that antibiotic therapy, advanced anesthetic techniques, and blood replacement therapy have had on this procedure and on medical science as a whole. These achievements paved the way for open surgical procedures and internal fixation, which have led to dramatic results and remarkable changes for individuals undergoing jaw wiring.

—*Karen A. Mattern*

See also Bones and the skeleton; Dentistry; Emergency medicine; Fracture and dislocation; Fracture repair; Hyperadiposis; Nutrition; Obesity; Oral and maxillofacial surgery; Orthodontics; Orthopedic surgery; Orthopedics; Orthopedics, pediatric; Plastic surgery.

For Further Information:

Fonseca, Raymond J., et al., eds. *Oral and Maxillofacial Trauma*. 3d ed. St. Louis, Mo.: Saunders/Elsevier, 2005.

Jones, Pamela. "Corrective Jaw Surgery." *Health Library*, March 15, 2013.

Niamtu, Joseph, III. "Cosmetic Oral and Maxillofacial Surgery Options." *Journal of the American Dental Association* 131, no. 6 (June, 2000): 756–764.

Proffit, William R., Raymond P. White, Jr., and David M. Sarver, eds. *Contemporary Treatment of Dentofacial Deformity*. St. Louis, Mo.: Mosby, 2003.

Rahpima, A., and A. Halaj Mofrad. "The Use of Maxillomandibular Fixation Screws with Essig Wiring in the Treatment of Symphyseal Fracture of Deep Bite Patients." *Journal of Maxillofacial and Oral Surgery* 8, no. 4 (2009): 375–376.

Reyneke, Johan P. *Essentials of Orthognathic Surgery*. Chicago: Quintessence, 2003.

Salter, Robert Bruce. *Textbook of Disorders and Injuries of the Musculoskeletal System*. 3d ed. Baltimore: Williams & Wilkins, 1999.

Watts, V., S. Madick, J. Pepperney, and C. Petras. "When Your Patient Has Jaw Surgery." *RN* 48 (October, 1985): 44–47.

Yadav, Santosh Kumar, and Gopendra Deo. "Submental Intubation Including Extubation: Airway Complications of Maxillomandibular Fixation." *Case Reports in Anesthesiology* (2012): 1–3.

JOINT DISEASES. *See* ARTHRITIS.

JOINT REPLACEMENT. *See* ARTHROPLASTY; HIP REPLACEMENT.

JOINTS
Anatomy

Anatomy or system affected: Bones, knees, ligaments, musculoskeletal system, tendons

Specialties and related fields: Geriatrics and gerontology, orthopedic surgery, podiatry, radiology, rheumatology, sports medicine

Definition: The connection where two or more bones come together, which may or not allow a range of movement.

Key terms:

articulation: also known as the joint; the area where different bones of the skeleton connect for motion purposes of its body parts

biomechanics: the application of mechanical principles to the living body, specifically of forces used by muscles and gravity on the skeletal structure and how biomaterials such as collagen or elastin behave under those conditions

cartilage: a strong flexible connective tissue that lines the end of a bone at a joint, providing a cushioning effect, and supports the nose, ears, or bronchial tubes

ligament: a tough fibrous tissue supporting organs or connecting bones or cartilages at a joint

muscle: contractile tissue controlling movement of body parts through contraction and relaxation

tendon: tensile connective tissue that connects muscle to bone

Structure and Functions

In the musculoskeletal system, the joints are structures that connect individual bones while allowing some type of movement and mechanical support. This skeletal articulation holds together distinct bones with strong but flexible soft tissues that enable movement on components of the skeleton by muscles on opposite sides of the joint that contract or relax. Joints occur between bones but also appear between bones and cartilage, between bones and teeth, and between cartilages. Based on their anatomical location, they are grouped between the joints of the trunk and the upper or lower extremity. They can be classified structurally, functionally, or biomechanically.

Structurally, joints may be classified as cartilaginous, fibrous, bony, or synovial, based on the composition of how these bones connect to each other. A cartilaginous joint is connected by hyaline cartilage or fibrocartilage. A fibrous joint is connected by a collagen- and elastin-rich connective tissue. In a bony joint, there is a fusion between bones. Synovial joints are not directly connected but are found within a synovial cavity full of synovial fluid that lubricates and cushions the joint.

Strength and flexibility are important functional features of joints but also contradictory concepts in which greater joint strength translates into less flexibility and otherwise. Functionally, joints are ranked based on the degree of mobility rendered: immobility (synarthrosis), slight mobility (amphiarthrosis), and free mobility (diarthrosis). Synarthroses are the immovable joints such as those located between the plates of the skull. Amphiarthroses are joints that allow slight movement such as in the vertebrae. Diarthroses are joints that move freely and are also known as synovial joints. These include the joints in the shoulder, hip, knee, and elbow.

The most common mobile joints present in the body are the hinge joint, pivot joint, ball-and-socket joint, saddle joint, and ellipsoidal joint. Joints allow four types of movement: gliding, angular, circumduction, and rotation. The shape of bones and their articular surfaces, in addition to the ligaments and muscles intersecting the joint, determines the degree of movement permitted at a specific joint.

Biomechanically, joints can be characterized according to number and configuration of articulating elements with regard to the movement that they allow. Therefore, joints are subdivided as simple and compound based upon the number of partaking bones and into combinational and complex joints.

Disorders and Diseases

Problems with joints range from minor injuries (sprains) to serious or chronic joint disease. Age, use, and overuse can diminish joint function or deteriorate this structure further to become diseased. Genetics, direct trauma, misalignment, dislocation, and mechanical loads may also play a role in damaging joints.

Several inflammatory conditions can affect the joints. Synovitis is the inflammation of the lining of the synovial joint, the synovial membrane. The swelling of this membrane causes pain especially when the joint moves. Treatment consists of anti-inflammatory drugs; in addition, cortisone injections directly to the joint may be used. Elevated levels of uric acid that deposit as crystals in joints cause a painful inflammation known as gout. Lifestyle changes, such as reducing the intake of protein and fats, can help gout symptoms. Bursitis (such as tennis elbow) is the inflammation of the bursa that rests between a tendon and skin or between a tendon and bone. The symptoms include joint pain, tenderness, swelling, stiffness, or warmth around the joint. When bursitis is not infected, treatment involves rest, elevation, ice, massage therapy, pain medication, or anti-inflammatory drugs; infected bursitis demands antibiotic therapy.

"Arthritis" is a generic term for a group of chronic medical conditions affecting the joints. The most common one is osteoarthritis (OA), which is characterized by the progressive wearing down of the cartilage in the joints. The symptoms of this degenerative joint disease include swelling, deep aching pain that gets worse after exercise or rainy weather, limited movement, loss of flexibility, stiffness, and grinding of the joint during movement. OA treatment might include anti-inflammatory medications, pain medications, creams or ointments to rub on the joint, cortisone or hyaluronic acid injections, glucosamine and chondroitin, physical therapy, exercise, weight loss, and braces or orthotics to stabilize the affected joint. For those patients who do not respond well to those treatments, surgical interventions are available.

Soft tissue problems can be corrected surgically using soft tissue techniques. Replacing damaged or missing cartilage is known as cartilage restoration and is performed in younger arthritis patients. In arthroscopy, a small fiber-optic instrument is used to evaluate the inner joint surface, to clean out debris around a degenerative joint, to biopsy synovial membrane, or to reconstruct anatomic joint anomalies such as a torn meniscus, damaged cartilage, or a cruciate ligament. Arthroplasty, or joint replacement surgery, is performed when damage is too severe and realigning or reconstruction is needed in the defective joint. Sometimes a joint is damaged to the point that the bone cannot support a prosthetic device. In this case, arthrodesis, the surgical fusion of the bones, is required; although the joint will lose its flexibility, it will be stable and painless.

Another type of medical condition that afflicts the joints is rheumatoid arthritis (RA), an autoimmune disease. In RA, the body produces an immunocellular reaction that targets the joints and causes inflammation. RA is a chronic autoimmune inflammatory joint disease afflicting the lining of the joints, resulting in painful swelling that will cause bone erosion and joint deformities. Since it is a systemic disease, it may involve other internal organs (lungs, kidneys, heart, or eyes) as well. Some of the associated symptoms are low-grade fever, weight loss, fatigue, morning stiffness, muscle aches, weakness, loss of appetite, skin redness or inflammation, hand and foot deformities, and numbness or tingling. Joint loss may appear within the first couple of years after diagnosis. RA frequently involves a lifetime of treatments—medications, ex-

ercise, physical therapy, education, and sometimes surgery. Medications that alleviate RA include nonsteroidal anti-inflammatory drugs (NSAIDs), steroids, immunosuppressants, and disease-modifying antirheumatic drugs (DMARDs).

An anterior cruciate ligament (ACL) injury occurs when there is a stretch or tear of the knee. These tears might be complete or partial. Football, soccer, skiing, basketball, and martial arts are risky sports that may result in ACL tears. Surgery is required to stabilize and repair the knee. A meniscus repair is needed when this shock-absorbing material is harmed. A graft is done to replace a torn ACL. In an autograft, the surgeon takes material from the patient's own tendon to restore the injured ACL. In an allograft, the original tendon material is derived from a donor cadaver. Proper rehabilitation follows ACL replacement.

Perspective and Prospects

Joint disorders and diseases were well-known ailments to physicians of ancient Greece and Rome. Evidence of joint problems has been discovered in Egyptian mummies and Roman gladiators. Today, one of every five adults in the United States has some type of joint disease. It is the primary cause of work disability in the United States. Although genetics and traumatic injuries may have a negative impact on joint health, this is a multifactorial disease and, as such, early diagnosis and proper management is essential to improve quality of life. The prevalence of joint disease, however, does not translate into total inevitability. It is possible to conserve joint function and mobility when knowledge, preventive measures, and correct treatments are implemented.

Aging thins the cartilage, which will eventually cause joint pain, stiffness, or disability. Microtraumatic injuries lead to low levels of inflammation, which over time will destroy the protective cartilage at the joints. Excess weight damages the joints in the long run as well, especially the knees, which support body weight. The loss of muscle mass during aging causes the joints to overcompensate by absorbing more of the beating from daily activities and aggravating the affected site.

While damaged cartilage is hard to repair or regain, joint movement and agility can be kept by adopting some simple steps for strong joints today and in the future. Preventing joint injuries is the best solution. Weight loss can lower stress on joints. Good stretching improves flexibility, and minor pains are relieved by muscle movement. Exercise reduces stiffness of the joints, and varying fitness routines avoids overtaxing any one area. Muscle and ligament strength training protects joints from damage. Omega-3 fatty acids not only relieve joint pain symptoms but also reduce the inflammation levels that cause more pain. Vitamin D is a protective agent for joints because of its anti-inflammatory properties. The popularity of glucosamine to alleviate joint pain and disability has grown beyond the controversy about its effectiveness. Still, future research is needed to determine the therapeutic mechanisms of glucosamine. Although established treatments or surgical procedures might help slow down or halt joint disease progression following early detection, it is the collaborative efforts of patients and health care providers that can ultimately restore joint health, achieve optimal quality of life, and reduce the financial burden on society.

—*Ana Maria Rodriguez-Rojas, M.S.*

See also Arthritis; Bone disorders; Bones and the skeleton; Bursitis; Cartilage; Fracture and dislocation; Gout; Hip fracture repair; Hip replacement; Inflammation; Juvenile rheumatoid arthritis; Ligaments; Massage; Muscle sprains, spasms, and disorders; Orthopedic surgery; Orthopedics; Orthopedics, pediatric; Osteoarthritis; Pain management; Physical rehabilitation; Rheumatoid arthritis; Rheumatology; Tendon disorders; Tendon repair; Tendons.

For Further Information:
Blockyz, J. A., et al. "The Effects of Oral Glucosamine on Joint Health: Is a Change in Research Approach Needed?" *Osteoarthritis and Cartilage* 18, no. 1 (January, 2010): 5–11.

Evans, Philip. "Aging, Degeneration, and Trauma in Joints." *Physiotherapy* 84, no. 11 (November, 1998): 564–566.

Firestein, Gary S., et al., eds. *Kelley's Textbook of Rheumatology*. 8th ed. Philadelphia: Elsevier, 2008.

Geipel, Udo. "Pathogenic Organisms in Hip Joint Infections." *International Journal of Medical Sciences* 6, no. 5 (September, 2009): 234–240.

Harms, S., et al. "Obesity Increases the Likelihood of Total Joint Replacement Surgery Among Younger Adults." *International Orthopaedics* 31, no. 1 (February, 2007): 23–26.

Huscher, D., et al. "Cost of Illness in Rheumatoid Arthritis, Ankylosing Spondylitis, Psoriatic Arthritis, and Systemic Lupus Erythematosus in Germany." *Annals of Rheumatic Diseases* 69, no. 9 (September, 2006): 1175–1183.

Leach, Robert E. "Sprain." *Health Library*, March 18, 2013.

Leondes, Cornelius T. *Biomechanical Systems: Musculoskeletal Models and Techniques*. Boca Raton, Fla.: CRC Press, 2001.

Miller, Carl W., et al. "Health Status, Physical Disability, and Obesity Among Adult Mississippians with Chronic Joint Symptoms or Doctor-Diagnosed Arthritis: Findings from the Behavioral Risk Factor Surveillance System, 2003." *Preventing Chronic Disease* 5, no. 3 (July, 2008): 1–9.

"Osteoarthritis." *MedlinePlus*, September 26, 2011.

"Rheumatoid Arthritis." *Health Library*, September 30, 2012.

Stillman, Barry C., et al. "Knee Joint Mobility and Position Sense in Healthy Young Adults." *Physiotherapy* 88, no. 9 (September, 2002): 553–560.

Watkins, James. *Structure and Function of the Musculoskeletal System*. 2d ed. Champaign, Ill.: Human Kinetics, 2010.

JUVENILE RHEUMATOID ARTHRITIS
Disease/Disorder

Anatomy or system affected: Back, circulatory system, eyes, heart, immune system, joints, musculoskeletal system

Specialties and related fields: Exercise physiology, family medicine, immunology, ophthalmology, orthopedics, pediatrics, psychology

Definition: A usually chronic autoimmune disease of unknown cause, characterized by joint swelling, pain, and sometimes the destruction of joints.

Key terms:

articular: of or relating to a joint or joints

autoimmune disease: a disease in which the body's immune system attacks itself

manifestation: an outward or visible expression

systemic: relating to the body as a whole, not limited to a particular part

Causes and Symptoms

Juvenile rheumatoid arthritis is an autoimmune disease of children that attacks the joints. It appears in three different subgroups that vary according to severity and type of extra-articular manifestation. Other significant variations within these subgroups include age at disease onset, the sex of affected children, genetic predisposition, and prognosis.

The first major clinical pattern is systemic disease, which includes about 10 percent of children with juvenile rheumatoid arthritis. This type has the most dramatic onset and is the least common form of the illness. It affects boys more than girls and can begin at any age. The most characteristic manifestations are high, intermittent fevers and a temporary red rash occurring during periods of fever. Occasionally, more serious complications are involved. In some cases, systemic onset is marked by polyarthritis, which affects large and small multiple joints, and moves subsequently to disease of the knee or hip with no further involvement of other joints. The systemic complaints, which are often sudden and explosive in nature, may recur months or years later. Some children with systemic onset, however, never develop lasting arthritis.

Polyarticular juvenile rheumatoid arthritis, the second subgroup, includes children in whom five or more joints have been involved in the first six months of illness. It affects more girls than boys and can begin at any age. This subgroup includes about 40 percent of children with juvenile rheumatoid arthritis and is frequently mild. Within this subgroup exists a smaller subgroup, which includes about 5 percent of children with juvenile rheumatoid arthritis and rarely begins before the eighth birthday. The arthritis is often severe, with joint destruction occurring within the first year. Polyarthritis may involve swelling of the joints over a period of time, in which pain is not a prominent feature, or a sudden articular swelling, in which pain can be severe. Weight-bearing joints, usually knees and ankles, are often involved initially.

The third major subgroup is pauciarticular disease, which involves about 50 percent of all children with juvenile rheumatoid arthritis. In the initial episode of this type, only one joint is involved. More joints usually become involved within a few weeks or months, although occasionally involvement is restricted to one joint. Most often, the knee is the primary

---

Information on Juvenile Rheumatoid Arthritis

Causes: Unknown

Symptoms: High, intermittent fevers; temporary red rash occurring during periods of fever; joint pain; occasionally polyarthritis

Duration: Acute and recurrent

Treatments: Alleviation of symptoms through medication (anti-inflammatory drugs), physical and occupational therapy, orthopedic treatment (e.g., splinting)

area, with the ankles and hips being the sites of minimal involvement.

Treatment and Therapy

The first step in treating juvenile rheumatoid arthritis is the identification of the child's problems and potential problems, which include active joint disease, disabilities, ocular disease, growth retardation, and psychosocial disability. Because the cause of chronic arthritis is not known, treatment suppresses the symptoms and does not cure the disease itself.

Drug therapy is used to relieve inflammatory pain and immobility. The main type of medication used are the standard nonsteroidal anti-inflammatory drugs (NSAIDs), such as aspirin, ibuprofen, and naproxen. If NSAIDs are ineffective, another pharmacological intervention is disease-modifying antirheumatic drugs (DMARDs), of which the most common is methotrexate. DMARDs slow the progression of the arthritis, but take a long time to act. Another powerful drug treatment is corticosteroids, administered either by mouth or injected directly into the joint; these are used sparingly, however, because of their serious side effects for children..

Physical and occupational therapy attempts to maintain strength and stamina and to preserve and increase the range of motion in the joints and in supporting muscles. All children with significant joint involvement should have a daily home program of activities and exercises directed toward the prevention and correction of disabilities that can be supervised by their parents. In addition to exercise, the program consists of the use of moist heat, adequate rest, and proper diet, which are aimed at maintaining strength. Children with severe disabilities may need hospitalization for intensive therapy.

Beyond physical therapy, orthopedic treatment for the joints may include splinting to preserve or repair joint motion. In the rehabilitation of older children who have suffered serious damage, the replacement of affected joints may provide good results.

Juvenile rheumatoid arthritis offers significant challenges for families. The family pediatrician or physician must act as teacher and adviser both to the patient and to family members. Other health care professionals who may be important to the care of a child with juvenile rheumatoid arthritis are ophthalmologists, pediatric nurses, social workers, and psychiatrists, as well as the child's schoolteachers.

Perspective and Prospects

George R. Still's finding in 1896 that juvenile rheumatoid arthritis includes at least three distinct joint afflictions first brought the subgroups to the attention of the medical profession and has fostered a greater understanding of the disease; in fact, systemic arthritis was originally known as Still's disease.

For most children with juvenile rheumatoid arthritis, early diagnosis and appropriate therapy point to a good prognosis. Of the children with systemic onset, at least 75 percent will enjoy a good outcome, whereas the rest may suffer severe arthritis, possibly resulting in disability. Between 80 and 90 percent of children with polyarthritis escape without permanent joint damage, although the disease itself may be chronic. The overall prospects for children with pauciarticular disease are not known.

Although most children suffering from juvenile rheumatoid arthritis eventually outgrow it, it is difficult for most parents to accept that accurate prediction for the ultimate outcome for their child is impossible. Nevertheless, a positive attitude, careful medical management, physical therapy, and psychological support can improve the quality of life for all children with juvenile rheumatoid arthritis.

—*Mary Hurd*

See also Arthritis; Autoimmune disorders; Exercise; Joints; Massage; Musculoskeletal system; Orthopedics, pediatric.

For Further Information:

Arthritis Foundation. http://www.arthritis.org.

Behrman, Richard E., Robert M. Kliegman, and Hal B. Jenson, eds. *Nelson Textbook of Pediatrics*. 19th ed. Philadelphia: Saunders/Elsevier, 2011.

Brewer, Earl J., Jr., and Kathy Cochran Angel. *The Arthritis Sourcebook*. 3d ed. Los Angeles: Lowell House, 2000.

Brewer, Earl J., Jr., Edward H. Giannini, and Donald A. Person. *Juvenile Rheumatoid Arthritis*. 2d ed. Philadelphia: W. B. Saunders, 1982.

"Childhood Arthritis." *Centers for Disease Control and Prevention*, August 1, 2011.

Judd, Sandra J. *Childhood Diseases and Disorders Sourcebook: Basic Consumer Health Information About the Physical, Mental, and Developmental Health of Pre-Adolescent Children*. 2d ed. Detroit, Mich.: Omnigraphics, 2009.

Melvin, Jeanne L., and Virginia Wright, eds. *Pediatric Rheumatic Diseases*. Vol. 3. Bethesda, Md.: American Occupational Therapy Association, 2000.

Merenstein, Gerald B., David W. Kaplan, and Adam A. Rosenberg. *Handbook of Pediatrics*. 18th ed. Stamford, Conn.: Appleton & Lange, 1999.

Parker, James N., and Philip M. Parker, eds. *Juvenile Rheumatoid Arthritis: The Official Patient's Sourcebook*. San Diego, Calif.: Icon Health, 2002.

"Questions and Answers About Juvenile Arthritis." *National Institute of Arthritis and Musculoskeletal and Skin Diseases*, October, 2012.

Rudis, Jacquelyn. "Juvenile Rheumatoid Arthritis." *Health Library*, February 5, 2013.

KAPOSI'S SARCOMA

Disease/Disorder

Anatomy or system affected: Intestines, liver, lungs, skin
Specialties and related fields: Internal medicine, oncology
Definition: A disease in which cancer cells are found in tissues, causing lesions on the skin and/or mucous membranes and spreading to other organs in the body.

Causes and Symptoms

It is uncertain whether Kaposi's sarcoma is actually cancer because, unlike cancer, it arises from several cell types. Although there is no accepted staging system for Kaposi's sarcoma, patients are grouped by the type that they have. The three types are classic, epidemic, and recurrent.

Classic Kaposi's sarcoma usually occurs in older men of Mediterranean heritage. It progresses slowly (over ten to fifteen years), with progression bringing lower limb swelling, impeded blood flow, possible spread to other organs, and other types of cancer in later life. Epidemic Kaposi's sarcoma, found in people with acquired immunodeficiency syndrome (AIDS), is a more virulent, fast-spreading, and fatal form, with symptoms of painless, either flat or raised, pink or purple plaques on the skin and mucosal surfaces. This type usually spreads to the lungs, liver, spleen, lymph nodes, digestive tract, and other internal organs. Recurrent Kaposi's sarcoma comes back after it has been treated in the original area where it started. Sometimes, it appears in another part of the body.

Treatment and Therapy

Four kinds of treatment are usually used: surgery (taking out

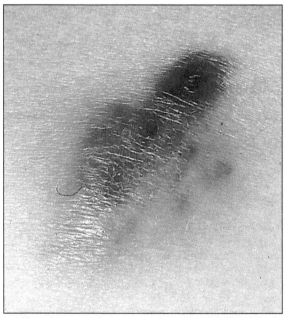

A Kaposi's sarcoma lesion on a patient with AIDS. (SIU School of Medicine)

**Information on
Kaposi's Sarcoma**

Causes: Unknown; epidemic type found in patients with AIDS
Symptoms: Flat or raised, pink or purple plaques on the skin and mucosal surfaces; lower limb swelling, impeded blood flow
Duration: Ranges from acute to chronic with recurrent episodes
Treatments: Surgery, chemotherapy, external beam radiation therapy, biological therapy

---

the cancer), chemotherapy (using drugs to kill cancer cells), external beam radiation therapy (using high-dose X rays to kill cancer cells), and biological therapy (using the body's immune system to fight the cancer).

Classic Kaposi's sarcoma may be treated by radiation therapy, local excision (cutting out the lesion and some of the tissue around it), systemic chemotherapy (in which the drug enters the bloodstream, travels through the body, and kills cancer cells outside the original site), intralesional chemotherapy (in which the drug is injected into the lesion), or a combination of these treatments.

Epidemic Kaposi's sarcoma is treated by surgery, including electrodesiccation and curettage (burning the lesion and removing it with a sharp instrument) and cryotherapy (killing the tumor by freezing it). It can also be treated with chemotherapy or biological therapy.

Perspective and Prospects

Until the early 1980s, Kaposi's sarcoma was found mainly in older male patients who had received organ transplants. The AIDS epidemic gave rise to cases in many other populations, such as homosexual men and African men. Recovery depends on the type of Kaposi's sarcoma, age, general health, and whether the condition is accompanied by AIDS.

—Patricia A. Ainsa, M.P.H., Ph.D.

See also Acquired immunodeficiency syndrome (AIDS); Biopsy; Cancer; Chemotherapy; Cryosurgery; Lesions; Malignancy and metastasis; Oncology; Opportunistic infections; Radiation therapy; Sarcoma.

For Further Information:
Alan, Rick. "Kaposi's Sarcoma." *Health Library*, April 10, 2013.
Dollinger, Malin, et al. *Everyone's Guide to Cancer Therapy*. 5th ed. Kansas City, Mo.: Andrews McMeel, 2008.
Feigal, Ellen G., Alexandra M. Levine, and Robert J. Biggar. *AIDS-Related Cancers and Their Treatment*. New York: Marcel Dekker, 2000.
Gottlieb, Geoffrey J., and A. Bernard Ackerman. *Kaposi's Sarcoma: A Text and Atlas*. Philadelphia: Lea & Febiger, 1988.
"Kaposi's Sarcoma." *MedlinePlus*, October 6, 2012.
Parker, James N., and Philip M. Parker, eds. *The Official Patient's Sourcebook on Kaposi's Sarcoma*. San Diego, Calif.: Icon Health, 2003.
Rutherford, George W., and James O. Kahn, eds. *The Epidemiology of AIDS-Related Kaposi's Sarcoma: A Symposium Sponsored by the San Francisco Center for AIDS Research, San Francisco,*

California, September 29, 1989. New York: Raven Press, 1990.

Shepherd, Frances A. *Management of Kaposi's Sarcoma Associated with Human Immunodeficiency Virus Infection*. Ottawa, Ont.: Health and Welfare Canada, 1991.

"What Is Kaposi Sarcoma?" *American Cancer Society*, February 20, 2013.

Karyotyping

Procedure

Also known as: Chromosome analysis

Anatomy or system affected: Cells

Specialties and related fields: Cytology, embryology, genetics, neonatology, obstetrics, oncology, pathology, perinatology

Definition: The photographing of all the chromosomes of a single cell to identify extra, missing, or abnormal chromosomes.

Key terms:

autosomes: all the chromosomes, except for the sex chromosomes

karyotype: an analysis of all the chromosomes in a single cell

mitosis: cell division

nondisjunction: a malfunction of mitosis, resulting in cells with an abnormal chromosome number

The Cell and Chromosomes

Every cell in the human body—except for red blood cells—contains a nucleus with rod-shaped structures called "chromosomes." The chromosomes, in turn, contain the genes, which are the units that transmit heredity from parents to offspring.

The forty-six individual chromosomes in a human cell exist as twenty-three pairs of so-called homologues. Homologous chromosomes are similar in size and appearance. The first twenty-two pairs of homologues are referred to as "autosomes," while pair number twenty-three contains two dissimilar chromosomes known as the X and Y chromosomes, which determine sex. Sperm and egg cells each have twenty-three chromosomes, or half the usual number. When a sperm fertilizes an egg, the normal chromosome number (forty-six) is reestablished in the first cell of life, the zygote.

Cells reproduce by mitosis, a process of simple division, the result being two identical daughter cells, each containing forty-six chromosomes. Since chromosomes contain the genetic information, it follows that mitosis must proceed with precision every time a cell divides. During the earliest stages of embryonic development, however, mistakes sometimes occur and the cells wind up with more or fewer chromosomes. This malfunction of mitosis is called "nondisjunction," and the incorrect number of chromosomes is passed to all the cells in the developing embryo. This leads to a variety of abnormal conditions, all of which can be diagnosed with the procedure known as "karyotyping."

Procedure and Interpretation

A karyotype is an analysis of all the chromosomes in a single cell. The prefix "karyo-" refers to the nucleus, the part of the cell where chromosomes reside; the suffix "-type" means characterization. Thus, a karyotype is a characterization of a nucleus in terms of its chromosomes.

Karyotypes are performed on embryos to diagnose chromosomal abnormalities and on adults who suspect chromosomal aberrations that could be passed on to offspring. Although a karyotype can be constructed from almost any cell in the body that contains a nucleus, it is most often performed on white blood cells, which are easily harvested from a routine blood sample.

The procedure is simple. Once the blood is collected, the white cells are separated from the red. In the laboratory, the white blood cells are then stimulated to undergo mitosis. At the stage of mitosis when the chromosomes are most visible, the process is chemically halted. The chromosomes are then stained to make them more visible, after which they are photographed and the individual chromosomes cut out and rearranged as homologous pairs in descending order by size. Each pair of chromosomes is also given a number, the largest pair being designated number 1. Then, another photograph is taken of the chromosomes in the rearranged format. The result is the karyotype. The entire process, from collecting the blood sample to growing the cells to preparing the karyotype, takes from one to three weeks.

Once the karyotype has been created, it is ready to be interpreted by a cytogeneticist, an expert in the study of chromosomes. The most common disorders visible with karyotyping are Down syndrome, an extra copy of chromosome number 21; Klinefelter syndrome, a male with an extra X chromosome, resulting in sterility and the development of some feminine features; and Turner syndrome, a female missing an X chromosome, resulting in sterility and a masculine body build.

Perspective and Prospects

Karyotyping was first reported in the mid-1950s when chromosomes were examined in fetal cells collected from amniotic fluid. This was the beginning of the discipline of prenatal genetic diagnosis. At the time, there was no ultrasound to guide the needle through the amniotic membrane, which increased the risk of damaging the fetus. The karyotyping itself required four or five weeks of cell culture and was not always successful.

Today, karyotyping is commonly used to diagnose chromosomal abnormalities in both fetuses and live individuals. It is considered an absolutely safe procedure, the only risks being those inherent in penetrating the amniotic sac with a needle. Also, although the advent of ultrasound has greatly reduced the risk to the fetus, the possibility always exists of inadvertently collecting maternal cells when the mother's tissues are penetrated.

Since the 1970s, dyes have been added to karyotypes to highlight the chromosomes for identification purposes. Today, when abnormalities are found on a karyotype, researchers can then examine the individual genes for deletions and duplications using molecular cytogenic procedures, such as fluorescence in situ hybridization (FISH) and comparative genomic hybridization (CGH). For instance, in the multicolor FISH method called "spectral karyotyping (SKY)," fluorescent dyes highlight specific regions of the chromosomes. A device called an "interferometer" is used to detect slight color variations invisible to the human eye and then assign visible colors to the homologous chromosomes. The SKY method is superior to traditional karyotyping with chemical stains because it more clearly identifies chromosomes that are damaged or that contain fragments of other, nonhomologous chromosomes.

Thanks to advances in computer technology and the Human Genome Project, digital karyotyping was developed in 2002. Unlike traditional karyotyping, digital karyotyping maps representative DNA fragments, known as "tags," and computationally models these tags to determine whether abnormalities are present in the sample. This genomic method is now being used for cancer research, among other applications.
—*Robert T. Klose, Ph.D.*

See also Amniocentesis; Biopsy; Cells; Chorionic villus sampling; Cytology; DNA and RNA; Gene therapy; Genetic engineering; Genetics and inheritance; Laboratory tests.

For Further Information:

A.D.A.M. Medical Encyclopedia. "Karyotyping." *MedlinePlus*, November 2, 2012.

Harris, Henry. *The Cells of the Body: A History of Somatic Cell Genetics*. Cold Spring Harbor, N.Y.: Cold Spring Harbor Laboratory Press, 1995.

Krogh, David. *Biology: A Guide to the Natural World*. 5th ed. San Francisco: Benjamin Cummings, 2010.

McGraw-Hill Concise Encyclopedia of Science and Technology. 6th ed. New York: McGraw-Hill, 2009.

National Human Genome Research Institute. "Frequently Asked Questions About Genetic Testing." *National Institutes of Health, US Department of Health and Human Services*, October 13, 2011.

National Human Genome Research Institute. "Spectral Karyotyping (SKY)." *National Institutes of Health, US Department of Health and Human Services*, April 30, 2013.

O'Connor, Clare. "Karyotyping for Chromosomal Abnormalities." *Nature Education*, 2008.

Tian-Li Wang, et al. "Digital Karyotyping: An Update of Its Applications in Cancer." *Molecular Diagnosis & Therapy* 10, no. 4 (2006): 231–237.

Vogel, F., and A. G. Motulsky. *Vogel and Motulsky's Human Genetics: Problems and Approaches*. 4th rev. ed. New York: Springer, 2010.

KAWASAKI DISEASE

Disease/Disorder

Also known as: Kawasaki syndrome, mucocutaneous lymph node syndrome (MLNS)

Anatomy or system affected: Brain, blood vessels, circulatory system, heart, immune system, lymphatic system, mouth, skin

Specialties and related fields: Cardiology, family medicine, immunology, pediatrics

Definition: An inflammatory disease that affects numerous organs and systems in the body and typically occurs in children under the age of five.

Causes and Symptoms

The exact cause of Kawasaki disease is unknown. Approximately 80 percent of the victims are aged five and under. Some doctors believe that the disease may be an allergic reaction to certain types of infection. Others think that it is produced by a virus or bacterium. Some researchers believe that the source is an interaction of T cells, white blood cells that help regulate the immune system's response to infections, with toxins produced by bacteria.

Kawasaki disease begins rather abruptly with a fever that persists for five days or longer and can reach 104 degrees Fahrenheit. A red, patchy rash typically spreads over the chest and genital area and may cover the entire body. The lips, mouth, tongue, and throat become very red. The lymph nodes in the neck may be swollen, as well as the hands and feet. The hands, feet, eyes, and mucous membrane linings of the eyelids turn red. These symptoms may be accompanied by diarrhea, vomiting, stomach pain, joint pain, and irritability. As the fever subsides, there is a characteristic peeling of the skin from the fingers and toes. The symptoms associated with Kawasaki disease may last for two weeks up to three months.

Treatment and Therapy

Kawasaki disease should be treated as soon as it is diagnosed. A variety of prescribed medications may be used. Aspirin can reduce the fever, ease joint pain, and relieve the rash. A physician should be consulted about the risk of Reyes syndrome before giving aspirin to children and teens. Gamma globulin, purified antibodies found in blood, is administered intravenously to help fight infection and reduce the risk of the development of coronary artery abnormalities or damage to the heart muscle. If the disease is treated within ten days of its onset, then less than 20 percent of the patients experience any heart problems.

A doctor may order an electrocardiogram (ECG or EKG), chest radiograph, and echocardiogram in order to monitor heart functions. If liver or gallbladder malfunction occurs, then ultrasonic imaging of those organs may be necessary.

Perspective and Prospects

Tomisaku Kawasaki first identified Kawasaki disease in 1967 when he reported the symptoms in fifty children in cases occurring between the years of 1961 and 1967. In

---

Information on Kawasaki Disease

Causes: Unknown; possibly allergic reaction, viral or bacterial infection, or immune system response

Symptoms: High fever; patchy rash; red lips, mouth, tongue, and throat; swollen lymph nodes in neck; swollen hands and feet; diarrhea; vomiting; stomach pain; joint pain; irritability; peeling skin on fingers and toes

Duration: Two weeks to three months; long-term heart damage possible

Treatments: Aspirin, gamma globulin

children under five, the disease has become the leading cause of acquired heart disease in the United States. About three thousand children are hospitalized with Kawasaki disease annually in the United States. Epidemics occurred in Japan in 1979, 1982, and 1985. Death from heart-related problems related to Kawasaki disease occurs in less than 2 percent of the victims. Less than 2 percent of children who experience Kawasaki disease have a reoccurrence.

—*Alvin K. Benson, Ph.D.*

See also Cardiology; Cardiology, pediatric; Childhood infectious diseases; Echocardiography; Electrocardiography (ECG or EKG); Epidemiology; Fever; Heart; Immune system; Immunology; Immunopathology; Joints; Lymphatic system; Rashes; Skin; Skin disorders.

For Further Information:

Hawker, Jeremy, et al. *Communicable Disease Control Handbook.* 2d ed. Malden, Mass.: Blackwell, 2006.

MedlinePlus. "Kawasaki Disease." *MedlinePlus*, May 19, 2013.

Parker, James N. and Philip M. Parker. *Kawasaki Disease: A Bibliography, Medical Dictionary, and Annotated Research Guide to Internet References.* San Diego, Calif.: ICON Health, 2004.

Powell, Michael, and Oliver Fischer. *101 Diseases You Don't Want to Get.* New York: Thunder's Mouth Press, 2005.

Safer, Diane A. "Kawasaki Disease." *Health Library*, November 26, 2012.

KERATITIS

Disease/Disorder

Anatomy or system affected: Eyes

Specialties and related fields: Family medicine, ophthalmology, optometry

Definition: An inflammation of the cornea caused most often by the herpes simplex virus.

Causes and Symptoms

Keratitis produces an inflammation or irritation of the cornea, the outer transparent layer of the eye. It is generally caused when the cornea has been scratched, cut, or injured so that a pathway is established for the entry of infectious agents. The resulting infection may be superficial or may involve deeper layers of the cornea. The most common cause of keratitis is the herpes simplex virus, the same virus that produces cold sores. Initially, the virus causes inflammation of the conjunctiva, the membrane lining the eyelid. Typically, it then produces infection of the cornea with branchlike ulcerations. Less common causes of keratitis include adenoviruses, varicella zoster virus, bacteria, fungi, parasites, excessive exposure to ultraviolet light, vitamin A deficiency, rheumatic diseases, surgery on the cornea, adverse reaction to broad-spectrum antibiotics, trauma to the eye that leaves scar tissue, allergic reactions to eye makeup or other irritants, and congenital syphilis (often termed interstitial keratitis). Bacterial keratitis usually results from improper cleaning or care of contact lenses.

The symptoms of keratitis typically include one or more of the following: eye redness, tearing and itching of the eye, a sensation that foreign matter is in the eye, blurred vision or re-

---

Information on Keratitis

Causes: Various; may include herpes or other viruses, congenital syphilis or other bacteria, fungi, parasites, excessive ultraviolet light, vitamin A deficiency, rheumatic diseases, eye surgery or other trauma, allergic reactions

Symptoms: Redness, tearing and itching, sensation of foreign matter, blurred or reduced vision, pain, discharge, light sensitivity, cloudy appearance of cornea

Duration: Acute

Treatments: Depends on cause; may include antiviral eyedrops, oral or eyedrop antibiotics, scraping away of diseased tissue, supplements for vitamin A deficiency

---

duction of vision clarity, eyelids sticking together, pain, eye discharge, sensitivity to light, and cloudy appearance of the cornea. If keratitis is left untreated, then corneal tissue can be destroyed, scar tissue can form, and feeling in the cornea may eventually be lost. At the first sign of eye infection, proper treatment should be administered.

Treatment and Therapy

Medical treatment of keratitis varies according to the cause. Antiviral eyedrops are administered for viral keratitis. Oral or eyedrop antibiotics are used for other infections. Some ophthalmologists prefer to scrape diseased tissue from the cornea, apply anesthetic eyedrops, and cover the eye temporarily with a patch. Later, the patient may wear a special type of contact lens to prevent a reoccurrence of the infection. For cases involving dry eyes, artificial tears are prescribed for lubrication. Contact lenses may need to be replaced. In the case of vitamin A deficiency, supplements and foods rich in vitamin A (such as carrots, mangoes, spinach, squash, and liver) are prescribed.

Perspective and Prospects

Approximately fifty thousand cases of keratitis are diagnosed worldwide each year. It is the most common cause of corneal blindness in the United States. If treatment for keratitis is started early, then it is typically very effective. In the treatment of keratitis caused by the herpes simplex virus, it is very important not to use topical corticosteroids, as they may worsen the infection and even lead to blindness. Because herpes simplex virus remains in the body after treatment, there is a 50 percent chance that keratitis may reoccur.

—*Alvin K. Benson, Ph.D.*

See also Blindness; Eye infections and disorders; Eyes; Herpes; Ophthalmology; Optometry; Optometry, pediatric; Viral infections; Vision disorders; Vitamins and minerals.

For Further Information:

Parker, James N. and Philip M. Parker. *Keratitis: A Bibliography, Medical Dictionary, and Annotated Research Guide to Internet References.* San Diego, Calif.: Icon Health, 2004.

Parker, James N., and Philip M. Parker, eds. *The Official Patient's*

Sourcebook on Keratitis. San Diego, Calif.: Icon Health, 2002.

Vorvick, Linda J. "Corneal Ulcers and Infections." *MedlinePlus*, March 22, 2013.

Wilhelmus, Kirk R., and Thomas J. Liesegang, eds. *Interstitial Keratitis*. Philadelphia: W. B. Saunders, 1994.

KIDNEY CANCER

Disease/Disorder

Also known as: Renal cancer, renal carcinoma

Anatomy or system affected: Kidneys, urinary system

Specialties and related fields: Nephrology, oncology, urology

Definition: A number of different malignant growths that occur in a kidney.

Key terms:

biological therapy: a type of medical treatment that stimulates the body's immune system or works with it to help it overcome disease

carcinoma: any cancer that begins in the skin or in tissues around body organs

chemotherapy: drug therapy for cancer, usually using multiple medications

embolization: a treatment that stops blood flow to a tumor by blocking small blood vessels

hematuria: blood in the urine, which may be visible (rust-colored or reddish urine) or microscopic (detectable only through laboratory tests)

kidney: one of a pair of abdominal organs that remove waste products from the blood and are involved in many regulatory processes of the body

magnetic resonance imaging (MRI): a radiologic technique that uses radio signals, magnets, and a computer to produce highly detailed images of tissues

malignant: cancerous; able to spread into and destroy nearby tissues and to spread to distant areas

metastasis: cancer that occurs at a distance from the primary location

nephrectomy: surgical removal of a kidney

radiation therapy: the use of high-energy rays to stop cancer cells from growing

renal: pertaining to the kidney

tumor suppressor gene: a gene that usually keeps tumors from growing

Causes and Symptoms

The most common type of kidney cancer is renal cell carcinoma (also known as hypernephroma or renal adenocarcinoma), which accounts for 90 to 95 percent of cases in adults. Renal cell carcinoma is about twice as common in men than in women and occurs most commonly between the ages of fifty and seventy.

The cause of kidney cancer is not known; however, various risk factors increase the chances of developing it. They include smoking, obesity, high blood pressure, chronic dialysis for kidney failure, and exposure to certain chemicals or industrial processes. Kidney cancer is also one part of a rare genetic disease called Von Hippel-Lindau syndrome.

Information on Kidney Cancer

Causes: Unknown; risk factors include smoking, obesity, high blood pressure, dialysis, carcinogens

Symptoms: Hematuria, abdominal pain, mass in abdomen or flank; sometimes fever and weight loss

Duration: Chronic

Treatments: Depends on severity; may include kidney removal, chemotherapy, radiation therapy

---

The most common symptom of kidney cancer is hematuria, which occurs in about two-thirds of cases. The patient may notice a change in the color of the urine, or urinalysis may detect microscopic blood in normally colored urine. About one-third of patients have abdominal pain, and another third have a mass (lump) in the abdomen or flank. These three symptoms form the classic triad of findings that suggest kidney cancer. Other, less common symptoms include fever and weight loss. If the cancer has spread to the lungs or bones, then the patient may cough or experience bone pain. On physical examination, a male patient may have a varicocele, a cluster of varicose veins in the scrotum. Laboratory studies may show elevated calcium in the blood, anemia, or, occasionally, an excess of red blood cells. Studies used to diagnose kidney cancer include intravenous pyelogram (IVP), an x-ray of the kidneys and urinary tract using a special dye; computed tomography (CT) scan, a technique that generates detailed pictures from a series of x-rays; and ultrasonography, the use of sound waves to create an image of the soft tissues of the body.

Less common types of adult kidney cancer include transitional cell cancer of renal pelvis, sarcoma, lymphoma, and metastases from other cancers such as melanoma (the deadliest form of skin cancer) and lung, breast, and stomach cancer. Kidney cancer itself may metastasize to the lungs, bones, liver, and the other kidney.

In children, the most common type of kidney cancer is Wilms" tumor, which is caused by the loss of a tumor suppressor gene called *WT1* found on chromosome 11. The most common finding is an abdominal mass. Other findings include abdominal pain, fever, hematuria, high blood pressure, or anemia. Unlike with adult kidney cancer, boys and girls have equal risk of developing Wilms" tumor. This cancer occurs most commonly in young children (three to four years), although it may be found in younger and older children and in teens.

Treatment and Therapy

The treatment of kidney cancer depends on the age and health of the patient, the exact location and size of the tumor, and whether it has metastasized. Size, location, and metastasis are determined through the process of staging that includes extensive studies such as bone scans, CT scans, and MRIs.

The main treatment for adult kidney cancer is nephrectomy to remove the diseased kidney. Embolization or radiation therapy may be used to shrink the tumor before surgery, which makes it easier to remove. In cases where the cancer is too advanced for surgical treatment, these techniques may be used to relieve symptoms and make the patient more comfortable.

The treatment for Wilms" tumor is a combination of surgery, chemotherapy, and radiation therapy. This has improved survival from about 60 percent in the 1950s to more than 90 percent in the early twenty-first century.

Perspective and Prospects

The American Cancer Society estimates that in the United States in 2013, approximately 65,150 new cases of kidney cancer will be diagnosed and 13,680 people will die of the disease. Since the 1990s, the rate of people who have kidney cancer has increased steadily, although it is unclear why this is the case.

Although chemotherapy has not been helpful in most adult kidney cancers, new drugs and new drug combination treatments are under investigation. Other new treatments include biological therapies with interferon alpha, interleukin-2, and other immune system modulators. Although the exact mechanism of these biological therapies is not entirely clear, they seem to slow, or even stop, the growth of cancer cells. They make it easier for the body's own immune system to destroy and remove cancer cells and appear to be particularly useful in treating metastatic disease.

Tumor vaccines and gene therapy are other biological treatments under development. The vaccines may prevent a cancer from starting, may treat a cancer that already exists, or may help rid the body of cancer cells that have not been eliminated by other forms of treatment. In the first decade of the twenty-first century, these vaccines are still being researched and are available only to patients who enroll in experimental studies. Gene therapy actually changes the genes that regulate cell growth and death. The goal is to improve the body's own ability to fight the cancer or to make the cancer more likely to respond to other forms of treatment. Researchers are also studying ablation (removal) of the cancer using radio frequencies or freezing.

—Rebecca Lovell Scott, Ph.D., PA-C

See also Cancer; Carcinoma; Chemotherapy; Dialysis; Gene therapy; Kidney disorders; Kidneys; Malignancy and metastasis; Nephrectomy; Nephrology; Nephrology, pediatric; Radiation therapy; Renal failure; Tumors; Urinary disorders; Urinary system; Urology; Urology, pediatric.

For Further Information:

Alan, Rick. "Kidney Cancer." *Health Library*, September 30, 2012.
American Cancer Society. "What Are the Key Statistics about Kidney Cancer?" *American Cancer Society*, January 18, 2013.
American Medical Association. *American Medical Association Family Medical Guide*. 4th rev. ed. Hoboken, N.J.: John Wiley & Sons, 2004.
Greenberg, Arthur, et al., eds. *Primer on Kidney Diseases*. 5th ed. Philadelphia: Saunders/Elsevier, 2009.
Komaroff, Anthony, ed. *Harvard Medical School Family Health Guide*. New York: Free Press, 2005.
MedlinePlus. "Kidney Cancer." *MedlinePlus*, May 20, 2013.
National Kidney Foundation. *National Kidney Foundation*, 2013.
Schrier, Robert W., ed. *Diseases of the Kidney and Urinary Tract*. 8th ed. Philadelphia: Wolters Kluwer Health/Lippincott Williams & Wilkins, 2007.
Stoppard, Miriam. *Family Health Guide*. London: DK, 2006.

KIDNEY DISORDERS
Disease/Disorder

Anatomy or system affected: Kidneys, urinary system

Specialties and related fields: Internal medicine, nephrology, urology

Definition: Disorders, from structural abnormalities to bacterial infections, that can affect the kidneys and may lead to renal failure.

Key terms:

creatinine: the breakdown product of creatine, a nitrogenous compound found in muscle, blood, and urine

cystinosis: a congenital disease characterized by glucose and protein in the urine, as well as by cystine deposits in the liver and other organs, rickets, and growth retardation

hematuria: the abnormal presence of blood in the urine

hydronephrosis: the cessation of urine flow because of an obstruction of a ureter, allowing urine to build up in the pelvis of the kidney; can cause renal failure

oliguria: the diminished capacity to form and pass urine, so that metabolic products cannot be excreted efficiently

reflux: the abnormal backward flow of urine

toxemia: blood poisoning

uremia: the presence of excessive amounts of urea and other nitrogenous waste products in the blood

Causes and Symptoms

Disorders of the kidney can occur for a variety of reasons. The cause may be congenital (present from birth) or may develop very quickly and at any age. Many of these problems and disorders can be easily treated. The main types of kidney disorder are malformations in the development of the kidney, part of the kidney, or the ureter; glomerular disease; tubular and interstitial disease or disruption; vascular (other than glomerular) disease; and kidney dysfunction that occurs secondary to another disease.

The kidney frequently exhibits congenital anomalies, some of which occur during specific developmental stages. Agenesis occurs when the ureteric bud fails to develop normally. When the tissue does not develop, the ureter itself fails to form. If there is an obstruction where the ureter joins the pelvis of the kidney, there may be massive hydronephrosis (dilation). One or both kidneys may be unusually small, containing too few tubules. The kidneys may be displaced, too high or offset to one side or the other. They may even be fused. All these conditions could seriously affect the manufacture of urine, its excretion, or both.

Glomerulonephritis refers to a diverse group of conditions that share a common feature: primary involvement of the glomerulus. The significance of glomerulonephritis is that it is the most common cause of end-stage renal failure. Its features include urinary casts, high protein levels (proteinuria), hematuria, hypertension, edema (swelling), and uremia. The two forms of glomerulonephritis are primary and secondary. In the primary form, only the kidneys are affected; in the secondary form, the lesion (affected area) is only one of a series of problems.

Nephrotic syndrome is usually defined as an abnormal condition of the kidney characterized by the presence of proteinuria together with edema and high fat and cholesterol levels. It occurs in glomerular disease, in thrombosis of a renal vein, and as a complication of many systemic diseases. Nephrotic syndrome occurs in a severe, primary form characterized by anorexia, weakness, proteinuria, and edema.

Interstitial nephritis is inflammation of the interstitial tissue of the kidney, including the kidneys. Acute interstitial nephritis is an immunologic, adverse reaction to certain drugs, especially nonsteroidal anti-inflammatory drugs (NSAIDs) and some antibiotics. Acute renal failure, fever, rash, and proteinuria are indicative signs of this condition. If the medication is stopped, normal kidney function returns. Chronic interstitial nephritis is defined as inflammation and structural changes associated with such conditions as ureteral obstruction, pyelonephritis, exposure of the kidney to a toxin, transplant rejection, and certain systemic diseases.

Kidney stones (calculi) are commonly manufactured from calcium oxalate or phosphate, triple phosphate, uric acid (urate), or a mixture of these. Calcium stones are not necessarily the result of high serum calcium, although they can be. Struvite calculi of magnesium ammonium (triple) phosphate mixed with calcium are bigger but softer than other types; they grow irregularly, filling much of the kidney pelvis. They arise from infection with urea-splitting organisms that cause alkaline urine. Urate stones are a complication of gout.

Those who have a tendency to develop stones may experience concomitant infection known as pyonephrosis. Pyonephrosis is a result of not only blockage at the junction of the ureter and kidney pelvis but also any constricture at this location. Bacteria from the bloodstream collect and cause an abscess to form. If the tube is completely blocked, the inflammation produces enough pus to rupture a portion of the kidney, and more of the abdominal cavity becomes involved.

Pyelonephritis is inflammation of the upper urinary tract. Acute pyelonephritis may be preceded by lower tract infection. The patient complains of lethargy, fever, and back pain. The major symptoms are fever, renal pain, and body aches,

accompanied by nausea and toxemia. Chronic pyelonephritis often affects the renal tubules and the small spaces within the kidney. Fibrous tissue may take over these areas and cause gradual shrinking of the functional kidney. The chronic form may also result from previous bacterial infection, reflux, obstruction, overuse of analgesics, x-rays, and lead poisoning.

Obstruction may be caused by inadequate development of the renal tissue itself, closing off one or both ureters. Other malformations and certain calculi can also obstruct urine flow. Reflux may occur when the contraction of the bladder forces urine backward, up toward and into the kidney. Lesser degrees of reflux do not damage the kidney, but the greater the reflux, the more likely damage will occur. Bacterial infection is often attributable to *Escherichia coli*, but other bowel bacteria may also infect the area. They generally move upward from outside the body through the urinary organs, but they may also move inward from the bloodstream.

Acute renal failure is defined as a sudden decline in normal renal function that leads to an increase in blood urea and creatinine. The onset may be fast (over days) or slow (over weeks) and is often reversible. It is characterized by oliguria and rapid accumulation of nitrogenous wastes in the blood, resulting in acidosis. Acute renal failure is caused by hemorrhage, trauma, burns, toxic injury to the kidney, acute pyelonephritis or glomerulonephritis, or lower urinary tract obstruction. Occasionally, it will progress into chronic renal failure.

Chronic renal failure may result from many other diseases as well. Its signs are sluggishness, fatigue, and mental dullness. Patients also display other systemic problems as a result of chronic renal failure. Almost all such patients are anemic, and three-fourths of them develop hypertension. The skin becomes discolored, a muddy coloration caused by anemia and the presence of excess melanin.

Renal symptoms suggestive of renal dysfunction include increases in frequency of urination, color changes in urine, areas of edema, and hypertension. The patient may experience only one symptom but is more likely to have a series of complaints. To determine the cause of renal disease, several diagnostic tools can be used to distinguish the type of pathogenic process affecting the kidney. The degree to which other body systems are involved determines whether the disease process is systemic or confined to the kidneys. Other valuable clues may be gathered from medical history, family history, and physical examination. The key factors, however, are renal size and renal histopathology.

Examination of the urine can reveal important data relative to renal health. Stick tests may show the abnormal presence of blood, glucose, or protein. Assaying the kind and amount of protein may pinpoint the cause of the disease. Urine contaminated with bacteria has always been used as an indication of some form of urinary tract infection. Microscopic examination of urine sediment may help diagnose acute renal failure. Blood tests may also indicate the source of a renal disorder. A series of blood tests might reveal rising urea and creatinine levels. The urea-to-creatinine ratio may aid in determining if and which type of acute renal failure may be present. A high red cell count might suggest kidney stones, a tumor, or glomerular disease; a high white cell count would hint at inflammation or infection. Cells cast from the kidney tubules may indicate acute interstitial nephritis, while red cell breakdown products may mean glomerulonephritis. The diagnostician should also be diligent in tracking down possible septic causes. Repeated cultures of blood and urine should help ascertain if there is an abscess anywhere near the kidney.

X-rays can provide useful information. An abdominal x-ray may show urinary stones and abnormalities in the renal outline. Ultrasound will measure renal size, show scarring, and reveal dilation of the tract, perhaps as a result of an obstructive lesion. Abdominal ultrasound has become the investigation of choice because it can be performed at the patient's bedside.

Renal biopsy can give an accurate diagnosis of acute renal failure but may be more dangerous to the patient than the condition itself. The main indications for biopsy would be suspected acute glomerulonephritis and renal failure that has lasted six weeks.

Treatment and Therapy

If glomerulonephritis is suspected or diagnosed, its treatment seeks to avoid complications of the illness. The patient is monitored daily for fluid overload; as long as the patient is retaining fluid, blood tests that measure urea, creatinine, and salt balance are also run daily. The patient should stay in bed and restrict fluid as well as potassium intake. Medications may be prescribed, including diuretics, vasodilators for hypertension, and calcium antagonists. If the cause is bacterial, a course of oral antibiotics may be given. If these measures are unsuccessful, short-term dialysis may be needed. Some urinary abnormalities may last for as long as a year.

The first measure undertaken to treat acute renal failure is to rebuild depressed fluid volumes: blood if the patient has hemorrhaged, plasma for a burn patient, and electrolytes for a patient who is vomiting and has diarrhea. If infection is suspected as the underlying cause, an appropriate antibiotic should be administered when blood cultures confirm the presence of bacteria. After fluid volumes have been replenished, a diuretic may be necessary to reduce swelling of tissues within the kidney.

In chronic renal failure, the major undertaking is to relieve the obstruction of the urinary tract. If the blockage is within the bladder, simple catheterization may relieve it. If a stone or some similar obstacle is blocking a ureter, however, surgery to remove it may be necessary. A tube may be inserted to allow urine drainage, and the stone will pass or be removed.

For those suffering from recurrent stones, maintaining a high urine output is important; this requires the patient to drink fluids throughout the day and even at bedtime. Patients enduring intense pain may need to be hospitalized. Analgesics for pain are administered, in addition to forced fluid intake to increase urine output so that the stone might be passed. If these measures do not work, surgical intervention may be necessary.

Patients suffering from progressive, incurable renal failure

need medical aid in managing conservation of, substitution for, and eventual replacement of nephron function. Conservation attempts to prolong kidney function for as long as possible; renal function is aided by drug treatment. Substitution means the maintenance of kidney function by dialysis, especially hemodialysis. Replacement is the restoration of renal function by a kidney transplant. By this third stage of treatment, urine formation is independent of further drug treatment, and kidney function must be achieved by other means. Patients suffering from end-stage renal failure have two options: dialysis and transplantation. A patient may go from dialysis to transplantation. In fact, if a compatible donor (preferably a sibling) is available, a transplant is advisable. For those without a suitable donor, long-term hemodialysis is the first option.

Dialysis is defined as the diffusion of dissolved molecules through a semipermeable membrane. Several types of dialysis are available. Hemodialysis filters and cleans the blood as it passes through the semipermeable membranous tube in contact with a balanced salt solution (dialysate). Hemodialysis can be performed in a dialysis unit of a hospital or at home. It must usually be done two or three times a week, with each session lasting from three to six hours, depending on the type of membranes used and the size of the patient. Hemodialysis can lead to acute neurological changes. Lethargy, irritability, restlessness, headache, nausea, vomiting, and twitching may all occur. In some patients, neurological complications occur after dialysis is terminated. Convulsions are the most common of these consequences. In continuous abdominal peritoneal dialysis, a fresh amount of dialysate is introduced from a bag attached to a permanently implanted plastic tube. Wastes and water pass into the dialysate from the surrounding organs; then the fluid is collected four to eight hours later. Peritoneal dialysis is performed by the patient. It is continuous, so the clearance rate of wastes is higher. The most important neurological complications of peritoneal dialysis are worsening of urea-induced brain abnormalities accompanied by twitching and, rarely, psychosis and convulsions.

Transplantation of a kidney is considered for patients with primary renal diseases as well as end-stage renal failure resulting from any number of systemic and metabolic diseases. Success rates are highest for those suffering from lupus nephritis, gout, and cystinosis. If a kidney is received from a close relative, there is a 97 percent one-year survival rate. Even if the organ transplant comes from a nonrelative, the survival rate is still 90 percent.

—Iona C. Baldridge

See also Dialysis; Diuretics; Edema; End-stage renal disease; Genital disorders, male; Hemolytic uremic syndrome; Incontinence; Kidney cancer; Kidney transplantation; Kidneys; Lithotripsy; Nephrectomy; Nephritis; Nephrology; Nephrology, pediatric; Polycystic kidney disease; Proteinuria; Pyelonephritis; Renal failure; Stone removal; Stones; Uremia; Urethritis; Urinary disorders; Urinary system; Urology; Urology, pediatric.

For Further Information:

Cameron, J. Stewart. *History of the Treatment of Renal Failure by Dialysis.* New York: Oxford University Press, 2002.

Catto, Graeme R. D., and David A. Power, eds. *Nephrology in Clinical Practice.* London: Edward Arnold, 1988.

Coffman, Thomas M., et al. *Schrier's Diseases of the Kidney.* 9th ed. Philadelphia: Wolters Kluwer Health/Lippincott Williams & Wilkins, 2013.

Daugirdas, John T., Peter G. Blake, and Todd S. Ing, eds. *Handbook of Dialysis.* 4th ed. Philadelphia: Lippincott Williams & Wilkins, 2007.

Dische, Frederick E. *Renal Pathology.* 2d ed. New York: Oxford University Press, 1995.

Greenberg, Arthur, et al., eds. *Primer on Kidney Diseases.* 5th ed. Philadelphia: Elsevier/Saunders, 2009.

"Kidney Diseases." *MedlinePlus,* March 25, 2013.

Morgan, Steven H., and Jean-Pierre Grunfeld, eds. *Inherited Disorders of the Kidney: Investigation and Management.* New York: Oxford University Press, 1999.

National Kidney Foundation. http://www.kidney.org.

O'Callaghan, C. A., and Barry M. Brenner. *The Kidney at a Glance.* Malden, Mass.: Blackwell Science, 2000.

Papadakis, Maxine A., Stephen J. McPhee, and Michael W. Rabow, eds. *Current Medical Diagnosis and Treatment.* 52d ed. New York: McGraw-Hill, 2013.

Parker, James N., and Philip M. Parker, eds. *The Official Patient's Sourcebook on Kidney Failure: A Revised and Updated Directory for the Internet Age.* San Diego, Calif.: ICON Health, 2005.

Parker, James N., and Philip M. Parker, eds. *The Official Patient's Sourcebook on Urinary Tract Infection.* San Diego, Calif.: ICON Health, 2002.

KIDNEY REMOVAL. *See* NEPHRECTOMY.

KIDNEY STONES. *See* KIDNEY DISORDERS; STONE REMOVAL; STONES.

KIDNEY TRANSPLANTATION

Procedure

Anatomy or system affected: Abdomen, kidneys, urinary system

Specialties and related fields: General surgery, nephrology

Definition: A surgical procedure that replaces the recipient's diseased, nonfunctioning kidney with a donated one.

Key terms:

end-stage renal disease: the final phase of long-standing kidney disease, characterized by a nearly complete loss of function

hemodialysis: the use of an external apparatus to filter the blood of patients with end-stage renal disease

immunosuppression: the use of a variety of drugs to depress the immune system's response to foreign tissue; lowers the probability of rejection of transplanted organs

rejection: a cellular and chemical attack by the immune system on a transplanted organ, which is recognized as foreign to the body

renal: referring to the kidneys

Indications and Procedures

Transplantation of a human kidney from a donor to a recipient

has been used since the middle of the twentieth century to improve the quality and length of life for people with renal failure. While hemodialysis—or the use of an artificial kidney machine, as it is commonly known—can be used satisfactorily for years, transplantation is often the ultimate goal because it can return the patient to a near-normal life.

The kidneys play a pivotal role in maintaining a stable internal environment by controlling fluid levels, excreting waste products, and regulating the blood concentration of acids and bases and of ions such as sodium and potassium. The kidneys are also responsible for regulating blood pressure by secreting substances that constrict the blood vessels. Clearly, the derangement of such complex functions, as occurs in renal disease, is life-threatening.

There are many reasons for renal failure, but the most frequent are inherited disorders, severe infections, toxic substances, allergic reactions, diabetes mellitus, and hypertension. The latter two, which are common illnesses in the United States, result in renal damage because of long-term injury to the blood vessels. The symptoms of minimally or nonfunctioning kidneys reflect an accumulation of toxic waste products and dramatic changes in the chemical composition of the blood. Every system is affected until coma and death ensue. The process of hemodialysis is used intermittently to cleanse the blood and maintain life. Transplantation in the otherwise healthy person, however, is preferred.

An extraordinary amount of cooperation and preparation is necessary for successful kidney transplantation. The donor organ may come from a living blood relative or from a cadaver within minutes of death. The organ is removed and maintained at low temperature in a special preservative solution for up to forty-eight hours. A suitable recipient is located through a national registry that can rapidly pair a cadaver organ to a waiting patient. The chosen candidate is immediately prepared for surgery, and through an abdominal incision, the kidney is placed in the abdomen and connected to the blood supply by its artery and vein. The ureter, the urine-collecting duct, is attached to the bladder. The recipient's own diseased kidneys may or may not be removed; their presence does not interfere with the transplanted organ. Within hours, the newly transplanted organ begins to form urine.

Uses and Complications

All transplanted organs and tissues face both immediate and long-term rejection by the recipient's immune system. Recognizing the donated kidney as foreign, or "nonself," the immune system attacks it both physically and chemically. The injury can be so severe as to result in the organ's death and the need for its surgical removal. In an attempt to prevent this reaction, certain steps are taken both before and after transplantation surgery.

Matching a donor and recipient involves careful selection that must minimize the physiological differences that exist between people. The blood types (the ABO and Rh systems) should be the same. Gene sequences on the sixth chromosome that code for immune system components are also matched as closely as possible in a process known as human leukocyte antigen (HLA) compatibility. Living, first-degree relatives, such as parents or siblings, often provide the best survival rates because of the genetic similarities between donor and recipient. The loss of one kidney in a healthy individual does not appear to affect the body.

The excellent success rates that have been achieved—over 80 percent—are attributable both to preoperative matching and to immunosuppression, which is begun shortly before surgery and continued for many months afterward. Potent drugs are used to inhibit the recipient's immune system, thereby protecting the new kidney from attack and significantly reducing rejection. Eventually, the drugs are tapered off and stopped, having allowed the body time to adjust to the foreign tissue and the kidney time to heal.

As can be expected in a procedure as difficult as kidney transplantation, the risks and complications are many. In the immediate postoperative period, hemorrhaging from the attached renal artery or vein, leakage from the ureter, organ malfunction, and immediate rejection can occur. Often, difficulties begin weeks or even months later, because of both rejection damage to the kidney and side effects related to severe immunosuppression. Immunosuppression leaves the body prey to bacterial, viral, and fungal infections, as well as cancer. Sometimes, a vicious cycle begins, in which life-threatening infections require the discontinuation of the immunosuppressive drugs, and the probability of organ rejection and irreparable kidney damage is heightened. Continual patient monitoring is absolutely essential to maintain the delicate balance between the risks and benefits involved in this procedure.

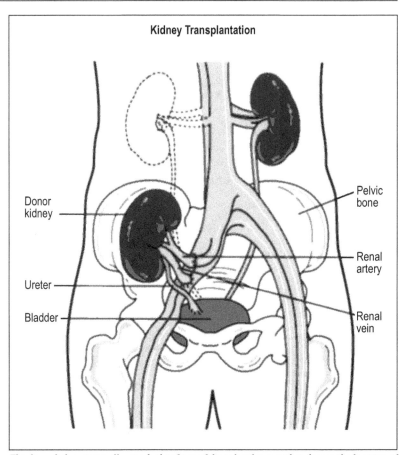

Kidney Transplantation

Donor kidney

Ureter

Bladder

Pelvic bone

Renal artery

Renal vein

The donor kidney is usually attached in front of the pelvic bone, rather than in the location of the nonfunctioning kidney, which is not removed in some cases.

Perspective and Prospects

Prior to 1962, when immunosuppressive drugs were unavailable and matching could only be based on blood type, kidney transplantation was an experimental procedure usually involving the organ of a living, first-degree relative. In the following decades, an extraordinary surge in information about the immune system and the genes that control the rejection response, as well as the discovery of powerful drugs, made transplantation a successful alternative for patients supported by hemodialysis. It also significantly increased the donor pool of organs by allowing unrelated cadaver kidneys to be used. It is in both areas, more precise matching and the development of less toxic postoperative drugs, that research continues. Contributions made in this field are readily used for research in all other organ transplantation as well.

—*Connie Rizzo, M.D., Ph.D.*

See also Circulation; Cysts; Dialysis; End-stage renal disease; Hemolytic uremic syndrome; Internal medicine; Kidney cancer; Kidney disorders; Kidneys; Nephrectomy; Nephritis; Nephrology; Nephrology, pediatric; Polycystic kidney disease; Renal failure; Transplantation; Urinalysis; Urinary disorders; Urinary system; Urology; Urology, pediatric; Xenotransplantation.

For Further Information:
American Kidney Fund. http://www.kidneyfund.org.
Brezis, M., et al. "Renal Transplantation." In *Brenner and Rector's The Kidney*, edited by Barry M. Brenner and Floyd C. Rector, Jr. 6th ed. Philadelphia: W. B. Saunders, 1999.
Carpenter, C., and M. Lazarus. "Dialysis and Transplantation in Renal Failure." In *Harrison's Principles of Internal Medicine*, edited by Dennis L. Kasper et al. 16th ed. New York: McGraw-Hill, 2005.
Danovitch, Gabriel, ed. *Handbook of Kidney Transplantation*. 5th ed. Philadelphia: Lippincott Williams & Wilkins, 2010.
Hoogland, E. R. Pieter, et al. "Improvements in Kidney Transplantation from Donors after Cardiac Death." *Clinical Transplantation* 27, no. 3 (May/June, 2013): E295–301.
"Kidney Transplant." *Health Library*, November 26, 2012.

"Kidney Transplant." *MedlinePlus*, June 13, 2011.

National Kidney Foundation. http://www.kidney.org.

Schrier, Robert W., ed. *Diseases of the Kidney and Urinary Tract*. 8th ed. Philadelphia: Wolters Kluwer Health/Lippincott Williams & Wilkins, 2007.

KIDNEYS
Anatomy

Anatomy or system affected: Abdomen, circulatory system, urinary system

Specialties and related fields: Hematology, nephrology, urology

Definition: The organs that control the amount and composition of body water by separating the blood into waste products (which leave the body as urine) and nutrients (which are returned to the blood).

Key terms:

Bowman's capsule: the group of renal cells that forms the cup of a nephron; fluids that seep from glomerular capillaries into the hollow wall of the capsule will be transformed into urine during their passage through the renal tubule leading from the capsule

glomerulus: a tuft or ball of capillaries contained within a Bowman's capsule

nephron: the almost-microscopic functional unit of the kidney, composed of special capillary blood vessels and of a Bowman's capsule connected to a renal tubule; each kidney has approximately 1.2 million nephrons

renal: of or relating to the kidneys

renal pelvis: the central pocket or sac of each kidney, which collects urine from all nephrons and channels it into the ureter

renal tubule: the tubular portion of a nephron that allows renal fluid to flow from the Bowman's capsule to the renal pelvis; these tubules, shaped like hairpins, are crucially important in the production of urine

ureter: the tube that transports urine from the renal pelvis to the urinary bladder

Structure and Functions

The normal human body has two kidneys, fist-sized organs located behind the abdomen and under the diaphragm. Each kidney, shaped like a bean, has a notch called the hilum, and the backbone separates the two kidneys. The kidneys make urine from blood. The renal artery transports blood into the kidney, while the renal vein transports blood out of the kidney. The blood vessels and the ureter connect with the kidney at its hilum.

The two kidneys are essentially identical in structure and function; consequently, kidney function can be discussed in the singular. The kidneys are a major functional unit of the circulatory system-unlike organs such as the brain, skin, or uterus, which are merely supported by that circulation. The kidney controls the environment of all cells of the body, an activity that is essential to life. That environment is salt water, and to understand the structure and function of the kidney, it is necessary to understand the nature of salt water in the body.

The human body is about 56 percent water, and the composition of this fluid is very important. One-third of this water is outside the cells; some of this extracellular fluid is between cells, and some of it is the liquid in blood vessels (blood is composed of liquid and cells). Two-thirds of the body's water is inside cells. The cell membrane surrounding each cell retains the intracellular fluid, but the water molecules move freely across the cell membrane. The size of each cell is determined by its water content. Cells swell or shrink based on the accumulation or loss of water molecules. The concentration of substances dissolved in the water determines whether water will accumulate inside or outside cells. Some of these dissolved substances are gases such as oxygen, hydrogen, and carbon dioxide; some are minerals such as sodium and calcium; some are sugars or proteins; and others are nutrients and waste products.

The amount and the composition of body water is controlled by the kidneys. Two other organs that aid in controlling the composition of body water are the lungs and the digestive tract; they can add or remove materials from the body water. The kidneys control the composition of body water primarily by removing materials from body water. Unlike the lungs and the digestive tract, however, the kidneys also regulate the amount of body water. The kidneys carry out both of these functions by acting on the blood. The kidney has three other important functions: It helps to control blood pressure, helps to control the manufacture of red blood cells, and participates in the manufacture of vitamin D. This article focuses on function of the normal kidney and what can make the kidney function abnormally.

Each kidney contains more than a million nephrons, its functional units, arranged in cones. A nephron is composed of blood vessels and a Bowman's capsule, a cup of renal cells containing the capillary tuft called a glomerulus and attached to a renal tubule.

A kidney has between eight and eighteen cones of nephrons. The base of each cone is near the surface of the kidney, and the peak of each cone is pointed at the renal pelvis, the central sac that collects and channels urine. Each nephron acts like a very sophisticated filtration system for the blood. Approximately 20 to 25 percent of all the blood in the body flows through the blood vessels of the kidneys every minute.

The action of the nephron actually begins with a porous filter, the glomerulus, that separates particles from a liquid. In this case, the liquid is blood plasma and the particles are blood cells and those protein molecules that are too large to pass through the glomerular pores. About 20 percent of the liquid in the blood seeps through the wall of glomeruli and into the inner space of Bowman's capsules. This liquid that crosses into a Bowman's capsule contains water, minerals, sugars, amino acids, and products of cell metabolism. The body needs to retain many of these substances, including water, so they must be recaptured by nephrons and returned to the blood.

The recapturing process occurs in the renal tubules. This is the process in which the nephron differs from an ordinary filter. The tubules have special cells that are capable of selectively reabsorbing those materials that must be retained by the body. These materials are passed from the liquid inside the tubules, through the tubule cells, and into blood capillaries that are laced or braided around the outside wall of the tubules. About 99 percent of the water molecules that seep into the renal tubules from the glomeruli are returned to the blood. The substances that do not need to be retained by the body continue to flow through the tubules and eventually leave the kidney as urine.

The mechanism in the renal tubular cells that selectively reabsorbs substances from the tubular liquid is quite special. The membrane of each cell contains proteins that act as chemical pumps. These pump proteins pick up substances to be reabsorbed from the tubular liquid and pass those substances into and through the tubular cells, where they enter renal capillaries. The reabsorbed substances may be salts or electrolytes, such as sodium or bicarbonate, or they may be sugars or even amino acids. As these substances are reabsorbed, much of the tubular water is also reabsorbed.

The pump proteins can work in the opposite direction as well. They can move substances from the renal capillaries surrounding the tubules, through the wall of the tubules, and into the tubular liquid. This process is called tubular secretion. Substances that commonly undergo tubular secretion are potassium, ammonium, and acid.

The remarkable action of the pump proteins requires fuel-in this case, adenosine triphosphate (ATP). ATP is made by living cells from oxygen, sugar, fatty acids, and nucleic acids in the blood. Pump proteins stop working when cells are unable to make ATP.

The pressure of the blood flow through the glomeruli and the reabsorption process of the renal tubules are closely controlled. This control takes place directly in the kidney, which contains sensing mechanisms that respond to changes in fluid composition. The kidney makes a hormone, called renin, that increases blood pressure. Other sensors that respond to changes in fluid composition are located in the brain. When these sensors detect changes that require action, the brain, acting through the pituitary gland, releases hormones, such as antidiuretic hormone (ADH), that act on the kidney. Another important hormone that controls kidney function, aldosterone, comes from the adrenal gland. The actual means by which these hormones control kidney function, however, is only partially understood.

By other mechanisms, the kidney detects whether the blood contains sufficient red blood cells (erythrocytes). Red blood cells are responsible for carrying oxygen to all the other cells in the body. When more red blood cells are needed, the kidney makes a hormone called erythropoietin, which stimulates the bone marrow and causes it to make more red blood cells.

Disorders and Diseases

The advantage of having a pair of kidneys becomes obvious if renal function becomes impaired. A person does quite well with one kidney; in fact, half of one kidney is sufficient to keep an individual alive.

A kidney problem may be suspected if an individual experiences changes in urination, such as pain on urination, changes in frequency of urination (more often or less often than usual), or changes in the urine that is formed (such as in its amount, appearance, or odor). Puffiness of the skin all over the body, but especially of the hands, feet, ankles, and face, may indicate abnormal renal function. This puffiness signifies water retention. Kidney disease can also be manifested by severe pain in the lower back, side, abdomen, or sex organs. The pain may be long-lasting or may occur with startling suddenness.

A person can be born with abnormal kidneys; this is a form of kidney disease. Normal kidneys, however, can malfunction because of a problem in the kidney itself, a problem in the blood circulation, or a problem in the flow of urine from the kidneys. Examples of abnormal kidneys at birth, abnormal urinary flow (kidney stones), and kidney infection will be discussed.

The formation of the kidneys by a fetus is quite complex and is controlled by genes. The development of the kidneys, other parts of the urinary tract (the ureters, bladder, and urethra), and the sex organs are all closely related. There are many opportunities for the developmental process to go wrong. Sometimes no kidneys are formed, sometimes the two kidneys are fused together, and sometimes more than one pair of kidneys is formed.

One of the most common malformations of the kidney is polycystic kidney disease, a hereditary (genetic) disorder affecting about 2 in 1,000 people. In the United States, it is ten times more common than sickle cell disease and fifteen times more common than cystic fibrosis. In polycystic kidney disease, each kidney contains numerous fluid-filled sacs, or cysts, scattered throughout the organ. The cysts are of different sizes, some very small and some the size of a grape. Polycystic kidneys are noticeably enlarged.

The cysts are caused by a malformation of the renal tubules. A cyst is formed when a renal tubule develops a branch from the main tubule. Tubules are not supposed to form branches; if this occurs, however, then the branch may become sealed off from the original tubule so that it has no entrance or exit. These sealed-off tubules are the cysts. They are capable of secretory activity because their cells contain pump proteins. The cysts enlarge as they accumulate fluid, putting pressure on the blood vessels, their capillaries, and the nephrons. The flow of blood and of urine is hindered. Patients with polycystic kidney disease often develop high blood pressure, kidney stones, and kidney infections. The disease can begin before birth, but symptoms may not occur until childhood or early adulthood. The intensity or severity of the disease varies greatly, from symptomless to life-threatening. Treatment of mild polycystic kidney disease may consist of relieving the pain, curing the infection, and controlling the blood pressure. Treatment of severe or life-threatening polycystic renal disease requires dialysis or kidney transplantation.

Stones in the urinary tract are very common. About 1 in 100 Americans has stones, and 1 in 1,000 adults experiences such severe symptoms that hospitalization is required. Kidney stones are caused by a prolonged high concentration of certain minerals in the urine, usually calcium, oxalate, or urate. The stones usually consist of crystals bound together by proteins.

The size and shape of kidney stones vary greatly. They may be microscopic or the size of a pea or even larger; they may be smooth or jagged. The stones may be passed from the urinary tract during urination, but some require removal by a urologist. Microscopic stones may not cause any symptoms, while larger stones can be very painful and may produce blood in the urine. Because stones hinder the flow of urine, their presence can allow bacteria to grow in the urinary tract, producing an infection.

Kidney stones that produce symptoms and are not passed by the patient must be removed. Some stones may be removed with a ureteroscope while the patient is under general anesthesia. A ureteroscope is a urological instrument like a hollow tube. It is inserted into the urinary tract through the external opening of the urethra and passed through the bladder and into the ureter. The tube can actually be inserted into the renal pelvis. The optical system of the ureteroscope allows the physician to see inside the urinary tract. Through the ureteroscope, kidney stones may be broken up by applying ultrasonic, laser, or electrohydraulic (acoustic shock-wave) energy.

An alternative means of removing large kidney stones is extracorporeal shock-wave lithotripsy, or ESWL. ESWL is desirable because it uses shock waves to break up the stones, thus eliminating the need to insert medical instruments into the patient. In one method of ESWL, the anesthetized patient is placed in a tub of water. X-ray imaging locates and monitors the stones as shock waves crush them. The patient's tissues are not damaged, and the sandy remains of the stones are then passed with urine. The development of ESWL has offered a useful means of treating kidney stones, but it has not eliminated the need for surgical or ureteroscopic removal of these stones from some patients. Each patient and each stone is different; they require the professional evaluation of a urologist.

Urinary tract infections are common, affecting 10 to 20 percent of women at some point in their lives; they are less common in men. Pathogens usually infect the kidneys by ascending the urinary tract via the urethra, bladder, and ureters. The normal bladder is an effective barrier to these infections, but any obstruction to the flow of urine, such as enlarged prostate, renal cysts, pregnancy, or a urinary stone, will weaken this barrier. Sometimes, pathogens infect the kidneys through the blood. Most urinary tract infections can be effectively treated with antibiotics. It is important for the physician to choose an antibiotic that is effective against the causative pathogen. Each antibiotic is effective against only a few types of bacteria, and many different bacteria can cause urinary tract infections.

Infections involving the kidney are especially serious. Because the kidneys are essential to life, these infections must be treated promptly and completely. Some infections affect the kidney even after the infection is cured. The body reacts to pathogens by producing proteins called antibodies, which circulate in the bloodstream. Antibodies in the blood can coat and damage the glomerular filters in Bowman's capsules. This reduces the effectiveness of the filters, allowing blood and protein to enter the urine and causing the body to become puffy. The medical term for this serious kidney disease is glomerulonephritis. Treatment is available, but it is better to prevent the disease from occurring. If left untreated, the kidney damage may be so extensive that dialysis or transplantation is required to prevent death.

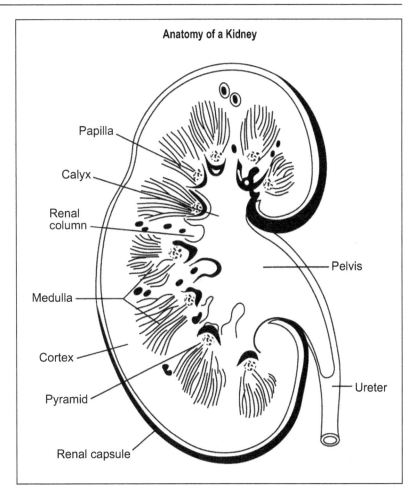

Anatomy of a Kidney

Papilla

Calyx

Renal column

Medulla

Cortex

Pyramid

Renal capsule

Pelvis

Ureter

Perspective and Prospects

The ancient Greeks seem to be the earliest people whose writings about the kidney have survived. They had no regard for the importance of this organ, mainly because their frame of reference consisted of four "humors." Even before 500 BCE, the Greeks were developing the doctrine of the four elements of the inanimate universe: air, fire, water, and earth. From this idea, Polybus, the son-in-law of Hippocrates, created the corollary of the four "humors" responsible for life: yellow bile (choler), blood, phlegm (pituita), and black bile (melancholia). The concept of humors dominated the thinking of Aristotle (384-322 BCE) when he wrote about his study of the anatomy of kidneys in several animals, including humans. This approach delayed an understanding of even the basic concept that kidneys and urine are related, an idea finally proposed about 290 BCE by Erasistratus of Ceos.

Knowledge of Erasistratus comes mainly from Galen (129-c. 199 CE). Galen, rather than applauding the advances of his forebears, ridiculed unfounded assertions. He conducted physiological experiments on living animals, such as observing the effect of cutting and tying one ureter while leaving the opposite one intact. His experiments yielded much information about renal physiology. The writings of Galen formed the foundation of medical knowledge for the next four hundred years. Students and teachers, rather than building upon the experimental process, accepted the proclamations of Galen as dogma.

The next great advance in renal knowledge came from the Italian anatomist Bartolommeo Eustachio (1520-1574), who, without the benefit of a microscope, discovered the renal tubules and their relationship to the renal vascular system. His descriptions and drawings of 1564 were lost in the Vatican library until 1714. In the meantime, another Italian, Lorenzo Bellini (1643-1704), independently discovered the renal tubules and discerned their function. A contemporary, Marcello Malpighi (1628-1694), discovered glomeruli and their relationship to tubules.

Subsequent advances had to wait until the nineteenth century, when knowledge of all aspects of human biology and medicine began a rapid advance. Many independent advances in the nineteenth and twentieth centuries-in surgery, pharmacology, and immunology-made the transplantation of kidneys and other major organs possible. General anesthesia was developed independently by two Americans: by Crawford Long in 1842 and by William T. G. Morton in 1846. Antiseptic procedures were originated in 1867 by the Englishman Joseph Lister, and vascular surgical techniques were developed in 1902 by the French surgeon Alexis Carrel and the Hungarian surgeon Emerich Ullman. Anticoagulants were developed in 1914 and 1915, and systemic antibiotics were developed in the 1930s and 1940s. Blood typing was begun in Europe by Karl Landsteiner (1868-1943). Tissue immunology was first explained in 1953, and tissue typing was introduced in France and the United States in the 1960s. Immunosuppressive drugs were developed during this same period. Kidney transplantation is also possible because of extracorporeal support devices such as the dialysis machine, the heart-lung machine, and the organ perfusion machine.

The first transplant of a human kidney between identical twins was performed on December 23, 1954, by Joseph E. Murray. He later performed the first human kidney transplant between unrelated persons on April 5, 1962. By the 1990s, tens of thousands of kidney transplants were being performed in the United States every year. There are many more persons waiting for a transplant than there are kidneys available for transplantation. The solution to this problem is unclear. Transplants between living persons in the same family may be encouraged, and transplants from animals to humans may be perfected. It is even possible that a transplantable artificial kidney can be developed, but this task will be enormously difficult, considering all the functions of a natural kidney.

—*Armand M. Karow, Ph.D.*

See also Adrenalectomy; Blood and blood disorders; Circulation; Corticosteroids; Cysts; Dialysis; Diuretics; End-stage renal disease; Hemolytic uremic syndrome; Internal medicine; Kidney cancer; Kidney disorders; Kidney transplantation; Laparoscopy; Lithotripsy; Nephrectomy; Nephritis; Nephrology; Nephrology, pediatric; Polycystic kidney disease; Proteinuria; Pyelonephritis; Renal failure; Stone removal; Stones; Systems and organs; Transplantation; Uremia; Urinalysis; Urinary disorders; Urinary system; Urology; Urology, pediatric.

For Further Information:

Andreoli, Thomas E., et al., eds. *Andreoli and Carpenter's Cecil Essentials of Medicine.* 8th ed. Philadelphia: Saunders/Elsevier, 2010. This paperback book, written for physicians, describes diseases and their treatment in humans. Contains a good section on the kidneys. Appropriate and helpful for nonscientists as well.

Brenner, Barry M., ed. *Brenner and Rector's The Kidney.* 8th ed. Philadelphia: Saunders/Elsevier, 2008. This treatise, at more than two thousand pages, is a comprehensive and authoritative source on the normal and diseased human kidney.

Eaton, Douglas C., and John D. Pooler. *Vander's Renal Physiology.* 7th ed. New York: McGraw-Hill, 2009. This paperback book, written for medical students, describes the anatomy and physiology of the normal human kidney. Provides extensive, exhaustive information in a comprehensible format. The text may be somewhat challenging for those who have not taken introductory college-level courses in chemistry and biology.

Gottschalk, Carl W., Robert W. Berliner, and Gerhard H. Giebisch, eds. *Renal Physiology: People and Ideas.* Bethesda, Md.: American Physiological Society, 1987. This collection of scholarly essays traces the historical development of renal physiology. While the work is exhaustive and comprehensive, emphasis is placed on the nineteenth and twentieth centuries.

Marieb, Elaine N. *Essentials of Human Anatomy and Physiology.* 9th ed. San Francisco: Pearson/Benjamin Cummings, 2009. This introductory anatomy and physiology textbook, easily accessible to those with little science background, is richly illustrated with diagrams and photographs, which help to illuminate body systems and processes.

O'Callaghan, C. A., and Barry M. Brenner. *The Kidney at a Glance.* Malden, Mass.: Blackwell Science, 2000. Covers a range of topics related to the kidneys, presenting text on one page and accompanying illustrations on the facing page. Covers basic anatomy and physiology and the pathologies and presentations of renal and urinary tract disease.

Voet, Donald, and Judith G. Voet. *Biochemistry.* 3d ed. Hoboken, N.J.: John Wiley & Sons, 2004. A good book to use for the description and explanation of the chemical processes taking place in the kidney and other areas of the body.

KINESIOLOGY
Specialty

Anatomy or system affected: Brain, cells, circulatory system, heart, lungs, muscles, musculoskeletal system, nervous system, psychic-emotional system, respiratory system, spine

Specialties and related fields: Cardiology, exercise physiology, orthopedics, physical therapy, psychology, sports medicine

Definition: The applied science of human movement, which combines the general areas of anatomy (the study of structure) and physiology (the study of function).

Science and Profession

In 1989, the American Academy of Physical Education endorsed the term *kinesiology* to describe the entire field traditionally known as physical education, which includes the following subdisciplines: exercise physiology, biomechanics, motor control and learning, sports nutrition, sports psychology, sports sociology, athletic training programs, pedagogy, adapted physical education, cardiac rehabilitation, and physical therapy.

Exercise physiology describes the body's muscular, cardiovascular, and respiratory functioning during both short-term and long-term exercise. Research has focused on muscle fiber typing, oxygen uptake assessment, lactic acid metabolism, thermoregulation, body composition, and muscle hypertrophy. Biomechanics applies Isaac Newton's laws of physics to improve the mechanical efficiency of muscle movement patterns; using high-speed video and computer analysis, flaws in joint and limb dynamics can be assessed and changed to optimize performance. Motor control and learning pinpoint the areas of the brain and spinal cord that are responsible for the acquisition and retention of motor skills. Understanding the neurological basis of reflex and voluntary muscle movements helps to refine teaching strategies and describe the mechanisms of fatigue.

Sportsnutrition describes how the body stores, circulates, and converts nutrients for aerobic and anaerobic energy production through carbohydrate loading and other strategies. Sports psychology explores the workings of the mind before, during, and after exercise and competition. Sports sociology examines aspects such as cultural, ethnic, and gender differences; dynamics in small and large groups; and the role of sports in ethical and moral development. Athletic trainers work with sports physicians and surgeons to prevent and rehabilitate injuries caused by overuse, trauma, or disease. Physical therapists use clinical exercise therapy and other modalities in a variety of rehabilitation settings.

Allied health areas under the kinesiology umbrella include pedagogy (teaching progressions for movement skills), adapted physical education (activities for the physically and mentally challenged), and cardiac rehabilitation (recovery stages for those disabled by heart disease). Professional organizations in the field of kinesiology include the American College of Sports Medicine, the American Physical Therapy Association, the National Athletic Trainers Association, the National Strength and Conditioning Association, and the American Alliance for Health, Physical Education, Recreation, and Dance.

—*Grace D. Matzen*

See also Genetic diseases; Genetics and inheritance; Gynecomastia; Hermaphroditism and pseudohermaphroditism; Hormone therapy; Puberty and adolescence; Reproductive system; Sexual differentiation.

For Further Information:

American Kinesiology Association. "Careers in Kinesiology." *American Kinesiology*, 2010.

American Medical Association. "Kinesiotherapist." *Health Care Careers Directory 2012–2013*. 40th ed. Chicago: American Medical Association, 2012. 15–16.

Brooks, George A., and Thomas D. Fahey. *Fundamentals of Human Performance*. Mountain View, Calif.: Mayfield, 2000.

Hamilton, Nancy, Wendi Weimar, and Kathryn Luttgens. *Kinesiology: Scientific Basis of Human Motion*. 12th ed. New York: McGraw-Hill, 2012.

Houglum, Peggy, Dolores B. Bertoti, and Signe Brunnstrom. *Brunnstrom's Clinical Kinesiology*. 6th ed. Philadelphia: Davis, 2012.

Lippert, Lynn. *Clinical Kinesiology and Anatomy*. 5th ed. Philadelphia: F. A. Davis, 2011.

McArdle, William, Frank I. Katch, and Victor L. Katch. *Exercise Physiology: Energy, Nutrition, and Human Performance*. 7th ed. Boston: Lippincott Williams & Wilkins, 2010.

Oatis, Carol A. *Kinesiology: The Mechanics and Pathomechanics of Human Movement*. 2d ed. Philadelphia: Lippincott Williams & Wilkins, 2009.

Plowman, Sharon A., and Denise L. Smith. 4th ed. *Exercise Physiology for Health, Fitness, and Performance*. Philadelphia: Wolters Kluwer/Lippincott Williams & Wilkins Health, 2014.

Powers, Scott K., and Edward T. Howley. *Exercise Physiology: Theory and Application to Fitness and Performance*. 8th ed. New York: McGraw-Hill, 2012.

Sharkey, Brian J., and Steven E. Gaskill. *Fitness and Health*. 7th ed. Champaign, Ill.: Human Kinetics, 2013.

KLINEFELTER SYNDROME
Disease/Disorder

Anatomy or system affected: Breasts, endocrine system, genitals, hair, psychic-emotional system, reproductive system

Specialties and related fields: Embryology, endocrinology, genetics, psychology

Definition: A male chromosomal disorder causing infertility and significant femaleness.

Causes and Symptoms

Klinefelter syndrome is caused by a variation in the number of sex chromosomes. Males normally possess one X and one Y chromosome, while females normally have two X chromosomes. When an embryo has two X chromosomes and one Y chromosome (XXY), normal development and reproductive function are hampered, and the boy shows the symptoms of Klinefelter syndrome. These symptoms include breast development, underdevelopment of sex organs, and school or social difficulties. The major symptom is sterility or very reduced fertility, although affected males have normal erections. The testes remain small after puberty and produce

---

Information on Klinefelter Syndrome

Causes: Genetic chromosomal disorder
Symptoms: Infertility, breast development, small testes that produce few, if any, sperm
Duration: Lifelong
Treatments: None; hormonal therapy for symptoms

---

few, if any, sperm. Sex drive may also be low.

In adolescence, breast tissue often develops significantly. In addition, normal facial and body hair may not develop in these boys. Although they usually grow quite tall, young men with Klinefelter syndrome often have disproportionate limbs and are less physically strong or coordinated than their peers. Some affected individuals exhibit some degree of subnormal intelligence. Others lack self-confidence or experience difficulties in learning language and speech or in concentrating.

Treatment and Therapy

Klinefelter syndrome is diagnosed using a karyotype, an analysis of the chromosomes from blood or cheek cells. It can determine the presence of forty-seven chromosomes, including one Y and two X. Although Klinefelter syndrome is genetic and cannot be cured, testosterone can be administered orally, intravenously, or transdermally to supplement the usually insufficient amount produced by the boy's own testes. This therapy should enhance male physical development by increasing the size of the penis, causing hair growth and greater muscle bulk, and deepening the voice. Other benefits may include increased concentration, greater physical strength and energy, and higher sex drive.

Hormone therapy cannot increase the size of the testes, cure sterility, or reverse breast tissue development, which can only be treated by surgical removal. It may, however, increase self-esteem and a sense of masculinity, thereby easing social interactions.

For children with Klinefelter syndrome who experience difficulty with language development, early speech therapy interventions and educational assistance are recommended. Counseling and behavioral training may help with social interaction.

Perspective and Prospects

Found in about one out of every five hundred born, Klinefelter syndrome is the most common human chromosomal variation. Described by Harry Klinefelter in 1942, its cause was discovered by Patricia Jacobs and John Strong in 1959.

Men with Klinefelter syndrome are at higher risk of developing heart or lung disease, diabetes, hypothyroidism, dental complications, osteoporosis, breast or lung cancer, venous disease, depression, and autoimmune disorders. Nevertheless, the average life expectancy for those with Klinefelter syndrome is about the same as men without the condition.

—*Grace D. Matzen*

See also Genetic diseases; Genetics and inheritance; Gynecomastia; Hermaphroditism and pseudohermaphroditism; Hormone therapy; Puberty and adolescence; Reproductive system; Sexual differentiation.

For Further Information:
A.D.A.M. Medical Encyclopedia. "Klinefelter Syndrome." *MedlinePlus*, November 2, 2012.
Bandmann, H.-J., and R. Breit, eds. *Klinefelter's Syndrome.* New York: Springer, 1984.
Klinefelter Syndrome and Associates. "Frequently Asked Questions Related to 47, XXY." *Genetic.org*, 2012.
Kronenberg, Henry M., et al., eds. *Williams Textbook of Endocrinology.* 12th ed. Philadelphia: Saunders/Elsevier, 2011.
Martin, Richard J., Avroy A. Fanaroff, and Michele C. Walsh, eds. *Fanaroff and Martin's Neonatal-Perinatal Medicine: Diseases of the Fetus and Infant.* 9th ed. St. Louis, Mo.: Mosby/Elsevier, 2010.
Milunsky, Aubrey, and Jeff Milunsky, eds. *Genetic Disorders of the Fetus: Diagnosis, Prevention, and Treatment.* 6th ed. Hoboken, N.J.: Wiley-Blackwell, 2010.
Morales, Ralph, Jr. *Out of the Darkness: An Autobiography of Living with Klinefelter Syndrome.* Louisville, Ky.: Chicago Spectrum Press, 2002.
National Institute of Child Health and Human Development. "Klinefelter Syndrome: Condition Information." *U.S. Department of Health and Human Services, National Institutes of Health*, November 30, 2012.
Parker, James N., and Philip M. Parker, eds. *The Official Parent's Sourcebook on Klinefelter Syndrome.* San Diego, Calif.: Icon Health, 2002.
Rosenblum, Laurie, and Kari Kassir. "Klinefelter Syndrome."*Health Library*, September 27, 2012.
SÃ¸rensen, Kurt. *Klinefelter's Syndrome in Childhood, Adolescence, and Youth: A Genetic, Clinical, Developmental, Psychiatric, and Psychological Study.* Park Ridge, N.J.: Parthenon, 1988.

KLIPPEL-TRENAUNAY SYNDROME
Disease/Disorder

Also known as: Angio-osteohypertrophy, nevus vasculosus osteohypertrophicus syndrome, hemangiectasia hypertrophicans, Klippel-Trenaunay-Weber syndrome
Anatomy or system affected: Blood vessels, circulatory system, gastrointestinal system, joints, lymphatic system
Specialties and related fields: Genetics, internal medicine, pediatrics, vascular medicine
Definition: A rare congenital syndrome characterized by hemangiomas of the vascular system that can affect bone or soft tissue throughout the body.

Causes and Symptoms

Klippel-Trenaunay syndrome was first described in 1900 in patients exhibiting a combination of varicose veins, multiple vascular nevi (birthmarks on the skin sometimes called port-wine stains), and excessive growth or development (hypertrophy) of limbs or soft tissue. Increased vascularity is common. At birth, a large vein may be observed running from the lower leg into the upper thigh, referred to as the Klippel-Trenaunay vein.

The molecular basis for the disease is unclear, as most cases appear as simply random occurrences. Among those few cases which appear to be heritable, it is believed that an autosomal dominant gene may be at fault, possibly linked to

---

Information on Klippel-Trenaunay Syndrome

Causes: Unknown, possibly genetic
Symptoms: Varicose veins, port-wine stains, limb or soft tissue hypertrophy, noticeable large vein running from lower leg into upper thigh, localized tumors, excessive bleeding
Duration: Lifelong
Treatments: Alleviation of symptoms, such as compression garments and leg elevation for varicose veins, surgery for limb hypertrophy, anticoagulants

---

chromosome numbers 5 or 11. Evidence suggests that, at the molecular level, deregulation of deoxyribonucleic acid (DNA) methylation of imprinted genes may play a role.

Whichever gene may be at fault, it is believed the mutation occurs early in embryonic development. The result is that the defect appears randomly among cells as they migrate and differentiate early during embryonic stages, resulting in the seemingly haphazard distribution of the trait as the fetus develops.

Diagnosis is based upon the triad of vascular or soft tissue defects, with venous or capillary malformations leading to localized, and often extensive, tumors. Preliminary diagnosis can be based upon any two of the characteristics. Another symptom may be excessive bleeding, especially from the rectum or detected in the urine.

Treatment and Therapy

If the disorder becomes apparent during the prenatal period, then the prognosis is generally poor. Treatment in the adult is generally symptomatic, although the possibility of internal organ involvement, as well as pulmonary embolisms, leaves the patient at risk even in the absence of symptoms.

Since varicose veins are generally apparent, the patient may wear compression garments, elevating the legs at intervals. Surgery may be necessary to correct limb hypertrophy. Because the formation of embolisms is a risk, the patient may utilize anticoagulants prophylactically, particularly prior to surgery. Corticosteroid use may help limit swelling in some cases. In the absence of significant malformations, the patient should simply be monitored on an annual basis.

Perspective and Prospects

The rare and sporadic nature of the disorder complicates routine screening. At best, proper prenatal care during pregnancy may result in diagnosis if the disorder does appear. Research into the molecular basis of the disorder may eventually determine its origins.

—*Richard Adler, Ph.D.*

See also Birthmarks; Blood vessels; Congenital disorders; Hypertrophy; Skin; Skin disorders; Varicose veins; Vascular medicine; Vascular system.

For Further Information:

Baskerville, P. A., et al. "The Etiology of the Klippel-Trenaunay Syndrome." *Annals of Surgery* 202 (November, 1985): 624–27.

Evans, Jeff. "Klippel-Trenaunay Stains Predict Complications." *Skin and Allergy News* 34, no. 2 (February 1, 2003): 40.

MedlinePlus. "Klippel-Trenaunay Syndrome." *MedlinePlus*, March 22, 2013.

Mulliken, John B., and Anthony E. Young, eds. *Vascular Birthmarks: Hemangiomas and Malformations*. Philadelphia: W. B. Saunders, 1988.

Telander, R. L., et al. "Prognosis and Management of Lesions of the Trunk in Children with Klippel-Trenaunay Syndrome." *Journal of Pediatric Surgery* 19 (1984): 417–22.

KLUVER-BUCY SYNDROME
Disease/Disorder

Anatomy or system affected: Brain, eyes, genitals
Specialties and related fields: Family medicine, ophthalmology, pediatrics, psychiatry, psychology
Definition: A behavioral disorder characterized by lack of emotional activity or responses similar to that often observed in patients with Alzheimer's disease.

Key terms:

agnosia: inability to recognize common objects
amygdala: the front portion of the temporal lobe of the brain
hyperorality: use of the mouth for the examination of objects
lobotomy: the severance of nerve fibers in the frontal lobe of brain
temporal lobes: lateral portions of the cerebrum of the brain

Causes and Symptoms

Kluver-Bucy syndrome was first observed in 1937 when German neuroanatomist Heinrich Kluver, working with American neuropathologist Paul Bucy at Northwestern University, observed that the removal of the temporal lobes, including the amygdala, of a rhesus monkey resulted in significant behavioral changes in the animal. More specifically, the monkey displayed visual agnosia, the inability to recognize objects while at the same time displaying excessive responses to visual stimulation (hypermetamorphosis). The animals also demonstrated a significantly increased tendency to orally examine objects (hyperorality) and heightened sexual responses.

The syndrome was first described in humans in 1955 by Sergio Dalle Ore and a colleague following a temporal lobectomy in a male being treated for epilepsy. Symptoms largely followed those previously observed by Kluver and Bucy in monkeys and are still considered valid for the diagnosis of the illness. Specific characteristics of the syndrome in humans include auditory, tactile, or visual agnosia; the inability to recognize familiar objects including other persons (psychic blindness); hyperorality; the examination of objects orally rather than visually; docility; complete lack of aggressiveness sometimes termed as placidity; and changes in diet that can include either overeating or the eating of inappropriate objects (hyperphasia). Hyperphasia has been reported to take the form of not only placing in the mouth unusual foods but also placing in the mouth dangerous objects such as cigarettes, razors, and nails or even excrement. Altered sexuality, attempting to achieve sexual satisfaction not through intercourse or masturbation but through comments or touching,

---

Information on Kluver-Bucy Syndrome

Causes: Malfunction in communication between left and right temporal lobes or damage to amygdala
Symptoms: Unusual fear response, use of mouth for examining objects, inability to recognize objects
Duration: Lifelong
Treatments: Symptomatic

---

has also been observed in persons diagnosed with Kluver-Bucy syndrome. Humans generally do not exhibit all the characteristics of the syndrome, with diagnosis based upon manifestation of three or more of these symptoms.

The underlying physiological basis for the syndrome remains unclear. Kluver-Bucy syndrome may be triggered by damage either to the temporal lobes or within the amygdala, the frontal portion of the temporal lobes. The function of the cells that constitute the amygdala includes production of a variety of neurotransmitters; the initial studies carried out by Kluver and Bucy that resulted in the description of the condition had involved investigation of the effect of mescaline on this region of the brain. Kluver-Bucy syndrome has been triggered by pathological conditions associated with, or secondary to, more than fifty different conditions, including encephalitis, strokes, tumors, and dementias such as Alzheimer disease or Pick's disease.

Specific diagnosis beyond the appearance of behavioral changes has been difficult and controversial. Radioimaging studies as well as positron emission tomography (PET) scans have shown the presence of damage to neural connections within the amygdala as well as other regions in the temporal lobes. The issue has been controversial, however, since not all patients diagnosed with the syndrome exhibit such changes or the presence of lesions.

Treatment and Therapy

Few effective treatments have been described. However, the use of anticholinergics, drugs that inhibit the activity of the neurotransmitter acetylcholine, have shown some success in causing regression of the syndrome. Several studies have reported that treatment of patients with carbamazepine, an anticonvulsant and analgesic prescribed for treatment of seizures that have their origin in the trigeminal ganglia region, has had some success, particularly in adults.

Treatments have also been directed toward the functioning of the amygdala directly. The region is associated with cognitive recognition and social behaviors, the result of its interconnections with other regions of the cortex of the brain. The amygdala is characterized by neural interactions involving the neurotransmitter serotonin. Inhibitors of serotonin uptake have shown some success in addressing the syndrome. This class of drugs has been categorized as selective serotonin reuptake inhibitors (SSRI) and includes at least eight major categories of drugs. SSRIs are frequently prescribed as antidepressants, and they function to increase serotonin levels within the nerve synapse, with the result that neurotransmitter action on nerves is increased.

Perspective and Prospects

No cure for Kluver-Bucy syndrome currently exists; fortunately, the syndrome is a relatively rare disorder with no more than several hundred cases being reported since it was first described in humans in 1955. Furthermore, Kluver-Bucy syndrome manifests itself in behavior difficulties rather than in life-threatening conditions. Therefore, management of the problem is the primary means of dealing with the condition. Since the syndrome most commonly manifests itself in the aftermath of other diseases or difficulties, prevention of the condition is indirect, reflecting the elimination or prevention of other underlying causes. They include recognition and rapid treatment of the causes of encephalitis or intervention during birth to address conditions that may result in oxygen deprivation (hypoxia).

Rare cases may evolve into Korsakow syndrome, a brain disorder characterized by significant encephalopathy. Korsakow syndrome is generally observed only among alcoholics.

—Richard Adler, Ph.D.

See also Alzheimer's disease; Brain; Brain damage; Brain disorders; Dementias; Encephalitis; Frontotemporal dementia (FTP); Neurology; Pick's disease; Psychiatric disorders; Psychiatry.

For Further Information:

Goscinski, I., et al. "The Kluver-Bucy Syndrome." *Journal of Neurosurgical Sciences* 41, no. 3 (1997): 269.

Jha, Sanjeev, et al. "Cerebral Birth Anoxia, Seizures and Kluver-Bucy Syndrome: Some Observations." *Journal of Pediatric Neurology* 3, no. 4 (2005): 227.

Kalat, James. *Biological Psychology.* Belmont, Calif.: Wadsworth, 2008.

Malloy, Paul, and Jeffrey Cummings. *The Neuropsychiatry of Limbic and Subcortical Disorders.* Washington, D.C.: American Psychiatric Press, 1997.

National Institute of Neurological Disorders and Stroke. "NINDS Kluver-Bucy Syndrome Information Page." *National Institute of Neurological Disorders and Stroke*, July 2, 2008.

Salim, Ali, et al. "Kluver-Bucy Syndrome as a Result of Minor Head Trauma." *Southern Medical Journal* 95, no. 8 (August 1, 2002): 929.

KNEECAP REMOVAL

Procedure

Also known as: Patellectomy

Anatomy or system affected: Bones, joints, knees, legs, musculoskeletal system, tendons

Specialties and related fields: General surgery, orthopedics

Definition: The surgical removal of the kneecap.

Indications and Procedures

The kneecap, or patella, is the triangular bone at the front of the knee. It is held in position by the lower end of the quadriceps muscle, which surrounds the patella and is attached to the upper part of the tibia by the patellar tendon. The role of the kneecap is to protect the knee.

Kneecap removal surgery, or patellectomy, is performed as a result of fracture, frequent dislocation, or painful arthritis in the kneecap. Fracture is usually caused by a direct or sharp blow to the knee. Dislocation of the patella is often linked to a congenital abnormality, such as the underdevelopment of the lower end of the femur or excessive laxity of the ligaments that support the knee. Painful degenerative arthritic conditions, such as retropatellar arthritis and chondromalacia patellae, inflame and roughen the undersurface of the kneecap. Arthritic pain often worsens with the climbing of stairs or bending of the knee.

Before surgery begins, a clinical examination is conducted including blood and urine studies, and X rays of both knees. The knee is thoroughly cleansed with antiseptic soap. Anesthesia is administered either by local injection or spinal injection or by inhalation and injection (general anesthesia).

Surgery begins with an incision made around the kneecap. The skin is pulled back, exposing the muscle-covered kneecap. Surrounding muscle and connecting tendons attached to the kneecap are cut, and the kneecap is carefully removed. The remaining muscle is then sewn back together with strong suture material. Surgery is completed with the closing of the skin with sutures or clips. Full recovery takes about six weeks.

Uses and Complications

Following surgery, a scar will form along the incision. As the incision heals, the scar will recede gradually. Pain from the incision can be alleviated with heating pads. The affected leg should be elevated with pillows. Frequent movement of legs while resting in bed will decrease the likelihood of deep vein blood clots. General activity and returning to work is encouraged as soon as possible. Standing for prolonged periods of time, however, is not recommended during recovery. Following the approximate six-week recovery time, physical therapy is often used to restore strength to the knee.

Possible complications associated with kneecap removal include excessive bleeding and surgical wound infection. Additional complications can occur during recovery if general postoperative guidelines are not followed. Some loss of function can be expected.

—Jason Georges

See also Arthritis; Bones and the skeleton; Fracture and dislocation; Joints; Lower extremities; Orthopedic surgery; Orthopedics; Orthopedics, pediatric; Physical rehabilitation.

For Further Information:

Cresse, Mary. "Patella Fracture." *Health Library*, September 28, 2012.

Doherty, Gerard M., and Lawrence W. Way, eds. *Current Surgical Diagnosis and Treatment*. 12th ed. New York: Lange Medical Books/McGraw-Hill, 2006.

Halpern, Brian. *The Knee Crisis Handbook: Understanding Pain, Preventing Trauma, Recovering from Knee Injury, and Building Healthy Knees for Life*. Emmaus, Pa.: Rodale Books, 2003.

Kwong, Yune, and Vikram V. Desai. "The Use of a Tantalum-Based Augmentation Patella in Patients with a Previous Patellectomy." *Knee* 15, no. 2 (March 2008): 91–94.

Mulholland, Michael W., et al., eds. *Greenfield's Surgery: Scientific Principles and Practice*. 4th ed. Philadelphia: Lippincott Williams & Wilkins, 2006.

Tapley, Donald F., et al., eds. *The Columbia University College of Physicians and Surgeons Complete Home Medical Guide*. Rev. 3d ed. New York: Crown, 1995.

Tierney, Lawrence M., Stephen J. McPhee, and Maxine A. Papadakis, eds. *Current Medical Diagnosis and Treatment 2007*. New York: McGraw-Hill Medical, 2006.

Yao, Reina, Matthew Lyons, James Howard, and James McAuley. "Does Patellectomy Jeopardize Function after TKA?" *Clinical Orthopaedics & Related Research* 471, no. 2 (February 2013): 544–553.

KNOCK-KNEES
Disease/Disorder

Also known as: Genu valgum

Anatomy or system affected: Bones, feet, hips, joints, knees, legs, ligaments, muscles

Specialties and related fields: Orthopedics, pediatrics, physical therapy

Definition: A deformity in which the knees are positioned close together or turn toward each other and the tibias and ankles are apart when the feet are placed in a normal standing position.

Causes and Symptoms

Knock-knees, affecting both knees or occasionally only one, are a normal condition as children mature. Infants" leg bones are slightly rotated because of uterine positioning. As toddlers" legs straighten after having bowlegs, their tibias and knees often temporarily rotate toward the body's axis, causing the feet to be several inches apart. When knock-knees are not representative of normal physical development, they occur because of health conditions such as infections, obesity, or fractured legs that disrupt knee growth. Knock-knees are sometimes a symptom of other conditions.

Mobility may be affected with knock-knees. Patients sometimes adjust leg and foot movement to compensate for altered knee positioning and imbalanced centers of gravity. Usually, children walk with their toes turned in for balance when they have knock-knees. Knock-kneed adults sometimes develop arthritis because of the strain on knee joints and ligaments. Knock-knees can also place stress on patients" backs and hips.

Treatment and Therapy

Medical professionals do not treat most knock-knees unless specific cases seem abnormal, cause pain, or impede movement. Growth usually corrects knee positioning. Physicians measure legs and the distance between ankles to assess the progress of natural correction. X-rays are useful to detect bone problems that may exacerbate knock-knees. Photographs can document leg alignment.

Stretching the leg muscles can aid the natural resolution of knock-knees. Shoes designed with inserts can mitigate the stress on feet and manipulate patients to walk straight. Physical therapy can alleviate cartilage and joint pain associated with knock-knees.

If young patients do not outgrow knock-knees, ankle distances increase to four inches or more, or the condition wors-

Information on Knock-Knees

Causes: Normal condition in infants; infections, obesity, or fractures in older individuals

Symptoms: Altered knee positioning, imbalanced center of gravity, sometimes arthritis

Duration: Usually temporary

Treatments: None, unless pain develops or movement is impeded; may include stretching, shoe inserts, physical therapy, orthopedic braces, surgery

ens, particularly in one knee, then medical intervention often becomes necessary to ensure that patients are capable of normal movement. Physicians sometimes advise patients to wear a brace. If such efforts are unsuccessful, then the patient may undergo surgery to adjust leg bones and growth plates.

Treatment is essential for diseases or conditions in which knock-knees is a symptom. Some patients seek medical correction for aesthetic reasons.

Perspective and Prospects

Beginning in the late nineteenth century, physicians routinely recommended therapeutic braces to treat knock-knees. During the 1950s, Soviet doctor Gavril Abramovich Ilizarov devised a fixator that encircles legs and uses tension to correct rotation problems associated with knock-knees. Italian doctor Antonio Bianchi-Maiocchi first used this device in Western countries in 1981. James Aronson brought the method to the United States in the 1980s. In that decade, Ukrainian doctor Veklich Vitaliy adapted Ilizarov's fixator for a procedure that is often used to correct severe knock-knees.

By the late twentieth century, however, physicians discouraged the use of braces to treat normal cases of knock-knees. Most advised patients to permit natural correction to occur, emphasizing that devices would not quicken that process.

—*Elizabeth D. Schafer, Ph.D.*

See also Bones and the skeleton; Growth; Joints; Lower extremities; Orthopedics; Orthopedics, pediatric.

For Further Information:

Atanda, Alfred Jr. "Common Childhood Orthopedic Conditions." *KidsHealth.org*. Nemours Foundation, Nov. 2011.

Bianci-Maiocchi, Antonio, and James Aronson, eds. *Operative Principles of Ilizarov: Fracture Treatment, Nonunion, Osteomyelitis, Lengthening, Deformity Correction*. Baltimore: Williams & Wilkins, 1991.

"Bowlegs and Knock-Knees." *HealthChildren.org*. American Academy of Pediatrics, Nov. 19, 2012.

England, Stephen P., ed. *Common Orthopedic Problems*. Philadelphia: W. B. Saunders, 1996.

Halpern, Brian. *The Knee Crisis Handbook: Understanding Pain, Preventing Trauma, Recovering from Knee Injury, and Building Healthy Knees for Life*. Emmaus, Pa.: Rodale Books, 2003.

Herring, John A., ed. *Tachdjian's Pediatric Orthopaedics*. 4th ed. 3 vols. Philadelphia: Saunders/Elsevier, 2008.

Kaneshiro, Neil K., et al. "Knock knees." *MedlinePlus*, Nov. 12, 2012.

Korsakoff's Syndrome

Disease/Disorder

Anatomy or system affected: Brain

Specialties and related fields: Addiction, neurology, nutrition, psychiatry, psychology

Definition: Korsakoff's syndrome is a neurological condition involving disturbances in the ability to form short-term memories, often resulting in confabulation and psychosis, and attributable to deficiencies in thiamine often associated with chronic alcohol use.

Key terms:

alcohol dependence: a substance use disorder where alcohol consumption leads to a sustained pattern of significant problems involving alcohol tolerance and/or withdrawal and which may impair health, relationships, or other functioning

alcohol-related dementia: a chronic condition of overall deterioration in all mental functions, such as memory, concentration, judgment, and which may involve personality change and mood problems, that is attributable to alcohol-related behavior

confabulation: verbal behavior reflecting that a person is making up a story to replace facts or information they do not recall or otherwise remember

intoxication: the condition of having consumed a drug and being under its influence to the point of experiencing a range of reactions from excitement to stupefaction

long-term memory: information stored in the mind and that refers to knowledge, experiences, thoughts, and perceptions over lengthier periods of time

psychosis: a mental state, that may be brief or lengthy, where a person has a loss of contact with reality, sees or hears or otherwise experiences things that are not truly present, and suffers from impaired social, emotional, and/or mental functioning

short-term memory: information stored in the mind that refers to knowledge, experiences, thoughts, and perceptions that may have just occurred recently

thiamine: a nutritional substance known as vitamin B1 derived from food sources like meats, yeasts, and the bran of grain, that is necessary for normal neurological activity and carbohydrate metabolism

Wernicke's encephalopathy: a condition associated with Korsakoff's syndrome characterized by confusion, problems of muscle coordination, and visual problems

Causes and Symptoms

Individuals are recognized as having Korsakoff's syndrome when they appear to be confused and have short-term memory problems, such as difficulty forming new memories. They may think it is the wrong year, for example, 10 years earlier than the present day. They may not understand why someone they know suddenly looks so old, because in their mind it is 10 years ago and the person should still look as they did then. Individuals with this syndrome also often tell stories that sound perfectly rationale to them and uninformed observers, but are complete fabrications. Confabulation is the term used to describe the process of telling such stories. In the absence of being able to recall the actual detail of certain memories, the individual will make up stories or segments of stories to fill in the blanks. This is not necessarily willful lying to cover up a failure to remember something. Instead, the person often fails to recognize that they have made up a story. This can in turn lead to more confusion and, as the condition worsens, to psychosis.

The cause of this syndrome is attributable to thiamine deficiency. Often this can happen with unusual eating habits, problems with the body absorbing thiamine (as can occur after certain illnesses or surgeries to the gastro-intestinal system), or a diet deficient in thiamine. Individuals with alcohol dependence sometimes will fail to eat properly and suffer nutritionally. Lack of thiamine in the diet can result in Korsakoff's syndrome.

Korsakoff's syndrome often occurs in conjunction with another disorder called Wernicke's encephalopathy. It is a separate condition, but the two occur so frequently together that they are known as Wernicke-Korsakoff syndrome. This combination of problems is associated with severe and chronic alcohol dependence. The typical presentation is that the symptoms of Wernicke's encephalopathy will present first, followed by the Korsakoff's syndrome.

Treatment and Therapy

The treatment for Korsakoff's syndrome generally begins with a thorough assessment of the symptoms presenting. There are many conditions that involve memory problems. Additionally, there are other health and mental health issues that can complicate the interpretation of memory issues. Thorough evaluation is the first step in any good treatment regimen.

Once the condition is identified, treatment relies on the replenishment of thiamine to the body. It is also necessary to keep the affected individual out of harm until they are stabilized and confusion and psychosis are minimized. Treatment efforts also will focus on decreasing any behaviors or conditions that may predispose an individual to be unable to consume or properly metabolize thiamine.

Shots of B1 vitamins are common and may reverse some of the symptoms, such as problems with coordination or vision. Memory may also improve if the condition has not yet become chronic. When chronic alcohol problems are present, however, often by the time the syndrome is discovered, memory problems can be permanent. As such, early attention to keeping a well-balanced diet is critical in individuals identified as being at risk for chronic alcohol problems to avoid Korsakoff's syndrome.

Perspective and Prospects

Historically discussed as Wernicke-Korsakoff syndrome, these conditions that often occur together in individuals with alcohol-related problems are now more appropriately discussed separately as Korsakoff syndrome and Wernicke's encephalopathy. This is partly because additional causes and associations have been drawn between these disorders. For example, Korsakoff syndrome also is associated with other problems resulting from thiamine deficiencies. One example in this regard is surgeries that remove sections of the gastrointestinal tract. Such surgeries may diminish the ability of the body to absorb varied vitamins, including thiamine, and result in Korsakoff's syndrome. Additionally, treatment professionals understand that high levels of glucose can trigger Wernicke's encephalopathy in individuals at risk. As such, a common practice now is to first administer thiamine to avoid triggering these additional symptoms. Future work on these problems is likely to focus on increasing methods of identifying individuals at risk for these problems, improving prevention efforts to stave off the problems, and improving therapies related to mitigating long-term memory loss.

—*Nancy A. Piotrowski, Ph.D.*

See also Amnesia; Neuropsychology; Addiction; Alcoholism; Thiamine

For Further Information:

Anderson, Kenneth, G. Alan Marlatt, and Patt Denning. *How to Change Your Drinking: A Harm Reduction Guide to Alcohol.* 2nd ed. Seattle: CreateSpace, 2010.
Inaba, Daryl S., William E. Cohen, Elizabeth von Radics, and Ellen K. Cholewa. *Uppers, Downers, All-Arounders: Physical and Mental Effects of Psychoactive Drugs.* 7th ed. Medford, OR: CNS Productions, 2011.
Schildkrout, Barbara. *Masquerading Symptoms: Uncovering Physical Illnesses that Present as Psychological Symptoms.* Hoboken, NJ: Wiley, 2013.

KWASHIORKOR
Disease/Disorder

Also known as: Malignant malnutrition, protein malnutrition, protein-calorie malnutrition, Mehl hrschaden

Anatomy or system affected: Gastrointestinal system, muscles, skin

Specialties and related fields: Family medicine, nutrition, pediatrics

Definition: A form of malnutrition caused by inadequate protein intake.

Causes and Symptoms

Kwashiorkor occurs most commonly in areas of famine, limited food supply, and low levels of education, which can lead to inadequate knowledge of diet and appropriate dietary intakes. Early symptoms are general and include fatigue, irritability, and lethargy. As protein deprivation continues, symptoms include failure to gain weight and linear growth. Other progressed symptoms include apathy, decreased muscle mass, edema, a large protuberant belly (resulting from decreased albumin in the blood), diarrhea, and dermatitis. Skin may lose pigment where it has peeled away or darken where it has been irritated or traumatized. Hair may become thin and brittle and may change color, becoming lighter or reddish. As a result of immune system damage, patients may suffer from increased numbers of infections and increased severity of

Information on Kwashiorkor

Causes: Protein deprivation
Symptoms: Fatigue, irritability, lethargy, poor growth, apathy, edema, decreased muscle mass, large belly, diarrhea, dermatitis, loss of skin pigmentation, changes in color and texture of hair, infections; may progress to shock, coma, and death
Duration: Progressive if untreated
Treatments: Depends on degree of malnutrition; may include treatment for shock and increased calorie intake (first as carbohydrates, simple sugars, and fats, then proteins)

what normally might be mild infections. In the final stages, shock and/or coma usually precede death.

Treatment and Therapy

A physical examination may show an enlarged liver and generalized edema. Treatment varies depending on the degree of malnutrition. Patients in shock will require immediate treatment. Often, calories are given first in the form of carbohydrates, simple sugars, and fats. Proteins are started after other caloric sources have provided increased energy. Vitamin and mineral supplements are essential. Many children will have developed intolerance to milk lactose (sugar intolerance) and will need to be supplemented with lactase (an enzyme) if they are to benefit from milk products. Adequate diet with appropriate amounts of carbohydrates, fat, and protein will prevent kwashiorkor.

Perspective and Prospects

Kwashiorkor means "deposed child" in one African dialect, referring to a child "deposed" from the mother's breast by a newborn sibling. Kwashiorkor is found largely in tropical and subtropical regions where the diet is high in starch (such as cereal grains or plantains) and low in protein. Treatment early in the course of kwashiorkor generally produces positive results. Treatment in later stages will improve a child's general health, but the child may be left with permanent physical ailments and mental disabilities. With delayed or no treatment, the condition is fatal.

—*Jason A. Hubbart, M.S.*

See also Dietary reference intakes (DRIs); Edema; Food biochemistry; Malnutrition; Nutrition; Protein.

For Further Information:

Champakam, S., S. G. Srikantia, and C. Gopalan. "Kwashiorkor and Mental Development." *American Journal of Clinical Nutrition* 21 (1968): 844.
Golden, M. H. N. "Severe Malnutrition." In *Oxford Textbook of Medicine*, edited by D. J. Weatherall, J. G. G. Ledingham, and D. A. Warrell. 3d ed. New York: Oxford University Press, 1996.
Kaneshiro, Neil K. "Kwashiorkor." *MedlinePlus*, February 1, 2012.
Kleinman, Ronald E., ed. *Pediatric Nutrition Handbook*. 6th ed. Elk Grove Village, Ill.: American Academy of Pediatrics, 2009.

KYPHOSIS

Disease/Disorder
Also known as: Dowager's hump
Anatomy or system affected: Back, bones
Specialties and related fields: Orthopedics
Definition: A marked increase of the normal curvature of the thoracic vertebrae or upper back, sometimes referred to as dowager's hump because of its prevalence in elderly women.

Causes and Symptoms

Patients with kyphosis appear to be looking down with their shoulders markedly bent forward. They are unable to straighten their backs and their body height is reduced, causing their arms to appear to be disproportionately long. The increased curvature of the thoracic vertebrae tilts the head forward, and the patient has to raise his or her head and hyperextend his or her neck in order to look forward. This posture increases the strain on the neck muscles and leads to discomfort in the neck, shoulders, and upper back. It limits the field of vision and increases the patient's chances of tripping over an object not directly in the line of vision. It also shifts forward the body's center of gravity and increases the chances of falling.

In severe cases, kyphosis limits chest expansion during breathing. As a result, less air gets into the lungs, which become underventilated and prone to infections. Pneumonia is a common cause of death in these patients. In very severe cases, the curvature of the thoracic vertebrae is so pronounced that the lower ribs lie over the pelvic cavity. Patients with severe kyphosis are not able to lie flat on their backs, and many spend most of their time sitting up in a chair or in bed, propped by a number of pillows. Unless the patient changes positions frequently, the pressure exerted by the vertebrae on the skin and subcutaneous tissue may precipitate pressure sores (bedsores) on the upper back. Pressure sores may also develop on the buttocks. The sores often become infected, and the infection may spread to the blood, leading to septicemia and death.

The most common cause of kyphosis is osteoporosis, a disease in which the bone mass is reduced. As a result, the bones become mechanically weak and are unable to sustain the pressure of the body weight. The vertebrae gradually become

Information on Kyphosis

Causes: Osteoporosis, tumors, infection
Symptoms: Inability to straighten one's back, reduced body height, appearance of disproportionately long arms, strain on neck muscles leading to discomfort, pain
Duration: Chronic
Treatments: Hormone therapy, drug therapy (e.g., Fosamax, teriparatide)

wedged and partially collapsed, more so in the front (anteriorly) than in the back (posteriorly), thus increasing the forward curvature of the thoracic vertebrae. Sometimes, the compression of a vertebra is associated with sudden, very severe and incapacitating pain that is usually relieved spontaneously after about four weeks. In most cases, however, the compression is a gradual process associated with slowly worsening back discomfort. The discomfort is caused by the strain imposed on the muscles on either side of the vertebrae. In rare instances, the nerves exiting the spinal cord become trapped by the wedged or collapsed vertebrae, and the patient experiences severe pain that tends to radiate to the area supplied by the entrapped nerve.

Less common causes of kyphosis include the compression of a vertebra as a result of tumors or infections. In these cases, the angulation of the thoracic curvature is very prominent.

Treatment and Therapy

The availability of medications to treat and prevent osteoporosis, including alendronate and teriparatide, should significantly reduce the prevalence of both that disease and kyphosis. Severe cases of kyphosis or cases due to infection or tumor may require surgery.

—Ronald C. Hamdy, M.D.

See also Aging; Back pain; Bone disorders; Bones and the skeleton; Braces, orthopedic; Orthopedic surgery; Orthopedics; Orthopedics, pediatric; Osteoporosis; Pneumonia; Safety issues for the elderly; Spinal cord disorders; Spine, vertebrae, and disks.

For Further Information:
Byyny, Richard L., and Leon Speroff. *A Clinical Guide for the Care of Older Women: Primary and Preventive Care*. 2d ed. Baltimore: Williams & Wilkins, 1996.

Currey, John D. *Bones: Structures and Mechanics*. 2d ed. Princeton, N.J.: Princeton University Press, 2006.

Heaney, Robert P. "Osteoporosis." In *Nutrition in Women's Health*, edited by Debra A. Krummel and Penny M. Kris-Etherton. Gaithersburg, Md.: Aspen, 1996.

Hodgson, Stephen F., ed. *Mayo Clinic on Osteoporosis: Keeping Bones Healthy and Strong and Reducing the Risk of Fractures*. Rochester, Minn.: Mayo Clinic, 2003.

Joseph, Thomas N., and David Zieve. "Kyphosis." *MedlinePlus*, September 4, 2012.

Meredith, C. M. "Exercise in the Prevention of Osteoporosis." In *Nutrition of the Elderly*, edited by Hamish Munro and Gunter Schlierf. Nestle's Nutrition Workshop Series 29. New York: Raven Press, 1992.

Nelson, Miriam E., and Sarah Wernick. *Strong Women, Strong Bones: Everything You Need to Know to Prevent, Treat, and Beat Osteoporosis*. Rev. ed. New York: Berkley Books, 2006.

Van De Graaff, Kent M. *Human Anatomy*. 6th ed. New York: McGraw-Hill, 2002.

LABORATORY TESTS

Procedures

Anatomy or system affected: Blood, cells

Specialties and related fields: Bacteriology, cytology, endocrinology, epidemiology, forensic medicine, genetics, hematology, histology, immunology, microbiology, oncology, pathology, pharmacology, serology, toxicology, virology

Definition: The collection and analysis of body fluids such as blood and urine to establish a diagnosis or to monitor a treatment regimen.

Key terms:

antibody: a protein produced in the body by the immune system that recognizes and binds selectively to foreign material (antigens) to facilitate their elimination; antibodies can be cultivated in animals or by artificial means in the laboratory and chemically altered for use as reagents in immunoassays

clinical chemistry: a chemistry specialty that deals with an analysis of the chemical components of body fluids

clinical laboratory: a general term for those areas of a medical facility where analyses of body fluids are performed

clinical microbiology: the scientific discipline involving the study of microscopic organisms (such as bacteria, fungi, and viruses) that cause disease

coagulation: the process of blood clotting, a very complicated process that can be affected by many disease states; the clotting process is inhibited for specimen collection purposes using substances called anticoagulants

hematology: the medical specialty dealing with the detection and diagnosis of blood-related diseases

immunoassay: the use of antibody-antigen recognition as the basis of a medically useful method of detecting and measuring a substance in body fluids

pathology: the medical specialty that deals with the structural and biochemical changes that are produced by disease

Indications and Procedures

Clinical laboratory testing is a vital element in diagnosis. After physical examination and the taking of the patient's medical history, the physician will often request that specific tests be performed on blood, urine, or other body fluids. Appropriate specimens are collected and forwarded to the laboratory for specimen processing.

Blood is the most common specimen submitted for testing in the clinical laboratory. In a hospital or large referral laboratory, there may be special personnel, called phlebotomists, employed to collect blood. In a small office laboratory, blood may be collected by the attending physician or nurse. Blood is collected in a syringe or in special tubes that may contain anticoagulants.

Urine is the next most common laboratory specimen and is collected as a result of a single void (random urine specimen) or for a time period of twenty-four hours or more. In the latter case, the collection container may also contain substances that act as a preservative. If a long-term urine specimen is

necessary, it is very important for the patient to follow the directions regarding collection. Failure to follow these directions can lead to erroneous laboratory results.

Less commonly collected specimens include cerebrospinal fluid, gastric (stomach) fluid, and amniotic fluid. Cerebrospinal fluid is usually collected by a physician by direct sampling with a needle (lumbar puncture, or spinal tap). Gastric fluid is obtained by the insertion of a gastric collection tube. Amniotic fluid is collected by an obstetrician in the process called amniocentesis, in which a sample of the fluid surrounding the fetus is removed by the insertion of a needle through the mother's abdomen. Frequently, laboratory tests are also ordered on infectious material associated with a wound or surgical incision.

A major aspect of specimen collection is ensuring that the sample is correctly labeled and that no mix-up of specimens has occurred. Part of this process may involve checking identification armbands or asking patients or nursing staff to confirm identification. While this procedure may be exasperating to the patient or nursing personnel, it is a necessary part of detecting errors.

Immediately after the specimen is received in the laboratory, documentation of time of receipt and the tests requested is made, which is referred to as logging in the specimen. Each sample receives a special code called an accession number. The test performance and results are tracked with this number, since multiple specimens can be received on a single patient in a given day. This process is usually computerized and may use bar code labeling in a process very similar to that used for automatic cash-register pricing of grocery items.

In large hospital or referral laboratories, the processing center is responsible for distributing the sample to the laboratory sections, where various tests are performed. Since each test requires a specific amount of sample, specimen processing also involves determining that the correct amount of fluid has been collected and reserved for proper performance of the test.

For blood specimens, many laboratory determinations are made regarding plasma, or serum, which is the liquid component of blood that contains no cells. The whole blood specimen is separated into cellular and liquid components by centrifugation. The sample is spun rapidly so that the force of the spin sediments the cells, with the serum or plasma layer on top.

Once the specimen is distributed to the pertinent laboratory sections, testing is done using a variety of analytical techniques. The testing methodology is almost as varied as the types of analyses requested. A few general statements, however, are applicable. Automation is the guiding force behind laboratory test methodology development. Routinely ordered tests are done with instruments specifically designed to perform a group or panel of tests, rather than each test being performed individually by a technologist using manual chemistry methods. Automation coupled with computerization has greatly increased laboratory efficiency, decreased turnaround time (the time required for a test to be performed and results to be reported to the physician), eliminated human errors, and allowed more tests to be performed on smaller sample material. The latter advantage is particularly important for pediatric specimens, in which sample size is usually an important consideration. Automation also eliminates much of the technologist's contact with the specimen, considerably reducing the risk of spreading infectious diseases.

Each section of the laboratory is responsible for a specific set of tests. The chemistry section performs chemical analyses of body fluids. Panels of tests related to kidney, heart, and liver function are also done. In addition, tests to measure amounts of therapeutic drugs, hormones, blood proteins, and cancer-related proteins are accomplished with immunoassay techniques. The development of antibody-related techniques has revolutionized testing in all areas of the clinical laboratory. The ability to customize antibody production and adapt it to specific analytical requirements has allowed the continual development of new tests and methodologies.

Thehematology section is responsible for monitoring the levels of blood cells and clotting factors. Other specialized tests to diagnose cancer of the blood cells may also be done. Blood typing and donor testing are technically hematology-related tests, but they are usually reserved for a separate section designated asblood bank or transfusion services. Transfusion service is a specialty in its own right and is almost always reserved for hospital-associated laboratories.

Microbiology is the section where body fluids are checked for infectious microorganisms. Once an organism is identified, the section can also determine which antibiotics may be useful for treatment by performing antibiotic susceptibility tests.

As the laboratory tests are performed, the results are recorded and reported to the physician. Computerization has permitted the transfer of patient results directly from the instrument performing the test to the patient's file, eliminating many tedious and error-prone clerical functions.

For hospital and reference laboratories, a laboratory director—either a physician (usually a pathologist) who specializes in laboratory medicine or a scientist with doctoral level training in a laboratory specialty—monitors the performance of the laboratory, helps physicians with the interpretation of ambiguous or complex laboratory results, and provides guidance on the introduction of new tests or instrumentation. Most laboratories also have a section supervisor or administrator who is an experienced medical technologist to oversee the daily laboratory routine.

Uses and Complications

Because of the variety of laboratory testing, it is impractical to cover its applications in depth in a brief review. Instead, a few illustrative tests that are performed often or are associated with familiar disorders will be presented. The most frequently ordered laboratory tests are serum glucose tests, serum electrolyte (salt) level measurements, and complete blood count (CBC) tests.

The maintenance of blood glucose (sugar) levels is essential

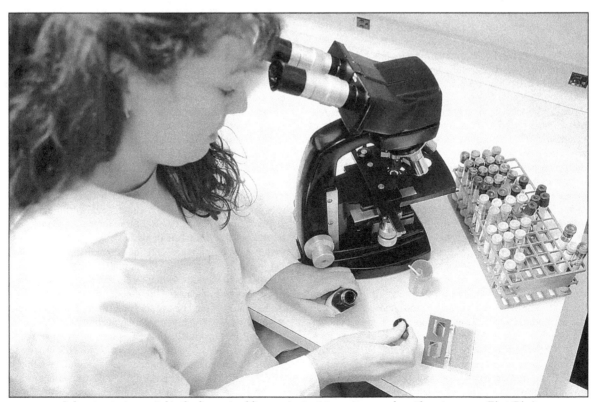

Laboratory tests are vital in the diagnosis of disease. A scientist examines samples with a microscope. (PhotoDisc)

for body activity and brain function. The laboratory measurement of blood glucose is one of the oldest known procedures performed in the clinical laboratory. It is part of the diagnostic procedures used to monitor and test for diabetes mellitus. Glucose and electrolyte testing are performed in the chemistry section of the laboratory, while a CBC takes place in hematology. Certain levels of electrolytes—sodium, chloride, potassium, and calcium—are needed for proper cardiac function. An abnormal level of these salts could also indicate possible hormonal or kidney malfunction. The CBC is a measure of the cell populations that carry oxygen (red blood cells), fight infection or invasion by foreign substances (white blood cells), and activate the blood-clotting mechanism (platelets). The white cell population is elevated in infections but also in cases of leukemia (malignant growth of a white cell population). More specialized testing is needed when leukemia is suspected. An instrument called a flow cytometer can be used to count and detect subtypes of white cells. These data, along with a pathologist's microscopic examination of a blood smear and the results of clinical examination, are used to arrive at a diagnosis of the specific type of leukemia present. The identification of the cell population causing the cancer is important for determining treatment and prognosis.

A deficiency of red cells or their oxygen-carrying hemoglobin molecule is called anemia. It can be caused by iron deficiency and other impairments of red cell production, chronic bleeding, or accelerated red cell destruction (hemolysis). Each of the causes must be either confirmed or ruled out through additional testing or by clinical examination.

Platelet deficiency is a major cause of clotting disorders, although many other causes of bleeding disorders exist. The specific defect can be determined by measuring the clotting time and by using special immunoassays to measure clotting substances in the blood.

Many hormonal (endocrine) disorders can be diagnosed through laboratory testing. For example, the thyroid, the regulator gland for body metabolism, can produce a variety of symptoms when it is not functioning properly. Thyroid testing is the most common endocrine-related laboratory procedure requested by physicians. The blood levels of thyroid hormone and of the pituitary factor that stimulates the thyroid gland are measured in the laboratory using immunoassay methods. These types of assays can also be used to monitor other hormones involved in fertility, growth, and the function of the adrenal gland (the gland that helps maintain sugar metabolism and electrolyte balance).

Immunoassay methodology has also permitted the routine laboratory testing of therapeutic drugs as well as of drugs of abuse. In the past, the technology for analyzing drugs in biological fluids involved expensive, labor-intensive techniques that were impractical for routine laboratory use. With the introduction of immunologically based testing for drugs, however, it became possible to monitor patients on antibiotics, immunosuppressive agents, cardiac drugs, and antiseizure medication. Testing has been automated so that these drug levels can be performed as routine laboratory procedures. Assay results can be used to establish an individual dosage

schedule so that dosage is maintained in the therapeutic range and does not exceed the concentration threshold, leading to toxic effects, or decline to values too low to achieve adequate treatment (subtherapeutic levels).

A continuing research effort is directed toward developing specific diagnostic cancer tests. These tests could be used to screen patients for tumors in order to detect them early, when therapy would be most effective. Substances that appear in body fluids coincident with the growth of tumors are referred to as tumor markers. The ideal tumor marker would appear only in patients afflicted with a specific type of cancer. Its concentration would reflect the size of the tumor as well as the presence of metastasis, in which tumor cells migrate from the initial cancer site to other sites in the body.

The ideal tumor marker has not yet been discovered. Most have not been specific or sensitive enough to use as a screening tool for detecting tumors, although they have been useful for monitoring the effects of therapy. One example of a useful marker is prostate-specific antigen (PSA). The level of this protein in serum is very low when the prostate gland is normal. When prostate cancer is present, however, the serum level, as measured by immunoassay, is elevated. The test can also be used for screening, provided that any positive result is confirmed by clinical examination. It is also used following prostate surgery or radiation therapy in order to determine the completeness of tumor removal. Continually high or rising levels of PSA in the serum following treatment indicate that residual tumor is still present.

In the microbiology department, the culturing of body fluids and antibiotic susceptibility studies allow the selection of the most appropriate antibiotic for treatment. The course and duration of treatment can then be followed in the chemistry laboratory using the therapeutic drug monitoring techniques discussed above. When an infection is suspected, body fluids are cultured or incubated with media selected to grow only specific microorganisms. Antibiotic susceptibility studies are performed by culturing the organism with various antibiotics until growth is arrested. Many strains of bacteria and other microorganisms will become resistant to an antibiotic that had proven effective previously, and patients who are allergic to some antibiotics may need to be treated with an alternative regimen.

The detection and identification of viruses has become a subspecialty in microbiology with distinctly different culturing techniques. Newer immunoassay methods and other biotechnologically based methods have made virus diagnosis easier. Acquired immunodeficiency syndrome (AIDS) testing is a prime example of the application of immunoassay techniques to virology testing. A detection technique that required growth of the human immunodeficiency virus (HIV) in the laboratory would be extraordinarily difficult and tedious. It would also be prohibitively expensive and time-consuming to screen large populations such as blood donors and high-risk groups. Instead, laboratory screening for HIV uses an automated immunoassay technique based on the detection of patient antibodies to virus-specific antigens. Although this test is very specific, the possibility of false positives is greatly minimized by confirming all positive screening results with

In the News: In-Home Medical Testing

In-home health testing has become increasingly popular as a result of its convenience, privacy, and affordability. Home tests can enable the consumer to determine the potential risk for developing a health problem even when no immediate signs or symptoms exist, or they can enable the consumer to follow a specific medical condition more accurately. Several home tests are available for over-the-counter purchase, including those that test for cholesterol levels, drugs of abuse, fecal occult blood, glucose levels, hepatitis C, human immunodeficiency virus (HIV), ovulation timing, pregnancy, prothrombin time screening, and vaginal pH. Home test kits should not be used as stand-alone measures to determine one's health care, but rather the results should be used in conjunction with proper medical advice in order to confirm the test results.

Most reports state that the test kits approved by the Food and Drug Administration (FDA) are either "about as accurate" or "fairly accurate," when compared to those that a doctor would use, provided that the instructions are carefully followed. The consumer should understand that no test is 100 percent accurate; test accuracy is improved when the consumer can read, understand, and follow the directions for test administration carefully. A home test kit will require accurate timing, specific collection materials, and typically a body fluid sample. Failure to comply with any of these factors could result in an inaccurate reading. If a product is not approved by the FDA, then the test's safety and efficacy is in question. Internet shopping for diagnostic test kits can be particularly misleading, since not all test kits available for purchase in this fashion are FDA-approved and some are illegal to sell over the Internet.

A search of the Clinical Laboratory Improvement Amendments (CLIA) database will inform the consumer if a home test has FDA approval. To use this search engine, the consumer must know if the test is considered a "test kit" (a consumer takes a sample, performs the test, and analyzes it, all on one's own) or a "collection kit" (a consumer takes a sample but sends it out to a laboratory for analysis). Collection kits are not currently listed on the CLIA database, although one can contact the FDA directly to find out if a kit is FDA-approved. The FDA maintains another database called Manufacturer and User Facility Device Experience (MAUDE), which lists reports on problems with kits and testing devices. *Consumer Reports* magazine and its Web site can also provide the consumer with additional product comparison information for a handful of home tests.

—*Bonita L. Marks, Ph.D.*

another antibody test called a Western blot. In this test, a serum sample from a suspected HIV-positive patient is applied to a membrane impregnated with virus proteins. The virus proteins are localized at a characteristic position determined by their migration rate when the membrane coated with virus proteins is subjected to an electric field in a process called protein electrophoresis. After the membrane has been treated with patient serum and color development reagents, the presence in the patient sample of an antibody to one or more of these proteins is revealed as a colored stripe on the membrane. A combination of the two tests is a cost-efficient and extremely accurate procedure to confirm a suspected diagnosis of HIV infection.

Perspective and Prospects

According to a 2002 study of the history of the clinical laboratory by J. Büttner, the concept of the modern hospital laboratory was first documented in 1791, when French physician and chemist Antoine-François de Fourcroy wrote that in hospitals, "a chemical laboratory should be set up not far away from a ward having twenty or thirty beds." Büttner asserts that the two suppositions necessary for the creation of these laboratories were the idea that the results of laboratory examinations can be used as "chemical signs" in medical diagnosis

and a new concept of disease that was the result of the "birth of the clinic" at the end of the eighteenth century.

During this phase of laboratory development, investigations were performed at patients" bedsides by physicians themselves. In the period from 1840 to 1855, clinical laboratories were established as operations distinct from hospitals and clinics. Most of these laboratories were developed in German-speaking countries and staffed by scientists who performed tests for the hospitals and taught medical students physiological chemistry. From 1855 onward, the concept of the clinical laboratory spread rapidly, with clinicians assuming directorship roles. The laboratory ultimately serving as a model for clinical laboratories in the United States was established by the renowned pathologist Rudolf Virchow at Berlin University. As the chair for pathological anatomy, he set up a "chemical department" within the institute for pathology in 1856. This laboratory represented a center of clinical chemistry research and established the clinical laboratory as integral to pathology.

Laboratories have evolved as essential but distinctly separate specialties of medical services. Although there is little or no participation in the analytical process by the physicians ordering the tests, a major part of a physician's diagnostic skill is knowing which tests to order as a supplement to examination and medical history. Laboratory tests cost money and time, and they may be useless in the diagnostic process if not ordered in a judicious fashion. The old medical admonishment to "treat the patient, not the laboratory result" is still an appropriate consideration. Moreover, responsibility for the correct interpretation of the results lies with the attending physician, who has access to all the pertinent patient data.

Laboratory results are usually interpreted with the help of a reference range. Reference ranges ideally represent laboratory values characteristic of a sample population that is free of known disease. If the results lie within this range, however, the laboratory result cannot always be assumed to rule out a specific diagnosis. Since considerable biological variation exists for most laboratory values, diseased individuals can sometimes yield test values in the normal range, and, conversely, healthy individuals can occasionally have low or elevated values.

To verify a diagnosis, all laboratory results and clinical impressions should complement one another. The detection of blood-clotting deficiencies by the hematology department could be related to a poorly functioning liver, which will also be reflected in changes in enzymes and blood proteins measured in the chemistry laboratory. Cardiac disorders are diagnosed not only by examining an electrocardiograph (EKG or ECG) but also by measuring the levels of specific cardiac-related enzymes that rise to abnormally high levels when cardiac blood supply is diminished (such as with myocardial infarction, or heart attack). In summary, the clinical laboratory provides a valuable tool for physicians, but it should never displace clinical examination and medical history as methods of determining the final diagnosis.

—*David J. Wells, Jr., Ph.D.*

See also Amniocentesis; Bacteriology; Biopsy; Blood and blood disorders; Blood testing; Breast biopsy; Cells; Cytology; Cytopathology; Diagnosis; DNA and RNA; Endometrial biopsy; Forensic pathology; Genetic engineering; Genetics and inheritance; Gram staining; Hematology; Hematology, pediatric; Histology; Hormones; Karyotyping; Lymph; Microbiology; Microscopy; Pathology; Screening; Serology; Toxicology; Urinalysis.

For Further Information:

Bennington, James L., ed. *Saunders Dictionary and Encyclopedia of Laboratory Medicine and Technology*. Philadelphia: W. B. Saunders, 1984.

Cavanaugh, Bonita Morrow. *Nurse's Manual of Laboratory and Diagnostic Tests*. 4th ed. Philadelphia: F. A. Davis, 2003.

Griffith, H. Winter. *Complete Guide to Symptoms, Illness, and Surgery*. Revised and updated by Stephen Moore and Kenneth Yoder. 5th ed. New York: Perigee, 2006.

Lab Tests Online. "Understanding Your Tests." *American Association for Clinical Chemistry*, November 5, 2012.

McPherson, Richard A., and Matthew R. Pincus, eds. *Henry's Clinical Diagnosis and Management by Laboratory Methods*. 21st ed. Philadelphia: Saunders/Elsevier, 2007.

MedlinePlus. "Laboratory Tests." *MedlinePlus*, June 20, 2013.

National Heart, Lung, and Blood Institute. "What Do Blood Tests Show?" *National Institutes of Health*, January 6, 2012.

Pagana, Kathleen Deska, and Timothy J. Pagana. *Mosby's Diagnostic and Laboratory Test Reference*. 9th ed. St. Louis, Mo.: Mosby/Elsevier, 2009.

Price, Christopher P., and David J. Newman, eds. *Principles and Practice of Immunoassay*. 2d ed. New York: Stockton Press, 1997.

Wu, Alan H. B., ed. *Tietz Clinical Guide to Laboratory Tests*. 4th ed. St. Louis, Mo.: Saunders/Elsevier, 2006.

LACERATION REPAIR

Procedure

Anatomy or system affected: Skin

Specialties and related fields: Emergency medicine, general surgery, plastic surgery

Definition: The closure of an irregular skin wound.

Indications and Procedures

A laceration is a jagged, torn, mangled, or ragged wound. This type of wound is most commonly encountered in the skin, although any tissue may be lacerated. Lacerations are caused by sharp objects such as a piece of metal, glass, or a stick. They may also occur in accidents involving machinery or animals.

The first priority in laceration repair is to stop the bleeding,

thereby minimizing blood loss. This is usually accomplished by pressure either directly on the wound or on the injured blood vessel nearest the injury site.

The second priority with a laceration is to clean the wound, which involves the removal of any foreign material or debris. With penetrating injuries, this cleaning must be done carefully, lest the removal of the object initiate bleeding. Tissue that has been destroyed beyond the body's ability to repair it must also be removed; this process is called debridement. Devitalized tissue is removed to prevent infection. The wound site is then cleaned via irrigation with saline and a disinfectant, usually a mild soap or a chemical.

After the laceration has been cleaned, it may then be treated for bacterial or other pathogenic contamination. Aqueous solutions containing an antibiotic are used with most wounds. If contamination with other pathogens is suspected, appropriate agents are used to rinse the wound. Antibiotic powders may be employed in field conditions, although this form of treatment is unusual in a hospital setting. Other than soap and water, there is no special treatment for viral contamination.

Closure of the wound is then completed. The edges are brought together and may be held in place with forceps. Sutures, or stitches, are inserted to hold the edges together while the tissue heals. On skin surfaces, these sutures are usually nonabsorbable and are later removed. The amount of time that sutures are kept in place varies with the location of the wound and the age of the patient; mucous membranes heal more quickly than the palm, for example, and children's skin

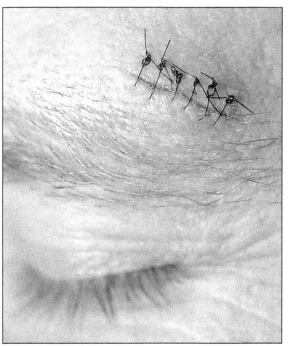

Stitches or sutures may be required to hold together the edges of lacerations that are large, deep, or ragged. (PhotoDisc)

heals more rapidly than that of adults. Removable sutures are made of nylon or a similar material. Sutures that are used beneath the skin cannot be removed and are made of material that will break down within the body. Wound closure may also be accomplished with wire, staples, or adhesive tape. These materials have both advantages—durability (wire), ease of placement (staples), and minimal pain (tape)—and disadvantages, such as potential contamination (wire) and accidental premature removal (tape). Lacerations should be rechecked by a physician when sutures or other means of wound closure are removed.

Uses and Complications

The techniques of laceration repair are used on all parts of the body where such wounds occur. Plastic surgery may be required to improve the appearance of the repaired tissue and to reduce scars when the patient believes that cosmetic results are an issue. In addition to scarring, other complications that may be associated with the repair of lacerations include infection and tetanus. All these problems can be minimized through good surgical techniques, the use of antibiotics, and careful postoperative care. The repair of lacerations to exposed facial skin is especially important. Careful technique minimizes scarring, as do some new methods of wound closure.

—*L. Fleming Fallon, Jr., M.D., Ph.D., M.P.H.*

See also Bleeding; Bruises; Emergency medicine; Grafts and grafting; Healing; Plastic surgery; Skin; Wounds.

For Further Information:

American Red Cross and Kathleen A. Handal. *The American Red Cross First Aid and Safety Handbook*. Boston: Little, Brown, 1992.

Barnes, Leaugeay, Joseph A. Ciotola, and Benjamin Gulli, eds. *Emergency Care and Transportation of the Sick and Injured*. 10th ed. Sudbury, Mass.: Jones and Bartlett, 2011.

Mulholland, Michael W., et al., eds. *Greenfield's Surgery: Scientific Principles and Practice*. 5th ed. Philadelphia: Lippincott Williams & Wilkins, 2011.

Rymaruk, Jen, and Michael Woods. "Laceration Repair." *Health Library*, November 26, 2012.

Thygerson, Alton L. *First Aid and Emergency Care Workbook*. Boston: Jones and Bartlett, 1987.

Vorvick, Linda J., and David Zieve. "Laceration: Sutures or Staples—At Home." *MedlinePlus*, May 13, 2012.

Vorvick, Linda J., and David Zieve. "Lacerations: Liquid Bandage." *MedlinePlus*, May 13, 2012.

Weedon, David. *Weedon's Skin Pathology*. 3d ed. New York: Churchill Livingstone/Elsevier, 2010.

LACTOSE INTOLERANCE

Disease/Disorder

Anatomy or system affected: Gastrointestinal system, intestines, stomach

Specialties and related fields: Gastroenterology, nutrition

Definition: Lactose intolerance is an inability to break down and absorb milk sugar, known as lactose, resulting in stomach pain, gas, and diarrhea if lactose is consumed.

Information on Lactose Intolerance

Causes: Insufficient lactase production
Symptoms: Gas, cramping, and diarrhea after consumption of lactose-containing food or drink
Duration: One to two days
Treatments: Avoidance of dairy products, lactase pills

Causes and Symptoms

Lactose is a complex sugar commonly found in dairy products. It is composed of two simple sugars, glucose and galactose. In babies and young children, a gene produces an enzyme called lactase that breaks down lactose into its two component sugars, which are then absorbed into the bloodstream through the intestinal wall. In many people, sometime after early childhood, the lactase gene is "turned off." It no longer synthesizes lactase, which prevents the digestion and absorption of lactose.

Normal bacterial inhabitants of the intestines synthesize lactase and break down the lactose molecules, producing large quantities of gas as a by-product. This can lead to cramping for the lactose-intolerant individual. The presence of lactose in the large intestine causes excessive amounts of water to move into the intestine, which can lead to diarrhea. Symptoms subside one to two days after the last lactose-containing food has been consumed.

Treatment and Therapy

Lactose intolerance can often be misdiagnosed as a host of gastrointestinal disorders, largely as a result of the commonness of its major symptoms, cramps and diarrhea. Typically, a dietary history must be kept. Patients with lactose intolerance will note an association between their symptoms and the consumption of milk products containing lactose. After elimination of these products from the diet, symptoms should not recur.

There is no cure for lactose intolerance; prevention of symptoms is the general course of action. Avoidance of foods that contain lactose—including milk, ice cream, and cheese—is usually the best recourse. For those who wish to indulge in these products, over-the-counter lactase pills are available; their use usually prevents symptoms of the disorder.

Perspective and Prospects

The vast majority of the world's population is lactose intolerant, yet this disorder was not recognized until later in the twentieth century. Today, lactase supplements are available to help prevent symptoms for lactose-intolerant people who choose to consume dairy products. Alternatively, more and more dairy products are being manufactured as lactose-free; they can be consumed safely by the lactose-intolerant population.

—*Karen E. Kalumuck, Ph.D.*

See also Acid reflux disease; Diarrhea and dysentery; Digestion; Enzymes; Gastroenterology; Gastroenterology, pediatric; Gastrointestinal disorders; Gastrointestinal system; Gluten intolerance; Irritable bowel syndrome (IBS); Metabolic disorders; Nutrition.

For Further Information:

Dobler, Merri Lou. *Lactose Intolerance Nutrition Guide*. Chicago: American Dietetic Association, 2002.

Gracey, Michael, ed. *Diarrhea*. Boca Raton, Fla.: CRC Press, 1991.

Greenberger, Norton J. *Gastrointestinal Disorders: A Pathophysiologic Approach*. 4th ed. Chicago: Year Book Medical, 1989.

Icon Health. *Lactose Intolerance: A Medical Dictionary, Bibliography, and Annotated Research Guide to Internet References*. San Diego, Calif.: Author, 2004.

Janowitz, Henry D. *Your Gut Feelings: A Complete Guide to Living Better with Intestinal Problems*. Rev. ed. New York: Oxford University Press, 1995.

"Lactose Intolerance." *MedlinePlus*, May 17, 2013.

"Lactose Intolerance." *National Digestive Diseases Information Clearinghouse*, Apr. 23, 2012.

Peikin, Steven R. *Gastrointestinal Health*. Rev. ed. New York: Quill, 2001.

Wood, Debra, and Brian Randall. "Lactose Intolerance." *Health Library*, Mar. 15, 2013.

LAMINECTOMY AND SPINAL FUSION
Procedures

Anatomy or system affected: Back, bones, spine

Specialties and related fields: General surgery, orthopedics

Definition: Surgical procedures that join two or more vertebrae, the arching bones that make up the spine.

Indications and Procedures

Laminectomies, which are designed to relieve pressure on the spinal cord, are often performed as the initial surgery in cases of extreme back pain caused by the compression of the spinal canal. An incision is made in the patient's back to expose the laminae, the flattened portions of the vertebral arch, and one or more adjacent laminae are chipped away. On occasion, several laminae are excised.

In such cases, spinal fusion, which involves the immobilization of the spine with steel rods or bone grafts, is indicated. Spinal fusion, like laminectomy a major surgery done under general anesthesia, is performed if x rays reveal unusual motion between adjacent vertebrae.

The causes of the severe back pain that usually precedes laminectomy or spinal fusion may be related to three conditions: osteoarthritis, which causes deterioration of the spinal joints; scoliosis caused by an injury or tumor that is destroying vertebrae; or spondylolisthesis, the dislocation of facet joints. In spinal fusion, when the damaged vertebrae are exposed, joint fusion is sometimes performed by using bone chips from the patient's pelvis. Following surgery, the vertebrae are held in place with plates or screws.

Uses and Complications

Both laminectomy and spinal fusion usually relieve the persistent back pain that has caused patients to seek treatment. Such surgery involves distinct risks, inasmuch as the spinal cord is exposed and there is often considerable blood loss. In the hands of a seasoned orthopedic surgeon, however, the risk is minimized.

Recovery from the surgery can be slow and often involves up to six weeks of confinement in bed. After this confinement, patients are usually required to wear a plaster cast until final vertebral fusion has occurred. This process can take half a year.

Fusion sometimes places an additional burden on the rest of the spinal column. In some cases, this pressure results in renewed back pain in other areas of the spine. Additional surgery may be indicated to control this pain.

—*R. Baird Shuman, Ph.D.*

See also Back pain; Bone grafting; Bones and the skeleton; Disk removal; Fracture and dislocation; Grafts and grafting; Orthopedic surgery; Orthopedics; Orthopedics, pediatric; Osteoarthritis; Scoliosis; Spinal cord disorders; Spine, vertebrae, and disks.

For Further Information:

Aldskogius, Hakan. *Animal Models of Spinal Cord Repair*. New York: Humana Press, 2013.

Benzel, Edward C., and Todd B. Francis. *Spine Surgery: Techniques, Complication Avoidance, and Management*. Philadelphia: Elsevier/Saunders, 2012.

Boden, Scott D., ed. *Spinal Fusion*. Philadelphia: W. B. Saunders, 1998.

Brewer, Sarah. *The Illustrated Surgery Guide: Twenty Common Operations Explained Step-by-Step*. London: Quercus, 2010.

Devlin, Vincent J., ed. *Spine Secrets*. Philadelphia: Hanley & Belfus, 2003.

Frymoyer, John W., and Sam W. Wiesel, eds. *The Adult and Pediatric Spine: Principles, Practice, and Surgery*. 3d ed. Philadelphia: Lippincott Williams & Wilkins, 2004.

Hitchon, Patrick W., Setti Rengachary, and Vincent C. Traynelis, eds. *Techniques in Spinal Fusion and Stabilization*. New York: Thieme Medical, 1995.

Lewandrowski, Kai-Uwe, et al., eds. *Advances in Spinal Fusion: Molecular Science, Biomechanics, and Clinical Management*. New York: Marcel Dekker, 2004.

Nakamura, K., Y. Toyama, and Y. Hoshino, eds. *Cervical Laminoplasty*. New York: Springer, 2003.

Vaccaro, Alexander R., and Eli M. Baron. *Spine Surgery*. Philadelphia: Elsevier/Saunders, 2012.

Wetzel, F. Todd, and Edward Nathaniel Hanley, Jr. *Spine Surgery: A Practical Atlas*. New York: McGraw-Hill, 2002.

LAPAROSCOPY
Procedure

Anatomy or system affected: Abdomen, gallbladder, gastrointestinal system, intestines, kidneys, reproductive system, urinary system, uterus

Specialties and related fields: Endocrinology, gastroenterology, general surgery, gynecology

Definition: The examination of the abdominal organs with a laparoscope, a fiber-optic tube that can also be used to perform surgery to correct several disease conditions.

Key terms:

abdomen: the area of the body between the diaphragm and the pelvis; it contains the visceral organs

cholecystectomy: the surgical removal of the gallbladder

ectopic pregnancy: the development of a fertilized egg in a

Fallopian tube instead of the uterus; can be fatal to the mother unless it is corrected surgically

endometriosis: a female reproductive disease in which cells from the uterine lining (the endometrium) grow outside the uterus, causing severe pain and infertility and sometimes the need for hysterectomy

Fallopian tubes: the two tubes through which eggs pass on the way from the ovaries to the uterus

general anesthesia: anesthesia that induces unconsciousness

implant: a section of endometrial tissue found outside the uterus

local anesthesia: anesthesia that numbs the feeling in a body part, administered by injection or direct application to the skin

Indications and Procedures

Laparoscopy is a surgical technique for examining the abdominal organs and for treating surgically many diseases of these organs. The instrument used is called a laparoscope. It is a flexible tube that contains fiber optics for visualization purposes and a channel through which physicians can pass special surgical instruments into the abdominal cavity.

Upon insertion of a laparoscope into the abdomen through a small surgical incision (usually near the navel), physicians can observe the liver, kidneys, gallbladder, pancreas, spleen, and exterior aspects of the intestines in both sexes. Hence the technique is useful for detecting cirrhosis of the liver, the presence of stones and tumors, and many other diseases of the abdominal organs. The female reproductive organs can also be examined in this manner.

Before laparoscopy can be carried out, the patient must fast for at least twelve hours. The patient is given a local or general anesthetic, depending on the purpose of the procedure. In exploratory abdominal examinations, the instrument is inserted into the abdomen through a small incision in the abdominal wall after local anesthesia has numbed it. Often, especially when extensive surgery is anticipated, the procedure begins after general anesthesia produces unconsciousness. Upon the completion of exploration or surgery, the laparoscope is withdrawn and the incision is closed.

Laparoscopic abdominal examination is often used to detect endometriosis, the presence of endometrial cells outside the uterus. This procedure begins with the administration of local anesthesia when only exploration or biopsy is planned. General anesthesia is used when the removal of implants (endometrial tissue) is anticipated. The entry incision is made near the navel, and the laparoscope is inserted. The fiber-optics system is used to search the abdominal organs for implants. Visibility of the abdominal organs is usually enhanced by pumping in a harmless gas, such as carbon dioxide, to distend the abdomen. After the confirmation of endometriosis, surgical implant removal is carried out immediately, unless the decision is made to institute drug therapy instead. Full recovery from this surgery requires only a day of postoperative bed rest and a week of curtailing activities.

Laparoscopy can also be employed for female sterilization. The patient is given a general anesthetic. After laparo-

scopic visualization of the Fallopian tubes in the gas-distended abdomen is achieved, surgical instruments for tube cauterization or cutting are introduced and the sterilization is carried out. The entire procedure often requires only thirty minutes, which is one reason for its popularity. In addition, patients can go home in a few hours and have fully recovered after a day or two of bed rest and seven to ten days of curtailing activities.

Uses and Complications

Common laparoscopic surgeries are cholecystectomy (the removal of the gallbladder), the removal of gallstones and kidney stones, tumor resection, female sterilization by cutting or blocking the Fallopian tubes, the treatment of endometriosis through the removal of implants from abdominal organs, and the removal of biopsy samples from abdominal organs. Traditional uses of laparoscopy in female reproductive surgery are to identify and correct pelvic pain resulting from endometriosis, ectopic pregnancy, and pelvic tumors.

Laparoscopy has several advantages. There is rarely a need for patients on chronic drug therapy to discontinue medication before laparoscopy. In addition, the use of laparoscopy dramatically lowers surgical incision size, surgical trauma, length of hospital stay, and recovery time. Laparoscopy should be avoided, however, in cases of advanced abdominal wall cancer, severe respiratory or cardiovascular disease, or tuberculosis. Extreme obesity does not disqualify a

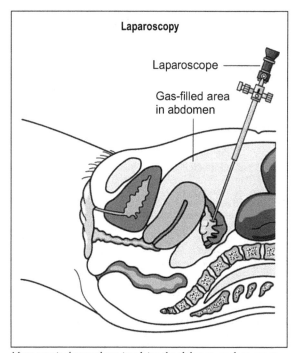

Laparoscopy

Laparoscope

Gas-filled area in abdomen

Many surgical procedures involving the abdomen, such as appendectomy or the removal of eggs from the ovaries for in vitro fertilization, can be performed using laparoscopy. Gas is pumped into the abdominal cavity, and a fiber-optic scope and instruments are inserted through a small hole in the skin.

patient from undergoing laparoscopy but makes the procedure much more difficult to perform.

As laparoscopic surgery has increased in scope, more procedures yield surgical tissues that are larger in size than the laparoscope channel (for example, the removal of gallbladders, gallstones, and ovaries). In many cases these organs and structures are cut into small pieces for removal. If potentially dangerous items are involved—such as malignancies that can spread on dissection—larger, more conventional incisions are often combined with laparoscopy.

Perspective and Prospects

Since the 1970s, the uses of laparoscopy have constantly expanded. Once confined to the exploratory examination of the abdomen, the methodology has been applied to a large number of different types of surgery in addition to those already mentioned. Such versatility is attributable to the development of better laparoscopes, advanced instrumentation for diverse surgeries, and improved fiber-optic and video technologies.

As a consequence of these advances, many surgeons predict that most future abdominal surgery will be laparoscopic. The driving force for such innovation includes the public demand for quicker recovery times. In the United States, this desire is intensified by the requirements of insurance companies, employers, and the federal government for shorter hospital stays. Both changes are made possible by decreased severity of surgical trauma in laparoscopy when compared to traditional surgery, a result of the smaller incisions. The dramatic trend toward laparoscopy can be seen with cholecystectomies: Of those done in 1992, 70 percent were laparoscopic, compared to less than 1 percent in 1989; according to a 2010 report, about 75 percent of cholecystectomies are done with laparoscopic surgery.

—*Sanford S. Singer, Ph.D.*

See also Abdomen; Abdominal disorders; Appendectomy; Appendicitis; Biopsy; Cholecystectomy; Ectopic pregnancy; Endometriosis; Endoscopy; Gynecology; Internal medicine; Sterilization; Stone removal; Stones; Tubal ligation; Tumor removal; Tumors.

For Further Information:

Graber, John N., et al., eds. *Laparoscopic Abdominal Surgery.* New York: McGraw-Hill, 1993.

Henderson, Lorraine, and Ros Wood. *Explaining Endometriosis.* 2d ed. St. Leonards, N.S.W.: Allen and Unwin, 2000.

Kapadia, Cyrus R., James M. Crawford, and Caroline Taylor. *An Atlas of Gastroenterology: A Guide to Diagnosis and Differential Diagnosis.* Boca Raton, Fla.: Pantheon, 2003.

Ost, Michael C. *Robotic and Laparoscopic Reconstructive Surgery in Children and Adults.* New York: Humana Press, 2011.

Reddick, Eddie Joe, ed. *An Atlas of Laparoscopic Surgery.* New York: Raven Press, 1993.

Terzicĺ, Hana. *Laparoscopy: New Developments, Procedures, and Risks.* Hauppauge, N.Y.: Nova Science, 2012.

Zollinger, Robert M., Jr., and Robert M. Zollinger, Sr. *Zollinger's Atlas of Surgical Operations.* 9th ed. New York: McGraw-Hill, 2011.

Zucker, Karl A., ed. *Surgical Laparoscopy.* 2d ed. Philadelphia: Lippincott Williams & Wilkins, 2001.

LARYNGECTOMY

Procedure

Anatomy or system affected: Respiratory system, throat

Specialties and related fields: General surgery, oncology, otorhinolaryngology

Definition: The removal of all or part of the voice box, or larynx.

Indications and Procedures

Continued hoarseness and coughing can indicate laryngeal disorders. Polyps, which may be caused by excessive smoking or drinking, can form on the larynx. Children sometimes develop warts on it. Although these polyps and warts are generally benign, they should be removed and subjected to biopsy to preclude the presence of cancer.

Polyps, warts, and tumors are all detected quite easily with a laryngoscopic examination carried out by an otorhinolaryngologist with a mirror, an endoscope (a flexible fiber-optic tube), or a combination of the two. Such an examination, in addition to determining whether a growth is benign or cancerous, can detect signs of cancer in the lining of the larynx.

If cancer is detected early enough, radiation can usually control it. If the disease has advanced significantly, however, a laryngectomy may be necessary. In this surgical procedure, performed under general anesthesia, an incision is made in the neck and the larynx is removed. The windpipe directly below the larynx is then sewn to the skin around the surgical opening to form a permanent opening, or stoma, through which the patient breathes.

Uses and Complications

This surgery is used when cancer is sufficiently advanced that radiation therapy cannot destroy it. The major complication is that the patient's air supply is now taken through the stoma, meaning that swimming is precluded and that bathing must be undertaken with considerable caution.

A more apparent complication is that, with the loss of the larynx, one cannot speak. Through an extensive and painstaking course of speech therapy, however, esophageal speech can be achieved. This involves swallowing air and expelling it in such a way that it can be shaped by the palate, lips, and tongue into understandable words and sentences. An electronic larynx is also available. It makes a buzzing sound that the patient can convert into words when the device is pressed against the top of the throat.

—*R. Baird Shuman, Ph.D.*

See also Cancer; Endoscopy; Esophagus; Head and neck disorders; Mouth and throat cancer; Otorhinolaryngology; Polyps; Speech disorders; Tumors; Voice and vocal cord disorders; Warts.

For Further Information:

Alan, Rick. "Laryngeal Cancer." *Health Library,* May 1, 2013.

Blom, Eric D., Mark I. Singer, and Ronald C. Hamaker, eds. *Tracheoesophageal Voice Restoration Following Total Laryngectomy.* San Diego, Calif.: Singular, 1998.

Casper, Janina K., and Raymond H. Colton. *Clinical Manual for Laryngectomy and Head/Neck Cancer Rehabilitation.* 2d ed. San Diego, Calif.: Singular, 1998.

Edels, Yvonne, ed. *Laryngectomy: Diagnosis to Rehabilitation.* Rockville, Md.: Aspen Systems, 1983.

Ferrari, Mario. *PDxMD Ear, Nose, and Throat Disorders.* Philadelphia: PDxMD, 2003.

Gadepalli, C., et al. "Functional Results of Pharyngo-Laryngectomy and Total Laryngectomy: A Comparison." *Journal of Laryngology & Otology* 126, no. 1 (January 2012): 52–57.

Griffith, H. Winter. *Complete Guide to Symptoms, Illness, and Surgery.* Revised and updated by Stephen Moore and Kenneth Yoder. 5th ed. New York: Perigee, 2006.

"Laryngectomy." *MedlinePlus*, February 28, 2011.

Montgomery, William W., ed. *Surgery of the Larynx, Trachea, Esophagus, and Neck.* Philadelphia: W. B. Saunders, 2002.

Zollinger, Robert M., Jr., and Robert M. Zollinger, Sr. *Zollinger's Atlas of Surgical Operations.* 8th ed. New York: McGraw-Hill, 2003.

LARYNGITIS

Disease/Disorder

Anatomy or system affected: Throat

Specialties and related fields: Otorhinolaryngology, speech pathology

Definition: Inflammation of the larynx (voice box), often associated with common colds, bacterial infection, or straining the voice. The throat is dry, swallowing becomes difficult, and speech is a hoarse whisper.

Causes and Symptoms

The larynx, located directly above the windpipe (trachea), is the short, hollow tube containing the vocal cords, two heavily lined slits in a mucous membrane. Voiced sounds, such as vowels, result when air from the lungs induces vocal fold vibration. Laryngitis occurs when the folds are obstructed or do not vibrate properly; depending on the cause, laryngitis is classified as simple, chronic, diphtheritic, tuberculous, or syphilitic.

Simple laryngitis may be caused by bacterial infection (common cold, typhoid fever), a virus (influenza), or nonbacterial irritants (chemical fumes, dust, or tobacco smoke). The primary infection site is the mucous membrane lining the larynx. It becomes red and swollen, secreting a viscous discharge that impedes vocal fold vibration. In severe cases of viral infection, the larynx may become completely obstructed, causing suffocation.

Chronic laryngitis often results from excessive smoking, alcoholism, or consistent strain or abuse of the voice. It is an occupational hazard of auctioneers, orators, singers, and those who frequently shout for long periods, such as cheerleaders. Nondisease-induced chronic laryngitis may also be instigated by hysteria, allergic reaction, remote disease of the nerves serving the voice, strong external pressure against the larynx, or irritation caused by tubes inserted down the throat to sustain breathing.

Diphtheritic laryngitis occurs when diphtheria afflicting the upper throat spreads to the larynx. The result may be a membrane of diseased cells infiltrating the mucous membrane and obstructing the vocal cords.

Tuberculous laryngitis is a secondary infection spread from the lungs. Tubular nodulelike growths are formed in larynx tissue, leaving ulcers on the surface. Starting at the vocal cords, this infection may spread over the entire larynx and eventually destroy the epiglottis and laryngeal cartilage.

Syphilitic laryngitis is one of the many complications of syphilis. Sores or mucous patches form in the larynx, eventually producing tissue destruction and scar formation. The mucous membrane becomes dry and covered with polyps (small bumps of tissue that project from the surface). These polyps distort the larynx, shorten the vocal cords, and produce persistent hoarseness.

Treatment and Therapy

Simple laryngitis is best treated by resting the voice. When it is absolutely necessary to speak, it should be with a soft, breathy voice, not a whisper. The throat should be kept well lubricated by frequent drinks of water and not cleared. Relative humidity in the recovery room should be maintained at 40 to 50 percent, and alcohol, tobacco, and decongestants should be avoided. Complete recovery usually occurs within several days.

A persistent hoarseness indicates a bacterial infection (usually curable by antibiotics) or polyps, cysts, or other fibrous growths on the vocal cords. These growths may become ulcerated and require surgical intervention. Although cancer of the larynx is not uncommon (2 percent of malignancies), it is usually completely curable if detected sufficiently early.

Systemic diseases not localized in the larynx, such as tuberculosis and syphilis, are best treated by antibiotics.

—*George R. Plitnik, Ph.D.*

See also Common cold; Laryngectomy; Multiple chemical sensitivity syndrome; Nasopharyngeal disorders; Otorhinolaryngology; Pharyngitis; Pharynx; Polyps; Sore throat; Strep throat; Tonsillectomy and adenoid removal; Tonsillitis; Voice and vocal cord disorders.

For Further Information:

Bellenir, Karen, and Peter D. Dresser, eds. *Contagious and Noncontagious Infectious Diseases Sourcebook.* Detroit, Mich.: Omnigraphics, 1996.

Colton, Raymond H., Janina K. Casper, and Rebecca Leonard. *Understanding Voice Problems: A Physiological Perspective for Diagnosis and Treatment.* 3d ed. Philadelphia: Lippincott Williams & Wilkins, 2006.

Information on Laryngitis

Causes: Bacterial infection (common cold, typhoid fever, diphtheria, syphilis), viral infection (influenza), irritants (chemical fumes, dust, smoke, alcohol), consistent strain or abuse of voice

Symptoms: Red and swollen larynx; discharge; obstruction that can cause suffocation if severe; polyps, cysts, or other fibrous growths on vocal cords

Duration: Acute or chronic

Treatments: Depends on cause; may include resting the voice, antibiotics, or surgery

Icon Health. *Laryngitis: A Medical Dictionary, Bibliography, and Annotated Research Guide to Internet References*. San Diego, Calif.: Icon Health, 2004.

LaRusso, Laurie. "Laryngitis." *Health Library*, January 9, 2013.

Mayo Clinic. "Laryngitis." *Mayo Clinic*, June 28, 2012.

Ossoff, Robert H., et al., eds. *The Larynx*. Philadelphia: Lippincott Williams & Wilkins, 2003.

Sataloff, Robert T., ed. *Reflux Laryngitis and Related Disorders*. 4th ed. San Diego, Calif.: Plural, 2013.

Swartzberg, John Edward. *Wellness Self-Care Handbook: The Everyday Guide to Prevention and Home Remedies to Over 150 Common Ailments*. New York: Times Books, 1999.

LASER USE IN SURGERY

Procedure

Anatomy or system affected: Eyes, skin

Specialties and related fields: Dermatology, oncology, ophthalmology, urology

Definition: The application of laser technology to surgical procedures, such as the vaporization of blood clots or arterial plaque, the breaking up of kidney stones into small fragments, the removal of birthmarks, and the stoppage of hemorrhaging in the retina of the eye.

Key terms:

ionization: a process in which a neutral atom loses one or more of its orbital electrons because of light, heat, or electrical collisions

laser: an acronym for light amplification by stimulated emission of radiation; a laser produces a very-high-intensity light beam at a single wavelength

optical fiber: a very thin thread made of high-purity glass, plastic, or quartz; used to transmit light from a laser into the body

photon: a particle of light whose energy depends on its wavelength (that is, its color); many billions of individual photons make up a light beam

pulsed laser: a laser technique used to deliver a light beam of high power for a very short time in order to localize the heating effect without damaging surrounding tissue

shock wave: a miniature explosion caused by intense local heating with a laser beam; used to fragment stones in the kidney or gallbladder

stimulated emission of radiation: the process in a laser whereby an avalanche of photons is created, all of which are synchronized in wavelength and direction of travel

wavelength: a property used to measure colors in the spectrum of light from infrared to ultraviolet; usually expressed in units of microns (one micron is equal to one-millionth of a meter)

The Fundamentals of Laser Technology

The first successful laser was built in 1960 by Theodore H. Maiman at the Hughes Aircraft Research Laboratory in Palo Alto, California. Since then, many applications have been developed for lasers. These include the compact disc player, telephone systems with fiber optics, guidance systems for military weapons, supermarket checkout scanners, quality control in industry, entertainment with laser light shows, and numerous medical applications.

Ordinary light sources such as flashlights, flames, and the sun do not emit laser light. The individual atoms emit their light waves in a random, uncoordinated manner, in the same way that water waves spread out at random when a handful of pebbles is thrown into a pool. In contrast, a laser beam consists of light waves that are all synchronized; they all have the same wavelength and remain in step as they travel in the same direction. Synchronizing the light emission from billions of atoms in a light source is the chief difficulty in building a laser.

The key idea for solving this problem had been proposed in an article on the general theory of light absorption and emission by atoms written by the famous physicist Albert Einstein in the 1920s. When an atom absorbs a burst of light energy (a photon), an electron in the atom is raised from a lower energy level to a higher one. A short time later, the electron spontaneously falls back down to the lower energy level, emitting a photon of light in the process. Einstein's contribution was to suggest a third mechanism in addition to ordinary absorption and emission. Based on theoretical arguments of symmetry and the conservation of energy, he proposed a new process called "stimulated emission of radiation." (The word "laser" is an acronym for light amplification by stimulated emission of radiation.)

To understand stimulated emission, consider an atom whose electron has been raised to a higher energy level, called an "excited state." This state is unstable, and the electron ordinarily will fall back down to the lower energy level in a short time. Suppose, however, that a photon of precisely the right energy strikes the atom while the electron is still in its temporary excited state. This photon cannot be absorbed because the electron is already in its excited state. Einstein reasoned that the incoming photon would cause the excited electron to fall to the lower energy level. A photon would then be emitted from the atom and would join the incoming photon. The two photons would be exactly synchronized in wavelength and direction.

If there were many atoms whose electrons had previously been raised to excited states, the process of stimulated emission would continue. The two photons could strike two other excited atoms and stimulate them to emit light energy, making a total of four photons. These four would trigger four more atoms, making eight photons, and so forth. Eventually, a so-called photon avalanche consisting of a huge number of synchronized light waves would be generated, which is the desired laser beam.

To make a successful laser, some additional requirements must be met. For one thing, a source of energy must be provided to raise most of the electrons to their excited states. For a gas laser, this energy is normally supplied by a high voltage. Examples of gas lasers are those using carbon dioxide, argon, or a mixture of helium and neon. A solid crystal, such as a clear ruby rod, would be excited by a bright burst of light from a device similar to a camera flash attachment. A solid-state diode laser is energized by a flow of electric current across a diode junction. In each case, it is necessary to

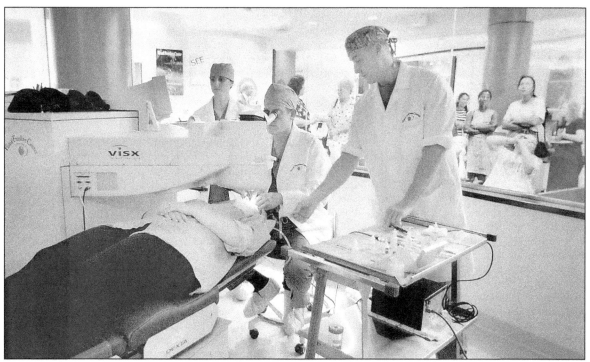

Lasers are taking a more prominent role in many procedures, especially eye surgery. Some worry that the popularity of laser vision correction—here a patient is treated at a shopping mall as spectators look on—has compromised safety. (AP/Wide World Photos)

"pump" the laser so that many atoms are in their excited state, ready and waiting to be triggered by an incoming photon to release their energy.

Another requirement for a successful laser is that the electrons must remain in their excited state for a longer-than-normal time. The problem with most materials is that electrons fall spontaneously to their lower energy level almost instantaneously, in less than one-millionth of a second. The photon avalanche effect requires that a substantial majority of the atoms be in their excited state. For very short-lived excited states, it is not possible to maintain this condition. Experimenters have no way to control the lifetime of excited states, so they must search for those atoms and molecules that already have the appropriate longer lifetime supplied by nature. It has not been possible to build a laser using hydrogen gas, for example, because hydrogen does not have any long-lived excited states. The spontaneous emission of light takes place so quickly that there is no time for a photon avalanche to develop.

Another condition for laser action is to have two parallel mirrors at the ends of the laser material. The laser beam bounces back and forth many times between the mirrors at the speed of light, gaining or maintaining its energy from the excited atoms of the laser material. One of the mirrors is made slightly less than 100 percent reflecting, so that a small portion of the laser energy is allowed to exit in a narrow beam. For most medical applications, a thin optical fiber is joined directly to the end of the laser in order to transmit the beam to the desired location in the body.

Much research has been done to develop good optical fibers. The fiber should transmit a laser beam with very little loss of energy along the way. The technology of drawing thin glass fibers with few impurities or imperfections has become quite sophisticated. A fiber must be thin and uniform so that the laser beam will be forced to travel down its center, thus avoiding the loss of light energy through the walls.

For an ultraviolet laser, glass fibers cannot be used because of absorption. (The sun's ultraviolet radiation is absorbed by ordinary eyeglasses.) Special quartz fibers with low absorption have been developed for lasers in the ultraviolet region of the spectrum. In the infrared region of the spectrum, new optical materials are still under continuing investigation.

The wavelength (color) of a laser is determined entirely by the energy levels of the atoms or molecules being used. For example, a carbon dioxide laser always has a wavelength of 10.6 microns, which is infrared. The helium-neon gas laser always produces visible red light at a wavelength of 0.63 microns. A wide range of laser wavelengths has become available as a result of extensive research efforts by physicists and optical engineers. Since 1960, lasers have become much more rugged and dependable in construction. Some lasers operate with a continuous beam, while others produce very short pulses, depending on the desired application. Also, lasers can be designed to operate at a low power level for diagnostic purposes or a high power level for surgery.

Safety precautions must be followed when working with a

laser. Not only the patient but also the surgical team must be protected from possible harmful radiation. The eyes must be protected from laser beam reflections from a shiny surface. Ultraviolet light is a special hazard because its high-energy photons can cause cell damage and genetic mutations. The great benefits of laser surgery can be negated by an inexperienced or careless surgeon.

Uses and Complications

The first medical use of a laser beam was for surgery on the retina of the eye, in 1963. Diabetic patients in particular frequently develop excessive blood vessels in the retina that give their eyes a typically reddish color. In advanced cases, the blood vessels can hemorrhage and eventually cause blindness. The green light of an argon laser will pass through the clear cornea and lens of the eye, but when it hits the dark brown melanin pigment of the retina, it will be absorbed and cause a tiny hot spot. The physician uses a series of laser pulses, carefully focused on affected areas of the retina, to burn away the extra blood vessels. The remarkable property of the laser beam in this procedure is that its energy penetrates to the rear of the eye, leaving the clear fluid unaffected.

In a greenhouse, light from the sun comes in through the glass but infrared radiation cannot get back out. This example illustrates that some materials, such as glass, are transparent for visible light but opaque for infrared light. Similarly, the front of the eye is transparent for visible light but absorbs infrared light. Therefore, an infrared laser such as the YAG (yttrium-aluminum-garnet) laser can be used for surgery near the front of the eye because its light energy is selectively absorbed there.

A particular problem following cataract surgery is that a secondary cataract may develop on the membrane behind the implanted artificial lens. About one-third of patients with such a lens implant require a second surgery to remove the secondary cataract. A YAG laser beam will pass through the cornea and artificial lens but can be focused to produce a hot spot at the site of the secondary cataract to destroy it. More than 200,000 such procedures are performed each year in the United States, and the result is a dramatic, almost instantaneous improvement of vision.

A third form of laser eye surgery, laser-assisted in situ keratomileusis (LASIK), became quite popular at the end of the twentieth century; it has, in fact, become the most commonly performed surgery in the country. In LASIK surgery, the cornea of the eyeball is reshaped to help patients overcome myopia (nearsightedness), hyperopia (farsightedness), or astigmatism. The procedure is done with a cool beam laser that can be used to remove thin layers of tissue from selected sites on the cornea to change its curvature. Success rates for the surgery are high: 95 to 98 percent of the patients get 20/40 vision. The surgery is not without its problems, however. Because of its popularity and the large fee charged for a quick and fairly simple procedure, unqualified or less experienced physicians are oftentimes performing the delicate procedure; approximately 5 percent of patients receiving LASIK surgery receive less-than-satisfactory results. Two other corrective procedures for eyesight involving lasers are the use of Keravision Intacs (intrastomal corneal rings), which involves placing a lens in the cornea, and PRK (photorefractive keratectomy), in which the cornea is scraped without actual incision into the cornea.

Another dramatic medical application of the laser is the breaking up of stones in the kidney, ureter, or gallbladder. Such calcified, hard deposits previously could be removed only by surgery. It is now possible, for example, to insert an optical fiber of less than half a millimeter in diameter through the urethra and then transmit the laser beam to the site of the stone. High-power light pulses of very short duration (less than one-billionth of a second) create a shock wave that breaks the stone into small fragments that the body can eliminate.

Another promising application of laser surgery that has received much publicity is laser angioplasty, which is used to open up a blood vessel near the heart that is partially or wholly blocked by a deposit of plaque. The hope is that the laser procedure may be able to replace heart bypass surgery, but the results are still preliminary.

Laser angioplasty involves inserting a catheter that contains a fiberscope, an inflation cuff, and an optical fiber into the artery of the arm and advancing it into the coronary artery. The fiberscope enables the physician to see the blockage, the cuff is used to stop the blood flow temporarily, and the optical fiber transmits the laser energy that vaporizes the plaque. Sometimes, the laser method is used only to open up a small channel, after which balloon angioplasty is used to stretch the walls of the blood vessel.

The main risk in using the laser beam is that the alignment of the optical fiber inside the artery may be deflected and cause a puncture of the blood vessel wall. Improvements in the imaging system are needed. Also, further work must be done to see which light wavelengths are most effective in removing plaque and preventing recurrence of the obstruction.

The heating effect of a laser beam has been used by surgeons to control bleeding. For example, bleeding ulcers in the stomach, intestine, and colon have been successfully cauterized with laser light transmitted through an optical fiber. A similar procedure has been used to treat emphysema patients. An optical fiber is inserted through the wall of the chest, and the laser's heat is used to shrink the small blisters that are present on the surface of the lungs. Also, the heat from a laser has been used during internal surgery to seal the surrounding capillaries that contribute to bleeding.

For the preceding procedures, a carbon dioxide gas laser that emits infrared light is normally used. The reason is that water molecules in the tissue absorb the infrared wavelengths most efficiently. The optical fibers used to transmit infrared light are not as efficient and reliable as those used for visible or ultraviolet light, however, so further research on fiber materials is in progress.

One notable success of laser surgery has been the removal of birthmarks. Because of their typically reddish-purple coloration, birthmarks are commonly called port-wine stains. They can be quite unsightly, especially when located on the face of a person with an otherwise light complexion. To remove such a birthmark, the laser beam has to burn out the network of extra blood vessels under the skin. A similar procedure can be used to remove unwanted tattoos.

The color of the laser must be chosen so that its wavelength will be absorbed efficiently by the dark purple stain. What would happen if a purple laser beam were used? Its light would be reflected rather than absorbed by a purple object, and it would not produce the desired heating. Yellow or orange is most effectively absorbed by a purple object. The surgeon must be careful that the laser light is absorbed primarily by the purple birthmark without harming the normal, healthy tissue around it.

Experimental work is being done to determine whether laser surgery can be applied to cancer. Small malignant tumors in the lungs, bladder, and trachea have been treated with a technique called photodynamic therapy. The patient is injected with a colored dye that is preferentially absorbed in the tumor. Porphyrin, the reddish-brown pigment in blood, is one substance that has been known for many years to become concentrated in malignant tissue. The suspected site is irradiated with ultraviolet light from a krypton laser, causing it to glow like fluorescent paint, which allows the surgeon to determine the outline of the tumor. To perform the surgery, an intense red laser is focused on the tumor to kill the malignant tissue. Two separate optical fibers must be used for this procedure, one for the ultraviolet diagnosis and one for the red laser therapy.

The three traditional cancer treatments of surgery, chemotherapy, and radiation therapy all seek to limit damage to healthy tissue surrounding a tumor. Photodynamic surgery by laser must develop its methodology further to accomplish the same goal.

Much has already been accomplished in applying laser surgery to various body organs. Future developments are likely to emphasize microsurgery on smaller structures, such as individual cells or even genetic material in DNA molecules.

Perspective and Prospects

Some inventions, such as the printing press, the steam engine, and the electric lightbulb, were made by innovators who were trying to solve a particular practical problem of their time. Other inventions, such as the microscope, artificial radio waves, and low-temperature superconductivity, initially were scientific curiosities arising from basic research, and their later applications were not at all anticipated. The laser belongs to this second category.

The first successful laser, built by Theodore Maiman, consisted of a small cylindrical ruby rod with shiny mirrored ends and a bright flash lamp to excite the atoms in the rod. Maiman's goal was to determine whether the separately excited atoms could be made to release their absorbed energy almost simultaneously in one coordinated burst of monochromatic (single-wavelength) light.

No one could have foreseen the wide range of technological applications that resulted from Maiman's experiment. It is important to appreciate that he did not set out to improve telephone communication or eye surgery; those developments came about after the laser became available.

It is worthwhile here to summarize some of the general uses for lasers in modern technology. The tremendous advances in medical applications could not have happened without the concurrent development of new types of lasers, with a variety of wavelengths and power levels, needed for other industrial products.

Among laser applications are the following: the compact disc (CD) player, in which the laser beam replaces the LP record needle; optical fibers that can carry several thousand simultaneous telephone calls; supermarket checkout scanners, in which a laser beam reads the universal product code on each item; three-dimensional pictures, called holograms, that are displayed at many art museums; military applications, such as guided weapons and Star Wars technology; surveying, bridge building, and tunneling projects in which exact alignment is critical; and nuclear fusion research, in which high-power lasers can produce nuclear reactions that may become a future source of energy as coal and oil resources are depleted. Sophisticated advances in using lasers to control specific chemical reactions and to predict earthquakes are under development.

Laser technology in medicine will continue to advance as biologists, electrical and optical engineers, physicians, biophysicists, and people from related disciplines share this common interest.

—*Hans G. Graetzer, Ph.D.;*
updated by Cassandra Kircher, Ph.D.

See also Angioplasty; Astigmatism; Bionics and biotechnology; Birthmarks; Bleeding; Blood vessels; Blurred vision; Cataract surgery; Cataracts; Cervical procedures; Dermatology; Electrocauterization; Eye surgery; Eyes; Melanoma; Myopia; Neurosurgery; Ophthalmology; Plaque, arterial; Plastic surgery; Refractive eye surgery; Skin; Skin disorders; Skin lesion removal; Stone removal; Stones; Tattoo removal; Ulcer surgery; Ulcers; Vision.

For Further Information:
Alster, Tina S., and Lydia Preston. *Skin Savvy: The Essential Guide to Cosmetic Laser Surgery.* New York: Cadogan, 2002.
American Society for Laser Surgery and Medicine. http://www.aslms.org.
Azar, Dimitri T., and Douglas D. Koch, eds. *LASIK: Fundamentals, Surgical Techniques, and Complications.* New York: Marcel Dekker, 2003.
Buettner, Helmut, ed. *Mayo Clinic on Vision and Eye Health: Practical Answers on Glaucoma, Cataracts, Macular Degeneration, and Other Conditions.* Rochester, Minn.: Mayo Foundation for Medical Education and Research, 2002.
Buratto, Lucio, Stephen Slade, and Marco Tavolato. *LASIK: The Evolution of Refractive Surgery.* Thorofare, N.J.: SLACK, 2012.
Goldberg, David J. *Laser Dermatology.* New York: Springer, 2013.
Goldman, Mitchel P., ed. *Cutaneous and Cosmetic Laser Surgery.* Philadelphia: Mosby/Elsevier, 2006.
Krueger, Ronald R., Jonathan H. Talamo, and Richard L. Lindstrom. *Textbook of Refractive Laser Assisted Cataract Surgery (ReLACS).* New York: Springer, 2013.
Narins, Rhoda S., and Paul Jarrod Frank. *Turn Back the Clock Without Losing Time: Everything You Need to Know About Simple*

Cosmetic Procedures. New York: Three Rivers Press, 2002.

Sutton, Amy L., ed. *Eye Care Sourcebook: Basic Consumer Health Information About Eye Care and Eye Disorders.* 3d ed. Detroit, Mich.: Omnigraphics, 2008.

Victor, Steven, and Ina Yalof. *Ageless Beauty: A Dermatologist's Secrets for Looking Younger Without Surgery.* New York: Crown, 2003.

LAW AND MEDICINE

Ethics

Definition: The use of medicine in legal contexts-to determine whether a person has been injured by the act of another, the extent of such an injury and its treatment, and whether a defendant was physically or emotionally capable of committing a crime or tort-and in related ethical and philosophical contexts-to determine when life begins (in the abortion debate) or how one evaluates "quality of life" (the euthanasia debate).

Key terms:

compensable injury: an injury for which damages may be awarded

competency: the capacity to understand and act reasonably under given circumstances

diminished capacity: partial insanity; a legal determination that a defendant does not have the ability to achieve the state of mind required to commit a crime

DNA testing: a technique for identifying a person based on matching unique gene-bearing proteins (deoxyribonucleic acid, or DNA) from an organic sample taken from that person (such as hair, blood, or tissue) with another organic sample

emotional distress: damage to a plaintiff's emotional state caused by fear, anger, anxiety, stress, depression, or other negative emotions; such damage may be judged compensable

euthanasia: the act of putting a person or other living being to death in order to end incurable pain or disease; popularly called mercy killing

forensic: having to do with a court of justice; forensic medicine and its various subspecialties apply medical science to the purposes of the law

insanity: a mental disease or defect that renders a person incapable of appreciating the wrongfulness of certain acts or of conforming to the requirements of the law

tort: a wrongful act for which civil courts, rather than criminal courts, are empowered to render justice

Medicine in Legal and Ethical Debates

Medicine as it relates to law is referred to as forensic medicine. Forensic medicine plays a part in three basic areas of the law. The first two involve the practical application of medicine in civil law and in criminal law. The third area involves the use of medical science to help in defining philosophical or ethical issues, such as when life begins and ends. Ethics in medicine, also called bioethics, refers to a set of moral standards and a code for behavior that govern people's interactions with one another and with society. Bioethics deals with moral issues and problems that have arisen as a result of modern medicine and research. Bioethical principles focus on autonomy (self-determination), beneficence (doing good), nonmaleficence (avoiding evil), and justice (the fair distribution of scarce resources).

In a civil case, a private party, the plaintiff, files a complaint in court against another party, the defendant, requesting that a judge or a jury settle a dispute between the two parties. A party to a civil suit can be an individual, a corporation, an association, a government organization, or any other group. A civil suit differs from a criminal case in that neither party is claiming that a crime (such as theft, kidnapping, or murder) was committed and that someone should be put in jail. Instead, the plaintiff in a civil suit can ask that the defendant pay some amount of money to the plaintiff to compensate for damages that the plaintiff has suffered because of something the defendant did.

In a criminal case, however, the government, on behalf of "the people," files a complaint with the court claiming that the defendant committed a crime, and the government seeks to have a judge or jury determine the guilt or innocence of that defendant. If the defendant is determined to be guilty, the judge has the authority to punish the defendant, usually by imposing a fine, by requiring community service, by setting a jail sentence, or rarely, in some states, by having the defendant put to death.

In both civil and criminal cases, medical science is called upon to provide evidence that can be used to prove or disprove a party's case. In a civil case, the parties will often turn to medical experts to determine the extent of a plaintiff's mental and physical injuries. These experts act as witnesses in their areas of expertise and testify in a court of law. For example, a plaintiff in a civil suit might claim that he or she was born with birth defects as a result of drugs that the mother had taken during pregnancy and may present evidence of that injury and its cause in the form of testimony of doctors and medical research experts specializing in those related areas of medicine. This testimony, supported by current medical knowledge, would be presented to the jury to bolster the plaintiff's claim that the drug caused the plaintiff's birth defect.

Medical science, through the discovery of disease causality and pathophysiology, has created more distinct medical specialties. This trend is reflected in the increasing number of expert witnesses: At the beginning of the twentieth century, a general practitioner was considered qualified to testify on most areas of medicine; today, the courts require expert witnesses to be specifically qualified in the area of medicine about which they testify.

The practice of using highly qualified and specialized doctors as expert witnesses has long been accepted by courts as an effective way to educate a jury regarding the extent, cause, and treatment of the injury in question. However, there are some limitations on the use of such testimony. In order for the court to allow a medical expert to testify as to specific facts from which conclusions are to be drawn, the facts must be outside what is considered to be the general or common knowledge of a lay jury. For example, a court may not allow a party to use a medical expert to explain commonplace injuries, such as sprained ankles. The court would, however, allow a medical expert to explain toxic shock syndrome, because the existence, causes, and effects of that impairment are not common knowledge. The reasoning behind this limitation is that the jury members are supposed to form their own opinions when such opinions do not involve or require specialized knowledge. Only when it is necessary or helpful to the jury to be educated in a specialized area of knowledge is expert testimony usually allowed. In contrast to a lay witness, an expert witness is permitted to testify about the ultimate issue in the case. The medical expert in an accident case, for example, may testify about the proximate cause of injury, that is whether the accident caused the plaintiff's injury that is subject of the lawsuit. Lay witnesses are not permitted to testify along these lines because they do not have the expertise to do so.

The court also recognizes a distinction between testimony from a medical expert and testimony from the plaintiff's treating doctor. Whereas the former educates the jury regarding an area of medicine that is relevant to the case, the latter does not. Instead, the treating doctor is called to testify to actual events or facts of the case that the doctor personally witnessed: that the plaintiff was examined on a certain date, the extent of his or her injuries, and so on. Thus, although an expert witness may not be allowed by the court to educate the jury on the subject of a sprained ankle or other topic of common knowledge, the fact that the plaintiff sustained a sprained ankle and was treated for it may be testified to by the treating doctor.

In a civil suit, the plaintiff must prove that he or she was injured by some act of the defendant. That injury can be economic (the loss of property or money), physical (such as a torn muscle or broken leg), or mental (stress or anxiety). Over the years, more and more types of injuries have become recognized as compensable injuries in civil cases. The term "pain and suffering" has been used to describe physical and emotional symptoms that a plaintiff may claim were caused by the defendant. Medical facts can help determine the existence and extent of all these types of injury.

Sometimes the expert will testify only hypothetically. In the hypothetical question, the expert may be asked to render an opinion based on certain assumptions concerning a hypothetical case that closely resembles the case at bar. The hypothetical question provides an opportunity for counsel to summarize his or her client's position. Sometimes, however, a medical expert will need to examine a plaintiff. It is not unusual for such examinations to take place years after the injury occurred, and the doctor will have to determine whether the injury exists, the extent of the injury, the cause of the injury, what (if any) limitations are caused by the injury, the treatment that is indicated, and the probable duration of the injury (perhaps based on the average rate of recovery for such an injury).

In the criminal justice system, medical experts may testify on a variety of scientific and medical issues. In the case of a murder, for example, it may be necessary to identify blood, tissue, bone, or some other human remains and to determine the source of those remains-namely, whether the remains belong to the alleged victim or perpetrator of the crime. Doctors who specialize in forensic medicine are often called upon to conduct special tests, such as DNA testing, to identify whose blood or tissue was found at the scene of a crime or on a murder weapon. Forensic experts can also determine the approximate time and cause of death. Testimony on these issues helps a jury determine the guilt or innocence of the accused.

Criminal cases occasionally also require the testimony of a forensic psychiatrist, who is an expert in mental and emotional disorders as they relate to legal principles. Testimony from such an expert assists in determining whether the defendant is "insane." According to section 4.01 of the Model Penal Code, a person is insane if he or she "lacks substantial capacity either to appreciate the criminality [wrongfulness] of his conduct or to conform his conduct to the requirements of the law." Not every state follows the Model Penal Code. Other variations of the insanity defense exist that deal with a person's ability to distinguish right from wrong. Psychiatric evaluations of the accused are performed to determine whether the defendant fit this definition at the time the crime was committed. Testimony regarding the defendant's insanity would significantly affect the case's outcome and sentencing.

A separate issue, unrelated to the defendant's mental condition at the time of the crime, is the defendant's "competency" to stand trial. According to Black's Law Dictionary (9th ed., 2008), a defendant is competent to stand trial if he or she has "the capacity to understand the proceedings, to consult meaningfully with counsel, and to assist in the defense." The law ensures that an accused person's rights are protected by requiring that the defendant be capable of understanding these proceedings and their implications before he or she is allowed to stand trial. If either of the attorneys, or the judge, asserts that the defendant is not competent to stand trial, the court will hold a competency hearing to decide whether the defendant is "competent." In determining the competency of the defendant, the court will hear the testimony of psychiatric experts. If the defendant is determined to be incompetent at the time of the trial, the defendant will not be tried but may instead be sent to a mental institution until such time as he or she is competent to stand trial.

In addition to being used in civil cases and criminal cases, medical science is used to provide scientific information to support or disprove wholly nonscientific determinations. Such philosophical and ethical issues include abortion and euthanasia. In the long-running debate over the legality of abortion, for example, many issues and circumstances come into play, including rape and the possibility that pregnancy may endanger the woman's life. One central and hotly contested question, however, is "When does life begin?" This question may also involve an equally difficult and controversial one: "What is life?" The courts and various state legislatures have turned to medical science to address these profound, and possibly unanswerable, questions. Medical science has identified two key concepts to answer these questions: the concept of "viability" (that is, the ability of the fetus to survive outside the womb) and the distinction between the first, second, and third trimesters of a pregnancy. The distinction of trimesters was originally based on the concept of viability: A fetus generally could not survive outside the womb during the first trimester (that is, was not viable), while a fetus was generally considered viable during the third trimester. Thus, the courts and legislature would often use the concept of trimesters in determining a cutoff date after which an abortion could not be performed.

These concepts have been used as the basis for legislation to regulate and authorize abortions. Medical science is, however, a rapidly evolving field. Because it is now possible for a human egg, once fertilized, to become viable outside the womb, the legal foundation upon which abortions are based is becoming unstable.

Another important area that has emerged from late twentieth and early twenty-first century technology concerns the use of human embryonic stem cells. Widely acknowledged as extremely valuable in assisting scientists in understanding basic mechanisms of embryo development and gene regulation, stem cell research holds the promise of enabling scientists to direct stem cells to grow into replacement organs and tissues to treat a wide variety of diseases. Embryos are valued in research for their ability to produce stem cells, which can be harvested to grow a variety of tissues for use in transplantation to treat serious illnesses such as cancer, heart disease, and diabetes.

The Applications of Medical Testimony

Medical experts in almost every field of medicine have played a part in civil cases, criminal cases, and controversies involving philosophical and ethical issues. Sometimes, the interaction between medicine and the law has spawned new medical or legal subspecialties. In fact, medical expert testimony has become a field and an occupation in itself, supporting an entire group of medical professionals to the exclusion of actual medical practice. This phenomenon has occurred in large part in response to the greater acceptance by the courts of medical expert testimony and the increased reliability of recent medical testing.

Personal injury cases afford a good example of all the different types of testimony that come into play in civil suits. A physical injury case, as the name suggests, is based on a physical (or mental) injury, as opposed to a purely financial injury, suffered by the plaintiff. A physical injury case may involve an automobile accident and its resulting injuries. In such a case, doctors who are experts in the field of muscle damage, neurology (for head and nerve injuries), orthopedic surgery, and countless other areas could be called as experts, depending on the extent of the injuries.

Another type of case, called a product liability case, will often use expert medical testimony. A product liability case is one in which a person has been injured by a specific product on the market and sues the manufacturer, and often the seller, claiming that the product was defective. Famous examples of product liability cases include claims filed against manufacturers of asbestos products, certain tampons (for causing toxic

shock syndrome), contraceptive devices such as the Dalkon Shield, and some generic or prescription drugs, such as thalidomide and Halcion. All these cases required medical experts in recently developed fields of medicine. Prior to the product liability suits filed against some tampon manufacturers, few people had heard of toxic shock syndrome. The testimony of medical experts was required to prove a link between an allegedly defective product and the resulting injury that was claimed. Without expert medical testimony in these cases, it would be impossible to prove that the defective products caused the injuries of which the defendants complained.

Another example of the medical profession developing to suit the law is in the area of workers' compensation. The California legislature, like the legislatures of many states, has established by statute (Labor Code section 3600 and following) a method by which to compensate any employee who has suffered a job-related injury. An employer is required by law to carry workers' compensation insurance, which will compensate an injured employee. If an employee is injured on the job in any manner, that employee is supposed to file a claim notifying his or her employer of the injury. The claim is then submitted to the workers' compensation insurance carrier. If the employer and the carrier accept liability, necessary treatment is provided to the employee. If the carrier denies further treatment or denies that an employee is disabled, the employee may file a claim with the Workers' Compensation Appeal Board. Once such a claim is filed, a judge will review all the medical reports of the injured worker. Additional medical evidence and testimony may be introduced to prove or disprove the employee's claim of injury or disability. The award of the Workers' Compensation Appeal Board is determined by the medical condition of the person claiming the injury. The growing popularity of workers' compensation has spawned an entire field of medicine, that of work-related injuries.

California courts routinely allow damages for "mental distress" in almost every type of tort action. Accordingly, psychiatrists and psychologists are routinely called upon to testify regarding whether a plaintiff has suffered such an injury. Emotional distress is not a specific medical condition, but rather a general emotional state, which may include anger, fear, frustration, anxiety, depression, and similar symptoms. Although psychiatric or psychological testimony is not required by the court for the plaintiff to recover damages for mental distress, it can be very effective in explaining to the jury the extent of the injuries and the effect of those injuries on the plaintiff's future life.

If a jury determines that the plaintiff suffered a physical or mental injury caused by the defendant, then, based on the medical testimony-of either the medical witness or the treating doctor-the jury may award any medical fees incurred, as well as anticipated medical fees and costs and compensation for the pain and suffering of the defendant. The jury may also award further damages not related to the medical condition of the plaintiff, if the case warrants such damages.

In a criminal case, particularly a case of homicide, forensic medicine often provides the key and fundamental evidence upon which the entire case is based. During the investigations of the assassination of President John F. Kennedy in the 1960s, the forensic evidence played a vital, although controversial, role. The testimony presented by the doctors who examined the president's body was used to reconstruct the crime. Forensic science was used to interpret the angle of entry of the bullets that killed Kennedy and thereby to extrapolate the source of the shots. Furthermore, forensic science was called upon to demonstrate how many shots were fired and the paths of the bullets upon entering the bodies of the president and Governor John Connally. Using medical evidence, along with other evidence, the Warren Commission concluded that the bullets all came from the book depository building behind the presidential caravan. Also using medical evidence and experts, critics of the Warren Commission's findings have alleged that the injuries suffered by the president could have been caused only by a bullet entering from the front of the president's neck and exiting the rear of the skull.

In another case, forensic evidence was able to reach a conclusive determination that certain bones were those of the Nazi war criminal Josef Mengele, known as the Angel of Death. In 1992, forensics experts discovered, using DNA testing, that some bones retrieved from a grave in Brazil were those of Mengele. To make this determination, doctors compared the DNA found in the blood of Mengele's son with DNA from the bones found in the grave. They found that the DNA from both sources matched. Because DNA constitutes a "genetic fingerprint" that remains the same from parent to offspring, the doctors were able to conclude that the remains found in Brazil were those of Mengele.

DNA testing is now also commonly used in suits to determine the father of an infant. According to the Genetics Institute, DNA testing is at least 99.8 percent accurate. Medical science has so refined its ability to chart DNA "fingerprints" that the chance of coming upon two identical DNA patterns is approximately one in six billion. Prior to DNA testing, a blood testing method called human leukocyte antigen (HLA) typing was used to determine paternity, but this typing was only 95 percent accurate.

Some medical or scientific tests, while accepted by the courts, remain subject to much controversy. The Breathalyzer test, used to determine blood alcohol levels, is one such test. While the courts regularly accept the results of such tests to determine whether a suspect was intoxicated, the test is based on several assumptions and averages. Based on the alcohol content in the suspect's breath, the test extrapolates a probable amount of alcohol in the suspect's blood. The reliability of this test depends on the correct calibration of the equipment and the care of the person taking the readings. Since the tests are taken by nonmedical or nonscientific personnel in the field, mistaken readings are not uncommon. Furthermore, if the suspect used a spray breath freshener just before the test, the readings may be skewed, since such breath fresheners are usually alcohol-based.

Perspective and Prospects

Medicine has always played some role in the outcome of court cases, but this relationship did not come into full flower until relatively recently. In the early twentieth century, courts placed strict limitations on the type and amount of medical testimony allowed into evidence. Often, certain types of medical evidence were not admissible because the science was not deemed reliable-there was too much room for error. The polygraph (lie detector), for example, could not be relied upon to reveal consistently whether a person was telling the truth, since it simply measured galvanic skin response, respiration rate, and other factors that only tend to be correlated with the subject's feelings of guilt. Most other evidence presented by medical experts concerned the likelihood of events or outcomes and therefore usually constituted opinion, rather than fact.

With the advent of new technologies in the later part of the twentieth century, medical science began to present "hard" (more precise) data that became more frequently accepted by the courts as reliable and relevant evidence. Even so, it took some time before medical scientists were able to present enough data to persuade the courts that the evidence of such methods as DNA "fingerprinting" was truly reliable. The acceptance of DNA testing, for example, was a long and hard-fought battle among legions of medical experts on both sides of the issue. Finally, DNA testing was accepted by the courts as a reliable source of evidence. As forensic medicine advances, no doubt its contribution to the law will also advance. The ability of the medical and other scientific professions to determine reliable conclusions relating to court cases is progressing rapidly with increases in scientific knowledge, methods, and technology.

Ironically, medical progress may cloud other areas of the law. In the early twentieth century, for example, few could have dreamed of the technology that makes life support possible. With the advent of kidney dialysis machines, pacemakers, respirators, and other life-support devices, medical science has achieved the ability to prolong an individual's bodily functioning. Whether this functioning alone is sufficient to define "life," however, remains a question that cannot be addressed by medical science alone but must be considered in the light of philosophical, ethical, and other values. Medicine is consequently becoming an area in which the law must adapt. Issues that have challenged existing laws include abortion and the point at which life begins, euthanasia, the individual's right not to have life extended, the right to reveal an individual's genetic predisposition toward disease, egg implantation, and genetic engineering. Medical science has propagated these dilemmas but may also be called upon to solve them.

Larry M. Roberts, J.D.;
updated by Joshua Lampert, MS-III,
and Amanda Grannis, B.A.

See also Abortion; Animal rights vs. research; Assisted reproductive technologies; Autopsy; Blood testing; Cloning; Environmental health; Ethics; Euthanasia; Forensic pathology; Genetic engineering; In vitro fertilization; Living will; Malpractice; Occupational health; Screening

For Further Information:

Boumil, Marcia M., Clifford E. Elias, and Diane Bissonnette Moes. *Medical Liability in a Nutshell.* 2nd ed. St. Paul, MN: Thomson/West, 2003. Succinctly discusses salient topics in medical liability: medical negligence, standard of care, intentional torts, informed consent and the right to refuse treatment, the duty of disclosure, causation and damages, and various defenses to liability.

Fremgen, Bonnie F. *Medical Law and Ethic.* 2nd ed. Upper Saddle River, NJ: Pearson/Prentice Hall, 2006. Essential legal and ethical principles for the health care provider. Contains case studies and legal citations.

Furrow, Barry R., et al. *Health Law: Cases, Materials, and Problems.* 6th ed. St. Paul, MN: Thomson/West, 2008. Covers a range of issues related to health and the law, including cost control, prospective payment, health care antitrust, and federal and state regulation of health care delivery; legal and ethical issues created by reproductive technology and by the dilemmas of death and dying; and the core topics of professional liability and the physician-patient relationship.

Garner, Bryan A., ed. *Black's Law Dictionary.* 9th ed. St. Paul, MN: Thomson/West, 2008. The fundamental legal dictionary, containing definitions and examples of how terms have been interpreted by courts.

James, Stuart H., and Jon J. Nordby, eds. *Forensic Science: An Introduction to Scientific and Investigative Techniques.* 2nd ed. Boca Raton, FL: CRC Press, 2005. An introductory text that covers a range of topics, including trace evidence, forensic toxicology, DNA analysis, crime scene investigation, fingerprints, traumatic death, forensic anthropology, bloodstain patterns, and criminal profiling, among many others.

Jonsen, Albert R., Mark Siegler, and William J. Winslade. *Clinical Ethics: A Practical Approach to Ethical Decisions in Clinical Medicine.* 6th ed. New York: McGraw-Hill, 2006. Discusses the whole range of medical ethics, including legal issues, confidentiality, care of the dying patient, and euthanasia and assisted suicide.

Lewis, Marcia A., and Carol D. Tamparo. *Medical Law, Ethics, and Bioethics for Ambulatory Care.* 6th ed. Philadelphia: F.A. Davis, 2007. Directed to the general health care provider, the book covers practical topics such as management, guidelines and regulations for medical and allied health professionals, public duties, medical records, collection, allocation of scarce resources, genetic engineering, abortion, and life-and-death issues from the legal and ethical perspectives.

Munson, Ronald, comp. *Intervention and Reflection: Basic Issues in Medical Ethics.* 7th ed. Belmont, CA: Thomson/Wadsworth, 2004. An undergraduate text that combines social context, case studies, readings, and decision scenarios for topics that include abortion, advances in gene therapy, genetic discrimination, and health care rights.

Pence, Gregory E. *Classic Cases in Medical Ethics: Accounts of Cases That Have Shaped Medical Ethics, with Philosophical, Legal, and Historical Backgrounds.* 4th ed. Boston: McGraw-Hill, 2004. Surveys important cases that have defined and shaped the field of medical ethics. Each case is accompanied by careful discussion of pertinent philosophical theories and legal and ethical issues.

Lead poisoning

Disease/Disorder

Also known as: Saturnism, plumbism, painter's colic

Anatomy or system affected: Brain, circulatory system, endocrine system, musculoskeletal system, nervous system, reproductive system

Specialties and related fields: Environmental health, pediatrics, preventive medicine, toxicology

Definition: A condition caused by high levels of lead in the blood. This major preventable environmental health problem is found in both children and adults, but more frequently in children.

Key terms:

arthralgia: severe joint pain, especially when inflammation is not present

chelation: the taking up or release of a metallic ion by an organic molecule

encephalopathy: any disease of the brain

lead: a limited naturally occurring element widely distributed throughout the environment by industrial uses and pollution

paresis: partial paralysis

paresthesia: an abnormal sensation, such as burning, tingling, tickling, or pricking

Causes and Symptoms

Lead poisoning is a major, preventable environmental health problem. Elevated lead levels in adults can increase blood pressure and cause fertility problems, nerve disorders, arthalgia, and problems with memory and concentration. Children under the age of six are at high risk for harm because their brains and nervous systems are still maturing. Blood lead levels as low as 10 micrograms per deciliter are associated with harmful effects on children's ability to learn. Very high blood lead levels of 70 micrograms per deciliter can cause devastating health consequences, including seizures and other neurological symptoms, abdominal pain, developmental delays, attention deficit, hyperactivity, behavior disorders, hearing loss, anemia, coma, and death.

Children can be exposed to lead in many ways. Sources of exposure include automobile exhaust, lead-based paint, and environmental contaminants released by industrial processes that use or produce lead-containing materials. Contributors to childhood lead exposure also include lead-contaminated containers, food, dust, soil, air, and water; toys contaminated with lead paint; lead-containing ceramics and hobby supplies; substance abuse such as gasoline sniffing; parental transfer from lead-rich occupational environments; and traditional medicines such as azarcon and greta. Deteriorating lead-based paint in older homes is the most important source of lead exposure in children (many homes built prior to 1960 contain some lead-basaed paint). Swallowing lead-based paint dust through normal hand-to-mouth activity and chewing directly on painted surfaces are major methods of lead ingestion. Children are often attracted to lead paint because of its sweet taste. Lead-based paint in homes, however, was banned from residential use in 1978, but families living in homes built before this time (especially before 1960) are at risk. Lead exposure in adults is usually a result of jobs in house painting, welding and smelting, the manufacturing of car batteries, and other occupations involving lead.

Upon entering the human body, inorganic lead is not metabolized but is directly absorbed, distributed, and excreted. The rate at which lead is absorbed depends on its chemical

---

Information on Lead Poisoning

Causes: Environmental exposure
Symptoms: Vary; can include abdominal discomfort, fatigue, muscle pain, tremor, difficulty concentrating, headache, vomiting, weight loss, constipation, hearing loss, changes in consciousness
Duration: Can be short-term or chronic
Treatments: Chelation drug therapy

---

and physical form and on the physiologic characteristics of the exposed person. Once in the blood, lead is distributed among three compartments: the blood; soft tissue zones such as the kidneys, bone marrow, liver, and brain; and mineralizing tissues such as bones and teeth. For lead poisoning to take place, major acute exposures to lead need not occur. The body accumulates lead and releases it slowly; therefore, even small doses over time can be toxic. It is the total body accumulation of lead that is related to the risk of adverse effects. Whether lead enters the body through inhalation or ingestion, the biologic effects are the same—interference with normal cell function and with certain physiologic processes.

By and large, children show a greater sensitivity to the effects of lead than do adults. Parents working in lead-related industries not only may inhale lead dust and lead oxide fumes but also may eat, drink, and smoke in or near contaminated areas, increasing the probability of lead ingestion and subsequent transfer to their children. Since lead readily crosses the placenta, the fetus is at risk. Fetal exposure can cause potentially adverse neurological effects in utero and during postnatal development. The incomplete development of the blood-brain barrier in very young children, up to thirty-six months of age, increases the risk of the entry of lead into the developing nervous system, which can result in prolonged neurobehavioral disorders. Children absorb and retain more lead in proportion to their weight than do adults. Young children also show a greater prevalence of iron deficiency, a condition that can increase the gastrointestinal absorption of lead.

Symptoms of lead poisoning and lead intoxication vary because of differences in individual susceptibility, and the severity of symptoms increases with increased exposure. Symptoms of mild lead toxicity include abdominal discomfort, fatigue, muscle pain, or paresthesia. Moderate toxicity is indicated by arthralgia, tremor, fatigue, difficulty concentrating, headache, abdominal pain, vomiting, weight loss, and constipation. Severe toxicity symptoms include paresis or paralysis, encephalopathy, seizures, severe abdominal cramps, hearing loss, changes in consciousness, and coma.

Treatment and Therapy

If a child is suspected of having lead poisoning, laboratory tests are necessary to evaluate lead intoxication levels. Laboratory techniques defining lead toxicity include blood lead level screening, erythrocyte protoporphyrin (EP) and zinc protoporphyrin (ZPP) screening, creatinine, urinalysis, and hematocrit and hemoglobin tests with peripheral smear. The Centers for Disease Control and Prevention (CDC) and the American Academy of Pediatrics (AAP) recommends that all children living in high-risk neighbourhoods or conditions should have their blood levels tested regularly until the age of five.

The physical examination for suspected lead poisoning cases includes special attention to hematologic, cardiovascular, gastrointestinal, and renal systems. Any neurological or behavioral changes are considered significant indicators. In addition, severe and prolonged lead poisoning may be indicated by a purplish line on the gums. A complete interview and medical evaluation of a suspected lead poisoning patient includes a full workup and medical history. Clues to potential exposure vectors can be obtained by discussing family and occupational history, use of traditional medicines, remodeling activities, hobbies, table and cookware, drinking water source, nutrition, proximity to industry or waste sites, and the physical condition and age of the patient's residence, school, and/or day care facility.

The treatment and management of lead poisoning first involves the separation of the patient from the source of lead. After a diagnosis of lead poisoning is made, local environmental health officials should be contacted to determine the lead source and what remediation action is necessary for its control. This may include testing a home's paint and water for lead, as well as identifying hobbies such as making stained glass, soldering electrical devices, fishing with lead-containing sinkers, all of which can expose children to lead poisoning. A diet high in calcium and iron may help to decrease the absorption of lead.

The Centers for Disease Control and Prevention recommends that children with blood lead levels of 45 micrograms per deciliter or greater should be referred for chelation therapy immediately. Several drugs are capable of binding or chelating lead, depleting both soft and hard (skeletal) tissues of lead and reducing its acute toxicity. All these drugs have potential side effects and must be used with caution. The most commonly used chelating agent is calcium disodium edetic acid, but several other agents are available.

—Randall L. Milstein, Ph.D.; updated by
Sharon W. Stark, R.N., A.P.R.N., D.N.Sc.

See also Developmental disorders; Environmental diseases; Environmental health; Learning disabilities; Mental retardation; Occupational health; Poisoning; Safety issues for children; Screening; Toxicology.

For Further Information:
Denworth, Lydia. *Toxic Truth: A Scientist, a Doctor, and the Battle Over Lead.* Boston: Beacon Press, 2009.
Goldstein, Inge F., and Martin Goldstein. *How Much Risk? A Guide to Understanding Environmental Health Hazards.* New York: Oxford University Press, 2002.
Kessel, Irene, and John T. O'Connor. *Getting the Lead Out: The Complete Resource on How to Prevent and Cope with Lead Poisoning.* Rev. ed. Cambridge, Mass.: Perseus, 2001.
Korfmacher, Katrina S., and Michael L. Hanley. "Are Local Laws the Key to Ending Childhood Lead Poisoning?" *Journal of Health*

1324 • LEARNING DISABILITIES

Politics, Policy and Law 38, no. 4 (August, 2013): 757–813.

Morgan, Monroe T. *Environmental Health.* 3d ed. Belmont, Calif.: Thomson/Wadsworth, 2003.

Roberts, J. R., et al. "Are Children Still at Risk for Lead Poisoning?" *Clinical Pediatrics* 52, no. 2 (February, 2013): 125–130.

Schmidt, Charles W. "Unsafe Harbor? Elevated Blood Lead Levels in Refugee Children." *Environmental Health Perspectives* 121, no. 6 (June, 2013): A190–A195.

Smoots, Elizabeth. "Lead Poisoning—Child." *Health Library,* March 18, 2013.

Vivier, Patrick, et al. "The Important Health Impact of Where a Child Lives: Neighborhood Characteristics and the Burden of Lead Poisoning." *Maternal and Child Health Journal* 15, no. 8 (November, 2011): 1195–1202.

Warren, Christian. *Brush with Death: A Social History of Lead Poisoning.* Baltimore: Johns Hopkins University Press, 2001.

LEARNING DISABILITIES

Disease/Disorder

Anatomy or system affected: Brain, nervous system, psychic-emotional system

Specialties and related fields: Neurology, pediatrics, psychology

Definition: A variety of disorders involving the failure to learn an academic skill despite normal levels of intelligence, maturation, and cultural and educational opportunity; estimates of the prevalence of learning disabilities in the general population range between 2 and 20 percent.

Key terms:

achievement test: a measure of an individual's degree of learning in an academic subject, such as reading, mathematics, and written language

dyslexia: difficulty in reading, with an implied neurological cause

intelligence test: a psychological test designed to measure an individual's ability to think logically, act purposefully, and react successfully to the environment; yields intelligence quotient (IQ) scores

neurological dysfunction: problems associated with the way in which different sections and structures of the brain perform tasks, such as verbal and spatial reasoning and language production

neurology: the study of the central nervous system, which is composed of the brain and spinal cord

perceptual deficits: problems in processing information from the environment, which may involve distractibility, impulsivity, and figure-ground distortions (difficulty distinguishing foreground from background)

standardized test: an instrument used to assess skill development in comparison to others of the same age or grade

Causes and Symptoms

An understanding of learning disabilities must begin with the knowledge that the definition, diagnosis, and treatment of these disorders have historically generated considerable disagreement and controversy. This is primarily attributable to the fact that people with learning disabilities are a highly diverse group of individuals with a wide variety of characteristics. Consequently, differences of opinion among professionals remain to such an extent that presenting a single universally accepted definition of learning disabilities is not possible. Definitional differences most frequently center on the relative emphases that alternative groups place on characteristics of these disorders. For example, experts in medical fields typically describe these disorders from a disease model and view them primarily as neurological dysfunctions. Conversely, educators usually place more emphasis on the academic problems that result from learning disabilities. Despite these differences, the most commonly accepted definitions, those developed by the United States Office of Education in 1977, the Board of the Association for Children and Adults with Learning Disabilities in 1985, and the National Joint Committee for Learning Disabilities in 1981, do include some areas of commonality.

Difficulty in academic functioning is included in the three definitions, and virtually all descriptions of learning disabilities include this characteristic. Academic deficits may be in one or more formal scholastic subjects, such as reading or mathematics. Often the deficits will involve a component skill of the academic area, such as problems with comprehension or word knowledge in reading or difficulty in calculating or applying arithmetical reasoning in mathematics. The academic difficulty may also be associated with more basic skills of learning that influence functioning across academic areas; these may involve deficits in listening, speaking, and thinking. Dyslexia, a term for reading problems, is the most common academic problem associated with learning disabilities. Because reading skills are required in most academic activities to some degree, many view dyslexia as the most serious form of learning disability.

The presumption of a neurological dysfunction as the cause of these disorders is included, either directly or indirectly, in each of the three definitions. Despite this presumption, unless an individual has a known history of brain trauma, the neurological basis for learning disabilities will not be identified in most cases because current assessment technology does not allow for such precise diagnoses. Rather, at least minimal neurological dysfunction is simply assumed to be present in anyone who exhibits characteristics of a learning disorder.

The three definitions all state that individuals with learning disabilities experience learning problems despite possessing normal intelligence. This condition is referred to as a discrepancy between achievement and ability or potential.

Finally, each of the three definitions incorporates the idea

Information on Learning Disabilities

Causes: Unclear; possibly neurological deficits, genetic and hereditary influences, exposure to toxins during pregnancy or early childhood

Symptoms: Difficulty in academic functioning (including deficits in listening, speaking, and thinking)

Duration: Often chronic

that learning disabilities cannot be attributed to another condition such as vision or hearing problems, emotional or psychiatric disturbance, or social, cultural, or educational disadvantage. Consequently, these conditions must be excluded as primary contributors to academic difficulties.

A number of causes of learning disabilities have been proposed, with none being universally accepted. Some of the most plausible causal theories include neurological deficits, genetic and hereditary influences, and exposure to toxins during fetal gestation or early childhood.

Evidence to support the assumption of a link between neurological dysfunction and learning disabilities has been provided by studies using sophisticated brain imaging techniques such as positron emission tomography (PET) and computed tomography (CT) scanning and magnetic resonance imaging (MRI). Studies using these techniques have, among other findings, indicated subtle abnormalities in the structure and electrical activity in the brains of individuals with learning disabilities. The use of such techniques has typically been confined to research; however, the continuing advancement of brain imaging technology holds promise not only in contributing greater understanding of the nature and causes of learning disabilities but also in treating the disorder.

Genetic and hereditary influences also have been proposed as causes. Supportive evidence comes from research indicating that identical twins are more likely to be concordant for learning disabilities than fraternal twins and that these disorders are more common in certain families.

A genetic cause of learning disabilities may be associated with extra X or Y chromosomes in certain individuals. The type and degree of impairment associated with these conditions vary according to many genetic and environmental factors, but they can involve problems with language development, visual perception, memory, and problem solving. Despite evidence to link chromosome abnormalities to those with learning disabilities, most experts agree that such genetic conditions account for only a portion of these individuals.

Exposure to toxins or poisons during fetal gestation and early childhood can also cause learning disabilities. During pregnancy nearly all substances the mother takes in are transferred to the fetus. Research has shown that mothers who smoke, drink alcohol, or use certain drugs or medications during pregnancy are more likely to have children with developmental problems, including learning disabilities. Yet not all children exposed to toxins during gestation will have such problems, and the consequences of exposure will vary according to the period when it occurred, the amount of toxin introduced, and the general health and nutrition of the mother and fetus.

Though not precisely involving toxins, two other conditions associated with gestation and childbirth have been linked to learning disabilities. The first, anoxia, or oxygen deprivation, occurring for a critical period of time during the birthing process has been tied to both developmental and learning disabilities. The second, and more speculative, involves exposure of the fetus to an abnormally large amount of testosterone during gestation. Differences in brain development are proposed to result from the exposure, causing learning disorders and other abnormalities. Known as the embryological theory, it may account for the large number of males with these disabilities, since they have greater amounts of testosterone than females.

The exposure of the immature brain during early childhood to insecticides, household cleaning fluids, alcohol, narcotics, and carbon monoxide, among other toxic substances, may also cause learning disabilities. Lead poisoning resulting from ingesting lead from paint, plaster, and other sources has been found in epidemic numbers in some sections of the United States. Lead poisoning can damage the brain and cause learning disabilities as well as a number of other serious problems.

The number and variety of proposed causes not only reflect differences in experts" training and consequent perspectives but also suggest the likelihood that these disorders can be caused by multiple conditions. This diversity of views also carries to methods for assessing and providing treatment and services to individuals with learning disabilities.

Treatment and Therapy

In 1975, the US Congress adopted the Education for All Handicapped Children Act, which, along with other requirements, mandated that students with disabilities, including those with learning disabilities, be identified and provided appropriate educational services. Since that time, much effort has been devoted to developing adequate assessment practices for diagnosis and effective treatment strategies.

In the school setting, assessment of students suspected of having learning disabilities is conducted by a variety of professionals, including teachers specially trained in assessing learning disabilities, school nurses, classroom teachers, school psychologists, and school administrators. Collectively, these professionals are known as a multidisciplinary team. An additional requirement of this educational legislation is that parents must be given the opportunity to participate in the assessment process. Professionals outside the school setting, such as clinical psychologists and independent educational specialists, also conduct assessments to identify learning disabilities.

Because the definition of learning disabilities in the 1975 act includes a discrepancy between achievement and ability as a characteristic of the disorder, students suspected of having learning disabilities are usually administered a variety of formal and informal tests. Standardized tests of intelligence, such as the third edition of the Wechsler Intelligence Scale for Children, are administered to determine ability. Standardized tests of academic achievement, such as the Woodcock-Johnson Psychoeducational Battery and the Wide Range Achievement Test, also are administered to determine levels of academic skill.

Whether a discrepancy between ability and achievement exists to such a degree as to warrant diagnosis of a learning disability is determined by various formulas comparing the scores derived from the intelligence and achievement tests.

The precise methods and criteria used to determine a discrepancy vary according to differences among state regulations and school district practices. Consequently, a student diagnosed with a learning disability in one part of the United States may not be viewed as such in another area using different diagnostic criteria. This possibility has been raised in criticism of the use of the discrepancy criteria to identify these disorders. Other criticisms of the method include the use of intelligence quotient (IQ) scores (which are not as stable or accurate as many assume), the inconsistency of students" scores when using alternative achievement tests, and the lack of correspondence between what students are taught and what is tested on achievement tests.

In partial consequence of these and other problems with standardized tests, alternative informal assessment methods have been developed. One such method that is frequently employed is termed curriculum-based assessment (CBA). The CBA method uses materials and tasks taken directly from students" classroom curriculum. For example, in reading, CBA might involve determining the rate of words read per minute from a student's textbook. CBA has been demonstrated to be effective in distinguishing among some students with learning disabilities, those with other academic difficulties, and those without learning problems. Nevertheless, many professionals remain skeptical of CBA as a valid alternative to traditional standardized tests.

Other assessment techniques include vision and hearing tests, measures of language development, and tests examining motor coordination and sensory perception and processing. Observations and analyses of the classroom environment may also be conducted to determine how instructional practices and a student's behavior contribute to learning difficulties.

Based on the information gathered by the multidisciplinary team, a decision is made regarding the diagnosis of a learning disability. If a student is identified with one of these disorders, the team then develops an individual education plan to address identified educational needs. An important guideline in developing the plan is that students with these disorders should be educated to the greatest extent possible with their peers, while still being provided with appropriate services. Considerable debate has occurred regarding how best to adhere to this guideline.

Programs for students with learning disabilities typically are implemented in self-contained classrooms, resource rooms, or regular classrooms. Self-contained classrooms usually contain ten to twenty students and one or more teachers specially trained to work with these disorders. Typically, these classrooms focus on teaching fundamental skills in basic academic subjects such as reading, writing, and mathematics. Depending on the teacher's training, efforts may also be directed toward developing perceptual, language, or social skills. Students in these programs usually spend some portion of their day with their peers in regular education meetings, but the majority of the day is spent in the self-contained classroom.

The popularity of self-contained classrooms has decreased significantly since the 1960s, when they were the primary setting in which students with learning disabilities were educated. This decrease is largely attributable to the stigmatizing effects of placing students in special settings and the lack of clear evidence to support the effectiveness of this approach.

Students receiving services in resource rooms typically spend a portion of their day in a class where they receive instruction and assistance from specially trained teachers. Students often spend one or two periods in the resource room with a small group of other students who may have similar learning problems or function at a comparable academic level. In the elementary grades, resource rooms usually focus on developing basic academic skills, whereas at the secondary level time is more typically spent in assisting students with their assignments from regular education classes.

Resource room programs are viewed as less restrictive than self-contained classrooms; however, they too have been criticized for segregating children with learning problems. Other criticisms center on scheduling difficulties inherent in the program and the potential for inconsistent instructional approaches and confusion over teaching responsibilities between the regular classroom and resource room teachers. Research on the effectiveness of resource room programs also has been mixed; nevertheless, they are found in most public schools across the United States.

Increasing numbers of students with learning disabilities have their individual education plans implemented exclusively in a regular classroom. In most schools where such programs exist, teachers are given assistance by a consulting teacher with expertise in learning disabilities. Supporters of this approach point to the lack of stigma associated with segregating students and the absence of definitive research supporting other service models. Detractors are concerned about the potential for inadequate support for the classroom teacher, resulting in students receiving insufficient services. The movement to provide services to students with learning disabilities in regular education settings, termed the Regular Education Initiative, has stirred much debate among professionals and parents. Resolution of the debate will greatly affect how individuals with learning disabilities are provided services.

No one specific method of teaching these students has been demonstrated to be superior to others. A variety of strategies have been developed, including perceptual training, multisensory teaching, modality matching, and direct instruction. Advocates of perceptual training believe that academic problems stem from underlying deficits in perceptual skills. They use various techniques aimed at developing perceptual abilities before trying to remedy or teach specific academic skills. Multisensory teaching involves presenting information to students through several senses. Instruction using this method may be conducted using tactile, auditory, visual, and kinesthetic exercises. Instruction involving modality matching begins with identifying the best learning style for a student, such as visual or auditory processing. Learning tasks are then presented via that mode. Direct instruction is based on the principles of behavioral psychology.

The method involves developing precise educational goals, focusing on teaching the exact skill of concern, and providing frequent opportunities to perform the skill until it is mastered.

With the exception of direct instruction, research has generally failed to demonstrate that these strategies are uniquely effective with students with learning disabilities. Direct instruction, on the other hand, has been demonstrated to be effective but has also been criticized for focusing on isolated skills without dealing with the broader processing problems associated with these disorders. More promisingly, students with learning disabilities appear to benefit from teaching approaches that have been found effective with students without learning problems when instruction is geared to ability level and rate of learning.

Perspective and Prospects

Interest in disorders of learning can be identified throughout the history of medicine. The specific study of learning disabilities, however, can be traced to the efforts of a number of physicians working in the first quarter of the twentieth century who studied the brain and its associated pathology. One such researcher, Kurt Goldstein, identified a number of unusual characteristics, collectively termed perceptual deficits, that were associated with head injury.

Goldstein's work influenced a number of researchers affiliated with the Wayne County Training School, including Alfred Strauss, Laura Lehtinen, Newell Kephart, and William Cruickshank. These individuals worked with children with learning problems who exhibited many of the characteristics of brain injury identified by Goldstein. Consequently, they presumed that neurological dysfunction, whether it could specifically be identified or not, caused the learning difficulties. They also developed a set of instructional practices involving reduced environmental stimuli and exercises to develop perceptual skills. The work and writings of these individuals through the 1940s, 1950s, and 1960s were highly influential, and many programs for students with learning disabilities were based on their theoretical and instructional principles.

Samuel Orton, working in the 1920s and 1930s, also was influenced by research into brain injury in his conceptualization of children with reading problems. He observed that many of these children were left-handed or ambidextrous, reversed letters or words when reading or writing, and had coordination problems. Consequently, he proposed that reading disabilities resulted from abnormal brain development and an associated mixing of brain functions. Based on the work of Orton and his students, including Anna Gilmore and Bessie Stillman, a variety of teaching strategies were developed that focused on teaching phonics and using multisensory aids. In the 1960s, Elizabeth Slingerland applied Orton's concepts in the classroom setting, and they have been included in many programs for students with learning disabilities.

A number of other researchers have developed theories for the cause and treatment of learning disabilities. Some of the most influential include Helmer Mykelbust and Samuel Kirk, who emphasized gearing instruction to a student's strongest learning modality, and Norris Haring, Ogden Lindsley, and Joseph Jenkins, who applied principles of behavioral psychology to teaching.

The work of these and other researchers and educators raised professional and public awareness of learning disabilities and the special needs of individuals with the disorder. Consequently, the number of special education classrooms and programs increased dramatically in public schools across the United States in the 1960s and 1970s. Legislation on both state and federal levels, primarily resulting from litigation by parents to establish the educational rights of their children, also has had a profound impact on the availability of services for those with learning disabilities. The passage of the Education for All Handicapped Children Act in 1975 not only mandated appropriate educational services for students with learning disabilities but also generated funding, interest, and research in the field. The Regular Education Initiative has since prompted increased efforts to identify more effective assessment and treatment strategies and generated debates among professionals and the consumers of these services. Decisions resulting from these continuing debates will have a significant impact on future services for individuals with learning disabilities.

—Paul F. Bell, Ph.D.

See also Aphasia and dysphasia; Asperger's syndrome; Attention-deficit disorder; Autism; Brain; Brain disorders; Developmental disorders; Down syndrome; Dyslexia; Mental retardation; Neuralgia, neuritis, and neuropathy; Neurology; Neurology, pediatric; Psychiatry; Psychiatry, child and adolescent; Speech disorders.

For Further Information:

Bender, William N. *Learning Disabilities: Characteristics, Identification, and Teaching Strategies.* 6th ed. Boston: Pearson/Allyn & Bacon, 2006.

Hallahan, Daniel P., et al. *Learning Disabilities: Foundations, Characteristics, and Effective Teaching.* 3d ed. Boston: Allyn & Bacon, 2005.

Healthy Children. "How Learning Problems Are Managed." *American Academy of Pediatrics*, May 11, 2013.

Jordan, Dale R. *Overcoming Dyslexia in Children, Adolescents, and Adults.* Austin, Tex.: Pro-Ed, 2002.

Learning Disabilities Association of America. http://www.ldanatl.org.

Levinson, Harold N. *Smart but Feeling Dumb: The Challenging New Research on Dyslexia—and How It May Help You.* Rev. ed. New York: Warner Books, 2003.

Lovitt, Thomas. *Introduction to Learning Disabilities.* Needham Heights, Mass.: Allyn & Bacon, 1989.

MedlinePlus. "Learning Disorders." *MedlinePlus*, August 14, 2013.

National Institute of Child Health and Human Development. "What Are the Symptoms of Learning Disabilities?" *National Institutes of Health*, November 30, 2012.

Rief, Sandra F. *The ADHD Book of Lists: A Practical Guide for Helping Children and Teens with Attention Deficit Disorders.* San Francisco: Jossey-Bass, 2003.

Swanson, H. Lee, Karen R. Harris, and Steve Graham, eds. *Handbook of Learning Disabilities.* New York: Guilford Press, 2006.

LEGIONNAIRES' DISEASE

Disease/Disorder

Anatomy or system affected: Chest, lungs, respiratory system

Specialties and related fields: Bacteriology, environmental health, epidemiology, internal medicine, public health

Definition: A rapidly progressing bacterial pneumonia caused by infection with an organism of the genus *Legionella* and characterized by influenza-like illness, with high fever, chills, headache, and muscle aches.

Key terms:

alveolus: an outpouching of lung tissue in which gas exchange takes place between air in the lungs and blood capillaries

legionellosis: another name for any infection caused by a member of the genus *Legionella*; generally denotes Legionnaires' disease

macrophage: any of a variety of phagocytic cells; macrophages are found in highest numbers in tissue; alveolar macrophages are found in lungs and function to remove respiratory pathogens

phagocytes: white cells capable of ingesting and digesting microbes, a process referred to as phagocytosis; primarily refers to neutrophils and macrophages

Pontiac fever: a self-limiting, nonpneumonic disease caused by *Legionella* bacteria; clinically and epidemiologically distinct from Legionnaires' disease

virulence factor: a bacterial factor that enhances the pathogenic potential of the organism; includes products such as toxins and capsules

Causes and Symptoms

Legionnaires' disease, or legionellosis, is an acute bacterial pneumonia that was unknown prior to 1976. In July and August of that year, an outbreak of pneumonia occurred among persons who had either attended an American Legion convention in Philadelphia or had been in the vicinity of the Bellevue-Stratford Hotel in the downtown area. The likely source of the epidemic was a contaminated air-conditioning unit in the hotel. Though speculation among the media and general public suggested all sorts of causes for the epidemic, the specific etiological agent was isolated by January, 1977. It turned out to be a somewhat common bacterium, which was subsequently given the genus and species names *Legionella pneumophila*; the genus name reflected the first known victims, while the species name meant "lung-loving."

Within several years, additional strains of *Legionella* bacteria were isolated from patients suffering from bacterial pneumonia. Through 2005, forty-one species have been identified, of which eighteen have been associated with human disease. Most cases of Legionnaires' disease have been linked to infection by *L. pneumophila* or, to a lesser degree, *L. micdadei*.

Genetic evidence confirmed that *Legionella* was indeed a newly isolated bacterium. Several factors contributed to its previous invisibility. First, Legionnaires' disease is similar in its characteristics to other forms of nonbacterial pneumonia,

---

Information on Legionnaires' Disease

Causes: Bacterial infection

Symptoms: Dry cough, muscle aches, rising fever, possible vomiting and diarrhea

Duration: Acute

Treatments: Antibiotics (erythromycin, rifampin)

---

such as that caused by viruses. Since no bacteria were readily isolated, there was no immediate reason to suspect a bacterium as the infectious agent. The second reason related to the initial difficulty of growing *Legionella* bacteria in the laboratory. Aspirates from pneumonia victims were inoculated onto routine laboratory media; most common bacteria grow quite readily on such media. No growth was observed, however, in the case of *Legionella*. Many nutrient supplements were tried. *Legionella* bacteria grew only on media that were supplemented with iron and the amino acid cysteine. Since the early 1980s, the medium of choice has been agar containing buffered charcoal yeast extract (BCYE). Nutrients such as amino acids, vitamins, and iron are included in the medium while the charcoal removes potentially toxic materials.

Legionellosis actually constitutes two separate clinical entities: Legionnaires' disease and Pontiac fever. Legionnaires' disease is potentially the more serious of the two. The victim is initially infected through a respiratory route. In general, the source of the infection is an aerosol generated by contaminated water supplies such as those found in the cooling units of building air-conditioning systems. Rarely, if at all, does the disease pass from person to person. Most infections are unapparent, with either mild disease or none at all. The estimate is that less than 5 percent of exposed individuals actually contract Legionnaires' disease. Certain factors seem to increase the chances that the infection will progress toward pneumonia. Often, the lungs of the victim have suffered from previous trauma, such as that caused by emphysema or smoking. The person is generally, though not always, middle-aged or older. These observations suggest that, in most instances, the person's immune system is quite capable of handling the infection.

The disease begins with a dry cough, muscle aches, and rising fever—symptoms that resemble the flu. The person may also suffer from vomiting and diarrhea. In serious cases, the disease becomes progressively more severe over the next three to six days. The alveoli, or air sacs, of the lung become necrotized, increasing the difficulty in breathing. Small abscesses may also form in the lungs, as phagocytes infiltrate the area. The mortality rate has ranged from 15 to 60 percent in various outbreaks, although with early treatment, these numbers can be significantly lowered. Patients with other underlying lung problems, or who may be immunosuppressed, are at particular risk.

Pontiac fever is a much less serious form of disease. Named for the Michigan city in which a 1968 outbreak occurred in the Public Health Department building, the disease is self-limiting, nonpneumonic, and not life-threatening.

Pontiac fever also seems to follow the inhalation of the etiological agent. Though the attack rate in exposed individuals appears to approach 100 percent, there is no infiltration of lung tissue and no abscess formation. A febrile period occurs one to two days following infection, with the individual progressing to recovery after several days. The difference between the two forms of disease remains obscure. There appears to be no obvious difference between the organisms associated with the two diseases, though strains associated with Pontiac fever may not replicate as readily inside human cells.

The mechanism by which infection by *Legionella* bacteria results in pneumonia is not altogether clear. Research into this area has centered on forms of virulence factors produced by the organism and their relationships to disease. Following their infiltration into the lung, *Legionella* bacteria are phagocytized by alveolar macrophages or other leukocytes (white blood cells). Unlike other ingested microbes, however, *Legionella* bacteria often survive the process and begin a process of intracellular replication. In this intracellular state, *Legionella* bacteria are shielded from many of the host's immune defenses.

Certain questions lend themselves to understanding this approach in elucidating the mechanisms of Legionnaires' disease. First, are intracellular survival and multiplication necessary factors in the development of the disease? Second, if these factors are indeed relevant, exactly how does the organism manage to evade the killing mechanisms that exist inside the cell?

The first question has been dealt with by various animal studies. Guinea pigs were exposed to a *Legionella* aerosol, and lung aspirates were prepared after forty-eight hours. Large numbers of viable organisms were found inside alveolar macrophages. Few live *Legionella* bacteria, however, were observed outside cells. In addition, mutant *Legionella* bacteria that were incapable of intracellular growth showed reduced virulence in guinea pigs. Therefore, initial intracellular infection and multiplication does appear to be necessary to initiate the disease process.

The mechanism of intracellular survival is less clear. Macrophages are phagocytes that have a wide variety of means for killing ingested microorganisms. These mechanisms range from the production of reactive oxygen molecules to the synthesis of oxidizing agents such as peroxides. In addition, after a foreign microbe has been phagocytized within the membrane-bound vessel called a phagosome, a cell organelle, the lysosome, will fuse with the phagosome. Contained within the lysosome are large numbers of digestive enzymes that proceed to digest the target. Under normal circumstances, foreign microbes are ingested and digested, eliminating the threat of infection.

Somehow, *Legionella* bacteria evade these defense mechanisms. Different strains of *Legionella* bacteria appear to have evolved a variety of mechanisms for survival. In particular, there are two types of molecules, a phosphatase and a cytotoxin, whose presence is correlated with intracellular survival. Both appear to act by preventing the phagocytes

from producing potentially lethal oxidation molecules such as hydrogen peroxide.

Another virulence factor that appears to be important for infectivity is a surface protein known as the macrophage infectivity potentiator, or MIP. The MIP proteins are apparently unique to *Legionella* bacteria; mutants that lack the MIP gene are significantly less virulent than wild-type strains. The MIP protein appears to be necessary for the internalization of *Legionella* bacteria by the macrophage, and for survival against the array of bacteriocidal activities.

A variety of other mechanisms may also exist that allow *Legionella* bacteria to escape the killing mechanisms of the macrophage. For example, in addition to the phosphatase, which removes phosphate molecules from host proteins or lipids, *Legionella* bacteria also produce protein kinases, which can add phosphate molecules to host cell proteins. In this manner, *Legionella* bacteria can potentially regulate the metabolism of the cells in which they find themselves by adding or subtracting phosphates from various sites or metabolic pathways.

Though a precise sequence of events that leads to the development of Legionnaires' disease remains to be worked out, certain steps appear to be necessary. Following the inhalation of a *Legionella* aerosol, probably from a contaminated water source, the organism lodges in the alveoli of the lung. Resident macrophages phagocytize the microbe, resulting in its internalization. Through a variety of virulence factors, *Legionella* survives, and multiplies within the macrophage. Death of the host cells along with the concomitant infiltration of other white cells results in the inflammation and lung damage recognized as Legionnaires' disease.

Treatment and Therapy

Despite the hysteria associated with the Philadelphia outbreak of Legionnaires' disease and the difficulty associated with the initial isolation of the etiological agent, there is nothing particularly unusual about the organism. The *Legionella* bacterium is a small, thin microbe some two to ten micrometers in length, about the size of most average bacteria. Because of its characteristic staining pattern, it is classified as a gram-negative organism. This results from the molecular nature of its cell wall, which has a high lipopolysaccharide (LPS) content.

Since legionellosis can resemble other forms of pneumonia, improper diagnosis can be a problem. Though the prognosis of the disease is generally favorable with early intervention, improper or delayed treatment can prove fatal. In general, legionellosis is suspected in a patient with a progressive pneumonia for which other organisms do not appear to be a factor.

Legionnaires' disease pneumonia may be diagnosed microbiologically in a number of ways. The simplest, most rapid, and least costly test is the urinary antigen. The test is available only for *L. pneumophila* serogroup 1, but this organism is responsible for 80 percent of pneumonia cases. The antigen is detectable in the urine three days after symptoms begin and persists for several weeks. Expectorated sputum or secretions obtained through bronchoscopy may be stained and cultured. A special stain to visualize the bacteria through the microscope, called direct fluorescent antibody (DFA), is very specific but not very sensitive, because it requires large numbers of bacteria to be positive and such number are usually present only in the most severe cases. The definitive diagnostic method is culture using BCYE media. The bacteria grow slowly and colonies become visible only after three to five days of incubation. Lastly, blood (sera) may be collected as acute and convalescent specimens. A fourfold rise in the antibody titer is considered diagnostic. A single specimen of high titer (1:128 dilution or higher) is considered presumptive, but not definitive, evidence of infection. In the case of Pontiac fever, serologic testing is the usual method for diagnosis.

There are several aspects of the clinical significance of the gram-negative character of the organism, one of which is that this type of bacteria responds poorly to penicillin or penicillin derivatives. This serves to limit the type of antimicrobial therapy available for treatment of severe cases of legionellosis. Other antibiotics exist, of course, that exhibit antibacterial characteristics similar to those of penicillin—for example, the cephalosporins. And, indeed, penicillin derivatives have been used to treat at least some types of gram-negative infections. Legionellosis patients did not respond well, however, to treatment with any of these agents. It was subsequently found that the basis for the resistance by *Legionella* bacteria to these antibiotics lay in a type of extracellular enzyme produced by these bacteria—a beta-lactamase.

The lack of pharmacologic activity associated with the penicillins, the cephalosporins, and certain other antibiotics is thus easy to explain. The activity of these antibiotics is associated with the presence of a structure in the molecule called a beta-lactam ring. The beta-lactamase produced by the *Legionella* bacterium causes a break in the ring, rendering the antibiotic harmless to the microbe, and thus useless as a form of treatment. Such resistance has become increasingly common among bacteria, since the genes encoding the beta-lactamase are passed from organism to organism.

Fortunately, other antibiotics did prove to be useful in the treatment of legionellosis. To a certain extent, the determination of the antibiotics of choice was fortuitous. During the Philadelphia outbreak, the nature of the illness was unknown. The primary assumption was that an infectious agent was at fault, but determination of the nature of that agent lay months beyond the extent of the epidemic. Therefore, as would be true in the treatment of any illness of unknown origin, various treatments were carried out. Two antibiotics in particular proved to be useful: erythromycin and rifampin. Erythromycin, which specifically inhibits bacterial protein synthesis, has continued to be useful. Though long-term use can result in liver damage and some individuals are hypersensitive to the drug, the intravenous administration of erythromycin remains the treatment of choice for legionellosis. Rifampin is used on occasion in association with other methods of treatment, but the high frequency of

bacterial resistance to the drug precludes its use as a treatment of first choice.

Since the virulent properties of the *Legionella* bacterium depend on its intracellular presence in the macrophage, those antimicrobial agents that exhibit intracellular penetration would be expected to be most effective. Erythromycin fits this requirement, as do a number of other antibiotics. Newer antibiotics with intracellular activity have replaced erythromycin and rifampin as first choices for treatment of Legionnaires' disease pneumonia. Azithromycin, a macrolide antibiotic similar to erythromycin, yields higher intracellular levels than erythromycin and has proven to be more effective. Alternative monotherapy can be employed using one of the new respiratory fluoroquinolones such as levofloxacin or moxifloxacin. The quinolones are used for those who have undergone transplantation, as they do not interfere with the immunosuppressive drugs used in these patients.

Other aspects of treatment center on maintaining the comfort of the individual. This may include the use of analgesics for relief of pain. Pontiac fever is a self-limiting disease and requires only such symptomatic therapy.

Prevention of the disease is obviously preferable to dealing with the sequelae of infection. Epidemiological studies have demonstrated that the *Legionella* bacterium is a common soil organism that is often found in bodies of water contaminated by soil. The organism has been found in lakes and pond water, and it can survive for long periods in unchlorinated tap water. In fact, contaminated water appears to have been the source of infection for most outbreaks of the illness. Problems have often been associated with cooling towers, evaporative condensers, and other water supplies found with air-conditioning units of buildings. Infectious aerosols may be generated from these units, allowing for a respiratory route of infection. Though the disease is thus spread in an airborne manner, there is no evidence that it can be passed from person to person.

The epidemiological evidence for the disease supports an airborne hypothesis. Most outbreaks have occurred in regions of soil disruption, such as that occurring during construction. Subsequent isolation of *Legionella* bacteria from the cooling towers confirmed such contamination. Though the air-conditioning unit of the Bellevue-Stratford Hotel in Philadelphia was replaced prior to isolation of the organism, the assumption is that the unit was contaminated. The outbreaks of the disease during the summer, when air-conditioning use has peaked, are consistent with the role of air-conditioning units in the spread of *Legionella* bacteria.

The method by which the *Legionella* bacterium survives in the environment has not been completely determined. The organism is somewhat resistant both to chlorine treatment and to heat as high as 65 degrees Celsius. It appears to grow best in the presence of biological factors secreted by other microflora in the environment; growth stimulation may also be enhanced by the presence of physical factors such as sediment, silicone, and rubber compounds. Its ability to survive, and indeed be transmitted, may also be related to its tendency to penetrate and multiply intracellularly within environmental protozoa or amoeba.

Prevention of disease transmission must take into account these problems. Contamination of water supplies must be minimized. The resistance of the *Legionella* bacterium to standard methods of decontamination has made the process more difficult, and methods of choice remain controversial. Chlorination at relatively high levels remains the preferred method, with subsequent treatment at lower concentrations over the long term. The disadvantages of this method include the cost of constant treatment and the eventual corrosion of the units. Continuous or intermittent heating of the water has also proved effective in decontamination.

Perspective and Prospects

Prior to August, 1976, Legionnaires' disease was unknown. From July 21 to 24 of that year, however, the Pennsylvania branch of the American Legion held its annual convention at the Bellevue-Stratford Hotel in Philadelphia. Some four thousand delegates and their families attended the festivities. Following the convention, as delegates returned to their homes, a mysterious illness began to appear among the attendees. A total of 149 conventioneers and 72 others became ill. Characterized by a severe respiratory infection that progressed into pneumonia, and high fever, the illness proved fatal to 34 of the victims.

By August, it became clear to the Pennsylvania Department of Health that an epidemic was at hand. The cause of the outbreak was not clear, and rumors began to circulate. At various times, the news media explained the outbreak as a Communist plot against former military men, a Central Intelligence Agency test gone awry, and even an infectious agent arriving from space. The truth was less dramatic. By the beginning of 1977, David Fraser, Joseph McDade, and their colleagues from the Centers for Disease Control isolated the etiological agent: a bacterium subsequently named *Legionella pneumophila*.

With the isolation and identification of the organism, it became possible to explain earlier outbreaks of unusual illness. For example, during July and August of 1965, an outbreak of pneumonia at a chronic-care facility at St. Elizabeth's Hospital in Washington, D.C., resulted in eighty-one cases and fourteen deaths. An outbreak among personnel at the Oakland County Health Department in Pontiac, Michigan, during July and August of 1968 of a disease that was subsequently called Pontiac fever was also traced to the same organism. In this case, however, though 144 persons were affected, none died. In fact, illness associated with the *Legionella* bacterium has been traced as far back as 1947. The 1976 outbreak was not new; it was merely the first time that medical personnel were able to isolate the organism that caused the disease.

The precise prevalence of the *Legionella* bacterium remains murky, but it is clearly more common than was at first realized. In 2013, the Centers for Disease Control and Prevention reported that between 8,000 and 18,000 people with the disease are hospitalized annually in the United States. These figures do not include cases that are undetected or unreported, however, so the actual number of cases might be much higher.

Despite the public's fear of the disease, in most instances it probably remains a mild respiratory infection, resembling nothing worse than a bad cold. Most cases remain undetected. A study of hospitalized community-acquired pneumonia patients conducted in Ohio showed that about 3 percent of cases were caused by *Legionella*. Estimates have suggested that as many as 25,000 persons in the United States develop infection. Based on seroconversions—the production of anti-*Legionella* antibody in the sera of persons—it has been estimated that more than 20 percent of the population of Michigan has been exposed to the organism. There is no reason to doubt that the same situation exists in many other states. In addition to sporadic cases, outbreaks continue to occur around the world. The most recent large outbreak was in Toronto. A colonized air-conditioning cooling tower atop the Seven Oaks Home for the Aged caused illness in 127 residents and workers, and 20 of the residents died.

The basis for the difference in severity between Legionnaires' disease and Pontiac fever is also unclear. There is no obvious difference between the two diseases that accounts for the differences in virulence. It also remains to be seen whether *Legionella* bacteria are associated with other illnesses.

The final lesson of Legionnaires' disease is as subtle as its initial appearance. Humans exist in an environment replete with infectious agents. Despite the battery of modern methods of treatment for illness, there always remains the potential for new outbreaks of previously unknown disease.

—*Richard Adler, Ph.D.;*
updated by H. Bradford Hawley, M.D.

See also Antibiotics; Bacterial infections; Epidemics and pandemics; Epidemiology; Lungs; Pneumonia; Pulmonary diseases; Pulmonary medicine; Pulmonary medicine, pediatric; Respiration.

For Further Information:

Alan, Rick. "Legionnaires' Disease." *Health Library*, March 15, 2013.

Brock, Thomas D., ed. *Microorganisms: From Smallpox to Lyme Disease*. New York: W. H. Freeman, 1990.

Centers for Disease Control and Prevention. "*Legionella* (Legionnaires' Disease and Pontiac Fever). *Centers for Disease Control and Prevention*, February 5, 2013.

Dowling, John N., Asish K. Saha, and Robert H. Glew. "Virulence Factors of the Family *Legionellaceae*." *Microbiological Reviews* 56 (March 1, 1992): 32.

Frank, Steven A. *Immunology and Evolution of Infectious Disease*. Princeton, N.J.: Princeton University Press, 2002.

Gorbach, Sherwood L., John G. Bartlett, and Neil R. Blacklow, eds. *Infectious Diseases*. 3d ed. Philadelphia: W. B. Saunders, 2004.

Hoebe, Christian J. P. A., and Jacob L. Kool. "Control of *Legionella* in Drinking-Water Systems." *The Lancet* 355, no. 9221 (June 17, 2000): 2093–2094.

Kasper, Dennis L., et al., eds. *Harrison's Principles of Internal Medicine*. 16th ed. New York: McGraw-Hill, 2005.

MedlinePlus. "Legionnaires' Disease." *MedlinePlus*, May 16, 2013.

Ryan, Kenneth J., and C. George Ray, eds. *Sherris Medical Microbiology: An Introduction to Infectious Diseases*. 4th ed. New York: McGraw-Hill, 2004.

Springston, John. "*Legionella* Bacteria in Building Environments." *Occupational Hazards* 61, no. 8 (August, 1999): 51–56.

LEISHMANIASIS
Disease/Disorder

Also known as: Kala-azar

Anatomy or system affected: Bones, immune system, lymphatic system, skin

Specialties and related fields: Family medicine, public health

Definition: A complex of diseases caused by protozoan parasites of the genus *Leishmania*.

Causes and Symptoms

Leishmaniasis, also known as kala-azar in its visceral form, is a parasitic disease that strikes nearly two million persons each year. At least 350 million persons, from more than ninety subtropical and tropical countries around the world, are at risk of contracting the disease. Leishmaniasis has received more attention among United States" medical authorities because of the risk of contracting the disease faced by US military personnel in Southwest Asia, including Iraq, and Central Asia, including Afghanistan. Leishmaniasis may be a contributor to the complex of illnesses called Gulf War syndrome reported from veterans of the first Persian Gulf War in 1991.

Leishmaniasis is caused by any of more than twenty species of the protozoan parasite *Leishmania*. They are transmitted by the bites of sandflies, small bloodsucking insects in the subfamily Phlebotominae. The parasite may also be transmitted by blood transfusion, sharing of needles by intravenous drug abusers, and other modes not requiring the bite of a sandfly. Humans are one of many mammalian hosts of these parasites. Infection can cause skin disease, called cutaneous leishmaniasis. *Leishmania* can also affect the mucous membranes, frequently resulting in ulcers, or cause systemic disease called visceral leishmaniasis, which is often fatal. Infection in children is usually sudden, with symptoms including vomiting, fever, abdominal discomfort, diarrhea, weight loss, and cough. Adults suffer from similar symptoms, but they may be accompanied by nonspecific symptoms such as fatigue, weakness, and loss of appetite. The skin may become darker, dry, and flaky, and the hair may begin to thin. Other signs include an enlarged spleen, liver, and lymph nodes.

Diagnosis is based on demonstration of the organism in spleen pulp, lymph nodes, liver, or peripheral blood. Species of *Leishmania* cannot be differentiated morphologically. They are distinguished on the basis of the disease produced, the host and its immune response, and geographical distribution.

Treatment and Therapy

Compounds containing the mineral antimony are the principal medications used to treat leishmaniasis. These compounds include meglumine antimonite and sodium stibogluconate. When these drugs are ineffective, other antiprotozoan medications may be utilized, including amphotericin B, pentamidine, flagyl, and allopurinol. With mucocutaneous leishmaniasis, plastic surgery may be needed to correct the disfigurement caused by destructive facial lesions. Removal of the spleen may be required in

---

Information on Leishmaniasis

Causes: Transmission of protozoa through sandflies

Symptoms: Skin infection and ulcers; vomiting, fever, abdominal discomfort, diarrhea, weight loss, and cough in children; also fatigue, weakness, and appetite loss in adults; darkening, dry, and flaky skin; thinning hair; enlargement of spleen, liver, and lymph nodes

Duration: Often chronic

Treatments: Medications containing the mineral antimony (meglumine antimonite, stibogluconate) and sometimes amphotericin B, pentamidine, flagyl, and allopurinol; plastic surgery to correct disfigurement; removal of spleen

---

drug-resistant cases of visceral leishmaniasis. Relapse may occur and infection may persist despite treatment.

Perspective and Prospects

Cases of infection by *Leishmania* have been reported on all the continents except Australia. In the Americas, *Leishmania* can be found from southern Mexico into the South American continent. The disease is widespread in the tropics. In the United States, cases have been reported in dogs, cats, and humans in Texas, Ohio, and Oklahoma.

The prognosis for leishmaniasis is quite variable and depends on the specific strain of infecting protozoan, as well as on the individual patient's immune system response to infection. Cure rates are high with antimony compounds. There are no preventive vaccines. Preventing sandfly bites is the most immediate form of protection. Insect repellent, appropriate clothing, screening of windows, and fine mesh netting will reduce exposure.

—*Jason A. Hubbart, M.S.;*
updated by David M. Lawrence

See also Bites and stings; Insect-borne diseases; Parasitic diseases; Protozoan diseases; Tropical medicine; Ulcers.

For Further Information:
Centers for Disease Control and Prevention. "Parasites—Leishmaniasis." *Centers for Disease Control and Prevention,* January 10, 2013.

Chang, K.-P., and R. S. Bray, eds. *Leishmaniasis.* New York: Elsevier, 1985.

Hide, G., et al. *Trypanosomiasis and Leishmaniasis: Biology and Control.* Wallingford, Oxon, England: CAB International, 1997.

Lane, R. P. "Sandflies (Phlebotominae)." In *Medical Insects and Arachnids,* edited by Richard P. Lane and Roger W. Crosskey. New York: Chapman & Hall, 1993.

MedlinePlus. "Leishmaniasis." *MedlinePlus,* April 5, 2013.

Raghunath, D., and R. Nayak, eds. *Trends and Research in Leishmaniasis: With Particular Reference to Kala Azar.* New York: Tata/McGraw-Hill, 2005.

Ryan, Kenneth J., and C. George Ray, eds. *Sherris Medical Microbiology: An Introduction to Infectious Diseases.* 4th ed. New York: McGraw-Hill, 2004.

LEPROSY

Disease/Disorder

Also known as: Hansen's disease

Anatomy or system affected: Immune system, nerves, nervous system, skin

Specialties and related fields: Bacteriology, epidemiology, immunology, internal medicine, public health

Definition: A bacterial infection that affects skin and nerves, causing symptoms ranging from mild numbness to gross disfiguration.

Key terms:

acid-fast: the ability of a bacterium to retain a pink stain in the presence of a mixture of acid and alcohol

antibody: a protein found in the blood and produced by the immune system in response to bodily contact with an antigen

antigen: a foreign substance (such as a bacterium, toxin, or virus) to which the body makes an immune response

Bacillus Calmette-Guérin (BCG): a vaccine for tuberculosis made from a harmless strain of *Mycobacterium bovis*

bacterium: microscopic single-celled organism that multiplies by simple division; bacteria are found everywhere; most are beneficial, but a few species cause disease

cellular immune response: the reaction of the body that produces active white blood cells that can destroy antigens associated with other body cells

humoral immune response: the reaction of the body that produces antibodies that can destroy antigens present in body fluids

hypersensitivity: an overreaction by the immune system to the presence of certain antigens; this overreaction often results in some damage to the person as well as the antigen

immune response: the working of the body's immune system to prevent or combat an infectious disease

Causes and Symptoms

Leprosy, also known as Hansen's disease, is caused by the bacterium *Mycobacterium leprae (M. leprae)*. Humans are the only natural host for this bacterium; it can be found only in leprosy victims. Most people who are exposed to this bacterium are unaffected by it; in the remainder, the bacterium grows inside skin and nerve cells, causing a wide range of symptoms that depend upon the person's immune response to the growth of the bacteria.

M. leprae is an obligate intracellular parasite, which means that it can grow only inside other cells. *M. leprae* has a unique waxy coating that helps to protect it while it is growing inside human skin and nerve cells. The bacterium grows very slowly, dividing once every twelve days, whereas the average bacterium will divide every twenty to sixty minutes. *M. leprae* grows best at temperatures slightly below body temperature (37 degrees Celsius). The leprosy bacterium is the only bacterium known to destroy peripheral nerve tissue (nerves that are not a part of the central nervous system) and will also destroy skin and mucous membranes. This bacterium is closely related to the bacterium that causes tuberculo-

---

sis: *Mycobacterium tuberculosis.*

Leprosy is not very contagious. Several attempts to infect human volunteers with the bacteria have been unsuccessful. It is believed that acquiring leprosy from an infected person requires prolonged intimate contact with that person, such as living in the same house for a long time. Although the precise mode of transmission of *M. leprae* bacteria is unclear, it is highly probable that the bacteria are transferred from the nasal or respiratory secretions of the victim to the nasal passages or a skin wound of the recipient.

Once inside a person, *M. leprae* will grow and reproduce inside skin and nerve cells and destroy tissue. The exact mechanism of tissue destruction is not understood, but it probably results from a combination of nerve damage, massive accumulation of bacteria, and immunological reactions. Because the bacteria grow so slowly, the length of time from infection to appearance of the symptoms (the incubation period) is quite long. The average incubation period is two to seven years, but incubation can range from three months to forty years. Since the bacteria prefer temperatures slightly lower than normal body temperature, symptoms appear first in the cooler parts of the body, such as the hands, fingers, feet, face, nose, and earlobes. In severe cases, symptoms also appear in the eyes and the respiratory tract.

The symptoms associated with leprosy can range from very mild to quite severe, and the symptoms that a person gets depend heavily on that person's ability to mount a cellular immune response against the bacteria. In a normal infection, the human body is capable of defending itself through two processes of the immune system; the humoral immune response and the cellular immune response. The humoral response produces chemicals called antibodies that can attack and destroy infectious agents that are present in body fluids such as the blood. The cellular response produces white blood cells that can destroy infectious agents that are associated with cells. Since *M. leprae* hides and grows inside human cells, a cellular response is the only type of immune response that can be of any help in fighting the infection. The ability to generate a cellular immune response against *M. leprae* is dependent upon the genetic makeup and overall health of the victim, as well as the number of infecting bacteria and their ability to invade the body and cause disease. A quick and strong cellular response by a person infected with *M. leprae* will result in no symptoms or in the mild form of the disease: tuberculoid leprosy. A slow or weak cellular response by a person exposed to leprosy may result in the more severe form of the disease: lepromatous leprosy.

Only one in two hundred people exposed to leprosy will get some form of the disease. The earliest symptom is a slightly bleached, flat lesion several centimeters in diameter that is usually found on the upper body or on the arms or legs. About three-fourths of all patients with an early solitary lesion heal spontaneously; the rest progress to tuberculoid or lepromatous leprosy or to one of the many forms that fall between these two extremes.

Tuberculoid leprosy is characterized by flat skin lesions five to twenty centimeters in diameter. The lesions are lighter in color than the surrounding skin and are sometimes surrounded by nodules (lumps). The lesions contain only a few bacteria, and they, along with the surrounding tissue, are numb. These lesions are caused by a hypersensitive cellular immune response to the bacteria in the nerves and skin. In an attempt to destroy the bacteria, the immune system overreacts, and some of the surrounding nerve and skin tissue is damaged while the bacteria are being killed. This causes the areas of the skin to lose pigment as well as sensation. Often, tuberculoid leprosy patients can experience more extensive physical damage if the numbness around the lesions leads to accidental loss of digits, skin, and so forth. Leprosy victims may burn and cut themselves unknowingly, since they have no feeling in certain areas of their bodies.

In lepromatous leprosy, the bacteria grow unchecked because of the weak cellular immune response. Often, there are more than 100 million bacterial cells present per square centimeter of tissue. These bacteria cause the formation of tumorlike growths called lepromas as well as tissue destruction of the skin and mucous membranes. Also, the presence of so many bacteria causes large numbers of antibacterial antibodies to be produced, but these antibodies are of no benefit in fighting off the infection. Instead, they can contribute to the formation of lesions and tissue damage both internally and on the skin through a process called immune complex hypersensitivity. This is a process whereby the large number of antibodies bind to the large number of bacteria in the body and form immune complexes. These complexes can be deposited in various parts of the body and trigger a chemical reaction that destroys the surrounding tissue. The large number of bacteria puts pressure on the nerves and destroys nerve tissue, which causes loss of sensation and tissue death.

The initial symptoms of lepromatous leprosy are skin lesions that can be spread out or nodular and are found on the cooler parts of the body, such as the inside of the nose, the front part of the eye, the face, the earlobes, the hands, and the feet. Often, the victim loses all facial features because the nodules enlarge the face, and the eyebrows and nose deteriorate, giving the victim a characteristic lionlike appearance. Severe lepromatous leprosy erodes bones; thus, fingers and toes become needlelike, pits form in the skull, nasal bones are destroyed, and teeth fall out. Also, the limbs become twisted and the hands become clawed. The destruction of the nerves leads to the inability to move the hands or feet, deformity of the feet, and chronic ulceration of the limbs. In addition, as is the case with tuberculoid leprosy, destruction of the small peripheral nerves leads to self-inflicted trauma and secondary infection (infection by another bacterium or virus). As the disease progresses, the growth of bacteria in the respiratory tract causes larynx problems and difficult breathing. Deterioration of the optic nerve leads to blindness. Bacteria can invade the bloodstream and spread infection throughout the whole body except the central nervous system. Death associated with leprosy usually results from respiratory obstruction, kidney failure, or secondary infection.

Treatment and Therapy

A physician can tell whether a person has leprosy by looking for characteristic symptoms (light-colored and numb lesions, nodules, and so forth) and by determining whether the patient may have been exposed to someone with leprosy. In addition, samples of scrapings from skin lesions, nasal secretions, fluid from nodules, or other tissue secretions can be examined for the presence of *M. leprae*. Samples are treated with a procedure called the acid-fast technique. Because of *M. leprae*'s waxy coating, these bacteria retain a pink stain after being washed in an acid-alcohol mixture, whereas all other bacteria

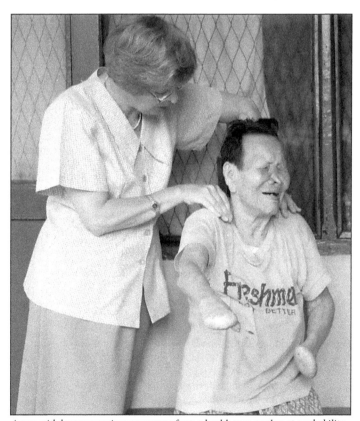

A man with leprosy receives a massage from a health care worker at a rehabilitation center in Thailand. (AP/Wide World Photos)

lose the pink stain. Therefore, pink, rod-shaped bacteria observed in samples treated with the acid-fast technique indicate the presence of *M. leprae*. It is easy to find the acid-fast *M. leprae* in lepromatous leprosy patients because they have so many bacteria in their lesions, but the bacteria are more difficult to find in the lesions of tuberculoid leprosy patients.

The lepromin test was originally developed to be used as a diagnostic tool for leprosy, in the same way that the tuberculin test is used as a diagnostic tool for tuberculosis. Lepromin, which is heat-killed *M. leprae* taken from nodules, is injected under the skin in the lepromin test. Two reactions are possible: an early reaction that appears twenty-four to forty-eight hours later and a late reaction that appears three to four weeks later. In both reactions, a hard red lump at the injection site indicates a positive lepromin test. This test is not specific for leprosy, however, because a person who has been exposed to *M. leprae*, *M. tuberculosis*, or the tuberculosis vaccine, Bacillus Calmette-Guérin (BCG), will show a positive early reaction. Even though this test is not useful as a diagnostic tool, it is useful in determining whether a patient has a strong or a weak cellular immune response to *M. leprae*. Tuberculoid leprosy patients show both the early and late reactions, while lepromatous leprosy patients show no reaction at all.

Leprosy can be treated with antibiotics. The antibiotic dapsone began to be used on a wide scale in the treatment of leprosy in 1950. Since that time, however, many dapsone-resistant strains of *M. leprae* have appeared. This means that, for some victims, this drug is no longer helpful in fighting the disease. In 1981, in response to the problem of dapsone-resistant strains, the World Health Organization (WHO) recommended a multidrug regimen for leprosy victims. For lepromatous leprosy patients, dapsone, rifampin, and clofazimine are recommended, whereas tuberculoid leprosy patients need take only dapsone and rifampin. For patients who are intolerant of one or more of the standard antibiotics or who suffer from infections unresponsive to these medications, doxycycline and moxifloxacin are additional antibiotics that have been found to be effective. Treatment is expected to continue until skin smears are free from acid-fast bacteria, which can last from two years up to the lifetime of the patient. Since 1989, the US recommendations for tuberculoid leprosy are six months of rifampin and dapsone daily, then dapsone alone for three years. For lepromatous leprosy, the recommendation is to use rifampin and dapsone daily for three years, then dapsone only for the rest of the person's life.

Often, antibiotics are given to family members of leprosy patients to prevent them from contracting the disease. Antibiotic therapy can make a leprosy victim noncontagious, stop the progress of the disease, and in some cases cause a reversal of some of the symptoms. Until treatment is complete, however, it is recommended that patients sleep in separate bedrooms, use their own linens and utensils, and not live in a house with children. Thus, leprosy victims can lead nearly normal lives without fear of infecting others in the community.

The best ways to keep from getting leprosy are to avoid exposure to leprosy bacteria and to receive antibiotic therapy

following exposure. It should be possible to control and, eventually, eliminate leprosy. If every case of leprosy were treated, the disease could not spread and the bacteria would die out with the last leprosy victim. Progress in this direction is slow, however, because of ignorance, superstition, poverty, and overpopulation in areas with many leprosy cases. The first strategy in controlling leprosy is to treat all leprosy cases with antibiotics. As of 1991, about 50 percent of all leprosy victims were not receiving drug therapy. Second, the early detection and rigid isolation of lepromatous leprosy patients are important, as is preventive antibiotic therapy for individuals in close contact with those patients. Finally, even in the early twenty-first century, too many countries lack adequate basic health resources, and too many patients disabled by leprosy are not receiving adequate care. The development of a vaccine for leprosy would aid control efforts.

A global effort for the production of a vaccine for leprosy is being made under the auspices of WHO. The first problem with vaccine development is that, until recently, it was not possible to grow *M. leprae* bacteria outside a leprosy victim; therefore, not much is known about the nature of the bacteria. Even though this bacterium was the first to be associated with a disease, it cannot be grown on an artificial laboratory medium, whereas nearly all other bacteria known can be grown artificially. It was not until 1960 that scientists at the Centers for Disease Control (CDC) discovered that the bacterium could be grown in the footpads of mice. Finally, in 1969, scientists at the National Hansen's Disease Center in Carville, Louisiana, found that the bacteria would grow in the tissues of the nine-banded armadillo. Several potential vaccines for leprosy have been tested since that time. One vaccine being tested is BCG, a live bacterial vaccine of the bacteria *Mycobacterium bovis*, which is a close relative of *M. leprae*. In four major trials with BCG, a range of 20 to 80 percent protection from leprosy was obtained. It is not known why there was such a wide variation in results. Recent strategies for vaccine development include making a modified BCG that contains *M. leprae* cell wall antigens. It is more advantageous to use BCG than *M. leprae* in a vaccine because BCG is much easier to grow. In addition, scientists are trying to find a way to grow *M. leprae* artificially so that larger quantities will be available to be used for a vaccine. In 1999, WHO set up a strategic plan titled "The Final Push Toward Leprosy Elimination: 2000–2005" and the Global Alliance for the Elimination of Leprosy was launched.

Perspective and Prospects

Leprosy is one of the oldest known diseases. References to leprosy are contained in Indian writings that are more than three thousand years old. The Bible refers to leprosy and the isolation of lepers, although the term refers to other skin diseases as well. The examination of ancient skeletons has provided insights into how leprosy spread in past centuries. Early evidence suggests that the disease was highly contagious and that leprosy was widespread in Europe during the Middle Ages. Leprosy was so prevalent, in fact, that both governments and churches moved to deal with the problem.

At that time, the cause of leprosy was unknown, and the disease was generally believed to be a punishment for some personal sin. Lepers were treated as outcasts and required to shout "unclean." They were required to wear gloves and distinctive clothes and carry a bell or clapper to warn people of their approach. They were forbidden to drink from public fountains, speak loudly, eat with healthy people, or attend church. Some lepers were even pronounced legally dead, burned at the stake, or buried alive. Later, they were isolated in asylums called leprosaria, and at one time about nineteen thousand leprosaria existed—mostly in France.

There was a sharp decrease in the number of leprosy cases in the sixteenth century. Several factors may have contributed to this decline, including the isolation of lepers, a better diet, warmer clothes, the plague epidemic, and the increase in tuberculosis, which may have provided resistance to leprosy. Leprosy is no longer as deadly or contagious as it once was, yet the stigma attached to this disease has remained. In an effort to alleviate the social stigma, the Fifth International Congress on Leprosy in 1948 banned the use of the word *leper* and encouraged the use of the term *Hansen's disease* instead of *leprosy. M. leprae*, the causative agent of leprosy, was first identified in the tissues of leprosy patients by the Norwegian physician Gerhard Armauer Hansen in 1873—hence the alternate name, Hansen's disease. Today, victims of leprosy are referred to as Hansenites or Hansenotic.

From the 1960s to the 1980s, estimates of the number of cases of leprosy worldwide ranged from 10 to 12 million. In 2001, at the Fifty-fourth World Health Assembly, it was announced that the global prevalence of leprosy had fallen to below one case per ten thousand by the end of 2000 and health experts believed that eliminating leprosy in all countries was an attainable goal by the year 2005. More than 600,000 new cases of leprosy were reported globally in 2002. A new combination of drugs known as multidrug therapy has been used to treat and completely cure patients. The drugs are donated free through foundations, and since these donations began in 2000, millions of the "blister packs," each of which provides one month's treatment to one patient, have been shipped. By 2008, some countries had achieved elimination, but leprosy remained endemic in others. And, although the disease has not been completely eliminated, its incidence has decreased dramatically. The World Health Organization reports that, worldwide, about 219,000 new cases of leprosy were reported in 2011 and that about 182,000 people had the disease in early 2012.

Leprosy is prevalent in tropical areas such as Africa, Southeast Asia, and South America. In the United States, most cases occur in Hawaii and small parts of Texas, California, Louisiana, and Florida. The number of new cases in the United States annually—mostly from foreign-born immigrants from leprosy-prone areas—has been very low in the last several decades.

—*Vicki J. Isola, Ph.D.*

See also Antibiotics; Bacterial infections; Immune system; Immunology; Necrosis; Nervous system; Numbness and tingling; Thalidomide; Tropical medicine; Tuberculosis; World Health Organization.

For Further Information:

Biddle, Wayne. *A Field Guide to Germs*. 3d ed. New York: Anchor Books, 2010.

Bloom, B. R. "Learning from Leprosy: A Perspective on Immunology and the Third World." *Journal of Immunology* 137 (July, 1986): i–x.

Donnelly, Karen J. *Leprosy (Hansen's Disease)*. New York: Rosen, 2002.

Frank, Steven A. *Immunology and Evolution of Infectious Disease*. Princeton, N.J.: Princeton University Press, 2002.

Hastings, Robert C., ed. *Leprosy*. 2d ed. New York: Churchill Livingstone, 1994.

Joklik, Wolfgang K., et al., eds. *Zinsser Microbiology*. 20th ed. Norwalk, Conn.: Appleton and Lange, 1997.

Mandell, Gerald L., John E. Bennett, and Raphael Dolin, eds. *Mandell, Douglas, and Bennett's Principles and Practice of Infectious Diseases*. 7th ed. New York: Churchill Livingstone/Elsevier, 2010.

National Institutes of Health. "Leprosy (Hansen's Disease)." *NIH: National Institute of Allergy and Infectious Disease*, April 25, 2011.

Sehgal, Alfica. *Leprosy*. Philadelphia: Chelsea House, 2006.

Vorvick, Linda. "Leprosy." *MedlinePlus*, March 22, 2013.

Weedon, David. *Weedon's Skin Pathology*. 3d ed. New York: Churchill Livingstone/Elsevier, 2010.

World Health Organization. "Leprosy." *World Health Organization Media Centre*, September 2012.

LEPTIN

Biology

Anatomy or system affected: All

Specialties and related fields: Biochemistry, cardiology, endocrinology, genetics, gynecology, nutrition

Definition: A protein hormone involved in regulation of food intake and obesity, with secondary effects on immunity, reproduction, and heart disease.

Structure and Functions

Leptin (from the Greek *leptos*, meaning "thin") is a protein hormone with important effects in regulating body weight, metabolism, and reproductive function. It is the product of the obese (*ob*) gene occurring on chromosome 7 in the human. Leptin is produced primarily by adipocytes (white fat cells). It is also produced by cells of the epithelium of the stomach and in the placenta. It appears that as adipocytes increase in size because of accumulation of triglycerides (fat molecules), they synthesize more and more leptin. However, the mechanism by which leptin production is controlled is largely unknown. It is likely that a number of hormones modulate leptin output, including corticosteroids and insulin.

Disorders and Diseases

At first leptin was assumed to be simply a signaling molecule involved in limiting food intake and increasing energy expenditure. Studies published as early as 1994 showed a remarkable difference in weight gain in mice deficient in leptin (mice with a nonfunctional ob gene). Daily injections of leptin into these animals resulted in a reduction of food intake within a few days and a 50 percent decrease in body weight within a month.

More recent studies in the human have not been as promising. It appears that leptin's effects on body weight are mediated through effects on hypothalamic (brain) centers that control feeding behavior and hunger, body temperature, and energy expenditure. If leptin levels are low, appetite is stimulated and use of energy limited. If leptin levels are high, appetite is reduced and energy use stimulated. The most likely target of leptin in the hypothalamus is inhibition of neuropeptide Y, a potent stimulator of food intake. However, this inhibition alone could not account for the effects seen, and studies looking at other hormones are under way.

Leptin also affects reproductive function in humans. It has long been known that very low body fat in human females is associated with cessation of menstrual cycles, and the onset of puberty is known to correlate with body composition (fat levels) as well as age. Several studies have suggested that leptin stimulates hypothalamic output of gonadotropin-releasing hormone, which in turn causes increases of luteinizing and follicle-stimulating hormones from the anterior pituitary gland. These hormones stimulate the onset of puberty. Prepubertal mice treated with leptin become thin and reach reproductive maturity earlier than control mice. One report has also indicated that humans with mutations in the *ob* gene that prevent them from producing leptin not only become obese but also fail to achieve puberty.

Leptin has been identified in placental tissues; newborn babies show higher levels than those found in their mothers. Leptin has also been found in human breast milk. Together, these findings suggest that leptin aids in intrauterine and neonatal growth and development, as well as in regulation of neonatal food intake.

Finally, leptin appears to have a role in immune system function. Studies have suggested a role for leptin in production of white blood cells and in the control of macrophage function. Mice that lack leptin have depressed immune systems, but the mechanisms for this remain unclear.

Perspective and Prospects

Although early reports claimed that leptin could be useful in treating human obesity, clinical reports to date have not looked promising. It appears that deficiencies in leptin production are a rare cause of human obesity. However, since most obese individuals have plenty of leptin available, additional leptin will have no effect. In those individuals with a genetic deficiency of leptin, clinical use would require either daily injections of leptin or gene therapy. At this point neither of these options looks particularly promising.

—*Kerry L. Cheesman, Ph.D.*

See also Appetite loss; Endocrinology; Endocrinology, pediatric; Hormones; Immune system; Obesity; Obesity, childhood; Puberty and adolescence; Reproductive system; Weight loss and gain.

For Further Information:

Barinaga, Marcia. "Obesity: Leptin Receptor Weighs In." *Science* 271 (January 5, 1996): 29.
Castracane, V. Daniel, and Michael C. Henson, eds. *Leptin*. New York: Springer, 2011.
Goodman, H. Maurice. *Basic Medical Endocrinology*. 4th ed.
Boston: Academic Press/Elsevier, 2009.
Hemling, Rose M., and Arthur t. Belkin. *Leptin: Hormonal Functions, Dysfunctions, and Clinical Uses*. New York: Nova Science, 2011.
Henry, Helen L., and Anthony W. Norman, eds. *Encyclopedia of Hormones*. 3 vols. San Diego, Calif.: Academic Press, 2003.
Holt, Richard I. G., and Neil A. Hanley. *Essential Endocrinology and Diabetes*. 6th ed. Chichester, West Sussex: Wiley-Blackwell, 2012.
Rink, Timothy J. "In Search of a Satiety Factor." *Nature* 372 (December 1, 1994): 372–373.
Society for Neuroscience. "Food for Thought: Obesity and Addiction." *BrainFacts*, April 20, 2012.

LEPTOSPIROSIS
Disease/Disorder

Also known as: Weil's disease

Anatomy or system affected: Blood vessels, brain, eyes, kidneys, liver, lungs, lymphatic system, nervous system, spleen, urinary system

Specialties and related fields: Bacteriology, epidemiology, internal medicine, microbiology, nephrology, occupational health, public health, pulmonary medicine, urology

Definition: A bacterial infection acquired from domestic animals and wildlife. Humans become infected through contact with animal urine or water and soil contaminated with animal urine. Potentially fatal complications arise from infection of the kidneys, liver, lungs, brain, and heart.

Key terms:

antibiotics: drugs that inhibit or kill bacteria and are used to treat bacterial infections

relapse: the recurrence of signs and symptoms after they have subsided or ceased

self-limiting: a disease that resolves without medical intervention

septicemia: blood-borne bacterial infection

vaccine: a substance, usually injected, that stimulates the immune system to protect the body against a specific infectious disease

zoonotic: an infection of animals that can be transmitted to humans

Causes and Symptoms

Leptospirosis is the most widespread zoonotic infectious disease. Zoonotic diseases are animal infections transmitted to humans but not normally transmitted among humans. Leptospirosis is caused by corkscrew-shaped bacteria in the genus Leptospira. The bacteria are transmitted by contact with urine from infected animals, especially rodents, raccoons, opossum, and domestic cattle, sheep, goats, and bison. Dogs and cats can transmit leptospirosis. Humans also acquire leptospirosis by contact with soil and water or by drinking water contaminated with urine or excretions from infected animals. The bacteria survive in soil or water a few weeks to several months, depending on climate conditions. Found throughout the world, leptospirosis is most common in temperate and tropical regions, where warm and wet conditions permit the bacteria to persist in water and soil.

The risk for leptospirosis is highest among farmers, miners, veterinarians, sewer workers, slaughterhouse and fisheries workers, and the military. Floods and hurricanes cause outbreaks of leptospirosis among residents and rescue workers. Swimming and wading expose people to infection, because the bacteria contact wounds and eyes, are aspirated (drawn into the lungs), or swallowed. Water sports such as rafting and kayaking are associated with leptospirosis. Campers acquire leptospirosis by bathing in or drinking contaminated water.

Contact with exposed skin, especially open wounds, offers entry for the bacteria. Other entry points include the mucous membranes, including the eye surface and inner linings of the nose, mouth, and lungs. Bacteria enter cells at these sites and migrate into the lymphatic system, a network of veins that filter and carry excess tissue fluid back to the blood vessels. The bacteria enter the bloodstream and move to nearly all organs of the body. Leptospira invade endothelial cells, those cells that line the inside of blood vessels, where they reproduce, damage vessels, and cause many of the characteristic signs and symptoms of leptospirosis. At first, the immune system controls the infection. However, many bacteria reside within cells and in organs that cannot be reached by the immune system. For this reason, the bacteria reproduce in the kidney, brain, and the eye. Bacteria can survive in these organs for sixty days after infection, where they damage blood vessels and cause the serious complications of leptospirosis.

Signs and symptoms of disease begin two to twenty-six days after infection. The disease may last a few days to one month or more. Two stages of disease are recognized. The first stage is called septicemic. Septicemia refers to the presence of blood-borne bacteria. Symptoms develop suddenly and include fever and chills, headache and muscle ache, vomiting and diarrhea. Some individuals develop red eyes, a rash, abdominal pain, jaundice (yellow eyes and skin), and a dry cough. Some of these symptoms suggest influenza (the flu). For that reason, some cases go unrecognized, undiagnosed, and untreated. In addition, leptospirosis can be asymptomatic, which means the infection triggers no symptoms. The septicemic stage often ends in recovery, sometimes in relapse (the return of symptoms after apparent recovery).

The second, less common stage of leptospirosis is called immune-delayed or Weil's disease. In Weil's disease, the immune system's response to the infection harms tissue in several organs. Kidney and liver damage lead to kidney and liver failure. Damage to blood vessels in the lungs causes pulmonary hemorrhage, uncontrolled bleeding in the lungs. Weil's disease is also characterized by meningitis, inflammation of the membranes covering the brain and spinal cord. Leptospirosis causes death in about one to five percent of cases, and most fatalities are related to respiratory complications.

Infected animals often show no sign of disease. However, they are able to pass the bacteria in urine for many months after infection. Dogs might have general symptoms such as a fever, vomiting, loss of appetite, weakness, and muscle pain, and may seem depressed and inactive. Infected, mature, apparently healthy dogs may not be able to have puppies.

Rapid diagnosis and treatment are important for full recovery without the serious complications associated with Weil's disease. Diagnosis is based on a physical exam, signs and symptoms, and a history of exposure to the bacteria. A blood test can detect antibodies to the bacteria. Antibodies are substances produced by white blood cells, and they defend the body by binding to specific infectious agents. Because the body makes specific antibodies in response to specific infectious agents, the presence of antibodies to leptospirosis bacteria are a reliable sign of infection. However, in leptospirosis antibodies are not detectable until two weeks after symptoms begin. Blood cultures allow the bacteria to be grown in the laboratory. A blood culture places a blood sample in nutrients that encourage the growth of bacteria so that they can be studied and identified. Blood culture also takes weeks to months. For these reasons, treatment usually does not wait for antibody or culture results; treatment often begins if signs, symptoms, and history are consistent with leptospirosis.

Treatment and Therapy

Fortunately many cases of leptospirosis turn out well and can be described as self-limiting infections. This type of infection produces disease until the immune system eliminates the bacteria. However, it is not possible to predict whether a mild infection will become severe. Therefore, leptospirosis is treated promptly to reduce the risk for severe disease. Leptospirosis is treated with antibiotics, which are drugs that kill bacteria, and usually penicillin, doxycycline, or third-generation cephalosporins are used. Given the presence of typical signs and symptoms, and a history of exposure to the bacteria, treatment with antibiotics begins as soon as possible. Treatment may last one week or more, depending on the severity of the disease. Severe infections are treated with antibiotics given intravenously, a method that delivers medicine through a needle inserted in a vein. Because intravenous drugs travel in blood throughout the body, antibiotics can reach bacteria in nearly every infected organ. Hospitalization is required to receive intravenous drugs.

Severe disease that affects the liver, kidney, heart, and lungs is treated with supportive therapy in addition to intravenous antibiotics. Supportive therapy does not cure disease, but it provides relief and reduces signs and symptoms of disease. In some cases, supportive therapy temporarily replaces the functions of a diseased organ. For example, severe leptospirosis causes inflammation and bleeding in the lungs, impairing their function. A ventilator assists the lungs if breathing becomes difficult or inefficient. A ventilator is a machine that pumps oxygen and air through a tube directly into a patient's windpipe. Severe leptospirosis damages the kidney's blood vessels and causes inflammation, which impairs the kidney's filtering function. This results in dangerously high levels of toxins in the blood. Dialysis removes these toxins from the blood by removing a patient's blood and passing it through a dialysis machine before returning it to the body. The dialysis machine pumps blood along a membrane, across which the toxins diffuse and are removed. While dialysis does not reverse kidney damage, it temporarily restores the blood's normal chemistry. Without dialysis, kidney failure is fatal. Meningitis is treated with anti-inflammatory drugs in addition to antibiotics. Anti-inflammatory drugs reduce swelling of the membranes around the brain and spinal cord.

Recreational and occupational exposure to leptospirosis can be prevented. Workers exposed to infected animals or contaminated soil or water should wear protective clothing such as gloves, shoes, and eye protection. Swimming or wading in contaminated water should be avoided. Water from natural sources should be treated, filtered, or boiled before consumption. In the community and at home, rodent populations should be controlled because infected rats excrete the bacteria in their urine. People who expect to be exposed, such as military personnel, can take antibiotics to prevent infection. No effective vaccine is available for humans. In the United States, a vaccine is used to prevent infection in livestock.

Perspective and Prospects

Leptospirosis was first described in 1886 as infectious jaundice by Adolf Weil. The signs and symptoms Weil described are now known to be associated with liver disease that occurs in the advanced, severe stage of leptospirosis. For this reason, the severe stage of leptospirosis is called Weil's disease or Weil's syndrome. Historical records report earlier outbreaks of infectious jaundice. An epidemic affected American Indians in Massachusetts during the seventeenth century. In 1812, infectious jaundice broke out among Napolean's armies during the siege of Cairo, Egypt. Infectious jaundice also affected soldiers in the trenches during World War I. Although an infectious cause was suspected, Leptospira was not linked to Weil's disease for many years. The bacteria were first described in kidney autopsy tissue in 1907. In 1908, Leptospira was shown to be the cause of Weil's disease. In 1917 scientists discovered that rats are a natural host for Leptospira and that they transmit the bacteria in urine.

Leptospirosis is uncommon in the United States, affecting about one hundred people each year. Half of all cases occur in Hawaii. Scientists are studying the role of feral pigs, wild boars, and rats in the transmission of leptospirosis in Hawaii. Livestock vaccination and occupational precautions have significantly reduced the number of cases in the United States, and most outbreaks are associated with floods, hurricanes, recreational water sports, and rat infestations. Hurricane Mitch hit Nicaragua in 1995, and associated flooding caused an outbreak of leptospirosis. In 1998, Ecuador and Peru experienced outbreaks following especially heavy rainfall. In 2006 several people became sick following an "ecochallenge" sporting event in Canada, in which contestants race through challenging terrain and water courses. Fortunately, although widespread, the disease continues to be mild in ninety percent of cases.

Scientists have uncovered some changes in the occurrence and transmission of leptospirosis. Occupational exposure on farms and in the agricultural industry seems to be increasing, while recreational exposure may be declining. In addition, one species of Leptospira may be losing its ability to survive and be transmitted in water, which suggests that the risk of acquiring leptospirosis from urine-contaminated water might decline. Computer models suggest that global warming will enable the infection to spread beyond the current temperate and tropical zones.

—*Mark Zelman, Ph.D.*

See also Bacteriology; Environmental health; Immunology; Immunopathology; Microbiology; Nephrology, Neurology; Ophthalmology; Vascular medicine

For Further Information:

Katz, Alan R., Arlene E. Buchholz, Kialani Hinson, Sarah Y. Park, and Paul V. Effle. "Leptospirosis in Hawaii, USA, 1999-2008." *Emerging Infectious Diseases* 17 (2011): 221-226.

Leggat, David. "Rowing: Rare Disease Kills Rowing Great." *The New Zealand Herald*. (October 27, 2010). This news story tells how Andy Holmes acquired leptospirosis. Holmes won Olympic gold for rowing in 1984 and 1988.

Marr, John S., and John T. Cathey. "New Hypothesis for Cause of an Epidemic among Native Americans, New England, 1616-1619." *Emerging Infectious Diseases* 2 (2010): 281-286. This study suggests that European rats probably brought leptospirosis to New England, causing an epidemic among American Indians. Previously, this epidemic was thought to be caused by plague or yellow fever.

Perez, Julie, Fabrice Brescia, Jérôme Becam, Carine Mauron, and Cyrille Goarant. "Rodent Abundance Dynamics and Leptospirosis Carriage in an Area of Hyper-Endemicity in New Caledonia." *Neglected Tropical Diseases.* 5 (2011): 1361. This article describes the role of rats in causing leptospirosis outbreaks, especially in poor urban communities.

Pommerville, Jeffrey C. *Alcamo's Fundamentals of Microbiology.* 9th ed. Sudbury, MA: Jones and Bartlett, 2011. An excellent, comprehensive college level text on the principles and practice of microbiology. Includes discussion of the fundamentals of many infectious diseases.

Professional Guide to Diseases. 10th ed. Springhouse, PA: Lippincott Williams & Wilkins, 2013. This book describes the cause, signs and symptoms, diagnosis, treatment, and prevention for human diseases.

World Health Organization. "Human Leptospirosis: Guidance for Diagnosis, Surveillance and Control." *Geneva: The World Health Organization, 2003.* This report describes the worldwide status of leptospirosis.

Lesions

Disease/Disorder

Anatomy or system affected: All

Specialties and related fields: Cardiology, dermatology, gastroenterology, general surgery, gynecology, internal medicine, nephrology, neurology, oncology, ophthalmology, otorhinolaryngology, podiatry, pulmonary medicine, urology, vascular medicine

Definition: Any tissue damaged by injury or disease.

Causes and Symptoms

"Lesion" is the general term describing any damage to tissue. Lesions result from some insult to the body, which may take many forms, including physical injury from an accident; intentional surgical incisions to treat a disorder; bacterial,

Information on Lesions

Causes: Disease, physical trauma, cancer, autoimmune action, genetic abnormality
Symptoms: Pain, reduced function
Duration: Various
Treatments: Medication, surgery

parasitic, or viral disease, such as ringworm or syphilis; stomach ulcers caused by excess acid production; an autoimmune reaction, such as arthritis; heart muscle damage during a heart attack; malformations in the circulatory system; or brain tissue damage caused by a stroke.

Because of this great variety, lesions are often classified by location and by whether they develop on their own (primary) or are related to another lesion (secondary). Primary skin lesions, for example, include cuts and scrapes, pustules, birthmarks, hives, and cancers—anything that changes the color and texture of the skin. Secondary lesions include such things as scabs, scratches from itching hives, or scars from removing or picking at a primary lesion. Most of these examples are benign, or at least more annoying than harmful. Skin cancers, on the other hand, can be deadly if left untreated.

Likewise, internal lesions vary from benign to deadly. Ulcers of the stomach or duodenum may heal on their own, but some worsen and can penetrate the bowel wall, leaking digestive fluid into the body cavity. In addition to cancerous lesions, some types are progressively dangerous, such as the scarring left by tuberculosis or the plaques of multiple sclerosis. Still others require immediate medical attention, such as an aneurysm in the brain or a puncture of a lung.

Treatment and Therapy

Therapy depends on the type of lesion. Topical ointments or creams, such a cortisol cream, soothe the effects of many skin lesions. Lesions caused by a specific disease clear up with the appropriate medication for the disease. Likewise, medications can clear up some internal lesions, such as the antacids or H$_2$-receptor antagonists that reduce stomach-acid production in an attempt to treat gastric ulcers.

Surgery, heat therapy, ultrasound, cautery, chemotherapy, radiation, and laser surgery are used to remove lesions or destroy damaged tissue. Classic examples include removing a polyp in the colon with a cauterizing snare, using radiation to destroy cancer cells and shrink a tumor, performing surgery to cut out a melanoma, and suturing a wound.

—*Roger Smith, Ph.D.*

See also Aneurysms; Birthmarks; Cancer; Dermatology; Dermatopathology; Disease; Electrocauterization; Grafts and grafting; Heart attack; Hives; Melanoma; Multiple sclerosis; Plastic surgery; Skin; Skin cancer; Skin disorders; Skin lesion removal; Strokes; Tuberculosis; Ulcers; Wounds.

For Further Information:

Anderson, Robin L. *Sources in the History of Medicine: The Impact of Disease and Trauma.* Upper Saddle River, N.J.: Pearson/Prentice Hall, 2006.
"Brain Lesions." *MayoClinic.com*, Oct. 25, 2011.
Beers, Mark H. *The Merck Manual of Medical Information.* New York: Pocket Books, 2003.
Feliciano, David, Kenneth Mattox, and Ernest Moore. *Trauma.* 7th ed. New York: McGraw-Hill Medical, 2013.
Habif, Thomas P., et al. *Skin Disease: Diagnosis and Treatment.* 3d ed. Philadelphia: Elsevier/Saunders, 2011.
Sompayrac, Lauren. *How Cancer Works.* Sudbury, Mass.: Jones and Bartlett, 2004.

LEUKEMIA

Disease/Disorder
Anatomy or system affected: Blood
Specialties and related fields: Hematology, internal medicine, serology, toxicology
Definition: A family of cancers that affect the blood, characterized by an increase in the number of white blood cells.
Key terms:

blast cell: an immature dividing cell

bone marrow: the tissue within bones that produces blood cells; in children, all bones have active marrow, but in adults, blood cell production occurs only in the trunk

bone marrow transplant: the removal of bone marrow from an immunologically matched individual for infusion into a patient whose bone marrow has been destroyed

chemotherapy: the use of drugs to kill rapidly growing cancer cells; this treatment will also kill some normal cells, producing undesirable side effects

granulocytes: white blood cells that generally help to fight bacterial infection; these cells are capable of passing from the blood capillaries into damaged tissues

hematopoiesis: the process by which blood cells develop in the bone marrow; this maturation is regulated by specific molecules called growth factors

immune system: the cells and organs of the body that fight infection; destruction of these cells leaves the body vulnerable to numerous diseases

lymphocytes: white blood cells that specifically target a foreign organism for destruction; the two classes of lymphocytes are B cells, which produce antibodies, and T cells, which kill infected cells

oncogenes: genes found in every cell that are capable of causing cancer if activated or mutated

Causes and Symptoms

The blood is essential for all the physiological processes of the body. It is composed of red cells called erythrocytes, white cells called leukocytes, and platelets, each of which has distinct functions. Erythrocytes, which contain hemoglobin, are essential for the transport of oxygen from the lungs to all the cells and organs of the body. Leukocytes are important for protecting the body against infection by bacteria, viruses, and other parasites. Platelets play a role in the formation of blood clots; therefore, these cells are critical in the process of wound healing. Blood cell development, or hematopoiesis, begins in the bone marrow with immature stem cells that can produce all three types of blood cells. Under the influence of

Information on Leukemia

Causes: Unclear; possibly environmental and genetic factors

Symptoms: Mild cold symptoms; fever; enlargement of lymph nodes, spleen, and liver; fatigue; paleness; weight loss; repeated infections; increased susceptibility to bleeding and bruising

Duration: Acute or chronic with recurrent episodes

Treatments: Chemotherapy, bone marrow transplantation

special molecules called growth factors, these stem cells divide rapidly and form blast cells that become one of the three blood cell types. After several further divisions, these blast cells ultimately mature into fully functional erythrocytes, leukocytes, and platelets. In a healthy individual, the number of each type of blood cell remains relatively constant. Thus, the rate of new cell production is approximately equivalent to the rate of old cell destruction and removal.

Mature leukocytes are the key players in defending the body against infection. There are three types of leukocytes: monocytes, granulocytes, and lymphocytes. In leukemia, leukocytes multiply at an increased rate, resulting in an abnormally high number of white cells, a significant proportion of which are immature cells. All forms of leukemia are characterized by this abnormally regulated growth; therefore, leukemia is a cancer, even though tumor masses do not form. The cancerous cells live longer than the normal leukocytes and accumulate first in the bone marrow and then in the blood. Since these abnormal cells crowd the bone marrow, normal hematopoiesis cannot be maintained in a person with leukemia. The patient will usually become weak as a result of the lack of oxygen-carrying red cells and susceptible to bleeding because of a lack of platelets. The abnormal leukocytes do not function effectively in defending the body against infection, and they prevent normal leukocytes from developing; therefore, the patient is immunologically compromised. In addition, once the abnormal cells accumulate in the blood, they may hinder the functioning of other organs, such as the liver, kidney, lungs, and spleen.

It has become clear that leukemia, which was first recognized in 1845, is actually a pathology that comprises more than one disease. Leukemia has been divided into four main types, based on the type of leukocyte that is affected and the maturity of the leukocytes observed in the blood and the bone marrow. Both lymphocytes and granulocytes can be affected. When the cells are mainly immature blasts, the leukemia is termed acute, and when the cells are mostly mature, the leukemia is termed chronic. Therefore, the four types of leukemia are acute lymphocytic (ALL), acute granulocytic (AGL), chronic lymphocytic (CLL), and chronic granulocytic (CGL). The granulocytic leukemias are also known as myologenous leukemias (AML, CML) or nonlymphoid leukemias (ANLL, CNLL). These are the main types of leukemia, although there are additional rarer forms. These four forms of leukemia account for about 5 percent of the cancer

cases in the United States. The incidence of acute and chronic forms is approximately equivalent, but specific forms are more common at different stages of life. The major form in children is ALL; after puberty, there is a higher incidence of AGL. The chronic forms of leukemia occur in the adult population after the fourth or fifth decade of life, and men are twice as likely to be affected as women.

The causes of leukemia are still not completely understood, but scientists have put together many pieces of the puzzle. It is known that several environmental factors increase the risk of developing leukemia. Among these are exposure to radiation, chemicals such as chloramphenicol and benzene, and possibly viruses. In addition, there is a significant genetic component to this disease. Siblings of patients with leukemia have a higher risk of developing the disease, and chromosomal changes have been found in the cells of most patients, although they disappear when the patient is in remission. For example, the genetic basis of certain forms of CML is an exchange of information (translocation) between chromosome 22 and chromosome 9; the shortened chromosome 22 is referred to as the Philadelphia chromosome. These different "causes" can be linked by understanding how oncogenes function. Every person, as part of his or her genetic makeup, has several oncogenes that are capable of causing cancer. In the healthy person, these oncogenes function in a carefully regulated manner to control cell growth. After exposure to an environmental or genetic influence that causes chromosome abnormalities, however, these oncogenes may become activated or deregulated so that uncontrolled cell growth occurs, resulting in the abnormally high number of cells seen in leukemia. The translocation associated with the Philadelphia chromosome results in abnormal expression of an oncogene encoding an enzyme that regulates cell division.

Leukemia is often difficult to diagnose in the early stages because the symptoms are similar to more common or less serious diseases. "Flulike" symptoms, sometimes accompanied by fever, may be the earliest evidence of acute leukemia; in children, the first symptoms may be less pronounced. The symptoms quickly become more pronounced as white cells accumulate in the lymph nodes, spleen, and liver, causing these organs to become enlarged. Fatigue, paleness, weight loss, repeated infections, and an increased susceptibility to bleeding and bruising are associated with leukemia. As the disease progresses, the fatigue and bleeding increase, various skin disorders develop, and the joints become painfully swollen. If untreated, the afflicted individual will die within a few months. Chronic leukemia has a more gradual progression and may be present for years before symptoms develop. When symptoms are present, they may be vague feelings of fatigue, fever, or loss of energy. There may be enlarged lymph nodes in the neck and armpits and a feeling of fullness in the abdomen because of an increase in the size of the spleen as much as tenfold. Loss of appetite and sweating at night may be initial symptoms. Often, chronic leukemia eventually leads to a syndrome resembling acute leukemia, which is ultimately fatal.

If these symptoms are present, a doctor will diagnose the

presence of leukemia in two stages. First, blood will be drawn and a blood smear will be analyzed microscopically. This may indicate that there are fewer erythrocytes, leukocytes, and platelets than normal, and abnormal cells may be visible. A blood smear, however, may show only slight abnormalities, and the number of leukemic cells in the blood may not correspond to the extent of the disease in the bone marrow. This requires that the bone marrow itself be examined by means of a bone marrow biopsy. Bone marrow tissue can be obtained by inserting a needle into a bone such as the hip and aspirating a small sample of cells. This bone marrow biopsy, which is done under local anesthetic on an outpatient basis, is the definitive test for leukemia. Visual examination of the marrow usually reveals the presence of many abnormal cells, and this finding is often confirmed with biochemical and immunological tests. After a positive diagnosis, a doctor will also examine the cerebrospinal fluid to see if leukemic cells have invaded the central nervous system.

Treatment and Therapy

The treatment and life expectancy for leukemic patients varies significantly for each of the four types of leukemia. Treatment is designed to destroy all the abnormal cells and produce a complete remission, which is defined as the phase of recovery when the symptoms of the disease disappear and no abnormal cells can be observed in the blood or bone marrow. Unfortunately, a complete remission may be only temporary, since a small number of abnormal cells may still exist even though they are not observed under the microscope. These can, with time, multiply and repopulate the marrow, causing a relapse of the disease. With repeated relapses, the response to therapy becomes poorer and the durations of the remissions that follow become shorter. It is generally believed, however, that a remission that lasts five years in ALL, eight years in AGL, or twelve years in CGL may be permanent. Therefore, the goal of leukemia research is to develop ways to prolong remission.

By the time acute leukemia has been diagnosed, abnormal cells have often spread throughout the bone marrow and into several organs; therefore, surgery and radiation are usually not effective. Treatment programs include chemotherapy or bone marrow transplants or both.

Chemotherapy is usually divided into several phases. In the first, or induction, phase, combinations of drugs are given to destroy all detectable abnormal cells and therefore induce a clinical remission. Vincristine, methotrexate, 6-mercaptopurine, L-asparaginase, daunorubicin, prednisone, and cytosine arabinoside are among the drugs that are used. Combinations that selectively kill more leukemic cells than they do normal cells are available for the treatment of ALL; however, in AGL no selective agents are available, resulting in the destruction of equal numbers of diseased and healthy cells. An alternative strategy does not rely on destroying the abnormal cells but instead seeks to induce immature leukemic cells to develop further. Once the cells are mature, they will no longer divide and will eventually die in the same way that a normal leukocyte does. Drugs such as cytarabine and

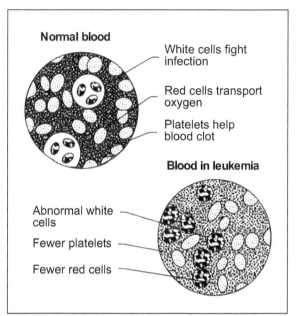

Leukemia is characterized by a high number of white blood cells and a reduced number of red blood cells and platelets; also, abnormal cells may be visible.

retinoic acid have been tested, but the results are inconclusive.

Although the induction phase achieves clinical remission in more than 80 percent of patients, a second phase, called consolidation therapy, is essential to prevent relapse. Different combinations of anticancer drugs are used to kill any remaining cancer cells that were resistant to the drugs in the induction phase. Once the patient is in remission, higher doses of chemotherapy can be tolerated, and sometimes additional intensive treatments are given to reduce further the number of leukemic cells so that they will be unable to repopulate the tissues. During these phases of treatment, patients must be hospitalized. The destruction of their normal leukocytes along with the leukemic cells makes them very susceptible to infection. Their low numbers of surviving erythrocytes and platelets increase the probability of internal bleeding, and transfusions are often necessary. The dosages of chemotherapeutic agents must be carefully calculated to kill as many leukemic cells as possible without destroying so many normal cells that they cannot repopulate the marrow. In general, children handle intensive chemotherapy better than adults.

Following the induction and consolidation phases, maintenance therapy is sometimes used. In ALL, maintenance therapy is given for two to three years; however, its benefit in other forms of leukemia is a matter of controversy.

A second form of therapy is sometimes indicated for patients who have not responded to chemotherapy or are likely to relapse. Bone marrow transplantation has been increasingly used in leukemic patients to replace diseased marrow with normally functioning stem cells. In this procedure, the patient is treated with intensive chemotherapy and whole-body irradiation to destroy all leukemic and normal cells. Then a small amount of marrow from a normal donor is infused. The donor can be the patient himself, if the marrow was removed during a previous remission, or an immunologically matched donor, who is usually a sibling. If a sibling is not available, it may be possible to find a matched donor from the National Marrow Donor Program, which has on file approximately ten million donors. Marrow is removed from the donor, broken up into small pieces, and given to the patient intravenously. The stem cells from the transplanted marrow circulate in the blood, enter the bones, and multiply. The first signs that the transplant is functioning normally occur in two to four weeks as the numbers of circulating granulocytes and platelets in the patient's blood increase. Eventually, in a successful transplant, the bone marrow cavity will be repopulated with normal cells.

Bone marrow transplantation is a dangerous procedure that requires highly trained caregivers. During this process, the patient is completely vulnerable to infection, since there is no functional immune system. The patient is placed in an isolation unit with special food-handling procedures. There is little chance that the patient will reject the transplanted marrow, because the immune system of the patient is suppressed. A larger problem remains, however, because it is possible for immune cells that existed in the donor's marrow to reject the tissues and organs of the patient. This graft-versus-host disease (GVHD) affects between 50 and 70 percent of bone marrow transplant patients. Even though the donor is immunologically matched, the match is not perfect, and the recently transplanted cells regard the cells in their new host as a "foreign" threat. Twenty percent of the patients who develop GVHD will die; therefore, drugs such as cyclophosphamide and cyclosporine, which suppress the immune system, are usually given to minimize this response. GVHD is not a problem if the donor is the patient. In 2012, the drug Prochymal was approved for use in children with GVHD; it was the stem-cell drug approved for usage. Since the availability of matching bone marrow cells is exceeded by the need, recent studies have involved the testing of hematopoietic umbilical cord cells from unrelated donors. The incidence of relapse as well as GVHD was similar to that when using matched bone marrow cells, suggesting that cord blood cells have the potential to serve as an alternative to conventional transplants.

Aggressive chemotherapy and bone marrow transplantation have dramatically increased the number of long-lasting remissions. For those who survive the therapy, it appears that, in ALL, approximately 40 percent of adults may be cured of the leukemia. The outlook for permanent remission is 10 to 20 percent in AGL and 65 percent for CGL patients. Statistics for chronic lymphocytic leukemia have been difficult to predict, because individual cases that have been similarly treated have had very different outcomes. The average lifespan after a diagnosis of CLL is three to four years; however, some patients live longer than fifteen years.

Perspective and Prospects

As the number of deaths from infectious disease has decreased, cancer has become the second most common cause of disease-related death. It is estimated that one of three people in the United States will develop a form of cancer and that the disease will kill one of five people. The search for causes and treatments of various cancers is perhaps the most active area of biological research today. Multiple lines of experimentation are being pursued, and significant advances have been made.

Leukemia is one of the cancers that scientists understand fairly well, but many unanswered questions remain. Leukemia research can be divided into two broad approaches. In the first, the researcher seeks to modify and improve the current methods for treatment: chemotherapy and bone marrow transplantation. In the second, an effort is being made to understand more about the disease itself, with the hope that completely different strategies for treatment might present themselves.

The risks involved in current therapy for leukemia have been discussed in the previous section. Treatment schedules, individually designed for each patient, will add to the understanding of how other physiological characteristics affect treatment outcome. Significant advances in reducing the risk of GVHD are likely to come quickly. In marrow transplants in which the donor is the patient, research is in progress to improve ways to screen out abnormal cells, even if they are present at very low levels, before they are infused back into the patient. In addition, for transplants in which the donor is not the patient, techniques that remove the harmful components of the bone marrow are being developed. Bone marrow cells can be partially purified, resulting in an enriched population of stem cells. Administering these to the leukemic patient should greatly reduce the risk of GVHD. Since bone marrow can be stored easily, the day may come when healthy people will store a bone marrow stem cell sample in case they contract a disease that would require a transplant.

Basic research in leukemia focuses on a simple question, "Why are leukemic cells different from normal cells?" This question is asked from a variety of perspectives in the fields of immunology, cell biology, and genetics. Immunologists are looking for markers on the surfaces of leukemic cells that would distinguish them from their normal counterparts. If such markers are found, it should be possible to target leukemic cells for destruction by using monoclonal antibodies attached to drugs. These "smart drugs" would be able to home in on the diseased cells, leaving normal cells untouched or only slightly affected. This would be a great advance for leukemia treatment, since much of the risk for the leukemic patient following chemotherapy or bone marrow transplant involves susceptibility to infection because the normal immune cells have been destroyed. Similarly, it may be possible to "teach" the patient's immune system to destroy abnormal cells that it had previously ignored. Similar forms of immunotherapy have shown promise in treating forms of cancer such as melanoma.

Cell biologists are seeking to understand the normal

hematopoietic process so that they can determine which steps of the process go awry in leukemia. Some of the growth factors involved in hematopoiesis have been identified, but it appears that the process is quite complex, and as yet scientists do not have a clear picture of normal hematopoiesis. When the understanding of the normal process becomes more complete, it may be possible to localize the defect in a leukemic patient and provide the missing growth factors. This might allow abnormal immature cells to complete the developmental process and relieve the symptoms of disease.

Geneticists are studying the chromosomal changes that underlie the onset of leukemia. As the oncogenes that are involved are identified, the reasons for their activation will also be determined. Once the effects of these genetic abnormalities are understood, it may be possible to intervene by genetically engineering stem cells so that they can develop normally.

These areas of research will likely converge to provide the leukemia treatments of the future. Leukemia is a cancer for which there is already a significant cure rate. It is not unreasonable to expect that this rate will approach 100 percent in the near future.

—*Katherine B. Frederich, Ph.D.;*
updated by Richard Adler, Ph.D.

See also Blood and blood disorders; Bone marrow transplantation; Cancer; Carcinogens; Chemotherapy; Malignancy and metastasis; Oncology; Radiation sickness; Stem cells.

For Further Information:

Bellenir, Karen, ed. *Cancer Sourcebook: Basic Consumer Health Information About Major Forms and Stages of Cancer.* 6th ed. Detroit, Mich.: Omnigraphics, 2012.

Dollinger, Malin, et al. *Everyone's Guide to Cancer Therapy.* 5th ed. Kansas City, Mo.: Andrews McMeel, 2008.

Eyre, Harmon J., Dianne Partie Lange, and Lois B. Morris. *Informed Decisions: The Complete Book of Cancer Diagnosis, Treatment, and Recovery.* 2d ed. Atlanta: American Cancer Society, 2002.

Goldman, John, and Junia Melo. "Chronic Myeloid Leukemia: Advances in Biology and New Approaches to Treatment." *New England Journal of Medicine* 349, no. 15 (October 9, 2003): 1451–64.

Henderson Edward S., T. A. Lister, and M. F. Greaves. *Leukemia.* 7th ed. Philadelphia: Saunders, 2002.

Keene, Nancy. *Childhood Leukemia: A Guide for Families, Friends and Caregivers.* 4th ed. Sebastopol, Calif.: O'Reilly, 2010.

Kimball, Chad T. *Childhood Diseases and Disorders Sourcebook: Basic Consumer Health Information About Medical Problems Often Encountered in Pre-adolescent Children.* Detroit, Mich.: Omnigraphics, 2003.

Leukemia and Lymphoma Society of America. http://www.leukemia.org.

Rennie, Ed. *Beginning of the End of My Life.* Philadelphia: Xlibris, 2005.

Wapner, Jessica, and Robert A. Weinberg. *The Philadelphia Chromosome: A Mutant Gene and the Quest to Cure Cancer at the Genetic Level.* New York: Workman, 2013.

Westcott, Patsy. *Living with Leukemia.* Austin, Tex.: Raintree-Steck-Vaughn, 1999.

Wiernik, Peter H., et al. *Neoplastic Diseases of the Blood.* New York: Springer, 2013.

Leukodystrophy

Disease/Disorder

Anatomy or system affected: Brain, ears, eyes, muscles, nerves

Specialties and related fields: Biochemistry, family medicine, genetics, neurology, nutrition, occupational health, pediatrics, physical therapy

Definition: A group of genetic disorders characterized by progressive deterioration of the white matter (myelin sheath) of the brain.

Causes and Symptoms

Leukodystrophy is caused by a breakdown in the enzyme systems that metabolize fats (lipids) in the nerve cells. As a result, the body can no longer break down very long chain fatty acids (VLCFA), which then accumulate. This causes the substance around nerve fibers, known as the myelin sheath, to degenerate. The myelin sheath protects and insulates the axons of nerve cells, allowing them to transmit impulses between the nerve cells in the brain and other parts of the body. Loss of the myelin sheath around nerve cells short-circuits nerve impulses. As a result, the victim can experience uncontrolled muscle stiffness, paralysis, speech difficulties, memory failures, personality changes, impaired reasoning, urinary incontinence, loss of vision, and loss of hearing. These symptoms may be difficult to recognize during the early stages of the disease. Leukodystrophy usually begins in the back of the brain, eventually spreading throughout the white matter of the cerebral hemispheres and often into the spinal cord. Leukodystrophy is typically diagnosed with a blood test that is used to determine the amount of VLCFA in the body.

The myelin sheath is a complex chemical substance made from a variety of lipids. Different types of leukodystrophy affect one of the particular constituents of myelin. Specific leukodystrophies include adrenoleukodystrophy (ALD), metachromatic leukodystrophy (MLD), Zellweger syndrome, and Alexander disease. Having one type of leukodystrophy does not increase the risk of having another type.

Treatment and Therapy

The effects of leukodystrophy may be tempered through the use of various medications, dietary supplements, exercise programs, and occupational and speech therapies. For ALD, the most common form of leukodystrophy, Lorenzo's oil helps the body bring VLCFA levels back to normal. To be effective, Lorenzo's oil should be coupled with a very-low-fat diet. Lovastatin, an anticholesterol drug, does the same thing as Lorenzo's oil without the patient needing to be on a low-fat diet.

For some types of leukodystrophy, particularly MLD, bone marrow transplants have shown promise in slowing down the disease. Gene therapy is being investigated. The hope is to deliver genes to the patient that will stimulate the oligodendrocyte cells in the brain to produce myelin once again.

Information on Leukodystrophy

Causes: Enzyme defect resulting in degeneration of the myelin sheath
Symptoms: Uncontrolled muscle stiffness, paralysis, speech difficulties, memory failures, personality changes, impaired reasoning, urinary incontinence, vision loss, hearing loss
Duration: Lifelong

Perspective and Prospects

Leukodystrophy is genetically inherited. Most types show up in early childhood, although there are some late childhood forms. Public awareness of the disease was greatly enhanced by the 1992 film *Lorenzo's Oil*, the true story of Augusto and Michaela Odone seeking a cure for ALD for their five-year-old son Lorenzo. They founded the Myelin Project, a research effort that continues to seek ways for victims of leukodystrophy to produce myelin that will insulate their nerve cells.

—*Alvin K. Benson, Ph.D.*

See also Adrenoleukodystrophy; Brain; Brain damage; Brain disorders; Multiple sclerosis; Nervous system; Neuralgia, neuritis, and neuropathy; Neuroimaging; Neurology; Neurology, pediatric.

For Further Information:

Canadian Agency for Drugs and Technologies in Health. *Newborn Screening for Krabbe Leukodystrophy: A Review of the Clinical and Cost Effectiveness and Guidelines*. Ottawa, Ont.: Author, 2012.

Icon Health. *Leukodystrophy: A Medical Dictionary, Bibliography, and Annotated Research Guide to Internet References*. San Diego, Calif.: Author, 2004.

Kimball, Chad T. *Childhood Diseases and Disorders Sourcebook: Basic Consumer Health Information About Medical Problems Often Encountered in Pre-adolescent Children*. Detroit, Mich.: Omnigraphics, 2003.

Lazzarini, Robert A. *Myelin Biology and Disorders*. San Diego, Calif.: Academic Press/Elsevier, 2004.

Raymond Gerald V., et al. *Leukodystrophies*. London: Mac Keith Press for the International Child Neurology Association, 2011.

Salvati, S., ed. *A Multidisciplinary Approach to Myelin Diseases II*. New York: Plenum Press, 1994.

LICE, MITES, AND TICKS

Disease/Disorder
Anatomy or system affected: Ears, genitals, hair, skin
Specialties and related fields: Dermatology, pediatrics, public health
Definition: Parasites that live on the human body, causing severe itching, skin rashes, and sometimes more serious diseases.

Key terms:

louse (pl. *lice*): a wingless insect that sucks blood and that can be involved in transmitting diseases

mite: a very small spider that is parasitic to humans and can carry disease

molt: to shed all or part of the skin or outer covering

parasite: an organism that lives off of another organism while contributing nothing to the survival of the host

tick: a wingless insect that sucks blood and can spread disease

Causes and Symptoms

Lice, mites, and ticks are parasites that live on human beings. Two species of lice survive on human blood: body lice and crab lice. Body lice are divided into two subspecies, the head louse (*Pediculus humanus capitis*) and the body louse (*Pediculus humanus corporis*). Head lice live on the scalp among the hairs of the head. Body lice actually live in and on clothing. They move off clothes and attach themselves to human skin to feed on blood frequently during the day. It is very difficult to tell the difference between these types of lice. They are both flat, wingless, grayish in color, and very small. The body louse is about .08 to .16 inch long, slightly larger than the head louse, which measures only .04 to .08 inch. Body lice are a slightly lighter shade of gray than are head lice.

Both subspecies of body lice live by sucking blood from their victims. These insects of the order *Anoplura* have three pointed tubes on their bodies called stylets that can jab into the skin and draw out blood. When not in use, the stylets are tucked away in a pouch. Body lice begin their lives as eggs dropped into the folds of clothing by mature adult females. Head lice eggs are glued to the base of a strand of hair on top of the head. The eggs, called nits, are about one-fourth the size of a mature female. After about seven to ten days, the nits hatch into young nymphs. Because hair grows about 0.3 millimeter a day, the nits hatch about 3 millimeters away from the scalp. After the nymph emerges, it leaves behind an empty egg shell still tightly cemented to the hair. Nymphs begin sucking blood as soon as they hatch. Within nine days, the nymph molts three times before a full adult louse is formed. Adults then live about two weeks, with females laying about ten eggs every day.

Lice are passed from head to head only by direct contact. This usually happens at school, often on the playground or in the gym. Head lice have different effects on different people. Some experience only slight itching, while others are terribly irritated and develop a swollen and inflamed scalp. An itching scalp is the most obvious symptom of head lice. Nits are visible upon inspection of hair near the scalp. On girls, they are usually found behind the ears, while on boys, they are most likely to be found attached near the top of the head. Parents should be very careful in treating head lice; they too can

Information on Lice, Mites, and Ticks

Causes: Bites or exposure to diseases through parasites
Symptoms: Severe itching, rashes, development of diseases
Duration: Acute to chronic
Treatments: Insecticidal shampoos, medications, lotions

Viral Diseases Spread by Ticks	
Disease	Principal Vector
Colorado tick fever	Dermacentor andersoni
Encephalitis, Far East Russian	Ixodes persulcatus
Louping ill	Isodes ricinus

be infected. Head lice can be the transmitters of several dangerous infectious diseases, such as epidemic typhus, relapsing fever, and trench fever.

Body lice are less often found on children than are head lice. They thrive in clothing and bodies that are unclean for long periods of time. Body lice are especially troublesome and numerous on homeless people, prisoners of war, and others living in dirty conditions. (Cleanliness, however, is not a factor with head lice; they can thrive in clean or dirty hair.) Body lice have helped spread a number of contagious diseases, the most deadly of which is typhus. This disease starts with flulike symptoms, followed by a high fever and rash. During World War II, more than three million Russian prisoners of war died from louse-spread typhus. In recent years, however, typhus has been rare.

Crab lice (*Phthirus pubis*) are usually found living in pubic hair and are most likely to infect adults. Like all lice, they are very small, .083 inch in length when fully grown, but they cause great discomfort. As adults, they firmly grab pubic hair with their crablike legs (six per louse), insert their barbed tongue into the skin, and suck blood. The female lays its eggs about .08 inch from the skin. When the eggs hatch, the nymphs begin to feed and stop only while molting. Feeding causes intense itching and a rash. Rarely, but occasionally, the lice spread to the chest, eyebrows, or armpits. They can be passed on only by human carriers through direct contact. Crab lice cannot live on any other species except humans, and about 3 percent of people have them. Crab lice do not carry sexually transmitted diseases but are often associated with them.

Ticks are members of a blood-sucking family of insects called Ixodidae. Several different species suck blood from warm-blooded vertebrates, such as human beings, cows, and dogs. Common species in the United States and Canada include hard ticks and the American dog tick. Ticks have a hard, shieldlike plate on their backs called a scutum that makes them very difficult to crush. A female tick can swell up to the size of a pea when ingesting blood and can lay from four thousand to six thousand eggs within four to ten days.

The eggs hatch after about a month, and six-legged larvae, called seed ticks, emerge. A seed tick waits on the tip of a leaf of grass or other low-growing plant until a suitable animal walks by. The seed tick grabs onto its meal and, after sucking enough blood, molts into its next stage, an eight-legged nymph called a yearling tick. It finds another host, sucks more blood, and then molts one more time into an adult. After another week of feeding, adults mate, the female produces its eggs, and the three-stage cycle begins all over again.

Ticks are very good survivors: Eight-legged nymphs can live more than a year without food, while adults can go without a meal of blood for more than two years. Ticks carry many dangerous diseases, including Rocky Mountain spotted fever, Colorado tick fever, tularemia, anaplasmosis, and Lyme disease.

Mites are actually related to spiders, rather than insects. Dust mites (*Dermatophagiodes pteronyssinus*), the chief living forms found in house dust, are among the most numerous inhabitants of human environments. One study of 150 houses in Holland found mites in every one of them. Dust mites measure about .01 inch in diameter. They have eight legs, like all spiders, and are closely related to ear mites found in dogs and cats and scab mites found in sheep. House dust mites spend all of their life stages, from birth to death, in dust. There can be as many as five hundred mites in every gram of house dust. This measures out to about fourteen thousand mites per ounce of dust. They survive by eating human skin that is shed daily, scabs that fall off, and dandruff, which is about 10 percent fat and which they digest with the help of a fungus also found in house dust. Dust mites are responsible for some allergies and asthma attacks. They can also invade the skin and cause allergic reactions such as dermatitis. Although dust mites cannot penetrate the surface of the skin, they can live in ulcers, fungal infections, scabs, and other skin openings.

The scabies mite (*Sarcoptes scabei*) does burrow into the skin in search of its preferred food, skin cells and intestinal fluids. Female scabies mites are about .016 inch long, while males are only about half as big. The female lays its eggs only a few hours after mating and can lay two to three eggs a day for up to four weeks. The eggs hatch after only three to four days. The larvae often move about on the skin surface until they find a suitable space, usually between the fingers or at the bend in the knee, elbow, or wrist. The underarms, breasts, and genitals can also be invaded by these travelers. Frequently, they travel all the way down to the ankles or between the toes. Sometimes it takes up to six weeks before the pests are noticed by the person acting as their host.

Children are especially sensitive to the feces and eggs of scabies mites, which can cause an agonizing itch that is particularly irritating at night. Scabies mites are most active in the fall and winter, but they are transmissible at any time. They can be spread by shaking hands, by touching the infected areas of another person, and even by having contact with the clothes or bedsheets of the infected individual. Scabies mites do not carry any major diseases, but they do cause a good deal of itching and discomfort.

Treatment and Therapy

Treatments for lice, mites, and ticks vary according to the type and severity of infestation. The only way to protect a child against head lice is through regular inspection of the head. The hair should be combed and brushed every night; this will injure the lice, which will not be able to survive. Treatment involves an insecticidal shampoo such as Proderm, which contains malathion, or Kwell, which contains lindane or gamma benzene hexachlorine. These

Bacterial and Rickettsial Diseases Spread by Lice, Mites, and Ticks

Disease	Disease Agent	Principal Vectors
Boutonneuse fever	Rickettsia conori	Ticks: Rhipicephalus sanguineus, R. secundus, and species of Haemaphysalis, Hyalomma, Amblyomma, Boophilis, Dermacentor, and Ixodes
Q fever	Coxiella burneti	Ixodid ticks
Relapsing fever	Borrelia	Ornithodoros ticks
Rickettsialpox	Rickettsia akari	Mite: Liponyssoides sanguineus
Rocky Mountain spotted fever	Rickettsia rickettsi	Ticks: Dermacentor andersoni, D. variabilis, Amblyomma americanus, Haemaphysalis leporispalustris (rabbit-to-rabbit transmission)
Trench fever	Rickettsia quintana	Human body louse Pediculus humanus humanus
Tularemia	Francisella tularensis	Deer flies and ticks
Typhus, louse-borne	Rickettsia prowazekii	Human body louse Pediculus humanus humanus
Typhus, murine	Rickettsia mooseri	The rat louse Polyplax spinulosa and the tropical rat mite Ornthonssus bacoti are zoonotic vectors
Typhus, scrub	Rickettsia tsutsugamushi	Mites: Leptotrombidium akamushi and L. deliensis

shampoos kill both the lice and the nits. Removing lice by hand or crushing them is a difficult and usually impossible task. The force required to remove a nit from a hair is greater than most parents can provide. Crushing a louse requires direct pressure of about five hundred thousand times the weight of a louse. The crushed body of a louse can also cause infection. The best treatment for body lice is washing clothes and infected areas with soap. Soap and hot water usually kill body lice. If an infection of either head or body lice is discovered, all members of a family should be checked, and a doctor should be consulted. If a child has head lice, his or her school should always be notified. If crab lice are discovered, a physician should be contacted immediately. Pubic lice can be treated with insecticides such as pyrethrin pediculicide. Pyrethrins are available over the counter in drugstores. Stronger treatments require a prescription. Crab lice can be controlled by washing clothing and bedding and drying them in a very hot dryer.

Ticks are very difficult to remove from the body. A tick should not be pulled or yanked out because its head, filled with jagged teeth, can remain in the wound and cause an infection. Ticks have to be removed so that their mouthparts do not break off. Unattached ticks can be brushed off with a hand, but an attached tick should not be removed with bare fingers. To remove a tick, the hands should be covered with a tissue or gloves. Then, the tick is grabbed with a pair of tweezers as close to its head as possible. Gentle, steady pres-

sure is applied until the tick comes out. The tick should not be twisted or crushed until it is fully out. Body fluids from the tick can carry Lyme disease organisms, which can enter the body through broken skin. The safest way to kill the tick is to drown it in soapy water or crush it with the tweezers, avoiding contact with the hands. The site of the bite should be washed and checked carefully to see if any part of the head is still embedded. Anything that remains should be removed with tweezers, which will help prevent infection. If all parts cannot be removed, the spot should be rubbed with an antiseptic. A doctor should be consulted if the site becomes inflamed or filled with pus.

Scabies mites can be controlled by insecticidal lotions containing lindane or sulfur. The pesticide lindane is the one most commonly used for scabies mites, but it has been linked to cancer in some tests. Sulfur is preferred by most physicians because it is safer and more widely available. Sulfur requires three applications over three days, however, and frequently leaves stains on bedding and clothes. The fastest-acting miticide is permethrin. It usually requires only one application to be effective, but it is more toxic than sulfur. Scabies mites can be controlled by washing the clothing, bedding, and towels used by the infected person. If scabies mites are found, other people with whom the child has had contact should be told so that they can seek treatment, even though they might not have started to itch. Scabies mites cannot live long if detached from their hosts, usually no more than two to three days. Sealing infected clothes in a plastic bag for a week or so will also kill most of the mites.

Dust mites can be controlled by reducing their sources of food. This can be accomplished by covering mattresses in plastic, keeping pets away from beds and sleeping areas, reducing humidity in the house, and vacuuming once a week. Killing dust mites requires vacuuming with a water vacuum or one with special dust filters, washing sheets and pillowcases in hot soapy water, freezing or heating blankets, or using pesticides such as mosquito repellents containing diethyl-m-toluamide (DEET) or products containing boric acid.

Perspective and Prospects

New chemicals have proven very effective in the treatment of diseases spread by lice, mites, and ticks. Louse-spread typhus, once responsible for millions of deaths, is no longer a great danger. Improved standards of cleanliness have done much to eliminate the problem of body lice in all but the poorest populations in the United States. Unfortunately, head lice cannot be controlled simply by keeping things clean, so they continue to cause itching and scratching when contracted even by the cleanest children. Lice, mites, and ticks will always be with humans, but the diseases that these parasites spread, with a few exceptions such as Rocky Mountain spotted fever and Lyme disease, are now much less deadly because of new medicines and drug treatments.

—*Leslie V. Tischauser, Ph.D.*

See also Allergies; Asthma; Babesiosis; Bites and stings; Dermatitis; Dermatology; Dermatology, pediatric; Ehrlichiosis; Insect-borne diseases; Itching; Lyme disease; Parasitic diseases; Rashes; Rocky Mountain spotted fever; Scabies; Skin; Skin disorders; Typhus.

For Further Information:

Ashford, R. W., and W. Crewe. *The Parasites of "Homo sapiens": An Annotated Checklist of the Protozoa, Helminths, and Arthropods for Which We Are Home*. 2d ed. New York: Taylor & Francis, 2003. A comprehensive checklist of all the animals naturally parasitic in or on the human body. Each parasite includes a complete summary of characteristics.

Berenbaum, May R. *Ninety-nine Gnats, Nits, and Nibblers*. Urbana: University of Illinois Press, 1989. A scientist describes how insects affect human lives. Offers an informative description of the life cycles and habits of lice, mites, ticks, and other troublemakers.

Goddard, Jerome. *Physician's Guide to Arthropods of Medical Importance*. 4th ed. Boca Raton, Fla.: CRC Press, 2003. Nontechnical description of a wide variety of arthropods and conditions related to their stings or bites. Topics include allergy to venoms and the signs and symptoms of arthropod-borne diseases.

Olkowski, William, Sheila Daar, and Helga Olkowski. *Common-Sense Pest Control*. Newton, Conn.: Taunton Press, 1996. A very useful book by a biologist that describes the best methods of dealing with all kinds of insect problems, including lice, mites, and ticks. Offers detailed descriptions of how to remove these pests from your children and the environment safely.

Robinson, William H. *Urban Entomology: Insect and Mite Pests in the Human Environment*. London: Chapman & Hall, 1996. Discusses household pests in urban areas, including how to control them. Provides a bibliography and an index.

Service, M. W., ed. *Encyclopedia of Arthropod-Transmitted Infections of Man and Domesticated Animals*. New York: CAB International, 2001. Offers basic information related to the transmission, symptoms, treatment, and control of infections transmitted by biting midges, ticks, lice, and related organisms.

Sheorey, Harsha, John Walker, and Beverley-Ann Biggs. *Clinical Parasitology*. Melbourne, Vic.: University of Melbourne Press, 2003. Reviews global parasitic diseases and includes information regarding classification and geographical distribution of parasites, details of diagnostic tests, availability and treatment regimens of drugs, and means of obtaining uncommon drugs.

Vanderhoof-Forschner, Karen. *Everything You Need to Know About Lyme Disease and Other Tick-Borne Disorders*. 2d ed. Hoboken, N.J.: John Wiley & Sons, 2003. A consumer guide that aims to provide basic knowledge and useful insights into the prevention and management of disease.

Weedon, David. *Skin Pathology*. 3d ed. New York: Churchill Livingstone/Elsevier, 2010. Text with extensive photographs, covering tissue reaction patterns; the epidermis, dermis and subcutis; the skin in systemic and miscellaneous diseases; infections and infestations; and tumors, among other topics.

LIGAMENTS

Anatomy

Also known as: Connective tissue

Anatomy or system affected: Joints, musculoskeletal system, reproductive system

Specialties and related fields: Exercise physiology, orthopedics, osteopathic medicine, pathology, physical therapy, rheumatology, sports medicine

Definition: White fibrous connective tissue that has a supportive role by attaching to the ends of bones to form movable joints. Ligaments also provide support for internal organs such as the kidneys and the spleen.

Key terms:

articular joint: a freely moving joint consisting of the joining of two bony surfaces covered by cartilage

collagen: a protein arranged in bundles to form the fibers of tendons and ligaments

elastin: a protein that forms the main substance of yellow elastic fibers within connective tissue such as ligaments

fibroblast: a cell in connective tissue that gives rise to other cells which form binding and supportive tissue of the body

osteoarthritis: a degenerative process where components of the joints undergo thinning, resulting in loss of motion, pain, and often inflammation in the later stages

synovium: a transparent fluid secreted by the synovial membrane acting as a lubricant for many joints

Structure and Functions

Structurally, ligaments appear to be strap-like bands or round cords. They are strong yet somewhat pliable. In terms of the musculoskeletal system, they serve to stabilize the adjoining bones making up what is referred to as an articulating joint. Ligaments consist of a cellular component called fibroblasts, making up 20 percent of their total tissue volume. The remaining 80 percent of the tissue volume is outside the fibroblast cells and consists of collagen and elastin. The relative proportion of collagen to elastin varies among ligaments. The degree of stabilization also varies and depends on each particular joint, such as shoulder and ankle joint ligaments. This degree of stabilization may be one which limits the amount of movement or prevents certain movements entirely. Some ligaments surround an entire joint filled with a lubricating fluid called synovium and are termed capsular ligaments. Ligaments located outside this joint capsule are called extracapsular and provide joint stability, while ligaments located inside the capsular ligament are called intracapsular and permit much more movement of the joint.

Other locations outside the musculoskeletal system that consist of ligaments for supporting structures include the broad ligament for the uterus and Fallopian tubes, which attaches these organs to the pelvic wall. Suspensory ligaments are also found in the body supporting a variety of organs, including the eyeball and breasts.

Disorders and Diseases

Ligaments are elastic, and they gradually lengthen when under tension. The term *sprain* describes an injury to a ligament caused by forces that stretch some or all of the ligament's fibers beyond their limit. This type of ligament injury can result in some degree of rupture of some or all of the fibers. In some instances, the ligament injury includes the possibility of pulling attachments from the bones. The classification for grading ligament injuries is based on two factors, the numbers of fibers ruptured and the resulting instability of the joint involved. Ligament injuries are also classified clinically as first degree (mild), second degree (moderate), or third degree (severe).

A consequence of a stretched or ruptured ligament can be instability of the joint. Not all injured ligaments require surgery, but if surgery is needed to stabilize the joint, the torn ligament can be repaired. Instability of a joint can, over time, lead to wear to the cartilage and eventually to osteoarthritis.

Joint inflammation from trauma or other medical reasons can stiffen the joint ligaments, resulting in restricted motion. In contrast, a group of rare inherited diseases called Ehlers-Danlos syndrome can lead to abnormal collagen, resulting in loss of joint stability because of laxity in the joint capsule.

Several immune diseases can affect the ligaments of the body's joints. Rheumatoid arthritis is a chronic disease that affects the synovial membrane of the joint, which produces the joint's lubricant synovium. This fluid becomes thickened and fleshy and erodes the joint structures, including the articular ligaments.

Perspective and Prospects

The discovery of joint structures is credited to early anatomists such as Andreas Vesalius, who published *De fabrica humana* in 1543. Until this time, his contemporaries had claimed that ligaments and tendons were types of nerve units. Three centuries later, in 1858, Henry Gray's writings on dissection, *Gray's Anatomy*, described and illustrated the anatomy and function of the human body, including the role of ligaments.

Advances in orthopedic medicine and the development of sports medicine have introduced specific braces to protect major joint ligaments during athletic and nonathletic activities. In addition, the continuing development of surgical procedures for the repair of damaged ligaments can help the individual return to an optimal level of function after the ligament injury. Research is ongoing to provide information to treat and find a cure for the many pathologies that affect ligaments and associated connective tissues.

—*Jeffrey P. Larson, P.T., A.T.C.*

See also Arthritis; Bones and the skeleton; Cartilage; Connective tissue; Joints; Osteoarthritis; Sports medicine; Tendon disorders; Tendons.

For Further Information:

Hoppenfeld, Stanley. *Physical Examination of the Spine and Extremities*. Norwalk, Conn.: Appleton-Century-Crofts, 1976.

Leach, Robert E. "Sprain." *Health Library*, March 18, 2013.

Malone, T. R., T. McPoil, and A. J. Nitz. *Orthopedic and Sports Physical Therapy*. 3d ed. St. Louis: Mosby Year Books, 1997.

MedlinePlus. "Sprains and Strains." *MedlinePlus*, June 24, 2013.

Norkin C. C. *Joint Structure and Function*. 4th ed. Philadelphia: F. A. Davis, 2005.

Scuderi, Giles R. *Sports Medicine: A Comprehensive Approach*. 2d ed. Philadelphia: Mosby/Elsevier, 2005.

Gray, Henry, H. V. Carter, et. al. *Gray's Anatomy*. 15th ed. London: Bounty, 2012.

Vorvick, Linda J. "Tendon vs. Ligament." *MedlinePlus*, August 14, 2012.

LIGHT THERAPY

Treatment

Anatomy or system affected: Brain, nervous system, psychic-emotional system, skin

Specialties and related fields: Dermatology, gerontology, oncology, ophthalmology, psychiatry, psychology

Definition: A noninvasive procedure using exposure to light as the mechanism for clinical treatment.

Indications and Procedures

Light therapy, or phototherapy, treats a variety of disorders. By exposing individuals to different kinds of light (for example, monochromatic, polychromatic, ultraviolet), symptoms can often be delayed, reduced, and eradicated. Immunological, neurotransmitter, and neuroendocrine systems play key roles in response to this type of treatment.

Best known in psychiatry, light therapy serves as a treatment for seasonal affective disorder (SAD), or winter depression; bulimia nervosa; sleep disorders; and "sundowner's syndrome," the late afternoon confusion and agitation sometimes accompanying Alzheimer's disease. Shift workers can also experience difficulties related to light exposure, and light therapies may provide some relief. Reduced environmental light is a factor in the etiology, onset, or maintenance of these problems. Thus, treatment involves exposing individuals to bright, full-spectrum light for specific time periods. Duration of exposure and light intensity vary by the disorder and the individual treated.

In dermatology and oncology, light therapy treats psoriasis, skin ulcers, tumors, and esophageal cancers. The type of light and the intensities used, however, vary considerably from those applied for the treatment of psychiatric disorders.

Uses and Complications

The side effects of light therapy are best documented in psychiatry: insomnia, mania, and (less frequently) morning hot flashes have been noted. Persons with other sensitivity to light, such as those prone to migraines, may also need to exercise caution with light therapy in order to avoid undesirable effects. Careful monitoring by medical providers of the patient's response to treatment is necessary. Additionally, professionals advise morning administrations of light therapy.

Users of light therapy must also be cautioned to adhere closely to recommended doses and intensity of exposure to light. Use of light outside prescribed parameters may be damaging to the eyes.

Light therapy is not effective universally; some patients may experience no improvement. For seasonal affective disorder, evidence suggests that younger individuals whose depression involves weight gain and increased sleep may be most likely to respond to treatment. For psoriasis, complementary treatments, such as psychotherapy, may facilitate a response to treatment.

Perspective and Prospects

Light and dark cycles are a biological reality; thus, it is no surprise that light affects physical, emotional, and mental well-being. As the interest in noninvasive interventions increases, the attention given to environmental treatments such as light therapy is likely to increase as well. Recent developments in the use of light therapy for sleep and behavioral disorders are fueling clinical, research, consumer, and other business interests in this procedure. Experimentation with different frequencies or colors of light, doses, intensities, and sites on the body for the application of light are ongoing and likely to increase the diversity of uses for this type of treatment. Additionally, applications of light-based interventions in the workplace and elsewhere may prove useful in preventing disorders related to light deprivation and in helping to affect productivity, directly and indirectly.

—*Nancy A. Piotrowski, Ph.D.*

See also Alternative medicine; Alzheimer's disease; Bulimia; Chronobiology; Depression; Dermatology; Psoriasis; Psychiatry; Seasonal affective disorder; Skin disorders; Sleep; Sleep disorders.

For Further Information:

Gold, Michael H. *Photodynamic Therapy in Dermatology*. New York: Springer Science, 2011.
Goldberg, Burton, John Anderson, and Larry Trivieri, eds. *Alternative Medicine: The Definitive Guide*. 2d ed. Berkeley, Calif.: Celestial Arts, 2002.
Hyman, Jane Wegscheider. *Light Book: How Natural and Artificial Light Affects Our Health, Mood, and Behavior*. Los Angeles: J. P. Tarcher, 1990.
"Is Phototherapy Right for Your Psoriasis?" *PsoriasisNet*. American Academy of Dermatology, Jan. 2010.
Jacobs, Jennifer, ed. *The Encyclopedia of Alternative Medicine: A Complete Family Guide to Complementary Therapies*. Rev. ed. Boston: Journey Editions, 1997.
Kastner, Mark, and Hugh Burroughs. *Alternative Healing: The Complete A-Z Guide to over 160 Different Alternative Therapies*. New York: Henry Holt, 1996.
Marshall, Fiona, and Peter Cheevers. *Positive Options for Seasonal Affective Disorder*. New York: Hunter House, 2003.
Palmer, John D. *The Living Clock: The Orchestrator of Biological Rhythms*. New York: Oxford University Press, 2002.
Rosenthal, Norman E. *Winter Blues: Everything You Need to Know to Beat Seasonal Affective Disorder*. 4th ed. New York: Guilfod Press, 2013.
Safer, Diane A., and Michael Woods. "Phototherapy." *Health Library*, Nov. 26, 2012.

LIPIDS

Biology

Anatomy or system affected: Cells, gastrointestinal system

Specialties and related fields: Biochemistry, cytology, nutrition, vascular medicine

Definition: Organic compounds found in the tissues of plants and animals that serve as energy-storage molecules, function as solvents for water-insoluble vitamins, provide insulation against the loss of body heat, act as a protective cushion for vital organs, and are structural components of cell membranes.

Key terms:

alcohol: an organic compound containing a hydroxyl (-OH) group attached to a carbon atom

carboxylic acid: an organic compound that contains the carboxyl ($-CO_2H$) group

ester: the relatively non-water-soluble compound formed when an alcohol reacts with a carboxylic acid

fatty acid: an organic compound that is composed of a long hydrocarbon chain with a carboxyl group at one end

glycerol: a three-carbon alcohol that has one hydroxyl compound on each carbon atom

hydrocarbon: an organic compound composed of only hydrogen and carbon atoms that does not dissolve in water (water-insoluble)

hydrophilic: "water-loving" or "water-attracting"; a term given to molecules or regions of molecules that interact favorably with water

hydrophobic: "water-hating" or "water-repelling"; a term given to molecules or regions of molecules that do not interact favorably with water

saponification: a reaction in which a strong basic solution splits a molecule into a carboxylic acid unit and an alcohol unit

Structure and Functions

Lipids are a class of bio-organic compounds that are typically insoluble in water and relatively soluble in organic solvents such as alcohols, ethers, and hydrocarbons. Unlike the other classes of organic molecules found in biological systems (carbohydrates, proteins, and nucleic acids), lipids possess a unifying physical property—solubility behavior—rather than a unifying structural feature. Fats, oils, some vitamins and hormones, and most of the nonprotein components of cell membranes are lipids.

There are two categories of lipids—those that undergo saponification and those that are nonsaponifiable. The saponifiable lipids can be divided into simple and complex lipids. Simple lipids, which are composed of carbon, hydrogen, and oxygen, yield fatty acids and an alcohol upon saponification. Complex lipids contain one or more additional elements, such as phosphorus, nitrogen, and sulfur, yielding fatty acids, alcohol, and other compounds on saponification.

The fatty acid building blocks of saponifiable lipids may be either saturated, which means that as many hydrogen atoms as possible are attached to the carbon chain, or unsaturated, which means that at least two hydrogen atoms are missing. Saturated fatty acids are white solids at room temperature, while unsaturated ones are liquids at room temperature, because of a geometrical difference in the long carbon chains. The carbon atoms of a saturated fatty acid are arranged in a zigzag or accordion configuration. These chains are stacked on top of one another in a very orderly and efficient fashion, making it difficult to separate the chains from one another. When carbons in the chain are missing hydrogen atoms, the regular zigzag of the chain is disrupted, leading to less efficient packing, which allows the chains to be separated more easily. Saturated fatty acids have a higher melting temperature because they require more energy to separate their chains than do unsaturated fatty acids. Unsaturated fatty acids can be converted into saturated ones by adding hydrogen atoms through a process called hydrogenation.

Simple lipids can be divided into triglycerides and waxes. Waxes such as beeswax, lanolin (from lamb's wool), and carnauba wax (from a palm tree) are esters formed from an alcohol with a long carbon chain and a fatty acid. These compounds, which are solids at room temperature, serve as protective coatings. Most plant leaves are coated with a wax film to prevent attack by microorganisms and loss of water through evaporation. Animal fur and bird feathers have a wax coating. For example, the wax coating on their feathers is what allows ducks to stay afloat.

Edible fats and oils such as lard (pig fat), tallow (beef fat), corn oil, and butter are triglycerides. Triglyceride molecules are fatty acid esters in which three fatty acids (all saturated, all unsaturated, or mixed) combine with one molecule of the alcohol glycerol. Oils are triglycerides that are liquid at room temperature, while fats are solid at room temperature. The fluidity of a triglyceride is dependent on the nature of its fatty acid chains; the more unsaturated the triglyceride, the more fluid its structure. The triglycerides found in animals tend to have more saturated fatty acids than do those found in plants. Vegetable oils and fish oils are frequently polyunsaturated.

Complex lipids are classified as phospholipids or glycolipids. Structurally, phospholipids are composed of fatty acids and a phosphate group. Glycerol-based lipids called phosphoglycerides contain glycerol, two fatty acids, and a phosphate group. The phosphoglyceride structure contains a hydrophilic (polar) head, the phosphate unit, and two hydrophobic (nonpolar) fatty acid tails. The polar head can interact strongly with water, while the nonpolar tails interact strongly with organic solvents and avoid water. Egg yolks contain a large amount of the phosphoglyceride phosphatidylcholine (also called lecithin). This lipid is used to form the emulsion mayonnaise from oil and vinegar. Normally, oil and water do not mix. The hydrophobic oil forms a separate layer on top of the water. Since lecithin's structure contains both a hydrophobic and a hydrophilic region, it can attach to the water with its polar head and the oil with its nonpolar tail, preventing the two materials from separating. Lipids derived from the alcohol sphingosine are called sphingolipids. They contain one fatty acid, one long hydrocarbon chain and a phosphate group. Like the phosphoglycerides, sphingolipids have a head-and-two-tail structure. Sphingolipids are important components in the protective and insulating coating that surrounds nerves.

Glycolipids differ from phospholipids in that they possess a sugar group in place of the phosphate group. Their structure is again the polar head and dual tail arrangement in which the sugar is the hydrophilic unit. Cerebrosides, which are sphingosine-based glycolipids containing a simple sugar such as galactose or glucose, are found in large amounts in the white matter of the brain and in the myelin sheath. Gangliosides, which are found in the gray matter of the brain, in neural tissue, and in the receptor sites for neurotransmitters, contain a more complex sugar component.

Nonsaponifiable lipids do not contain esters of fatty acids as their basic structural feature. Steroids are an important class of nonsaponifiable lipids. All steroids possess an identical four-ring framework called the steroid nucleus, but they differ in the groups that are attached to their ring systems. Examples of steroids are sterols such as cholesterol, the bile acids secreted by the liver, the sex hormones, corticosteroids secreted by the adrenal cortex, and digitoxin from the digitalis plant, which is used to treat heart disease.

Lipids constitute about 50 percent of the mass of most animal cell membranes. Biological membranes control the chemical environment of the space they enclose. They are selective filters controlling what substances enter and exit the cell, since they constitute a relatively impermeable barrier against most water-soluble molecules. The three types of lipids involved are phospholipids (most abundant), glycolipids, and cholesterol. Phospholipids, when surrounded by an aqueous environment, tend to organize into a double layer of lipid molecules, a bilayer, allowing their hydrophobic tails to be buried internally and their hydrophilic heads to be exposed to the water. These phospholipids have one saturated and one unsaturated tail. Differences in tail length and saturation influence the packing efficiency of the molecules and affect the fluidity of the membrane. Short, unsaturated tails increase the fluidity of the membrane. Cholesterol is important in maintaining the mechanical stability of the lipid bilayer, thereby preventing a change from the fluid state to a rigid crystalline state. It also decreases the permeability of small water-soluble molecules.

The lipid bilayer provides the basic structure of the membrane and serves as a two-dimensional solvent for protein molecules. Protein molecules are responsible for most membrane functions; for example, they can provide receptor sites, catalyze reactions, or transport molecules across the membrane. These proteins may extend across the bilayer (transmembrane proteins) or be associated with only one face of the bilayer. Cell membranes also have carbohydrates attached to the outer face of the bilayer. These carbohydrates are bound to membrane proteins or part of a glycolipid. Typically, 2 to 10 percent of a membrane's total weight is carbohydrate. Evidence exists that cell-surface carbohydrates are used as recognition sites for chemical processes.

Lipids play an important role in health and well-being. The body acquires lipids directly from dietary lipids and indirectly by converting other nutrients into lipids. There are two fatty acids, linoleic and linolenic acids, which are called essential fatty acids. Since these fatty acids cannot be synthesized in the body in sufficient amounts, their supply must come directly from dietary sources. Fortunately, these acids are widely found in foodstuffs, so deficiency is rarely observed in adults.

About 95 percent of the lipids in foods are triglycerides, which provide 30 to 50 percent of the calories in an average diet. Triglycerides produce 4,000 calories of energy per pound, compared to the 1,800 calories per pound produced by carbohydrates or proteins. Since the triglyceride is such an efficient energy source, the body converts carbohydrates and proteins into adipose (reserve fatty) tissue for storage to be used when extra fuel is required.

While carbohydrates and proteins undergo major degradation in the stomach, triglycerides remain intact, forming large globules that float to the top of the mixture. Fats spend a longer time than other nutrients in the stomach, slowing molecular activity before continuing into the intestines. Thus, a fat-laden meal gives longer satiety than a low-fat one.

In the small intestine, bile salts split fat globules into smaller droplets, allowing enzymes called lipases to saponify the triglycerides. In some instances, the fatty acids at the two ends are removed, leaving one attached as a monoglyceride. About 97 percent of dietary triglycerides are absorbed into the bloodstream; the remainder are excreted. Although glycerol and fatty acids with short carbon chains are water-soluble enough to dissolve in the blood, the long-chain fatty acids and monoglycerides are not. These insoluble materials recombine to form new triglycerides. Since these hydrophobic triglycerides would form large globules if they were dumped directly into the blood, small triglyceride droplets are surrounded with a protective protein coat that can dissolve in water, taking the encapsulated triglyceride with it. This structure is an example of a lipoprotein.

Cholesterol is found in relatively small (milligram) quantities in foods, compared to triglycerides. Cholesterol supplies raw materials for the production of bile salts and to be used as a structural constituent of brain and nerve tissue. Since these functions are important to animals but serve no purpose in plants, cholesterol is found only in animals. Only about 50 percent of dietary cholesterol is absorbed into the blood; the rest is excreted. Much of the body's supply of cholesterol is produced in the liver. For most individuals, the amount of cholesterol synthesized in the body is larger than the amount absorbed directly from the diet.

Digested lipids released from the intestine and those synthesized in the liver compose the lipid content of the blood. The fatty acids required by the liver are obtained directly from the bloodstream or by synthesis from sources such as glucose, amino acids, and alcohol. Liver-synthesized triglycerides are incorporated into lipoprotein packages before entering the bloodstream. There are three types of lipoprotein packages that transport lipids to and from the liver. Very-low-density lipoproteins (VLDLs) transport triglycerides to tissues; low-density lipoproteins (LDLs) transport the cholesterol from the liver to other cells; and high-density lipoproteins (HDLs) transport cholesterol from other tissues to the liver for destruction.

Disorders and Diseases

Lipid consumption is an important dietary concern. Lipid deficiency is rarely observed in adults but can occur in infants who are fed nonfat formulas. Since fatty acids are essential for growth, lipid consumption should not be restricted in individuals under two years of age. Excess lipid consumption is associated with health problems such as obesity and cardiovascular disease. Although excess calories from any dietary source can lead to obesity, the body must expend less energy to store dietary fat than to store dietary carbohydrate as body fat. Thus, high-fat diets produce more body fat than do high-carbohydrate, low-fat diets.

Atherosclerosis, or "hardening of the arteries," is the leading cause of cardiovascular disease. A strong correlation exists between diets high in saturated fats and the incidence of atherosclerosis. In this condition, deposits called plaques, which have a high cholesterol content, form on artery walls. Over time, these deposits narrow the artery and decrease its elasticity, resulting in reduced blood flow. Blockages can occur, resulting in heart attack or stroke. High serum cholesterol levels (total blood cholesterol content) often result in increased plaque formation. Since dietary cholesterol is not efficiently absorbed into the bloodstream and the serum cholesterol level is largely determined by the amount of cholesterol synthesized in the liver, high serum cholesterol levels are frequently related to high saturated fat intake.

Since the measurement of the serum cholesterol level gives the total cholesterol concentration of the blood, it can be a somewhat misleading predictor of atherosclerosis risk; cholesterol is not free in blood, but is encapsulated in lipoproteins. Since the cholesterol packaged in the LDL, cholesterol that can be deposited in plaques ("bad" cholesterol), has a very different fate from that in the HDL, which is transporting cholesterol for destruction ("good" cholesterol), measuring the ratio of LDL cholesterol to HDL cholesterol has been found to be a better indicator of atherosclerosis risk. Decreasing dietary intake of cholesterol and saturated fats, increasing water-soluble fibers in the diet, removing excess body weight, and increasing the amount of aerobic exercise will all serve to improve the LDL-C/HDL-C ratio.

A number of hereditary diseases are known that result from abnormal accumulation of the complex lipids utilized in membranes. These diseases are called lipid (or lysosomal) storage diseases, or lipidoses. In normal individuals, the amount of each complex lipid present in the body is relatively constant; in other words, the rate of formation equals the rate of destruction. The lipids are broken down by enzymes that attack specific bonds in the lipid structure. Lipid storage diseases occur when a lipid-degrading enzyme is defective or absent. In these cases, the lipid synthesis proceeds normally, but the degradation is impaired, causing the lipid or a partial degradation product to accumulate, with consequences such as an enlarged liver and spleen, mental disability, blindness, and death.

Niemann-Pick, Gaucher's, and Tay-Sachs diseases are examples of lipidoses. Niemann-Pick disease is caused by a defect in an enzyme that breaks down sphingomyelin. The disease becomes apparent in infancy, causing mental retardation and death normally by age four. Gaucher's disease, a more common disease involving the accumulation of a glycolipid, produces two different syndromes. The acute cerebral form affects infants, causing severe nervous system abnormalities, retardation, and death before age one. The chronic form, which may become evident at any age, causes enlargement of the spleen, anemia, and erosion of the bones. In Tay-Sachs disease, a partially degraded lipid accumulates in the tissues of the central nervous system. Symptoms include progressive loss of vision, paralysis, and death at three or four years of age. Although Tay-Sachs disease is relatively rare (1 in 300,000 births), it has a high incidence in individuals of Eastern European Jewish descent (1 in 3,600 births). This defect is a recessive genetic trait that is found in one of every twenty-eight members of this population. For two parents who are both carriers of this trait, there is a one in four chance that their child will develop Tay-Sachs disease. Tests have been developed to detect the presence of the defective gene in the parent, and the amniotic fluid of a developing fetus can be sampled using a technique called amniocentesis to detect Tay-Sachs disease. Lipid storage diseases have no known cures; however, they can be prevented through genetic counseling.

Perspective and Prospects

The ability of a cell to discriminate in its chemical exchanges with the environment is fundamental to life. How the cell membrane accomplishes this feat has been a subject of intense biochemical research since the beginning of the twentieth century.

In 1895, Ernst Overton observed that substances that are lipid-soluble enter cells more quickly than those that are lipid-insoluble. He reasoned that the membrane must be composed of lipids. About twenty years later, chemical analysis showed that membranes also contain proteins. Irwin Langmuir prepared the first artificial membrane in 1917 by mixing a phospholipid-containing hydrocarbon solution with water. Evaporation of the hydrocarbon left a phospholipid film on the surface of the water, which showed that only the hydrophilic heads contacted the water. When the Dutch biologists E. Gorter and F. Grendel deposited the lipids from red blood cell membranes on a water surface and decreased the occupied surface area with a movable barrier, a continuous

film resulted that occupied an area approximately twice the surface area of the original red blood cells. In 1935, all these observations, along with the fact that the surfaces of artificial membranes containing only phospholipids are less water-absorbent than the surfaces of true biological membranes, were combined by Hugh Davson and James Danielli into a membrane model in which a phospholipid bilayer was sandwiched between two water-absorbent protein layers.

The technological advances of the 1950s in x-ray diffraction and electronmicroscopy allowed the structures of membranes to be probed directly. Such studies revealed that membranes are indeed composed of parallel orderly arrays of lipids, although many of the proteins are attached to one of the faces of the bilayer: The Davson-Danielli model was too simplistic. The freeze-fracture technique of preparing cells for electron microscopy has provided the most information about the nature of membrane proteins. In this technique, the two layers are separated so that the inner topography can be studied. Instead of the smooth surface predicted by the Davson-Danielli model, a cobblestone-like surface was observed that resulted from proteins penetrating into the interior of the membrane. All experimental evidence supports the fluid mosaic model for biological membranes, a model first proposed by Seymour Singer and Garth Nicholson in 1972. In this model, proteins are dispersed and embedded in a phospholipid bilayer that is in a fluid state. How membranes function was the next question to be considered.

Although most of the small molecules needed by cells cross the barrier via protein channels, some essential nutrients, such as cholesterol in its LDL package, are too large to pass through a small channel. In 1986, Michael Brown and Joseph Goldstein received the Nobel Prize for their discovery of specific protein receptors on the membranes of liver cells to which LDL molecules attach. These receptors move across the surface until they encounter a shallow indentation or pit. As the pit deepens, the membrane closes behind the LDL, forming a coating allowing transport across the hydrophobic membrane interior. The presence of insufficient numbers of these receptors causes abnormal LDL-cholesterol buildup in the blood.

Many questions remain unanswered concerning the roles of proteins and glycolipids in membranes. Membranes are involved in the movement, growth, and development of cells. How the membrane is involved in the uncontrolled multiplication and migration in cancer is one medically important question. Experiments that will answer questions about how membrane structure affects functioning should lead to the development of new medical treatments.

—*Arlene R. Courtney, Ph.D.*

See also Arteriosclerosis; Carbohydrates; Cholesterol; Digestion; Fluids and electrolytes; Food biochemistry; Gaucher's disease; Heart disease; Hypercholesterolemia; Hyperlipidemia; Metabolic disorders; Metabolic syndrome; Metabolism; Niemann-Pick disease; Nonalcoholic steatohepatitis (NASH); Obesity; Obesity, childhood; Plaque, arterial; Protein; Steroids; Tay-Sachs disease.

For Further Information:

Bettelheim, Frederick A., et al. *Introduction to General, Organic, and Biochemistry.* 10th ed. Belmont, Calif: Brooks/Cole Cengage Learning, 2013.

Bloomfield, Molly M., and Lawrence J. Stephens. *Chemistry and the Living Organism.* 6th ed. New York: John Wiley, 1996.

Brown, Michael S., and Joseph L. Goldstein. "How LDL Receptors Influence Cholesterol and Atherosclerosis." *Scientific American* 251 (November, 1984): 58–66.

Carlson, Emily. "The Big, Fat World of Lipids." *NIH National Institute of General Medical Sciences: Inside Life Science*, August 9, 2012.

Christian, Janet L., and Janet L. Greger. *Nutrition for Living.* 4th ed. Redwood City, Calif.: Benjamin/Cummings, 1994.

Cornatzer, W. E. *Role of Nutrition in Health and Disease.* Springfield, Ill.: Thomas, 1989.

MedlinePlus. "Dietary Fats." *MedlinePlus*, June 28, 2013.

National Institute of General Medical Sciences. "You Are What You Eat." *NIH National Institute of General Medical Sciences: ChemHealthWeb*, August 9, 2012.

Sikorski, ZdzisÅ‚aw E., and Anna KoÅ‚akowska, eds. *Chemical and Functional Properties of Food Lipids.* Boca Raton, Fla.: CRC Press, 2002.

Vance, Dennis E., and Jean E. Vance, eds. *Biochemistry of Lipids, Lipoproteins, and Membranes.* 5th ed. Boston: Elsevier, 2008.

LIPOSUCTION
Procedure

Anatomy or system affected: Abdomen, arms, hips, knees, legs

Specialties and related fields: General surgery, plastic surgery

Definition: The removal of fat deposits with a cannula and a suction pump in order to recontour body areas.

Key terms:

abdomen: the area of the body between the diaphragm and the pelvis; it contains the visceral organs

adipose tissue: the tissue that stores fat

cannula: a tube used to drain body fluids or to administer medications

general anesthesia: anesthesia that induces unconsciousness

local anesthesia: anesthesia that numbs the feeling in a body part; administered by injection or direct application to the skin

subcutaneous: under the skin

Indications and Procedures

The fat contained in adipose tissue makes up 15 to 20 percent of the body weights of most healthy individuals. Much adipose tissue is found inside the abdominal cavity, but significant amounts are located under the skin of the abdomen, arms, breasts, hips, knees, legs, and throat. The quantity of this subcutaneous fat at any such site is based on individual heredity, age, and eating habits. When excessive eating greatly elevates body fat, a patient becomes obese, a condition that can be life-threatening. Until recently, the sole means for decreasing fat content resulting from obesity was time-consuming dieting, which requires much patience and will power. In addition, the positive consequences of long diets can be easily obliterated if dieters begin to overeat again. Recurrent overeating is common and often followed by the rapid regaining of the fat.

Persons who have undesired, unattractive fat deposits as a result of age, heredity, or obesity may undergo cosmetic surgery, such as so-called tummy tucks, to remove them. Such major procedures, however, often remove muscle along with fat and cause considerable scarring. Liposuction is a relatively easy way to lose unattractive body fat; it also is seen as a fast way to reverse obesity and is touted as more permanent than dieting. A cannula connected to a suction pump is inserted under the skin in the desired area. Then a chosen amount of fat is sucked out, the cannula is withdrawn, and the incision is closed. The result is a recontouring of the body part. Hence, liposuction has become a very popular cosmetic surgery procedure for the abdomen, arms, breasts, hips, knees, legs, and throat; many pounds can be removed from large areas such as the abdomen.

Liposuction begins with the administration of antibiotics and the anesthesia of the area to be recontoured. Local anesthesia is safer, but general anesthesia is used when necessary. The process usually begins after a 1.3-centimeter (0.5-inch) incision is made in a fold of the treated body region, so that the scar will not be noticeable after healing. At this time, a sterile cannula is introduced under the skin of the treatment area. Next, the surgeon uses suction through the cannula to remove the fat deposits. Liposuction produces temporary tunnels in adipose tissue. Upon completion of the procedure, the incision is closed and the surgical area is wrapped with tight bandages or covered with support garments. This final stage of recontouring helps the tissue to collapse back into the desired shape during healing. In most patients, the skin around the area soon shrinks into the new contours. When this does not happen easily, because of old age or other factors, liposuction is accompanied by surgical skin removal.

Uses and Complications

Liposuction can be used for body recontouring only when undesired contours are attributable to fat deposits; those attributable to anatomical features such as bone structure cannot be treated in this manner.

A major principle on which liposuction is based is the supposition that the body contains a fixed number of fat cells and that, as people become fatter, the cells fill with droplets of fat and expand. The removal of fat cells by liposuction is deemed to decrease the future ability of the treated body part to become fat because fewer cells are available to be filled. Dieting and exercise are less successful than liposuction because they do not diminish the number of fat cells in adipose tissue, only decreasing fat cell size. Hence, when dieters return to eating excess food again or exercise stops, the fat cells expand again.

Another aspect of liposuction which is becoming popular is the ability to remove undesired fat from some body sites and insert it where the fat is wanted for recontouring. Most often, this transfer involves enlarging women's breasts or correcting cases in which the two breasts are of markedly different size. Liposuction also can be used to repair asymmetry in other body parts as a result of accidents.

The Use of Liposuction

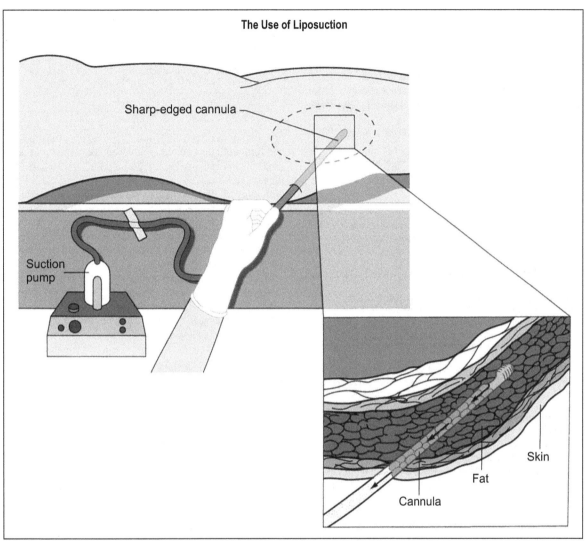

Sharp-edged cannula

Suction pump

Skin

Fat

Cannula

When unwanted areas of fat seem resistant to dieting and exercise, some patients turn to liposuction, the physical removal of fat deposits with a tube and a suction pump. The cosmetic results of this procedure may vary considerably.

Liposuction, as with any other surgery, has associated risks and complications. According to reputable practitioners, however, they are temporary and relatively minor, such as black-and-blue marks and the accumulation of blood and serum under the skin of treated areas. These complications are minimized by fluid removal during surgery and by the application of tight bandages or garments after the operation. Another related complication is that subcutaneous fat removal leads to fluid loss from the body. When large amounts of fat are removed, shock occurs if the fluid is not replaced quickly. Therefore, another component of successful liposuction is timely fluid replacement.

The more extensive and complex the liposuction procedure attempted, the more likely it is to cause complications. Particularly prone to problems are liposuction procedures in which major skin removal is required. Hence, surgeons who

perform liposuction suggest that potential patients be realistic about the goals of the surgery. It is also recommended that patients choose reputable practitioners.

Perspective and Prospects

Liposuction, currently viewed as relatively safe cosmetic surgery, originated in Europe in the late 1960s. In 1982, it reached the United States. Since that time, its use has burgeoned, and about a half million liposuction surgeries are carried out yearly. Although its first use was as a purely cosmetic procedure, liposuction is now done for noncosmetic reasons, including repairing injuries sustained in accidents. Women were once the sole liposuction patients. Men make up about 15 percent of treated individuals; liposuction is the most popular form of cosmetic surgery among men.

In the United States, liposuction is not presently accepted

by insurance companies or considered tax deductible. This situation may change because several studies have found that obese people have a greater chance of developing cardiovascular disease and cancer. It must be noted, however, that liposuction offers only temporary relief from body fat. Although it does decrease fat deposition in a treated region, lack of proper calorie intake and exercise will deposit fat elsewhere in the body.

—Sanford S. Singer, Ph.D.

See also Bariatric surgery; Dermatology; Lipids; Nutrition; Obesity; Obesity, childhood; Plastic surgery; Skin; Weight loss and gain.

For Further Information:

Rubin, J. Peter, et al. *Body Contouring and Liposuction*. New York Elsevier Saunders, 2013.

Schafer, Jeffry B. *A Patient's Guide to Liposuction: How to Make an Informed Decision*. Denver, Colo.: Outskirts Press, 2011.

Schein, Jeffery R. "The Truth About Liposuction." *Consumers Digest* 30 (January/February, 1991): 71–74.

Shelton, Ron M., and Terry Malloy. *Liposuction*. New York: Berkley, 2004.

Shiffman, Melvin A., and Alberto Di Giuseppe, eds. *Liposuction: Principles and Practice*. New York: Springer, 2006.

Wilkinson, Tolbert S. *Atlas of Liposuction*. Philadelphia: Saunders/Elsevier, 2005.

US Food and Drug Administration. "The Skinny on Liposuction." Author, April 12, 2013.

Zollinger, Robert M., Jr., and Robert M. Zollinger, Sr. *Zollinger's Atlas of Surgical Operations*. 8th ed. New York: McGraw-Hill, 2003.

Lisping
Disease/Disorder
Anatomy or system affected: Mouth, teeth
Specialties and related fields: Dentistry, speech pathology
Definition: The defective pronunciation of the sibilants "s" and "z," usually substituted with a "th" sound.

Causes and Symptoms

A central or frontal lisp is caused by a child pushing the tongue past the teeth while speaking, which tends to occur in cases of an open bite. This produces the familiar lisp in which s and z sounds are pronounced like *th*. Sometimes, the child tries to correct the protrusion of the tongue by pulling it in, but lisping still occurs because the correct position of the tongue has not been learned.

A lateral lisp involves the escape of air on both sides of the tongue, yielding an unpleasant "blubbering" sound. A possible cause is missing teeth, particularly the two upper front teeth.

A recessive lisp is caused by holding the tongue too far back in the mouth. The s and z sounds come out sounding more like *sh*. This mild lisp is often associated in the popular media with the speech of an intoxicated person.

Treatment and Therapy

Speech therapists work with lisping children in two ways. In the phonetic placement method, the child is asked to pronounce the *t* sound and then prolong it. Once this is learned, the bite is closed, and the child then practices moving the lips

---

> ## Information on Lisping
>
> **Causes:** Physiological defects, dental problems, missing teeth
> **Symptoms:** Mispronunciation of sibilants *s* and *z*
> **Duration:** Typically short-term but may be chronic
> **Treatments:** Speech therapy

in a slightly protracted position; the tongue is moved back and forth until the *s* sound is achieved. This same process is used in learning to pronounce *z*; the *d* sound, however, is used in practice instead of a *t*. In some cases, asking the child to pronounce *sh* first and then move the tongue forward along the roof of the mouth will produce an *s* sound.

In the auditory stimulation method, the speech therapist pronounces the correct sound repeatedly and compares it to the incorrect articulation. This method is very successful in young children with lisps.

After a sound has been practiced by itself, the child attaches it to nonsense syllables and practices pronouncing them. Gradually, the sound is introduced in familiar words, followed by sentences. The final test is the use of the newly acquired sound in spontaneous conversation.

—Rose Secrest

See also Developmental disorders; Developmental stages; Motor skill development; Speech disorders; Stuttering; Voice and vocal cord disorders.

For Further Information:

Bleile, Ken M. *Manual of Articulation and Phonological Disorders: Infancy Through Adulthood*. 2d ed. Clifton Park, N.Y.: Thomson/Delmar Learning, 2004.

Gordon-Brannan, Mary E., and Curtis E. Weiss. *Clinical Management of Articulatory and Phonologic Disorders*. 3d ed. Philadelphia: Lippincott Williams & Wilkins, 2007.

Hamaguchi, Patricia McAleer. *Childhood Speech, Language, and Listening Problems: What Every Parent Should Know*. 3d ed. New York: Wiley, 2010.

Rogers, Kara. "Articulation Disorders." In *Ear, Nose, and Throat*. New York: Britannica Educational, 2012.

"Speech and Language Impairments: NICHCY Disability Fact Sheet #11." *National Dissemination Center for Children with Disabilities*, April, 2013.

Williams, A. Lynn. *Speech Disorders Resource Guide for Preschool Children*. Clifton Park, N.Y.: Thomson/Delmar Learning, 2003.

Listeria infections
Disease/Disorder
Also known as: Listeriosis, *Listeria monocytogenes*
Anatomy or system affected: Brain, nerves, nervous system
Specialties and related fields: Bacteriology, obstetrics, pediatrics
Definition: Infections caused by the bacterium *Listeria monocytogenes*.

Causes and Symptoms

Infection with *Listeria* bacteria is relatively rare and primarily affects pregnant women, newborn infants, and people

Information on *Listeria* Infections

Causes: Consumption of unpasteurized dairy products, uncooked meats, unwashed vegetables

Symptoms: Can be asymptomatic or include fever, abdominal pain, diarrhea, seizures, headache, death

Duration: Begins a day after ingestion of contaminated food, can last two to three days; more serious central nervous system infections can last much longer, with permanent damage

Treatments: Antibiotics

with compromised immune systems. *Listeria* infection is a foodborne illness, meaning that infection occurs after eating a contaminated food product. Foods most commonly contaminated with *Listeria* are unpasteurized dairy products, uncooked meats, and raw, unwashed vegetables. For this reason, most pregnant women are advised by their doctors to make sure that all susceptible foods consumed during pregnancy are pasteurized and cooked thoroughly. Listeria monocytogenes is the cause of about 260 deaths a year.

The symptoms of *Listeria* infection include fever, abdominal pain, diarrhea, and muscle aches, though some infections are completely asymptomatic. If infection progresses to reach the central nervous system, then symptoms can involve dizziness, headache, seizures, and death. Pregnant women who become infected can pass the bacteria to their unborn children. Shortly after birth, the newborn can become acutely ill and exhibit fever, irritability, and poor feeding. *Listeria* infection in the newborn is an emergency and can progress to death quickly. If the newborn survives the infection, then the child may suffer lifelong neurological damage.

Treatment and Therapy

Diagnosis of *Listeria* infection is performed with a blood test or analysis of the spinal fluid through a spinal tap (lumbar puncture). Treatment for infection may require hospitalization and involves antibiotics. Ampicillin or penicillin G, often in conjunction with gentamicin, are the most commonly used antibiotics for these infections, but others such as trimethoprim-sulfamethoxazole and meropenem may be used in cases where the patient is allergic to penicillin or first-line treatments fail. Antibiotic treatment may last anywhere from ten days to eight weeks, depending on the patient's immune system and response to therapy.

Since the damage to newborn infants can be devastating, most infants presenting with fever, seizures, or other neurological symptoms receive a lumbar puncture to aid in diagnosis and are placed on prophylactic antibiotics that include ampicillin to treat *Listeria*. Ampicillin may be discontinued two to three days after treatment initiation if the spinal fluid is free of *Listeria* infection.

—*Jennifer Birkhauser, M.S., M.D.*

See also Bacterial infections; Botulism; *E. coli* infection; Enterocolitis; Food poisoning; Gastroenteritis; Gastroenterology; Gastroenterology, pediatric; Gastrointestinal disorders; Gastrointestinal system; Intestinal disorders; Intestines; Nausea and vomiting; Poisoning; Rotavirus; Salmonella infection; Shigellosis; Trichinosis; Tularemia.

For Further Information:

Edelstein, Sari. "Foodborne Illness-Causing Pathogens." In *Food and Nutrition at Risk in America: Food Insecurity, Biotechnology, Food Safety, and Bioterrorism*, edited by Sari Edelstein. Sudbury, Mass.: Jones and Bartlett, 2008.

Greenwood, David. *Medical Microbiology: A Guide to Microbial Infections—Pathogenesis, Immunity, Laboratory Diagnosis, and Control.* 18th ed. Oxford: Churchill Livingstone, 2012.

Romano, Andino, and Carmine F. Giordano. *Listeria Infections: Epidemiology, Pathogenesis, and Treatment.* Hauppauge, N.Y.: Nova Science, 2012.

Ryser, Elliot T., and Elmer H. Marth *Listeria, Listeriosis, and Food Safety.* 3d ed. Boca Raton, Fla.: CRC Press, 2007.

Stone, Joanne. "Pregnancy in Sickness and in Health." In *Pregnancy for Dummies*, edited by Mary Duenwald. Indianapolis: Wiley, 2008.

World Health Organization, ed. *Risk Assessment of Listeria Monocytogenes in Ready-to-Eat Foods: Interpretative Summary.* Rome: Food & Agricultural Organization of the United Nations, 2004.

LITHOTRIPSY

Procedure

Anatomy or system affected: Abdomen, bladder, kidneys, urinary system

Specialties and related fields: Nephrology, urology

Definition: A method of breaking up stones in the kidneys, ureters, and urinary bladder using shock waves or high-frequency sound waves.

Indications and Procedures

Stone fragmentation using shock waves or ultrasonic waves is less invasive, less painful, and less time consuming than conventional open surgery to remove stones or the organs that contain them. With lithotripsy, blood loss is minimal and recovery is quick, with a low morbidity (injury rate).

Methods of Lithotripsy

Kidney stones can be removed or broken into fragments using lithotripsy. In extracorporeal shock-wave lithotripsy (top), an emitter sends shock waves into tissues above the kidney stones, breaking the stones into very small fragments that can then be passed through the urine. In percutaneous lithotripsy (bottom), a nephroscope is inserted through the skin and into the kidney, where an ultrasonic probe breaks up and removes the stones.

In extracorporeal shock-wave lithotripsy (ESWL), the patient is given either local or general anesthesia. A machine called a lithotripter is placed on the abdomen over the site of the stones. An emitter in the lithotripter sends out shock waves that break the stones into fine fragments that can pass through the urinary tract without harm to the patient, who is encouraged to drink copious amounts of fluid following the procedure.

In ultrasonic lithotripsy, an incision is made in the skin. The stone is approached and visualized with an endoscope, a

Methods of Lithotripsy

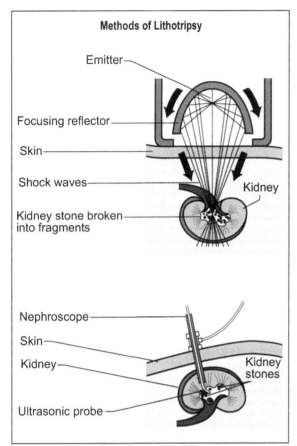

Emitter

Focusing reflector

Skin

Shock waves

Kidney stone broken into fragments

Kidney

Nephroscope

Skin

Kidney

Kidney stones

Ultrasonic probe

Kidney stones can be removed or broken into fragments using lithotripsy. In extracorporeal shock-wave lithotripsy (top), an emitter sends shock waves into tissues above the kidney stones, breaking the stones into very small fragments that can then be passed through the urine. In percutaneous lithotripsy (bottom), a nephroscope is inserted through the skin and into the kidney, where an ultrasonic probe breaks up and removes the stones.

hollow instrument with a telescope at one end for visualization. The other end of the instrument is introduced via the urethra into the bladder or ureter or via a small skin hole into the kidney. For kidney stones, a small needle is introduced into the kidney through the back under X-ray control, and a nephrostomy tract is established between the skin and the kidney. The ultrasonographic lithotripsy probe is introduced through the endoscope and brought in contact with the stone.

A piezoceramic crystal is electrically stimulated, which generates ultrasonic waves that will fragment the stone. The design of the probe allows it to suction out the broken stone particles simultaneously. Larger stones can be fragmented into smaller pieces, which can then be grasped with forceps and pulled out. When a ureteral stone is treated by this method, a plastic tube (a double-J stent) is left in the ureter to prevent postoperative blockage and future scar formation. When a kidney stone is treated by this method, a large-caliber tube is left in the kidney (a nephrostomy tube) to drain the

kidney and secure a tract for future X-ray studies and reinspection of the kidney for possible residual stone fragments.

Uses and Complications

The main morbidity associated with this procedure occurs during the establishment of the nephrostomy tract to gain access to the kidney, which can lead to bleeding, or during the introduction of the endoscope into the ureter, which can lead to perforation and future scarring. During stone fragmentation, it is imperative that the probe be in direct contact with the stone at all times, or it may cause ureteral perforation and bleeding. Overall, however, ultrasonographic lithotripsy is a safe and effective method of stone treatment, with few injuries and a quick recovery.

As with ultrasonic lithotripsy, few serious complications are associated with shock-wave lithotripsy. The presence of blood in the urine (hematuria) may be noted but is usually only temporary, as the stone fragments pass through the ureters, bladder, and urethra. Abdominal bruising may also occur, but this complication is minor in comparison to more invasive techniques. Severe pain that is unresponsive to medication may rarely signal perirenal hematoma. Other rare complications include pancreatitis and nerve palsy. Research is ongoing regarding the possibility of an association of ESWL with the development of hypertension in some patients.

—Saeed Akhter, M.D.;
updated by Victoria Price, Ph.D.

See also Cholecystectomy; Gallbladder; Gallbladder diseases; Kidney disorders; Kidneys; Nephrology; Stone removal; Stones; Ultrasonography; Urinary disorders; Urinary system; Urology.

For Further Information:
Alexander, Ivy L., ed. *Urinary Tract and Kidney Diseases and Disorders Sourcebook: Basic Consumer Health Information About the Urinary System.* 2d ed. Detroit, Mich.: Omnigraphics, 2005.
El-Assmy, Ahmed, et al. "Kidney Stone Size and Hounsfield Units Predict Successful Shockwave Lithotripsy in Children." *Urology* 81, no. 4 (April 2013): 880–884.
"Kidney Stone Treatment: Shock Wave Lithotripsy." *National Kidney Foundation,* 2009.
Leikin, Jerrold B., and Martin S. Lipsky, eds. *American Medical Association Complete Medical Encyclopedia.* New York: Random House Reference, 2003.
"Lithotripsy." *MedlinePlus,* September 16, 2011.
McCoy, Krishna. "Extracorporeal Shock Wave Lithotripsy for Kidney Stones." *Health Library,* May 21, 2013.
Parker, James N., and Philip M. Parker, eds. *The 2002 Official Patient's Sourcebook on Kidney Stones.* San Diego, Calif.: Icon Health, 2002.
Tanagho, Emil A., and Jack W. McAninich, eds. *Smith's General Urology.* 17th ed. New York: McGraw-Hill, 2008.
Tierney, Lawrence M., Stephen J. McPhee, and Maxine A. Papadakis, eds. *Current Medical Diagnosis and Treatment 2006.* New York: McGraw-Hill Medical, 2006.
Walsh, Patrick C., et al., eds. *Campbell-Walsh Urology.* 4 vols. 9th ed. Philadelphia: Saunders/Elsevier, 2007.

LIVER
Anatomy

Anatomy or system affected: Abdomen, blood, circulatory system, endocrine system, gastrointestinal system, glands

Specialties and related fields: Endocrinology, gastroenterology, hematology, internal medicine, toxicology

Definition: A vital organ that contributes to control of blood sugar levels; metabolizes carbohydrates, lipids, and proteins; stores blood, iron, and some vitamins; degrades steroid hormones; and inactivates and/or excretes certain drugs and toxins.

Key terms:

cirrhosis: a condition of the liver in which injured or dead cells are replaced with scar tissue

endoplasmic reticulum: a component of cells which in the liver is responsible for, among other things, the metabolism of xenobiotics

hepatitis: an infectious disease of the liver that is caused by a virus; at least three different types of hepatitis exist

hepatocyte: the functional cell of the liver; the liver contains only one type of functional cell

plasma proteins: any proteins found in the plasma of blood, which include those proteins necessary for blood clotting and some necessary for the transport of other molecules; most are produced by the liver

subclinical: referring to an infection in which the patient has no symptoms of disease; the infection is detected by other indicators, such as the presence of antibodies

virus: a subcellular particle that enters cells and causes cellular damage; it uses the cells' mechanisms to reproduce itself

xenobiotic: a nonbiological chemical that can enter a biological system; it could be a prescribed drug, a pollutant, or another substance

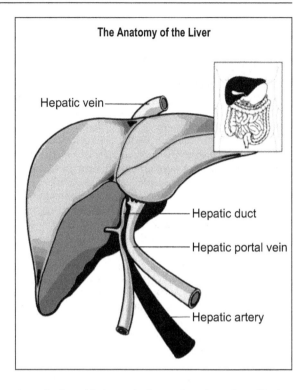

The Anatomy of the Liver

Hepatic vein

Hepatic duct

Hepatic portal vein

Hepatic artery

Structure and Functions

The liver, an accessory gland of the digestive system, is the largest organ in the human body. Located in the upper-right quadrant of the abdominal cavity, it abuts the diaphragm on the anterior surface. The liver is composed of two lobes of unequal size, with the large right lobe further divided into two smaller lobes. The organ is protected by the ribs, which cover nearly the entire surface. The liver contains only one type of functional cell, known as a hepatocyte. Closely associated with the organ is the gallbladder, a saclike structure that holds bile, a product of the hepatocytes. Bile is continually produced by the hepatocytes but is stored in the gallbladder until it is required for digestive products.

The liver is unique in that it receives blood from two different sources. The hepatic artery delivers blood to the liver from the systemic circulation. The liver also receives blood via the portal vein, which collects blood that has previously passed through the small intestine and has absorbed nutrients from the digestive system. As the blood enters the liver, it flows into dilated capillaries called sinusoids. Blood flow through sinusoids is much slower than through capillaries, and the exchange of materials between hepatocytes and the bloodstream is accomplished with little difficulty. This slower process also allows the liver to serve as a storage organ for blood, which gives the organ its characteristic dark red appearance.

The liver is essential to the normal functioning of the body. Its activities are many and varied: It regulates the metabolism of carbohydrates, lipids, and proteins; synthesizes proteins, particularly those of blood plasma that control clotting; serves as a storage site for some vitamins and iron; degrades steroid hormones; and inactivates and/or excretes certain drugs and toxins.

The liver plays a major role in carbohydrate metabolism. As carbohydrates are absorbed from the small intestine, they are transported to the liver through the portal vein. The liver regulates blood sugar levels by removing excess quantities. If the diet includes too much glucose, this substance is stored in the liver or skeletal muscle as glycogen. If the blood sugar levels are low, the glycogen is broken down into glucose and released to the bloodstream. The liver is also capable of converting amino acids, lipids, or simple carbohydrates into glucose.

The principal functions of the liver in lipid metabolism are twofold. First, it is responsible for the breakdown of large fat molecules into small compounds that can be used for energy. Second, it synthesizes triglycerides, cholesterol, and phospholipids from other fats. All three of these compounds play important roles in cellular function.

The synthesis of proteins by the liver is of major importance for the body. The liver is capable of synthesizing not only a variety of proteins but also the nonessential amino acids that are the building blocks of proteins. Many of the proteins that the liver synthesizes are found in blood plasma, including those factors responsible for blood clotting. To protect the body against deficiencies in these substances, the liver stores vitamins A, D, and B_{12}. It is also capable of storing iron, the mineral necessary for the production of hemoglobin.

Located in the smooth endoplasmic reticulum of hepatocytes are nonspecific enzymes called the mixed-function oxidases. They are capable of metabolizing a wide variety of hormones, including some polypeptide hormones and the steroid hormones, such as cortisol, estrogen, and testosterone. These same enzymes are responsible for the degradation of many foreign substances that enter the body, such as prescription medications, illegal drugs, and toxins. Most of the materials metabolized are made more water-soluble, and therefore more easily excreted, by the kidney. Others are removed from the hepatocytes in the bile that the cells produce.

Production of bile by the hepatocytes is of utmost importance to the digestive system. Bile is composed of lecithin, cholesterol, bile pigments, proteins, and bile acids, along with an isotonic solution similar to blood plasma. Bile is produced continually and stored in the gallbladder. Several minutes after a meal begins, the gallbladder releases bile to the duodenum of the small intestine. The highest rate of bile release occurs during the duodenal digestion of food and is controlled by the hormone cholecystokinin. In the duodenum, bile acts as an emulsifier of fat in the diet. It breaks large lipid droplets into many small lipid droplets, which can more easily be digested by enzymes in the small intestine. About 95 percent of the bile is reabsorbed and returned to the liver, and the other 5 percent is excreted with the feces. This provides one mechanism for the body to use the digestive system for the removal of waste products. One important product that is excreted in this manner is bilirubin, a by-product of the normal destruction of old red blood cells.

Disorders and Diseases

The liver is unique among body organs because it has the ability to regenerate in cases of injury or disease. It is estimated that in a young, healthy individual a liver that has suffered a physical injury could regenerate as much as 80 percent of the total organ. Many important organs are paired, such as the lungs and kidneys. Though the liver is a single organ, its ability to regenerate ensures normal function even in cases of severe injury.

The presence of liver disease is detectable in many ways. With some diseases, the liver becomes enlarged and can be felt below the ribs. This swelling may be associated with localized discomfort or pain in the region. In more severe cases of liver disease, the organ may actually shrink and recede further under the ribs, a condition easily detected by a physician.

The pathophysiology of the liver is characterized by certain physiologic events that occur regardless of the underlying cause. Within the liver, disease may result in portal hypertension, blockage of bile ducts, and cellular injury or death.

Cellular injury may be manifest by fatty infiltration and by interference with cellular functions, including the synthesis of proteins necessary for blood clotting, the metabolism of drugs or toxins, the regulation of glucose, and the production of bile. Any or all of these physiologic changes can lead to effects in other parts of the body.

Disease of the liver is often detectable by routine blood tests that include liver function tests. The patient may show decreased levels in the blood serum of proteins that are normally produced by the liver, an increased blood-clotting time, or increased serum levels of enzymes that are normally found only in the liver. A yellow skin tone known as jaundice has been associated with liver disease. This discoloration of skin and the sclera of the eye is a result of excessively high levels of bilirubin in the blood. Bilirubin is a by-product of the breakdown of red blood cells that are near the end of their 120-day life cycle.

The injury or death of liver cells may present a pathology unique to the liver, the disease cirrhosis. When hepatocytes are injured or diseased, they begin to accumulate lipids in vacuoles, giving the liver a whitish appearance. Associated with the development of a fatty liver, the cells may divide to produce more cells that will ensure normal function. Sometimes, however, this stimulation of cell division leads to an excess of hepatocytes, a condition that may result in abnormal patterns of blood flow through the liver. In addition, this phenomenon may include the production of large nodules of connective tissue to replace dead or dying cells, a condition comparable to scarring. The development of scars may cause increased blood pressure in the portal veins and may block bile ducts. Cirrhosis may be caused by a variety of conditions, including alcoholism, exposure to toxic substances, or infection. It is irreversible and ultimately causes the death of the patient.

Diseases of the liver can be classified according to the following scheme: congenital liver disorders, viral and nonviral infections, drug-induced and toxin-induced disease, vascular disorders, metabolic disorders, iron accumulation, alcoholic liver disease, and tumors.

The most common types of congenital diseases of the liver involve abnormalities of the bile ducts or of the portal vein, which may be associated with portal hypertension. More important, however, are those diseases that lead to the formation of cysts, such as polycystic liver disease or hepatic fibrosis. Jaundice of the newborn, a discoloration of the skin at birth, usually clears within a week or so with no long-term effects.

Viral infections of the liver may be associated with the hepatitis viruses or other viruses less specific for the liver. The four most common hepatitis viruses are hepatitis A, hepatitis B, hepatitis C, and hepatitis D. Hepatitis can also be associated with yellow fever, infectious mononucleosis, cytomegalovirus infection, and herpes simplex.

Hepatitis A is also known as infectious hepatitis. It is generally transmitted via fecal contamination of milk, water, or seafood. It is most common in the areas of the world where untreated sewage may come into contact with the water supply or food sources. It has a short incubation period and is usually not fatal; it does not lead to chronic hepatitis. Hepatitis B, also known as serum hepatitis, is transmitted from persons with an active form of the disease or from carriers via contaminated blood or blood products. It is particularly prevalent among drug users who share needles. The threat of contraction of hepatitis B from a transfusion has been greatly reduced by the screening of blood products. Hepatitis B has a long incubation period, up to six months. The severity of the disease varies greatly from subclinical hepatitis (showing no symptoms) to chronic hepatitis and in some cases may result in death. The course of hepatitis C disease resembles that of hepatitis B and may lead to chronic hepatitis. Hepatitis D is believed to be a defective virus that is found only in the presence of hepatitis B. It is transmitted via the same route and can result in chronic hepatitis.

Hepatitis from any cause may show subclinical or mild, influenza-like symptoms. Acute hepatitis may cause loss of appetite, vomiting, fever, jaundice, and enlargement of the liver. The viruses that cause hepatitis replicate within the liver cells, which could be the cause of the injury to these cells. Hepatocyte injury could also be a result of the immune system's attempt to fight the virus, which may injure the cells of the liver in the process. In either case, the damaged cells swell before they die. The liver can also be infected by bacterial cells, which usually reach the liver as a result of a systemic infection.

Many toxins or drugs can injure the liver, in a general pattern that is similar to the effects of infectious agents. The assault on the cell often leads to fatty infiltration, followed by swelling and finally by the death of the hepatocyte. Even in less severe cases of injury, those that do not lead to death of the hepatocyte, there is often impairment of the metabolic activities of the liver that can lead to diverse systemic effects. One of these effects is the ability to metabolize foreign compounds or naturally occurring steroids; the accumulation of these compounds throughout the body can have wide-ranging consequences.

The liver is adversely affected by the constant intake of excessive quantities of ethyl alcohol. In the early stages of alcoholism, the physiologic changes may be a result of improper nutrition or of vitamin deficiencies. During the more advanced stages of alcoholism, the patient is likely to suffer from a fatty liver and, ultimately, from cirrhosis. While those who stop drinking may slow down the advancement of cirrhosis, the disease appears to be irreversible.

There are more than five thousand metabolic enzymes in the liver, each of which is controlled genetically. Important in the treatment of metabolic disease is early diagnosis, which may prevent damage to other organs or to the liver. Dietary control may be used to minimize the effects of such conditions, leading to a near-normal life. Examples of treatable metabolic diseases are galactosemia, a condition that prevents the conversion of galactose to glucose; fructosemia, a condition that leads to the accumulation of fructose-1-phosphate; and Wilson disease, an accumulation of copper in vital organs as a result of a defect in copper metabolism. In each case, the accumulation of a certain substance can lead to cel-

lular damage, but dietary control of the substance can minimize the effects. Hemochromatosis is a similar disease that leads to accumulation of iron in the liver. As with Wilson disease, the deposition of this element is not limited to the liver and can accumulate in other vital tissues of the body as well.

Cancer of the liver is usually caused by its spread from another site. Primary liver cancers are rare and usually do not occur until late in life. Risk factors may include exposure to hepatotoxins, chronic liver disease, or hepatitis B. There are two types of primary carcinomas of the liver: hepatocellular carcinoma, which develops in hepatocytes, and cholangiocellular carcinoma, which develops in bile ducts.

Perspective and Prospects

The liver is a vital organ that plays a major role in the homeostasis of the body. Any condition that adversely influences the liver will have wide-ranging effects on other organs and the patient as a whole.

Because one of its functions is the metabolism of pollutants, drugs (including alcohol), and hormones, the liver is often exposed to substances that are toxic to its hepatocytes. When these compounds are encountered, the liver efficiently alters them for excretion. Sometimes, however, these substances may do damage to the cells before the liver can metabolize them.

When a liver cell is injured, the end result may be the death of the cell. Fortunately, liver cells are efficient at cell division and can replace those cells that have been injured or that have died. With continued damage to liver cells, however, the body can no longer replace them, and the resulting decrease in liver function leads to extensive complications throughout the body. A decrease in liver function will not only have an effect on the digestive system but will have wide-ranging effects on glucose and lipid metabolism (normal functions of the blood whose proteins are synthesized by the liver) and on the ability to remove certain foreign substances or toxins from the blood. For example, if the ability to metabolize medication is impaired by liver disease, the patient's body may accumulate high, even toxic, levels of drugs. These substances can have pronounced effects, particularly on the nervous system. With liver injury, the once-simple act of determining a medication dosage can become a critical problem.

Despite the liver's regenerative capacity, liver injury or disease can have permanent effects. However, some conditions previously thought incurable, such as chronic hepatitis B and C, can now be treated successfully in many cases with antiviral drugs and interferon. The medical community can treat the symptoms of hepatitis.

Cancer of the liver is also difficult to treat. Because it is not easily detected, the diagnosis is rarely early. Unless the cancer is restricted to one lobe that can be removed, surgery is rarely the answer. Treatment is further complicated by the fact that the liver cells are particularly sensitive to radiation and that the doses needed to treat the cancer would be deadly to hepatocytes. Chemotherapy has been the mainstay of treatment for both metastatic and primary liver cancer, but transplantation is increasingly recommended for patients with primary liver cancer.

With the discovery of immunosuppressive drugs, liver transplantation has become a positive procedure in the treatment of liver disease, and the results are promising. The availability of healthy livers for transplant, however, makes this an option limited to a small percentage of patients.

—Annette O'Connor, Ph.D.

See also Abdomen; Abdominal disorders; Alcoholism; Anatomy; Bile; Blood and blood disorders; Circulation; Cirrhosis; Gastroenterology; Gastroenterology, pediatric; Gastrointestinal disorders; Gastrointestinal system; Hematology; Hematology, pediatric; Hepatitis; Internal medicine; Jaundice; Liver cancer; Liver disorders; Liver transplantation; Metabolism; Nonalcoholic steatohepatitis (NASH); Systems and organs; Transplantation; Wilson's disease.

For Further Information:

Chandrasoma, Parakrama, and Clive R. Taylor. *Concise Pathology.* 3d ed. Stamford, Conn.: Appleton & Lange, 1998.

Clavien, Pierre-Alain, et al. *Malignant Liver Tumors: Current and Emerging Therapies.* 3d ed. Hoboken, NJ: Wiley-Blackwell, 2010.

Dollinger, Malin, et al. *Everyone's Guide to Cancer Therapy.* 5th ed. Kansas City, Mo.: Andrews McMeel, 2008.

Feldman, Mark, Lawrence S. Friedman, and Lawrence J. Brandt, eds. *Sleisenger and Fordtran's Gastrointestinal and Liver Disease: Pathophysiology, Diagnosis, Management.* New ed. 2 vols. Philadelphia: Saunders/Elsevier, 2010.

Guyton, Arthur C., and John E. Hall. *Guyton and Hall Textbook of Medical Physiology.* 12th ed. Philadelphia: Saunders/Elsevier, 2011.

McCance, Kathryn L., and Sue M. Huether. *Pathophysiology: The Biologic Basis for Disease in Adults and Children.* 6th ed. St. Louis, Mo.: Mosby/Elsevier, 2010.

Reau, Nancy, and Fred Poordad. *Primary Liver Cancer: Surveillance, Diagnosis, and Treatment.* New York: Humana Press, 2012.

Scanlon, Valerie, and Tina Sanders. *Essentials of Anatomy and Physiology.* 6th ed. Philadelphia: F. A. Davis, 2012.

Schiff, Eugene R., et al. *Schiff's Diseases of the Liver.* 11th ed. New York: John Wiley & Sons, 2012.

LIVER CANCER

Disease/Disorder

Anatomy or system affected: Liver

Specialties and related fields: Gastroenterology, immunology, oncology, radiology

Definition: Malignancies of the liver, which may be primary (arising in the organ itself) but are more likely to be secondary (metastasizing from another site).

Causes and Symptoms

The liver filters the blood supply, removing and breaking down (metabolizing) toxins and delivering them through the biliary tract to the intestines for elimination with other wastes. Because of the large volume of blood flowing through the liver (about a quarter of the body's supply), blood-borne toxins or cancer cells migrating from tumors elsewhere (the process called metastasis) pose a constant threat. In fact, in the United States most liver cancers are

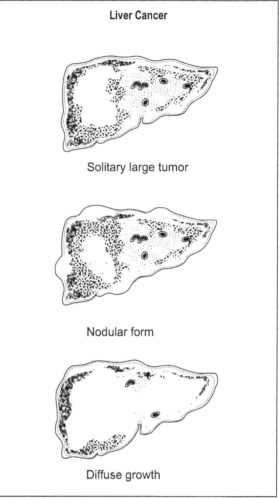

Liver Cancer

Solitary large tumor

Nodular form

Diffuse growth

The liver is a frequent site of cancer, most commonly from malignancies that have spread from their original site. The particular form the cancer takes depends on several factors, notably the primary source and its possible cause.

metastatic; only about 1 percent actually originate in the liver. In Southeast Asia and sub-Saharan Africa, primary liver cancer is the most common type, accounting for as much as 30 percent of all cancers.

Two major types of cancer affect the liver: those involving liver cells (hepatocellular carcinomas) and those involving the bile ducts (cholangiocarcinomas). The first is by far the more common, although tumors may contain a mixture of both, and their development is similar. Tumors may arise in one location, forming a large mass; arise in several locations, forming nodes; or spread throughout the liver in a diffuse form. Liver cancers occur in men about four to eight times more frequently than in women and in African Americans slightly more than in Caucasians, although the proportions vary widely among different regions of the world. In the United States, most cancers arise in people fifty years old or older; in other areas, people older than forty are at risk.

Primary liver cancer has so much regional and gender variation because causative agents are more or less common in different areas and men are more often exposed. A leading risk factor in the United States and Europe is cirrhosis, a scarring of liver tissue following destruction by viruses, toxins, or interrupted blood flow. In the United States, long-term alcohol consumption is the most common cause of cirrhosis, and men have long been more likely than women to become alcoholics. Likewise, hemochromatosis, a hereditary disease leading to the toxic buildup of iron, is a cancer precursor and more common in men than in women. In Africa and Southeast Asia, the hepatitis B and C viruses are leading precancer diseases because hepatitis has long been endemic in those areas, whereas in the United States it is not widespread (although the number of infected people began to rise in the 1980s).

Diet and medical therapies have also been implicated as liver carcinogens. Food toxins, especially aflatoxin from mold growing on peanuts (which are a staple in parts of Africa and Asia); oral contraceptives; anabolic steroids; and the high levels of sex hormones used in some treatments are thought to increase the likelihood of hepatobiliary tumors. Genetic factors, radiation, and occupational exposure to volatile chemicals may also play a minor role.

Although researchers generally agree about which agents are liver cancer precursors, the exact mechanism leading to tumor development is not thoroughly understood. Nevertheless, one factor may be universal. Viruses and toxins injure or destroy liver and bile duct cells; the body reacts to repair the damage with inflammation and an increased rate of new cell growth, a condition called regenerative hyperplasia. If the toxin damage continues, triggering ever more hyperplasia, as is the case with hepatitis and alcoholic cirrhosis, formation of a tumor becomes almost inevitable.

Like lymph nodes, the liver collects migrating cancer cells, so the cancers that physicians detect there often are metastases from cancers arising elsewhere in the body. In fact, liver involvement may be found before the primary cancer has been recognized. Colorectal cancer is especially given to metastasizing to the liver, since the digestive tract's blood supply is directly linked to the liver through the portal vein; similarly, lung and breast cancer may spread to the liver. Such metastases indicate advanced cancers that do not bode well for the patient's survival.

Symptoms may be ambiguous. Two common symptoms are jaundice and enlargement of the liver, with accompanying tenderness. Jaundice, a yellowing of the skin and eyes, is caused by an accumulation of bilirubin. Bilirubin builds up because a tumor has blocked the bile duct that normally empties it into the small intestine. (Both symptoms may also occur as a result of either gallstones or cirrhosis.) Patients with liver cancer may also have a fever and retain fluid in the abdominal cavities.

Treatment and Therapy

Doctors suspecting liver cancer conduct tests designed to distinguish this disease from other disorders. Palpation of the liver may reveal that the organ is enlarged or contains an unusual tissue mass, which is likely to be a tumor. A rubbing sound heard through the stethoscope may also come from a tumor. Hepatocellular carcinoma often elevates the alpha-fetoprotein level in blood. Abdominal ultrasound or computed tomography (CT) scans can provide good evidence of a tumor in the liver, and a biopsy will supply a tissue sample capable of proving the presence of cancer, especially if the biopsy is done with CT scan or ultrasound guidance. A tumor can also disrupt normal biochemical action in the body, which

---

In the News:
Percutaneous Hepatic Perfusion (PHP)

In 2009, a much-anticipated clinical trial, sponsored by the National Cancer Institute, completed enrollment for testing percutaneous hepatic perfusion (PHP) as an improved method for treating liver cancer. PHP diverts the blood going into and out of the liver so that high doses of toxic drugs can be added without harming the rest of the body. This "regional chemotherapy" is used for cancers that are especially difficult to treat, which is frequently the case with liver cancer.

By the time that liver cancer has been diagnosed, it has typically spread to the whole organ, making it impossible to remove surgically (resection). Chemotherapy by that time is often futile as well, and any hope of success requires extreme measures. One such measure that has been around for nearly fifty years is to surgically reroute the blood vessels so that blood circulates through the liver via a pump that delivers the anticancer drug. After about thirty minutes, clean blood is reintroduced, and blood flow is rerouted back to normal. About ten years ago, investigators began experimenting with a nonsurgical procedure for rerouting the blood flow. The latest incarnation, and the subject of the clinical trial, is a system patented by Delcath Systems, Inc., that uses special catheters (ultra-fine tubing that can snake through veins and arteries) threaded up from the groin until they reach the liver. One catheter is then inflated to block normal blood flow into the liver while serving at the same as an artificial blood vessel for delivering the chemotherapy. The other catheter blocks the blood flow exiting the liver and provides a channel for sending the toxic blood through a filter that removes the drug. The filtered blood is returned to the patient through a third catheter in the neck. The big advantage of using catheters is that inserting them is relatively quick and easy. The absence of surgical trauma also permits repeated rounds of treatment so that oncologists can treat the cancer as aggressively as possible.

—*Brad Rikke, Ph.D.*

doctors may detect in blood tests. Liver function blood tests may be abnormal with both primary and secondary liver cancer.

Under even the most favorable circumstances, the outlook for patients with liver cancer is still not good. If a primary cancer is found while still fairly small, surgical removal is the surest and fastest treatment, although it is a difficult, risky procedure because of the liver's complex, delicate structure. Radiation and chemotherapy have not succeeded in shrinking tumors effectively. Because symptoms usually appear late in the development of primary liver cancer, it seldom is found early enough for surgical cure; patients usually live only one to two months after detection. Those found with small, removable cancers live an average of twenty-nine months. Most liver cancers are metastases, however, and removal of the liver tumor will not rid the patient of cancer. In general, hepatobiliary cancer patients have low chance of living five years after diagnosis.

Liver cancer screening tests can locate tumors while they are still treatable, although routine physical examinations in Western nations seldom include such tests. Usually only patients with cirrhosis or chronic hepatitis are screened. The best ways to ward off liver cancer are to avoid viral infection and to abstain from alcohol. For those at risk for infection, such as health care workers, the most effective primary prevention is vaccination for hepatitis B. US cases of liver cancer are expected to rise by a factor of four during the second decade of the twenty-first century, primarily because of hepatitis C infections and "fatty liver" (which occurs in patients with diabetes and obesity).

—*Roger Smith, Ph.D.*

See also Alcoholism; Cancer; Carcinogens; Chemotherapy; Cirrhosis; Hepatitis; Jaundice; Liver; Liver disorders; Liver transplantation; Malignancy and metastasis; Oncology; Radiation therapy; Tumor removal; Tumors.

For Further Information:

Abou-Alfa Ghassan K., and Ronald DeMatteo. *One Hundred Questions and Answers About Liver Cancer.* 3d ed. Burlington, Mass.: Jones & Bartlett Learning, 2012.

Curley, Steven A., ed. *Liver Cancer.* New York: Springer, 1998.

Dollinger, Malin, et al. *Everyone's Guide to Cancer Therapy.* 5th ed. Kansas City, Mo.: Andrews McMeel, 2008.

Eyre, Harmon J., Dianne Partie Lange, and Lois B. Morris. *Informed Decisions: The Complete Book of Cancer Diagnosis, Treatment, and Recovery.* 2d ed. Atlanta: American Cancer Society, 2002.

Gu, Jianren. *Primary Liver Cancer: Challenges and Perspectives.* New York: Springer, 2012.

Liver Cancer Network. http://www.livercancer.com.

Parker, James N., and Philip M. Parker, eds. *The Official Patient's Sourcebook on Adult Primary Liver Cancer.* San Diego, Calif.: Icon Health, 2002.

Reau, Nancy, and Fred Poordad. *Primary Liver Cancer: Surveillance, Diagnosis, and Treatment.* New York: Humana Press, 2012.

Sachar, David B., Jerome D. Waye, and Blair S. Lewis. *Pocket Guide to Gastroenterology.* Rev. ed. Baltimore: Williams & Wilkins, 1991.

Shannon, Joyce Brennfleck. *Liver Disorders Sourcebook.* Detroit, Mich.: Omnigraphics, 2000.

Steen, R. Grant. *A Conspiracy of Cells: The Basic Science of Cancer.* New York: Plenum Press, 1993.

LIVER DISORDERS

Disease/Disorder

Anatomy or system affected: Liver

Specialties and related fields: Gastroenterology, internal medicine

Definition: As one of the most complex organs in the body, the liver is the target of a wide variety of toxins, infectious agents, and cancers that lead to hepatitis, cirrhosis, abscesses, and liver failure.

Key terms:

abscess: a localized collection of pus and infectious microorganisms

ascites: the presence of free fluid in the abdominal cavity

bilirubin: a major component of bile, derived from the breakdown products of red blood cells

cirrhosis: the fibrous scar tissue that replaces the normally soft liver after repeated damage by viruses, chemicals, and/or alcohol

hepatitis: inflammation of the liver, such as that caused by viruses or toxins

jaundice: a yellow discoloration of the skin, eyes, and membranes caused by excess bilirubin in the blood

portal hypertension: elevated pressures in the portal veins caused by resistance to blood flow through a diseased liver; produces many regional problems, including ascites

portal system: a system of veins, unique to the liver, that carry nutrient-rich blood from the digestive organs to the liver

Causes and Symptoms

The liver is the largest internal organ, lying in the upper-right abdominal cavity. Intricately attached to it by a system of ducts on its lower surface is the pear-shaped gallbladder. Unique to the liver is a blood supply that derives from two separate sources: the hepatic artery, carrying freshly oxygenated blood from the heart, and the portal vein, carrying blood rich in the products of digestion from the digestive organs. The liver cells, or hepatocytes, are arranged in thin sheets that are separated by large pores, blood vessels, and ducts. The result is a very soft, spongy organ filled with a large volume of blood.

The liver performs a wide variety of complex and diverse functions, more so than any other organ. Most commonly known is the production of bile, which is formed from the breakdown of red blood cells, cholesterol, and salts, stored in the gallbladder, and used in the small intestine to digest fats. The liver also serves the all-important purpose of detoxification by chemically altering harmful substances such as alcohol, drugs, and ammonia from protein digestion. Additionally, the liver is involved in the formation of such essential materials as blood proteins, blood-clotting factors, and sugar and fat storage compounds.

Because of the liver's many responsibilities and unique position as an intermediary between the digestive process and the blood (via the portal vein), it easily falls prey to many disease-causing agents. Chemicals, illegal drugs, alcohol, viruses, parasites, hormones, and even medical drugs can dam-

Information on Liver Disorders

Causes: Cirrhosis, infection, disease, abscess, liver failure, injury, genetic factors, tumors
Symptoms: Vary; can include pain, swelling, nausea and vomiting, jaundice, easy bruising, excessive bleeding, blood clotting problems
Duration: Acute to chronic
Treatments: Drug therapy, surgery, transplant; most often symptomatic relief and supportive care

age the liver and have widespread effects on the rest of the body. The liver is also the most frequent target of cancer cells that have spread beyond their primary site. In the United States and other industrialized countries, liver disease is usually related to alcoholism and cancer, while in the developing world, it is often the result of infectious contamination by viruses and parasites.

There are two simplified methods of classifying liver disorders. The first is based on cause: infections (viruses and parasites), injury (alcohol and other toxins), inheritance (inability to perform certain functions), infiltration (iron and copper deposits), and tumors (both benign and malignant). The second method of classification is based on the result, such as hepatitis (inflammation), cirrhosis (permanent injury from alcohol or other toxins), or cancer.

Each of these liver diseases produces a particular set of signs and symptoms depending on the length of time and the specific disruption of structure and function. Pain and swelling rarely occur alone and are usually associated with one or more of the following: nausea and vomiting, jaundice, ascites, blood-clotting defects, and encephalopathy. Indeed, in some cases liver failure ensues, leading to coma and death.

Jaundice, a yellow discoloration of the skin and whites (sclera) of the eyes, is caused by the secretion of bile precursors (bilirubin) from the damaged liver cells directly into the blood rather than into the ducts leading to the gallbladder. Consequently, bilirubin accumulates in the body's tissues, including the skin and eyes. Ascites, the collection of fluid beneath the liver in the abdomen, is an important sign of liver disease. This fluid comes primarily from the portal vein system, which lies between the liver and the digestive organs. As the liver becomes congested and enlarged in response to injury or infection, blood flow becomes difficult and pressure begins to build, causing liquid to leak from the blood vessels into the abdominal cavity. Easy bruising, excessive bleeding, and other problems with blood clotting are important signs that reflect the failure of the liver to produce essential blood proteins. Neuropsychiatric symptoms such as asterixis (flapping hand tremor) and encephalopathy (a state of mental confusion and disorientation that can quickly progress to coma) are not well understood, but it is likely that they result from an accumulation of toxic substances that would normally be cleared from the blood by the liver. Several other problems, such as the enlargement of male breasts, atrophy of the testicles, and other sexual changes, derive from the inability of the

liver to clear the blood of hormones.

Hepatitis, an inflammation of the liver generally caused by viruses, is one of the most common diseases in the world. Hepatitis A, B, and C; Epstein-Barr virus (the causative agent of mononucleosis); and herpes are a few of the organisms that can infect the liver. Hepatitis A, transmitted through contaminated food, water, and shellfish, is usually a self-limited disease that resolves itself. Hepatitis B, transmitted through contact with infected blood and body secretions, is much more serious, with a carrier state, progressive organ damage, cancer, and death as possible sequelae. Hepatitis C is transmitted by intravenous drug use or blood transfusion. Infection most often causes no symptoms initially but leads to chronic infection in about 80 percent of individuals. Chronic infection progresses to cirrhosis in 20 to 30 percent of cases and may lead to liver cancer. Noninfectious causes of hepatitis in susceptible people include such frequently used substances as acetaminophen (Tylenol), halothane (general anesthesia), and oral contraceptives. Nonalcoholic steatohepatitis (NASH) is a disease that causes chronic inflammation and, upon biopsy, resembles alcoholic hepatitis. It is diagnosed in patients with persistent abnormal liver function tests, no evidence of hepatitis B or C, and consumption of less than 40 grams of ethanol per week. NASH is most often found in patients with obesity, type 2 diabetes, and hyperlipidemia.

Cirrhosis is the result of continuous toxic exposure that injures the liver beyond repair. Fibrous scar tissue replaces the normally soft, spongy organ, making it small and firm, with few hepatocytes capable of functioning normally. Chronic alcohol abuse is by far the most frequent factor in the development of cirrhosis. Severe ascites, bleeding disorders, encephalopathy, and sex organ changes often herald imminent liver failure and death from this disease.

In the Western world, liver cancer is most often secondary to malignancies that have spread from other sites. In Asia and Africa, primary tumors of the liver itself are much more common due to high incidences of hepatitis B infection, food toxins, and parasite infestation, among other factors. Chronic injury appears to play the critical role in liver cancer, with the main risk factors established thus far being cirrhosis, hepatitis B and C, and long-term exposure to a variety of chemicals, hormones, and drugs. Benign tumors may occur in young women who use oral contraceptives, but they are relatively infrequent.

Several other hepatic diseases warrant mention. Liver abscesses, or encapsulated areas filled with infectious material, can be caused by bacteria, fungi, or parasites. These organisms enter the bloodstream through ingestion, skin puncture, or even intestinal rupture (as in cases of appendicitis and diverticulitis) and travel to the liver. Two unusual but notable disorders of iron and copper metabolism—hemochromatosis and Wilson's disease, respectively—have prominent liver involvement. While the disease mechanisms are not well understood, these essential metals are retained in excess and deposited in body tissues in toxic levels, causing damage. Finally, several genetic disorders of bile production run the gamut from mere nuisances to potentially fatal in infancy.

Bilirubin metabolism, in which red blood cell waste products are incorporated into bile, is affected or disrupted to varying degrees. Severe jaundice reflects the accumulation of toxic levels of bilirubin in all body tissues, including the brain.

Treatment and Therapy

The diagnosis of a patient with suspected liver disease is an orderly process that begins with a thorough history and physical examination, supported by a number of valuable blood tests and imaging techniques. Liver biopsy, in which a tissue sample is obtained for microscopic analysis, is often a final and definitive procedure if the disorder remains ambiguous. Both the cause and the chronology or state of the disease— that is, whether it is of recent onset or advanced—determine treatment and outcome. While many signs and symptoms are nonspecific, including nausea, vomiting, pain, hepatic enlargement, and jaundice, others such as ascites,

encephalopathy, blood-clotting defects, and sex organ changes reflect significant organ damage and an advanced stage of disease.

Careful questioning regarding the recent and past history of a patient can elicit facts that may point to a diagnosis, including exposure to known liver toxins such as alcohol, anesthetics, certain medications, and occupational chemicals; travel to countries with known contaminated water supplies (hepatitis A); blood transfusions, kidney dialysis, sexual promiscuity, or intravenous drug use (hepatitis B and C); unexplained weight loss (cancer); or even a history of gallstones (blocked bile ducts between the liver and gallbladder). Armed with suspicions from the history, the physician performs a physical examination to look for signs that confirm or reject the possibilities. A small and firm liver with ascites, tremor, enlarged male breasts, and small, shrunken testicles all point to an advanced stage of cirrhosis, for example. An

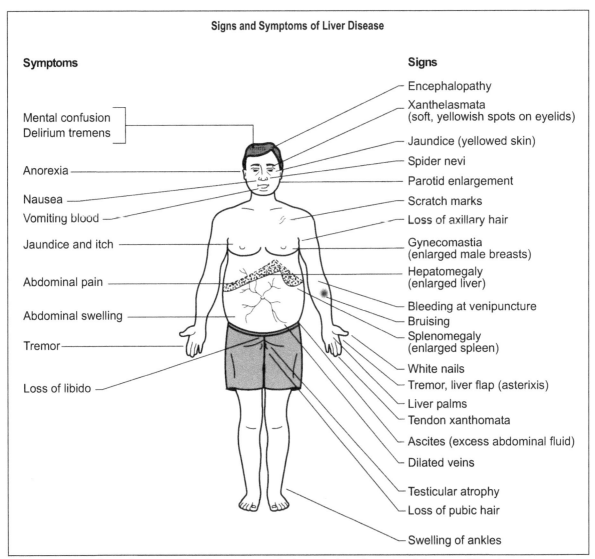

Signs and Symptoms of Liver Disease

Symptoms

Mental confusion
Delirium tremens

Anorexia

Nausea

Vomiting blood

Jaundice and itch

Abdominal pain

Abdominal swelling

Tremor

Loss of libido

Signs

Encephalopathy

Xanthelasmata
(soft, yellowish spots on eyelids)

Jaundice (yellowed skin)

Spider nevi

Parotid enlargement

Scratch marks

Loss of axillary hair

Gynecomastia
(enlarged male breasts)

Hepatomegaly
(enlarged liver)

Bleeding at venipuncture

Bruising

Splenomegaly
(enlarged spleen)

White nails

Tremor, liver flap (asterixis)

Liver palms

Tendon xanthomata

Ascites (excess abdominal fluid)

Dilated veins

Testicular atrophy

Loss of pubic hair

Swelling of ankles

Particular combinations of these factors can provide clues to both the diagnosis and the extent of liver damage.

Liver Disorders

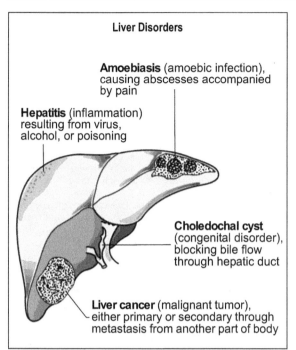

Amoebiasis (amoebic infection), causing abscesses accompanied by pain

Hepatitis (inflammation) resulting from virus, alcohol, or poisoning

Choledochal cyst (congenital disorder), blocking bile flow through hepatic duct

Liver cancer (malignant tumor), either primary or secondary through metastasis from another part of body

The liver's unique structure and functions leave it vulnerable to a wide range of diseases.

enlarged and painful liver, vomiting, jaundice, and fever following recent ingestion of raw shellfish would likely suggest hepatitis A.

Blood tests play a critical role in evaluating liver disease. An elevated bilirubin level would correlate with the severity of jaundice. Blood protein levels (albumin) and blood-clotting factors (prothrombin) may be dangerously low, revealing a near inability of the hepatocytes to synthesize these vital substances. Special chemicals that exist primarily in liver cells (hepatic enzymes and the aminotransferases) may be quite high, indicating that these cells are dying and releasing their contents into the blood. Finally, elevated white blood cell counts and special tests for individual infections (viruses, bacteria, fungi, and parasites) can positively establish the diagnosis.

Depending on the suspected disease, confirmation may be needed from various imaging techniques, chosen specifically for a particular diagnosis. Plain x-rays do little to visualize the liver, although they can reveal air in the abdomen, a consequence of a perforated intestine, appendix, or ulcer. A much more advanced method, thecomputed tomography (CT) scan, combines computer-generated views of multiple cross-sectional x-rays, providing a highly detailed examination of the liver and thereby establishing a diagnosis in the majority of cases. Two other techniques that have more specific uses are ultrasound, which uses sound-wave transmission, and magnetic resonance imaging (MRI), which uses magnetic fields to create an image. Ultrasound can readily distinguish solid masses from those that are fluid filled (tumors versus

abscesses) and can view the bile ducts. MRI is quite helpful in determining blood-flow problems such as portal hypertension.

Finally, if a precise diagnosis remains elusive, a biopsy is performed. A sample of liver tissue is obtained using a large needle inserted through the skin, under the guidance of an ultrasound image. The sample is then viewed microscopically, which should make both the cause and the extent of liver damage readily apparent.

Treatment options for the majority of liver diseases are improving. If drug toxicity is suspected, especially from alcohol, immediate withdrawal of the agent can prevent further damage, as has been shown in cases of cirrhosis. Obstructing gallstones can be surgically removed to relieve pressure in the bile ducts. Combinations of surgery, radiation, and chemotherapy are used in cases of liver cancer, but the prognosis is poor. Little can be done for the inherited diseases of bilirubin metabolism, while some success has been achieved in treating the iron- and copper-storage diseases.

Infections of viral origin have specific treatment regimens. Prevention of hepatitis A and B is possible if pooled serum immunoglobulin is given immediately after exposure. This substance is a concentrated form of antibodies obtained from infected individuals whose diseases have completely resolved; essentially, it is a method of giving passive immunity. Chronic hepatitis B may be effectively treated with several antiviral medications or interferon. Chronic hepatitis C is treated with a combination of an antiviral medication (ribavirin) and interferon. Response rates to therapy range between 50 and 80 percent, depending on the viral load, the genotype of the virus, and compliance with treatment. There are no specific therapies proven effective for treatment of NASH. Treatment is recommended for associated medical conditions, including weight loss, reduction of lipids (cholesterol and triglycerides), and control of diabetes. One area in which effective treatment does exist is in bacterial, fungal, and parasitic infections and abscesses. Appropriate antibiotics and surgical drainage yield dramatic improvement in most cases.

In many cases of liver disease, symptom relief and nutritional support, often carried out in the hospital, are the only options. Pain relief and the administration of intravenous fluid and nutrients to counteract vomiting and dehydration are the first steps. Ascites is relieved through bed rest, salt restriction, diuretics, and paracentesis, a procedure that uses ultrasound to guide a needle into the abdomen and withdraw fluid. Attempts to correct encephalopathy by removing toxins such as ammonia from the blood are generally ineffective, and mental changes, along with other intractable symptoms, often herald complete liver failure and imminent death.

Clearly, preventive measures are the most important factor in liver disease. One effective measure that is widely available is the hepatitis B vaccine, which is recommended during childhood in a three-injection series. Hepatitis A vaccine is available and recommended in children older than one year. Hepatitis A and B vaccines are recommended to any non-immune adult with chronic liver disease.

Perspective and Prospects

Liver transplantation offers approximately four thousand patients per year replacement of the diseased organ with a normal, donated one. The procedure was begun experimentally in the early 1960s, and after decades of low success rates (less than 20 percent), it has finally been accepted as a lifesaving operation, with five-year survival rates approaching 75 percent as of 2012. Technical improvements, especially intraoperative blood circulation and cadaver organ preservation, have been combined with refined patient selection and timing and advances in immunosuppressive therapy that counteract rejection. The result is that liver transplantation has become the method of choice for patients whose liver disease is life-threatening, progressive, and unresponsive to other treatments.

Specific guidelines exist for both children and adults to be considered candidates for the procedure. It is imperative that the person is otherwise healthy and that the heart, lungs, kidneys, and brain are functioning well. Malignancy, human immunodeficiency virus (HIV) infection, incorrectable congenital defects, and continuing drug or alcohol abuse are obvious contraindications. Infants with inherited, inevitably fatal liver disorders are good candidates for transplantation, as are adults with end-stage liver failure, such as from chronic hepatitis. Controversial indications, requiring case-by-case evaluation, include advanced viral hepatitis (as recurrent infection in the donated organ often occurs) and alcohol-induced cirrhosis (because of the likelihood of damage to other organs and the high relapse rate after surgery). Relapse is also very common if the transplantation is done for a primary liver cancer.

Careful donor selection is equally important. The principal source of cadaver organs is victims of head trauma who are declared brain-dead. Organs are accepted from those sixty years of age or younger who have no viral, bacterial, or fungal infections and who were otherwise healthy up to the time of death. In the United States, recipient-donor matches are made through a nationwide organ transplantation registry, with highest priority going to those most critically ill. Only twelve to eighteen hours can elapse between organ retrieval and implantation; beyond that, liver tissue begins to degenerate.

The use of immunosuppressive therapy, drugs that keep the recipient's immune system in check, has contributed significantly to success and survival. Rejection of the transplanted organ remains one of the most feared postoperative complications, along with hemorrhaging. Because the body recognizes the organ as foreign tissue, the immune system's white blood cells attack and damage the implanted donor liver. The use of drugs to counteract this process allows the new liver to heal and the body to adapt to the presence of foreign tissue. Despite the use of these potent drugs, which themselves have serious side effects, rejection continues to be a problem. Nevertheless, one-year survival rates are 87 percent, and at five years, 73 percent of transplant patients are alive.

—Connie Rizzo, M.D., Ph.D.
updated by James P. McKenna, M.D.

See also Abdomen; Abdominal disorders; Alcoholism; Cirrhosis; Hepatitis; Jaundice; Liver; Liver cancer; Liver transplantation; Nonalcoholic steatohepatitis (NASH); Wilson's disease.

For Further Information:

American Liver Foundation. http://www.liverfoundation.org.
Blumberg, Baruch S. *Hepatitis B: The Hunt for a Killer Virus.* Princeton, N.J.: Princeton University Press, 2003.
Chopra, Sanjiv. *Dr. Sanjiv Chopra's Liver Book: A Comprehensive Guide to Diagnosis, Treatment, and Recovery.* New York: Simon & Schuster, 2002.
Feldman, Mark, Lawrence S. Friedman, and Lawrence J. Brandt, eds. *Sleisenger and Fordtran's Gastrointestinal and Liver Disease: Pathophysiology, Diagnosis, Management.* 9th ed. 2 vols. Philadelphia: Saunders/Elsevier, 2010.
Fishman, Mark, et al. *Medicine.* 5th ed. Philadelphia: Lippincott Williams & Wilkins, 2004.
Goldman, Lee, and Dennis Ausiello, eds. *Cecil Textbook of Medicine.* 23d ed. Philadelphia: Saunders/Elsevier, 2007.
"Liver Diseases." *MedlinePlus,* October 2, 2012.
Longstreth, George F., and David Zieve. "Hepatic Encephalopathy." *MedlinePlus,* October 16, 2011.
Yamada, Tadataka, et al., eds. *Textbook of Gastroenterology.* 5th ed. Hoboken, N.J.: Blackwell, 2009.

LIVER TRANSPLANTATION

Procedure

Anatomy or system affected: Abdomen, gallbladder, liver
Specialties and related fields: Gastroenterology, general surgery
Definition: Surgery performed to replace a diseased, nonfunctional liver with one that is healthy and capable of carrying out normal liver functions.

Key terms:

bile: fluid produced by the liver and stored in the gallbladder to be secreted into the intestine; contains salts, bile pigments (bilirubin), cholesterol, and other waste products

cirrhosis: a severe degenerative condition in which healthy liver tissue is replaced with nonfunctional scar tissue; alcohol and drug abuse are the most common causes

hepatic: of or referring to the liver

hepatitis: inflammation of the liver

jaundice: a yellowish coloration of the skin and mucous membranes caused by high levels of bilirubin in the blood; the result of liver malfunction

Indications and Procedures

Liver transplantation is performed on individuals whose livers are severely diseased and unable to carry out normal liver functions. The most common cause of liver failure in adults is cirrhosis, which results from alcohol and/or drug abuse. In this condition, the liver becomes filled with tough, nonfunctional scar tissue. Symptoms of cirrhosis, as well as other liver diseases, include abnormal levels of liver enzymes in the blood, jaundice, a lack of blood-clotting factors, the inability to dispose of bile, and the failure to detoxify metabolic by-products and other poisons, which can lead to coma and death. Other conditions that can lead to liver disease include hepatic cancer, long-term hepatitis B infection, and obstruction of the bile passages in the liver.

The donor liver may be obtained from a recently deceased individual, or a section of the liver can be obtained from a living donor. In either case, the donated organ must be a close immunological match to reduce the chance of transplant rejection. A preoperative injection is given to the recipient to dry up internal fluids and promote drowsiness, and general anesthesia is administered. A vertical incision is made from just below the breastbone to the navel. Muscles are moved aside, and a second incision is made through the outer membranous lining of the body cavity, revealing the internal organs. Bypass tubes are inserted into the hepatic veins and connected to veins in the arm to divert the flow of blood from the liver. When this is completed, the hepatic veins are cut, and the liver and gallbladder are removed from the body cavity. The veins of the donor liver are connected to the recipient veins, and the bypass tubes are removed. The new liver is then connected to the intestine, and the incisions are closed.

Uses and Complications

Liver transplantation is performed only when the individual has no other chance for survival. Typically, there is a long waiting list for available organs. Certain factors such as blood type and protein markers on cell surfaces must be matched as closely as possible in order to avoid rejection by the recipient's immune system. A liver from a recently deceased donor may be kept functioning only for five hours with specific cooling fluid, thus limiting its ability to be transported long distances. Because of the lack of available transplant organs and the necessity of compatibility, many people die before an appropriate organ becomes available. It is possible to transplant a segment of liver from a close relative; the liver can grow considerably and regenerate itself. This is a preferable situation and eliminates the pressure of transporting a donor liver between hospitals while attempting to keep it functioning.

After liver transplantation, the patient is kept in an intensive care unit for several days and in bed for at least a week. Pain from the incisions is alleviated with drugs. Rejection is the major danger, even with closely matched donor organs. Drugs such as cyclosporine are administered to suppress the immune system and, in most cases, must be taken for life. These immunosuppressive drugs inhibit the normal functioning of the immune system, thus making the individual much more susceptible to frequent—and more severe—infections, including bacterial, fungal, and viral infections. Other possible complications of the long-term use of immunosuppressive drugs include cataracts, impaired wound healing, peptic ulcers, and steroid-induced diabetes mellitus. About 20 percent of patients suffer graft rejection, obstruction of the arteries, or infection. In the case of serious complications, another transplantation may be the patient's only hope for survival. In successful surgeries, patients are able to return to normal, active lives within a few weeks of the surgery.

Perspective and Prospects

The first successful liver transplantation procedure was performed in 1967. Nevertheless, this surgery was considered an experimental procedure until 1983, when a National Institutes of Health (NIH) conference on liver transplantation accepted it as a routine procedure. In 1984, more than 250 liver transplantations were performed in the United States. Within five years, that number increased dramatically, to 2,188 transplantation procedures performed in 1989; by 2002, the number had climbed to more than 5,300 transplants and has risen to an average of about 6,000 per year. Long-term results are steadily improving; about 70 percent of recipients survive for five years or more. Improvements in survival rates are attributable to improved methods of preserving donor livers, the advent of living donor transplantation, better methods to prevent graft rejection, more suitable selection of recipients (for example, hepatic cancer patients typically have a high rate of recurrence of the disease in their transplanted liver), and improved surgical techniques.

Future prospects include further improvements in surgical techniques and advanced drug therapy to prevent graft rejection but not totally compromise the disease-fighting ability of the patient's immune system. Efforts at public education regarding the need for donor organs may cause more individuals to contact donor organ societies, family, and friends regarding their wishes to donate organs in the event of untimely death. In addition, improved treatments for the diseases that lead to liver failure may help to decrease the need for this surgical procedure.

—*Karen E. Kalumuck, Ph.D.*

See also Abdomen; Abdominal disorders; Alcoholism; Circulation; Cirrhosis; Gastroenterology; Gastroenterology, pediatric; Gastrointestinal disorders; Gastrointestinal system; Hepatitis; Internal medicine; Jaundice; Liver; Liver disorders; Nonalcoholic steatohepatitis (NASH); Transplantation.

For Further Information:

Ahmed, Moustafa. *Surviving Liver Diseases: Life with a Liver Transplant*. London: MegaZette, 1999.

Belzer, Folkert O., and Hans W. Sollinger. "Immunology and Transplantation." In *Basic Surgery*, edited by Hiram C. Polk, Jr., H. Harlan Stone, and Bernard Gardner. 5th ed. St. Louis, Mo.: Quality Medical, 1995.

Griffith, H. Winter. *Complete Guide to Symptoms, Illness, and Surgery*. 6th ed. New York: Perigee, 2012.

Haerens, Margaret. *Organ Donation*. Detroit: Greenhaven Press, 2013.

Mulholland, Michael W., et al., eds. *Greenfield's Surgery: Scientific Principles and Practice*. 5th ed. Philadelphia: Lippincott Williams & Wilkins, 2011.

National Digestive Diseases Information Clearinghouse. "What I Need to Know About Liver Transplantation." *US Department of Health and Human Services*, May 10, 2012.

United Network for Organ Sharing. http://www.unos .org.

Youngson, Robert M. *The Surgery Book: An Illustrated Guide to Seventy-three of the Most Common Operations*. New York: St. Martin's Press, 1997.

Zaman, Atif. *Managing the Complications of Cirrhosis: A Practical Approach*. Thorofare, N.J.: SLACK, 2012.

Zollinger, Robert M., Jr., and Robert M. Zollinger, Sr. *Zollinger's Atlas of Surgical Operations*. 9th ed. New York: McGraw-Hill, 2011.

LOCAL ANESTHESIA

Procedure

Also known as: Peripheral nerve block

Anatomy or system affected: Nerves, nervous system

Specialties and related fields: Anesthesiology, dentistry, dermatology, emergency medicine

Definition: A method of numbing a small area of the body for pain relief or prevention during surgical procedures.

Key terms:

anesthetic: a pharmacologic agent used to block nerve conduction and reduce sensations

injection: administration into the skin, muscle, or blood vessels via needle

local: for a drug effect, confined to a small area near the administration site

neurotoxicity: an excessive or unwanted effect of too much anesthetic drug on the nerves

topical: applied directly onto the skin to be absorbed into the area around the nerve tips

Indications and Procedures

Local anesthesia is the application of numbing agents to temporarily reduce or remove transmission of nerve sensations for short surgery or other localized procedures. A secondary use is continuous infusion administration for temporary relief of acute or chronic pain conditions. Local anesthesia in its truest form is limited to small body areas; conduction, or regional, anesthesia simply extends localized administration to a larger body area. The anesthetic agents can be applied to the skin topically or can be injected under the skin into tissue directly around a nerve ending. Both methods provide short-term blockage of sensations between peripheral nerve endings or bundles and the brain by interacting with sodium ion channels around the nerve-conduction pathways; the local anesthetics alter ion gradients across cell walls at the site to prevent nerves from conducting sensory information. Local anesthetics in any form do not provide sedation or whole-body effects, because they affect the peripheral nervous system, in contrast with the sedative effects of general anesthesia on the central nervous system. The duration of the nerve block may be proportional to the amount or rate of drug administered and the potency of the anesthetic selected; however, the intensity and duration of effect also may vary depending on type of drug, administration site and method (for example, topical administration is less intense than tissue injection), size of the nerve sheaths affected (for example, smaller sheaths or individual, rather than bundled, nerves may react more intensely to similar doses), and interactions with other drugs (for example, antihypertensive medications) or conditions.

The two main classes of local anesthetics are the esters and the amides, which have similar aromatic and amine groups in the chemical structures but differ in the intermediate group. Esters, which include procaine (Novocaine) and benzocaine, are hydrolyzed during breakdown, whereas amides, which include lidocaine and bupivicaine, are broken down by cytochrome enzymes in the liver. Both types come as sprays, patches, creams or lotions, and injections that generally have half-lives of less than two hours. Both can be given with vasoconstrictors, such as epinephrine, to slow blood-vessel distribution of the anesthetic away from local tissue and to improve the duration of the numbing effect at the application site.

Uses and Complications

In a surgical context, local anesthesia is most often used for dental, minor surgical, and emergency procedures. Emergency-department techniques such as sutures may require topical agents or an injection into the tissue for deeper or longer suturing. Many types of invasive dental procedures, such as cavity fillings and root canals, require anesthetic injection over a large area of nerve bundles in the oral cavity. Dermatologic procedures such as mole removal require topical or injected anesthetic nerve block at nerve endings. Topical skin numbing prior to drug injections is also common, such as topical lidocaine/prilocaine cream applied before vaccines given to children. Spinal anesthesia procedures block the peripheral nervous system conduction directly where the peripheral and central nervous systems meet to prevent sensation during cesarean section deliveries, cytoscopies, and other pelvic procedures for which general anesthesia is not required. After the anesthetic is administered by skin absorption or injection, nerve block typically occurs within approximately fifteen minutes and ranges from blockage of pain sensations only to full blockage of pain and temperature sensitivity. The extent of numbness is proportional to the potency and dose administered, with pain inhibition followed sequentially by touch, heat, and muscle-control inhibition.

Use of local anesthesia for pain is less common. Continuous catheter infusion with low doses of local anesthetics provides relief of acute pain, such as during treatment of a patient who has experienced trauma, and may have fewer side effects than analgesic treatments. Chronic pain may be successfully numbed by similar use of anesthesia, but as yet there is no evidence of long-term effects beyond the time of administration.

Although topical or local injected applications are safer than generalized anesthesia, or sedation, risks are still present. Allergy to para-aminobenzoic acid (PABA) can cause a cross-reaction to ester anesthetics, because hydrolysis of an ester anesthetic releases PABA as a breakdown product. Although rare, allergy to amide anesthetics is also possible; both allergies can manifest as a rash, wheezing, or even anaphylactic shock. Common side effects of both anesthetic drug classes are shallow breathing, altered heart rate, anxiety, tremors, dizziness, prolonged numbness, and tinnitus (ringing sensation in the ear). Although unlikely, central nervous system depression with associated bradycardia and cardiac depression are possible, especially with extremely high doses or rates of administration. Potentially irreversible nerve-conduction block can occur within five minutes of toxic doses of anesthesia, and methemoglobinemia—evidenced by shortness of breath, fatigue, dizziness, and weakness—has occurred with benzocaine in particular. Such extreme side effects are more likely to occur if the patient has preexisting renal or liver problems that prevent adequate drug clearance, is pregnant, or is very young or very old. Improper injection into the vascular system or directly into a nerve sheath can also lead to these toxicities. Typically, however, nerve block from the correct application of local anesthetics will reverse on its own within a few hours.

Perspective and Prospects

Since the isolation of cocaine from coca plants in the late 1800s, interest in using chemical agents to reduce sensory effects without sedation has grown substantially. Procaine was derived from cocaine in 1904 by Alfred Einhorn to reduce toxicity associated with cocaine use; the more concentrated amide drug lidocaine, still one of the most widely used local anesthetic agents, followed in 1943, and others in the amide class have improved upon the potency of lidocaine. Local anesthetics have since played an expanding role in medicine, from large-area nerve blocks for cesarean deliveries to short-term relief as a treatment for chronic pain via catheter infusion. In the twenty-first century, efforts to standardize office-based anesthesia are developing because of the prevalence of local anesthesia administration for routine outpatient skin, dental, and minor surgical procedures.

Long-term local anesthesia is being developed that could provide numbing effects for as long as two to three days, with research focused mainly on the natural agent saxitoxin. Such extended localized numbness would provide pain relief throughout a procedure and afterward during the period of most acute pain and recovery time. Saxitoxin is unrelated to cocaine and the other amide and ester agents; it is found in many varieties of fish and works by blocking transmission at extracellular, rather than intracellular, sodium channels.

—*Nicole M. Van Hoey, Pharm.D.*

See also Acupuncture; Anesthesia; Anesthesiology; Dermatology; Narcotics; Nervous system; Neurology; Neurology, pediatric; Pain; Pain management; Pharmacology; Surgery, general; Surgical procedures.

For Further Information:

"Anesthesia." *MedlinePlus*, May 2, 2013.

Auletta, Michael J., and Roy C. Grekin. *Local Anesthesia for Dermatologic Surgery*. New York: Churchill Livingstone, 1991.

Dinehart, Scott M. "Topical, Local, and Regional Anesthesia." In *Cutaneous Surgery*, edited by Ronald G. Wheeland. Philadelphia: W. B. Saunders, 1994.

Epstein-Barash, Hila, et al. "Prolonged Duration Local Anesthesia with Minimal Toxicity." *Proceedings of the National Academy of Sciences* 106, no. 17 (April 28, 2009): 7125–7130.

Feldman, J. M., J. S. Gravenstein, and I. Kalli, eds. *Office-Based Anesthesia Safety*. Special issue of *Anesthesia Patient Safety Foundation Newsletter* 15, no. 1 (Spring, 2000).

Huang, Wilber, and Allison Vidimos. "Topical Anesthetics in Dermatology." *Journal of the American Academy of Dermatology* 43, no. 2 (August, 2000): 286–298.

Larson, Merlin D. "History of Anesthetic Practice." In *Miller's Anesthesia*, edited by Ronald D. Miller et al. 7th ed. New York: Churchill Livingstone/Elsevier, 2010.

Malamed, Stanley F. *Handbook of Local Anesthesia*. 6th ed. St. Louis, Mo.: Mosby/Elsevier, 2013.

Marx, John A., et al., eds. *Rosen's Emergency Medicine: Concepts and Clinical Practice*. 7th ed. Philadelphia: Mosby/Elsevier, 2009.

McCoy, Krisha, and Rosalyn Carson-DeWitt. "Regional Anesthesia." *Health Library*, December 30, 2011.

LOCKJAW. *See* TETANUS.

LOU GEHRIG'S DISEASE. *See* AMYOTROPHIC LATERAL SCLEROSIS.

LONGEVITY

Also known as: Life span, life expectancy
Anatomy or system affected: All
Specialties and related fields: Gerontology, ethics, philosophy
Definition: A broad concept that encompasses the progressive biopsychosocial changes associated with advancing age. The average lifespan expected under ideal conditions.
Key term:
life expectancy: the average lifespan expected of a group

Overview

Lifespan or life expectancy are terms that are often used synonymously with longevity, although life expectancy is used more commonly when referring to demographics and population data, while longevity is a more philosophical term and perhaps less well-defined.

It has been speculated that with age comes wisdom: the culmination of years of experience, memories, and lessons learned informs a person's perspective on life and what kind of legacy one wants to leave behind. Conversely, the process of aging also increases a person's risk of dying: Many theories suggest that years of physical and emotional (internal), and environmental (external) influences render a person more susceptible to acute illness or the development of chronic disease. Today, modern medicine-pharmaceuticals, therapies, technology-has the capability to extend life well beyond previously held norms: The average life expectancy in the United States is eighty-one for women and seventy-six for men, and the eighty-five-year-old and older population is now the fastest growing population in much of the developed world. With the technological advances that have been made, it begs the relevant question: Can aging be cured? And if it can, should it?

The concept of longevity, the progression from birth to death, has been recognized by human beings for hundreds of years, but the ethical discussion of whether or not we should exercise the right to live as long as possible is a relatively new one. Charles Darwin, the English naturalist and major contributor to the theory of human evolution, would argue that death is the result of natural selection; a process that is expected and a natural happenstance when adverse events suffered outmatch the ability of the body to sustain life. Longevity has also been explored in fictional literature. Shakespeare often depicted a person's life as a series of "roles" acted out on the societal stage, roles that are gradually lost as old age progresses until death finally arrives-the final act. Less metaphorically, Jonathan Swift's popular novel Gulliver's Travels relates the story of the Struldbrugs, a nation of humans that never die but still suffer the ravages of time and advancing age, eventually sightless, demented, crippled, as the body deteriorates but death never arrives-living but not living. While graphic and extreme, perhaps modern-day Struldbrugs can be identified in hospitals across the developed world as machines and technology are often utilized to sustain quantity of life but do little to preserve quality of life.

Further inquiry in the fields of population biology, psychology, ethics, and anthropology will undoubtedly lend new insights into the evolving concept of longevity.

—*Christopher J. Norman, B.A., B.S.N., R.N.-B.C., B.C.*

See also Aging; Aging, Extended care; Chronobiology; Death and Dying; Developmental stages; Epidemiology; Euthanasia; Extended care; Geriatrics and gerontology; Hospice; Palliative medicine; Resuscitation; Terminally ill

For Further Information:
Albert, Steven M., and Vicki A. Freedman. *Public Health and Aging: Maximizing Function and Well-Being.* 2nd ed. New York: Springer, 2010.
Moody, H.R. *Aging: Concepts and Controversies.* 6th ed. Los Angeles: Pine Forge Press, 2010.
Thomas, William H. *What Are Old People For? How Elders Will Save the World.* Acton, MA: Vanderwyk & Burnham, 2007.

LOWER EXTREMITIES
Anatomy
Anatomy or system affected: Bones, feet, hips, knees, legs, lymphatic system, musculoskeletal system, nerves, nervous system, skin
Specialties and related fields: Neurology, orthopedics, physical therapy, podiatry
Definition: The thighs, lower legs, and feet; the lower extremities are attached to the pelvis at the hip joint and consist of muscles, bones, blood vessels, lymph vessels, nerves, skin, and toenails.
Key terms:
distal: farther away from the base or attached end
femur: the thigh bone
fibula: the smaller of the two bones in the lower leg, on the lateral side
knee: the joint between the thigh and the lower leg
lateral: on the outer side; toward the little toe when in reference to the leg
leg: the lower extremity, excluding the foot; the lower leg runs from the knee to the ankle
medial: on the side toward the midline; toward the big toe when in reference to the leg
proximal: closer to the base or attached end
tarsus: the ankle
thigh: the upper segment of the leg, from the hip joint to the knee
tibia: the larger of the two bones in the lower leg, on the medial side

Structure and Functions
The lower extremities consist of the thighs, lower legs, and feet. Each extremity attaches to the pelvis (innominate bone) at the hip joint. The lower extremity is made mostly of bones and muscles, but it also contains blood vessels, lymphatics, nerves, skin, toenails, and other structures. Important directional terms for the lower extremity include proximal (closer to the base or attached end), distal (further from the base or attached end), medial (on the same side as the tibia and big toe), and lateral (on the same side as the fibula and little toe). Along the foot, the lower surface is called plantar; the upper surface is called dorsal. The lower extremity is clothed in skin (or integument). The sole or plantar surface of the foot is unusual, along with the palm of the hand, in being completely hairless; it also contains the thickest outer skin layer (the stratum corneum) of any part of the body. Each toe has a hardened toenail on its dorsal surface.

The pelvic girdle that supports the lower extremity develops as three separate bones: the ilium, ischium, and pubis. All three help form the acetabulum, a socket into which the femur fits. Below the acetabulum, the ischium and pubis surround a large opening called the obturator foramen. The right and left pubis meet to form a pubic symphysis. The bones of the lower extremity include the femur, tibia, fibula, tarsals, metatarsals, and phalanges. The femur (thigh bone) is the largest bone in the body. Its rounded upper end, or head, fits into the acetabulum and is attached by a short neck. A rough-surfaced greater trochanter lies just beyond this neck and serves for the attachment of many muscles. The lesser trochanter, also for muscle attachments, lies just below the neck. The knee joint is covered and protected by the kneecap, or patella, the largest of the sesamoid bones formed within tendons at points of stress. The lower leg, from the knee to the ankle, contains two bones: the tibia on the medial side and the more slender fibula on the lateral side. The tarsus, or ankle, includes the talus, calcaneus, and five smaller bones. The talus (or astragalus) has a pulleylike facet for the tibia and other curved surfaces for articulation with the calcaneus and navicular. The calcaneus, or heel bone, is vertically enlarged in humans; the Achilles tendon attaches to its roughened lower tuberosity. Smaller tarsal bones include the navicular, the medial (or inner) cuneiform, the intermediate cuneiform, the lateral (or outer) cuneiform, and the cuboid. Beyond the tarsal bones, the foot is supported by five metatarsal bones. The big toe, or hallux, contains two phalanges; each of the remaining toes contains three phalanges.

The muscles of the lower extremity include extensors, which straighten joints, and flexors, which bend joints. Abductor muscles move the limbs sideways, away from the midline, while adductors pull the limbs back, toward the midline. The muscles of the iliac region attach the lower extremity to the body. The psoas major runs from the lumbar vertebrae to the lesser trochanter of the femur. The iliacus runs from the ilium and part of the sacrum to the femur, including the lesser trochanter. The anterior muscles of the thigh include the sartorius, the quadriceps femoris, and the articularis genus. The sartorius, the longest muscle in the body, flexes both hip and knee joints. It runs obliquely from the anterior border of the ilium across the front of the thigh to insert onto the medial side of the knee at the upper end of the tibia. The quadriceps femoris consists of the rectus femoris and the three vastus muscles; all four are strong extensors of the knee. The rectus femoris originates from the region surrounding the acetabulum. The vastus lateralis, vastus medialis, and vastus intermedius muscles all originate along the shaft of the femur. All four quadriceps muscles insert onto a common tendon that runs over the knee and inserts onto the top of the tibia. The patella is a sesamoid bone enclosed within this tendon where it runs over the front of the knee. The smaller articularis genus muscle originates on the anterior side of the shaft of the femur; it inserts onto the kneecap.

The extensor muscles of the hip and thigh help to maintain upright posture. The gluteus maximus, the largest of these muscles, originates from the posterior portion of the ilium and inserts high on the femur, especially onto the greater trochanter. The gluteus medius and gluteus minimis both originate from the outer surface of the ilium and insert onto the greater trochanter. The tensor fasciae latae originates along the iliac crest; it inserts onto a broad, sheetlike tendon (the fascia lata) which covers much of the lateral surface of the thigh. The piriformis runs from the sacrum to the greater trochanter of the femur. The obturator internus runs from the inner surface of the pelvis through the obturator foramen to the greater trochanter of the femur. The gemellus superior and the gemellus inferior originate from the rear margin of the ischium; they both insert onto the greater trochanter. The quadratus femoris originates from the lateral surface of the ischium; it inserts between the greater and lesser trochanters of the femur. The obturator externus originates along the outer surface of the pelvis below the obturator foramen and inserts near the greater trochanter.

The muscles on the medial (or inner) side of the thigh are all abductors of the thigh. The gracilis is a long, thin muscle that originates from the pubis, runs along the medial side of the thigh, and inserts high on the tibia. The pectineus originates anteriorly on the pubis and inserts onto the shaft of the femur below the lesser trochanter. The adductor longus originates from the pubis and inserts onto the posterior edge of the femur. The adductor brevis originates from the pubis and inserts onto the posterior edge of the femur. The adductor magnus is a large, triangular muscle that originates from the lower portion of the ischium and pubis; it expands to a long, thin insertion along the posterior edge of the femur.

The hamstring muscles run along the posterior side of the femur; they flex the knee and extend the hip joint. The biceps femoris originates from the posterior portion (the tuberosity) of the ischium and separately from the posterior edge of the femur. Both portions converge onto a common tendon that inserts primarily onto the top of the fibula. The semitendinosus originates from the posterior end of the ischium; it inserts by a long tendon onto the medial side of the tibia. The semimembranosus runs from the ischium to the posterior surface of the tibia.

The muscles on the front (anterior) side of the lower leg raise the foot by flexing it dorsally. At the ankle, their tendons are all held in place by two transverse bands, the extensor retinacula. The tibialis anterior originates along the anterior edge of the tibia; it inserts by a tendon onto the medial cuneiform and the base of the first metatarsal. The extensor hallucis longus originates from the anterior surface of the fibula; its tendon passes beneath the extensor retinacula to insert onto the distal phalanx of the big toe. The extensor digitorum longus originates near the top of the tibia and along the anterior side of the fibula. Its tendon passes beneath the extensor retinacula and splits into four tendons, inserted onto the second and third phalanges of the second through fifth digits. The peroneus tertius originates along the anterior edge of the fibula and runs alongside the extensor digitorum longus. It inserts onto the base of the fifth metatarsal bone.

The muscles on the posterior surface of the lower leg are mostly extensors of the foot; some also flex the knee. The gastrocnemius originates in two heads from opposite sides of the femur. It inserts onto the Achilles tendon, which attaches to the calcaneus. The soleus originates from the posterior surface of the fibula; it inserts onto the Achilles tendon. The plantaris originates from the posterior surface of the femur and inserts onto the posterior portion of the calcaneus. The popliteus runs from the lateral side of the femur across the back of the knee to insert onto the tibia. The flexor hallucis longus originates along the posterior surface of the fibula; its tendon runs around to the medial side of the ankle and inserts onto the base of the big toe. The flexor digitorum longus originates from the posterior surface of the tibia; its tendon crosses the sole of the foot obliquely and divides into four tendons that insert onto the distal phalanges of the second through fifth toes. The tibialis posterior originates from the posterior surfaces of the tibia, the fibula, and the interosseous membrane that joins them; its tendon passes around to insert onto the navicular bone. The peroneus longus originates along the lateral surface of the fibula; its tendon runs along a groove on the bottom of the cuboid to insert obliquely onto the base of the first metatarsal. The peroneus brevis originates along the lateral margin of the fibula; its tendon inserts onto the fifth metatarsal. The extensor digitorum brevis originates from the calcaneus and runs obliquely across the dorsal side of the foot, dividing into four tendons. One tendon inserts onto the base of the big toe; the remaining tendons insert onto the tendons of the extensor digitorum longus.

Several flexor muscles of the foot are attached to the plantar aponeurosis, a flat ligament that runs from the calcaneus along the sole of the foot to the bases of the toes and to several flexor tendons. The abductor hallucis originates from the calcaneus and the plantar aponeurosis; it inserts onto the base of the big toe. The flexor digitorum brevis originates from the plantar aponeurosis and the calcaneus; it divides into four portions, each of which gives rise to a tendon. These tendons run into the second through fifth toes, each splitting in half to insert onto opposite sides of the second phalanx, separated by the tendons of the flexor digitorum longus, which emerge between them. The abductor digiti quinti originates from the calcaneus and the plantar aponeurosis; it inserts onto the base of the fifth toe. The quadratus plantae originates from the calcaneus and inserts onto the tendons of the flexor digitorum longus. The four small lumbricals run from the tendons of the flexor digitorum longus to the corresponding tendons of the extensor digitorum longus. The flexor hallucis brevis originates from the cuboid and lateral cuneiform bones; its two portions insert onto the big toe from opposite sides. The adductor hallucis originates from the second through fourth metatarsals and also from the bases of the third through fifth toes. Its tendon inserts onto the base of the big toe. The flexor digiti quinti originates from the base of the fifth metatarsal and inserts onto the base of the fifth toe. The four dorsal interossei originate from the bases of the metatarsal bones; they insert onto the bases of the second through fourth toes. The three plantar interossei originate from the third through fifth metatarsals and run beneath these bones to insert onto the bases of the corresponding toes.

Blood vessels of the lower extremity include both arteries and veins. The common iliac arteries arise from the dorsal aorta; each divides into an internal and an external iliac. The internal iliac artery supplies many muscles of the thigh region and pelvis. The external iliac artery branches into an inferior epigastric artery and a deep iliac circumflex artery; it then continues along the femur as the femoral artery. The femoral artery gives rise to a deep femoral artery running to the medial and posterior regions of the thigh; the base of this artery also gives rise to two circumflex arteries that send branches upward into many thigh muscles. Near the knee, the femoral artery branches into a descending geniculate artery to the knee, then continues as the popliteal artery, forming several branches to the thigh muscles and other small branches to the knee before splitting into anterior and posterior tibial arteries.

The anterior tibial artery descends along the front of the tibia, forming several small branches. It then continues into the foot as the dorsalis pedis artery, giving rise to a lateral tarsal artery and an arcuate artery, both of which form arches by joining with branches of the peroneal artery. The deep plantar artery and hallucis dorsalis artery also branch from the dorsalis pedis artery, while individual arteries to the second through fourth metatarsals arise from the arcuate artery. Arterial branches to all the toes arise from the individual metatarsal arteries, including the hallucis dorsalis, forming a system of collateral circulation in which multiple alternate routes permit blood flow even if one of the routes is temporarily blocked.

The posterior tibial artery gives rise to a peroneal artery; the two arteries then run down the posterior side of the lower leg, forming small branches to the muscles of the lower leg and nutrient arteries to the tibia and fibula. The posterior tibial artery branches to the calcaneus before it splits into a medial plantar artery, which runs along the medial margin of the foot into the big toe, and a much larger lateral plantar artery. The lateral plantar artery runs across the foot obliquely to the lateral side, then turns and runs obliquely in the other direction to the base of the big toe, where it runs into the deep plantar artery to form a loop. From this loop arise a series of plantar metatarsal arteries to all five toes. Blood can reach each toe from either side, and the arch that supplies this blood can receive its blood either by way of the posterior tibial and lateral plantar arteries or by way of the anterior tibial and deep plantar arteries, providing another example of collateral circulation.

There are several important veins draining the lower extremity. The deep veins originate from a series of plantar digital veins draining the individual toes into a deep plantar venous arch. This arch is drained to either direction by a lateral plantar vein and a medial plantar vein, which later unite to form a posterior tibial vein; this vein and the peroneal vein run parallel to the corresponding arteries along the posterior side of the lower leg. An anterior tibial vein drains the anterior side of the lower leg and the dorsal side of the foot. Near the knee, the peroneal vein and the anterior and posterior tibial veins unite to form the popliteal vein, which continues into the thigh as the femoral vein. The femoral vein receives the deep femoral vein as a tributary, then the saphenous vein. The femoral vein then continues as the external iliac vein.

The lower extremity is also covered with a network of superficial veins that lie just beneath the skin. The vessels of this network are drained along the medial side of the lower leg and thigh by the great saphenous vein, which runs into the femoral vein just below the groin. The lateral side of the foot and the posterior surface of the lower leg are drained by the small saphenous vein, which drains into the popliteal vein.

The nerves to the lower extremity arise from two series of complex branchings, the lumbar plexus and sacral plexus. The largest nerve formed from the lumbar plexus is the femoral nerve, supplying muscles on the anterior side of the thigh and part of the lower leg. Other branches to the muscles include the obturator nerve to the adductor muscles and separate muscular branches to the psoas and iliacus muscles. Cutaneous sensory nerves to the skin include the lateral femoral cutaneous nerve to the lateral side of the thigh, the anterior cutaneous branches of the femoral nerve to the medial side of the thigh, and the saphenous nerve, a branch of the femoral nerve to the medial side of the lower leg.

The sacral plexus gives rise to the very large sciatic nerve and to several smaller nerves, including the superior gluteal and inferior gluteal nerves to the gluteal muscles, and separate muscular branches to the piriformis, quadratus femoris, obturator internus, and gemelli. Cutaneous branches such as the posterior femoral cutaneous nerve supply sensory fibers to the skin on the posterior surface of the thigh. The sciatic nerve, the largest nerve in the body, branches off to the hamstring muscles before splitting into tibial and peroneal nerves. The tibial nerve supplies the muscles on the posterior side of the lower leg and then runs onto the sole of the foot, where it splits into the medial and lateral plantar nerves, which together supply both cutaneous sensation and muscular innervation to the sole of the foot. The peroneal nerve divides into deep and superficial portions. The deep peroneal nerve supplies the muscles on the anterior side of the lower leg and the dorsal surface of the foot. The superficial peroneal nerve supplies cutaneous sensation to the lateral surface of the lower leg and the dorsal surface of the foot.

Disorders and Diseases

Many medical conditions and disorders affect the lower extremity; these include animal bites (including snakebites), injuries, fungus infections such as athlete's foot, contact dermatitis (including poison ivy), and an assortment of neuromuscular disorders, including nerve paralyses, muscular atrophies, and muscular dystrophies. Nerve paralyses of the lower extremities usually arise from traumatic injury.

Muscular atrophies are diseases in which muscle tissues become progressively weaker and smaller, usually beginning after the age of forty. Spastic movements sometimes occur. The small muscles of the hands and feet are usually affected sooner and more severely in comparison to the larger muscles of the legs and thighs. Amyotrophic lateral sclerosis (ALS), commonly known as Lou Gehrig's disease, is one such disease that usually begins with weakness and deterioration of the distal muscles. The disease proceeds to affect the rest of the extremities, then other parts of the body; it is usually fatal within three to five years after onset. A more rare type of atrophy, myelopathic muscular atrophy (or Aran-Duchenne atrophy), affects both upper and lower extremities and eventually spreads to the trunk. A degenerative lesion of the gray matter in the cervical region of the spinal cord is usually responsible.

Muscular dystrophy is a series of inherited diseases that begin in early childhood, affecting males more often than females. The most common type, Duchenne muscular dystrophy, is caused by a sex-linked recessive trait that impairs the body's ability to synthesize a large protein called dystrophin. Muscular dystrophy primarily affects the large muscles of the thigh and lower leg, impairing the ability to stand unassisted or to walk. The affected muscles become very weak but remain approximately normal in size and may even increase as muscle tissue is replaced by fatty and fibrous tissue. Progressive weakening makes walking and similar motor functions impossible, but, with proper care, patients can live for decades.

Sports injuries often occur in the lower extremities and are generally treated by orthopedic specialists. Fractured bones are generally set in casts and kept immobile until they heal. Injured or ruptured ligaments often require surgical treatment. Snakebites and other animal bites occur more often to the lower extremities than to other parts of the body. The bites of poisonous snakes must be treated quickly, before the venom reaches the heart. The patient must be kept calm and quiet, and experienced medical attention should be sought as soon as possible.

Perspective and Prospects

The major muscles and bones of the lower extremities were studied in ancient societies by such individuals as Galen (or Caius Galenus), the physician to the Roman army in the second century. The science of anatomy took many great strides because of the efforts of artists, who studied the human body in order to create realistic sculptures and paintings. During the Renaissance, Leonardo da Vinci (1452–1519) and Michelangelo (1475–1564) dissected human corpses illegally in their quest for this knowledge. Andreas Vesalius (1514–64) produced the first well-illustrated anatomical texts, containing information that corrected many of the errors made by Galen.

Injuries to the leg are generally treated surgically. Whenever possible, broken bones are set in place, immobilized in a cast, and then allowed to heal. Muscles (or their tendons) must be sewn together. Nerve endings must be matched with their former locations if they are to grow back correctly. Gangrene, or tissue death from lack of circulation, occurs more often in the lower extremities than in the upper extremities. When the lower extremity is gangrenous or is injured beyond repair, an amputation is often performed. Artificial legs or partial legs are sometimes attached to the lower extremity.

—*Eli C. Minkoff, Ph.D.*

See also Amputation; Arthritis; Arthroplasty; Arthroscopy; Bone cancer; Bone disorders; Bone grafting; Bones and the skeleton; Bowlegs; Braces, orthopedic; Bunions; Bursitis; Casts and splints; Deep vein thrombosis; Feet; Flat feet; Foot disorders; Fracture and dislocation; Fracture repair; Frostbite; Grafts and grafting; Hammertoe correction; Hammertoes; Heel spur removal; Hemiplegia; Hip fracture repair; Hip replacement; Joints; Kneecap removal; Knock-knees; Ligaments; Liposuction; Motor skill development; Muscle sprains, spasms, and disorders; Muscles; Nail removal; Nails; Orthopedic surgery; Orthopedics; Orthopedics, pediatric; Osgood-Schlatter disease; Osteoarthritis; Osteochondritis juvenilis; Osteogenesis imperfecta; Osteopathic medicine; Paralysis; Paraplegia; Physical rehabilitation; Pigeon toes; Podiatry; Poliomyelitis; Prostheses; Quadriplegia; Restless legs syndrome; Rheumatoid arthritis; Rheumatology; Rickets; Tendon disorders; Tendon repair; Upper extremities; Varicose vein removal.

For Further Information:

Agur, Anne M. R., and Arthur F. Dalley. *Grant's Atlas of Anatomy*. 13th ed. Philadelphia: Wolters Kluwer Health/Lippincott Williams & Wilkins, 2013.

Brummett, Chad M., and Steven P. Cohen. *Managing Pain: Essentials of Diagnosis and Treatment*. New York: Oxford University Press, 2013.

Crouch, James E. *Functional Human Anatomy*. 4th ed. Philadelphia: Lea & Febiger, 1985.

Currey, John D. *Bones: Structures and Mechanics*. 2d ed. Princeton, N.J.: Princeton University Press, 2006.

Iyer, K. Mohan. *Orthopedics of the Upper and Lower Limb*. New York: Springer, 2013.

Kim, Daniel H., Alan R. Hudson, and David G. Kline. *Atlas of Peripheral Nerve Surgery*. Philadelphia: Elsevier/Saunders, 2013.

Marieb, Elaine N. *Essentials of Human Anatomy and Physiology*. 10th ed. San Francisco: Pearson/Benjamin Cummings, 2012.

Rosse, Cornelius, and Penelope Gaddum-Rosse. *Hollinshead's Textbook of Anatomy*. 5th ed. Philadelphia: Lippincott-Raven, 1997.

Standring, Susan, et al., eds. *Gray's Anatomy*. 40th ed. New York: Churchill Livingstone/Elsevier, 2008.

Van De Graaff, Kent M. *Human Anatomy*. 6th ed. New York: McGraw-Hill, 2002.

LUMBAR PUNCTURE
Procedure

Also known as: Spinal tap

Anatomy or system affected: Brain, nerves, nervous system, spine

Specialties and related fields: Anesthesiology, biochemistry, critical care, general surgery, neurology, oncology, pathology

Definition: A process in which the physician places a hollow needle into the lower part of the spinal canal, either to harvest cerebrospinal fluid for diagnosis or to inject substances into the spinal canal.

Key terms:

aneurysm: ballooning within an artery or vein that protrudes through a weak spot

angiogram: film on which images of blood vessels treated with a medium that is opaque to X rays become visible

cerebrospinal fluid (CSF): watery fluid that surrounds the brain and the spinal cord

meningeal irritation: inflammation of the meninges, or membranes surrounding the brain and spinal cord

meningitis: inflammation of the membranes of the brain or spinal cord

myelography: X-ray examination of the spinal cord, tissues, and nerves within the spinal canal

subarachnoid hemorrhage: a condition in which blood from a ruptured cranial blood vessel invades the surface of the brain

vertebrae: pieces of bone or cartilage of which the backbone or spine is composed

xanthochromic spinal fluid: yellowish CSF, indicating either an abnormally high protein level or a brain hemorrhage

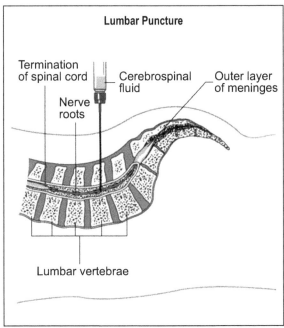

A lumbar puncture, commonly known as a spinal tap, is a diagnostic procedure in which cerebrospinal fluid is extracted from the meninges of the spine and analyzed for the presence of infection.

Indications and Procedures

A lumbar puncture, often referred to as a spinal tap, is indicated for the diagnosis of meningitis because it is the best method for detecting meningeal irritation. A laboratory examination of the cerebrospinal fluid (CSF) harvested through a lumbar puncture can detect problems relating to the brain and spinal cord. Meningitis cannot be diagnosed through imaging methods such as computed tomography (CT) scanning.

Similarly, some subarachnoid (brain) hemorrhages involve the loss of so little blood that they are not detectable radiologically. When this is the case, the CSF may contain small amounts of blood that continues to be present in successive testing. If diagnosis is delayed, then the blood from a subarachnoid hemorrhage may have dissipated, making the CSF yellowish. This signifies that the blood in it is being metabolized. When this is the case, an immediate angiogram is indicated.

CSF withdrawn through a lumbar puncture should be examined immediately by a pathologist or hematologist to determine if blood is present or, if it is xanthochromic or yellowish, to ascertain if the protein level is abnormally high or a subarachnoid hemorrhage exists and blood is spreading over the surface of the brain. Such leakage may indicate an aneurysm and generally requires prompt surgery.

Although lumbar puncture is essentially a diagnostic tool, it is sometimes indicated when CSF has built up to dangerous levels in the spinal canal and the patient is hydrocephalic. In such instances, excess CSF can be withdrawn from the spinal canal, but it is imperative that the cause of the buildup be immediately determined and treated.

Patients undergoing lumbar punctures lie on their side, with their chin down and their knees drawn up to separate the vertebrae. Local anesthetic is used to numb the area surrounding the lower vertebrae. A hollow needle is inserted between two lower vertebrae and pushed into the spinal canal. The entire procedure takes about twenty minutes and involves minimal discomfort. The puncture wound left by the needle is covered with a sterile bandage. Patients may experience a headache following the procedure, but it usually disappears quickly. If it does not disappear within a few days, a small amount of the patient's blood can be injected into the site, creating a patch that should eliminate the headache.

Uses and Complications

Lumbar puncture is used to inject dyes into the spinal canal to serve as a contrast medium in diagnostic procedures involving x-rays, particularly myelography. It is also used to introduce medications into the CSF for the treatment of certain types of cancer. This use, often appropriate in cases of leukemia and carcinomas of the nervous system, is frequently employed in pediatric care.

Some surgical procedures require that patients be awake during surgery. In such cases, local anesthetics are introduced into the spinal canal through lumbar puncture, allowing patients to remain conscious while rendering them insensate.

As with any invasive procedure, there is risk of infection, but it is minimal. The procedure is performed under sterile conditions. One danger, in the case of a subarachnoid hemorrhage, is blood loss. Bleeding, in rare cases, may become uncontrollable and result in death. One cautionary note is that a lumbar puncture should never be performed in cases where a brain abscess is suspected unless reliable CT scans or other tests have failed to reveal a mass or reveal only a small mass.

Lumbar puncture in and of itself is not a high-risk procedure, although the conditions that require its use often involve high risks for the patient. It is advisable in most cases that the procedure be performed in a location where immediate surgery can be carried out if the patient's condition deteriorates suddenly.

Perspective and Prospects

The earliest use of CSF in diagnosis was in the nineteenth century, when such primitive tools as sharpened bird quills were used to penetrate the lumbar region. The technique came into its own in the mid-twentieth century, when most problems of the central nervous system were diagnosed through an examination of the CSF.

Because of the importance of CSF in diagnosing meningitis, cerebral hemorrhages, and other dangerous conditions, the lumbar puncture procedure has seen considerable progress and become increasingly sophisticated. However, the imaging tools currently available to surgeons, neurologists, hematologists, and pathologists are so advanced and accurate that lumbar puncture is used as a diagnostic tool less often than in the past.

—*R. Baird Shuman, Ph.D.*

See also Anesthesia; Anesthesiology; Bacterial infections; Bacteriology; Biopsy; Bleeding; Diagnosis; Fluids and electrolytes; Infection; Invasive tests; Meningitis; Nervous system; Neuroimaging; Neurology; Neurology, pediatric; Neurosurgery; Spine, vertebrae, and disks; Viral infections.

For Further Information:

Bowden, Vicky R., and Cindy Smith Greenberg. *Pediatric Nursing Procedures*. 3d ed. Philadelphia: Wolters Kluwer Health/ Lippincott Williams & Wilkins, 2012.

Colyar, Margaret R. *Well-Child Assessment for Primary Care Providers*. Philadelphia: F. A. Davis, 2003.

Doherty, Gerard M., ed. *Current Diagnosis and Treatment: Surgery*. 13th ed. New York: Lange Medical Books/McGraw-Hill, 2010.

Dougherty, Lisa, and Sara E. Lister, eds. *The Royal Marsden Hospital Manual of Clinical Nursing Procedures*. 8th ed. Ames, Iowa: Wiley-Blackwell, 2011.

Dugdale, David C., Kevin Sheth, and David Zieve. "Cerebral Spinal Fluid (CSF) Collection." *MedlinePlus*, June 18, 2011.

Lukas, Rimas, and Michael Woods. "Lumbar Puncture." *Health Library*, May 20, 2013.

McAllister, Leslie D., et al. *Practical Neuro-oncology: A Guide to Patient Care*. Boston: Butterworth-Heinemann, 2002.

LUMPECTOMY. *See* MASTECTOMY AND LUMPECTOMY.

LUMPS, BREAST. *See* BREAST CANCER; BREAST DISORDERS; BREASTS, FEMALE.

LUNG CANCER
Disease/Disorder
Anatomy or system affected: Chest, lungs, lymphatic system, respiratory system

Specialties and related fields: Environmental health, immunology, occupational health, oncology, pulmonary medicine, radiology

Definition: The appearance of malignant tumors in the lungs, which is usually associated with cigarette smoking.

Causes and Symptoms

Most forms of lung cancer fall within one of four categories: squamous cell (or epidermoid) carcinomas and adenocarcinomas , small or oat cell carcinomas (accounting for about 15 percent of lung cancers), and large cell carcinomas. Each of these forms can be further categorized on the basis of cell differentiation within the tumor: either well differentiated (resembling the original cell type) or moderately or poorly differentiated. Upon biopsy, stage groupings are also determined on the basis of size, invasiveness, and possible extent of metastasis.

Oat or small cell carcinomas usually consist of small, tightly packed, spindle-shaped cells, with a high nucleus-to-cytoplasm ratio within the cell. Oat cell carcinomas tend to metastasize early and widely, often to the bone marrow or brain. As a result, by the time that symptoms become apparent, the disease is generally widely disseminated within the body. Coupled with a resistance to most common forms of radiation and chemotherapy, oat cell carcinomas present a particularly poor prognosis. In general, patients diagnosed with this form of cancer have a survival period measured, at most, in months.

Adenocarcinomas are tumors of glandlike structure, presenting as nodules within peripheral tissue such as the bronchioles. Often these forms of tumors may arise from previously damaged or scarred tissue, such as has occurred among smokers. The development of adenocarcinoma of the lung is not as dependent upon smoke inhalation, however, as are other forms of lung cancer.

Squamous cell, also called epidermoid, carcinomas tend to be slower-growing malignancies which form among the flat epithelial cells on the surface of a variety of tissues, including the bladder, cervix, or skin, in addition to the lung. The cells are often polygonal in shape, with keratin nodes on the surface of lesions. Squamous cell carcinomas tend to metastasize less frequently than other forms of lung cancer, allowing for a more optimistic prognosis.

Large cell carcinomas are actually a more general form of cancer in which the cells are relatively large in size, with the cell nucleus being particularly enlarged. Often these carcinomas have arisen as either squamous cell carcinomas or

---

Information on Lung Cancer

Causes: Smoking, exposure to other environmental toxins (asbestos, hydrocarbon products, nickel, vinyl chloride, uranium, pitchblende)

Symptoms: Persistent cough (sometimes accompanied by blood), difficulty breathing, chest pain, repeated and long-lasting attacks of bronchitis or pneumonia

Duration: Progressive and usually fatal

adenocarcinomas. Metastasis, when it occurs, is frequently within the gastrointestinal tract.

There is no question that the single leading cause or factor resulting in lung cancer is smoking. Persons who do not smoke, and indeed even smokers who smoke fewer than five cigarettes per day, are at relatively low risk of developing any form of lung cancer. Those who smoke more than five cigarettes per day run an increased risk of developing lung cancer at rates approaching two hundred times that of the non-smoker. This risk is greatest for oat cell carcinomas and least for adenocarcinomas (but still approximately a tenfold risk over that for nonsmokers). The relative risk is related to the number of cigarettes smoked: The more cigarettes, the greater the risk. In addition, though other environmental hazards can be related to the development of lung cancers, the risk associated with those hazards is without exception amplified by cigarette smoke.

Exposure to other specific environmental factors has also been associated with the formation of certain forms of pulmonary cancers. Individuals chronically exposed to materials such as asbestos, hydrocarbon products (coal tars or roofing materials), nickel, vinyl chloride, or radiochemicals (uranium and pitchblende) are at increased risk. Chronically damaged lungs, for whatever reason, are at significantly increased risk for development of cancer.

The symptoms of lung cancer may represent the damage caused by the primary tumor or may be the result of metastasis to other organs. The most common symptom is a persistent cough, sometimes accompanied by blood in the sputum or difficulty breathing. Chest pain may be present, especially upon inhalation. There may also be repeated attacks of bronchitis or pneumonia that tend to persist for abnormal periods of time.

Treatment and Therapy

Diagnosis of a tumor in the lung generally includes a chest x ray, along with use of a variety of diagnostic tests: bronchography (x-ray observation of the bronchioles following application of an opaque material), tomography (cross-sectional observation of tissue), and cytologic examination of sputum or bronchiole washings. Recent evidence indicates that low-dose CT scans can be effective in early detection of lung cancer, detecting the cancer earlier that x rays are able to. Confirmation of the diagnosis, in addition to determination of the specific type of tumor and its clinical stage, generally requires a needle biopsy of material from the lung.

The treatment of the tumor is dependent on the form of the disease and on the extent of its spread. Surgery remains the preferred method of treatment, but because of the nature of the disease, less than half the cases are operable at the time of diagnosis. Of these, a large proportion are beyond the point at which the surgical removal of the cancer and resection of remaining tissue are possible. A variety of chemotherapeutic measures are available and along with the use of radiation therapy can be used to produce a small number of cures or at least temporary alleviation of symptoms. Nevertheless, only

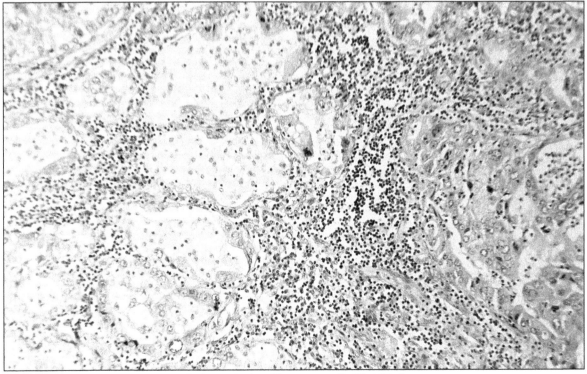

A microscopic view of lung cancer cells. (PhotoDisc)

In the News:
Lack of Lung Cancer Symptoms in Some Women

In 2006, media stories reporting the death from lung cancer of Dana Reeve, widow of actor Christopher Reeve, focused on nonsmoking women who developed that disease. Reports concentrated on risk factors, including studies addressing the possible connection of estrogen with lung cancer, to educate women regarding screening. News accounts stressed that because lung cancer was often asymptomatic in women, female patients should not rely solely on symptoms to seek medical help, noting the work of researchers striving to develop effective methods to locate early-stage lung cancer. Articles noted the limitations of chest X rays, which do not detect most early-stage lung cancer tumors.

During 2005, the media had reported development of a potentially accurate lung cancer test in which dentists, physicians, or patients scraped samples of cheek cells inside the mouth to submit to medical laboratories for automated quantitative cytometry (AQC) evaluation. Researchers emphasized the low cost of this test, which did not need special equipment to take samples.

In the spring of 2006, the media reported on findings published in the journal *Chest* that indicated tests for chronic obstructive pulmonary disease (COPD) might not reveal women had lung cancer because their lungs seemed to function normally during those tests and no symptoms were apparent. Researchers emphasized women at risk of having lung cancer should undergo other types of tests and that physicians should consider patients' age, smoking history, and environment when screening for that disease.

The media discussed the October, 2006, issue of the *New England Journal of Medicine*, which printed information regarding a New York-Presbyterian Hospital/Weill Cornell Medical College study evaluating the benefits of computed tomography (CT) scanning to detect lung cancer in asymptomatic subjects who smoked or were exposed to risk factors. This method, using low radiation dosages, alerted researchers to cancerous lung tumors in 484 of the 31,567 subjects scanned, enabling surgical removal before the cancer spread. Reports noted that because physicians could focus on small tumors, healthy lung tissue could be preserved during surgery.

Critics expressed concerns that the study lacked a control group to evaluate whether CT scans helped extend patients' life spans. They criticized the approach for resulting in unnecessary biopsies and surgeries for scan-detected tumors which later were determined to be benign, stressing that additional studies examining the role of CT scanning for lung cancer should be considered. The Lung Cancer Alliance, however, endorsed CT scans.

—Elizabeth D. Schafer, Ph.D.

a small proportion of lung cancers, perhaps 10 percent, respond with a permanent remission or cure.

Lung cancer represents the leading cause of cancer deaths among American men and women. In 2006, there were approximately 365,000 cases of lung cancer, and lung cancer accounted for 31 percent of male cancer deaths and 26 percent of female cancer deaths. The American Cancer Society predicted there would be 228,190 new cases of lung cancer in the United States in 2013. The prognosis for most forms of lung cancer remains poor.

—Richard Adler, Ph.D.

See also Addiction; Asbestos exposure; Bronchi; Bronchitis; Cancer; Carcinogens; Carcinoma; Chemotherapy; Lungs; Malignancy and metastasis; National Cancer Institute (NCI); Nicotine; Occupational health; Oncology; Pneumonia; Pulmonary diseases; Pulmonary medicine; Radiation therapy; Respiration; Smoking; Tumor removal; Tumors; Wheezing.

For Further Information:

Dollinger, Malin, et al. *Everyone's Guide to Cancer Therapy.* 5th ed. Kansas City, Mo.: Andrews McMeel, 2008.

Eyre, Harmon J., Dianne Partie Lange, and Lois B. Morris. *Informed Decisions: The Complete Book of Cancer Diagnosis, Treatment, and Recovery.* 2d ed. Atlanta: American Cancer Society, 2002.

Falk Stephen A., and C. J. Williams. *Lung Cancer.* 3d ed. New York: Oxford University Press, 2010.

Henschke, Claudia I. *Lung Cancer: Myths, Facts, Choices—and Hope.* New York: W. W. Norton, 2003.

Kernstine, Kemp H., and Karen L. Reckamp. *Lung Cancer: A Multidisciplinary Approach to Diagnosis and Management.* New York: Demos Medical, 2011.

Lung Cancer Online Foundation. http://www.lungcanceronline.org.

Parles, Karen, and Joan H. Schiller. *One Hundred Questions and Answers About Lung Cancer.* 2d ed. Sudbury, Mass.: Jones and Bartlett, 2010.

Pass, Harvey I., et al., eds. *Lung Cancer: Principles and Practice.* 4th ed. Philadelphia: Lippincott Williams & Wilkins, 2010.

Steen, R. Grant. *A Conspiracy of Cells: The Basic Science of Cancer.* New York: Plenum Press, 1993.

Stewart David J. *Lung Cancer: Prevention, Management, and Emerging Therapies.* New York: Humana, 2010.

LUNG DISEASES. *See* PULMONARY DISEASES.

LUNG SURGERY
Procedure

Anatomy or system affected: Lungs, respiratory system

Specialties and related fields: Emergency medicine, general surgery, pulmonary medicine

Definition: The correction and treatment of such lung problems as bronchiectasis, cancer, emphysema, and pneumothorax.

Key terms:

catheter: a flexible tube inserted into a body cavity to distend it or maintain an opening

diaphragm: the muscular partition that separates the abdomen and the thorax

expiration: the act of breathing out, which partly collapses the lungs

inspiration: the act of breathing in, which expands the lungs

trachea: a cartilaginous, air-carrying tube that runs from the larynx to the bronchi of the lungs

Indications and Procedures

Located in the chest (or thoracic) cavity, the lungs rest on the diaphragm. Each lung is connected to the trachea, which brings air in on inspiration and carries it away on expiration. Prior to its entry into the lungs, the trachea forms two bronchi. Each enters a lung near its middle and subdivides into smaller and smaller passages called bronchioles. The smallest tubes open into tiny air sacs called alveoli. Each alveolus contains blood vessels called capillaries that take up oxygen and release carbon dioxide into the lungs to be expelled as waste. Alveoli are arranged into lobules, which are united into lung lobes. The left lung contains two such lobes, and there are three in the larger right lung. Appropriate alveolar function is essential to life. To optimize their action, the lungs are surrounded by a double membrane, the pleura, and supplied by nerves that control expansion on inspiration and contraction on expiration. This size change, accomplished by muscular action, normally occurs eighteen times per minute throughout life. It slows during sleep and accelerates during exercise.

Good health requires adequate lung operation, which can be compromised in many ways. The best-known lung disorders are abscesses, asthma, bronchiectasis, bronchitis, cancer, emphysema, pneumonia, pneumothorax, and tuberculosis. Of these, lung cancer, abscesses, bronchiectasis, and pneumothorax can be corrected surgically.

Lung cancer is a leading cause of cancer death among both men and women. The disease has been attributed primarily to smoking, although causative agents such as asbestos, radioactive substances, and other air pollutants also have been implicated. The development of lung cancer is slow until severe symptoms appear. An early warning is a persistent cough unassociated with asthma or emphysema, chest pain, shortness of breath, fatigue, and general listlessness. The detection of lung cancer in its beginning stages requires regular chest x rays. Early detection greatly enhances long-term survival.

Lung cancer is best treated by surgery. This requires the removal of a small wedge of lung tissue, a lobectomy (lobe removal), or a pneumonectomy (lung removal), depending on the stage of the cancer. During surgery, general anesthesia is followed by an incision around the rib cage on the affected side, along a lower rib. The rib is then detached to produce a gap, and the tumor and/or section of the lung is removed. Postsurgical patients are kept in an intensive care unit for several days, where they are fed and given therapeutic drugs intravenously. Chest drainage tubes are used to drain the incision site. Convalescence takes several months after leaving the hospital. Complications can include infection at the site of the incision and lung collapse.

Lung abscesses most often result from the inhalation of food or tooth fragments. The symptoms are chills, fever, chest pain, and a severe cough that brings up phlegm containing blood and pus. Abscesses are often located using x rays. In many cases, antibiotics are curative. Severe and/or large lung abscesses, however, require surgical drainage or—in extreme cases—the surgical removal of affected lung tissue. For lung abscesses to require surgery, the affected tissue must be thick-walled and antibiotic-resistant. The simplest such cases involve the placement of a catheter in the abscess to act as a drain. In very severe cases, the affected lung portion (usually a wedge) is removed surgically, as with lung cancer.

Bronchiectasis, the distortion of air tubes, is often the result of childhood lung infections and takes years to develop. In most cases, it causes the production of large amounts of foul-smelling phlegm and predisposes the patient to repeated severe lung infections following colds. Diagnosis is by x ray, and treatment is often the use of antibiotics at the first sign of any cold. In some cases, the problem is severe enough to require lung surgery. Bronchiectasis that is severe enough to cause recurrent pneumonia in the same lung segment is treated by surgery when the air tube involved can be removed as well. The potential dangers of this procedure are infection and lung collapse, but they are uncommon.

Pneumothorax occurs when air enters the space between the pleura layers around a lung, causing the afflicted lung parts to collapse. It may be attributable to chest injury (such as knife wounds) or to air from ruptured blisters on the surface of the lungs. The symptoms of pneumothorax are breathlessness, chest pain, and chest tightness. Minor pneumothorax often cures itself, but severe pneumothorax can be fatal if left untreated. Surgery to correct major pneumothorax, although rare, must be carried out quickly. Minor pneumothorax cases that require surgical intervention usually involve the insertion of a catheter to remove the intrapleural air. Patients are then monitored for several days to ensure proper healing. In cases in which the leakage of air persists or a pleural tear is responsible for the pneumothorax, surgical repair of the pleura is required.

Uses and Complications

Lung surgery is straightforward but potentially dangerous because it can lead to death as a result of respiratory failure. After major operations, it is important for patients to convalesce slowly and to comply with the physician's instructions. It is particularly important for the patient to ensure that infection does not occur, to report pain and other danger signs, and to convalesce carefully. The resumption of work and physical activity should be as directed by a physician.

Major advances in treating problems associated with lung surgery include better diagnosis of their extent via computed tomography (CT) scanning and magnetic resonance imaging (MRI). Furthermore, the use of cytotoxic drugs and radiotherapy to treat cancer, including lung cancer, seems to minimize the severity of the surgical treatment of these lesions.

—*Sanford S. Singer, Ph.D.*

See also Abscess drainage; Abscesses; Cancer; Chest; Edema; Embolism; Heart transplantation; Internal medicine; Lung cancer; Lungs; Pleurisy; Pneumothorax; Pulmonary diseases; Pulmonary medicine; Pulmonary medicine, pediatric; Respiration; Resuscitation; Thoracic surgery; Thrombosis and thrombus; Transplantation; Tumor removal; Tumors.

For Further Information:

American Cancer Society. *Lung Cancer: What You Need to Know—Now.* Atlanta, Ga.: Author, 2013.

Beers, Mark H., et al., eds. *The Merck Manual of Diagnosis and Therapy.* 18th ed. Whitehouse Station, N.J.: Merck Research Laboratories, 2006.

Griffith, H. Winter. *Complete Guide to Symptoms, Illness, and Surgery.* 6th ed. New York: Perigee, 2012.

Matthews, Dawn D. *Lung Disorders Sourcebook.* Detroit, Mich.: Omnigraphics, 2002.

MedlinePlus [Internet]. Bethesda (MD): National Library of

Medicine (US); [updated 2013 Mar 22]. Lung surgery; [updated 2013 Mar 22; cited 2013 June 26]; [about 2 p.]. Available from: http://www.nlm.nih.gov/medlineplus/ency/article/002956.htm.

Professional Guide to Diseases. 9th ed. Philadelphia: Lippincott Williams & Wilkins, 2008.

Terry, Peter B. *Lung Disorders: Your Annual Guide to Prevention, Diagnosis, and Treatment*. New York: Remedy Health Media, 2013.

Tierney, Lawrence M., Stephen J. McPhee, and Maxine A. Papadakis, eds. *Current Medical Diagnosis and Treatment*. 50th ed. New York: McGraw-Hill Medical, 2012.

LUNGS

Anatomy

Anatomy or system affected: Chest, respiratory system

Specialties and related fields: Environmental health, exercise physiology, oncology, pulmonary medicine, vascular medicine

Definition: Vital organs that allow gas exchange between an organism and its environment.

Key terms:

aerobic respiration: the chemical reactions that use oxygen to produce energy; some small organisms do not use oxygen and are called anaerobic

alveoli: small, thin-walled sacs at the end of the airways; most gas exchange with the blood occurs here

cellular respiration: the chemical reactions that produce energy in the cell; these reactions can be aerobic or anaerobic

cilia: hairlike structures on cells that sweep mucus containing bacteria and foreign particles out of the airways

diffusion: the constant motion of molecules that tends to spread them from places of high concentration to those of lower concentration; gases move across the alveoli by diffusion

gas exchange: the movement of oxygen and carbon dioxide across the membrane of the lungs; other gases, such as nitrogen, may also cross the membrane

mucus: a thick, clear, slimy fluid produced in many parts of the body; in the lungs, mucus catches foreign material and provides lubrication to allow smooth airflow

respiration: the exchange of gases in breathing or the cellular chemistry that involves the same gases in the cell and produces energy

Structure and Functions

Efficient gas exchange with the environment is critical for larger organisms because oxygen is required for the last step in a series of cellular chemical reactions which processes nutrients from food. These reactions, called aerobic respiration, provide most of the energy that maintains life. Furthermore, as these reactions proceed, parts of larger carbon molecules are removed. Carbon dioxide is produced as a by-product and must be removed from the body. Hence, oxygen and carbon dioxide must be exchanged.

Small aerobic organisms can simply absorb the oxygen from air or water across their moist membranes or skins. The oxygen travels from where it is more concentrated to where it is less concentrated, a process called diffusion. The carbon dioxide inside the cells also diffuses across the membrane in the opposite direction to the environment. Larger organisms, however, have relatively less outside surface area and require special structures for their gas exchange. Various types of gills, swim bladders, and lungs are all examples of ways to absorb more oxygen and release more carbon dioxide.

This article focuses on one of these specialized structures: the lung. The lung is found in air-breathing land creatures. It allows oxygen to enter the blood and carbon dioxide to be removed. Form reflects function: The lung provides large amounts of moist surface area, close to many small blood vessels for gas exchange. Humans have a joined pair of lungs suspended in the chest cavity. The two lungs are somewhat different in size: The left lung is divided into two lobes, while the right has three lobes. This difference reflects the fact that the left side of the chest cavity has less room because of the position and shape of the heart.

The pathway to the lungs begins with the nose. The air entering each nostril is temporarily divided among three pathways (nasal conchae) and then warmed and moisturized by contact with a mucous membrane containing many blood vessels. Bacteria and particles get caught on the sticky mucus on this membrane. If objects pass this point they can be trapped by mucus lower in the tract and be swept out by waving cilia, hairlike fibers extending from cells of the airway that move in unison to push particles backward. Large particles that irritate the mucous membranes can cause a sneeze, which may eject the offending particle at speeds up to 169 kilometers per hour.

The air then continues to the pharynx (throat), where the nasal passageways and the mouth meet, and moves into the larynx, the organ that produces the voice. Swallowing pulls the larynx upward, allowing the epiglottis to flip over the opening and prevent food from entering this part of the airway. This movement of the larynx during swallowing can be felt by light touch with the fingers.

The trachea, or windpipe, follows. It is 11 centimeters long and made rigid by rings of cartilage. The inside of the trachea has cilia and also produces mucus. As the trachea approaches the lungs, it branches into two bronchi, which enter sides of the lungs at a midpoint between top and bottom. The walls of the bronchi contain cartilage rings and smooth muscles. Irritation in the larynx, the trachea, or the bronchi may cause coughing. Coughing is a reflex, like sneezing, that attempts to cast out impurities.

The bronchi continue to branch until they contain only smooth muscle; at this point, they are called bronchioles. The smooth muscle can contract or relax to allow the diameter of the bronchioles to adjust. Hence, the airflow can be changed according to the needs of the body. The pathways inside the lungs resemble an upside-down tree. Millions of cilia line the bronchial "tree" and constantly beat to remove particles. Each bronchial tube branches into several alveolar ducts. Each duct ends with a grapelike cluster of sacs called alveoli. The irregular branching that has led to this point ranges from eight to twenty-five divisions, with an average of twenty-three. Each alveolus has walls that are only one cell thick. Because of the large number of these air sacs, the lungs are very light in weight.

Gas exchange occurs in the alveoli. These structures are closely associated with the body's smallest blood vessels, the capillaries. Oxygen dissolves into the moisture on the vast surface of the alveoli. It then crosses the thin tissue of the lungs and moves into the capillaries to enter the blood. Carbon dioxide moves in the other direction to the lungs. Direction is maintained by the principle of diffusion: Flow is always from a higher to a lower concentration. The surface tension of the watery film inside the alveoli can cause a problem in gas exchange. Water molecules have a strong attraction for one another and can cause the alveoli to collapse to a smaller volume, reducing the surface area available for gas exchange. Fortunately, among the regular cells of the lining of the alveoli is found a second type of cell, called the type II cell. Type II cells produce surfactant, a mixture of chemicals that lowers the overall surface tension in the alveoli by separating the water molecules. Therefore, the alveoli stay fully inflated.

Roaming white blood cells called macrophages are a final defense against foreign objects at the alveolar level. Macrophages protect the lungs by attacking and eating bacteria and particles. They can be found elsewhere in the body performing the same function.

The pleural membrane is a double covering, one layer lining the outside of the lungs and the other lining the inside of the chest cavity. These two layers, which are really the same membrane, move over each other as breathing occurs, reducing friction. If air enters the space between the double membrane, however, the lung will collapse, a condition known as pneumothorax.

Air enters the entire airway by expansion of the chest cavity, or thorax. The cavity can be thought of as a box in which the top cannot be moved upward but the bottom and the sides may move outward. The arched diaphragm muscle at the base of the cavity contracts to lower the bottom of the box. Muscles between the ribs, called intercostals, contract to elevate the chest. The ribs, which slant downward when relaxed, move outward. This expansion pushes the walls out, increases the volume of the chest cavity, and lowers its internal pressure, causing air to be pushed into the lungs. Exhalation results when the muscles relax and allow the natural recoil of the lungs to expel the air.

Young children breathe differently than do older children or adults. Babies and toddlers have ribs that are nearly horizontal. They depend mainly on the descent of the diaphragm muscle for breathing. By two years of age, the ribs have moved to the adult position and rib muscles increase in importance. In addition, a sexual difference in breathing has been observed. Females tend to rely mainly on rib movement, while males tend to use both rib and diaphragm movement, with an emphasis on the diaphragm.

The rate of breathing is controlled by the medulla of the brain, which checks the carbon dioxide content of the blood. Activity produces more carbon dioxide and affects the rate. The normal relaxed breathing rate is about twelve times a minute. A person resting in bed may inhale 8 liters of air per minute, while a runner may reach 50 liters per minute. If a person relaxes and falls into a very shallow rhythm, a yawn attempts to break the pattern. A yawn is a deeper breath that causes more gas exchange.

Disorders and Diseases

The lungs are the only major internal organs exposed to the outside environment, and they tend to show the effects of both age and type of use. A child's lungs are pink, but with age this color becomes darker and mottled because of particles that are trapped inside the macrophages of the lung. The lungs of city dwellers and coal miners show the greatest effects because of the poor quality of the air being inhaled. Understanding the pathologies of the lungs is linked to understanding the function of the lung itself.

For example, smoking and air pollution are known to cause chronic bronchitis. The repeated irritation of the bronchi by pollutants causes the linings of the air tubules to thicken, closing down the airways. Muscles contract, and the secretion of mucus increases. Poor drainage may lead to pneumonia. Smoking tobacco can also lead to cancer of the lung, mouth, pharynx, and esophagus. Tobacco smoke may contain as many as forty-three carcinogenic (cancer-causing) chemicals. Lung cancer usually begins with changes in the lining of the bronchi among the cells with cilia and those that produce mucus. The long-term irritation of smoking eventually destroys these cells faster than the bronchi can replace them. Abnormal cells, without cilia or the ability to produce mucus, begin to take their place. These cells offer less protection and, as irritation and replacement continues, may become cancerous. In the United States, lung cancer is the leading cause of cancer deaths in both men and women, and evidence has revealed the danger of inhaling smoke from someone else's cigarette. Smoking also leads to greater risk of various other lung diseases.

Pneumonia is a general term for any inflammation that produces a fluid buildup in the lungs. The excess fluid makes breathing difficult by blocking the alveoli. The cause of the inflammation can be bacterial, viral, fungal, or chemical. For example, Legionnaires' disease is a type of pneumonia caused by a bacterium that lives in air conditioners, humidifiers, and other water-storage devices. Because it causes a lack of oxygen in the body, pneumonia can be fatal if it is not controlled: More than 70,000 deaths attributed to pneumonia occur in the United States each year. The very young and the very old are in the most danger, especially if they have already been weakened by other illnesses. Since the discovery of antibiotics, however, the majority of those infected recover.

Bronchitis is an inflammation of the mucous membrane of the bronchi that often follows a cold. A telltale symptom is a deep cough that eventually brings up gray or greenish phlegm. Bronchitis may be viral or bacterial; if the cause is bacterial, antibiotics can help in recovery. Chronic bronchitis can result from repeated attacks of bronchitis and is aggravated by smoking and air pollution.

Another lung disease is emphysema, which is usually caused by smoking. This condition is often seen in advanced cases of chronic bronchitis. In emphysema, the alveoli over-inflate and break. Nearby alveoli are damaged and merge into larger units, leaving less surface area for gas exchange. Therefore, less of the air coming into the lungs comes into contact with the membrane. The increase in dead air space requires deeper breaths to obtain oxygen, and the lungs suffer further damage. Because the air sacs are permanently broken down, the damage is irreversible.

Tuberculosis is a highly contagious bacterial infection that damages the lungs and can spread to the kidneys and the bones. Immunization, screening for exposure, and antibiotics have controlled the number of cases found in countries with modern medical care systems. Worldwide, however, tuberculosis remains a major danger, and millions of lives are still lost to this disease every year.

According to the Mayo Clinic, cases of asthma appear to be increasing in the United States population. Asthma involves a hyperactive response of the airways. During an attack, the smooth muscles of the bronchi and bronchioles contract, and excess mucus is produced. In other cases, the airways may become inflamed and swollen. The cause may be allergies or other stimuli. Asthma is rarely fatal but interferes with normal functioning, as breathing becomes difficult. The blockage of breathing can be reversed with proper medications. Asthma does not lead to emphysema.

Respiratory distress syndrome occurs in about 50,000 premature infants every year. These infants have not yet developed the ability to produce sufficient surfactant in their alveoli to prevent collapse. The importance of surfactant can be illustrated by the difficulty of a baby's first breath. To inflate the alveoli requires up to twenty times the force of a normal breath. Without surfactant, the alveoli would collapse again and the next breath would be just as difficult. In 1990, a surfactant treatment derived from calf lungs became available. Treatment of premature babies with this surfactant before symptoms develop has resulted in an 88 percent survival rate.

Cystic fibrosis is a severe genetic problem in which the mucus produced in the airways (and the gastrointestinal tract) is abnormally thick. This thick mucus interferes with gas exchange, causing the heart to work harder and the valves to be damaged. As a result, the lung may collapse. Serious infections are more likely to occur. While about 50 percent of those with cystic fibrosis live only until their late teens and twenties, an increasing number of children and young adults with this disease are living into adult life. Progress on curing cystic fibrosis is being made: Researchers working in this area have located the gene that causes the condition.

If air is allowed to enter between the pleural membrane, the lungs will instantly collapse. The two lungs are independent enough so that one lung can be collapsed for healing while the other performs the gas exchange for the body. Furthermore, each lung subdivides into its lobes and then into ten bronchopulmonary segments. Each of these segments is a structural unit that can be removed surgically if diseased.

Perspective and Prospects

The ancient Greeks established the first understandings of lung function. They rightly accepted that life depended on air but overgeneralized that air carried all disease. Empedocles of Agrigentum (c. 500-430 BCE) demonstrated that air was a real substance by filling a wineskin with it. Empedocles erred, however, in explaining the mechanism of breathing. He compared the body to a pipe and thought that the movement of air in and out of the lungs caused vital air to move in and out of pores in the body's skin.

The writings of Galen of Pergamum (129-c. 199 CE) came to dominate Western medicine until the Renaissance. In his physiology, Galen attempted to connect the function of the lungs with the blood. He believed, however, that the liver produced a "vegetative" blood that traveled to the vena cava and then took different pathways. Some then flowed to other veins to nourish the whole body for growth. The rest entered the right side of the heart. Some of this substance entered the pulmonary artery into the lungs to allow impurities to be exhaled. The rest filtered to the left side of the heart through imagined pores in the septum.

In Galen's complicated scheme, the lungs were not only for exhaust: Vital air was inhaled there to be modified. The heart then pumped the modified air through the pulmonary vein to its left side. Here the air joined the blood to become "vital spirit," which traveled by arteries to warm the whole body. The brain converted this vital spirit into "animal spirit," distributing it by the nerves to cause movement and sensation. Galen did not know that blood traveled from one side of the heart to the other by moving through the lungs. He believed that the lungs acted as a reservoir of air for the heart. Galen also thought that breathing cooled the heart.

William Harvey (1578-1657) studied the position of valves in the veins and realized that Galen's vegetative blood traveled backward. Harvey then argued for a single blood that must go through the lungs to reach the other side of the heart. Blood travels in a circle, he bravely suggested. He was supported when the new microscopes discovered the necessary small vessels that connect arteries to veins.

Antoine-Laurent Lavoisier (1743-1794) noted that the lungs take in oxygen and that carbon dioxide is exhaled. He concluded that a slow combustion must occur in the lungs to warm the blood, while opponents noted that the lungs are not warmer than other parts of the body. By the 1790s, the idea was accepted that the lungs exchange Lavoisier's gases with the blood. Many believed that blood was the essence of life. In the 1850s, however, Georg Liebig and Hermann von Helmholtz showed that muscle tissue uses oxygen and releases carbon dioxide and heat. It was finally realized that the cells are the location of Lavoisier's slow fire of respiration and that the blood is the carrier of gases between the cells and the lungs.

—Paul R. Boehlke, Ph.D.

See also Abscess drainage; Abscesses; Allergies; Altitude sickness; Anatomy; Apnea; Asbestos exposure; Aspergillosis; Asphyxiation; Asthma; Avian influenza; Bacterial infections; Bronchi; Bronchiolitis; Bronchitis; Cancer; Chest; Childhood infectious diseases; Choking; Chronic obstructive pulmonary disease (COPD); Common cold; Coughing; Croup; Cyanosis; Cystic fibrosis; Diphtheria; Edema; Embolism; Emphysema; Environmental diseases; Environmental health; Exercise physiology; Heart transplantation; Hyperventilation; Influenza; Internal medicine; Interstitial pulmonary fibrosis (IPF); Kinesiology; Legionnaires' disease; Lung cancer; Lung surgery; Measles; Multiple chemical sensitivity syndrome; Nicotine; Occupational health; Oxygen therapy; Physiology; Plague; Pleurisy; Pneumonia; Pneumothorax; Pulmonary diseases; Pulmonary edema; Pulmonary hypertension; Pulmonary medicine; Pulmonary medicine, pediatric; Respiration; Respiratory distress syndrome; Resuscitation; Smoking; Systems and organs; Thoracic surgery; Thrombolytic therapy and TPA; Thrombosis and thrombus; Toxoplasmosis; Transplantation; Tuberculosis; Tumor removal; Tumors; Wheezing; Whooping cough.

For Further Information:

Corrin, Bryan, and Andrew G. Nicholson. *Pathology of the Lungs*. 2d ed. New York: Churchill Livingstone/Elsevier, 2006. This volume discusses such topics as lung development, infectious diseases, vascular disease, tumors, and transplantation.

Levitzky, Michael G. *Pulmonary Physiology*. 7th ed. New York: McGraw-Hill Medical, 2007. A clinical text that describes the structure and function of the respiratory system. Covers topics such as the physical process of respiration from the interrelationship of basic lung mechanics, the microscopic changes at the alveolar level of gas exchange, the "nonrespiratory" functions of the lungs, and how the lungs respond to stress.

Mason, Robert J., et al., eds. *Murray and Nadel's Textbook of Respiratory Medicine*. 5th ed. Philadelphia: Saunders/Elsevier, 2010. Details basic anatomy, physiology, pharmacology, pathology, and immunology of the lungs.

Sarosi, George A., and Scott F. Davies, eds. *Fungal Diseases of the Lung*. 3d ed. Philadelphia: Lippincott Williams & Wilkins, 2000. This resource covers a wide range of topics, including blastomycosis, coccidioidomycosis, cryptococcosis, and sporotrichosis.

Tapley, Donald F., et al., eds. *The Columbia University College of Physicians and Surgeons Complete Home Medical Guide*. Rev. 3d ed. New York: Crown, 1995. A comprehensive, practical health guide explaining all aspects of illness and treatment in common language. The section on respiratory diseases and lung health covers both the causes and the prevention of various diseases and problems.

West, John B. *Pulmonary Pathophysiology: The Essentials*. 7th ed. Philadelphia: Wolters Kluwer/Lippincott Williams & Wilkins, 2008. Examines lungs afflicted with obstructive, restrictive, vascular, and environmental diseases. Bronchoactive drugs, the causes of hypoventilation, and the pathogenesis of asthma and pulmonary edema are new topics covered in this edition.

Lupus. *See* Systemic lupus erythematosus (SLE).

Lyme disease

Disease/Disorder

Also known as: Lyme borreliosis

Anatomy or system affected: Eyes, heart, joints, knees, nerves, nervous system, skin

Specialties and related fields: Bacteriology, cardiology, dermatology, epidemiology, neurology, ophthalmology, rheumatology

Definition: Lyme disease is caused by bacteria transmitted by ticks. Initial symptoms include a spreading rash at the site

of the tick bite; later, the central nervous system, heart, or joints may be affected.

Key terms:

ectoparasite: an external parasite

seronegative Lyme disease: Lyme disease in which serum lacks a reaction with antibodies

spirochete: a long, helically coiled bacterial cell

Causes and Symptoms

Lyme disease is the most common tick-borne disease in the United States and Europe. It is caused by spirochete bacteria of the species complex *Borrelia burgdorferi sensu lato*. (This name refers to all bacteria causing Lyme disease.) *Borrelia burgdorferi sensu stricto* is the predominant cause of Lyme disease in the United States, while *Borrelia afzelii* and *Borrelia garinii* more often cause Lyme disease in Europe. The hard-bodied (Ixodes) tick transmits *Borrelia burgdorferi* to humans. Lyme disease is endemic in parts of New England, the upper Midwest, and Northern California. The tick species *Ixodes scapularis* (the black-legged tick or deer tick) transmits Lyme disease in the East and Midwest, while *Ixodes pacificus* (the Western black-legged tick) is the vector for Lyme disease in the West. In Europe, *Ixodes ricinus* (the sheep tick) is the vector.

Ticks are arachnid, obligate, blood-feeding ectoparasites with mouth parts that pierce the host skin. The tick saliva contains analgesics, anti-inflammatories, antihistamines, and anticoagulants that make it less likely that the tick bite will be detected. A tick takes three blood meals—as a larva, a nymph, and an adult—typically from different host species. The spirochete does not pass from the adult tick into the tick eggs. When a tick larva feeds on a host infected with *Borrelia burgdorferi*, that larva becomes infected, molts to the nymph stage, and passes on the spirochete when it takes its next blood meal. In the eastern United States, the hosts infected with *Borrelia burgdorferi* on which the tick feeds are white-footed mice (the reservoirs of infection) and deer. There is a receptor that binds an outer membrane protein of the bacterium to maintain the bacteria in the tick gut. When the tick begins feeding on another host, a bacterial protein is produced that aids in detaching the bacteria from the receptor, and bacteria begin multiplying. The bacteria then go to the salivary glands and via saliva go to the host skin. Initially, there is little or no transmission of bacteria to the host. It takes at least twelve hours and perhaps as long as three days before the efficient transfer of bacteria. Even though the adult tick is twice as likely as the nymph to be infected with the Lyme spirochete, most cases of Lyme disease are noted in the late spring and summer, when nymphs seek blood meals from hosts. This may be because the smaller nymph is more difficult to notice.

Within a month after *Borrelia burgdorferi* bacteria enter the skin, a bull's-eye-shaped, rapidly expanding rash may form at the bite site. Bacteria travel through the bloodstream to other organs. Viral infection-like symptoms may develop, such as fatigue, headache, and neck pain. Respiratory symptoms, such as coughing, and vomiting or diarrhea do not oc-

---

Information on Lyme Disease

Causes: Bacterial infection from bite of infected ticks
Symptoms: Fatigue, malaise, chills and fever, headache, muscle and joint pain, swollen lymph nodes, rash, arthritis, nervous system abnormalities
Duration: Acute
Treatments: Oral antibiotics

---

cur. Not all who have the viral infection-like symptoms develop the rash or note a tick bite. About 60 percent of those who had the skin rash and were not treated develop arthritis, usually of the knee. About 10 percent develop neurological problems, usually facial nerve palsy. About 5 percent develop a cardiac complication as a result of atrioventricular block. The eyes may also be affected.

Lyme disease experts disagree about other possible effects. In some individuals, months after initial infection and treatment, symptoms such as muscle pain and fatigue seem to develop. Bacteria in some parts of the body may be resistant to antibiotic treatment, causing a persistent infection. Such infections would benefit from additional antibiotic treatment. A Lyme infection may be more severe because of coinfection from the tick with other pathogens, such as the rickettsial infection human granulocytic anaplasmosis and the protozoan disease babesiosis.

Treatment and Therapy

To prevent Lyme disease, avoiding exposure to ticks is key. In a tick-infected area, one should wear protective clothing, use tick repellent such as DEET, check daily for ticks, and promptly remove any ticks. To reduce the population of ticks around a house, the lawn should be kept mowed and brush cleared.

The rash of Lyme disease is treated with antibiotics such as doxycycline, amoxicillin, or cefuroxime axetil. For those under eight years of age and pregnant women, however, doxycycline is not recommended.

In the late 1990s, a vaccine against Lyme disease was available. This vaccine induced the production of antibodies to a *Borrelia burgdorferi* outer cell membrane surface lipoprotein. In 2002, the manufacturers of the vaccine withdrew it from the market because of problems involving postvaccination fatigue. In its 2012 report to the Africa, Global Health and Human Rights Subcommittee's Hearing on Global Challenges in Diagnosing and Managing Lyme Disease, the Infectious Diseases Society of America (IDSA) stated that the withdrawal of the vaccine had been misguided and was caused by what it considers to be unsubstantiated claims about the vaccines' side effects; currently, there is no human vaccine available. In 2008, the National Institutes of Health and the Center for Disease Control started a serum reference repository to house serum samples that can be used to compare different tests for the diagnosis of Lyme disease; in 2011, the samples became available to the scientific community at large.

Perspective and Prospects

The clinical symptoms of Lyme disease have been documented in European medical literature as early as the 1880s, but each clinical sign was considered a separate illness. In the 1970s, an outbreak of apparent juvenile rheumatoid arthritis, in some cases preceded by a rash, occurred in Old Lyme and Lyme, Connecticut. In 1975, this range of different symptoms was recognized as a single illness. *Borrelia burgdorferi* was identified in 1982 by Willy Burgdorfer, a tick-borne disease expert from the Rocky Mountain Labs in Montana.

In 2006, the IDSA released updated diagnosis and treatment guidelines for Lyme disease. These guidelines recommend a bull's-eye, or erythema migrans (EM), rash or positive laboratory tests to diagnose Lyme disease. The IDSA guidelines do not recognize a chronic form of Lyme disease, nor do they recognize seronegative Lyme disease except in early infections. This stance has generated a great deal of controversy. Both the International Lyme and Associated Disease Society (ILADS), a professional medical society, and the Lyme Disease Association, an all-volunteer association, have expressed concern about the stricter guidelines. They worry that patients with chronic Lyme disease will continue to suffer. However, as of 2013, the IDSA continues to stand behind its initial diagnosis guidelines, stating that there is not sufficient evidence for the existence of "chronic Lyme disease." There is much more to learn about the Lyme bacteria in order to aid patients.

—*Susan J. Karcher, Ph.D.*

See also Antibiotics; Arthritis; Bacterial infections; Bites and stings; Epidemiology; Lice, mites, and ticks.

For Further Information:

American Lyme Disease Foundation. http://www.aldf .com.
Edlow, Jonathan A. *Bull's-Eye: Unraveling the Medical Mystery of Lyme Disease*. 2d ed. New Haven, Conn.: Yale University Press, 2004.
Edlow, Jonathan A., and Robert Moellering, Jr., eds. "Tick-Borne Diseases, Part 1: Lyme Disease." *Infectious Disease Clinics of North America* 22, no. 2 (June, 2008).
Horowitz, Richard. *Why Can't I Get Better? Solving the Mystery of Lyme and Chronic Disease*. New York: St. Martin's Press, 2013.
International Lyme and Associated Disease Society. http://www.ilads.org.
Lyme Disease Association. http://www.lymedisease association.org.
Plotkin, Stanley A. *The Need for a New Lyme Disease Vaccine*. Chicago: University of Chicago Press, 2011.
Stricker, Raphael B., Andrew Lautin, and Joseph J. Burrascano. "Lyme Disease: The Quest for Magic Bullets." *Chemotherapy* 52 (2006): 53–59.
Wormser, Gary P., et al. "The Clinical Assessment, Treatment, and Prevention of Lyme Disease, Human Granulocytic Anaplasmosis, and Babesiosis: Clinical Practice Guidelines by the Infectious Diseases Society of America." *Clinical Infectious Diseases* 43, no. 9 (2006): 1089–134.

LYMPH

Biology

Anatomy or system affected: Blood, circulatory system, immune system, lymphatic system, spleen
Specialties and related fields: Hematology, immunology, in-

ternal medicine, oncology, serology

Definition: A milky fluid that carries cellular waste, nutrients, and pathogens for processing in the lymphatic system.

Structure and Functions

Blood flows from the heart through smaller and smaller arteries until it reaches capillaries. There the plasma (blood without red blood cells) oozes into the surrounding tissue, bathing the cells in oxygen, nutrients, and hormones. About 90 percent of this tissue fluid (also known as intercellular fluid or interstitial fluid) is absorbed back into the blood system via the veins. The remaining 10 percent enters the lymphatic system, and this is the milky fluid known as lymph. It carries with it cellular debris, minerals, proteins, and pathogens, such as viruses, bacteria, and cancer cells.

The lymphatic system is a network of vessels, similar to blood vessels, and lymph nodes. At some point, lymph passes through one of the hundred lymph nodes in the body, where it is cleansed of debris. White blood cells, primarily lymphocytes and macrophages, attack cancer cells and cells infected by microorganisms. Lymph therefore helps the immune system combat disease. The lymphatic system also plays a role in balancing the body's fluid load. Lymph exits the lymphatic system at the subclavian veins at the base of the neck, reentering the blood.

Disorders and Diseases

Problems associated with lymph arise when the lymphatic system fails to circulate it or when the fluid carries pathogens that cause an infection in the system. Lymphedema is the accumulation of lymph, which causes swelling. Congenital lymphedema is caused by an inadequate number of lymph vessels. It results in swelling in the legs, for the most part. The more common acquired lymphedema is usually the result of major surgery that involves removal of lymph nodes—as occurs, for instance, during surgery for breast cancer. Filariasis, a parasitical infection, can cause scarring and constriction in the lymphatic vessels and lymphedema. It may so distend the legs that they look like elephant legs, a rare condition known as elephantiasis.

Lymphadenitis is the inflammation of lymph nodes by a pathogen, typically bacteria or viruses spread from the skin or an orifice. Similarly, acute lymphangitis involves inflamed lymph vessels because of bacteria, usually streptococcus, in the skin.

—*Roger Smith, Ph.D.*

See also Blood and blood disorders; Circulation; Elephantiasis; Immune system; Immunology; Immunopathology; Lymphadenopathy and lymphoma; Lymphatic system; Vascular medicine; Vascular system.

For Further Information:

Abrahams, Peter H., et al. *McMinn and Abrahams' Clinical Atlas of Human Anatomy.* Edinburgh: Mosby, 2013.

Beers, Mark H., ed. *The Merck Manual of Medical Information: Second Home Edition.* Whitehouse Station, N.J.: Merck Research Laboratories, 2003.

Faiz, Omar, and David Moffat. *Anatomy at a Glance.* 3d ed. Malden, Mass.: Blackwell, 2011.

McDowell, Julie, and Michael Windelsprecht. *The Lymphatic System.* Santa Barbara, Calif.: Greenwood, 2004.

Olteanu, Horatiu, Alexandra M. Harrington, and Steven H. Kroft. *Lymph Nodes.* New York: Demos Medical, 2013.

Parker, Steve. *The Human Body Book.* 2d ed. New York: DK Adult, 2013.

Thibodeau, Gary A., and Kevin T. Patton. *Structure and Function of the Human Body.* 14th ed. St. Louis: Mosby/Elsevier, 2012.

Lymphadenopathy and Lymphoma

Disease/Disorder

Anatomy or system affected: Lymphatic system

Specialties and related fields: Hematology, internal medicine, oncology, vascular medicine

Definition: Lymphadenopathy, or enlarged lymph nodes, refers to any disorder related to the lymphatic vessels of lymph nodes; lymphoma is a group of cancers consisting of unchecked multiplication of lymphatic tissue cells.

Key terms:

B lymphocyte: a blood and lymphatic cell that plays a role in the secretion of antibodies

Hodgkin's disease: a malignant disorder of lymphoid tissue, generally first appearing in cervical lymph nodes, which is characterized by the presence of the Reed-Sternberg cell

lymphoma staging: a classification of lymphomas based upon the stage of the disease; used in the determination of treatment

non-Hodgkin's lymphoma: any malignant lymphoproliferative disorder other than Hodgkin's disease

Reed-Sternberg cell: a large atypical macrophage with multiple nuclei; found in patients with Hodgkin's disease

T lymphocyte: a blood and lymphatic cell that functions in cell-mediated immunity, which involves the direct attack of diseased tissues; subclasses of T cells aid B lymphocytes in the production of antibodies

Causes and Symptoms

The lymphatic system consists of a large complex of lymph vessels and groups of lymph nodes ("lymph glands"). The lymph vessels include a vast number of capillaries that collect fluid and dissolved proteins, carbohydrates, and fats from tissue fluids. The lacteals of the intestinal villi are lymph vessels that serve to absorb fats from the intestine and transport them to the bloodstream.

Information on Lymphadenopathy and Lymphoma

Causes: Disease, allergies, infection, viruses, genetic factors

Symptoms: Enlarged lymph nodes, fatigue, mild fever, night sweats, weight loss

Duration: Varies from acute to long-term

Treatments: Vary; may include antibiotics, radiation therapy, chemotherapy, bone marrow transplantation

Lymph nodes are found throughout the body but are concentrated most heavily in regions of the head, neck, armpits, abdomen, and groin. Nodes function to filter out foreign materials, such as bacteria or viruses, which make their way into lymphatic vessels.

The sizes of lymph nodes vary: some are as small as a pinhead, some as large as a bean. In general, they are shaped much like kidney beans, with an outer covering. Internally, they consist of a compartmentalized mass of tissue that contains large numbers of B and T lymphocytes as well as antigen-presenting cells (APC). The lymphatic circulation into the lymph nodes consists of a series of entering, or afferent, vessels, which empty into internal spaces, or sinuses. A network of connective tissue, the reticulum, regulates the lymph flow and serves as a site of attachment for lymphocytes and macrophages. The lymphatic circulation leaves the node through efferent, or exiting, vessels in the lower portion of the organ, the hilum.

Among the functions of lymph nodes are those of the immune response. B and T lymphocytes tend to congregate in specialized areas of the lymph nodes: B cells in the outer region, or cortex, and T cells in the underlying paracortex. When antigen is presented by an APC, T- and B-cell interaction triggers B-cell maturation and proliferation within the germinal centers of the cortex. The result may be a significant enlargement of the germinal centers and subsequently of the lymph node itself.

Lymphadenopathy, or enlarged lymph nodes, may signify a lymphoma, or cancer of the lymphatic system. More commonly, however, the enlarged node is secondary to other phenomena, usually local infections. For example, an ear infection may result in the entrance of bacteria into local lymphatic vessels. These vessels drain into regional nodes of the neck. The result is an enlargement of the nodes in this area, as an immune response is carried out.

Enlarged nodes caused by infections can, in general, be easily differentiated from those caused by malignancies. Infectious nodes are generally smaller than 2 centimeters in diameter, soft, and tender. They usually occur in areas where common infections occur, such as the ears or the throat. Malignant lymph nodes are often large and occur in groups. They are generally firm and hard, and they often appear in unusual areas of the body (for example, along the diaphragm). To confirm a malignancy, a biopsy of material may be necessary.

Infectious nodes can also be caused by diseases such as infectious mononucleosis, tuberculosis, and acquired immunodeficiency syndrome (AIDS). Lymphadenopathy syndrome (LAS), a generalized enlargement of the lymph nodes, is a common feature of the prodromal AIDS-related complex (ARC).

Since lymphadenopathy can be caused by any immune proliferation in the germinal centers, allergy-related illnesses may also cause enlargement of the lymph nodes. Consequently, immune disorders such as rheumatoid arthritis, systemic lupus erythematosus, and even hay fever allergies may show enlarged nodes as part of their syndromes.

As is the case for any cell in the body, cells constituting the

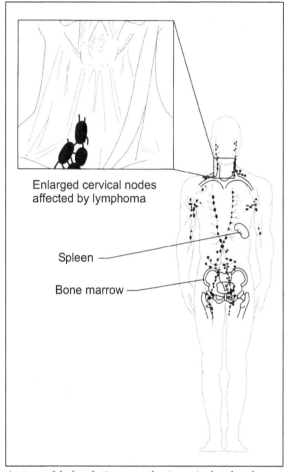

Anatomy of the lymphatic system, showing major lymph nodes; enlarged lymph nodes may occur for a wide variety of reasons, including but not limited to lymphoma (cancer).

lymphatic system may undergo a malignant transformation. The broadest definition of these lymphoproliferative diseases, or lymphomas, can include both Hodgkin disease and Hodgkin lymphomas, in addition to acute and chronic lymphocytic leukemias (ALL and CLL). With the understanding of, and ability to detect, specific cell markers, it is possible to classify many of these lymphomas on the basis of their cellular origin. Such is the case for ALL, CLL, Burkitt lymphoma, and many other forms of non-Hodgkin lymphomas. The cell type that ultimately forms the basis for Hodgkin disease remains uncertain.

Hodgkin disease is a malignant lymphoma that first manifests itself as a painless enlargement of lymphoid tissue. Often, this is initially observed in the form of swollen lymph nodes in the neck or cervical region. Occasionally, the victim may exhibit a mild fever, night sweats, and weight loss. Untreated, the disease spreads from one lymphatic region to another, resulting in diffuse adenopathy. An enlarged spleen (splenomegaly) is a common result. As the disease spreads, other organs such as the liver, lungs, and bone marrow may be involved.

The disease is characterized by the presence of a characteristic cell type—the Reed-Sternberg cell. Reed-Sternberg cells appear to be of macrophage origin, with multilobed nuclei or multiple nuclei. They may also be present in other lymphatic disorders, but their presence is considered to be indicative of all cases of Hodgkin disease. The precise relationship of the cell to the lymphoma is unclear, but some researchers in the field believe that the Reed-Sternberg cell is the actual malignant cell of the disease. The other infiltrative cells present in the node, including many B and T lymphocytes, may simply represent the reaction to the neoplasm. This interpretation, however, has been disputed.

Lymphoma staging is a system of classifying lymphomas according to the stage of development of the disease. Staging is important in that the prognosis and basis for treatment are in part determined by the stage of disease. Characterizing the form of Hodgkin disease, therefore, involves two forms of classification. The first is a four-part classification based on the histology or cell type (Rye Conference classification). This scheme is based upon the proportion of Reed-Sternberg cells, ranging from their being "hard to find" to their being the predominant type. The prognosis becomes less favorable as the proportion of these cells increases.

Clinical staging, like that based on histology, is a four-part classification scheme (it is actually six parts, since stage III can be divided into subclasses). In this system, classification is based upon the extent of spread or extralymphatic involvement. For example, stage I features the involvement of a single lymph node region or a single extralymphatic site. Stage IV involves multiple disseminated foci. Early-stage disease is more easily treated and has a better prognosis than late-stage disease.

Non-Hodgkin lymphomas (NHLs) represent a multitude of malignant disorders. Unlike Hodgkin disease, they frequently arise in lymphatic tissue that is not easily observed; for example, in the gastrointestinal tract, tonsils, bone, and central nervous system. They have a tendency to spread rapidly, with malignant cells being released into the bloodstream early in the disease. Consequently, by the time diagnosis of NHL is made, the disease has often spread and the prognosis may be poor.

Though the etiology of most forms of NHL remains unknown, certain characteristics are evident in some forms of these diseases. For example, a portion of chromosome 14 is elongated in about 60 percent of NHL patients. Nearly one-third of patients with NHLs of B-cell origin demonstrate a chromosomal translocation, often involving a piece of chromosome 14 being translocated to chromosome 18. Though the relationship of these changes to disease is unclear, one can surmise that chromosomal defects play at least some role in the development of some forms of these disorders.

At least two forms of NHL are either caused by viruses or related to their presence: Burkitt lymphoma and adult T-cell lymphoma/leukemia. Burkitt lymphoma, which was first described by Denis Burkitt in central Africa, is a B-cell tumor that occurs primarily in children. It is generally manifested as a large tumor of the jaw. This type of lymphoma is associated with early infection by the Epstein-Barr virus, or EBV (also the etiological agent of infectious mononucleosis). The relationship of the disorder to the virus remains unclear, and EBV may be either a specific cause or a necessary cofactor.

Specific chromosomal abnormalities are also associated with Burkitt lymphoma. In 75 percent of cases, a translocation from chromosome 8 to chromosome 14 is evident, while in most other cases, a portion of chromosome 8 is translocated to either chromosome 2 or chromosome 22. Each of these translocations involves the transfer of the same gene from chromosome 8, the c-myc gene. The site to which the c-myc is translocated is in each instance a region that encodes protein chains for antibody production, proteins that are produced in large quantities. The c-myc gene product normally plays a role in committing a cell to divide. By being translocated into these specific regions, the c-myc gene product is overproduced, and the B cell undergoes continual replication.

Approximately 80 percent of NHL tumors are of B-cell origin; the remainder are primarily of T-cell origin. Those lymphomas that arise within the thymus, the organ of T-cell maturation, are called lymphoblastic lymphomas. Those that originate as more differentiated and mature T cells outside the thymus include a heterogeneous group of diseases (for example, peripheral T-cell lymphomas and Sézary syndrome). Often, by the time of diagnosis, these disorders have spread beyond the early stage of classification and have become difficult to treat.

Treatment and Therapy

Treatment and other means of dealing with lymphadenopathy depend on the specific cause. In the case of lymph node enlargement that is secondary to infections, treatment of the primary cause is sufficient to restore the normal appearance of the node. For example, in a situation in which nodes in the neck region are enlarged as the result of a throat infection, antibiotic treatment of the primary cause—that is, the bacterial infection—is sufficient. The nodes will resume their normal size after a short time.

Dealing with lymph node enlargement caused by lymphoma requires a much more aggressive form of treatment. There are many kinds of lymphomas, which differ in type of cell involvement and stage of differentiation of the involved cells. The manifestations of most lymphomas, however, are similar. In general, these disorders first present themselves as painless, enlarged nodes. Often, this occurs in the neck region, but in many forms of NHL, the lymphadenopathy may manifest itself elsewhere in the lymphatic system. As the disease progresses, splenomegaly (enlarged spleen) and hepatomegaly (enlarged liver) may manifest themselves. Frequently, the bone marrow becomes involved. If the enlarged node compresses a vital organ or vessel in the body, immediate surgery may be necessary. For example, if one of the veins of the heart is compressed, the patient may be in immediate, life-threatening danger. Treatment generally includes radiation therapy and/or chemotherapy.

As is true for lymphomas in general, Hodgkin disease is found more commonly in males than in females. In the United States, it occurs at a rate of 3.2 per 100,000 population per year for men and 2.4 per 100,000 for women, with more than nine thousand cases expected to be diagnosed in 2013. More than one thousand persons die of the disease each year. The cause of the disease is unknown, though attempts have been made to assign the Epstein-Barr virus to this role.

Hodgkin disease has an unusual age incidence. The age-specific incidence exhibits a bimodal curve. The disease shows an initial peak among young adults between fifteen and thirty years of age. The incidence drops after age thirty, only to show an additional increase in frequency after age fifty. This is in contrast to NHL, which shows a sharp increase in incidence only after age forty-five. The reasons are unknown.

As noted earlier, the staging of Hodgkin disease is important in determining methods of treatment; the earlier the stage, the better the prognosis. Patients in stage I (single node or site of involvement) or stage II (two or more nodes on the same side of the diaphragm involved, or limited extralymphatic involvement) have a much better prognosis than patients in stages III and IV (splenic or disseminated disease). Prior to the mid-1960s, a diagnosis of Hodgkin disease was almost a death sentence. The development of radiation therapy and chemotherapy has dramatically increased the chances for survival; long-term remission can be achieved in nearly 70 percent of patients, and the "cure" rate may be higher than 90 percent with early detection. In part, this has been the result of understanding the progression of the disease (reflected in the process of staging) and utilizing a therapeutic approach to eradicate the disease both at its current site and at likely sites of spreading.

Radiation therapy is the treatment of choice for patients in stages I and II; spreading beyond local nodes is still unlikely in these stages. The body is divided into three regions to which radiation may be delivered: The mantle field covers the upper chest and armpits; the para-aortic field is the region of the diaphragm and spleen; and the third field is the pelvic area. For example, a patient manifesting lymphadenopathy in a single node in the neck region may undergo only "mantle" irradiation. As noted above, with early detection, such treatment is effective 90 percent of the time (based on five-year disease-free survival).

Beyond stage II, a combination of radiation therapy and chemotherapy treatment is warranted. A variety of chemotherapy programs have been developed, the most common of which is known by the acronym MOPP (nitrogen mustard/ Oncovin/procarbazine/prednisone). With combined radiation therapy and chemotherapy, even stage III disease may go into remission 60 to 70 percent of the time, while 40 to 50 percent of stage IV patients may enter remission. In general, therapy takes six to twelve months.

Non-Hodgkin lymphomas represent a heterogeneous group of malignancies. Eighty percent are of B-lymphocyte origin. The wide variety of types has made classification difficult. The most useful method of classification for clinical purposes is based on the relative aggressiveness of the disease, low-grade being the slowest growing, followed by intermediate-grade and high-grade, which is the most aggressive.

NHLs often arise in lymphoid areas outside the mainstream. For example, the first sign of disease may be an abdominal mass or pain. Fever and night sweats are uncommon, at least in the early stages. Consequently, once the disease is manifested, it is often deep and widespread. Because the disorder is no longer localized by this stage, radiation therapy by itself is of limited use. For comparison, nearly half of Hodgkin disease patients are in stage I at presentation; not quite 15 percent of NHL patients are in stages I and II. Consequently, treatment almost always involves extensive chemotherapy.

A variety of aggressive forms of chemotherapy may be applied. These may include either single drugs such as alkaloids (vincristine sulfate) and alkylating agents (chlorambucil) or combination programs such as that of MOPP. Low-grade types of NHL are frequently slow growing and respond well to less aggressive forms of therapy. Low-grade NHL patients often enter remission for years. Unfortunately, the disorder often recurs with time and may become resistant to treatment; remission may occur in 50 percent of the patients, but only about 10 percent survive disease-free after ten years. High-grade lymphomas are rapidly growing, and the prognosis for most patients in the short term is not good. Those patients who do achieve remission with aggressive therapy, however, often show no recurrence of disease. As many as 50 percent of these persons may be "cured." The difference in prognosis between low-grade and high-grade disease may relate to the characteristics of the malignant cell. A rapidly growing cancer cell may be more susceptible to aggressive therapy than a slow-growing cancer and more likely to die as a result. Thus, if a patient enters remission following therapy, there is greater likelihood that the cancer has been eradicated.

Perspective and Prospects

What was likely Hodgkin disease was first described in 1666 as an illness in which lymphoid tissues and the spleen had the appearance of a "cluster of grapes." The disorder was invariably fatal. In 1832, Thomas Hodgkin published a thorough description of the disease, including its progression from the cervical region of the body to other lymphatic regions and organs. The unusual histological appearance of the cellular mixture characteristic of Hodgkin disease was noted during the nineteenth century. It was early in the twentieth century, however, that Dorothy Reed and Karl Sternberg described the cell that is characteristic of the disorder: the Reed-Sternberg cell. As noted earlier, the number and proportion of such cells are the bases for the classification of the disease.

Two forms of non-Hodgkin lymphoma are known to be associated with specific viruses: Burkitt lymphoma (BL) and adult T-cell leukemia (ATL). BL was described by Denis Burkitt, who studied the pattern of certain forms of lymphomas among Ugandan children during the late 1950s. He noted that nearly all cases were found in children between the ages of two and fourteen, and noted that most cases in Africa were found in the malarial belt. Burkitt suspected that a mosquito might be involved in the transmissions of BL. Though no link has been found with arthropod transmission, the idea that BL might be associated with a viral agent bore fruit. In 1964, Michael Epstein and Yvonne Barr reported the presence of a particle in BL tissue that resembled the herpes virus. The Epstein-Barr virus was eventually linked to BL, though the specific role played by the virus remains elusive.

Adult T-cell leukemia was first noted in Japan during the 1970s. Japanese scientists observed that the majority of NHLs there were of T-cell origin and exhibited a similar clinical spectrum. The disease was later observed in the Caribbean basin, the southeastern United States, South America, and central Africa. In 1980, Robert Gallo isolated the etiological agent, the human T-cell lymphotrophic type I virus (HTLV-I).

The treatment of Hodgkin disease represents one of the few success stories in dealing with cancers. In addition, some forms of NHL—notably, Burkitt lymphoma—respond well to treatment. The prognosis for most patients with NHL, however, is less than optimal. In addition, the specific causes of most NHL syndromes are not known. Those with which a virus is linked may, in theory, be prevented by means of vaccination. The etiological agents or factors associated with the development of other forms of lymphomas remain elusive.

—*Richard Adler, Ph.D.*

See also Burkitt's lymphoma; Cancer; Carcinogens; Chemotherapy; Epstein-Barr virus; Hodgkin's disease; Infection; Lymph; Lymphatic system; Malignancy and metastasis; Oncology; Radiation therapy.

For Further Information:

Cerroni, Lorenzo, Kevin Gatter, and Helmut Kerl. *Skin Lymphoma: The Illustrated Guide.* 3d ed. Hoboken, N.J.: Wiley-Blackwell, 2009.

Delves, Peter J., et al. *Roitt's Essential Immunology.* 12th ed. Malden, Mass.: Blackwell, 2011.

Greer, John, et al., eds. *Wintrobe's Clinical Hematology.* 12th ed. Philadelphia: Wolters Kluwer/Lippincott Williams & Wilkins Health, 2009.

Holman, Peter, and Jodi Garrett. *One Hundred Questions and Answers About Lymphoma.* 2d ed. Sudbury, Mass.: Jones and Bartlett, 2011.

Jacobs, Charlotte. *Henry Kaplan and the Story of Hodgkin's Disease.* Stanford, Calif.: Stanford University Press, 2010.

Jandl, James H. *Blood: Textbook of Hematology.* 2d ed. Boston: Little, Brown, 1996.

Knowles, Margaret A., and Peter J. Selby. *Introduction to the Cellular and Molecular Biology of Cancer.* 4th ed. New York: Oxford University Press, 2006.

Leukemia and Lymphoma Society. http://www.leuke mia.org.

Lymphoma Information Network. http://www.lym phomainfo.net.

National Cancer Institute. *What You Need to Know About Non-Hodgkin's Lymphoma.* Rev. ed. Bethesda, Md.: Department of Health and Human Services, Public Health Service, National Institutes of Health, 2007.

Schwab, M. *Encyclopedia of Cancer.* 3d ed. Philadelphia: Springer, 2012.

Specht, Lena, and Joachim Yahalom. *Radiotherapy for Hodgkin Lymphoma.* New York: Springer, 2011.

LYMPHATIC DISORDERS. *See* LYMPHADENOPATHY AND LYMPHOMA.

LYMPHATIC SYSTEM
Anatomy
Anatomy or system affected: Circulatory system, immune system, spleen

Specialties and related fields: Hematology, immunology, vascular medicine

Definition: A network of vessels, paralleling those of the circulatory system, and nodules that collects extravascular materials and fluids from tissue in order to return them to the bloodstream.

Key terms:

antigen-presenting cell (APC): a type of macrophage or interstitial cell that initiates the immune response by "presenting" processed antigen to B and T lymphocytes

edema: an abnormal accumulation of fluids around tissues

lacteals: lymphatic capillaries in the villi of the small intestine that absorb fat, producing a milky substance called chyle

lymph: the straw-colored fluid of the lymphatic system; as much as 1 to 2 liters is collected from tissue each day and returned to the bloodstream

lymph node: a small, oval structure that filters tissue fluids; lymph nodes are found in areas such as the armpits, groin, mouth, and neck, and serve as sites of immune response

lymphocytes: cells of the lymphatic system; B lymphocytes function in antibody production, while T lymphocytes function in cellular immunity

Peyer's patches: lymphatic nodules in the ileum of the intestine; Peyer's patches are one kind of mucosal associated lymphoid tissue (MALT), which, unlike lymph nodes, are not enclosed by tissue capsules

spleen: a lymphatic organ found between the stomach and the diaphragm; destroys old blood cells and filters foreign material from the blood

thoracic duct: the largest lymphatic vessel, which collects lymphatic fluid and returns it to the bloodstream at the left subclavian vein in the region of the neck

thymus: the lymphatic gland in which T lymphocytes mature; located in humans just below the thyroid

Structure and Functions

The lymphatic system is a complex of capillaries, ducts, nodes, and organs that filters and maintains interstitial fluid—that is, fluid from body tissues. Fluid is collected from body tissues and returned to the bloodstream. In addition, the system functions as a site of the immune response, primarily in the spleen and the lymph nodes, and transports fat and protein to the bloodstream.

The organs of the lymphatic system are divided into primary lymphoid organs and secondary organs. The primary organs include the thymus and the bone marrow, which are sites where lymphocytes are produced and mature. Secondary lymphoid organs are those in which the immune response is carried out. These include both encapsulated organs such as the spleen and lymph nodes and unencapsulated organs such as the mucosal associated lymphoid tissue, which includes Peyer's patches in the intestine and Waldeyer's ring in the throat (the tonsils and adenoids), which encircles the pharnyx. Lymph nodes are found throughout the body, but they occur in large numbers in the head, neck, armpits (the axillary nodes), and abdomen and groin (the inguinal nodes).

The lymphatic vessels essentially parallel those of the bloodstream. The system originates in peripheral tissue as small openings, or sinuses, within the tissue. Fluid that drains from the tissue collects in these sinuses and forms lymph. In addition, a significant amount of liquid (1 to 2 liters) that is lost from blood capillaries each day also collects in the interstitial fluid. The lymph is physiologically similar to blood plasma in that it is a balanced solution of electrolytes containing some carbohydrates, lipids, and proteins. In general, the protein level is about half that found in blood, since most blood proteins are too large to pass through the endothelial walls of blood capillaries. Arguably, the major function of the lymphatic system is the return of this fluid, and its constituent materials, to the blood. The buildup of abnormal amounts of fluid in tissue results in swelling, or edema. Approximately 60 percent of lost fluid is returned to the blood through the lymphatics, and the remainder is collected directly into small blood capillaries.

Generally speaking, the peripheral portion of the lymphatic system is completely separate from that of the blood. Once the interstitial fluid is collected, it begins to move toward the thoracic duct. Since the duct is found in the neck region, this movement is primarily in an upward direction. The fluid moves through regional lymph nodes, such as those found in the groin or armpits, and gradually collects in the larger ducts of the major lymphatics. Though an extensive system of valves is found in the lymphatic system to prevent the movement of lymph in the wrong direction, no internal pumping mechanism analogous to the heart exists. The movement of the lymph is mediated by the musculature of the body: respiratory pressure, muscular movement, and the pulsing or motion of nearby organs. Lymphatic fluids from all portions of the body, except for the upper-right quadrant, eventually collect in the thoracic duct. Lymph from the upper-right quadrant of the body collects in the right lymphatic duct. The endothelia of these major lymphatic ducts are contiguous with those of the veins in the neck, and it is here that the fluid is returned to the bloodstream. Valves present in the lymphatic ducts serve to prevent the backup of blood from the bloodstream into the lymphatic system.

In addition to the electrolytes and proteins that collect in lymph, foreign materials such as infectious agents may also penetrate the skin or internal surfaces of the body. These materials pass into tissue fluids and also collect in the lymphatic system. From here, they travel to regional lymph nodes, where they are filtered out by phagocytic cells such as macrophages. In addition, antigen-collecting cells in the skin, including dendritic cells, may transport foreign materials such as bacteria to these regional nodes. These cells may intercalate, or interdigitate, among the lymphocytes of the lymph nodes and, along with the macrophages, "present" antigen to B and T cells. In this manner, the immune response is initiated.

An analogous situation exists in the blood system. In this case, however, it is the macrophages of the spleen that serve to filter foreign material, such as infectious agents, from the blood. Damaged or old red blood cells are removed in a similar manner. The macrophages then degrade the foreign material and "present" it to B and T lymphocytes in the spleen.

Most of the immune response occurs in the lymph nodes and the spleen. Once the interaction has occurred between the APCs and the lymphocytes, differentiation of the B and T cells begins. The B cells develop into plasma cells, which are essentially antibody-producing factories, while T cells may undergo proliferation. Within the nodes, B and T cells are generally confined to specific areas: the outer cortex for B cells and the underlying paracortex for T cells. Embedded within the cortex are collections of primary nodules, which consist primarily of B cells. Once antigenic stimulation oc-

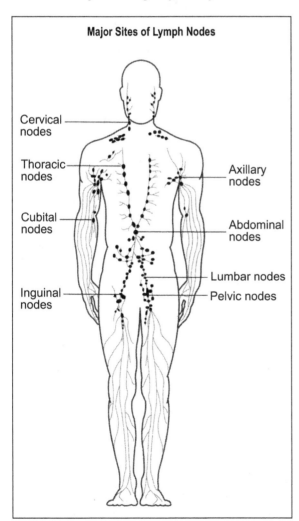

Major Sites of Lymph Nodes

Cervical nodes

Thoracic nodes

Cubital nodes

Inguinal nodes

Axillary nodes

Abdominal nodes

Lumbar nodes

Pelvic nodes

curs, the cells within the nodules enlarge and proliferate, forming secondary follicles that surround germinal centers. These germinal centers enlarge as B lymphocytes mature and proliferate, and they account for the enlargement of regional lymph nodes in the event of infection. In addition, blood vessels within the node may become enlarged, increasing blood flow. Though some of the activated lymphocytes eventually find their way to the bloodstream, most remain within the lymphatic system. Antibodies produced in response to an infection, however, are transported to the blood.

Since lymph nodes serve as regions of drainage for local tissue, they also represent a route through the body for cancer cells that break away from a tumor. For example, cells from a breast cancer may lodge in regional lymph nodes of the neck or armpit and travel from there to other areas of the body. Although specialized types of lymphocytes capable of killing tumor cells are found in the nodes, some cancer cells may survive. It is for this reason that, during the removal of tumors, localized nodes are examined for evidence of metastasis. If no cancer cells are observed in the nodes, the chances are high that the cancer has not spread.

Mucosal associated lymphatic tissue (MALT) is found along mucosal membranes in regions of the intestines (Peyer's patches and the appendix) and the throat (tonsils). The tonsils actually consist of a network of three groups of tissues that are located at the base of the tongue, at the back of the throat, and at the roof of the nasopharynx (adenoids). Like the spleen and the lymph nodes, MALT tissues may be sites of germinal centers. Unlike the spleen and lymph nodes, however, these tissues are not enclosed by defined capsules of connective tissue. They may be loosely organized, like the mucosa of the intestinal villi, or they may form organized regions like those of the tonsils and adenoids.

MALT appears to function to protect the body against respiratory or gastrointestinal agents. For example, agents such as bacteria or viruses that enter through the oral or respiratory route may stimulate an immune response by the tonsils. The swelling of the tonsils, tonsillitis, is the result of a localized immune response much like that found in the spleen or the lymph nodes. Germinal centers within the tissue represent areas of B cell maturation and proliferation. In the same way, the Peyer's patches consist of approximately thirty to forty nodules along the wall of the intestines. Gastrointestinal antigens that penetrate the intestinal wall stimulate germinal centers in these regions.

Digestion products of carbohydrates and proteins are actively transported into the villi of the small intestine and enter the bloodstream directly. Fats, however, enter the blood in a more roundabout way through the lymphatic system. Fats are digested in the small intestine and diffuse into underlying cells. There they are assembled into triglycerides and, along with cholesterol, are enclosed in protein envelopes; the resulting bodies are called chylomicrons. Once these bodies pass into the lacteals of the lymphatic system, the whitish fluid, chyle, is transported to a region at the beginning of the thoracic duct called the cisterna chyli. It is here that the fat enters the bloodstream.

Disorders and Diseases

If the interstitial fluid—that is, the fluid in the tissues—increases beyond the capacity of the lymphatic system to handle the situation, an abnormal accumulation of fluid will build up in the tissue. This creates a situation known as edema. A variety of etiological factors can cause edema. For example, burns, inflammation, and certain allergic reactions may increase the level of capillary permeability. This is particularly true if a large amount of protein is lost as the result of a serious burn.

An increase in capillary hydrostatic pressure may also increase the rate of fluid buildup in the tissues. This may be a by-product of several conditions: congestive heart failure, renal failure, or the use of a variety of drugs (estrogen, phenylbutazone). For example, an increase in the sodium concentration of the blood caused by retention resulting fromrenal failure or simply an excess of salt in the diet may cause water retention and increased blood volume. The sequelae include increased fluid leakage and edema. It is for this reason that a reduction in sodium intake is often recommended for those who suffer from this problem. Diuretics may be prescribed to promote the excretion of sodium and water. Similarly, venous obstruction as serious as phlebitis or as minor as the pressure from a tight bandage or clothing may increase hydrostatic pressure and lead to edema.

A buildup of fluid in the lungs, orpulmonary edema, may occur as a result of congestive heart failure. Hydrostatic pressure in the capillaries of the lungs is relatively low when compared with that of the circulation elsewhere. As a result, the "wetness" of lung tissue is minimal. In patients with serious congestive heart disease, capillary fluid is backed up into the lung (and, indeed, in tissues of the extremities). The result is fluid leakage into the alveoli and bronchioles. Though the lymphatics are capable of removing small amounts of excess fluids, at some point the leakage of plasma and dissolved proteins exceeds the capacity of the lymphatic system to handle the problem. The result is a vicious circle. Since less oxygen is taken up through the lungs, capillary permeability increases. More fluid and protein are then lost. Unless intervention is carried out, the patient may eventually drown in his or her own fluids.

Intervention for pulmonary edema generally involves elevating the head and knees of the patient (Fowler's position) and the administration of diuretics. A low-sodium diet, allowing for decreased fluid retention, may also relieve some of the stress on the lymphatic system. With time, the number of lymphatic vessels in the lungs may increase, allowing for a greater capacity to remove fluids.

A variety of disorders may directly involve the lymphatic system itself. Lymphedema, or the accumulation of lymph in tissue with subsequent swelling, may result from the absence of lymphatic vessels or from obstructions within the vessels. The symptoms of lymphedema, particularly in the lower extremities, include mild swelling that becomes increasingly severe with time. The problem may be exacerbated by menstruation or pregnancy. In some instances, lymphatic vessels may be absent, either congenitally or because of surgical removal. Diagnosis of the problem often requires the use of lymphangiography (lymphography). In this procedure, a contrast medium is injected, and the lymphatic vessels are examined by means of x-rays.

The etiologic factors associated with lymphatic obstruction may either be congenital or have external causes. Milroy disease is a hereditary lymphedema characterized by chronic obstructions. The obstruction of lymphatic vessels may also be caused by the presence of tumor cells or the infiltration of parasites. For example, elephantiasis is caused by an infestation of a parasitic worm that obstructs the flow of fluid. The affected limb or region of the body may swell to an astounding degree.

The treatment of most of these disorders is essentially symptomatic. An obstruction may be treated or removed. Often, lymphedema may be treated by having the patient sleep with the feet elevated. A low-salt diet or diuretics may be indicated, and a light massage in the direction of lymph flow may also be helpful.

As is true for all tissues in the body, the cells and organs of the lymphatic system may also undergo malignant transformation. Any neoplasm of lymphoid tissue is referred to as a lymphoma. In general, these are malignant. Though lymphomas may be of different forms and involve different types of cells, they are characterized by enlarged lymph nodes (generally in the neck), fever, and weight loss. Among the more common forms of lymphomas are Hodgkin's disease and non-Hodgkin lymphomas, a mixed collection of malignant solid tumors originating among the secondary lymphoid tissues of the lymph nodes. Hodgkin disease generally appears first among the cervical or axillary lymph nodes. Its manner of presentation usually allows for early diagnosis and treatment. As a result, the prognosis with early intervention has significantly improved since the 1960s.

Non-Hodgkin lymphomas often develop in less obvious areas of the lymphatic system, such as the gastrointestinal tract, the central nervous system, and the oral and nasal pharynx. The result is that diagnosis is often delayed until the disease has spread, and therefore the prognosis is less optimistic. According to the Lymphoma Research Foundation, 85 percent of non-Hodgkin lymphomas are of B-lymphocyte origin; they often arise within the follicles of the lymph node. There is some evidence that neoplastic transformation may be related to antigen exposure. In some instances, molecular defects of the cell DNA may result in the neoplastic event. Non-Hodgkin lymphomas may also be of T-lymphocyte or, less commonly, macrophage origin. Most treatments of lymphomas include both radiation therapy and chemotherapy.

Perspective and Prospects

The first description of the lymphatic system was made by the Italian anatomist Gasparo Aselli in 1622. Aselli observed the lacteals in the intestinal walls of dogs that he had dissected, and he included diagrams of the lacteals in his text *De Lactibus* (1627), the first anatomical medical text with color plates.

The role of the lymphatic system in maintaining the fluid dynamics of the body was understood by the beginning of the twentieth century. Much of this knowledge resulted from the early work of the British physiologist Ernest Henry Starling.

Beginning about 1900, Starling's research centered on the secretion and circulation of lymph. It was known that the lymphatic system as a parallel to blood circulation was found only among the higher vertebrates. This indicated that it had developed relatively late during the course of evolution. There occurred, along with the increasing development of the body's circulatory system as organisms evolved, an increase in the hydrostatic pressure within the system—that is, as the circulatory system became more complex, blood vessels branched into smaller and thinner capillaries. The pressure within those capillaries became higher. Starling pointed out the significance of the hydrostatic pressures within the capillaries: Fluids and dissolved materials leak out of the capillaries into the tissues.

Starling did not believe, however, that protein was able to leak through the capillary walls. In the 1930s, Cecil Drinker demonstrated that protein is a major constituent of dissolved material in lymph and suggested that an important role of the lymphatic system is the return of this protein to the bloodstream. Drinker was unable to prove definitively that the protein in lymph originated with the blood, and it remained for H. S. Mayerson to confirm this point in the 1940s.

Lymphocytes had been observed in the blood as early as the nineteenth century. Their role in the immune process was not readily apparent, however, and various functions were assigned to them. In 1948, Astrid Fagraeus demonstrated that lymphocytes mature into antibody-producing plasma cells. It remained unclear whether this was the sole purpose of these cells.

In 1956, Bruce Glick and Timothy Chang, working with chickens, discovered that an organ called the bursa, found near the cloaca in the region of the tail, was the site of the production of antibody-producing cells. Their discovery, along with those of Robert Good and Jacques Miller some years later, showed that lymphocytes are not all identical; at least two distinct populations exist. It remained for Henry Claman and his coworkers, in 1966, to demonstrate that these two populations of lymphocytes act cooperatively in the production of antibodies.

In 1969, Ivan Roitt called those lymphocytes that mature in the thymus gland T cells. The lymphocytes that mature in the bursa, an organ found only in birds, were called B cells. Since mammals lack the bursa, B cells in these organisms mature within the bone marrow (considered a bursa equivalent). Once the cells are released from the marrow, they migrate into both the lymphatic system and the bloodstream.

—*Richard Adler, Ph.D.*

See also Angiography; Bacterial infections; Bladder cancer; Blood and blood disorders; Breast cancer; Breast disorders; Burkitt's lymphoma; Cancer; Cervical, ovarian, and uterine cancers; Chemotherapy; Circulation; Colon cancer; DiGeorge syndrome; Edema; Elephantiasis; Epstein-Barr virus; Gallbladder cancer; Histology;

Hodgkin's disease; Immune system; Immunology; Immunopathology; Kawasaki disease; Kidney cancer; Liver cancer; Lower extremities; Lung cancer; Lymph; Lymphadenopathy and lymphoma; Malignancy and metastasis; Mononucleosis; Mouth and throat cancer; Oncology; Prostate cancer; Pulmonary edema; Skin cancer; Sleeping sickness; Splenectomy; Stomach, intestinal, and pancreatic cancers; Systems and organs; Testicular cancer; Tonsillectomy and adenoid removal; Tonsillitis; Tumors; Upper extremities; Vascular medicine; Vascular system.

For Further Information:

Delves, Peter J., et al. *Roitt's Essential Immunology*. 12th ed. Malden, Mass.: Blackwell, 2011.

Dwyer, John M. *The Body at War: The Story of Our Immune System*. 2d ed. London: J. M. Dent, 1993.

Eales, Lesley-Jane. *Immunology for Life Scientists*. Hoboken, N.J.: John Wiley & Sons, 2003.

Gold, John C. *Learning About the Circulatory and Lymphatic Systems*. Berkeley Heights, N.J.: Enslow, 2013.

Janeway, Charles A., Jr., et al. *Immunobiology: The Immune System in Health and Disease*. 7th ed. New York: Garland Science, 2007.

Kindt, Thomas J., Richard A. Goldsby, and Barbara A. Osborne. *Kuby Immunology*. 6th ed. New York: W. H. Freeman, 2007.

Santambrogio, Laura. *Immunology of the Lymphatic System*. New York: Springer, 2013.

Venuta, Federico, and Erino A. Rendina. *The Lymphatic System in Thoracic Oncology*. Philadelphia: Saunders, 2012.

LYMPHOMA. *See* LYMPHADENOPATHY AND LYMPHOMA.

MACRONUTRIENTS

Biology

Anatomy or system affected: All

Specialties and related fields: Biochemistry, nutrition, public health, sports medicine

Definition: The dietary ingredients required in large quantities for health and activity.

Key terms:

carbohydrates: organic substances with the general formula of $(CH_2O)n$; the primary dietary carbohydrates are starches and sugars

fiber: organic substances resistant to digestion by human enzymes; a common dietary fiber is cellulose

gluconeogenesis: the synthesis within the body of glucose from noncarbohydrate precursors

kwashiorkor: a condition caused by inadequate dietary protein intake

lipids: organic substances insoluble in water but soluble in alcohol, ether, chloroform and other fat solvents; the primary dietary lipids are triglycerides

marasmus: a condition caused by inadequate dietary macronutrient intake, both protein and energy

proteins: organic substances consisting of linked amino acids, nitrogen-containing molecules

triglycerides (triacylglycerides): three fatty acids covalently attached to a glycerol moiety

Structure and Functions

Macronutrients are generally considered to include carbohydrates, lipids, and proteins; these are dietary constituents consumed in the largest quantities. While water and oxygen are also needed in large amounts, they are not usually considered to be food. Although fiber ingested in substantial quantity is desirable for optimum health, it is, by definition, a non-nutritive dietary constituent. In addition, calcium, sodium and chloride (salt), magnesium, potassium, phosphorus, and sulfur are sometimes added to the list of macronutrients because they are needed in large amounts compared to vitamins and other minerals; however, they are best referred to as macrominerals.

Carbohydrates, lipids, and proteins provide the energy (calories) needed for maintenance, growth, thermoregulation, and physical activity, as well as pregnancy and lactation. All three also provide for other needs: Carbohydrates are components of structural polysaccharides inside cells and on their surfaces; lipids are important in cellular membrane structure and function and as precursors of some hormones; and proteins are a source of amino acids needed for the synthesis of body proteins, nucleic acids, and other hormones. Lipids also facilitate the uptake of the fat-soluble vitamins A, D, E, and K. As sources of energy, all three macronutrients are virtually interchangeable, although the nitrogen of the amino acid constituents of proteins must be concomitantly disposed of, mostly in the form of urinary urea. The carbon in these substances is combusted with oxygen, producing carbon dioxide, and during the process the metabolic energy and heat are generated that support living processes. Total dietary intake of macronutrients (and hence energy) should be kept in balance with energy expenditure. Excess intake over expenditure will lead to overweight and eventually obesity, which is detrimental to health, as it is associated with some cancers, coronary heart disease, diabetes, and other chronic diseases. Acceptable macronutrient distribution ranges in human diets have been set for carbohydrates, lipids, and proteins to prevent frank deficiencies and minimize incidences of chronic diseases from overconsumption.

Dietary carbohydrates, primarily starches and sugars, are digested to monosaccharides (primarily glucose and fructose), and transported into the blood. Carbohydrate uptake in excess of that needed for immediate use is stored as glycogen, principally in liver and skeletal muscle, or is converted to fatty acids and stored as triglycerides in adipose depots. Subsequently, glycogen can be broken down to glucose for use as a ready fuel source for the body. Humans do not have a dietary requirement for carbohydrates. However, a diet devoid of carbohydrates would have to compensate with much larger quantities of protein. Some amino acids can be converted to the glucose needed in the body by a process termed gluconeogenesis, whereas little of the fat content can be so converted. However, a high-protein diet would be ketotic, disrupting mineral balance. Because the brain and nervous tissue have a requirement for glucose, an acceptable macronutrient distribution range for carbohydrates has been set at 45 to 65 percent of the energy content of the diet. Furthermore, no more than 25 percent of the energy needs should be met with added sugar, which is metabolized rapidly and can thereby disrupt whole body metabolism. Added sugar is also associated with a lower intake of essential vitamins and minerals, as well as with a high risk of dental caries (cavities).

Dietary lipids, primarily triglycerides, are essentially digested to their constituent fatty acids for absorption and then are reconstituted to triglycerides in intestinal tissue. Because triglycerides are insoluble in water, they are transported in the body via a complex system of lipoproteins—chylomicra, low-density lipoproteins (LDLs), and high-density lipoproteins (HDLs). Their constituent fatty acids are used as fuel by various tissues, and any excess triglycerides are stored in adipose tissue. Two fatty acids, linoleic and α-linolenic, termed essential fatty acids because they cannot be synthesized by the human body, are required in small quantities. Human diets should contain a minimum of 10 percent diversified lipids (linoleic is found in a variety of plant oils and α-linolenic in fish oil) to ensure that the requirement for these essential fatty acids is met. The acceptable macronutrient distribution range for lipids has been set at 20 to 35 percent of the energy content of the diet for adults. Lipid intake should be slightly higher for infants and children because of the demands of growth.

Dietary proteins generally serve as energy sources once the need for their constituent amino acids as precursors of body protein has been met. Dietary proteins are digested to their constituent amino acids and absorbed across the intestinal tract into the blood, where they are taken up by various tissues for synthesis of body proteins, which are continually being broken down and resynthesized. Amino acids absorbed in excess of that need are used as fuel, either directly or after conversion to glucose by gluconeogenesis. Adult humans have a requirement for 0.8 grams (g) of well-balanced protein per kilogram (kg) of body weight each day; this corresponds to 56 g of protein per day for the average man and 46 g per day for the average woman. The acceptable macronutrient distribution range for proteins has been set at 10 to 35 percent of the energy content of the diet. Protein intake should be slightly lower for infants and children to compensate for the higher proportion of lipid intake and to minimize the need to dispose of excess nitrogen.

Disorders and Diseases

The main disorders associated with macronutrients result from their inadequate or excess consumption, namely starvation and obesity. The former is particularly problematic for infants and children because of their higher demands for growth and brain development; some early deficits lead to permanent impairment. Two general types of starvation are recognized; marasmus is due to a general deficiency of macronutrients, also referred to as protein-calorie malnutrition, whereas kwashiorkor is primarily attributed to a deficiency of dietary protein.

Anorexia nervosa (restricted intake) and bulimia nervosa (binge eating followed by purging, vomiting, or misuse of laxatives or diuretics) are two eating disorders with complex and variable etiologies that can lead to reduced macronutrient intake, starvation, and even death.

Ironically, calorie-restricted diets that reduce macronutrient intakes by 20 to 40 percent primarily from carbohydrate and lipids, while maintaining adequate intakes of protein and other nutrients, appear to be associated with increased longevity and decreased incidence of some cancers and other diseases of aging. However, few people are willing to restrict their intake voluntarily to such an extent and to live with a continuous feeling of hunger.

Obesity is a modern epidemic largely because of the ready availability and consumption of inexpensive food coupled with a sedentary lifestyle. While particularly a problem in Western societies, it is making inroads in the rest of the world. Obesity is associated with increased risk of coronary heart disease, some cancers, and type 2 diabetes. Excessive weight also puts added stress on knee and ankle joints. Obesity is, by definition, an energy imbalance, where energy intake (from macronutrients) exceeds energy expenditure, as from physical exercise. Obesity is a multifactorial disease, however, influenced by both genetic and environmental factors. Some people appear to be more susceptible to weight gain, as genetic factors have an impact on appetite, endocrinology, metabolism, and activity. The environmental factors include access to palatable food and lack of exercise. While not a major contributor to the current epidemic, binge eating disorder can lead to obesity.

Perspective and Prospects

The ancient Greeks noted that a wide variety of foods were converted into the organs and tissues of people consuming them. They concluded that the differences between food and human protoplasm must be superficial and that they must be made from the same substance. They also assumed that the need for food after growth had ceased was caused by the wearing out of organs and tissues and the continuous need to replace them. In the late 1700s, Antoine Lavoisier demonstrated that carbon dioxide expiration increased with exercise and that the oxidation of fats and carbohydrates accounted for most of the energy needed for animal heat production. In the nineteenth century, the need for nitrogen in the diet was demonstrated for dogs and by analogy for humans; proteins were first described as the main nitrogen-containing substances in food. Sophisticated calorimetry equipment large enough for humans to live in for several days made it possible to quantitate energy balance and, by 1900, permitted the conclusion that the metabolism of lipids and carbohydrates could be used for mechanical work with similar efficiency. In that same period, dietary proteins were shown to be broken down to amino acids in the digestive tract, absorbed, and used to rebuild body protein.

Relative to macronutrient consumption, the dilemma of undernutrition and overnutrition in the world, often within a country and even within the same household, makes it difficult for nutritionists and public health professionals to tailor recommendations and to inform political decisions. The concept of an optimum intake of macronutrients, while easy to grasp, is difficult to enact. A further complication is the individual variation in metabolism and taste, even within the same culture. Cases have been confirmed where individuals with distinct genotypes respond differently, even oppositely, to the same macronutrient intervention. In the future, one can foresee personalized genomic-based nutrition advice.

—*James L. Robinson, Ph.D.*

See also Anorexia nervosa; Antioxidants; Beriberi; Carbohydrates; Cholesterol; Digestion; Eating disorders; Enzymes; Food biochemistry; Gastroenterology; Gastroenterology, pediatric; Gastrointestinal system; Kwashiorkor; Lactose intolerance; Lipids; Malabsorption; Malnutrition; Metabolism; Obesity; Obesity, childhood; Phytonutrients; Protein; Supplements; Vitamins and minerals; Weight loss and gain.

For Further Information:

Gibney, Michael J., et al. *Clinical Nutrition.* Malden, Mass.: Blackwell Science, 2005.

Mahan, L. Kathleen, and Sylvia Escott-Stump. *Krause's Food, Nutrition, and Diet Therapy.* 11th ed. Philadelphia: W. B. Saunders, 2004.

Otten, Jennifer J., Jennifer Pitzi Hellwig, and Linda D. Meyers. *Dietary Reference Intakes: The Essential Guide to Nutrient Requirements.* Washington, D.C.: National Academies Press, 2006.

Shils, Maurice E., et al. *Modern Nutrition in Health and Disease.* 10th ed. Baltimore: Lippincott Williams & Wilkins, 2006.

United States Department of Agriculture National Agricultural Library. "Macronutrients." *USDA*, July 12, 2013.

Webster-Gandy, Joan, Angela Madden, and Michelle Holdsworth. *Oxford Handbook of Nutrition and Dietetics.* New York: Oxford

University Press, 2012.

Whitney, Eleanor Noss, and Sharon Rady Rolfes. *Understanding Nutrition*. Belmont, Calif.: Wadsworth, Cengage Learning, 2011.

MACULAR DEGENERATION
Disease/Disorder
Anatomy or system affected: Eyes
Specialties and related fields: Ophthalmology
Definition: A degenerative disease of the central portion of the retina that results primarily in loss of central vision.

Information on Macular Degeneration

Causes: Unclear; possibly aging, genetic factors, nutrition, smoking, sunlight exposure
Symptoms: Dependent on form; can include blurred or distorted central vision, bleeding within and beneath retina, development of scar tissue, eventual blindness
Duration: Typically long-term
Treatments: Vision aids (e.g., magnifying glasses, special lenses, electronic systems); laser photocoagulation; surgery; low-level radiation; injection of photosensitive chemicals into bloodstream

---

Causes and Symptoms

The macula is located in the center of the retina, the light-sensitive tissue at the back of the eye. The retina instantly converts light, or an image, into electrical impulses. The retina then sends these impulses, or nerve signals, to the brain. One of the earliest signs of age-related macular degeneration (ARMD) seen by physicians during a dilated eye examination is deposits of tiny, bright yellow material called drusen, which is harder as a result of aging or softer and larger if associated with ARMD and vision loss. As parts of the eye in the retina and choroid become thinner or lose tissue, central vision and/or peripheral vision is affected, depending on the area of damage. Central vision is needed to see clearly and to perform everyday activities such as reading, writing, driving, and recognizing people and things.

Peripheral vision, needed for walking, is much less commonly affected.

There are two forms of ARMD: early and advanced. About 90 percent of cases are early ARMD, although the advanced type affects 7 percent of those seventy-five years or older. Advanced ARMD is further categorized into two distinct types based on their clinical features: dry and wet. The dry form involves thinning of the macular tissues and disturbances in its pigmentation. About 70 percent of patients have the dry form. The remaining 30 percent have the wet form, which can involve bleeding within and beneath the retina, opaque deposits, and eventually scar tissue. The wet form accounts for 90 percent of all cases of legal blindness in macular degeneration patients.

Neither dry nor wet macular degeneration causes pain. The most common early sign of dry macular degeneration is blurring vision that prevents people from seeing details clearly that are in front of them, such as faces or words in a book. In the early stages of wet macular degeneration, straight lines appear wavy or crooked. This is the result of fluid leaking from blood vessels and lifting the macula, distorting vision.

A number of risk factors can affect the initial development of ARMD: age, smoking, genetic predisposition, and ethnicity. Two risk factors have also been studied and suggested in causing a progression of ARMD: nutrition and high blood pressure. Age is the most important risk factor for macular degeneration: The older the patient, the higher the risk. Studies have shown that having a family with a history of macular degeneration raises the risk factor. Because macular degeneration affects most patients later in life, however, it has proven difficult to study cases in successive generations of a family. Heavy smoking, at least a pack of cigarettes a day, can double a person's risk of developing ARMD. The more a person smokes, the higher the risk of macular degeneration. Moreover, the adverse effects of smoking persist, even fifteen to twenty years after quitting. Those with a family history of ARMD are more likely to develop the disease due to a genetic mutation of part of a gene called the complement factor H gene. With a family history of the disease, the risk is greater for developing the wet type than the dry type of ARMD. Studies have shown that non-Hispanic Caucasians have a greater risk of developing ARMD than do African Americans or Hispanics.

Poor dietary habits contribute to ARMD as well. A diet high in saturated fats may clog the vessels leading to the eyes, thus reducing the flow of nutrient-rich blood. Excess fat may deposit itself directly in the membrane behind the retina. In this case, nutrients might not be able to reach the cells that nourish the retina. High blood pressure has also been shown to increase the risk of developing ARMD in the second eye in those having ARMD in one eye.

An effective test to determine if a person has wet macular degeneration is fluorescent angiography. A special dye is injected into a vein in the patient's arm and then flows to the blood vessels in the eye. Photographs are taken of the retina. The dye highlights any problems in the blood vessels and allows the doctor to determine if they can be treated. Annual eye examinations that include dilation of the pupils are also useful in early detection. Early detection is important because a person destined to develop macular degeneration can sometimes be treated before symptoms appear, which may delay or reduce the severity of the disease. Anyone who notices a change in vision should contact an ophthalmologist immediately.

Treatment and Therapy

New and exciting treatments are in development for ARMD as extensive research is being done. Currently, there is no cure, and no treatment recommendations exist for those with dry type ARMD, the type that is much less threatening to vision. Some treatments, however, can slow the progression of wet type ARMD. Research has shown that stopping smoking is the most effective preventive measure in regard to developing ARMD and slowing its progression.

Antioxidants have proved promising in recent studies which show that they can lower the risk of progression to more advanced ARMD in those who have moderate or advanced disease. In a major clinical trial called the Age-Related Disease Study (AREDS), it was shown that patients with moderate or severe ARMD taking antioxidants vitamin C, vitamin E, and beta carotene plus zinc and copper had a lower risk of progression among both nonsmokers and smokers. Since the group of smokers who took zinc alone had the same lowered risk of progression as those smokers taking antioxidants plus zinc and copper, it was recommended that smokers with ARMD take zinc alone, as some antioxidants have shown to increase the risk of lung cancer and coronary heart disease when used at high doses.

Although no treatments can reverse the actual pathologic process of the disease of wet type ARMD, some treatments used by ophthalmologists are aimed at containing the damaged vessels that cause the loss of vision. They include laser photocoagulation, photodynamic therapy, intravitreous injections, and, as a last resort, macular translocation surgery.

Laser photocoagulation involves using a high-intensity thermal laser to burn off the blood supply to abnormal choroidal membranes. The benefits of this treatment are that it is done in the outpatient setting using only topical anesthetic drops and that it prevents the formation of new abnormal vessels associated with ARMD for two or three years. It is limited, however, to only those patients with well-defined abnormal areas (only about 15 percent of patients with ARMD). It cannot restore lost vision and may actually destroy normal retinal tissue along with the neovascular formation that is targeted.

Photodynamic therapy involves the injection of a dye called verteporfin which, when activated by a photo laser, forms substances that destroy the abnormal newly formed vessels associated with wet type ARMD. Thus, by the use of this dye and laser combination, the normal vessels are protected and the abnormal vessels are destroyed. It has also been shown that this treatment can be repeated safely.

The vascular endothelial growth factor (VEGF) inhibitors are a class of agents that block a factor involved in the disease process of ARMD. VEGF is essential for the formation of the new abnormal vessels that cause the loss of vision and the anatomic destruction associated with ARMD. The VEGF inhibitors block this factor, thereby limiting those destructive effects. Studies involving these agents have shown that a majority of patients showed improvement in their vision and marked anatomic improvement of their retinas.

Macular translocation surgery involves surgically removing the macula from a diseased area and attaching it to a healthier area of the retina. Although currently an experimental therapy and not well studied, it can be used for those patients in which no other treatment options are left. If performed successfully, macular translocation surgery can improve central vision and allow a majority of patients to read. Great risks are associated with this type of treatment, however, including detachment of the retina and the development of double vision. In addition, use of a steroid injection into the vitreous and/or the posterior sub-Tenon's space has shown short-term improvement in vision.

Many visual aids have been developed for patients with ARMD to make the most of their remaining vision, including magnifying glasses, powerful special lenses, and large-print books and reading materials. Voice synthesizers in electronic devices such as calculators, clocks, and phones are also very helpful. Maximizing room lighting by the use of stronger lights, opening windows, and painting walls brighter colors can help patients see better at home.

Perspective and Prospects

Blindness or low vision affects 2.6 million Americans aged forty and over, according to the National Eye Institute. This figure is projected to reach 7.1 million by the year 2030 and 13 million by 2050. The study reports that low vision and blindness increase significantly with age, particularly in people over age sixty-five. People eighty years of age and older account for 67 percent of blindness. ARMD affects about 15 percent of the US population by age fifty-five and more than 30 percent by age seventy-five. It is the most common cause of legal blindness in people over the age of fifty-five.

Although there is no cure for ARMD, many treatments are available to curtail progression of the disease. As extensive research continues in this area, advances in the diagnosis and treatment of this debilitating condition are anticipated by many in the field of ophthalmology. Currently, the National Eye Institute is studying the possibility of transplanting healthy cells into a diseased retina, evaluating families with a history of ARMD to understand genetic and hereditary factors that may cause the disease, and looking at certain anti-inflammatory treatments for the wet form of ARMD.

Kenneth Dill, M.D.

See also Aging; Blindness; Blurred vision; Cataracts; Eye infections and disorders; Eye surgery; Eyes; Laser use in surgery; Myopia; Ophthalmology; Smoking; Vision; Vision disorders.

For Further Information:

American Macular Degeneration Foundation. http://www.macular.org.

D'Amato, Robert, and Joan Snyder. *Macular Degeneration: The Latest Scientific Discoveries and Treatments for Preserving Your Sight*. New York: Walker, 2000.

Heier, Jeffrey S. *One Hundred Questions and Answers About Macular Degeneration*. Sudbury, Mass.: Jones and Bartlett, 2011.

Ho Allen C., and Carl D. Regillo. *Age-Related Macular Degeneration Diagnosis and Treatment*. New York: Springer, 2011.

Kansai, Jack. *Diseases of the Macula*. New York: Elsevier, 2002.

Macular Degeneration Foundation. http://www.eye sight.org.

MayoClinic.com. "Macular Degeneration." http://www.mayoclinic.com/health/macular-degeneration/DS00284.

Samuel, Michael A. *Macular Degeneration: A Complete Guide for Patients and Their Families*. Laguna Beach, Calif.: Basic Health, 2008.

Sardegna, Jill, et al. *The Encyclopedia of Blindness and Vision Impairment*. 2d ed. New York: Facts On File, 2002.

Sutton, Amy L., ed. *Eye Care Sourcebook: Basic Consumer Health Information About Eye Care and Eye Disorders*. 3d ed. Detroit, Mich.: Omnigraphics, 2008.

MAGNETIC FIELD THERAPY
Treatment

Anatomy or system affected: Cells, immune system
Specialties and related fields: Alternative medicine
Definition: A practical and inexpensive modality that uses magnets to relieve chronic and acute pain incurred through overuse or trauma.

Indications and Procedures

In this treatment method, which is based on physics principles called the Hall effect and Faraday's law, magnetic pads are placed on or near the site of injury or soreness in order to stimulate local circulation by attracting positive and negatively charged ions in the blood and lymph. This biomagnetic attraction of electrolytes utilizes an alternating pattern of polarities that penetrate 5 to 20 centimeters into the body's tissues, depending on field strength (which is normally between 300 and 950 gauss). A common magnet will not produce this effect because only the ions and fluid in vessels that are precisely in line with the north-south poles will be attracted. Many advocates claim that magnetic therapy works faster than diathermies such as ultrasound. A warm tingling sensation is often felt minutes after application because of the increase of microcirculation, which brings more oxygen, nutrients, white blood cells, and antibodies to the damaged tissues and which removes metabolic waste products.

Uses and Complications

Several forms of magnetic field therapy (including pulsed electromagnetic therapy) have been used for years in Japan, Germany, and other countries, and double-blind studies are being conducted in the United States to determine the validity of numerous testimonials. Disorders that are regularly treated with magnetic therapy in other countries include carpal tunnel syndrome, osteoarthritis, tendinitis, bursitis, migraine headaches, and energy problems such as chronic fatigue syndrome and malaise. Magnetic deficiency syndrome is now documented in Japanese medical literature, and many American physicians agree that proper magnetic balance in the tissues is an overlooked ingredient of health.

Magnetic pads come in several sizes and shapes to allow for comfortable attachment to any area of the body, including silver-dollar-sized pads that are one-eighth of an inch thick, for concentrated force, and 5-by-7-inch pads for larger areas such as the back. Magnetic massage balls, mattress pads, pillows, seat cushions, and orthotic insoles are also sold. The magnets are permanently charged and have no harmful side effects, although they are not recommended for pregnant women or patients wearing pacemakers. In 2005 and 2006, some respected medical journals reported positive treatment outcomes for the healing of surgical wounds. Because this result defies conventional medical wisdom, however, the use of magnetic field therapy in mainstream medicine remains controversial.

—Daniel G. Graetzer, Ph.D.;
updated by LeAnna DeAngelo, Ph.D.

See also Alternative medicine; Bursitis; Carpal tunnel syndrome; Chronic fatigue syndrome; Circulation; Fatigue; Migraine headaches; Osteoarthritis; Pain management; Tendon disorders.

For Further Information:

Burroughs, Hugh, and Mark Kastner. *Alternative Healing: The Complete A-Z Guide to Over 160 Different Alternative Therapies*. La Mesa, Calif.: Halcyon, 1996.
Jacobs, Jennifer, ed. *The Encyclopedia of Alternative Medicine: A Complete Family Guide to Complementary Therapies*. Rev. ed. Boston: Journey Editions, 1997.
National Center for Complementary and Alternative Medicine. "Magnets for Pain Relief." *National Institutes of Health*, February, 2013.
Null, Gary. *Healing with Magnets*. New York: Carroll & Graf, 2006.
Pelletier, Kenneth. *The Best Alternative Medicine*. New York: Fireside, 2002.
Trivieri, Larry, Jr., and John W. Anderson, eds. *Alternative Medicine: The Definitive Guide*. 2d ed. Berkeley, Calif.: Ten Speed Press, 2002.
Vegari, G. *Magnetic Therapy*. Christchurch, New Zealand: Caxton, 2004.
White, R., K. Cutting, and P. Beldon. "Magnet Therapy: Opening the Debate." *Journal of Wound Care* 15, no. 5 (May, 2006): 208-209.

MAGNETIC RESONANCE IMAGING (MRI)
Procedure

Anatomy or system affected: All
Specialties and related fields: Biotechnology, nuclear medicine, radiology
Definition: A noninvasive, nonradiological method of obtaining detailed information concerning normal and diseased tissue.

Key terms:

electromagnetic waves: a convenient way of understanding energy as a wave; visible light, X rays, and radiowaves, which have the longest wavelength and lowest energy, are the most familiar examples
Fourier transform: a mathematical method which allows MRI to utilize one radio frequency pulse and thereby examine all wavelengths, as opposed to examining each wavelength individually with a continuous wave
nucleus: the dense, positively charged, central core of an atom, containing its massive protons and neutrons
zeugmatography: a name applied to MRI characterizing the close relationship of nuclear magnetic forces and electromagnetic waves (from the Greek *zeugma*, meaning "to yoke together")

Indications and Procedures

In 1901, Wilhelm Conrad Röntgen won the first Nobel Prize in Physics for his discovery of x-rays. Twenty-first-century applications of this radiation have produced medical miracles. Magnetic resonance imaging (MRI), often called nuclear magnetic resonance (NMR) imaging, differs in fundamental ways from x-rays and other imaging methods. It is capable of producing a far richer array of three-dimensional images without the dangers attendant on ionizing radiation or the introduction of radioactive chemicals. MRI allows both safe diagnosis and study in healthy subjects. Furthermore, the method can be used to examine flowing matter, such as in the circulatory system.

MRI Scanning

This diagnostic imaging technique employs a powerful magnet to generate a magnetic field that is capable of aligning the protons in the body's hydrogen atoms, which are then knocked out of alignment by radio-wave pulses; as the protons realign, they emit radio signals that can be detected and used to create a cross-sectional image of the body.

The nuclei of hydrogen atoms behave like tiny magnets when they are placed in a magnetic field. When radio waves are superimposed on the magnetic waves, hydrogen atoms can be made to change their alignment with the magnetic field. The time required for the atoms to return to their original orientation, after the radio waves cease, varies with the nature of the tissue in which the hydrogen atoms reside. This combination of natural circumstances together with the marvels of modern electronics have made it possible to obtain detailed images of brain tumors, spinal fluid, and blood vessels.

The discovery, in the mid-1940s, by Edward M. Purcell and Felix Bloch of the basic techniques of nuclear magnetic resonance won for them the 1952 Nobel Prize in Physics. Their innovation changed dramatically the practice of chemistry, biochemistry, and biology. Following new theoretical and practical contributions, diagnostic medicine is participating fully in this revolution.

Both permanent magnets and electromagnets are used, and each has advantages, but the superconducting magnet is rapidly becoming the standard. The essential factors in producing detailed images are constant field strength and a highly uniform field. A transmitter, connected to a radio frequency transmitter-receiver, is used to broadcast the signal and to receive the signal returned from the patient. A short but intense pulse of radio frequency power is required, and its duration is critical to control electronic noise, which obscures the signal required to form the final image. These signals must be processed by complex computer methods to allow the final image to be displayed.

During the 1970s, several innovations were introduced that allowed broad application of the MRI technique. Paul Lauterbur demonstrated the generation of spatial maps by rotating the object to obtain a series of projections from which an image can be reconstructed. His method, called NMR zeugmatography, introduced a radically new approach to MRI. By superimposing a magnetic field gradient on the main magnetic field, it is possible to make the resonance frequency a function of the spatial origin of the signal. Later, Richard R. Ernst built on his earlier introduction of Fourier-transform NMR to develop methods of two-dimensional NMR. Such techniques provide detailed information concerning the local structure of large molecules of biological importance. He was awarded the 1991 Nobel Prize in Chemistry because this same method laid the groundwork for the clinical use of MRI. Methods are now available for the creation of three- and four-dimensional MRI, which are impor-

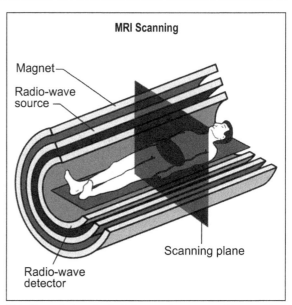

MRI Scanning

Magnet—
Radio-wave source
Scanning plane
Radio-wave detector

This diagnostic imaging technique employs a powerful magnet to generate a magnetic field that is capable of aligning the protons in the body's hydrogen atoms, which are then knocked out of alignment by radio-wave pulses; as the protons realign, they emit radio signals that can be detected and used to create a cross-sectional image of the body.

tant in protein studies and which will pave the way for future applications in nonchemical research.

Uses and Complications

MRI has been used in the evaluation of a wide variety of medical situations. The earliest uses involved the brain and the spinal cord, where it is absolutely necessary to avoid high-energy radiation or radioactivity. Since MRI is capable of providing excellent soft-tissue images and of penetrating bony and air-filled structures, it is also well suited to examination of the chest and abdomen. In these applications, it was first necessary to overcome problems associated with motion. A further important modification, the flow imaging technique, allows the use of MRI in studies of the vascular system and has led to magnetic resonance angiography. This latter approach has clear advantages over the invasive x-ray procedure. Additional modifications allow the direct study of tissues of various living organisms under physiological conditions.

Functional MRI is a developing technique that allows neuroradiologists and neurosurgeons to evaluate the activity of the brain and cerebral blood vessels in real time, observing brain activity while the patient is asked questions or asked to perform various functions. This technique is especially helpful in coma patients or in patients in a persistent vegetative state. There are even rare instances of functional MRI demonstrating active brain function in paralyzed patients who were thought to be brain dead or comatose.

Despite the broad applicability of MRI, there are limitations. Patients on life-support systems or with unstable physi-

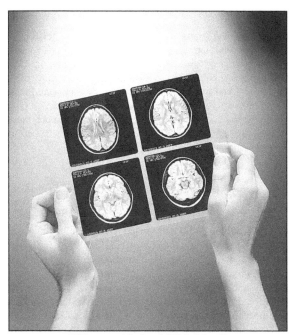

MRI scans of the head. (Digital Stock)

ological conditions must be evaluated with other imaging techniques. The presence of a magnetic metal apparatus in the body is another limitation. There have also been discussions concerning effects that might be related to the electrical currents induced by magnetic gradient fields.

—*K. Thomas Finley, Ph.D.*

See also Computed tomography (CT) scanning; Imaging and radiology; Neuroimaging; Noninvasive tests; Nuclear medicine; Positron emission tomography (PET) scanning; Radiopharmaceuticals; Single photon emission computed tomography (SPECT); Ultrasonography.

For Further Information:

A.D.A.M. Medical Encyclopedia. "MRI." *MedlinePlus*, November 9, 2012.

Bongard, Frederick, and Darryl Y. Sue, eds. *Current Critical Care Diagnosis and Treatment*. 3d ed. New York: McGraw-Hill Medical, 2008.

Bushong, Stewart C. *Magnetic Resonance Imaging: Physical and Biological Principles*. 3d ed. St. Louis, Mo.: Mosby, 2003.

Buxton, Richard B. *An Introduction to Functional Magnetic Resonance Imaging: Principles and Techniques*. 2d ed. New York: Cambridge University Press, 2009.

Cahill, Donald R., Matthew J. Orland, and Gary M. Miller. *Atlas of Human Cross-Sectional Anatomy: With CT and MR Images*. 3d ed. New York: Wiley-Liss, 1995.

Griffith, H. Winter. *Complete Guide to Symptoms, Illness, and Surgery*. Revised and updated by Stephen Moore and Kenneth Yoder. 5th ed. New York: Perigee, 2006.

"Magnetic Resonance Imaging." *Health Library*, March 27, 2013.

Pagana, Kathleen Deska, and Timothy J. Pagana. *Mosby's Diagnostic and Laboratory Test Reference*. 9th ed. St. Louis, Mo.: Mosby/Elsevier, 2009.

Smith, Michael B., K. Kirk Shung, and Timothy J. Mosher. "Magnetic Resonance Imaging." In *Principles of Medical Imaging*, edited by Shung, Smith, and Benjamin M. W. Tsui. San Diego, Calif.: Academic Press, 1992.

US Food and Drug Administration. "MRI (Magnetic Resonance Imaging)." *US Department of Health and Human Services*, June 6, 2012.

MALABSORPTION
Disease/Disorder

Anatomy or system affected: Gallbladder, gastrointestinal system, intestines, liver, pancreas, stomach

Specialties and related fields: Biochemistry, biotechnology, family medicine, gastroenterology, genetics, neonatology, nutrition, pediatrics

Definition: The impaired absorption of nutrients from food into the bloodstream.

Causes and Symptoms

The nutritive components of food—carbohydrates, protein, fats, vitamins, and minerals—must be digested in the gastrointestinal tract and absorbed into the circulatory system to be of use to the body. Malabsorption of these nutrients is caused by specific defects in any one of the many separate processes involved in the digestion and absorption of food. It is also the result of general impairment of the structure or function of the gastrointestinal tract.

Malabsorption leads to poor growth when it affects the uptake of any essential nutrient, which is one that must be obtained from the diet. It may cause diarrhea if one of the more abundant constituents of food is not absorbed; carbohydrate malabsorption will usually lead to a watery diarrhea, while protein and fat malabsorption will cause a foul-smelling diarrhea that is dark or whitish, respectively. Diarrhea itself may reduce the absorption of nutrients.

Cystic fibrosis is one of the most common causes of malabsorption in children. The mucus accompanying this disease is secreted into the gastrointestinal tract; it is largely indigestible and can obstruct the passage of nutrients.

Treatment and Therapy

Treatment for malabsorption depends entirely on its cause. In the case of bacterial infections that affect intestinal function, treatment with appropriate antibiotics will return this function to normal. In celiac sprue, an intolerance to the gluten found in wheat and other grains that alters the absorptive surface of the intestines, the removal of gluten from the diet restores normal activity. Some specific defects can be cured by the elimination or replacement of the dietary constituent that is not well digested or absorbed. Incidence of celiac disease rose during the first decade of the twenty-first century. In other cases, no curative treatment is known, as with cystic fibrosis.

Perspective and Prospects

In 1825, William Beaumont, a US Army surgeon, was the first to study human digestion in the stomach. Since then, the processes of digestion and absorption have become well understood, as have many of the causes of acquired and

```
┌─────────────────────────────────────────────┐
│          Information on Malabsorption         │
│                                               │
│  Causes: Cystic fibrosis, infection, physio-  │
│    logical defects                            │
│  Symptoms: Diarrhea, poor growth              │
│  Duration: Ranges from acute to chronic       │
│  Treatments: Depends on form; may include     │
│    antibiotics, dietary changes               │
└─────────────────────────────────────────────┘
```

inherited malabsorption. Effective treatment has been developed in all but the most intractable cases. It is hoped that progress in understanding the genetic basis for inherited malabsorption will lead to earlier and definitive identification of affected individuals and eventually to suitable therapies.

—James L. Robinson, Ph.D.

See also Allergies; Bariatric surgery; Carbohydrates; Celiac sprue; Cystic fibrosis; Diarrhea and dysentery; Digestion; Gastroenterology; Gastroenterology, pediatric; Gastrointestinal system; Gluten intolerance; Malnutrition; Nutrition; Protein; Vitamins and minerals.

For Further Information:

Bonci, Leslie. *American Dietetic Association Guide to Better Digestion*. New York: Wiley, 2003.

Christian, Janet L., and Janet L. Greger. *Nutrition for Living*. 4th ed. Redwood City, Calif.: Benjamin/Cummings, 1994.

Green, Peter H. R. *Celiac Disease: A Hidden Epidemic*. Rev. ed. New York: William Morrow, 2010.

Jackson, Gordon, and Philip Whitfield. *Digestion: Fueling the System*. New York: Torstar Books, 1984.

Janowitz, Henry D. *Indigestion: Living Better with Upper Intestinal Problems, from Heartburn to Ulcers and Gallstones*. New York: Oxford University Press, 1994.

Mayo Clinic. *Mayo Clinic on Digestive Health: Enjoy Better Digestion with Answers to More than Twelve Common Conditions*. 2d ed. Rochester, Minn.: Author, 2004.

Peikin, Steven R. *Gastrointestinal Health*. Rev. ed. New York: Quill, 2001.

Sharon, Michael. *Complete Nutrition: How to Live in Total Health*. London: Prion, 2001.

Wilson, Hannah M. *Diarrhea: Causes, Types, and Treatments*. New York: Nova Science, 2010.

Wu George Y., Nathan Selsky, and Jane M. Grant-Kels. *Atlas of Dermatological Manifestations of Gastrointestinal Disease*. New York: Springer, 2013.

MALARIA

Disease/Disorder

Also known as: Paludism

Anatomy or system affected: Blood, immune system, liver, spleen

Specialties and related fields: Biochemistry, immunology, internal medicine, pathology, public health

Definition: One of the world's most serious and potentially fatal diseases, malaria is the result of a parasite transmitted into the bloodstream by mosquito bites. It is most common in subtropical zones, especially in Africa, Asia, and Latin America.

Key terms:

Anopheles: the genus of mosquitoes that, by depositing infected saliva into the blood of humans, serves as a vector for transmission of the parasite that causes malaria

merozoites: products of a multistage reproductive process in the malarial parasite's life span; released into the bloodstream, where they destroy red blood cells

Plasmodium falciparum: one of several parasites that cause malarial symptoms; the species that is most dangerous, and lethal, for humans

Causes and Symptoms

Malaria in humans is caused by transfer into the bloodstream, through the saliva of the *Anopheles* mosquito, of the protozoan (single-cell) *Plasmodium* parasite. There are several different strains of the malaria parasite, all belonging to the phylum Sporozoa, a classification connected with the importance of spores in the organism's reproductive cycle. Serious and potentially lethal malarial infections in humans are primarily associated with *P. falciparum*. Other *Plasmodium* parasites that can produce infection are *P. vivax* (formerly present in temperate climate zones but now found only in the subtropics), *P. malariae* (also only subtropical), and *P. ovale* (quite rare, and mainly limited to West Africa). Other *Plasmodium* parasites infect only nonhuman primates (*P. knowlesi* and *P. cynomolgi*, for example), only rodents (four different species), or only birds (*P. cathemerium* and *P. gallinaceum*). The latter two species have been used widely in experimental testing of antimalarial vaccines.

It is important to note that only one mosquito genus, *Anopheles*, and only the female *Anopheles* mosquito, serves the vector function in transmitting malaria. The explanation of the female's role is surprisingly simple: Only the female *Anopheles* nourishes itself (usually in the night hours) by piercing the skin of its victim and sucking small quantities of blood. The male of the species feeds mainly on fruit juices.

In the most common scenario, the mosquito ingests the *Plasmodium* parasite when it sucks the blood of an already infected human. This phase is followed by several others—all connected with the reproductive processes of the same organism (both sexual and asexual)—until subsequent generations of the parasite are passed on by the mosquito to another human host, who then becomes infected. The protozoan's first, sexual stage of reproduction occurs when male gametes emit flagella that seek out and join their female counterpart, producing a fertilized zygote. Once lodged in the gut tissue of the mosquito in the form of an oocyst, a further, asexual stage of reproduction occurs through what is called sporogony: the release from the oocyst of myriad spores. They spread rapidly throughout the body of the mosquito. Many enter the insect host's salivary glands, from which they are transferred into the blood of the next human bitten by the mosquito. It is the further development of the spores in the human organism that produces the disease symptoms associated with malaria.

Once transmitted into the human host through the mosquito saliva, the parasite spores flow quickly through the blood, entering the liver. Their next transformation occurs

Information on Malaria

Causes: Transmission of parasitic infection via mosquitoes
Symptoms: Recurrent bouts of severe fever, chills, sweating, vomiting; damage to kidneys, blood, brain, and liver
Duration: Acute to long-term
Treatments: Drug therapy (chloroquine, mefloquine)

once they lodge themselves in the cells of the liver, becoming what are called hepatic trophozoites. As they feed off of the liver cells, the trophozoites grow and burst open. This process of asexual multiplication in the liver is referred to as hepatic schozogony. At that stage, the parasite has multiplied many hundreds of times, producing the actual agent of malarial disease, merozoites. If the parasite is *P. vivax*, then this phase may not occur immediately, as a result of a state of dormancy in the parasitic trophozoites. In this case, months or even years can pass before the merozoites are released. Even then, the delayed release is still not final. This explains why some malaria-infected individuals experience a cyclical disappearance of symptoms, followed some time later by a resurgence of the latent disease.

When released from the trophozoites, the merozoites quickly invade the red blood cells of the host. The damage that they inflict leads to anemic reactions as the number of healthy blood cells in the organism decreases. It is not only the liver that is affected; the disease can also spread to the spleen.

Once the effects of malaria begin to take hold in the blood and various organs of the body, certain symptoms will appear. There is an onset of fever, probably caused by the release of a pyrogen (a fever-inducing agent) by the white blood cells reacting to the diseased situation of red blood cells that have been attacked by the malaria parasite. Since this release of pyrogens may follow an irregular pattern, fever can come and go, seemingly sporadically. Meanwhile, as the number of parasitized red blood cells increases, infected red blood cells begin to attach themselves to the inside tissue of capillaries of the internal organs. The effect is blockage of the necessary free flow of blood. If pressure builds because of this blockage, then blood vessels themselves may burst. Such internal hemorrhages allow the directionless dispersion of infected blood within the body, increasing the anemic symptoms that are characteristic of malaria. Perhaps the most dramatic sign of blocked blood vessels occurs if and when the parasitized cells affect the blood flow to the brain. In such cases, convulsions occur, eventually leading to coma.

Treatment and Therapy

Long before researchers were able to explain the causes of malaria, treatment of its symptoms, primarily manifested in spells of fever, involved giving the patient doses of quinine. As knowledge of the disease increased, different forms of treatment evolved. Such developments occurred not only as new discoveries emerged; they also became necessary as the

malaria parasite itself evolved genetically, in effect developing its own immunity to quinine-based treatment.

Several compounds were developed in the later decades of the twentieth century to complement or, more recently, to replace complete dependence on quinine.

Depending on the *Plasmodium* species coming into contact with it, the alkaloid quinine could kill the parasitical organism at key stages in its reproductive activity. Sometimes, however, toxic side effects accompanied the use of quinine in malaria cases. These negative effects eventually sparked research aimed at producing synthetic drugs that could be as effective as quinine in preventing malaria, even though they might not be as effective in treating the disease once contracted. The earliest synthetic antimalarials, introduced between 1926 and the early 1950s, included pamaquine, the first synthetic; mepacrine; and chloroquine and primaquine, two well-known drugs from the mid-1940s through the 1950s. These synthetic agents intervened to stop reproduction of the malaria parasite at different points in its life span. Depending on which preventive drug was taken, treatment might have to begin well before expected exposure, during the period of exposure, or for a certain period after being present in a malaria-infected area. Several generations of antimalarial drugs are on the market, but such progress in pharmaceutical options has not effectively resolved the problem of endemic malaria in regions of the world where those most in need lack either public health information programs or the financial means to obtain necessary drugs.

Research involving vaccination to protect against malarial infection has tended to follow one of two main approaches: vaccines to combat the diffusion of spores directly, and vaccines to block one or several stages of the parasite's life cycle. Some vaccines have been developed by extracting spores from the blood of infected patients and using methods such as radiation to reduce their potency. Injection of these weakened agents into the blood can induce formation of antibodies that are able to fight invasive spores coming from an outside source (mosquito saliva) into a potential host organism. Commercial production of such vaccines, however, would require finding an economically viable way of obtaining and treating large quantities of *Plasmodium* spores, not only from *P. falciparum* but also from other malaria parasites that are less deadly but an important threat to large numbers of people around the world. For this reason, researchers have tended to concentrate more on isolating antigens that the body produces naturally to fight invasive spores and merozoites, analyzing them, and attempting to use biotechnology to produce effective synthetic antigens.

Observation over a long period of time has provided statistical evidence that, in a number of subtropical areas where malaria is endemic, fatalities from the disease are more frequent among children than among adults. The reason for this is linked to the adult population's prior exposure to one or more nonlethal malarial infections. In essence, the adult body's production of natural antigens seems to neutralize the effects of blood cells that have become carriers. If they remain in the bloodstream, these antigens reduce the susceptibility to what, in children, takes the form of a sudden invasion of infected and (for the body's immune system) unrecognizable blood cells transmitted through *Anopheles* mosquito bites.

There is, therefore, an entire field of malaria research dealing with the body's own immune responses. Where malaria is concerned, researchers pay particular attention not only to the challenge of understanding how immunity can build in populations living in endemic zones but also to the possibility of increasing the efficiency of certain body organs that naturally affect the bloodstream in ways that can impede the spread of the parasite's damage. Attention has focused, for example, on the internal functions of the spleen. The spleen can prevent the progress of intravascular pathogens in general by reducing the flow of infected red blood cells to other organs and isolating them in a chemical state that renders them less directly dangerous to the body. This capacity is called splenic filtration. Although research has not yet identified an effective way to use externally applied medications to enhance this facet of the spleen's natural defense system, it is agreed that here there is a serious prospect for another area of

treatment to complement, if not replace, preventive drugs and synthetic antigens.

Once it was clear that malaria was transmitted by mosquitoes, the most logical tactic to prevent spread of the disease involved campaigns to eradicate, or at least diminish the life chances of, *Anopheles*. Thus, drainage of swamp areas (a costly but effective measure where possible), public health measures to guard against insalubrious concentrations of stagnant water, and insecticide spraying have been practiced throughout the world to combat *Anopheles*. During World War II and until the late 1950s, DDT was the insecticide of choice. When the harmful side effects of DDT for humans and the environment became apparent, legislation in most but not all countries banned the chemical. Research has since aimed at, but not fully succeeded in, developing safer insecticides that can approach DDT's levels of efficiency.

Perspective and Prospects

Research in the field of malarial disease and its biological origins advanced rather slowly, with most major advances occurring fairly late in the nineteenth century. It was in 1897

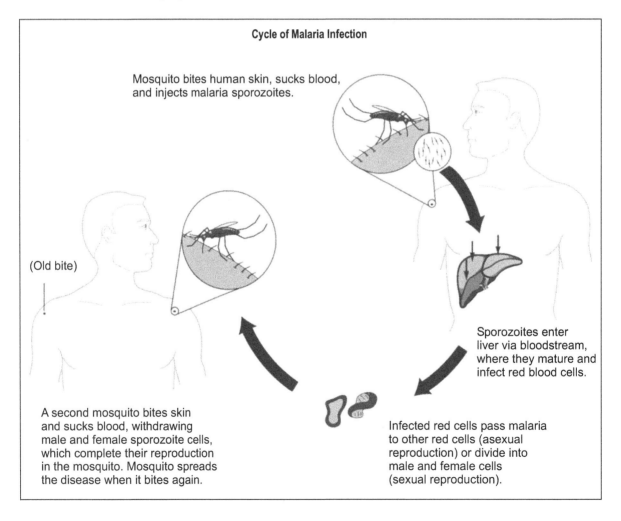

Cycle of Malaria Infection

Mosquito bites human skin, sucks blood, and injects malaria sporozoites.

(Old bite)

Sporozoites enter liver via bloodstream, where they mature and infect red blood cells.

A second mosquito bites skin and sucks blood, withdrawing male and female sporozoite cells, which complete their reproduction in the mosquito. Mosquito spreads the disease when it bites again.

Infected red cells pass malaria to other red cells (asexual reproduction) or divide into male and female cells (sexual reproduction).

that a surgeon in the British Indian army, Sir Ronald Ross, following British tropical disease expert Sir Patrick Manson's suggestions, announced his discovery that malaria was transmitted to humans by mosquitoes. There had been earlier theories concerning the role of mosquitoes, some going back as far as the early eighteenth century in Italy (where the term "malaria," meaning "bad air," had originated). It took the work of a French military doctor in Algeria, Alphonse Laveran, to show, under a microscope, the ongoing activity of parasites in the blood of malaria patients. Laveran also did postmortem studies of malaria victims" blood and organs and found a dark pigment composed mainly of iron which came from the parasites" apparent digestion and waste disposal of vital hemoglobin in the red blood cells. He became the first to posit that malaria was a disease of red blood cells and that it was caused by an invasion of parasites.

From there, it was a question of finding how the parasites entered the human bloodstream. This was the result of Ross's observation in India of a particular variety of mosquito larvae (later identified as the small brown *Anopheles*, distinct from *Culex* varieties commonly observed in the daytime) collected from stagnant waters in the region. When Ross followed Manson's suggestion that mosquitoes hatched from these larvae should be induced to feed from a known malaria patient, he found that only a few insects survived the next few days. When these were dissected, he found oocysts embedded on the wall of the mosquitoes" gut. Microscopic analysis showed that they contained the same dark pigment that Laveran had found in the blood of malaria victims in Algeria.

Both Ross (in 1902) and Laveran (in 1907) received Nobel Prizes in recognition of their work, Ross in medicine and Laveran in physiology or medicine. Other contributors, notably the Italian Giovanni Batista Grassi, carried on significant work in the same first decade of the twentieth century that paralleled (or, according to Grassi, may have been accomplished before) Ross's studies. The most important suggestion by Grassi—which was correct but which took much more work to prove in the laboratory—was that there must be significant transformations, in fact multiple stages of reproduction, between the sporozoite phase of dissemination of the parasite via mosquito saliva and the merozoite phase, when the actual attacking parasite can destroy red blood cells in the human host. Later researchers finally provided, in 1934, convincing evidence that there was a sequence of sexual and asexual phases of reproduction (the later labeled "schizogony") in the life cycle of the *Plasmodium* parasite.

Over the years, other researchers helped broaden the understanding of malaria, its causes, and treatment. Despite the obvious costs paid during the first half of the twentieth century involving debilitation and loss of human lives in areas where malaria was endemic, truly major breakthroughs occurred only during the extraordinary conditions created by World War II. The fact that large numbers of troops were sent to areas in East, South, and Southeast Asia as well as Africa meant that the danger of widespread malarial infection could hamper strategic operations. Distribution of all forms of preventive equipment, including both mosquito nets and insect repellents, was destined to become standard procedure in tropical zones. Doses of quinine were also part of each soldier's medical supply packet.

—*Byron D. Cannon, Ph.D.*

See also Bites and stings; Centers for Disease Control and Prevention (CDC); Epidemics and pandemics; Epidemiology; Fever; Insect-borne diseases; Parasitic diseases; Protozoan diseases; Tropical medicine; Zoonoses.

For Further Information:
Carlton, Jane M., Susan L. Perkins, and Kirk W. Deitsch. *Malaria Parasites: Comparative Genomics, Evolution, and Molecular Biology*. Norfolk, England: Caister Academic Press, 2013.

Farmer, Paul. *Infections and Inequalities: The Modern Plagues*. Berkeley: University of California Press, 2001.

Honigsbaum, Mark. *The Fever Trail: In Search of the Cure for Malaria*. New York: Farrar, Straus and Giroux, 2002.

Malaria Foundation International. http://www.malaria .org.

Rocco, Fiammetta. "Corrections and Clarification: The Global Spread of Malaria in a Future, Warmer World." *Science* 289 (September, 2000): 2283–284.

Rocco, Fiammetta. *The Miraculous Fever-Tree: Malaria and the Quest for a Cure That Changed the World*. New York: HarperCollins, 2003.

World Health Organization. *Defeating Malaria in Asia, the Pacific, Americas, Middle East, and Europe*. New York: Author, 2013.

MALIGNANCY AND METASTASIS
Disease/Disorder
Anatomy or system affected: All

Specialties and related fields: Internal medicine, oncology, pathology, plastic surgery

Definition: "Malignancy" is the uncontrolled growth of tumor cells that invade and compress surrounding tissues and break through the skin or barriers within the body; "metastasis" describes the tendency of malignant cells to break loose from their tumor of origin to travel to other locations within the body.

Key terms:
benign tumors: tumors that grow relatively slowly, do not interfere with normal body functions, and do not metastasize

carcinogen: a natural or artificial substance inducing the transformation of cells toward the malignant state

chemotherapy: the use of chemicals to kill or inhibit the growth of cancer cells

multistep progression: the typical pathway of induction of cancer, beginning with an initial alteration to a gene and progressing to the fully malignant state

oncogene: a gene directly or indirectly inducing the transformation of cells from the normal to the malignant state; most oncogenes have normal counterparts in body cells

retrovirus: a virus infecting mammalian and other cells that sometimes carries and introduces oncogenes into host cells

transfection: a technique used to introduce genes into cells by exposing the cells to fragmented deoxyribonucleic acid (DNA) under conditions that promote the uptake and incorporation of DNA

tumor suppressor gene: a gene that, in its normal form, inhibits cell division

Causes and Symptoms

Cancer cells are characterized by two primary features. One of these is uncontrolled cell division, in which cells enter an unregulated, rapid growth phase by losing the controls that normally limit division rates to the amount required for normal growth and maintenance of body tissues. The second feature is metastasis, in which tumor cells lose the connections that normally hold them in place in body tissues, break loose, and spread from their original sites to lodge and grow in other body locations. Tumor cells with these characteristics are described as malignant.

The detrimental effects of solid malignant tumors are caused by the interference of rapidly growing masses of cancer cells with the activities of normal tissues and organs or by the loss of vital functions due to the conversion of cells with essential functions to nonfunctional forms. Some malignant tumors of glandular tissue upset bodily functions by producing and secreting excessive quantities of hormones.

As solid malignant tumors grow, they compress surrounding normal tissues, destroying normal structures by cutting off blood supplies and interrupting nerve function. They may also break through barriers that separate major body regions, such as internal membranes and epithelia or the gut wall. They may also break through the skin. Such breakthroughs cause internal or external bleeding and infection, and they destroy the organization and separation of body regions necessary for normal function. Both compression and breakthroughs can cause pain that, in advanced cases, may become extreme.

Malignant tumors of blood tissues involve cell lines that normally divide to supply the body's requirements for red and white blood cells. Cancer in these cell lines crowds the bloodstream with immature, nonfunctional cells that are unable to accomplish required activities, such as the delivery of oxygen to tissues or the activation of the immune response.

When the total mass of actively growing and dividing malignant cells becomes large, their demands for nutrients may deprive normal cells, tissues, and organs of needed supplies, leading to generally impaired functions, fatigue, weakness, and weight loss.

Not all unregulated tissue growths are malignant. Some tumors, such as common skin warts, are benign—they do not usually interfere with normal body functions. They grow relatively slowly and do not metastasize. Often, benign tumors are surrounded by a closed capsule of connective tissue that prevents or retards expansion and breakup. Some initially benign tumors may change to malignant forms, however, including even common skin warts.

Individual cells of a malignant tumor exhibit differences from normal cells in activity, biochemistry, physiology, and structure. First and foremost is the characteristic of uncontrolled division. Cancer cells typically move through the division cycle much more rapidly than normal cells. This rapid division is accompanied by biochemical changes characteristic of dividing cells, such as high metabolic rates; increases in the rate of transport of substances across the plasma membrane; increases in protein phosphorylation; raised cytoplas-

---

Information on Malignancy and Metastasis

Causes: Genetic factors, carcinogens, retroviruses
Symptoms: Vary; can include loss or impairment of normal bodily functions, interrupted nerve function, internal or external bleeding and infection, pain, swelling, fatigue, weakness, weight loss
Duration: Often chronic with recurrent episodes
Treatments: Surgery, radiation, chemotherapy

---

mic concentrations of sodium, potassium, and calcium ions; and an elevated pH. Often chromosomal abnormalities are present, including extra or missing chromosomes, exchanges of segments between chromosomes, and breakage.

Cancer cells also typically fail to develop all the characteristics and structures of fully mature cells of their type. They may lose mature characteristics if these were attained before conversion to the malignant state. Frequently, loss of mature characteristics involves disorganization or disappearance of the cytoskeleton. Alterations are also noted in the structure and density of surface carbohydrate groups. Cancer cells lose tight attachments to their neighbors or to supportive extracellular materials such as collagen; some cancer cells secrete enzymes that break cell connections and destroy elements of the extracellular material, aiding their movement into and through surrounding tissues. If removed from the body and placed in test-tube cultures, most cancer cells have the capacity to divide indefinitely. In contrast, most normal body cells placed in a culture medium eventually stop dividing.

The conversion of normal cells to malignant types usually involves multiple causes inducing a series of changes that occur in stages over a considerable length of time. This characteristic is known as the multistep progression of cancer. In most cases, the complete sequence of steps leading from an initiating alteration to full malignancy is unknown.

The initial event in a multistep progression usually involves the alteration of a gene from a normal to an aberrant form known as an oncogene. The gene involved is typically one that regulates cell growth and division or takes part in biochemical sequences with this effect. The alteration may involve the substitution or loss of DNA sequences, the movement of the gene to a new location in the chromosomes, or the movement of another gene or its controlling elements to the vicinity of the gene. In some cases, the alteration involves a gene that in normal form suppresses cell division in cells in which it is active. Loss or alteration of function of such genes, known as tumor suppressor genes, can directly or indirectly increase growth and division rates.

An initiating genetic alteration may be induced by a long list of factors, including exposure to radiation or certain chemicals, the insertion of viral DNA into the chromosomes, or the generation of random mutations during the duplication of genetic material. In a few cancers, the initiating event involves the insertion of an oncogene into the DNA by an infecting virus that carries the oncogene as a part of its genetic makeup.

In some cases, about 5 percent in humans, an initiating oncogene or faulty tumor suppressor gene is inherited, producing a strong predisposition to the development of malignancy. Among these strongly predisposed cancers are familial retinoblastoma, familial adenomatous polyps of the colon, and multiple endocrine neoplasia, in which tumors develop in the thyroid, adrenal medulla, and parathyroid glands. In addition to the strongly predisposed cancers, some, including breast cancer, ovarian cancer, and colon cancers other than familial adenomatous polyps, show some degree of disposition in family lines, meaning that members of these families show a greater tendency to develop the cancer than individuals in other families.

Subsequent steps from the initiating change to the fully malignant state usually include the conversion of additional genes to oncogenic form or the loss of function of tumor suppressor genes. Also important during intermediate stages are further alterations to the initial and succeeding oncogenes that increase their activation. The initial conversion of a normal gene to oncogenic form by its movement to a new location in the chromosomes may be compounded at successive steps, for example, by sequence changes or the multiplication of the oncogene into extra copies. The subsequent steps in progression to the malignant state are driven by many of the sources of change responsible for the initiating step. Because genetic alterations often occur during the duplication and division of the genetic material, an increase in the cell division rate by the initiating change may increase the chance that further alterations leading to full malignancy will occur.

A change advancing the progression toward full malignancy may take place soon after a previous change or only after a long delay. Moreover, further changes may not occur, leaving the progression at an intermediate stage, without the development of full malignancy, for the lifetime of the individual. The avoidance of environmental factors that induce genetic alterations, including overexposure to radiation sources such as sunlight, x-rays, and radon gas and chemicals such as those in cigarette smoke, increases the chance that progression toward malignancy will remain incomplete.

The last stage in progression to full malignancy is often metastasis. After the loss of normal adhesions to neighboring cells or to elements of the extracellular matrix, the separation and movement of cancer cells from a primary tumor to secondary locations may occur through the development of active motility or through breakage into elements of the circulatory system.

Relatively few of the cells that break loose from a tumor survive the rigors of passage through the body. Most are destroyed by various factors, including deformation by passage through narrow capillaries and destruction by blood turbulence around the heart valves and vessel junctions. Furthermore, tumor cells often develop changes in their surface groups that permit detection and elimination by the immune system as they move through the body. Unfortunately, the rigors of travel through the body may act as a sort of natural selection for the cells that are most malignant—that is, those most able to resist destruction—which can then grow uncontrollably and spread further by metastasis.

Many natural and artificial agents trigger the initial step in the progression to the malignant state or push cells through intermediate stages. Most of these agents, collectively called carcinogens, are chemicals or forms of radiation capable of inducing chemical changes in DNA. Some, however, may initiate or further this progression by modifying ribonucleic acids (RNAs) or proteins, or they may act by increasing the rate of DNA replication and cell division.

Treatment and Therapy

Cancer is treated most frequently by one or a combination of three primary techniques: surgical removal of tumors, radiation therapy, and chemotherapy. Surgical removal is most effective if the growth has remained localized so that the entire tumor can be detected and removed. Often, surgery is combined with radiation or chemotherapy in an attempt to eliminate malignant cells that have broken loose from a primary tumor and lodged in other parts of the body. Surgical removal followed by chemotherapy is presently the most effective treatment for most forms of cancer, especially if the tumor is detected and removed before extensive metastasis has taken place. Most responsive to surgical treatments have been skin cancers, many of which are easily detected and remain localized and accessible.

Radiation therapy may be directed toward the destruction of a tumor in a specific body location. Alternatively, it may be used in whole-body exposure to kill cancer cells that have metastasized and lodged in many body regions. In either case, the method takes advantage of the destructive effects of radiation on DNA, particularly during periods when the DNA is under duplication. Because cancer cells undergo replication at higher rates than most other body cells, the technique is more selective for tumors than for normal tissues. The selection is only partial, however, so that body cells that divide rapidly, such as those of the blood, hair follicles, and intestinal lining, are also affected. As a consequence, radiation therapy often has side effects ranging from unpleasant to serious, including hair loss, nausea and vomiting, anemia, and suppression of the immune system. Because radiation is mutagenic, radiation therapy carries the additional disadvantage of being carcinogenic; the treatment, while effective in the destruction or inhibition of a malignant growth, may also initiate new cancers or push cells through intermediate stages in progression toward malignancy.

When possible, radiation is directed only toward the body regions containing a tumor in order to minimize the destruction of normal tissues. This may be accomplished by focusing a radiation source on the tumor or by shielding body regions outside the tumor with a radiation barrier such as a lead sheet.

Chemotherapy involves the use of chemicals that retard cell division or kill tumor cells more readily than normal body cells. Most of the chemicals used in chemotherapy have been discovered by routine screening of substances for their effects on cancer cells in cultures and test animals. Several hundred thousand chemicals were tested in the screening effort that produced the thirty or so chemotherapeutic agents available for cancer treatment.

Many of the chemicals most effective in cancer chemotherapy alter the chemical structure of DNA, produce breaks in DNA molecules, slow or stop DNA duplication, or interfere with the natural systems repairing chemical lesions in DNA. These effects inhibit cell division or interfere with cell functions sufficiently to kill the cancer cells. Because DNA is most susceptible to chemical alteration during duplication and cancer cells duplicate their DNA and divide more rapidly than most normal tissue cells, the effects of these chemicals are most pronounced in malignant types. Normal cells, however, are also affected to some extent, particularly those in tissues that divide more rapidly. As a result, chemotherapeutic chemicals can produce essentially the same detrimental side effects as radiation therapy. The side effects of chemotherapy are serious enough to be fatal in 2 to 5 percent of persons treated. Because they alter DNA, many chemotherapeutic agents are carcinogens and carry the additional risk, as with radiation, of inducing the formation of new cancers.

Not all chemicals used in chemotherapy alter DNA. Some act by interfering with cell division or other cell processes rather than directly modifying DNA. Two chemotherapeutic agents often used in cancer treatment, vinblastine and taxol, for example, slow or stop cell division through their ability to interfere with the spindle structure that divides chromosomes. The drugs can slow or stop tumor growth as well as the division of normal cells.

Tumors frequently develop resistance to some of the chemicals used in chemotherapy, so that the treatment gradually becomes less effective. Development of resistance is often associated with random duplication of DNA segments, commonly noted in tumor cells. In some, the random duplication happens to include genes that provide resistance to the chemicals employed in chemotherapy. The genes providing resistance usually encode enzymes that break down the applied chemical or its metabolic derivatives or transport proteins of the plasma membrane capable of rapidly excreting the chemical from the cell. One gene in particular, the multidrug resistance gene (MDR), is frequently found to be duplicated or highly activated in resistant cells. This gene, which is normally active in cells of the liver, kidney, adrenal glands, and parts of the digestive system, encodes a transport pump that can expel a large number of substances from cells, including many of those used in chemotherapy. Overactivity of the MDR pump can effectively keep chemotherapy drugs below toxic levels in cancer cells. Cells developing resistance are more likely to survive chemotherapy and give rise to malignant cell lines with resistance. The chemotherapeutic agents involved may thus have the unfortunate effect of selecting cells with resistance, thereby ensuring that they will become the dominant types in the tumor.

Success rates with chemotherapy vary from negligible to about 80 percent, depending on the cancer type. For most, success rates do not range above 50 to 60 percent. Some cancer types, including lung, breast, ovarian, and colorectal tumors, respond poorly or not at all to chemotherapy. The overall cure rate for surgery, radiation, and chemotherapy combined, as judged by no recurrence of the cancer for a period of five years, is between 50 and 60 percent.

It is hoped that full success in the treatment of cancer will come from the continued study of the genes controlling cell division and the regulatory mechanisms that modify the activity of these genes in the cell cycle. An understanding of the molecular activities of these genes and their modifying controls may bring with it a molecular means to reach specifically into cancer cells and halt their growth and metastasis.

Perspective and Prospects

Indications that malignancy and metastasis might have a basis in altered gene activity began to appear in the nineteenth century. In 1820, a British physician, Sir William Norris, noted that melanoma, a cancer involving pigmented skin cells, was especially prevalent in one family under study. More than forty kinds of cancer, including common types such as breast cancer and colon cancer, have since been noticed to occur more frequently in some families than in others. Another indication that cancer has a basis in altered gene activity was the fact that the chromosomes of many tumor cells show abnormalities, such as extra chromosomes, broken chromosomes, or rearrangements of one kind or another. These abnormalities suggested that cancer might be induced by altered genes with activities related to cell division.

These indications were put on a firm basis by research with tumors caused by viruses infecting animal cells, most notably those caused by a group of viruses called retroviruses. Many retroviral infections cause little or no damage to their hosts, but some are associated with induction of cancer. (Another type of pathogenic retrovirus is responsible for acquired immunodeficiency syndrome, or AIDS.) The cancer-inducing types of retroviruses were found to carry genes capable of transforming normal cells into malignant ones. The transforming genes were at first thought to be purely viral in origin, but DNA sequencing and other molecular approaches revealed that the viral oncogenes had normal counterparts among the genes directly or indirectly regulating cell division in cells of the infected host. Among the most productive of the investigators using this approach were J. Michael Bishop and Harold E. Varmus, who received the 1989 Nobel Prize in Physiology or Medicine for their research establishing the relationship between retroviral oncogenes and their normal cellular counterparts.

The discovery of altered host genes in cancer-inducing retroviruses prompted a search for similar genes in nonviral cancers. Much of this work was accomplished by transfection experiments, in which the DNA of cancer cells is extracted and introduced into cultured mouse cells. Frequently, the mouse cells are transformed into types that grow much more rapidly than normal cells. The human oncogene responsible for the transformation is then identified in the altered cells. Many of the oncogenes identified by transfection turned out to be among those already carried by retroviruses, confirming by a different route that these genes are capable of contributing to the transformation of cells into a cancerous state. The transfection experiments also identified some additional oncogenes not previously found in retroviruses.

In spite of impressive advances in treatment, cancer remains among the most dreaded of human diseases. Recognized as a major threat to health since the earliest days of recorded history, cancer still counts as one of the most frequent causes of human fatality. In technically advanced countries, it accounts for about 15 to 20 percent of deaths each year. Smoking, the most frequent single cause of cancer, is estimated to be responsible for about one-third of these deaths.

—*Stephen L. Wolfe, Ph.D.*

See also Biopsy; Cancer; Carcinogens; Carcinoma; Cytology; Cytopathology; Imaging and radiology; Laboratory tests; Lymphadenopathy and lymphoma; Mammography; Oncology; Pathology; Radiation therapy; Tumor removal; Tumors.

For Further Information:

Alberts, Bruce, et al. *Molecular Biology of the Cell.* 5th ed. New York: Garland, 2008.

"Cancer." *MedlinePlus*, May 2, 2013.

Eyre, Harmon J., Dianne Partie Lange, and Lois B. Morris. *Informed Decisions: The Complete Book of Cancer Diagnosis, Treatment, and Recovery.* 2d ed. Atlanta: American Cancer Society, 2002.

Ko, Andrew, Malin Dollinger, and Ernest H. Rosenbaum. *Everyone's Guide to Cancer Therapy.* 5th ed. Kansas City, Mo.: Andrews McMeel, 2008.

Lackie, J. M., ed. *The Dictionary of Cell and Molecular Biology.* 4th ed. Boston: Academic Press, 2007.

Lodish, Harvey, et al. *Molecular Cell Biology.* 7th ed. New York: W. H. Freeman, 2012.

"Metastatic Cancer Fact Sheet." *National Cancer Institute*, March 28, 2013.

Weinberg, Robert. "Finding the Anti-Oncogene." *Scientific American* 259 (September, 1988): 44-51.

Wolfe, Stephen L. *Molecular and Cellular Biology.* Belmont, Calif.: Wadsworth, 1993.

MALNUTRITION

Disease/Disorder

Anatomy or system affected: Gastrointestinal system, intestines, nails, stomach, all bodily systems

Specialties and related fields: Gastroenterology, nutrition, pediatrics, public health

Definition: Impaired health caused by an imbalance, either through deficiency or excess, in nutrients.

Key terms:

anemia: a condition in which there is a lower-than-normal concentration of the iron-containing protein in red blood cells, which carry oxygen

famine: a lack of access to food in a population, the cause of which can be a natural disaster, such as a drought, or a situation created by humans, such as a civil war

kwashiorkor: the condition that results from consuming a diet that is sufficient in energy (kilocalories) but inadequate in protein content

marasmus: the condition that results from consuming a diet that is deficient in both energy and protein

osteoporosis: a bone disorder in which the bone's mineral content is decreased over time, resulting in a weakening of the skeleton and susceptibility to bone fractures

protein energy malnutrition (PEM): a deficient intake of energy (kilocalories) and/or protein, the most common type of undernutrition in developing countries; the two major types of PEM are kwashiorkor and marasmus

undernutrition: continued ill health caused by a long-standing dietary deficiency of the energy (kilocalories) and the nutrients that are required to maintain health and provide protection from disease

Causes and Symptoms

Malnutrition literally means "bad nutrition." It can be used broadly to mean an excess or deficiency of the nutrients that are necessary for good health. In industrialized societies, malnutrition typically represents the excess consumption characterized by a diet containing too much energy (kilocalories), fat, and sodium. Malnutrition is most commonly thought, however, to be undernutrition or deficient intake, the consumption of inadequate amounts of nutrients to promote health or to support growth in children. The most severe form of undernutrition is called protein energy malnutrition, or PEM. It commonly affects children, who require nutrients not only to help maintain the body but also to grow. Two types of PEM occur: kwashiorkor and marasmus.

Kwashiorkor is a condition in which a person consumes adequate energy but not enough protein. It usually is seen in children between one and four who are weaned so that the next baby can be breast-fed. The weaning diet consists of gruels made from starchy foods that do not contain an adequate supply of amino acids, the building blocks of protein. These diets do, however, provide enough energy.

Diets in many developing countries are high in bulk, making it nearly impossible for a child to consume a sufficient volume of foods such as rice and grain to obtain an adequate amount of protein for growth. The outward signs of kwashiorkor are a potbelly, dry unpigmented skin, coarse reddish hair, and edema in the legs. Edema results from a lack of certain proteins in the blood that help to maintain a normal fluid balance in the body. The potbelly and swollen limbs often are misinterpreted as signs of being "fat" among the developing world cultures. Other signs requiring further medical testing include fat deposits in the liver and decreased production of digestive enzymes. The mental and physical growth of the child are impaired. Children with kwashiorkor are apathetic, listless, and withdrawn. Ironically, these children lose their appetites. They become very susceptible to upper respiratory infection and diarrhea. Children with kwashiorkor also are deficient in vitamins and minerals that are found in protein-rich foods. There are symptoms caused by these specific nutrient deficiencies as well.

Marasmus literally means "to waste away." It is caused by a deficiency of both calories and protein in the diet. This is the most severe form of childhood malnutrition. Body fat stores are used up to provide energy, and eventually muscle tissue is broken down for body fuel. Victims appear as skin and bones, gazing with large eyes from a bald head with an aged, gaunt appearance. Once severe muscle wasting occurs, death is imminent. Body temperature is below normal. The immune sys-

---

Information on Malnutrition

Causes: Limited diet, possibly related to poverty, famine, or war; chronic diarrhea; vitamin and mineral deficiency; iron-deficiency anemia; certain diseases

Symptoms: Vary; may include dry and unpigmented skin, coarse reddish hair, swollen limbs, impaired mental and physical development, apathy, listlessness, increased susceptibility to upper respiratory infection and diarrhea, gaunt appearance, muscle wasting

Duration: Can be short-term or chronic

Treatments: Refeeding with diet adequate in protein, calories, and other essential nutrients; fluid restoration; vitamin and mineral supplements

---

tem does not operate normally, making these children extremely susceptible to respiratory and gastrointestinal infections.

A vicious cycle develops once the child succumbs to infection. Infection increases the body's need for protein, yet the PEM child is so protein deficient that recovery from even minor respiratory infections is prolonged. Pneumonia and measles become fatal diseases for PEM victims. Severe diarrhea compounds the problem. The child is often dehydrated, and any nourishment that might be consumed will not be adequately absorbed.

The long-term prognosis for these PEM children is poor. If the child survives infections and is fed, PEM returns once the child goes home to the same environment that caused it. Children with repeated episodes of kwashiorkor have high mortality rates.

Children with PEM are most likely victims of famine. Typically, these children either were not breast-fed or were breast-fed for only a few months. If a weaning formula is used, it has not been prepared properly; in many cases, it is mixed with unsanitary water or watered down because the parents cannot afford to buy enough to use it at full strength.

It is difficult to distinguish between the cause of kwashiorkor and that of marasmus. One child ingesting the same diet as another may develop kwashiorkor, while the other may develop marasmus. Some scientists think this may be a result of the different ways in which individuals adapt to nutritional deprivation. Others propose that kwashiorkor is caused by eating moldy grains, since it appears only in rainy, tropical areas.

Another type of malnutrition involves a deficiency of vitamins or minerals. Vitamin A is necessary for the maintenance of healthy skin, and even a mild deficiency causes susceptibility to diarrhea and upper respiratory infection. Diarrhea reinforces the vicious cycle of malnutrition, since it prevents nutrients from being absorbed. With a more severe vitamin A deficiency, changes in the eyes and, eventually, blindness result. Night blindness is usually the first detectable symptom of vitamin A deficiency. The blood that bathes the eye cannot regenerate the visual pigments needed to see in the dark. Vitamin A deficiency, the primary cause of childhood blindness, can result from the lack of either vitamin A or the protein that transports it in the blood. If the deficiency of vitamin A occurs during pregnancy or at birth, the skull does not develop normally and the brain is crowded.

An older child deficient in vitamin A will suffer growth impairment.

Diseases resulting from B-vitamin deficiencies are rare. Strict vegetarians, called vegans, who consume no animal products are at risk for vitamin B_{12} deficiency resulting in an anemia in which the red blood cells are large and immature. Too little folate (folic acid) in the diet can cause a similar anemia. Beriberi is the deficiency disease of thiamine (vitamin B_1) in which the heart and nervous systems are damaged and muscle wasting occurs. Ariboflavinosis (lack of riboflavin) describes a collection of symptoms such as cracks and redness of the eyes and lips; inflamed, sensitive eyelids; and a purple-red tongue.

Pellagra is the deficiency disease of niacin (vitamin B_3). It is characterized by "the Four Ds of pellagra": dermatitis, diarrhea, dementia, and death. Isolated deficiency of a B vitamin is rare, since many B vitamins work in concert. Therefore, a lack of one hinders the function of the rest.

Scurvy is the deficiency disease of vitamin C. Early signs of scurvy are bleeding gums and pinpoint hemorrhages under the skin. As the deficiency becomes more severe, the skin becomes rough, brown, and scaly, eventually resulting in impaired wound healing, soft bones, painful joints, and loose teeth. Finally, hardening of the arteries or massive bleeding results in death.

Rickets is the childhood deficiency disease of vitamin D. Bone formation is impaired, which is reflected in a bowlegged or knock-kneed appearance. In adults, a brittle bone condition called osteomalacia results from vitamin D deficiency.

Malnutrition of minerals is more prevalent in the world, since deficiencies are observed in both industrialized and developing countries. Calcium malnutrition in young children results in stunted growth. Osteoporosis occurs when calcium reserves are drawn upon to supply the other body parts with calcium. This occurs in later adulthood, leaving bones weak and fragile. General loss of stature and fractures of the hip, pelvis, and wrist are common, and a humpback appears. Caucasian and Asian women of small stature are at greatest risk for osteoporosis.

Iron-deficiency anemia is the most common form of malnutrition in developing societies. Lack of consumption of iron-rich foods is common among the poor, and this problem is compounded by iron loss in women who menstruate and who thus lose iron monthly. This deficiency, which is characterized by small, pale red blood cells, causes weakness, fatigue, and sensitivity to cold temperatures. Anemia in children can cause reduced ability to learn and impaired ability to think and to concentrate.

Deficiencies of other minerals are less common. Although these deficiencies are usually seen among people in developing nations, they may occur among the poor, pregnant

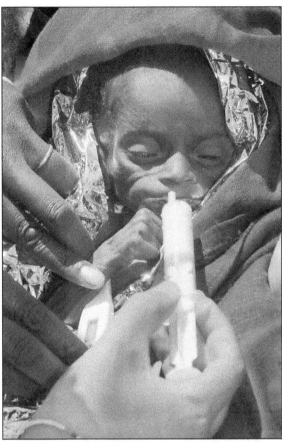

A seven-month-old child suffering from severe malnutrition is helped by a medic in Angola in 2002. (AP/Wide World Photos)

women, children, and the elderly in industrialized societies. Severe growth retardation and arrested sexual maturation are characteristics of zinc deficiency. With iodine deficiency, the cells in the thyroid gland enlarge to try to trap as much iodine as possible. This enlargement of the thyroid gland is called simple or endemic goiter. A more severe iodine deficiency results from a lack of iodine that leads to a deficiency of thyroid hormone during pregnancy. The child of a mother with such a deficiency is born with severe mental and/or physical retardation, a condition known as congenital hypothyroidism or cretinism.

The causes of malnutrition, therefore, can be difficult to isolate, because nutrients work together in the body. In addition, the underlying causes of malnutrition (poverty, famine, and war) often are untreatable.

Treatment and Therapy

Treatment for PEM involves refeeding with a diet adequate in protein, calories, and other essential nutrients. Response to treatment is influenced by many factors, such as the person's age, the stage of development in which the deprivation began, the severity of the deficiency, the duration of the deficiency, and the presence of other illnesses, particularly infections.

Total recovery is possible only if the underlying cause that led to PEM can be eliminated.

PEM can result from illnesses such as cancer and acquired immunodeficiency syndrome (AIDS). Victims of these diseases cannot consume diets with enough energy and protein to meet their body needs, which are higher than normal because of the illness. Infections also increase the need for many nutrients. The first step in treatment must be to cure the underlying infection. People from cultures in which PEM is prevalent often believe that food should not be given to an ill person.

Prevention of PEM is the preferred therapy. In areas with unsafe water supplies and high rates of poverty, women should be encouraged to breast-feed. Education about proper weaning foods provides further defense against PEM. Other preventive efforts involve combining plant proteins into a mixture of high-quality protein, adding nutrients to cereal products, and using genetic engineering to produce grains with a better protein mix. The prevention of underlying causes such as famine and drought may not be feasible.

Prekwashiorkor can be identified by regular plotting of the child's growth. If treatment begins at this stage, patient response is rapid and the prognosis is good. Treatment must begin by correcting the body's fluid imbalance. Low potassium levels must be corrected. Restoration of fluid is followed by adequate provision of calories, with gradual additions of protein that the patient can use to repair damaged immune and digestive systems. Treatment must happen rapidly yet allow the digestive system to recover—thus the term "hurry slowly." Once edema is corrected and blood potassium levels are restored, a diluted milk with added sugar can be given. Gradually, vegetable oil is added to increase the intake of calories. Vitamin and mineral supplements are given. Final diet therapy includes a diet of skim milk and other animal protein sources, coupled with the addition of vegetables and fat.

The residual effects of PEM may be great if malnutrition has come at a critical period in development or has been of long duration. In prolonged cases, damage to growth and the digestive system may be irreversible. Mortality is very high in such cases. Normally, the digestive tract undergoes rapid cell replacement; therefore, this system is one of the first to suffer in PEM. Absorptive surfaces shrink, and digestive enzymes and protein carriers that transport nutrients are lacking.

Another critical factor in the treatment of PEM is the stage of development in which the deprivation occurs. Most PEM victims are children. If nutritional deprivation occurs during pregnancy, the consequence is increased risk of infant death. If the child is carried to term, it is of low birth weight, placing it at high risk for death. Malnutrition during lactation decreases the quantity, but not always the nutritional quality, of milk. Thus, fewer calories are consumed by the baby. Growth of the child is slowed. These babies are short for their age and continue to be shorter later in life, even if their diet improves.

During the first two years of life, the brain continues to grow. Nutritional deprivation can impair mental development and cognitive function. For only minimal damage to occur, malnutrition must be treated in early stages. Adults experiencing malnutrition are more adaptive to it, since their protein energy needs are not as great. Weight loss, muscle wasting, and impaired immune function occur, and malnourished women stop menstruating.

Successful treatment of a specific nutrient deficiency depends on the duration of the deficiency and the stage in a person's development at which it occurs. Vitamin A is a fat-soluble vitamin that is stored in the body. Thus, oral supplements or injections of vitamin A can provide long-term protection from this deficiency. If vitamin A is given early enough, the deficiency can be rapidly reversed. By the time the patient is blind, sight cannot be restored, and frequently the patient dies because of other illnesses. Treatment also is dependent upon adequate protein to provide carriers in the blood to transport these vitamins. Treatment of the B-vitamin deficiencies involves oral and intramuscular injections. The crucial step in treatment is to initiate therapy before irreversible damage has occurred. Scurvy (vitamin C deficiency) can be eliminated in five days by administering the amount of vitamin C found in approximately three cups of orange juice. Treatment of vitamin D deficiency in children and adults involves an oral dose of two to twelve times the recommended daily allowance of the vitamin. Halibut and cod liver oils are frequently given as vitamin D supplements.

Successful treatment of a mineral deficiency depends on the timing and duration of the deficiency. Once the bones are fully grown, restoring calcium to optimal levels will not correct short stature. To prevent osteoporosis, bones must have been filled to the maximum with calcium during early adulthood. Estrogen replacement therapy and weight-bearing exercise retard calcium loss in later years and do more than calcium supplements can.

Iron supplementation is necessary to correct iron-deficiency anemia. Iron supplements are routinely prescribed for pregnant women to prevent anemia during pregnancy. Treatment also includes a diet with adequate meat, fish, and poultry to provide not only iron but also a factor that enhances absorption. Iron absorption is also enhanced by vitamin C. Anemias caused by lack of folate and vitamin B_{12} will not respond to iron therapy. These anemias must be treated by adding the appropriate vitamin to the diet.

Zinc supplementation can correct arrested sexual maturation and impaired growth if it is begun in time. In areas where the soil does not contain iodine, iodine is added to salt or injections of iodized oil are given to prevent goiter. Cretinism cannot be cured—only prevented.

In general, malnutrition is caused by a diet of limited variety and quantity. The underlying causes of malnutrition—poverty, famine, and war—are often untreatable. Overall treatment lies in prevention by providing all people with a diet that is adequate in all nutrients, including vitamins, minerals, and calories. Sharing the world's wealth and ending political strife and greed are essential elements of the struggle to end malnutrition.

Perspective and Prospects

Over the years, the study of malnutrition has shifted to include the excessive intake of nutrients. In developing countries, the primary causes of death are infectious diseases, and undernutrition is a risk factor. In industrialized societies, however, the primary causes of death are chronic diseases, and overnutrition is a risk factor. The excessive consumption of sugar is linked to tooth decay. Also, overnutrition in terms of too much fat and calories in the diet leads to obesity, high blood pressure, stroke, heart disease, some cancers, liver disease, and one type of diabetes.

Historically, the focus of malnutrition studies was deficiencies in the diet. In the 1930s, classic kwashiorkor was described by Cicely Williams. Not until after World War II was it known that kwashiorkor was caused by a lack of protein in the diet. In 1959, Derrick B. Jelliffe introduced the term *protein-calorie malnutrition* to describe the nutritional disorders of marasmus, marasmic kwashiorkor, and kwashiorkor.

PEM remains the most important public health problem in developing countries. Few cases are seen in Western societies. Historically, the root causes have been urbanization, periods of famine, and the failure to breast-feed or early cessation of breast-feeding. Marasmus is prevalent in urban areas among infants under one year old, while kwashiorkor is prevalent in rural areas during the second year of life.

Deficiencies of specific nutrients have been documented throughout history. Vitamin A deficiency and its cure were documented by Egyptians and Chinese around 1500 BCE. In occupied Denmark during World War I, vitamin A deficiency, caused by dairy product deprivation, was common in Danish children. Beriberi, first documented in Asia, was caused by diets of polished rice that were deficient in thiamine. Pellagra was seen in epidemic proportions in the southern United States, where corn was the staple grain, during World War I.

Zinc deficiency was first reported in the 1960s. The growth and maturation of boys in the Middle East were studied. Their diets were low in zinc and high in substances that prevented zinc absorption. Consequently, the World Health Organization recommended increased zinc intake for populations whose staple is unleavened whole grain bread. Goiter was documented during Julius Caesar's reign. Simply adding iodine to salt has virtually eliminated goiter in the United States.

If classic malnutrition is observed in industrialized societies, it usually is secondary to other diseases, such as AIDS and cancer. Hunger and poverty are problems that contribute to malnutrition; however, the malnutrition that results is less severe than that found in developing countries.

Specific nutrients may be lacking in the diets of the poor. Iron-deficiency anemia is prevalent among the poor, and this anemia may impair learning ability. Other deficiencies may be subclinical, which means that no detectable signs are observed, yet normal nutrient pools in the body are depleted. Homelessness, poverty, and drug or alcohol abuse are the major contributing factors to these conditions. In addition, malnutrition as a result of poverty is exacerbated by lack of nutritional knowledge and/or poor food choices.

—Wendy L. Stuhldreher, Ph.D., R.D.

See also Anemia; Anorexia nervosa; Appetite loss; Bariatric surgery; Beriberi; Breast-feeding; Bulimia; Carbohydrates; Celiac sprue; Cholesterol; Congenital hypothyroidism; Eating disorders; Failure to thrive; Food biochemistry; Fructosemia; Galactosemia; Gluten intolerance; Goiter; Growth; Hirschsprung's disease; Hypercholesterolemia; Hyperlipidemia; Kwashiorkor; Lactose intolerance; Lead poisoning; Macronutrients; Malabsorption; Metabolism; Nutrition; Osteoporosis; Protein; Scurvy; Supplements; Thyroid disorders; Vitamins and minerals; Weaning; Weight loss and gain; Weight loss medications.

For Further Information:

Barasi, Mary E. *Human Nutrition: A Health Perspective*. 2d ed. New York: Oxford University Press, 2003.

Christian, Janet L., and Janet L. Greger. *Nutrition for Living*. 4th ed. Redwood City, Calif.: Benjamin/Cummings, 1994.

Garrow, J. S., W. P. T. James, and A. Ralph, eds. *Human Nutrition and Dietetics*. 10th ed. New York: Churchill Livingstone, 2000.

Healey, Justin. "Global Food Crisis." In *Issues in Society*. Thirroul: Spinney Press, 2011.

Knight, Lindsay, and International Federation of Red Cross and Red Crescent Societies. "World Disasters Report 2011: Focus on Hunger and Malnutrition." In *Focus on Hunger and Malnutrition*. Geneva: International Federation of Red Cross and Red Crescent Societies, 2011.

Kreutler, Patricia A., and Dorice M. Czajka-Narins. *Nutrition in Perspective*. 2d ed. Englewood Cliffs, N.J.: Prentice Hall, 1987.

MedlinePlus. "Malnutrition." *MedlinePlus*, July 20, 2013.

Nemours. "Hunger and Malnutrition." *KidsHealth*, 1995-2013.

Wardlaw, Gordon M., and Anne M. Smith. *Contemporary Nutrition*. 9th ed. New York: McGraw-Hill, 2013.

Whitney, Eleanor Ross, and Sharon Rady Rolfes. *Understanding Nutrition*. 13th ed. Belmont, Calif.: Wadsworth, Cengage Learning, 2013.

Zieve, David, and David R. Eltz. "Malnutrition." *MedlinePlus*, June 14, 2011.

MAMMOGRAPHY

Procedure

Anatomy or system affected: Breasts

Specialties and related fields: Gynecology, oncology, preventive medicine, radiology

Definition: The use of X rays of the female breast, primarily in the detection and diagnosis of malignant breast tumors.

Indications and Procedures

X-ray mammography is a complicated procedure. The quality of the mammographic image is proportionately dependent upon the imaging equipment in use and the way in which it is utilized.

Critical factors include compression and positioning of the breast, the use of the right image receptor, and exposure of the x-ray tube. Improper use of equipment and procedures contributes to an image that is suboptimal. With proper care and thorough knowledge in the use of instruments designed for mammography, however, excellent image quality can be obtained.

In mammography, four physical constraints must be considered when evaluating the performance of the systems. First, contrast is of utmost importance because minute differences in soft tissue density are essential. Second, resolution is important because of the need to identify microcalcifications

as small as 100 micrometers, which are often associated with abnormalities. Third, an adequate x-ray dose is vital to obtain an image with the proper signal-to-noise ratio. Too much radiation, however, means added risk for the patient. Fourth, a decrease in noise (background) is important to achieve an image with an adequate signal-to-noise ratio for proper diagnosis.

The examination can be conducted with the patient standing or sitting. To achieve the desired radiographic projection, the x-ray tube is set at an optimal angle. The mammography unit has a support plate onto which the breast is positioned. A plastic paddle assists in compressing the breast onto this plate. The pressure applied to achieve proper compression can be applied manually, but most mammography technicians prefer power-assisted compression, as this permits the radiographer to use both hands to position the breast properly. The shape, rigidity, and composition of the compression or support plate are crucial factors. The support plate is composed of a carbon-fiber composite capable of a high x-ray transmission. The support is in front of the tunnel, and the tunnel receives the image receptor. The standard image receptor uses a high-resolution mammographic screen-film combination. With receptor technology advancing rapidly, however, digital receptors are fast becoming available. The big advantage of digital receptors is that they offer either a limited field of view for stereotactical localization or a full field of view for standard mammographic imaging.

Since all mammography units are intended to show the soft tissue of the breast while displaying differences in contrast and since proper compression is vital, the natural mobility of the breast should be considered. The breast is easiest to compress from the inferior and lateral aspects. The preliminary automatic compression between the paddle and the support plate should never go beyond forty-five pounds of pressure, and the patient should not be in pain. Nevertheless, the breast must be taut to the touch.

Improper compression can lead to erroneous results. The outcome of proper compression is a reduction of x-ray radiation to the breast by reducing tissue thickness; the bringing of lesions closer to the film, thus facilitating an accurate reading; a reduction in movement blurriness because the breast is held immobile; increased contrast as a result of flattened breasts, thereby decreasing thickness; elimination of confusion caused by superimposition shadows; and easier visualization of the borders of circumscribed lesions.

It is helpful if magnification of the image is possible, particularly if small areas are being examined. Magnification is of greater importance in areas of suspicious microcalcifications or at surgical sites. Unfortunately, the greater the magnification, the higher the patient's radiation dose because the breast is placed much closer to the source of radiation.

In addition to compression, image quality depends on a number of factors: positioning, radiation exposure, contrast, sharpness, noise, artifacts, and labeling. The craniocaudal position (compression of the breast from top to bottom) and the mediolateral oblique position (compression of the breast from side to side) are the two standard positions employed in mammography. Each position provides specific views, and proper positioning reveals as much of the tissue as possible for diagnosis. Any area that is omitted will create false results that may endanger the patient's life. Adequate exposure to radiation is essential. If this is not achieved, then it is difficult to identify the skin and subcutaneous tissue. Usually, contrast is highest for thinner breasts and lowest for thicker breasts; this is primarily the result of more scattered radiation and greater tissue absorption of low radiation in thicker breasts. Without contrast, particularly in thicker breast tissue, different tissue densities will have very similar appearances.

Sharpness, or the visualization of fine details in the image, is one of the central factors in achieving a correct diagnosis. If the desired sharpness is not obtained, then the image is referred to as "unsharp." Unsharpness may be the result of motion blur, poor screen-film contrast, or other technical factors. Noise and sharpness are closely linked. "Noise" is defined as increased background and a decreased ability to see tiny structures, such as calcifications. The major contributors of noise are scatter and quantum mottle, which is fluctuation in the number of x-ray photons needed to form the image. Examples of artifacts are scratches, fingerprints, dirt, lint, and dust. Standardized labeling in mammography to identify the left side from the right side, so that the films cannot be subject to misinterpretation, is vital, especially because mammograms can be legal documents.

A slightly different approach is used to screen women with breast implants. Two craniocaudal views are obtained, one with the implant in the field of view and one with the implant as much out of the field as possible. In a similar way, two mediolateral oblique views are imaged.

Digital mammography differs from regular mammography in that in the former, electronic detectors capture and facilitate the display of the x-ray signals on a computer or laser-printed film. In all other aspects, it is still the same procedure—proper positioning and compression of the breast are still critical for obtaining quality digital images. The goal of digital mammography also remains the same: to detect and localize breast abnormalities.

As exposure to radiation is a major concern with traditional mammography, the primary force to developing digital x-ray mammography is the idea that it has the potential to enhance image quality—and therefore lesion detection, especially for dense breasts—with a lower dose of radiation. The greatest advantage in digital mammography is its ability to separate image acquisition from image display, thus providing the ability to manipulate contrast, brightness, and magnification with one exposure.

Dynamic or real-time imaging, especially with biopsies, is possible with digital mammography, providing a better understanding of breast tumors with regard to localization and boundaries. This procedure can also facilitate the direct use of computers for detection and diagnosis. Such computer-aided detection (CAD) programs can identify areas of abnormal or suspicious tissue for the radiologist. In addition, with digital technology, it is possible to form three-dimensional (3-D) images by combining x-rays images from all angles along an arc

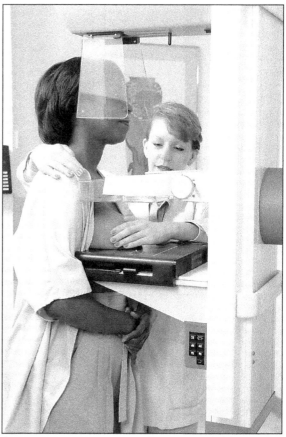

A woman receives a mammogram. It is recommended that regular screenings take place beginning in middle age. (PhotoDisc)

around the breast. The ease of digital image archiving, retrieval, and transmission is another advantage. One disadvantage is that while digital mammograms require lower doses of radiation than traditional film mammograms, 3-D imaging is often conducted simultaneous to traditional 2-D mammography, thus elevating the total radiation administered.

Uses and Complications

There are two basic types of mammographic examinations: screening mammography and diagnostic mammography. "Screening mammography" refers to examinations of women with no obvious symptoms to detect breast cancers. A standard screening examination includes two views of each breast, sometimes referred to as the "standard views."

General agreement has been reached that screening mammography reduces mortality from breast cancer in women fifty years of age or older, but an ongoing debate exists over the effectiveness of screening mammography in women aged forty to forty-nine. Randomized clinical trials have confirmed the validity of screening mammography. Deaths attributable to breast cancer have been reduced. The American Cancer Society and most other well-known professional societies have continued to recommend screening mammography for women in the younger age group because of the results of several studies that advocate the benefits of screening in this age group. Likewise, the frequency of screening mammography remains a subject of debate. Since 2009, the US Preventative Services Task Force has recommended biennial screening for women over fifty, while most other major organizations continue to recommend annual screening. The National Cancer Institute also recommends that screening mammography begin earlier and be conducted more frequently in women who have a family history of breast cancer.

A negative result produced by screening mammography would not include straight lines, unless there is a history of surgery or trauma, and would not show bulging contours from tissue into fatty areas. Characteristics in a screening view that suggest the need for follow-up diagnostic screening are masses, microcalcifications, architectural distortion, and parenchymal asymmetry. Palpable abnormalities described by the patient, focal tenderness, and spontaneous nipple discharge also warrant diagnostic screening.

As with all preventive measures, screening mammography cannot eliminate all deaths from breast cancer, for several reasons. It does not detect all types of cancers, including some that are actually detected by physical examination. Also some tumors may appear and develop too quickly to be detected and identified at an early, more curable stage. Mammograms are particularly difficult to interpret for women with dense breast tissue, which is especially common in young women. The dense tissue prevents the identification of abnormalities associated with tumors, thereby leading to a higher rate of false-positive and false-negative test results.

Diagnostic mammography, also referred to as "consultative mammography" or "problem-solving mammography," is the type of study preferred when there are clinical findings, such as a palpable lump or an abnormal screening mammogram requiring additional analysis. Additionally, each diagnostic mammography examination is performed to suit the individual patient who has symptoms or abnormal findings. Diagnostic mammography may warrant additional views of the breast (such as spot compression and magnification), a correlative clinical examination, and ultrasonography. In almost all instances, barring a few exceptions, a radiologist is present during a diagnostic mammography study.

Diagnostic mammography should be carried out when a biopsy is being considered for a palpable lump in a woman over thirty years of age. The reason for doing a mammogram preceding a biopsy is to better define the nature of the clinical abnormality and to find other unexpected lesions.

Mammographic characteristics of possible benign lesions are a cluster of small round or oval calcifications; nonpalpable, noncalcified, solid round or oval, and predominantly well-circumscribed masses; nonpalpable focal symmetry with concave margins and interspersed fat; asymptomatic single dilated duct (no nipple discharge); and multiple (three or more) similar findings, distributed randomly and often bilaterally. Mammographic characteristics of malignant lesions are a mass with no history of previous surgery,

trauma, or mastitis that is ill defined and microtubulated; malignant microcalcifications; skin thickening and retraction; nipple retraction; and architectural distortion with no history of previous surgery or trauma.

The ruling concern in mammography is the amount of radiation to which the patient is exposed. Therefore, an automatic radiation exposure control device is necessary to avoid overexposure. The radiation detector is placed behind the image receptor so that its image does not appear on the mammogram. Exposure is terminated when the signal recorded by the monitor reaches a predefined level. Unfortunately, the x-ray photons reaching the detector fluctuate considerably depending on the size and composition of the breast. As a result, the signal recorded by the detector is only an approximate indication of the energy absorbed. Therefore, it is unlikely that an accurate reading will be available.

In any therapeutic model that is considered a source of risk to the patient, it is essential to bear in mind the number of deaths caused by the technique as opposed to the number of deaths that it actually prevents. Fortunately, the benefits of mammography supersede the risk of radiation exposure. Furthermore, risk estimates have decreased following the adoption of a relative risk model and allowance for the variation of risk with age at exposure.

Perspective and Prospects

Though much progress has been made in the field of cancer medicine, early detection remains the best approach in the war against breast cancer. Ample clinical data have shown that women diagnosed with breast cancers in the early stages are more likely to survive than those diagnosed with more advanced stages of the same disease. A systematic physical breast examination by a clinician once a year may help in identifying tumors that are fairly small and that may go unnoticed in the absence of such examinations. The relative benefits and risks of regular breast self-examination remain a subject of debate among medical experts.

Nearly all medical experts agree that in women over fifty, routine x-ray mammography, with or without clinical examination, has been valuable in detecting tumors and at earlier stages. This has been very effectively shown in randomized clinical trials to reduce disease-specific mortality. Consequently, routine mammographic screening, especially for women over fifty years of age, has been actively promoted in many countries and nongovernmental agencies.

Breast imaging technologies that are being developed are progressing with three distinct goals in mind: to identify the most minute tumor lesions; to localize abnormalities to aid further examination, analysis, or treatment; and to characterize the abnormalities and assist in the decision-making process following identification. Radiologists and patients alike dream of an ideal imaging modality that would achieve all three goals in a single use. In reality, most current technologies fail to do so; hence, many developers are intent on perfecting one goal at a time. In addition to these technical goals, developers hope to generate methods that are more practical, inexpensive, harmless, and appealing to the patient.

—*Giri Sulur, Ph.D.*

See also Breast biopsy; Breast cancer; Breast disorders; Breast surgery; Breasts, female; Cancer; Cyst removal; Cysts; Glands; Gynecology; Imaging and radiology; Mastectomy and lumpectomy; Mastitis; Noninvasive tests; Oncology; Pathology; Screening; Tumor removal; Tumors; Women's health.

For Further Information:

A.D.A.M. Medical Encyclopedia. "Mammography." *MedlinePlus*, November 17, 2012.

Bassett, Lawrence W., et al. *Film-Screen Mammography: An Atlas of Instructional Cases*. New York: Raven Press, 1991.

Gamagami, Parvis. *Atlas of Mammography: New Early Signs in Breast Cancer*. Cambridge, Mass.: Blackwell Science, 1996.

Kopans, Daniel B. *Breast Imaging*. 3d ed. Baltimore: Lippincott Williams & Wilkins, 2007.

Love, Susan, and Karen Lindsey. *Dr. Susan Love's Breast Book*. 5th ed. Cambridge, Mass.: Da Capo Press, 2010.

"Mammography." *Health Library*, October 31, 2012.

National Cancer Institute. "Mammograms." *National Institutes of Health*, July 24, 2012.

Mitchell, George W., Jr., and Lawrence W. Bassett, eds. *The Female Breast and Its Disorders*. Baltimore: Williams & Wilkins, 1990.

RadiologyInfo.org. "Mammography." *Radiological Society of North America*, May 7, 2013.

Sutton, Amy L., ed. *Cancer Sourcebook for Women: Basic Consumer Health Information About Leading Causes of Cancer in Women*. 3d ed. Detroit, Mich.: Omnigraphics, 2006.

MANAGED CARE

Health care system

Specialties and related fields: Organizations and programs, public health

Definition: A health insurance system that oversees or manages the access, quality, and cost of medical care of its participants.

Structure and Subtypes

Managed care organizations are health insurance plans that aim to provide efficient, quality health care by management of services. The main goals of managed care organizations include providing quality health care services and providing the services at the best cost to the insurance company. These goals are met by direct oversight over an individual's care, such as determining medical necessity of health services and evaluating the appropriateness of specialists" referrals.

There are three general types of managed care organizations: the health maintenance organization (HMO), the preferred provider organization (PPO), and the point-of-service organization (POS). Each type of insurance plan has its own distinct characteristics and carries its own advantages and disadvantages to its participants. HMOs focus on preventive medicine and place strong emphasis on the role of the primary care physician. HMOs are structured into networks of providers, or physicians and hospitals that participate in their program. Patients pay a set monthly fee and, in order to be covered by the insurance company, must see only physicians within the approved network. HMOs are unique in that they serve as the insurance company (the payer) and the provider at the same time; the physicians, hospitals, and insurers that participate in the HMO are also employed by the organization. The primary care physician serves as a gatekeeper to other physicians in the system. Therefore, the primary care physician must approve and coordinate all contact with any medical care for his or her patients. This includes access to specialists (such as cardiologists, dermatologists, or psychiatrists) and any medical procedures. The only exception to this rule is during an emergency or crisis situation. In this way, HMOs are considered the strictest and most restricting type of managed care organization available.

One advantage of HMOs is low out-of-pocket costs for the patient. The fixed monthly fee that is charged to the patient does not depend on the amount of care given and cannot increase with increased visits. Similarly, HMOs do not have maximum lifetime payouts, unlike some other health insurance structures. Therefore, any amount of care that is deemed necessary will be provided to the patient with no maximum cap. Another advantage of an HMO plan is the focus on preventive medicine and wellness, encouraging visiting a physician regularly and healthy lifestyle choices. However, there are some disadvantages to HMO plans. These can include a limited access to specialty care in a timely manner and no coverage for physicians outside the network.

Health maintenance organizations operate in a variety of subtypes. These subtypes may overlap in style and operation. In the staff model, physicians are salaried and are direct employees of the HMO. Their offices are typically in buildings that belong exclusively to the HMO company and are operated by other physicians in the system. In this type of system, the physicians only see patients under the specific managed care of the HMO. In the group model of the HMO, the company does not employ the physicians directly; they are contracted together. Physicians practice under a group practice format, and the group practice is employed itself by the HMO. Traditionally, the group practice model physicians also only see patients who are part of the HMO program. The last subtype of HMO structure is an independent practice association (IPA), in which the association serves as an intermediate between the physician and the HMO. In this model, the physician may see his or her own patients as well as patients with the HMO plan.

The PPO, also called an open-access HMO, is managed differently than a health maintenance organization. In a PPO, the physicians and hospitals are contracted to provide services only to a specific group of individuals who participate in the PPO. The system is similar to the HMO in that the group of physicians and hospitals form a network for care, but there is no primary care physician who serves as a gatekeeper in the PPO. A patient may see a specialist without approval or management from another physician. Also, in a PPO, patients are permitted to visit a physician outside the network for an increased cost. Therefore, seeing a physician who is in the network usually has a lower out-of-pocket cost for the patient than seeing a physician out of the network. Unlike the HMO, in a PPO the patient does not pay monthly regardless of the services provided but pays out of pocket in deductibles and copays based on how many visits they incur.

One advantage of the PPO system is more freedom in choosing the provider of choice, as well as the ability to see a specialist without prior approval of a primary care physician. Also, out-of-pocket expenses, such as deductibles, are capped each year, limiting the amount a patient or family has to pay for health care services. However, a disadvantage of a PPO system is that there is limited coverage for providers who are outside the network. Also, significant paperwork and time may be involved in reimbursement for services out of the network.

A POS plan is a type of managed health care that integrates features of both the HMO and the PPO. These systems involve in-network (contracted) physicians and hospitals but also enable patients to visit physicians outside of the network. In this type of insurance plan, similar to an HMO, there is no deductible paid by the patient and usually only a minimal copayment when a health care provider in network is used. Also, a primary care physician is chosen who makes referrals to specialists. If one chooses to go outside the network for health care, POS coverage functions more like a PPO. When using an out-of-network provider, the patient may have an annual deductible and be responsible for copays to the out-of-network physician. The advantages of the POS system include the maximum amount of freedom in choosing which physician to see and allowing the patient to control out-of-pocket costs. Out-of-network costs can be significant, however, and serve as a disadvantage to POS systems.

Operation and Cost Containment

Health maintenance organizations manage their costs by restricting covered medical care to their in-network providers. The participating providers, as employees of the HMO, have agreed to practice medicine in accordance with the HMO's guidelines and restrictions. These guidelines and restrictions may be incorporated into primary care physicians" decisions regarding approval for specialty care visits.

Another way that HMOs manage costs is through utilization review, a process by which the HMO monitors the physicians" practice. By comparing the physician's practices with other physicians, such as number of referrals and cost of services, the HMO can measure the most efficient practice techniques.

Another technique for cost containment in HMO systems is case management. In case management, the goal is preventive medicine before a catastrophic event can occur. The theory behind case management is that it is cheaper to prevent a disease than to treat it. Case management may also include disease management, such as management of chronic conditions to prevent them from progressing into worsening conditions.

While many professionals argue that one main goal of health maintenance organizations is to save money, many HMOs themselves argue that they do not have a significant increase in profit over their PPO or POS plans. The research supporting this theory suggests that although the out-of-pocket expense is smaller for the patient, the patient may take advantage of the unlimited use of in-network providers and visit more often than those patients who participate in other programs. Therefore, with increased utilization from some patients, the cost to the HMO rises to that of other plans.

Perspective and Prospects

In 1929, the first health maintenance organization in the United States was organized by Michael Shadid. Shadid was a medical and business pioneer who provided medical care for rural farmers in Elk City, Oklahoma. The members who enrolled in his plan paid a predetermined fee and received medical care from Dr. Shadid. In the same year, the Ross-Loos Medical Group was established in Los Angeles to provide prepaid medical services to county employees and employees of the city's department of water and power. In 1982, the Ross-Loos Medical Group was purchased by CIGNA. The enactment of Medicare and Medicaid legislation in 1965 served as a landmark in the history of managed health care by extending coverage to millions of additional Americans who could otherwise not afford medical coverage.

The first mandated health care act by government was the Health Maintenance Organization Act of 1973, which required employers with twenty-five or more employees to offer federally certified HMO options. Dr. Gordon K. Macleod served as the first director of this program and also performed many research studies in other countries regarding health maintenance organization and structure. In 2010, the United States Congress passed the Patient Protection and Affordable Care Act, which introduced further requirements for health care organizations.

—*Leah M. Betman, M.S., C.G.C.*

See also Allied health; Ethics; Health care reform; Health maintenance organizations (HMOs); Law and medicine; Malpractice; Medicare.

For Further Information:

Andresen, Elena, and Erin DeFries Bouldin, eds. *Public Health Foundations: Concepts and Practices*. Malden: Wiley-Blackwell, 2010.

Dorsey, J. L. "The Health Maintenance Organization Act of 1973 and Prepaid Group Practice Plan." *Medical Care* 13 (January, 1975): 1–9.

Kongstvedt, Peter R. *Essentials of Managed Health Care*. 6th ed. Burlington: Jones & Bartlett, 2013.

Kongstvedt, Peter R. *The Managed Health Care Book*. 4th ed. Aspen, Colo.: Aspen, 2001.

Longest, B. B. "Health and Health Policy." In *Health Policymaking in the United States*. 4th ed. Chicago: Health Administration Press, 2006.

Samuels, David I. *Managed Health Care in the New Millennium*. Boca Raton: CRC Press, 2012.

MANIC-DEPRESSIVE DISORDER. *See* BIPOLAR DISORDERS.

MAPLE SYRUP URINE DISEASE (MSUD)
Disease/Disorder
Also known as: Branched-chain ketoaciduria
Anatomy or system affected: Nervous system

Information on Maple Syrup Urine Disease (MSUD)

Causes: Genetic defect resulting in accumulation of amino acids leucine, isoleucine, and valine
Symptoms: Within three to seven days after birth, poor weight gain, high-pitched cry, irritability, lethargy, characteristic maple syrup smell of urine; if untreated, mental retardation, seizures, and death
Duration: Lifelong
Treatments: Diet with controlled amounts of isoleucine, leucine, and valine

---

Specialties and related fields: Family medicine, genetics, neonatology, pediatrics
Definition: A recessive autosomal genetic disease resulting in the absence, partial activity, or inactivity of a multisubunit enzyme responsible for metabolizing the branched-chain amino acids leucine, isoleucine, and valine.

Causes and Symptoms

As a result of deficient branched-chain alpha-ketoacid dehydrogenase (BCKD), the essential branched chain amino acids leucine, isoleucine, and valine are not metabolized in patients with maple syrup urine disease (MSUD). The branched-chain amino acids and their ketoacid products accumulate in the blood and interfere with brain function. High levels of leucine are especially toxic. The classic form of the disease results in little (less than 2 percent) or no BCKD activity. Symptoms develop within three to seven days after birth and include poor weight gain, a high-pitched cry, irritability, lethargy, and a characteristic maple-syrup smell to the urine. If the disease is untreated, then intellectual and developmental disabilities, various neurological symptoms such as seizures, and even death can result.

Variant forms of the disease, in which there is some (3 to 12 percent) BCKD activity, result in milder symptoms. A rare variant form of the disease called thiamine-responsive MSUD responds to high doses of thiamine.

Treatment and Therapy

The treatment of severe MSUD, which should begin immediately after diagnosis, involves a special diet with controlled amounts of isoleucine, leucine, and valine to ensure metabolic control. Enfamil, a special dietary formula, provides leucine but may have to be supplemented with isoleucine and valine to provide adequate intake of all three amino acids and permit normal growth and development.

Treatment of the milder forms of MSUD also involves management through diet therapy. Diet therapy should be continued throughout life, and the levels of the branched-chain amino acids should be monitored often.

Perspective and Prospects

MSUD was first described in 1954. The name derives from the sweet, maple-syrup smell of the patient's urine. Because MSUD is caused by a recessive gene, there is a one in four chance that two heterozygous carriers will have an affected child. MSUD affects about 1 in 185,000 newborns in the United States, but in some populations, such as Mennonites, it may be as high as 1 in 176.

Some hospitals test for the disease in their newborn screening programs. Testing should be done within the first twenty-four hours after birth, since early diagnosis is essential. Some of the milder variant forms are missed in the screening programs. The detection of alloisoleucine is diagnostic for MSUD but may not appear until the sixth day of life. Carrier testing is available for the Mennonite variant of the disease.

—*Charles L. Vigue, Ph.D.*

See also Enzyme therapy; Enzymes; Food biochemistry; Genetic counseling; Genetic diseases; Metabolic disorders; Metabolism; Neonatology; Nutrition; Screening.

For Further Information:

Clarke, Joe T. R. *A Clinical Guide to Inherited Metabolic Diseases.* 3d ed. New York: Cambridge University Press, 2006.
Icon Health. *Maple Syrup Urine Disease: A Medical Dictionary, Bibliography, and Annotated Research Guide to Internet References.* San Diego, Calif.: Author, 2004.
Jorde, Lynn B., et al. *Medical Genetics.* 4th ed. St. Louis, Mo.: Mosby, 2009.
Mescka, Caroline P., et al. "Protein and Lipid Damage in Maple Syrup Urine Disease Patients: l-Carnitine Effect." International Journal of Developmental Neuroscience 31, no. 1 (February, 2013): 21–24.
Pritchard, Dorian J., and Bruce R. Korf. *Medical Genetics at a Glance.* 2d ed. Malden, Mass.: Blackwell Science, 2008.
Scaini, Giselli, et al. "DNA Damage in an Animal Model of Maple Syrup Urine Disease." Molecular Genetics and Metabolism 106, no. 2 (June, 2012): 169–174.
VeriMed Healthcare Network. "Maple Syrup Urine Disease." *Medline Plus,* May 15, 2011.

Marburg virus

Disease/Disorder

Also known as: Green monkey fever
Anatomy or system affected: Immune system
Specialties and related fields: Epidemiology, virology
Definition: Marburg hemorrhagic fever is a rare, highly lethal disease caused by Marburg filovirus.

Causes and Symptoms

Marburg hemorrhagic fever is caused by a filovirus. Filoviruses are separated into two distinct types, Marburg and Ebola. All filoviruses are classified as biosafety level 4 agents based on their high mortality rate, potential transmissibility, and the absence of effective vaccines or treatments. The systemic nature of filovirus infections suggest they may have immunosuppressive effects.

Human-infecting viruses usually appear as small, round, or oval organisms. Filoviruses are unique among human viruses, appearing as long, cylindrical organisms with twists and loops. The natural reservoir for filoviruses is unknown but is presumed to be wild animals (zoonotic). Research suggests that filoviruses may possibly be linked to fruit bats,

---

Information on Marburg Virus

Causes: Infection with a filovirus
Symptoms: High fever, headache, sore throat, rashes, muscle pain, inflamed lymph nodes, dementia, bloody vomiting and diarrhea, bleeding from gums and nose, small hemorrhages in eyes
Duration: Up to three weeks, often fatal
Treatments: None; alleviation of symptoms

---

from which the viruses are occasionally introduced into primate populations. The primary transmission of Marburg filovirus from its natural reservoir appears to occur only in sub-Saharan Africa within five degrees of the equator.

Human transmission of Marburg hemorrhagic fever is by direct contact with infected blood, semen, urine, mucus, and organs. Some evidence suggests that aerosol transmission may also occur. The virus enters the body through lesions and initially infects the lymph nodes, spleen, and liver. Marburg filovirus can survive several weeks in corpses and blood samples.

The incubation period of Marburg hemorrhagic fever is two to twenty-one days after infection, and symptoms include high fever, severe headache, painful sore throat, rashes, muscle pain (myalgia), inflamed lymph nodes, dementia, and bloody vomiting and diarrhea from internal hemorrhaging. Symptoms usually progress to bleeding from the gums and nose, puncture openings in the skin, small hemorrhages in the whites of the eyes, and eventual red blood cell immobilization. Hair, skin, and nail loss, as well as searing body pain from inflamed nerves, occur in later stages of infection. The infection may last as long as three weeks and is often described as agonizing. In fatal cases, the patient's blood pressure undergoes a final severe drop resulting in shock prior to death.

Treatment and Therapy

There is no vaccine or specific therapy available for filoviral infections, although several vaccines and drug therapies are currently being tested. Specific symptoms are treated during the course of infection; the patient either responds or does not. Secondary prevention requires total isolation of infected patients. Primary infected patients show a higher mortality rate than do secondary infected patients. The mortality rate for humans infected with Marburg hemorrhagic fever ranges from 24 to 88 percent, with some outbreaks being more deadly than others.

Perspective and Prospects

Marburg hemorrhagic fever was first described in 1967 during outbreaks at research laboratories in Marburg and Frankfurt, Germany, and Belgrade, Yugoslavia, and linked to African green monkeys imported for research purposes from Uganda. Since the initial outbreaks, sporadic cases of Marburg hemorrhagic fever have been identified in eastern and southern Africa, with the largest outbreaks occurring in the Democratic Republic of the Congo in 1998 and in Uganda in

2012. One of the most frightening aspects of Marburg hemorrhagic fever is its ongoing inclusion in some nations" biological weapons programs.

—*Randall L. Milstein, Ph.D.*

See also Bleeding; Centers for Disease Control and Prevention (CDC); Ebola virus; Epidemiology; Hemorrhage; Tropical medicine; Viral hemorrhagic fevers; Viral infections; Zoonoses.

For Further Information:
Garrett, Laurie. *The Coming Plague: Newly Emerging Diseases in a World out of Balance*. New York: Penguin, 1995.
Klenk, Hans-Dieter, ed. *Marburg and Ebola Viruses*. New York: Springer, 1999.
Levy, Elinor, and Mark Fischetti. *The New Killer Diseases: How the Alarming Evolution of Mutant Germs Threatens Us All*. New York: Crown, 2003.
"Marburg Haemorrhagic Fever." *World Health Organization*, November 2012.
"Marburg Hemorrhagic Fever Fact Sheet." *Centers for Disease Control and Prevention*, April 23, 2011.
Mayo Clinic Staff. "Ebola Virus and Marburg Virus." *Mayo Clinic*, June 18, 2011.
McCormick, Joseph B., Susan Fisher-Hoch, and Leslie Alan Horvitz. *Level 4: Virus Hunters of the CDC*. Rev. ed. New York: Barnes & Noble, 1999.

MARFAN SYNDROME
Disease/Disorder

Anatomy or system affected: Bones, eyes, heart, musculoskeletal system, spine

Specialties and related fields: Cardiology, genetics, ophthalmology, orthopedics

Definition: A condition in which the connective tissue does not form correctly and tends to be too flexible. The abnormal chemical composition, especially of the skeleton and heart, leads to major medical characteristics that are sometimes in evidence only at puberty.

Causes and Symptoms

Studies have located the gene that causes the inherited form of Marfan syndrome. About 25 percent of Marfan syndrome cases result from spontaneous mutation. While this knowledge promises better future recognition of the condition, the range and severity of the condition is so variable that diagnosis remains difficult.

Usually, Marfan syndrome is discovered through a detailed family history. The observation that a person is tall and

---

Information on Marfan Syndrome

Causes: Genetic mutation
Symptoms: Tall and slender appearance, long fingers or arms, loose joints, heart problems, dislocation of eye lens, scoliosis, crowded teeth
Duration: Lifelong
Treatments: Dependent on severity and structures affected; may include surgery and medications

---

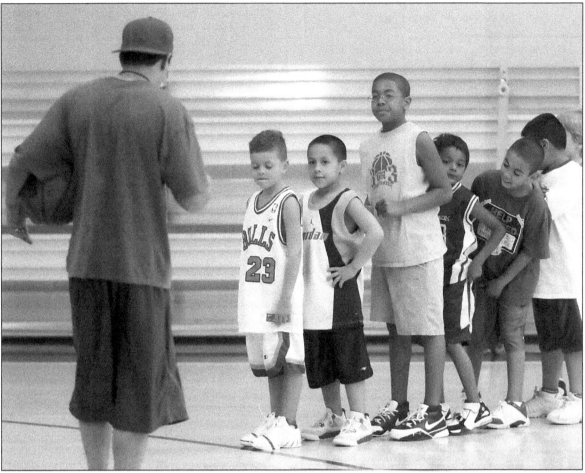

A seven-year-old (third child from left) who was born with Marfan syndrome, an inherited connective tissue disease that causes defects in the skeleton, eyes, and heart. (AP/Wide World Photos)

slender and has unusually long fingers or arms is often an early clue. The presence of loose joints with great suppleness is characteristic of the disease. Manifestations of this condition may occur in any part of the body, but the heart, eyes, and spinal column are the most common.

Treatment and Therapy

Because a variety of organs may be involved in Marfan syndrome, it is essential that several specialists form a team to evaluate and monitor the patient during his or her lifetime. The most serious, and most common, problem area is the heart. Mitral valve problems may lead to leakage or regurgitation of blood. The aortic valve can develop a backflow into the heart.

In the eyes, a characteristic sign is the dislocation of the lens. This symptom is difficult to detect and, like many others, can vary widely in intensity. Cataracts are also associated with this condition.

Other characteristics are found in the skeleton. Spinal curvature, or scoliosis, and a breastbone that either protrudes or indents are observed. Crowded teeth and an arched palate are not uncommon.

Any of these symptoms can lead to serious consequences and should be discovered as early as possible. Regular examinations by specialists in cardiology, ophthalmology, and orthopedics are essential. Most of the possible progressive aspects of the condition can be treated effectively.

—*K. Thomas Finley, Ph.D.*

See also Bones and the skeleton; Cardiology; Cardiology, pediatric; Eye infections and disorders; Eyes; Genetic diseases; Growth; Heart; Joints; Mitral valve prolapse; Optometry; Optometry, pediatric; Orthopedics; Orthopedics, pediatric; Scoliosis; Vision disorders.

For Further Information:
Alan, Rick. "Marfan Syndrome." *Health Library*, March 15, 2013.

Hetzer, R., P. Gehle, and J. Ennker, eds. *Cardiovascular Aspects of Marfan Syndrome*. New York: Springer, 1995.

"Learning about Marfan Syndrome." *National Human Genome Research Institute*, November 14, 2012.

"Marfan Syndrome." *Genetics Home Reference*, March 2012.

Parker, James N., and Philip M. Parker, eds. *The Official Patient's*

Sourcebook on Marfan Syndrome. San Diego, Calif.: Icon Health, 2002.

Pyeritz, Reed E., and Julia Conant. *Marfan Syndrome*. 5th ed. Port Washington, N.Y.: National Marfan Foundation, 2001.

Robinson, Peter N., and Maurice Godfrey, eds. *Marfan Syndrome: A Primer for Clinicians and Scientists*. New York: Kluwer Academic/Plenum, 2004.

MARIJUANA
Disease/Disorder

Also known as: Cannabis sativa, hemp, various popular names (pot, ganja, and weed)

Anatomy or system affected: Brain, circulatory system, eyes, gastrointestinal system, heart, lungs, musculoskeletal system, nerves, nervous system, psychic-emotional system, respiratory system

Specialties and related fields: Alternative medicine, ethics, neurology, pharmacology, psychiatry, psychology, public health

Definition: A plant containing a psychoactive substance with the potential for both recreational abuse and medical use.

Introduction

The term "marijuana" refers to both the illegal drug and the plant itself. Marijuana is the most commonly used illicit drug (17.4 million past-month users) according to the 2010 National Survey on Drug Use and Health (NSDUH). That year marijuana was used by 76.8 percent of current illicit drug users (defined as having used the drug at some time in the 30 days before the survey.

The hemp plant, Cannabis sativa, is a fast-growing (to fifteen feet) bushy annual with finely branched leaves further divided into lance-shaped, saw tooth-edged leaflets. The species was first classified in 1735 by the Swedish botanist Carolus Linnaeus. Both male and female plants produce tetrahydrocannabinol (THC), the psychoactive ingredient in the drug. THC collects in tiny droplets of sticky resin produced by glands located at the base of fine hairs covering most of the plant's surface, with the most highly concentrated THC found in the female flower heads. When pollinated, however, the female flower heads produce highly nutritious seeds containing no THC.

The Effects of Marijuana

When marijuana is smoked, THC rapidly passes from the lungs to the bloodstream, which carries the chemical to organs throughout the body including the brain. The effects of smoked marijuana can last from 1 to 3 hours. If marijuana is consumed in foods or as beverage (e.g., tea) the effect can appear between 30 to 60 minutes later. Interestingly, this effect can last up to one hour. Smoking by far delivers more THC to the bloodstream than eating or drinking. When it enters the brain, it binds to specific sites called cannabinoid receptors (CBRs) located on the surface of nerve cells, affecting the way those cells work. CBRs are abundant in parts of the brain that regulate movement, coordination, learning and memory, higher cognitive functions such as judgment and pleasure.

As THC enters the brain, it causes the user to feel euphoric or high by acting on the brain's reward system. This system controls the body's response to pleasurable things like sex and chocolate as well as to most drugs of abuse.

Recreational and Medicinal Uses

Responses vary according to dosage and experience using the drug, but most people experience a mild euphoria, or "high." Mood, short-term memory, motor coordination, thought, sensation, and time sense can all be affected. Hunger, known as "the munchies," frequently occurs soon after exposure.

Marijuana can impede a person's ability to form new memories. In fact, people who have taken large doses of the drug may experience hallucinations, delusions, and loss of personal identity. All these symptoms encompass acute psychosis. The heart rate increases, the blood pressure increases while supine but drops when standing, and the eyes can become bloodshot. The most rapid onset with most temporary effect occurs with smoked marijuana. Unlike alcohol or tobacco, no deaths have been directly attributed to marijuana use alone.

Marijuana has been cultivated and used as a medicine for thousands of years. The Food and Drug Administration (FDA) has approved a synthetic formulation of THC, Marinol (brand name of the generic drug dronabinol), that doctors can prescribe legally for the treatment of nausea and vomiting associated with cancer chemotherapy and the loss of appetite and weight loss characteristic of patients with acquired immunodeficiency syndrome (AIDS). In addition, both Marinol and marijuana are used to alleviate pain, muscle spasms, neurological disorders, and glaucoma. Many users of medicinal THC prefer to smoke marijuana despite its illegality rather than take the legal pill because orally delivered THC is not well absorbed by the body. Previously classified among drugs such as cocaine and morphine with a high potential for abuse, Marinol was moved to a less restricted category that includes anabolic steroids in July 1999.

Today, 25 years after Marinol was approved, the development of a THC-based mouth spray has been approved in the UK and Canada for relief of cancer associated pain and neuropathic pain in multiple sclerosis.

Perspective and Prospects

Despite the FDA's tacit acknowledgment of the medicinal value of marijuana by the approval of Marinol, marijuana itself is classified as a substance with high potential for abuse and no accepted medical use under federal drug laws, stifling research into other potential medical benefits. Scientific evidence, including the 1990 report of the National Academy of Sciences *Marijuana and Medicine: Assessing the Science Base*, strongly supports further research.

—Sue Tarjan;
updated by Stephen Henry, D.O.

See also Addiction; Alcoholism; Alternative medicine; Chemotherapy; Club drugs; Eye infections and disorders; Glaucoma; Herbal medicine; Intoxication; Narcotics; Nausea and vomiting; Pain management; Pharmacology; Self-medication; Smoking; Substance abuse; Tobacco

For Further Information:

Earleywine, Mitch. *Understanding Marijuana: A New Look at the Scientific Evidence.* New York: Oxford University Press, 2002.

ElSohly, Mahmoud A., ed. *Marijuana and the Cannabinoids.* Totowa, NJ: Humana Press, 2007.

Iversen, Leslie L. *The Science of Marijuana.* New York: Oxford University Press, 2000.

Mack, Alison, and Janet Joy. *Marijuana as Medicine? The Science Beyond the Controversy.* Washington, DC: National Academy Press, 2001.

National Institute on Drug Abuse. *NIH Research Report Series: Marijuana Abuse.* Rev. ed. Washington, DC: National Institutes of Health, 2012.

Onaivi, Emmanuel S., ed. *Marijuana and Cannabinoid Research: Methods and Protocols.* Totowa, NJ: Humana Press, 2006.

Shohov, Tatiana, ed. *Medical Use of Marijuana: Policy, Regulatory, and Legal Issues.* New York: Nova Science, 2003.

MASSAGE

Treatment

Anatomy or system affected: All

Specialties and related fields: Alternative medicine, exercise physiology, geriatrics and gerontology, oncology, pediatrics, physical therapy, preventive medicine, sports medicine

Definition: The intentional and systematic manipulation of the soft tissues of the body to promote health and healing.

Indications and Procedures

Massage is used in both wellness and treatment models of health care. Wellness implies the achievement of an optimal state of well-being. The health enhancing effects of massage such as relaxation, stress reduction, and increased body conditioning or awareness contribute to general wellness. In the treatment model, massage is considered a modality indicated to alleviate the symptoms and/or pain of a specific condition. A particular massage technique may be more or less effective for each illness or injury. The treatment model includes the subspecialty of sports massage, a beneficial intervention for athletes and people engaged in strenuous physical activity.

Two men were instrumental in the development of classic Western massage: Pehr Henrik Ling (1776–1839) and Johann Mezger (1838–1909). Ling developed an approach for treating medical conditions called the "Swedish movement cure" in the nineteenth century. Mezger defined four categories of massage using French terminology: *effleurage, petrissage, tapotement,* and *frictions.* The work of these men was further developed by their students and incorporated into both regular and alternative medicine. Other common techniques of massage are deep-tissue massage and trigger-point massage.

The physical effects of massage include healthy skin, relaxation, increased blood circulation and immune system functioning, metabolic balance in the muscles, connective tissue pliability, increased joint mobility and flexibility, and pain reduction. The mental and emotional benefits include increased mental clarity, reduced anxiety, and emotional release.

Uses and Complications

Massage has proven benefits for mind and body health. Research in the twentieth century showed a positive relationship between the reduction of pain and stress after massage. Other studies revealed that massage promoted weight gain in premature infants and reduced anxiety in adolescents hospitalized for psychiatric conditions. It may help slow the aging process among older adults and bring comfort to the terminally ill.

A basic tenet of massage practice is "Do no harm." Massage practitioners are trained to identify "endangerment sites." These are areas of the body that are less protected and more vulnerable to damage. "Contraindications" are conditions under which receiving massages are not advisable, such as when it could worsen a condition or spread infection. Health history information is essential for a safe massage session.

Perspective and Prospects

Massage has been used for centuries in native and folk cultures all over the world. It has periodically lost and regained popularity in the Western world. After a decline in the 1950s, it experienced a revival of credibility and value during the human potential movement of the late 1960s. Since then, it has been increasingly incorporated into medical treatment and prevention programs.

—*Susan L. Sandel, Ph.D.*

See also Acupressure; Alternative medicine; Headaches; Muscle sprains, spasms, and disorders; Muscles; Pain; Pain management; Physical rehabilitation; Stress; Stress reduction.

For Further Information:

American Massage Therapy Association. http://www.amtamassage.org.

Beck, Mark F. *Theory and Practice of Therapeutic Massage.* 5th ed. Clifton Park, N.Y.: Milady, 2010.

Fritz, Sandy. *Mosby's Fundamentals of Therapeutic Massage.* 5th ed. Maryland Heights, Mo.: Mosby/Elsevier, 2012.

"Massage: Get in Touch with Its Many Benefits." *Mayo Foundation for Medical Education and Research,* January 30, 2013.

"Massage Therapy." *Health Library,* March 26, 2013.

National Center for Complementary and Alternative Medicine. "Massage Therapy: An Introduction." *National Institutes of Health, US Department of Health and Human Services,* August, 2010.

Salvo, Susan G., and Maureen Pfeiffer, eds. *Massage Therapy: Principles and Practice.* 4th ed. St. Louis, Mo.: Saunders/Elsevier, 2011.

Trivieri, Larry, Jr., and John W. Anderson, eds. *Alternative Medicine: The Definitive Guide.* 2d ed. Berkeley, Calif.: Ten Speed Press, 2002.

Werner, Ruth. *A Massage Therapist's Guide to Pathology.* 4th ed. Philadelphia: Wolters Kluwer/Lippincott Williams & Wilkins, 2009.

MASTECTOMY AND LUMPECTOMY

Procedures

Anatomy or system affected: Breasts

Specialties and related fields: General surgery, oncology, pathology, plastic surgery, radiology

Definition: Mastectomy involves the surgical removal of one or both breasts, whereas lumpectomy involves the removal of one or more tumors and surrounding tissue from the breast.

Key terms:

BRCA1: an abbreviation for breast cancer 1; the mutant chromosomal factor, when found in chromosome 17, which indicates that a woman is vulnerable to developing breast cancer

estrogen: any of several hormones produced by the ovaries that regulate some female reproductive processes and maintain secondary sex characteristics in the female

fibrocystic breasts: the lumpy breasts that some women routinely develop, particularly in the seven or eight days before menstruation

mammography: an X-ray examination of the breasts, the purpose of which is to reveal tumors and other abnormalities

metastasis: the spreading of cancer cells from the original site to other parts of the body

palpation: a digital examination of affected parts of the body

quadrantectomy: a form of lumpectomy that removes more tissue than the usual lumpectomy, leaving little visible scarring but slightly diminishing the size of the affected breast

sonogram: an image of body organs produced through focusing sound waves on the part to be examined

ultrasound: a method of diagnostic imaging that focuses sound waves inaudible to humans on a given organ to produce detailed images of that organ

Indications and Procedures

The early indications of breast cancer are often quite subtle, although in this stage it may be revealed by routine mammograms. In some cases, no overt symptoms exist until the cancer is well advanced. Women between forty and fifty years of age without risk factors are advised to have a mammogram every two years. Women over fifty or in the high-risk category because of a family history of breast cancer should have a mammogram once every year. If palpation of the breast reveals a lump, then immediate mammography is indicated.

It is necessary to be constantly vigilant for any sign that an abnormality exists in the breast. Clear indications of possible breast cancer include lumps or thickening of the tissue in the breast or in the area under the arms. Symptoms such as discoloration of the breasts or dimpling, thickening, scaling, or puckering of one or both breasts may also arouse suspicion of breast cancer. A significant change in the shape of the breast or a swelling of it are also symptomatic. A bloody discharge from the nipple, scaly skin on the nipple or surrounding area, inversion of the nipple, or discoloration of the area surrounding the nipple may presage the presence of breast cancer.

Monthly palpation of the breasts, preferably seven or eight days after menstruation, may reveal lumps that could be harmless growths but that might be cancerous. This procedure is referred to as breast self-examination (BSE). Because the female breast contains many glands, it is not uncommon in some women for lumps to appear regularly—often profusely—particularly in the week prior to menstruation. Women with notably lumpy breasts are said to have fibrocystic breasts. Often, the lumps diminish in size in the week following menstruation. If they do not recede, however,

then these lumps should be regarded with suspicion and the patient should be examined by a physician, preferably a surgeon, gynecologist, or oncologist.

Once a problem is detected, a number of procedures must be considered for dealing with it. The initial procedure in treating suspected breast cancer usually involves a mammogram to reveal irregularities in the breast. If the results of the mammogram are negative and the patient is still convinced that there is a lump in the breast, an ultrasound or sonographic examination may be indicated. In such tests, harmless sound waves are focused on the breast. These sound waves are reflected so that they create an image of formations within the breast. Although ultrasound cannot definitively indicate whether a lump is cancerous, it can at least verify whether a lump exists. It can also show whether the lump is hollow and filled with fluid, in which case it is usually a benign cyst rather than a cancerous growth.

If a growth is detected, the next, least-invasive means of determining whether it is cancerous is through a needle biopsy. In this procedure, the patient, under local anesthetic, has a hollow needle inserted into the growth. Fluids and cells are then harvested from it. If the growth is a cyst, a clear or light yellow fluid will be withdrawn, causing the cyst to collapse. This may be all the treatment required. In all cases, however, the substances withdrawn from the growth are examined by a pathologist for the presence of cancer cells.

Not all growths are so positioned that needle biopsies are possible. In such cases, a surgical biopsy is probably necessary. If the lump is small, then a lumpectomy, or the removal of the entire lump, may occur. Larger lumps often cannot be removed at this stage, so portions are excised for pathological examination. A pathologist carefully studies the tissue removed to determine whether it contains cancer cells.

In the past, biopsies often occurred while patients were anesthetized and, if the pathological report was positive for cancer, then a radical mastectomy was performed immediately while the patient was still under anesthetic. Since the late twentieth century, however, a two-step procedure has usually replaced this one-step method. If cancer is detected, then surgery is delayed, giving physicians the opportunity to consult with their patients about the treatments available to them.

The major decision in such cases usually is whether a total mastectomy or a partial mastectomy, commonly referred to as a lumpectomy, should be performed. Total mastectomy involves the total removal of the breast and the surrounding lymph nodes.

A radical mastectomy, done under general anesthetic, involves making a large, elliptical incision on the breast, including the nipple and often the entire breast. The incision normally extends into the armpit. All the breast tissue is excised, including the skin and the fat down to the chest muscles. The incision extends into the armpit to remove as much of the breast tissue as possible, including the lymph nodes, which may be cancerous. Once the bleeding has been controlled, a drainage tube is inserted and the incision is closed with sutures, clips, or adhesive substances.

This drastic form of treatment can be traumatic both physically and psychologically to patients. Many women fear the disfigurement that follows it. Some women, especially those with a family history of breast cancer, may decide that the total removal of the breast is their safest option. In some cases, to prevent future threats of breast cancer, they demand the removal of both breasts.

A lumpectomy, usually performed under local anesthetic, involves the removal only of cancerous tissue. The incision is made under the breast, and the lump, with surrounding tissue, is removed. The appearance of the breast remains much the same as it was before the surgery. In some cases, physicians recommend a quadrantectomy, which involves the removal of the cancerous tissue as well as significant amounts of the surrounding tissue. Quite often, the lymph nodes are removed as well. When this treatment is used, the breast will appear slightly smaller than it previously was, but it can be enhanced through plastic surgery.

Subcutaneous mastectomy is frequently indicated in situations in which the tumor is small. In this procedure, the surgeon makes an incision under the breast. Most of the skin and the nipple remain intact, although the milk ducts that lead into the nipple are cut. Following the surgery, sometimes immediately, a breast implant can be inserted, restoring the breast to its normal appearance. Mastectomy and lumpectomy are routinely followed by a course of radiation and/or chemotherapy designed to kill any fugitive cancer cells that the surgery has missed.

While the goal of mastectomy is to create as little scarring as possible, considerable scarring may occur, particularly with radical mastectomy, and the absence of one or both breasts usually requires significant psychological adjustments on the part of women who have undergone the procedure. The breast reconstruction performed by a plastic surgeon following a mastectomy is often accompanied by treatment from a psychologist or psychiatrist.

Some women with family histories of breast cancer, particularly if the disease has occurred in first-level relatives (mother or sisters), may opt for a mastectomy rather than a lumpectomy to relieve themselves of the fear of contracting the disease, although most oncologists make such women fully aware of other, less drastic procedures available to them.

Certainly a consideration in reaching a decision about whether to have a lumpectomy or the more drastic mastectomy must include many factors. High on the list of such factors is heredity. In many patients who suffer from this disease, *BRCA1* and *BRCA2*, mutated genes, are an early indication that breast cancer may eventually occur. The *BRCA* gene is frequently present in the female members of families with histories of breast cancer and ovarian cancer. About 85 percent of women with the *BRCA* gene will develop breast cancer if they live a normal life span. Women who have the *BRCA* gene may decide to have a prophylactic mastectomy before symptoms occur, although many women in this situation prefer treatment with tamoxifen, which appears to hold breast cancer at bay.

Advances in treating cancers of all kinds progressed rapidly during the last half of the twentieth century, and even greater impetus characterizes current advances. The four major treatments—often used in combination with each other—are surgery, radiation therapy, chemotherapy, and hormonal therapy. In the treatment of breast cancer, radiation may be used initially to shrink existing tumors that, once reduced in size, will be removed surgically. However, when surgeons remove cancerous tumors, they also remove large numbers of surrounding cells that might be affected; such a procedure is usually followed by additional radiation aimed at killing any lingering cancer cells the surgery has missed.

Uses and Complications

The salient use of surgery in cases of breast cancer is to remove its source, not only clearing away any tumors that may be found but also removing additional cancerous tissue as well as lymph nodes that might be affected.

Cancer cells can exist either in the breast's lobules, which contain the cells that produce milk, or in the ducts that carry the milk to the nipples. Cancer cells in either of these locations can be of two types, invasive or noninvasive (also called in situ). The major complication with invasive cancer is that it can and usually does metastasize, spreading often to the lymph nodes, into the lungs and to other parts of the body. In such cases, a radical mastectomy is indicated. It must be performed as quickly as possible and followed by a strenuous course that typically includes radiation or chemotherapy. Noninvasive cancer is less likely to metastasize, although it sometimes does. Lumpectomy or quadrantectomy is often used to treat such cancers, but these procedures must be followed by close monitoring over the rest of the patient's life and by radiation or chemotherapy following surgery.

Chemotherapy is used less often than radiation in the postsurgical treatment of breast cancer but is occasionally used along with it. Some physicians use anticancer drugs to reduce the possibility of recurrence. This treatment, as well as hormone treatment, is designed to kill any fugitive cancer cells that have strayed from the immediate site of the cancer that has been removed. Whereas surgery and radiation are local, affecting only the part of the body being focused upon, chemotherapy is systemic: the drugs used in chemotherapy travel through the bloodstream to all parts of the body. The disadvantage of chemotherapy is that it nearly always has significant side effects. In rare cases, complications are so extreme that they result in death. Usually, chemotherapy is indicated only for women who have not yet undergone the menopause and whose tumors are an inch or larger in size. It may also be employed in cases in which the patient's tumor shows signs of growing rapidly and aggressively invading and attacking other parts of the body.

Related to chemotherapy is hormonal therapy. Hormones are chemicals produced by the body for various purposes. For example, when one is under sudden, undue stress, the body produces adrenaline, which provides a rush of energy and causes the heartbeat to accelerate. In women, the body produces estrogen every month during the menstrual cycle. Estrogen causes the cells in the milk ducts and lobules to grow in preparation for pregnancy. This chemical stimulates the growth of normal cells but can also stimulate the growth of cancer cells. Hormonal therapy is systemic. It involves introducing into the bloodstream a synthetic chemical, usually tamoxifen, which makes it impossible for the body's natural estrogen to find its way to cancer cells that would be nourished by it. A complete biopsy report can determine whether hormonal therapy is appropriate in individual cases.

Perspective and Prospects

Until the middle of the twentieth century, a diagnosis of cancer, particularly of breast cancer, was viewed as a death sentence. Diagnosis generally occurred after the cancer had metastasized. In the first half of the century, general practitioners were much more prevalent than the specialists who, working as a team, are now generally mustered to provide cancer treatment once a diagnosis is made.

With the proliferation of sophisticated medical equipment, including the highly sensitive X-ray machines used in mammography and the various forms of ultrasound and sonograph equipment that are part of nearly every hospital's arsenal of diagnostic equipment, an increasing number of cancers are discovered before they become symptomatic, so that they can be treated with considerable success.

Historically, mastectomies have been performed for centuries. President John Adams's daughter underwent this excruciating surgery early in the nineteenth century, enduring this procedure without the benefit of anesthesia. As was usually true in such cases, the surgery extended her life for only a little while because her cancer was discovered in an advanced stage and had metastasized.

By the late nineteenth and early twentieth centuries, accepted treatment for breast cancer was a radical mastectomy that involved the removal of the affected breast and of as many surrounding cancer cells and lymph nodes as possible. William Halsted, a pioneer in the field of breast cancer surgery and a professor of surgery at the highly respected Johns Hopkins University Medical School, championed the cause of the radical mastectomy, which he viewed as a procedure that could extend substantially the survival of his patients. Little was said about curing breast cancer patients of their cancers. The radical surgery that physicians across the country performed following Halsted's lead was viewed simply as a means of adding months or years to the life of the cancer patient. Until 1970, about 70 percent of women in the United States who had breast cancer were subjected to radical mastectomy.

Several factors brought about a major change in the treatment of breast cancer during the 1960s and 1970s, when social activism was very much in the forefront of American life. Feminists pointed out that most of the surgeons treating breast cancer were men. As an increasing number of women entered medical schools and eventually established medical practices, greater attention was paid to treating breast cancer in less disfiguring ways than had been common earlier.

Along with this change came advances in medical technology that made early diagnosis and more focused treatment a reality. As the chemical treatment of all cancers came to be better understood and more widely employed, the focus was more on preventing and curing cancer than on merely prolonging the lives of those who suffered from it.

Laboratory tests for detecting a woman's predisposition for breast cancer have become increasingly sophisticated and accurate. Where the *BRCA1* or *BRCA2* gene is present, the possibility of developing breast cancer is greatly increased; women shown to possess this gene have been made more vigilant than ever before in monitoring their conditions and in seeking immediate medical intervention if even the slightest symptom appears.

Shortly after the end of World War II, some oncologists rejected Halsted's emphasis on radical mastectomy. Surgeon Jerome Urban garnered numerous followers in his call for superradical surgeries in cancer cases. His procedures involved the removal of ribs, various internal organs, and even limbs in order to find and destroy every cancer cell. Surgeon Bernard Fisher stood in opposition to Urban, championing the effectiveness of smaller surgeries, such as the simple mastectomy, which involved the removal of one breast but not of all the lymph nodes and, in some cases, the lumpectomy, involving the removal only of the tumor and its surrounding cells.

The lumpectomy has gained acceptance through the intervening years. It is less disfiguring than either the radical or the simple mastectomy, leaving only a small scar on the underside of the breast. In cases where lumpectomy is viewed as a viable option, survival rates and cure rates are comparable to those of patients who have undergone more radical surgery.

Advances in medical science are accelerating substantially. Stem cell research offers great promise in the treatment and cure of diseases such as breast cancer. Researchers appear to be on the threshold of developing cells designed to destroy specific errant cells, such as those that cause cancer, while leaving healthy cells intact.

—*R. Baird Shuman, Ph.D.*

See also Breast biopsy; Breast cancer; Breast disorders; Breast surgery; Breasts, female; Cancer; Chemotherapy; Gender reassignment surgery; Gynecology; Malignancy and metastasis; Mammography; Oncology; Plastic surgery; Radiation therapy; Tumor removal; Tumors; Women's health.

For Further Information:

Abouzied, Mohei. "Lumpectomy." *Health Library*, Nov. 26, 2012.

"Breast Cancer." *MedlinePlus*, June 12, 2013.

Chisholm, Andrea. "Mastectomy." *Health Library*, Oct. 31, 2012.

Fowble, Barbara, et al. *Breast Cancer Treatment: A Comprehensive Guide to Management*. St. Louis: Mosby Year Book, 1991.

Friedewald, Vincent, and Aman U. Buzdar, with Michael Bokulich. *Ask the Doctor: Breast Cancer*. Kansas City, Mo.: Andrews McMeel, 1997.

Hirshaut, Yashar, and Peter I. Pressman. *Breast Cancer: The Complete Guide*. 5th ed. New York: Bantam Books, 2008.

Lange, Vladimir. *Be a Survivor: Your Guide to Breast Cancer Treatment*. 5th rev. ed. Los Angeles: Lange Productions, 2010.

Lerner, Barron H. *The Breast Cancer Wars: Hope, Fear, and the Pursuit of a Cure in Twentieth-Century America*. New York: Oxford University Press, 2001.

Link, John S. *The Breast Cancer Survival Manual: A Step-by-Step Guide*. 5th ed. New York: Henry Holt, 2012.

"Mastectomy." *MedlinePlus*, May 24, 2013.

Mayer, Musa. *Examining Myself*. London: Faber & Faber, 1994.

Morris, Peter J., and William C. Wood, eds. *Oxford Textbook of Surgery*. 2d ed. New York: Oxford University Press, 2000.

Phippen, Mark L., and Maryann Papanier Wells, eds. *Patient Care During Operative and Invasive Procedures*. Philadelphia: W. B. Saunders, 2000.

Sproul, Amy, ed. *A Breast Cancer Journey: Your Personal Guidebook*. 2d ed. Atlanta: American Cancer Society, 2004.

"Surgery for Breast Cancer." *American Cancer Society*, Feb. 26, 2013.

Sutton, Amy L., ed. *Breast Cancer Sourcebook: Basic Consumer Health Information About Breast Cancer*. 4th ed. Detroit: Omnigraphics, 2012.

MASTITIS

Disease/Disorder

Anatomy or system affected: Breasts, glands

Specialties and related fields: Bacteriology, family medicine, gynecology, nutrition, obstetrics

Definition: A bacterial infection of the mammary gland.

Causes and Symptoms

Mastitis is usually caused by a staphylococcal infection of the breast. The bacteria may enter the breast through a sore or crack in the nipple, although some patients do not report having sore or cracked nipples. Generally, mastitis occurs in women who are breast-feeding babies, but women who are not breast-feeding may also experience the disease. Onset of the infection is often associated with stress, reduced immunity, or missed or increased intervals between breast-feedings of a baby.

Common symptoms of mastitis are swelling, redness, hotness, tenderness, an area of hardness, and pain in part or all of the infected breast. In some cases, there is a localized area of soreness in the breast, while in other cases, the entire breast may be inflamed. The victim typically has flulike symptoms, such as tiredness, aches, chills, fever, and fatigue. These feelings often occur prior to breast soreness. If the cause is simple engorgement with breast milk or a plugged duct, then the patient will start feeling better instead of worse. Blocked ducts usually resolve themselves naturally within twenty-four to forty-eight hours, although a blocked duct may sometimes lead to mastitis.

Treatment and Therapy

Alternate hot and cold packs applied to the sore area of the infected breast help reduce the inflammation and pain and provide comfort. Gently massaging the tender area increases circulation and helps loosen any plugged ducts. Fever can be treated with acetaminophen or ibuprofen without any harm to a breast-feeding baby. Patients should also drink plenty of fluids. For nursing mothers, unless the pain is too intense, breast-feeding should be continued during the treatment of mastitis. If breast-feeding is discontinued, then the breast should be drained regularly with a breast pump.

Once a diagnosis of mastitis is made, proper antibiotics should be administered, if necessary. Cephalexin, cloxacillin, erythromycin, and flucloxacillin are effective drugs against

---

Information on Mastitis

Causes: Bacterial infection (usually staphylococcal) typically through cracks in nipples during breast-feeding; also, engorgement with breast milk or plugged duct

Symptoms: Breast swelling, redness, hotness, tenderness, hard area, pain; typically begins with flulike symptoms (tiredness, aches, chills, fever, fatigue)

Duration: Two to five days for bacterial infection; one to two days for blocked duct

Treatments: Alternate hot and cold packs, gentle massage, acetaminophen or ibuprofen for fever; continued breast-feeding; antibiotics if necessary (cephalexin, cloxacillin, erythromycin, flucloxacillin)

---

the *Staphylococcus* bacteria. Once they are administered, the soreness usually starts to disappear within two to five days. Redness may continue for up to a week or more. Bed rest helps relieve stress and builds up the immune system. If not treated properly and in a timely manner, mastitis can lead to a breast abscess that requires surgical draining.

Perspective and Prospects

Mastitis is most common among nursing mothers during the first three months postpartum. The most important preventive measure against mastitis for these women is regular breast-feeding. Recurrent mastitis is associated with irregular breast-feeding patterns, fatigue, and stress. Frequent breast-feeding and lifestyle changes that promote good health and a strengthened immune system are key ingredients for reducing the occurrence of mastitis.

If antibiotics are prescribed for treatment, it is important that the full course be taken even though the patient improves quickly; otherwise, the risk of mastitis returning increases. Two newer drugs, clindamycin and ciprofloxacin, have proven effective in treating mastitis if the patient is allergic to penicillin-derived medication.

—Alvin K. Benson, Ph.D.

See also Abscess drainage; Abscesses; Antibiotics; Bacterial infections; Breast biopsy; Breast disorders; Breast-feeding; Breasts, female; Hormones; Mammography; Women's health.

For Further Information:

Alan, Rick. "Mastitis." *Health Library*, May 11, 2013.

Colson, Jenni Lynn, ed. *Breastfeeding Sourcebook*. Detroit: Omnigraphics, 2002.

Hunt, K. M., et al. "Mastitis is Associated with Increased Free Fatty Acids, Somatic Cell Count, and Interleukin-8 Concentrations in Human Milk." *Breastfeeding Medicine* 8, no. 1 (2013): 105–110.

Icon Health. *Mastitis: A Medical Dictionary, Bibliography, and Annotated Research Guide to Internet References*. San Diego: ICON Health Publications, 2004.

Jahanfar, S., et al. "Antibiotics for Mastitis in Breastfeeding Women." *The Cochrane Database of Systematic Review* 2 (2013).

Marz, Russell B. *Medical Nutrition from Marz*. 2d ed. Portland, Oreg.: Quiet Lion Press, 1999.

Reddy, Pavani. "Postpartum Mastitis and Community-Acquired Methicillin-Resistant *Staphylococcus aureus* ." *Emerging*

Infectious Diseases 13, no. 2 (2007): 298.

Swenson, Deborah E. *Telephone Triage for the Obstetric Patient: A Nursing Guide*. Philadelphia: W. B. Saunders, 2001.

MASTURBATION
Development
Anatomy or system affected: Genitals
Specialties and related fields: Psychiatry
Definition: A manual stimulation of one's own or another person's genital organs usually resulting in orgasm without engaging in sexual intercourse.

Physical and Psychological Factors

Masturbation is the first sexual experience for a great majority of people. Some young people inadvertently stumble on sexual arousal and orgasm in the course of engaging in some other physical activity. Others purposely stimulate themselves, aroused by curiosity after reading erotic literature, watching sexually explicit films, or listening to the imaginary or real sexual adventures of their peers.

Most men and women practice masturbation to relieve sexual tension, achieve sexual pleasure, enjoy sexual stimulation in the absence of an available partner, and experience relaxation. When masturbating, men tend to focus on the stimulation of the penis. Stimulation of the clitoral shaft and clitoral area, and/or the vagina, with a hand or an object is the method that women most commonly employ. Some women masturbate by using a vibrator. Mutual masturbation provides a satisfying and pleasurable form of sexual intimacy and release for many couples. It is also one of the most common techniques that gay and lesbian couples use during sexual intimacy.

Disorders and Effects

Under certain circumstances, masturbation may result in some undesirable consequences. If a child masturbates constantly, it may be an indication of excessive anxiety and tension. Compulsive and frenzied masturbation may reflect abuse or maltreatment in a child's home life. Frequent masturbation may be a child's way of relieving tension or unconsciously reenacting past or present traumatic sexual episodes. Among adults, excessive masturbation may point toward a lack of self-esteem and the resultant fear and inability to develop healthy intimate relationships with others. Psychiatry, psychotherapy, and sex therapy have proven helpful in successfully alleviating these problems.

Perspective and Prospects

Throughout history, attitudes toward the practice of masturbation have been riddled with misconceptions, guilt, and fear. Fear of masturbation and its supposed harmful effects, such as loss of memory and intelligence, was widespread through the nineteenth century. Semen was considered a vital fluid important for bodily functioning, and wasting it through masturbation was thought to contribute to a weakening of the body and production of illness. Medical authorities today do not find any evidence of physical damage from masturbation.

In fact, many modern sex therapists encourage self-stimulation as part of healthy sexuality. In modern sex therapy, masturbation has become part of the therapeutics used in treating certain sexual dysfunctions. Patients with difficulties or inability to have orgasm are encouraged by their therapists to engage in masturbation. It is widely believed that orgasm once achieved through masturbation will eventually generalize and transfer to satisfactory sexual intercourse.

—Tulsi B. Saral, Ph.D.

See also Aphrodisiacs; Domestic violence; Men's health; Puberty and adolescence; Rape and sexual assault; Reproductive system; Sexual dysfunction; Sexuality; Women's health.

For Further Information:
Bockting, Walter, and Eli Coleman, eds. *Masturbation as a Means of Achieving Sexual Health*. New York: Haworth Press, 2003.
Dodson, Betty. *Sex for One: The Joy of Selfloving*. New York: Harmony Books, 1996.
Laqueur, Thomas Walter. *Solitary Sex: A Cultural History of Masturbation*. New York: Zone Books, 2003.
Marcus, Irwin M., and John J. Francis, eds. *Masturbation: From Infancy to Senescence*. New York: International Universities Press, 1975.
"Masturbation." *HealthyChildren.org*, May 11, 2013.
"Masturbation." *InteliHealth*, June 10, 2008.
Rowan, Edward L. *The Joy of Self-Pleasuring: Why Feel Guilty About Feeling Good?* Amherst, Mass.: Prometheus Books, 2000.
Sarnoff, Suzanne, and Irving Sarnoff. *Masturbation and Adult Sexuality*. Bridgewater, N.J.: Replica Books, 2001.

MEASLES
Disease/Disorder
Also known as: Morbilli, rubeola
Anatomy or system affected: Ears, lungs, mouth, nervous system, respiratory system, skin
Specialties and related fields: Family medicine, internal medicine, pediatrics, public health, virology
Definition: A highly contagious disease contracted through a virus transmitted in respiratory secretions and characterized by a spreading skin rash.
Key terms:
desquamation: the sloughing off of the outer layers of skin
Koplik's spots: small red spots with white centers generally found in the mouth during early stages of measles
maculopapular rash: reddish skin eruptions characterized by small, flat discolorations that may progress into small pimples
otitis media: infection or inflammation of the middle ear, an occasional complication of measles infection
paramyxoviruses: a group of ribonucleic acid (RNA) viruses that includes the etiological agents for measles, mumps, and a variety of respiratory infections
pharyngitis: infection or inflammation of the pharynx, or throat
photophobia: abnormal sensitivity of the eyes to light, a condition common to a variety of illnesses, including measles
prodromal stage: the early stage of a disease during which symptoms first appear

viremia: a condition characterized by the presence of a virus in the bloodstream

Causes and Symptoms

Measles is a highly contagious viral disease characterized by a maculopapular (pimply) rash that develops on the skin and spreads rapidly over much of the cutaneous surface of the body. Measles virus is classified with the paramyxoviruses, a class of viruses in which ribonucleic acid (RNA) serves as the genetic material. Closely related viruses in the same group include rinderpest and distemper virus, agents associated with disease in ruminants such as cows and in dogs or cats, respectively. It is likely that measles originated when one of these other animal viruses became adapted to humans several thousand years ago.

In modern times but before the advent of measles vaccination, measles was a common disease of childhood, usually appearing between the ages of five and ten. The illness is among the most contagious of infections, and the virus was generally spread among children in schools. Widespread immunization of children, begun in the 1960s, tended to push the age of exposure into the teenage years. Most outbreaks since the 1980s have occurred among college students. Since recovery from the disease confers lifelong immunity, infection among older adults is infrequent. In developing nations, places where vaccination may be haphazard, measles is still a disease of early childhood; malnutrition and related problems of poverty have resulted in a significant level of mortality among infected children.

Exposure generally follows an oral-oral means of transmission, as the person inhales contaminated droplets from an infected individual. The incubation period for active measles ranges from seven to fourteen days. During this early stage, the infected individual becomes increasingly contagious. The lack of any obvious symptoms during these early stages lends itself to the spread of the disease.

Contact by the virus with the surface cells of the respiratory passages, or sometimes the conjunctiva (the outer surface of the eye), allows the infectious agent to enter the body. The virus spreads through the local lymph nodes into the blood, producing a primary viremia. During this period, the virus replicates both in the lymph nodes and in the respiratory sites through which the virus entered the body. The virus returns to the bloodstream, resulting in a secondary viremia and widespread passage of the virus throughout the body by the fifth to seventh day after the initial exposure. Viral levels in the blood reach their peak toward the end of the incubation period, some fourteen days after infection. Once symptoms begin, the virus is widely disseminated throughout the body, including sites in small blood vessels, lymph nodes, and even the central nervous system.

The initial incubation period is followed by a prodromal stage, in which active symptoms appear. This stage is characterized by a fever that may reach as high as 103 degrees Fahrenheit, coughing, sensitivity of the eyes to light (photophobia), and malaise. Koplik's spots appear on the buccal mucosa in the mouth one to two days prior to development of the characteristic measles rash.

Information on Measles

Causes: Viral infection
Symptoms: Spreading rash, malaise, fever, respiratory difficulty
Duration: One to two weeks
Treatments: Alleviation of symptoms

The maculopapular rash first appears on the head and behind the ears and gradually spreads over the rest of the body during the course of twenty-four to forty-eight hours. Clear signs of respiratory infection appear, including a cough, pharyngitis, and occasional involvement of the bronchioles or even pneumonia. While malaise and anorexia (appetite loss) are common during the fever period, diarrhea and vomiting generally do not occur. Over time, the rash becomes increasingly dense, exhibiting a blotchy character. Desquamation is common in many affected areas of the skin. Gradually, over a period of three to five days, the rash begins to fade, usually following the sequence by which it first appeared. The rash fades first on the forehead, then on the extremities.

Complications, while they do occur, are unusual in otherwise healthy individuals. Most result from secondary bacterial infections. Occasionally, these complications may manifest themselves as infections of the ear. Pulmonary infections are common among cases of measles and account for most of the rare deaths that follow development of the disease. Photophobia is also common, accounting for the former belief that measles patients had to be kept in a dark room; as long as the patient is comfortable, this step is unnecessary.

The obvious manifestations of measles infection make the isolation of the virus unnecessary for diagnosis. Ironically, the near disappearance of measles in the United States has made most physicians there unfamiliar with the disease; it is not unusual for an attending physician to mistake the rash for another illness. For this reason, laboratory diagnosis is often useful. Laboratory confirmation is generally based on a serological assay for measles antibodies in the blood of infected persons.

A rare sequela to measles infection is the development of subacute sclerosing panencephalitis, a disease characterized by progressive neurological deterioration. The specific mechanism by which measles infection may develop into this disease remains unclear, but it may be the result of a rare combination of events in the victim. Since spread of the virus into the central nervous system is common during measles infection whereas the development of subacute sclerosing panencephalitis is rare (approximately one case per 100,000 measles infections), it is likely that some form of immune impairment is at the root of this disease. Diagnosis of subacute sclerosing panencephalitis is difficult and is based on developing dementia accompanied by unusual levels of measles antibodies in cerebrospinal fluid.

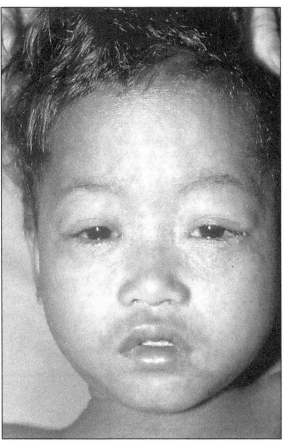

A child with measles. (CDC/Barbara Rice)

Treatment and Therapy

No specific treatment for measles is available; therapy consists of symptomatic intervention. Bed rest is recommended, and the patient should not come into contact with persons not previously exposed to the virus through either natural infection or immunization.

Itching of the rash is common and may be treated with cool water or the standard regimen of cornstarch or baking soda applications. The most common complications result from secondary bacterial infections, which generally take the form of otitis media (middle-ear infection), pharyngitis, or pneumonia. Appropriate use of antibiotics is usually sufficient to prevent or treat such complications.

Immunization with the measles virus may be either passive or active. Children less than one year of age and patients who are immunocompromised or chronically ill may be protected if human immunoglobulin is administered within a week after exposure. While effective immunity is short term, it is capable of protecting these individuals during this period. Since no active disease or infection develops, however, immunity to future infection remains minimal in these cases.

During the early 1960s, an effective vaccine was developed to immunize children against measles. The vaccine consists of an attenuated form of the virus. Although early forms of the vaccine were inconsistent in producing a lifelong immunity, they were effective in decreasing the prevalence of the disease. Later generations of the attenuated vaccine proved more effective in developing long-term immunity among the recipients.

Since maternal antibodies are present in newborns, it is recommended that measles immunization begin between twelve and fifteen months of age. Often, this program is part of a combination MMR vaccine, for measles, mumps, and rubella (German measles). A second booster is given following elementary school. The American Academy of Pediatrics does not consider a third vaccination to be necessary if the approved routine has been followed. It is recommended that children who were first immunized prior to their first birthday should receive boosters at fifteen months of age and again at age twelve. Indications are that immunity from vaccination is long term, if not lifelong. Recovery from natural infection results in a lifelong immunity to measles.

Inconsistency of the first generation of vaccine resulted in ineffective immunity among some individuals vaccinated during the 1960s. A number of small outbreaks during the 1980s were the result. Most cases of measles, however, have occurred in individuals who failed to be immunized.

Perspective and Prospects

The origin and early history of measles is uncertain, as the first authentic description of measles as a specific entity was that by the Arab physician al-Razi (Rhazes) in a 910 CE. treatise on smallpox and measles. Rhazes quoted earlier work by the Hebrew physician El Yehudi, so it is likely that familiarity with these respective illnesses had existed for some time.

Measles is entirely a human disease, with no known animal reservoir. Consequently, the paucity of human populations of sufficient size to maintain transmission means that the spread of such an epidemic disease would have been unlikely before 2500 BCE. It is probable that the disease entered the human species through adaptation of the similar animal viruses of rinderpest or distemper. The absence of any description of a disease like measles in the writings of Hippocrates (c. fourth century BCE) likewise renders it unlikely that the disease was widespread before that date.

Epidemic disease with a rash characteristic of measles is known to have spread through the Roman Empire during the early centuries of the common era. The difficulty in differentiating measles from smallpox by the physicians of the time contributes to the difficulty in understanding the history of the illness. It is certain that by the time of Rhazes, measles had become common in the population.

The terminology of measles lent further confusion during the Middle Ages. Measles was often referred to as *morbilli*, a Latin term meaning "little disease," to distinguish it from *il morbo*, or plague. The word *measles* first appeared in the fourteenth century treatise *Rosa Anglica*, by John of Gaddesden. The term may have been applied initially to the sores on the legs of lepers (*mesles*), and it was only later that illnesses characterized by similar rashes (measles, smallpox, and rubella) were clearly differentiated by European physicians. The significance of a rash with a white center in the mouth was probably recognized by John Quier in Jamaica and Richard Hazeltine in New England during the latter portion of the eighteenth century, but it was in 1896 that the American pediatrician Henry Koplik firmly reported its role in early stages of the disease.

Measles followed the path of European explorers to the Americas during the sixteenth century. Repeated outbreaks of measles devastated American Indian populations, which had minimal immunity to the newly introduced disease. The most thorough epidemiological investigation of measles newly introduced into a population was that by Peter Panum in his study *Observations Made During the Epidemic of Measles on the Faroe Islands in the Year 1846* (1940). In the population of 7,864 persons, 6,100 became ill, with 102 deaths. Mortality rates as high as 25 percent were not unusual in previously unexposed populations. In Hawaii in 1848, about 40,000 deaths occurred among the population of 150,000 persons following the introduction of measles. Even higher mortality rates probably occurred among the populations of Peru and Mexico in 1530–1531, following their exposure to infected Spanish explorers.

The earliest attempt at immunization was probably that of Francis Home of Edinburgh in 1758. Home soaked cotton in the blood of measles patients and placed it on the small cuts on the skin of children. The viral nature of measles was first demonstrated by John Anderson and Joseph Goldberger of the United States Public Health Service, who in 1911 induced the disease in monkeys using filtered extracts from human tissue. In 1954, the virus itself was isolated by John Enders, who grew the agent in human and monkey tissue in a laboratory.

The first effective vaccine was developed by Enders in 1958 using an attenuated (live) form of the virus. The vaccine was tested and then licensed in 1963. Several variations of the vaccine that proved superior in producing long-term immunity were developed in the decades that followed. In 1974, the World Health Organization (WHO) introduced a widespread vaccination program within developing countries.

The absence of any natural reservoir for measles other than humans has made the eradication of the disease possible. Active immunization of children in the United States reduced the annual incidence of the disease from 482,000 reported cases in 1962 to fewer than 1,000 in the late 1990s. The Measles and Rubella Initiative, a collaboration between the WHO, UNICEF, American Red Cross, US Centers for Disease Control and Prevention, and UN Foundation, has vaccinated one billion children worldwide since 2000. While widespread vaccination and worldwide surveillance has made global eradication of the disease a realistic possibility, the WHO reports that more than 20 million people contract measles each year and that it remains one of the top killers of children around the world, causing 158,000 deaths in 2011. Most of these fatalities occurred in children younger than five.

—*Richard Adler, Ph.D.*

See also Childhood infectious diseases; Epidemics and pandemics; Fever; Immunization and vaccination; Mumps; Rashes; Rubella; Viral infections.

For Further Information:

Alan, Rick. "Measles." *Health Library*, September 27, 2012.

American Medical Association. *American Medical Association Family Medical Guide*. 4th rev. ed. Hoboken, N.J.: John Wiley & Sons, 2004.

Bernstein, David, and Gilbert Schiff. "Viral Exanthems and Localized Skin Infections." In *Infectious Diseases*, edited by Sherwood L. Gorbach, John G. Bartlett, and Neil R. Blacklow. Philadelphia: W. B. Saunders, 2004.

Biddle, Wayne. *A Field Guide to Germs*. 2d ed. New York: Anchor Books, 2002.

Kiple, Kenneth F., ed. *The Cambridge World History of Human Disease*. New York: Cambridge University Press, 1999.

Madigan, Michael T., and John M. Martinko. *Brock Biology of Microorganisms*. 12th ed. San Francisco: Pearson/Benjamin Cummings, 2009.

MedlinePlus. "Measles." *MedlinePlus*, May 2, 2013.

Wagner, Edward K., and Martinez J. Hewlett. *Basic Virology*. 3d ed. Malden, Mass.: Blackwell Science, 2008.

Woolf, Alan D., et al., eds. *The Children's Hospital Guide to Your Child's Health and Development*. Cambridge, Mass.: Perseus, 2002.

World Health Organization. "Measles (Fact Sheet Number 286)." *World Health Organization Media Centre*, February 2013.

MECKEL'S DIVERTICULUM
Disease/Disorder

Also known as: Meckel diverticulum

Anatomy or system affected: Gastrointestinal system, intestines

Specialties and related fields: Embryology, gastroenterology, general surgery, oncology, radiology

Definition: A pouch on the wall of the lower part of the intestine that persists from embryonic development.

Key terms:

heterotopic tissue: tissue formed in an abnormal location

midgut: the portion of the embryonic gut from which most of the intestines develop

primitive gut: a tubular structure in the embryo that differentiates into the gastrointestinal tract and its associated structures

vitelline duct: a narrow tube that joins the midgut to the yolk sac in the early embryo

yolk sac: a sac-like membrane outside the embryo that serves as the early site for the formation of blood and blood vessels and is connected to the midgut by the vitelline duct

Causes and Symptoms

By the fourth week of embryonic development, an extraembryonic membrane known as the yolk sac (or umbilical vesicle) has formed. At this time, the embryo, which has formed insipient nervous and circulatory systems, lies above the yolk sac. Inside the embryo is a tube that eventually becomes the gastrointestinal tract (primitive gut). The primitive gut consists of three parts; the foregut, midgut, and hindgut.

Information on Meckel's Diverticulum

Causes: Persistence of an embryological structure that forms an intestinal pouch and sometimes causes complications
Symptoms: Usually asymptomatic but can cause rectal bleeding, recurrent abdominal pain, nausea, and vomiting
Duration: Lifetime duration unless surgically extirpated
Treatments: Surgery

The foregut forms the pharynx, lower respiratory system, esophagus and stomach, the liver and its associated structures, the pancreas, and the first part of the small intestine. The midgut forms the rest of the small intestine and over half the colon, and the hindgut forms the rest of the colon. Initially, the midgut opens directly into the yolk sac, but as development progresses, the front and back of the embryo bend downwards, constricting the connection of the midgut to the yolk sac. By the sixth week of gestation, the link between the midgut and the yolk sac has narrowed to a slim stalk known as the vitelline duct, and by the seventh week, all connections between the midgut and the yolk sac have completely disappeared.

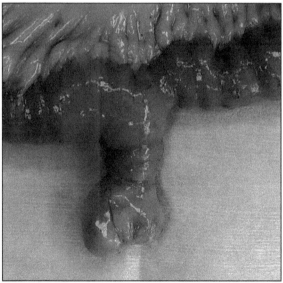

A Meckel's diverticulum. (Surgical-tutor.org.uk)

Occasionally, the vitelline duct persists and produces various structural abnormalities, the most common of which is a blind pouch that bulges from the small intestine known as Meckel's diverticulum (MD). In over half the cases, Meckel's diverticula harbor out-of-place or heterotopic gastrointestinal tissues; most commonly stomach tissue, or less frequently pancreatic tissue, or stomach combined with pancreatic tissue, and even less frequently, upper small intestinal, large

intestinal, or even liver tissue.

MD occurs in 2 percent of the population, but the vast majority of cases are asymptomatic. Children who do show symptoms most commonly experience rectal bleeding (hematochezia). Acid secreted by heterotopic stomach tissue erodes the intestinal lining and produces bleeding ulcers. This rectal bleeding tends to be painless and starts and stops on its own. However, in those patients who do suffer pain, their symptoms can mimic those of appendicitis.

Adults rarely show rectal bleeding, but more commonly experience intestinal obstruction as a result of MD wrapping around the intestine (incarcerated) or inverting and internally blocking it. In cases of intestinal obstruction, the most common symptoms include abdominal pain, tenderness, distention, and vomiting. In older patients, MD may become clogged with food and become infected and inflamed (diverticulitis). In this case the symptoms include diffuse abdominal tenderness and pain with distention.

Treatment and Therapy

Diagnosing MD represents a challenge, and it has been said that "MD is frequently suspected, often looked for and seldom found." Laparoscopy remains one of the best ways to diagnose MD. Laparoscopy uses a thin, lighted tube (laparoscope) that is inserted through a small incision in the abdomen to examine the organs. MD appears as a small pouch extending from the small intestine, about two feet from the junction between the small and large intestines (ileocecal valve). An alternative method for MD diagnosis uses a radioactive compound that concentrates in stomach tissue called technetium-99m pertechnate. Technetium scans are very accurate in children, but less accurate in adults. Computerized tomographic scans can effectively detect Meckel's diverticulitis, but not uninfected MD.

The treatment of choice for symptomatic MD is surgery. For patients with bleeding, incarcerated or obstructed intestines, laparoscopic removal of Meckel's diverticulum and the adjacent intestine (small bowel resection) cures the patient. Meckel's diverticulitis is treated with antibiotics such as clindamycin (Cleoncin), gentamicin (Gentacidin or Garamycin), or cefotetan (Cefotan).

Patients who bleed excessively may become anemic. Severe anemia may require a blood transfusion, but in most cases taking iron and folic acid supplements can restore normal hemoglobin levels and red blood cell numbers.

Five percent of all complicated cases of MD contain malignant tissue and should be referred to an oncologist.

Perspective and Prospects

The description of MD dates to 1598 by Fabricus Hildanus. Later, the German surgeon Lavater reported blind pouches that extended from the lower part of the small intestine (ileum) in 1671. In 1707, Ruysch augmented Lavater's anatomical descriptions by providing accurate illustrations of MD. In the eighteenth century, Morgagni correctly discerned that MD resulted from structures that persisted from human development, but the precise embryonic structures eluded him.

However, in 1809, Johann Friedrich Meckel examined twenty-two different pediatric cadavers and identified the vitelline duct (also known as the omphalomesenteric duct) as the persistent structure that causes MD. For this reason, MD is named after Meckel in his honor.

MD is the most common congenital malformation of the gastrointestinal tract, but because it tends to produce rather nonspecific symptoms, properly diagnosing it remains the greatest challenge facing clinicians with regard to this condition.

—*Michael A Buratovich, Ph.D.*

See also Embryology; Gastroenterology; Hematology; Oncology; Pediatrics

For Further Information:

Uppal, Kiranjit, R. Shane Tubbs, Petru Matusz, Kitt Shaffer, and Marios Loukas. "Meckel's Diverticulum: A Review." *Clinical Anatomy* 24, no. 4 (May 2011): 416-422.

Moore, Keith L., T. V. N. Persuad, and Mark G. Torchia. *Before We Are Born: Essentials of Embryology and Birth Defects.* 8th ed. Philadelphia: Elsevier/Saunders, 2012.

Sadler, Thomas W. *Langman's Medical Embryology.* 12th ed. Philadelphia: Lippincott Williams & Wilkins, 2011.

MEDICAL HOME

Treatment

Anatomy or system affected: All

Specialties and related fields: All

Definition: The base for children's medical and non-medical care.

In 1967, the American Academy of Pediatrics (AAP) coined the term "medical home," which was at first a center of a child's medical records. Since then, the idea of a medical home has transitioned.

Healthcare today is a multi-disciplinary approach encompassing patient, family, primary care provider and other disciplines providing care for the patient, such as specialists and community support. Within this model, the patient and patient's family is the focus around which the medical home is built. In addition, medical homes now encompass pediatrics as well as adults.

In 2007 the AAP, the American Academy of Family Physicians (AAFP), the American College of Physicians (ACP) and the American Osteopathic Association (AOA) united to form the Joint Principles of the Patient Centered Medical Home. These combined organizations now state that a medical home possesses the seven following characteristics:

Personal physician. Each patient has a continuous relationship with an individual physician who provides first contact, comprehensive and continuous care.

Physician directed medical practice. The personal physician coordinates and leads a team of colleagues at the practice that together works to provide continuing care for the patient.

Whole person orientation. The personal physician supplies direct care to the patient, or orchestrates care from other providers. This encompasses healthcare demands for all different pathologies and stages of life, including acute care,

chronic care, end-of-life care and preventive care. In addition, coordinating with the patient and their families necessitates understanding each patient's different needs, values and cultural backgrounds. The medical home assists patients to manage their own care at the level the patient desires. By perceiving the patients and families as integral parts of the health care team, the medical home facilitates their role as knowledgeable allies in creating the care plan.

Care is coordinated and/or integrated. It is done so across the various modalities of health care and across the patient's community. This can include hospitals, specialty care, home health care and community services and supports. The medical home practice involves the entire health care team, which can include physicians, advanced practice nurses, physician assistants, nurses, pharmacists, nutritionists, social workers, educators, and care coordinators, to build open and clear communication. Other smaller practices may use virtual tools to link various types of providers with patients.

Quality and safety. By using evidence-based medicine and clinical decision-support tools, the primary care medical home is committed to quality and safety. Patients and families share in the decision-making process in order to attain best outcomes that are patient-centered. Informational technology assists in providing best patient care, reviewing performance outcomes, providing patient education and strengthening communication with patients. Providers and staff seek feedback to make sure that patients are satisfied with their care and outcomes. The medical home demonstrates a continuous dedication to improvement by conducting performance measurements. A non-governmental organization reviews the medical home to ensure that it is maintaining patient-centered services that align with the model of a medical home.

Enhanced access to care. The medical home delivers accessible care. This is made possible by longer clinical hours, shorter waiting times for urgent needs, and additional modes of communication between patients and a member of the care team, such as after-hours email and telephone care. The medical home is receptive to patients' choices about access.

Payment. Because patient-centered medical homes provide added value to patients, payment is based on the below guidelines:

- It should recognize the work by the health-care team that falls outside of the face-to-face visit.
- It should pay for coordinating care across various different specialties.
- It should pay for implementing new health information technologies.
- It should pay for care provided through enhanced communication options, such as email and phone.
- It should support physician work, including remote monitoring of clinical data through new technology
- It should grant payment to separate fee-for-service payments.
- It should recognize case-mix differences in patient population
- It should allow grant savings to healthcare providers for re-

duced hospitalizations that are associated with their care

- It should allow for additional payments for achieving measurable and continuous quality improvements.

—*Samar Post Jamali*

For Further Information:

American College of Physicians. "What is the Patient-Centered Medical Home?" http://www.acponline.org/running_practice/delivery_and_payment_models/pcmh/understanding/what.htm

Patient Centered Medical Home Resource Center: http://pcmh.ahrq.gov/

MEDICARE

Health care system

Definition: A federal health insurance program for persons over sixty-five, persons with end-stage renal disease, and some disabled individuals. Medicare is part of the Social Security system, and participation is closely tied to Social Security eligibility.

Key terms:

beneficiary: the person who receives the benefits of an insurance policy; for health insurance, the beneficiary is the patient receiving health care

coinsurance: an arrangement in which a percentage of the total bill for health services is paid by the insurer and the rest is paid by the beneficiary

deductible: the amount that the patient must pay before the insurance pays any amount

managed care organization: a health care organization that combines the functions of insurer and provider; it reduces redundancy of services and uses primary care providers as gatekeepers to reduce cost

medically necessary: services and supplies that are appropriate and needed for the diagnosis or treatment of the person's medical condition

Medicare Trust Fund: accumulated contributions from Social Security payroll taxes that are used to pay for the Medicare program

premiums: periodic payments for insurance coverage

primary care provider: a doctor or nurse practitioner who is trained to provide basic medical care

skilled nursing care: a level of care that requires the skills of a registered nurse

Introduction

Medicare is a federal health insurance program for individuals who are sixty-five or older, persons who have end-stage renal disease (irreversible kidney failure), and some individuals who have disabilities. In addition to age and special conditions, eligible individuals or their spouses must have been employed for at least ten years in a job in which they paid Social Security payroll taxes and must be citizens or permanent residents of the United States. Medicare was passed into law as Title XVIII of the Social Security Act of 1965. The intent of the Medicare law was to provide financial protection to elderly individuals against the high cost of illness and hospitalization.

According to the US Census Bureau, in 2011, 46.9 million Americans were covered by Medicare services. Medicare is administered through the Centers for Medicare and Medicaid Services (CMS), formerly the Health Care Financing Administration (HCFA). CMS is an agency of the Social Security Administration within the Department of Health and Human Services (DHHS).

Medicare is financed through a combination of Social Security payroll tax, premiums, and general revenue funds. Services for the Original Medicare Plan are available nationwide, and the insured person can go to any provider that accepts Medicare. The original program operates in the same way as other fee-for-service medical insurance plans, which means the insured person is charged a fee each time that person receives health care services. The person providing the service files a claim for payment. These fees, or claims, are paid fully or partially by Medicare. The Social Security Administration does not pay the claims directly; it has contractual arrangements with private insurance organizations that handle all payments. Fiscal intermediaries process claims from hospitals and other inpatient facilities, and carriers process claims from physicians and suppliers.

CMS has the responsibility to interpret and clarify the provisions of the laws and regulations governing Medicare. Its responsibility includes making determinations as to whether a particular service will be approved for payment by Medicare. However, the majority of decisions about whether a specific type of service will be covered are made at the local level by the fiscal intermediaries or carriers who process claims.

The structure of the Medicare program has remained basically unchanged since its inception. There are two parts to the Original Medicare Plan: Part A and Part B. Part A, called Hospital Insurance (HI), pays for inpatient services. Most people do not pay for Medicare Part A; it is generally financed through the Social Security payroll taxes that are earmarked for the Medicare Trust Fund. At age sixty-five, individuals receive Part A automatically if they are already receiving Social Security retirement benefits or retirement benefits through the Railroad Retirement Board, or if they are eligible to receive either of these benefits but have not yet filed for them. Individuals who had Medicare-covered government employment also receive Part A without paying premiums, as do their spouses. Individuals under sixty-five can receive Part A benefits without paying if they have had Social Security or Railroad Retirement Board disability benefits for twenty-four months. Other individuals entitled to Part A benefits without paying are those with end-stage renal disease (ESRD) who are receiving kidney dialysis or who have had a kidney transplant.

Part A benefits include a semiprivate room in a hospital or skilled nursing facility as well as related services and supplies, including laboratory and diagnostic procedures, nursing care, surgical care, and rehabilitative services. Skilled nursing home services are paid for after the person has been hospitalized for three days for a related health condition. Medicare pays for medications given to the patient while in the hospital or skilled nursing facility. In situations of medical necessity, a private room is allowed. Part A also pays for part-time skilled nursing care in the home as well as for physical, occupational, and speech-language therapy. Hospice care for terminally ill patients is paid for through Part A. Hospice care includes medical and support services such as drugs for the control of pain or other symptoms and skilled nursing care.

Part B, called Medical Insurance (MI), pays for outpatient services, including services from primary care providers, specialist physicians, clinical psychologists, and social workers. Part B also pays for outpatient mental health services, surgical services and supplies, diagnostic tests, procedures, outpatient therapies, and durable medical equipment such as canes, wheelchairs, walkers, and oxygen-delivery equipment. These services and supplies are covered when they are medically necessary. Medicare helps pay for ambulance services when other sources of transportation would endanger the person's health, artificial limbs and prosthetic devices, braces, chiropractic services, emergency care, immunosuppressive drugs for patients who have undergone organ transplantation, kidney dialysis, nutritional therapy services for diabetics or patients with ESRD, and telemedicine in rural areas. Medicare pays for approved medications that are administered as part of physicians" services.

Preventive services are also covered under Part B. These preventive services include bone density tests, colorectal cancer screening, diabetes services and supplies, glaucoma screening, mammography, clinical breast examinations, Pap tests and pelvic examinations, prostate cancer screening, and vaccinations. Rules apply as to who qualifies and the frequency of these services.

A provider or supplier must inform the beneficiary if a specific service will likely not be paid for by Medicare. If the person still chooses to receive the service, the person will be asked to sign an advance beneficiary notice (ABN). By signing the ABN, the person is agreeing to pay out-of-pocket if Medicare does not pay.

Part B is optional, and individuals have a choice of whether to enroll in Part B at the same time that they enroll in Part A. Most people do have to pay for coverage under Part B. A portion of the total cost for these services is financed through premiums, and the remainder is financed through general federal revenue funds. The charge for the premium is adjusted yearly; in 2013, the monthly premium for Part B was $104.90, which is deducted from the person's Social Security, railroad retirement, or civil service retirement check. If individuals do not receive a retirement check, then Medicare bills them for the Part B premiums on a quarterly basis. Eligible persons can postpone enrolling in Part B if they or their spouses are working and have group health insurance through their employment. However, if they do not have group health insurance and delay enrolling in Part B, then their monthly payments may be increased by 10 percent for every year that they did not enroll but could have done so.

For services under both Part A and Part B, the insured person is responsible for paying the deductible, coinsurance, and copayment. The deductible for Part B was $147 per year in 2013. As an example, a patient has surgery on January 2 costing $547. Since he has not paid his deductible for the year, he must first pay that amount ($147); then Medicare pays its share, which is usually 80 percent, of the remaining amount ($320). The patient pays the remainder ($80). One exception to the usual 20 percent paid by beneficiaries is in the case of outpatient mental health services, in which beneficiaries paid 35 percent of the Medicare-approved amount in 2013. This percentage was scheduled to decrease to 20 percent in 2014.

Private insurance can be purchased separately to help pay coinsurance amounts, deductibles, and other out-of-pocket expenses for individuals who have the Original Medicare Plan. Such insurance policies are called Medigap policies, since they are used to fill the gaps in the Original Medicare Plan. Medigap policies are regulated by federal and state laws. Different Medigap plans offer different benefits, and some Medigap policies pay a portion of prescription medication fees.

In 2013, Medicare Part A had a $1,184 deductible for a hospital stay for each benefit period. A benefit period begins the day the person becomes an inpatient in either a hospital or a skilled nursing facility and ends when the person has not received inpatient care for sixty consecutive days. If the person is hospitalized after one benefit period has ended, then a new benefit period begins. In 2013, for each benefit period the costs were an initial deductible of $1,184 for days one through sixty and $246 for days sixty-one through ninety. After ninety days, the person can use lifetime reserve days, which means that Medicare will pay all covered costs, except for a coinsurance payment of $592 per day, for up to sixty days. These reserve days can be used only once during the person's lifetime. For care in a skilled nursing facility, for each benefit period the beneficiary pays nothing for the first twenty days, up to $148 per day for days twenty-one through one hundred, and all costs after one hundred days.

Medicare beneficiaries sometimes have additional health care coverage that pays bills first, after which Medicare pays the remainder; this is called Medicare Secondary Payer. Examples of primary payers are veterans" benefits, workers" compensation, union health coverage, or employer-sponsored insurance. To conserve Medicare funds, the Coordination of Benefits program monitors and manages the payment process when beneficiaries have more than one policy.

Physician services and supplies will cost more if the physician or supplier does not accept assignment. Assignment is an agreement from a physician, other health care provider, or supplier of medical equipment whereby they accept the Medicare-approved fee as full payment for rendered services. The approved fee is the cost that has been established by Medicare as reasonable for the particular service. Even if the physician or other providers do not accept assignment, a maximum is placed on what they can charge, called the limiting charge. The maximum, or limit, is 15 percent over Medicare's approved amount.

To reflect the changes occurring in health care delivery,

Medicare law was amended in 1997 to allow beneficiaries to choose among several different health insurance plans based on their needs. The Original Medicare Plan remained as it was originally implemented. Another option, Medicare Advantage (originally known as Medicare+Choice), enables beneficiaries to enroll in a managed care plan or private fee-for-service plan. In managed care plans, a specified group of providers render services to all members enrolled in the plan. All Medicare+Choice plans must include services covered by Parts A and B of the Original Medicare Plan. These plans can also provide additional services such as prescription medication, dental care, preventive care, and glasses. The cost for additional services depends on the specific plan. Under these plans, the beneficiary may be required to pay a premium, in addition to what is paid for Part B, and a copayment when services are rendered. All Medicare beneficiaries, regardless of the type of plan, have the right to appeal a decision related to the amount of payment for a service, whether a particular service or item should be covered, or the length of time that a service should be provided.

In addition to the right to appeal decisions, beneficiaries have a right to information, to know their treatment choices and be involved in treatment decisions, to file complaints, and to nondiscriminatory treatment that reflects sensitivity to cultural differences. Medicare is required by law to protect the privacy of medical information as set forth in the Health Insurance Portability and Accountability Act (HIPAA) of 1996.

If a person qualifies for Medicare but cannot afford to pay for Medicare deductibles and coinsurance, that person may be eligible for the Medicare Savings Programs available through the State Medical Assistance Office. If the person's income and resources are severely limited, then the individual may qualify for Medicaid in addition to Medicare.

In 2011, total Medicare expenditures were $549.1 billion. Since 1965, benefits have expanded, and there has been an increase in both expenditures per person and the number of beneficiaries in the program. These factors have caused continuing concern in Congress regarding the cost and financing of Medicare. Cost-containment measures over the years have included instituting a prospective payment system for hospitals, nursing home care, and home care; providing more options through managed care organizations; and shifting services previously covered by Part A to Part B.

Perspective and Prospects

In June 2003, Congress passed bills to amend Medicare to include coverage for prescription medications and give individuals more choice in the selection of health insurance plans. These bills reflected Congress's attempt to monitor and improve the quality of health care services for Medicare recipients while maintaining the integrity of the Medicare Trust Fund. The resulting Part D drug benefit received mixed reviews. The US government further reformed Medicare through the passage of the Patient Protection and Affordable Care Act in March of 2010. This act implemented additional prescription drug coverage for some Medicare recipients and

stipulated that Medicare must cover additional preventive services, such as mammograms and wellness exams, without charging a deductible.

—*Roberta Tierney, M.S.N., J.D., A.P.N.*

See also Aging: Extended care; American Medical Association (AMA); Department of Health and Human Services; Geriatrics and gerontology; Health care reform; Hospice; Hospitals; Terminally ill: Extended care.

For Further Information:
Barr, Donald A. *Introduction to US Health Policy.* 3d ed. Baltimore: Johns Hopkins University Press, 2011.

Béland, Daniel, and Alex Waddan. *The Politics of Policy Change.* Washington, DC: Georgetown University Press, 2012.

Medicare: The Official US Government Site for Medicare. http://www.medicare.gov.

Rettenmaier, Andrew J., and Thomas R. Saving. *The Economics of Medicare Reform.* Kalamazoo, Mich.: W. E. Upjohn Institute for Employment Research, 2000.

US Census Bureau. "Health Insurance." *US Department of Commerce,* 2011.

US Department of Health and Human Services. Centers for Medicare and Medicaid Services. *Medicare and You 2010.* Washington, DC: Author, 2010.

Weissert, William G. *Governing Health: The Politics of Health Policy.* 4th ed. Baltimore: Johns Hopkins University Press, 2012.

MEDITATION
Treatment

Anatomy or system affected: All

Specialties and related fields: Alternative medicine, preventive medicine

Definition: Techniques involving controlled breathing, visualization, and repeated words or phrases that are used to achieve relaxation and reduce muscle tension, which may have health benefits.

Indications and Procedures

One of the most popular techniques used in meditation is concentration, in which one focuses attention on a single object such as the function of breathing, a candle flame, or a visualized image. When attention wanders, the practitioner brings it gently back to the original focus. Sometimes a mantra, a chosen word or phrase given by a teacher or chosen by the practitioner (such as the om mantra of Tibetan Buddhism), is repeated silently or aloud.

Guided imagery utilizes listening to a voice, recorded or live, that guides the practitioner to visualize a beautiful and peaceful place, where one feels calm and secure. Walking meditation, tai chi, and qi gong focus on movement, breathing, and ritual, and the practice of yoga incorporates breathing and movement or physical postures to help relax body and mind. Soothing music may also be used with any of the techniques. Prayer and silent reading of and reflection on inspirational texts are other common forms of meditation. Teachers recommend starting slowly with five-minute sessions, working up to twenty minutes once or twice a day.

Uses and Complications

Meditation techniques, which are thousands of years old, are being promoted as a benefit to health and well-being, primarily in stress-related conditions. Meditation traditionally has been and is used in a religious sense to deepen one's understanding and involvement with the spiritual, mystical, and sacred aspects of life. It is also used as an exercise in self-discovery and revelation, helping the practitioner turn inward, temporarily shutting out worldly cares and strife to find inner peace and calm. Being religious, however, is not essential to meditation; in fact, most everyone can learn the techniques and reap the health benefits of this age-old practice. Physical limitations and preexisting mental health concerns should be taken into consideration before undertaking specific meditative practices, and practitioners should make their instructors aware of these conditions.

Numerous studies confirm that prolonged or interpersonal stress can produce such conditions as constriction of blood vessels, pain and swelling in joints, suppression of the immune system, decreases in white blood cells and changes in their function, and high cholesterol levels. Chemicals such as adrenaline, produced when the body is under stress, can raise blood pressure, increase heart rate, and cause other harmful physiological responses when stress is persistent or sustained. Stress is also linked to many diseases and conditions, including heart attacks, diabetes, cancer, allergies, and skin disorders.

Meditation, in helping the patient to relax, reduces muscle tension and decreases the release of these harmful chemicals. A number of stress-related conditions have been shown to benefit from meditation, including chronic pain, arthritis, infertility, psoriasis, respiratory conditions such as asthma and emphysema, premenstrual syndrome (PMS), tension headaches, irritable bowel syndrome (IBS), ulcers, insomnia, and fibromyalgia.

—*Martha Oehmke Loustaunau, Ph.D.*

See also Alternative medicine; Anxiety; Biofeedback; Hypnosis; Stress; Stress reduction; Yoga.

For Further Information:

Benson, Herbert, and Miriam Z. Klipper. *The Relaxation Response.* 25th anniversary ed. New York: Avon Books, 2000.

Harmon, Robert, and Mary Ann Myers. "Prayer and Meditation as Medical Therapies." *Physical Medicine and Rehabilitation Clinics of North America* 10, no. 3 (August, 1999): 651–662.

Kabat-Zinn, Jon. *Wherever You Go, There You Are: Mindfulness Meditation in Everyday Life.* 10th anniversary ed. New York: Hyperion, 2005.

"Meditation: A Simple, Fast Way to Reduce Stress." *Mayo Foundation for Medical Education and Research*, April 21, 2011.

National Center for Complementary and Alternative Medicine. "Meditation: An Introduction." *National Institutes of Health, US Department of Health and Human Services*, February 21, 2013.

"Relaxation Therapies." *Health Library*, September 17, 2012.

Scholten, Amy, and Brian Randall. "How to Meditate." *Health Library*, November 14, 2012.

Trivieri, Larry, Jr., and John W. Anderson, eds. *Alternative Medicine: The Definitive Guide.* 2d ed. Berkeley, Calif.: Ten Speed Press, 2002.

MELANOMA

Disease/Disorder

Anatomy or system affected: Skin

Specialties and related fields: Dermatology, internal medicine, pathology

Definition: A malignant disease which originates with the melanocytes in the skin. While there may be a variety of causes, the primary risk factor is extent of exposure to sunlight.

Key terms:

dysplasia: the aberrant growth or development of cells

melanocytes: cells in the upper layer of skin which produce the pigment melanin

metastasis: the spread of cells from a primary site of cancer to areas throughout the body

nevus: a pigmented site on the skin which is composed of melanocytes

Causes and Symptoms

Melanocytes are cells in the skin that produce melanin, most commonly recognized as the basis of skin color. Following exposure to ultraviolet (UV) light, particularly that found in sunlight, melanocytes begin the synthesis of increased levels of pigment, some of which is transferred to the surrounding cells. The process is a response to the potential damage induced by UV light and helps disperse the damaging effects of the rays.

Ultraviolet light is relatively high in energy, and significant exposure, especially exposure sufficient to cause sunburn, is damaging to deoxyribonucleic acid (DNA), the genetic material in the cell. The genetic changes that result have the potential to produce mutations that develop into cancer. Much of current research into the biology of melanomas has involved an understanding of these molecular changes.

The first alteration in physical appearance of the site is the formation of a nevus (mole), a benign lesion consisting of replicating melanocytes. Generally speaking, nevi do not often evolve beyond the benign stage, and they rarely progress to cancer. Depending upon the extent of mutation or the accumulation of genetic changes over time with continued exposure to sunlight, however, melanocytes within the lesion may grow increasingly dysplastic. Growth regulation is disrupted, and, on a microscopic level, they no longer appear normal. It is during this period that the first symptoms of an abnormal condition may appear.

Information on Melanoma

Causes: Exposure to ultraviolet light and resulting mutations

Symptoms: Nevus (usually a mole) that changes in shape, size, or pigmentation; may spread to lymphatic system and other regions

Duration: Chronic, sometimes fatal

Treatments: Surgery, chemotherapy, radiation, biological therapy using protein extracts from the melanoma

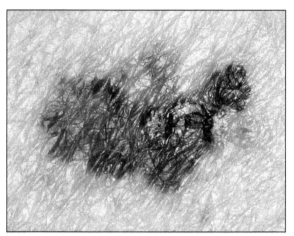

Melanoma. (National Cancer Institute)

Most melanomas start at the site of a mole. Often the initial indication a mole has progressed to a malignant form is a change in its shape, size, or pigmentation. The phrase "ABCDE" is often recommended as a means to remember the symptoms: *a*symmetry, in which one side of the mole differs from the other; *b*order, in which the edge is no longer sharp but ragged and pigmentation begins to spread; *c*olor, in which the pigmentation may develop hues of different shades; *d*iameter, in which the size of the mole changes, usually increasing; and *e*volving, in which the mole has changed during the past few weeks or months.

Analysis of what have become malignant cells, and therefore the decision as to the course of treatment, is indicated by a staging designation ranging from stage 0 to stage IV. Stage 0 designates a melanoma that is limited to the outer layer of skin, the epidermis. Stage IV indicates that a cancer has undergone metastasis, spreading into the lymphatic system and other regions of the body.

Treatment and Therapy

Initial treatment remains the surgical removal of the melanoma itself. Since this is an aggressive form of cancer, early diagnosis, prior to the stage at which metastasis has begun, is critical. The National Cancer Institute recommends four methods of treatment, the choice dependent upon the stage of the disease. If surgery is insufficient, usually because of metastasis, then chemotherapy remains the second choice. Chemotherapeutic drugs are either taken orally or injected directly into the bloodstream. If the tumor is localized, then the drug may be perfused directly into the local tissue. The relatively nonspecific nature of the chemotherapy often produces severe side effects.

An alternative treatment may involve radiation. Radiation therapy may be directed into the cancer either externally or from an implanted radiation source within the cancerous region itself. This form of directed treatment may help avoid the side effects of chemotherapy, but it is most effective only if the cancer is in a limited area.

In recent years, some success has been achieved using new forms of biological treatment. A cancer "vaccine" is prepared using protein extracts from the melanoma itself, the idea being that by allowing the immune system to react against the vaccine, the cancer itself may also be targeted. Other drugs that may be used in biological treatments are interferon, which is is injected intravenously to slow the growth of melanoma, and interleukin-2, which is given intravenously to kill cancer cells.

Another treatment option used for milder types of skin cancer, namely early-stage basal cell cancer and squamous cell cancer, is photodynamic therapy. In this treatment, a drug is absorbed by cancer cells; either several hours or several days later, a light source such as a laser is focused on the cancer, activating the drug and destroying the cancer cells.

Perspective and Prospects

Melanoma is a particularly deadly form of skin cancer. While only approximately 4 percent of skin cancers are actually melanomas, this form of cancer accounts for some 80 percent of skin cancer deaths.

While research into the molecular nature of melanoma has provided significant insight into the cause and progress of the disease, at least at the molecular level, prevention remains of primary importance. Most cases result from exposure to the UV light found in sunlight. Since sensitivity to sunlight is in part a function of the level of pigmentation of the skin, individuals, especially those with light skin, must be more cognizant of the danger of overexposure to the sun. If sun exposure cannot be avoided or is desired, then people must be careful to use proper sunscreens to at least limit the level of exposure to UV rays. Whether it is the myth of the "healthy tan" or simply the psychological desire to show a tanned body, however, people will continue to expose themselves to the sun. Until such behaviors change, it remains likely that the incidence of melanoma will remain at current levels.

Since the earlier the stage of development, the better the prognosis, recognition of the ABCDE warning signs is critical for those who have had extensive exposure to the sun. Current treatments for advanced or recurrent melanoma are primarily palliative, an attempt to prolong and improve the quality of life. Improved prognosis depends upon the effectiveness of new and combined forms of therapy, most notably combinations of immune therapy and chemotherapy.

—*Richard Adler, Ph.D.*

See also Cancer; Carcinogens; Chemotherapy; Dermatology; Dermatopathology; Lesions; Malignancy and metastasis; Moles; Oncology; Radiation therapy; Skin; Skin cancer; Skin disorders; Skin lesion removal.

For Further Information:
"About Melanoma." *Melanoma Research Foundation*, 2011.

Gilchrest, B., et al. "The Pathogenesis of Melanoma Induced by Ultraviolet Radiation." *New England Journal of Medicine* 340, no. 17 (April 29, 1999): 1341–1348.

Gore, Martin, and Julie Newton-Bishop. *Melanoma: Critical Debates*. Malden, Mass.: Blackwell, 2002.

LaRusso, Laurie,a nd Brian Randall. "Melanoma." *Health Library*, Apr. 9, 2013.

"Melanoma." *MedlinePlus*, May 10, 2013.

"Melanoma Skin Cancer." *American Cancer Society*, Jan. 17. 2013.

Miller, Arlo, and Martin C. Mihm, Jr. "Melanoma." *New England Journal of Medicine* 355, no. 1 (July 6, 2006): 51–65.

Poole, Catherine. *Melanoma: Prevention, Detection, and Treatment.* 2d ed. New Haven, Conn.: Yale University Press, 2005.

Sharfman, William. *Melanoma*. New York: Demos Medical, 2012.

"What You Need to Know about Melanoma and Other Skin Cancers." *National Cancer Institute*, June 2010.

Melatonin

Biology

Anatomy or system affected: Brain, endocrine system, glands

Specialties and related fields: Alternative medicine, endocrinology, neurology, pharmacology, preventive medicine

Definition: A substance produced by the pineal gland that has been used as a controversial therapeutic agent.

Key terms:

endocrine system: the glands that produce hormones

hormone: a substance produced in one part of the body that has effects in other parts of the body

melatonin: the hormone produced by the pineal gland

pineal gland: a small organ inside the brain that produces melatonin

Structure and Functions

Melatonin, also known as N-acetyl-5-methoxytryptamine, is a hormone found in a wide variety of living organisms. In vertebrates (animals with backbones), including humans, it is produced by the pineal gland. The pineal gland is located deep within the center of the brain. Although it is inside the brain, it is considered part of the endocrine system rather than the nervous system. In humans, the pineal gland is a gray or white organ less than 1 centimeter long and shaped like a pinecone.

The pineal gland produces varying amounts of melatonin in response to changes in light. Light inhibits the production of melatonin, and darkness stimulates it. In some small animals, light reaches the pineal gland directly through the skull. In larger animals, including humans, information about lightness and darkness is transmitted by the nervous system from the eyes to the suprachiasmatic nucleus, a cluster of nerve cells in a region of the brain known as the hypothalamus. The suprachiasmatic nucleus regulates the secretion of melatonin by the pineal gland.

Melatonin is believed to be involved in regulating the sleep cycle in response to changes in light. Because the amount of melatonin produced by the pineal gland declines sharply at puberty, it is believed to be involved in the development of the reproductive system. Because melatonin production continues to decline with age, some researchers believe that it is associated with the process of aging.

Disorders and Diseases

Disorders of melatonin production other than its normal decline with age are rare. Tumors of the pineal gland may reduce melatonin production. Some evidence suggests that this may lead to premature aging. Children with tumors of the pineal gland may reach puberty at a very early age.

Some researchers suggest that the normal decline in melatonin production with age is associated with diseases of the elderly. Animal studies suggest that loss of melatonin is associated with increased cell damage. Melatonin is believed to act as an antioxidant, a substance that protects cells from free radicals, which are produced when cells use oxygen. Cell damage has been linked to a large number of diseases of the elderly, including various forms of cancer, heart disease, and Alzheimer's disease.

Based on this evidence, melatonin has been used to treat and prevent a wide variety of illnesses. In the 1990s, melatonin became widely used in the United States. Because it was classified as a dietary supplement rather than as a drug, it was available without a prescription and with little government regulation. While some researchers suggested caution until more was known about melatonin, others suggested taking small daily doses of the hormone to slow down the aging process. Popular books such as *The Melatonin Miracle* (1995), by Walter Pierpaoli, William Regelson, and Carol Colman, claim that melatonin can stimulate the immune system, prevent cancer and heart disease, improve sexual relations, reduce the effects of stress, act as a contraceptive, and add years to the human life span. Critics argue that these claims are greatly exaggerated.

The least controversial suggested use for melatonin is as a sleeping aid. Human studies have indicated that melatonin is safe and effective for this use. Unlike many other sleeping pills, melatonin seems to have no effect on normal sleep patterns and few side effects. Melatonin has also been shown to be effective in treating jet lag, the difficulty that travelers have adjusting to a new time zone.

Critics of routine melatonin use point out that little is known about its long-term effects. They also point to evidence that some people may experience short-term side effects such as nightmares, headaches, daytime sleepiness, and mild depression. A major concern is the lack of regulation of melatonin products, leading to the possibility that other, unknown substances may be present.

Even the most optimistic proponents of melatonin suggest certain precautions. Many products contain more melatonin than researchers believe is necessary, leading to the possibility of a greater risk of side effects with no increase in benefit. Melatonin should only be taken at bedtime to avoid unwanted sleepiness. It should not be used by children, who already produce high levels of melatonin. It should not be used by pregnant women because its effect on the fetus is unknown. Because it is believed to stimulate the immune system, melatonin should be avoided in people with severe allergies, autoimmune disorders, or cancer of the immune system.

Perspective and Prospects

The pineal gland was known to exist in ancient times. It was first described scientifically by the Greek physician Galen in the second century. The French philosopher René Descartes (1596–1650) suggested that it was the location of the human soul. The true function of the pineal gland remained unknown until the middle of the twentieth century.

Melatonin was discovered in 1958 and first described as a hormone in 1963. Research into its effects began in the 1970s and 1980s. Interest in this hormone increased dramatically in 1995, with the publication of several books and articles publicizing its possible benefits. Research on melatonin is expected to continue for many years, particularly in regard to its long-term effects.

—Rose Secrest

See also Aging; Antioxidants; Brain; Chronobiology; Endocrine disorders; Endocrine glands; Endocrinology; Endocrinology, pediatric; Glands; Hormone therapy; Hormones; Light therapy; Pharmacology; Sleep disorders.

For Further Information:

AHFS Consumer Medication Information [Internet]. Bethesda (MD): American Society of Health-System Pharmacists, Inc.; ©2008. Melatonin; [update 2013 June 13; reviewed 2011 Dec 24; cited 2013 July 12]; [about 4 p.]. Available from: http://www.nlm.nih.gov/medlineplus/druginfo/meds/a604025.html.

Brzezinski, Amnon. "Melatonin in Humans." *New England Journal of Medicine* 336, no. 3 (January 16, 1997): 186–95.

Goodman, H. Maurice. *Basic Medical Endocrinology.* 4th ed. Boston: Academic Press/Elsevier, 2009.

Holt, Richard I. G., and Neil A. Hanley. *Essential Endocrinology and Diabetes.* 6th ed. Malden, Mass.: Blackwell, 2012.

"Melatonin: Questions, Facts, Mysteries." *University of California, Berkeley, Wellness Letter* 16, no. 8 (May, 2000): 1–2.

Olcese, James, ed. *Melatonin After Four Decades: An Assessment of Its Potential.* New York: Kluwer Academic/Plenum, 1999.

Pandi-Perumal, S. R., and Daniel P. Cardinali, eds. *Melatonin: Biological Basis of Its Function in Health and Disease.* Georgetown, Tex.: Landes Bioscience, 2006.

Turget, Mehmet, and Raj Kumar. *The Pineal Gland and Melatonin: Recent Advances in Development, Imaging, Disease, and Treatment.* New York: Nova Science, 2012.

Watson, Ronald R. *Melatonin in the Promotion of Health.* 2d edition. Boca Raton, Fla: CRC Press, 2012.

MEMORY LOSS
Disease/Disorder
Anatomy or system affected: Brain, nervous system, psychic-emotional system
Specialties and related fields: Geriatrics and gerontology, neurology, psychiatry, psychology
Definition: Total or limited impairment of memory that may be sudden or gradual.

Causes and Symptoms

Memory impairment is a common problem, and often a concern among older individuals. Memory problems are not, however, restricted to older adults. They may occur at any age and may be attributable to numerous conditions and behaviors, including the use of alcohol and other drugs. Memory loss occurs in various degrees and may be associated with other evidence of brain dysfunction and other physical and emotional problems. Memory loss may be partial, limited to events immediately before or after a traumatic event. Memory loss may also be complete. Amnesia is the term used to describe complete memory loss. Memory loss may also be

permanent or temporary, or may vacillate, with a person slipping in and out of being able to remember appropriately.

Benign senescent forgetfulness. In this condition, the memory deficit affects mostly recent events, and although a source of frustration, it seldom interferes with the individual's professional activities or social life. An important feature of benign forgetfulness is that it is selective and affects only trivial, unimportant facts. For example, one may misplace the car keys or forget to return a phone call, respond to a letter, or pay a bill. Cashing a check or telephoning someone with whom one is particularly keen to talk, however, will not be forgotten. The person is aware of the memory deficit, and written notes often are used as reminders. Patients with benign forgetfulness have no other evidence of brain dysfunction and maintain their ability to make valid judgments.

Dementia. In dementia, the memory impairment is global, does not discriminate between important and trivial facts, and interferes with the person's ability to pursue professional or social activities. Patients with dementia find it difficult to adapt to changes in the workplace, such as the introduction of computers. They also find it difficult to continue with their hobbies and interests.

The hallmark of dementia is no awareness of the memory deficit, except in the very early stages of the disease. This is an important difference between dementia and benign forgetfulness. Although patients with early dementia may write themselves notes, they usually forget to check these reminders or may misinterpret them. For example, a man with dementia who is invited for dinner at a friend's house may write a note to that effect and leave it in a prominent place. He may then go to his host's home several evenings in succession because he has forgotten that he already has fulfilled this social engagement. As the disease progresses, patients are no longer aware of their memory deficit.

In dementia, the memory deficit does not occur in isolation but is accompanied by other evidence of brain dysfunction, which in very early stages can be detected only by specialized neuropsychological tests. As the condition progresses, these deficits become readily apparent. The patient is often disoriented regarding time and may telephone relatives or friends very late at night or not realize the time of day. As the disease progresses, the disorientation affects the patient's environment: A woman with dementia may wander outside her house and be unable to find her way back, or she may repeatedly ask to be taken back home when she is already there. In later stages, patients may not be able to recognize people whom

---

Information on Memory Loss

Causes: Aging, head trauma, certain diseases, repeated strokes, depression
Symptoms: Vary; can include benign forgetfulness, disorientation and impaired judgment, weakness or paralysis in body part
Duration: Acute to chronic
Treatments: Varies; can include medication, surgery

they should know: A man may think that his son is his father or that his wife is his mother. In fact, it is possible for the patient to not even recognize his or her own reflection in a mirror. This stage is particularly distressing to the caregivers. Patients with dementia may often exhibit impaired judgment. They may go outside the house inappropriately dressed or at inappropriate times, or they may purchase the same item repeatedly or make donations that are disproportional to their funds. Alzheimer's disease is one of the most common causes of dementia in older people.

Multiple infarct dementia. Multiple infarct dementia is caused by the destruction of brain cells by repeated strokes. Sometimes these strokes are so small that neither the patient nor the relatives are aware of their occurrence. When many strokes occur and significant brain tissue is destroyed, the patient may exhibit symptoms of dementia. Usually, however, most of these strokes are quite obvious because they are associated with weakness or paralysis in a part of the body. One of the characteristic features of multiple infarct dementia is that its onset is sudden and its progression is by steps. Every time a stroke occurs, the patient's condition deteriorates. This is followed by a period during which little or no deterioration develops until another stroke occurs, at which time the patient's condition deteriorates further. Very rarely, the stroke affects only the memory center, in which case the patient's sole problem is amnesia. Multiple infarct dementia and dementia resulting from Alzheimer's disease should be differentiated from other treatable conditions which also may cause memory impairment, disorientation, and poor judgment. It is important to recognize, however, that both conditions may exist in the same person.

Depression. Depression may cause memory impairment as a result of problems related to concentration and attention. This condition is quite common and at times is so difficult to differentiate from dementia that the term "pseudo-dementia" is used to describe it. One of the main differences between depression that presents the symptoms of dementia and dementia itself is insight into the memory deficit. Whereas patients with dementia are usually oblivious of their deficit and not distressed (except those in the early stages), those with depression are nearly always aware of their deficit and are quite distressed. Patients with depression tend to be withdrawn and apathetic and to show a marked disturbance of affect. In contrast, those with dementia demonstrate emotional blandness and some degree of emotional lability, or a lack of stableness in expressed emotion. One of the problems characteristic of depressed patients is their difficulty in concentrating. This is typified by poor cooperation and effort in carrying out tasks with a variable degree of achievement, coupled with considerable anxiety. Further, anxiety may disrupt memory, compounding any other problems.

Head trauma. Amnesia is sometimes seen in patients who have sustained a head injury. The extent of the amnesia is usually proportional to the severity of the injury. In most cases, the complete recovery of the patient's memory occurs, except for the events just preceding and following the injury. With traumatic brain injury, however, amnesia may not be the only symptom. Other memory deficits can be observed and experienced. As such, following any head injury, evaluation is advisable, even if the injury is a closed head injury.

Perspective and Prospects

Memory impairment is a serious condition that can interfere with one's ability to function independently. Any time that memory loss develops, identification of underlying causes should occur because a treatable cause may be found, preventing further memory loss or perhaps reducing the amount of memory loss. In some cases, proper treatment may even reverse memory loss, such as in some conditions related to alcohol-related memory loss. Research examining memory continues to differentiate among conditions involving memory loss. Efforts to better assess conditions and make distinctions earlier in the process of such conditions remain important. The earlier that problems such as dementia can be identified, for instance, the earlier treatment may be able to occur, potentially increasing quality of life.

Research has also identified ways to slow the progression of some diseases related to memory loss. According to the Alzheimer's Association, there are currently five medications approved by the FDA to temporarily reduce the symptoms of Alzheimer's disease—cholinesterase inhibitors and N-methyl-D-aspartate (NMDA), for example. None of these drugs, however, prevent or cure the disease. As the root causes of memory impairment and brain changes are understood, future research may be able to arrest the progress of amnesia and memory loss and even to treat dementias now considered irreversible, such as Alzheimer's disease and multiple infarct dementia. Exciting research in the area of inflammation and immunological functioning may prove to be productive.

—Ronald C. Hamdy, M.D. and Louis A. Cancellaro, M.D.;
updated by Nancy A. Piotrowski, Ph.D.

See also Addiction; Aging; Alcoholism; Alzheimer's disease; Amnesia; Anxiety; Brain; Brain damage; Brain disorders; Club drugs; Concussion; Dementias; Depression; Geriatrics and gerontology; Head and neck disorders; Intoxication; Marijuana; Pick's disease; Psychiatry; Psychiatry, geriatric; Shock therapy; Strokes; Substance abuse.

For Further Information:

Carson-DeWitt, Rosalyn. "Dementia." *Health Library*, September 27, 2012.

Hamdy, Ronald C., J. M. Turnbull, and M. M. Lancaster, eds. *Alzheimer's Disease: A Handbook for Caregivers*. 3d ed. St. Louis, Mo.: Mosby Year Book, 1998.

Masoro, Edward J., and Steven N. Austad, eds. *Handbook of the Biology of Aging*. 6th ed. Boston: Academic Press/Elsevier, 2007.

Mendez, Mario F., and Jeffrey L. Cummings. *Dementia: A Clinical Approach*. 3d ed. Philadelphia: Butterworth-Heinemann, 2003.

O'Brien, John, et al., eds. *Dementia*. 3d ed. New York: Oxford University Press, 2006.

Savage, Kimberly R., and Eva Svoboda. "Long-Term Benefits of the Memory-Link Programme in a Case of Amnesia." *Clinical Rehabilitation* 27, no. 6 (2013): 521–526.

Shan, Yaso. "Treatment of Alzheimer's Disease." *Primary Health Care* 23, no. 6 (July, 2013): 32–38.

West, Robin L., and Jan D. Sinnott, eds. *Everyday Memory and Aging*. New York: Springer, 1992.

MÉNIÈRE'S DISEASE
Disease/Disorder

Also known as: Endolymphatic hydrops

Anatomy or system affected: Inner ear, nervous system

Specialties and related fields: Audiology, otologist, otolaryngology

Definition: A chronic inner ear disorder associated with endolymphatic hydrops causing sensorineural hearing loss, tinnitus, and vertigo.

Overview

Ménière's disease is an inner ear disorder associated with endolymphatic hydrops, or abnormal fluid and dilation of the endolymphatic sac. The etiology of Ménière's disease is unclear, and the presence of endolymphatic hydrops does not always cause the symptoms of Ménière's disease. Ménière's disease presents with a typical triad of symptoms including fluctuating sensorineural hearing loss, vertigo, and tinnitus. Ménière's syndrome presents with similar symptomatology but is caused secondarily by other known ear disorders. The disease can present at any age but is most common between ages 20-50. Risk factors for Ménière's disease include family history of Ménière's, autoimmune disorders, viral infection, syphilis (rare), excess salt in diet, barometric pressure changes, stress, allergies, vascular abnormalities (such as migraine syndrome), chronic exposure to loud noise, and head trauma.

Signs and Symptoms

The clinical features of Ménière's disease are characterized by recurrent attacks of tinnitus, vertigo, hearing loss, and sensations of aural fullness, though in early stage disease symptoms may not present concurrently. Patients can experience prolonged symptom-free periods lasting greater than one year. Vertigo is sudden onset and severe, lasting from 20 minutes to 24 hours. Hearing loss in early-stage disease is mild and episodic. Late-stage disease is defined by progressive and permanent hearing loss, often within 10-15 years from onset. Persistent tinnitus can be a sign of late stage disease. Symptoms are typically unilateral, but bilateral symptoms can occur in up to 50 percent of patients. Associated symptoms include nausea, vomiting, diaphoresis, diarrhea, and a poor sense of balance.

Diagnosis

Ménière's disease is a diagnosis of exclusion, as there is no definitive diagnostic test to detect the pathology. Other causes of sensorineural hearing loss must be ruled out. Differential diagnoses include ototoxic drugs, multiple sclerosis, late onset hereditary hearing loss, presbycusis, noise induced hearing loss, brain stem stroke, acoustic neuroma or cochlear damage from infection, trauma, vascular occlusion or fistula. Audiometry should be ordered in a patient with these presenting symptoms to differentiate sensorineural from conductive hearing loss. Rinne and Weber tests can also be useful in differentiating the type of hearing loss. A gadolinium enhanced magnetic resonance imaging (MRI) should be ordered to rule out acoustic neuroma.

Information on Ménière's Disease

Causes: Excess fluid in inner ear as result of infection, allergies, blood vessel spasm, or small hemorrhage in cochlear duct

Symptoms: Ringing and fullness in ears, dizziness, hearing impairment, rapidly progressing hearing loss, vertigo, loss of equilibrium, nausea and vomiting, rhythmic jerking motion of eyes, sometimes deafness

Duration: Often chronic with recurrent attacks lasting thirty minutes to several hours

Treatments: Diuretics, blood vessel dilators, low-salt diet, motion sickness medications, antihistamines, bed rest; in severe cases, destruction of cochlea through surgery or ultrasound

---

Treatment

Ménière's disease is often self-limited, and treatment should be focused on symptomatic relief. Lifestyle education and management should encourage stress reduction, avoidance of caffeine, alcohol, monsodium glutamate (MSG) and allergy control. A low sodium diet (less than 1.5g/day) should be recommended.

Antiemetics or anticholinergics can be used as pharmacological treatment for nausea. Antihistamines and benzodiazepines can be useful in sedating the vestibular system and controlling vertigo. A prednisone burst can also be used. Diuretics and a low sodium diet may decrease frequency and severity of episodes. If symptoms are not controlled by medical management, intratympanic injection of gentamicin may be effective. In patients with severe and debilitating episodes refractory to previous treatment, surgery may be recommended.

Perspective and Prospects

Ménière's disease was first described and recorded in detail in 1861 by French physician Prosper Ménière. Formerly only the most severe and disabling cases were treated surgically because the operation required destruction of the hearing nerve. Since the advent of microsurgical instruments, it has become possible to separate the hearing and balance filaments in the main nerve and clip only the balance filaments when the problem is in the semicircular canals. It is also now possible to utilize ultrasonic beams to selectively destroy balance filaments without damaging the sensitive auditory nerves.

—George R. Plitnik, Ph.D.;
updated by Nicole Mitchell and Sarah Acker

See also Audiology; Balance disorders; Dizziness and fainting; Ear infections and isorders; Ears; Hearing; Hearing loss; Nausea and vomiting; Otorhinolaryngology; Tinnitus.

For Further Information:

Dinces, Elizabeth A., and Steven D. Rauch. "Meniere Disease." *UpToDate,* edited by Daniel G. Deschler and H. Nancy Sokol. Retrieved from http://www.uptodate.com/contents/meniere-disease?detectedLanguage=en&source=search_result&search=meniere%27s+disease&selectedTitle=1~28&provider=noProvider.

"Meniere's Disease." *The Merck Manual,* 19th ed., edited by R. Porter and J. Kapan, 455-456. Whitehouse Station, NJ: Merck Sharp and Dohme Corporation, 2011.

"Meniere's Disease." *Goldman's Cecil Medicine,* 24th ed., edited by Lee Goldman and Andrew I. Schafer, 2463. Philadelphia: Elselvier Saunders, 2012.

MENINGITIS
Disease/Disorder

Anatomy or system affected: Brain, head, nervous system, spine

Specialties and related fields: Emergency medicine, neurology, public health

Definition: An inflammation of the meninges of the brain and spinal cord.

Causes and Symptoms

The meninges is the three-layered covering of the spinal cord and brain. The layers are the outer dura mater, inner pia mater, and middle arachnoid. Meningitis is the inflammation or infection of the arachnoid and pia mater. It is characterized by severe headaches, vomiting, and pain and stiffness in the neck. These symptoms may be preceded by an upper respiratory infection. The age of the patient may affect which signs and symptoms are displayed. Newborns may exhibit either fever or hypothermia, along with lethargy or irritability, disinterest in feeding, and abdominal distension. In infants, examination may find bulging of the fontanelles (the soft areas between the bones of the skull found in newborns). The elderly may show lethargy, confusion, or disorientation. As pressure in the skull increases, nausea and vomiting may occur. With meningococcal meningitis, a rash of pinpoint-sized or larger dots appears.

Most cases of meningitis are the result of bacterial infection. These cases are sometimes referred to as septic meningitis. The bacteria invade the subarachnoid space and may have traveled from another site of infection, having caused pneumonia, cellulitis, or an ear infection. It is unclear if the bacteria make their way from the original area of infection to the meninges by the bloodstream or the lymphatic system. Once they have entered the subarachnoid space, they divide without inhibition since there is no impediment posed by defensive cells. In other words, the cerebrospinal fluid (CSF) contains very few white blood cells to inactivate the bacteria. More rarely, some bacteria may be introduced into the area by neurological damage or surgical invasion.

The most common cause of bacterial meningitis in adults and older children is meningococcus (*Neisseria meningitidus*). It is a diplococcus that typically does its damage inside the cell. The incidence of meningococcal meningitis is 2 to 3 cases per 100,000 people per year, and it most often affects schoolchildren and military recruits. *Haemophilus*

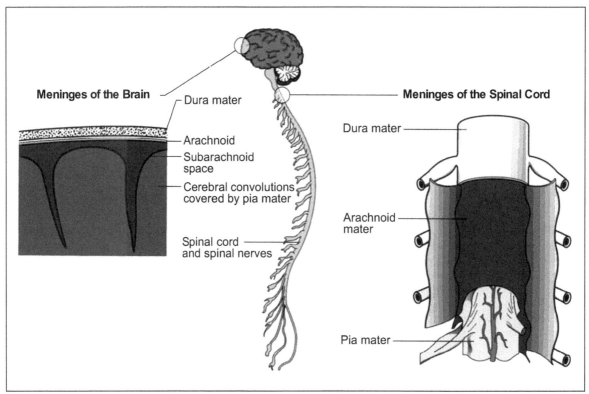

Meningitis attacks the meninges of the brain or the spinal cord or both.

Information on Meningitis

Causes: Bacterial or viral infection
Symptoms: Severe headaches, vomiting, pain and stiffness in the neck, upper-respiratory infection, lethargy, confusion, disorientation
Duration: Acute
Treatments: Antibiotics, surgery, supportive therapy (blood transfusions, subdural taps)

influenzae is the most common culprit infecting babies between two months and one year of age. Complications or residual effects often follow bacterial meningitis. These may include deafness, delayed-onset epilepsy, hydrocephalus, cerebritis, and brain abscess. In addition, for several weeks after resolution of the disease the patient may experience headaches, dizziness, and lethargy.

Aseptic meningitis is meningitis attributable to causes other than bacteria. These causes include neurotropic viruses, such as those that cause poliomyelitis or encephalitis; other viruses such as those that cause mumps, herpes, mononucleosis, hepatitis, chickenpox, and measles; spirochetes; bacterial products from brain abscesses or previous cases of bacterial meningitis; and foreign bodies, such as those found in the air or chemicals, in the CSF. Most cases of aseptic meningitis are viral in origin. The signs and symptoms are similar to those of bacterial meningitis. Onset is usually gradual, with symptoms starting mildly. The slight headache becomes worse over the course of several days, the neck becomes characteristically stiff, and photophobia (dislike of bright light) occurs.

Tuberculous meningitis is different from most other forms of meningitis because it lasts longer, has a higher mortality rate, and affects the CSF less. It mostly strikes children and is usually the result of a bacillus infection from the respiratory tract or the lymphatic system that has relocated to the meninges. When the bacilli are translocated to the central nervous system, they form tubercles that release an exudate. If tuberculous meningitis is left untreated, death may occur within three weeks. Even with treatment, it may result in neurologic abnormalities.

Treatment and Therapy

If meningitis is suspected, the first testing procedure is an examination of the CSF. To obtain CSF, a lumbar puncture, sometimes called a spinal tap, is made. Opening pressure, protein and glucose concentrations, total cell count, and cultures of microbes are determined. In cases of meningitis, the CSF is almost always cloudy and generally comes out under higher-than-normal pressure. An elevated white blood cell count in the CSF would be one indication that the patient has bacterial meningitis; another would be lowered serum glucose but slightly raised protein concentration, especially albumin. About 90 percent of bacterial meningitis cases show gram-positive staining. The examination of this slightly atypical fluid, along with presenting symptoms and signs, gives

the diagnostician some confidence in diagnosing meningitis accurately. Further cultures and a repeat puncture are necessary to pinpoint the kind of meningitis and to check the effect of the treatment.

Bacterial meningitis should be treated promptly with antibiotics specific for the causative bacteria. The success of treatment is contingent on the magnitude of the bacterial count and the quickness with which the bacteria can be controlled. Virtually all bacterial cases are treated with ampicillin or penicillin. Cases aggressively treated with very large doses of antibiotics are the most successful. If antibiotics do not destroy the areas of infection, surgery should be considered. Surgery is especially effective if meningitis is recurrent or persistent. Viral meningitis may be treated with adenine arabinoside if the cause is herpes simplex. No medication will kill other viruses causing the infection. The condition usually resolves itself in a few days, even without treatment. When necessary, supportive therapy should be employed, including blood transfusions. Young children with open fontanelles often undergo subdural taps to relieve pressure caused by CSF buildup.

Mortality rates in meningitis vary with age and the pathogen responsible. Those suffering from meningococcal meningitis (without overwhelming bacterial numbers) have a fatality rate of only 3 percent. Newborns suffering from gram-negative meningitis, however, have a 70 percent mortality rate. In addition, the younger the patient, the more likely the incidence of lasting neurological damage.

There are two basic ways to prevent meningitis: chemoprophylaxis for likely candidates of the disease and active immunization. Those exposed to a known case are usually treated with rifampin for four days; rifampin is especially useful in inactivating *H. influenzae*. Active immunization is suggested for toddlers eighteen to twenty-four months of age, especially for those in situations where there is a high risk of exposure (such as day care centers).

—*Iona C. Baldridge*

See also Abscesses; Antibiotics; Bacterial infections; Brain; Brain damage; Brain disorders; Chickenpox; Encephalitis; Hepatitis; Herpes; Immunization and vaccination; Lumbar puncture; Measles; Mononucleosis; Mumps; Nervous system; Neuroimaging; Neurology; Neurology, pediatric; Poliomyelitis; Spinal cord disorders; Spine, vertebrae, and disks; Viral infections; West Nile virus.

For Further Information:
American Medical Association. *American Medical Association Family Medical Guide.* 4th rev. ed. Hoboken, N.J.: John Wiley & Sons, 2004.
Bloom, Floyd E., M. Flint Beal, and David J. Kupfer, eds. *The Dana Guide to Brain Health.* New York: Dana Press, 2006.
Ferreiros, C. *Emerging Strategies in the Fight Against Meningitis.* New York: Garland Science, 2002.
Meningitis Research Foundation. http://www.meningitis.org.
Shmaefsky, Brian. *Meningitis.* Rev. ed. Philadelphia: Chelsea House, 2010.
Tunkel, Allan R. *Bacterial Meningitis.* Philadelphia: Lippincott Williams & Wilkins, 2001.
Wilson, Michael, Brian Henderson, and Rod McNab. *Bacterial Disease Mechanisms: An Introduction to Cellular Microbiology.* New York: Cambridge University Press, 2002.

MENOPAUSE
Biology

Anatomy or system affected: Psychic-emotional system, reproductive system, uterus

Specialties and related fields: Endocrinology, gynecology

Definition: The time during a woman's life when her ability to conceive ends; menopause is marked by irregular, and eventually complete cessation of, menstruation, accompanied by hormonal changes such as the dramatic reduction in the body's production of estrogen.

Key terms:

climacteric: that phase in the aging process of women marking the transition from the reproductive stage of life to the nonreproductive stage

estrogen: the female hormones estradiol and estrone, produced by the ovaries and responsible for the development of secondary sex characteristics

exogenous: originating outside an organ or part

osteoporosis: a condition characterized by a loss of bone density and an increased susceptibility to fractures

progesterone: a hormone, released by the corpus luteum and placenta, responsible for changes in the uterine endometrium

Process and Effects

The word "menopause" comes from two Greek words meaning "month" and "cessation." It is used medically to mean a cessation of, not a "pause" in, menstrual periods. Technically, the menopause begins the moment a woman has had her final menstrual period; until then, her menstrual periods may have shown a wide variety of irregularities, including missed periods.

Medical experts refer to the time when the body is noticeably preparing for the menopause as the perimenopause, which can begin anywhere from five to ten years before the menopause. While estrogen levels begin to decrease gradually, periods are normal but memory may be less sharp and mood swings may occur. During that time, a woman still experiences menstrual periods, but they are erratic. Some women stop menstruating suddenly, without irregularities; however, they are in the minority. For some women, signs of the menopause, such as hot flashes, may begin during the perimenopause. For even more women, such signs begin, or at least increase in intensity, at the menopause.

The term "climacteric" covers a longer span and includes all the years of diminishing estrogen production, both before and after a woman's last menstrual period. Some experts believe that women may undergo declines in their levels of estrogen even when they are in their late twenties; almost all experts believe that estrogen levels drop at least by a woman's mid-thirties, and the process accelerates in the late forties.

The average age at which the menopause occurs is fifty-one years, with the usual range between ages forty-five and fifty-five. For some it occurs much earlier, for others much later. Only 8 percent of women reach the menopause before age forty, and only 5 percent continue to menstruate after age fifty-three. A very few have menstrual periods until they are sixty.

Even after the menopause, the climacteric continues. Declining hormonal levels bring more changes, until the situation stabilizes. A decade or more of noticeable changes can take place before the climacteric is completed. Unlike the climacteric, the menopause itself is usually considered completed after one full year without a period. After two years, a woman can be reasonably certain that her periods have ceased permanently. The signs and symptoms of the menopause, however, can linger for years longer.

Starting in her mid-forties, a woman's ovaries gradually lose their ability to respond to the follicle-stimulating hormone (FSH), which is released by the pituitary into the blood, triggering the release of estrogen from the ovaries. A few eggs do remain even after menstrual flows have ceased, and the production of estrogen does not stop completely after the menopause; in much smaller amounts, it continues to be released by the adrenal glands, in fatty tissue, and in the brain. At the menopause, however, the blood levels of estrogen are drastically reduced—by about 75 percent.

About two to four years before the menopause, many women stop ovulating or ovulate irregularly or only occasionally. Although almost all the follicles enclosing the eggs are depleted by this time, the ovaries continue to produce estrogen. Estrogen continues to build up the endometrium (the lining of the uterus), but without ovulation no progesterone is produced to shed the extra lining. Therefore, instead of regular periods, a woman may bleed at unexpected times as the extra lining is shed sporadically.

During the perimenopause, menstrual periods may be late or early, longer than usual or shorter, and lighter than before or heavier. They may disappear for several months, then reappear for several more. It has been noted that in 15 to 20 percent of women the typical menopausal symptoms, sometimes accompanied by noticeable mood swings similar to premenstrual tension, begin during the perimenopausal period.

According to the National Institutes of Health (NIH), about 80 percent of women experience mild or no signs of the menopause. The rest have symptoms troublesome enough to seek medical attention. The two most important factors in determining how a woman will fare are probably the rate of decline of her female hormones and the final degree of hormone depletion. A woman's genes, general health, lifetime quality of diet, level of activity, and psychological acceptance of aging are also major influences. The most severe symptoms occur in women who lose their ovaries through surgery or radiation when they are perimenopausal.

When only the uterus is removed (hysterectomy) and the ovaries remain intact, menstrual periods stop but all other aspects of the menopause occur in the same way and at the same age. When only one ovary is removed, the menopause occurs normally. If both ovaries are removed, a complete menopause takes place abruptly, sometimes with intense effects. Women who have had a tubal ligation to prevent pregnancy will experience a normal menopause because tubal ligation does not affect ovaries, the uterus, or hormonal secretions.

Although experts disagree about the causes of a variety of symptoms that may appear at the menopause, there is no dis-

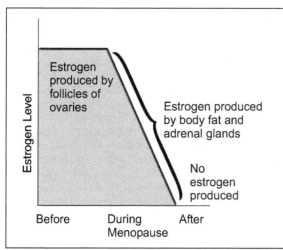

During the menopause, which may last for several years, estrogen production diminishes; after the menopause, estrogen is no longer produced by the body.

agreement about the fact that the majority of women experience hot flashes, or flushes. For two out of three women, hot flashes can start well before the last menstruation. Generally, however, hot flashes increase dramatically at menopause and continue to occur, with intermittent breaks (sometimes lasting several months), for five years or so.

While hot flashes are not dangerous, they are uncomfortable. Many women have only three or four episodes a day—or even a week—and hardly notice them. Others have as many as fifty severe flashes a day. The intense waves of heat generally last several minutes, but some unusual flashes have been reported to last as long as an hour. Usually there is some perspiration; with a severe flash, there is heavy perspiration. Because the blood vessels dilate (expand) and then contract, the hot flash is often followed by chills, even intense shivering. Since the flashes are usually worse at night, they can cause insomnia.

Other vasomotor symptoms can also appear with the menopause. Experts believe that they are the result of disruptions of the same mechanisms—vasomotor instability—that are manifested as hot flashes. Palpitations, which are distinct and rapid heartbeats, may also occur. A woman may experience dizziness or may feel faint or nauseated at times. She may have peculiar sensations in her arms and hands, especially her fingers. Some feel these sensations as tingling, or pins and needles, while others say that their fingers occasionally feel numb. One of the oddest, most frightening sensations associated with the menopause is formication, a feeling of insects crawling over the skin.

Headaches, depression, mood swings, insomnia, and weight gain often affect women at the menopause and may be related to the body's hormonal readjustments. Insomnia is second only to hot flashes as the symptom that causes women to seek out their doctors" help at the menopause. The hypothalamus controls sleep as well as temperature and hormone production; insomnia is caused by changes in sleep patterns and brain waves from the same hypothalamic disturbances that result in the hot flashes and an overstimulated central nervous system.

Complications and Disorders

During the menopause, the walls of the vagina become smooth and dry and produce less lubrication, producing a condition called atrophic vaginitis. It has been assumed that this condition is attributable to a lack of estrogen. Despite doubts concerning the relationship between circulating estrogen and objective measures of vaginal atrophy, estrogen (often topical) is frequently prescribed and effectively used in the alleviation or elimination of symptoms.

One of the problems that women encounter with the menopause is calcium deficiency. Many experts believe that before the menopause a woman requires a minimum of 1,000 milligrams of calcium a day in food or supplements. At the menopause, however, a woman who is not taking estrogen needs 1,500 milligrams of calcium a day. Since it is very difficult to obtain these daily allotments from food without consuming considerable amounts of milk or milk products, calcium supplements are often recommended for menopausal and postmenopausal women.

If the calcium deficiency is allowed to persist, osteoporosis, a loss of bone density that can lead to dangerous fractures, can result. Osteoporosis is known to have less of a damaging effect on women who are somewhat overweight because estrogen continues to be produced in fatty tissues after the menopause. Cigarettes, alcohol, and caffeine increase bone loss because they interfere with the body's ability to absorb calcium. A well-balanced diet, calcium supplements, and regular exercise—especially weight-bearing exercise—are effective ways of controlling osteoporosis. Hormone therapy is another means of coping with osteoporosis brought on by the menopause. Since nearly half of all women do not develop osteoporosis, however, many physicians do not believe that administering estrogen therapy to combat this disease is worth the risks, except in women at high risk for osteoporosis.

Although estrogen was isolated as a substance in the 1920s, the modern study of hormones—how they work, where they are produced, and what their benefits are—began in the 1940s. Originally, estrogen was administered cautiously to women who had lost their ovaries through surgery and to those with severe distress after the menopause. It was not until the 1960s that estrogen replacement therapy became widespread, however, when books such as Robert A. Wilson's *Feminine Forever* (1966) promoted its use as the newfound "fountain of youth" for women. The replacement of estrogen was suddenly fashionable, with the hormone being viewed as a miracle drug that could keep women looking and feeling youthful well into their later years. Physicians began prescribing it for women well before the menopause, and it was recommended for use throughout life. Often, large doses were prescribed.

By the mid-1970s, millions of women were taking estrogen. A decade later, however, the numbers had fallen. Beginning in 1975, research studies began documenting dramatic increases—sometimes as high as 500 percent—in cases of cancer of the lining of the endometrium among women taking estrogen, compared with those not taking it. Other studies at that time found higher rates of breast cancer as well as other problems, such as gallbladder conditions, among women taking estrogen.

Some studies found the overall risk of contracting uterine cancer increased 350 percent for women who took estrogen for a year or more. Some women who were on the therapy for long periods were judged to be as much as 100 percent more likely to contract uterine cancer. Furthermore, contrary to expectations, some studies claimed that the risk persisted even ten years after the estrogen use was discontinued. Other studies also found that the risk of cancer persisted, though for a shorter period.

These studies were based on replacement therapy using estrogen only. Estrogen stimulates the growth of cells in the endometrium, which is one of the aspects of the development of cancer. Consequently, a treatment was developed in which estrogen was combined with a form of progesterone in an effort to reduce the risk of uterine cancer and other diseases. Today, the most widely used regimen calls for estrogen in the lowest effective dose. A form of progesterone called progestin is added to this therapy, and then both hormones are stopped. Uterine bleeding, similar to that of a menstrual period, may occur, allowing the progesterone to break down any excess buildup of cells in the endometrium.

In the past, a number of women were given hormone therapy to alleviate menopausal symptoms, and they may have received longer-term therapy with the intention of preventing cardiac disease and osteoporosis. Some clinicians prescribed estrogen therapy for women with severe symptoms after a surgical menopause.

In the early twenty-first century, however, the use of hormone therapy—either long-term or short-term—was questioned. A study called the Women's Health Initiative, funded by the NIH, compared thousands of women who took combination hormone therapy to women who were given placebos. Those on the combination treatment had an increased risk for heart disease, stroke, and blood clots in the lungs. As a result, organizations such as the American Heart Association, the American College of Obstetricians and Gynecologists, and the North American Menopause Society recommended that combination therapy not be used for the prevention of cardiac disease, osteoporosis, or dementia. Today, combination hormone therapy is offered only to women with vasomotor symptoms (hot flashes and associated discomforts) that are severe enough to negatively impact life, and dosages are intended to be the lowest possible dose for the shortest period of time. Other drugs can be used to prevent or treat osteoporosis, drugs such as bisphosphonates and estrogen agonists/antagonists, which do not carry the same risks as hormone therapy.

Anecdotal evidence and some research studies suggest that stress reduction and exercise can relieve some of the symptoms of the menopause, including hot flashes and mood swings. In addition, a host of herbal remedies on the market claim to improve menopausal symptoms, although caution should be used in choosing these products. A double-blind pilot study of women using soy as a natural estrogen replacement therapy turned out positive; hot flashes decreased significantly in women taking soy powder for six weeks. The isoflavones in soy are chemically similar to estrogens. However, other studies involving the effects of soy have been inconsistent. Vitamin E, which is structurally similar to estrogen at the molecular level, decreases hot flashes in some women. Evidence of this is anecdotal, however, as no large studies have been conducted that prove the claim. Black cohosh is the best documented of all the herbal remedies. Studies suggest that it can relieve menopause-related headaches, depression, anxiety, hot flashes, night sweats, heart palpitations, and vaginal dryness and thinning. Black cohosh suppresses the secretion of luteinizing hormone, a hormone that is believed to be at the root of many menopausal symptoms. One European study of eighty women found that black cohosh relieved menopausal symptoms more effectively than estrogen replacement therapy. Other studies had mixed results.

Perspective and Prospects

The menopause, in various guises, was referred to in many early cultures and texts. Initially, an association was made between age and the loss of fertility. By the sixth century, written records on the cessation of menstruation were well documented. At that time, it was believed that menstruation does not cease before the age of thirty-five, nor does it usually continue after the age of fifty. It was thought that obese women cease menstruation very early and that periods remain normal or abnormal and increase in flow or become diminished depending on age, the season of the year, the habits and peculiar traits of women, the types of food eaten, and complicating diseases. Similar descriptions of menstrual cessation and its age of onset continued for another thousand years. It was not until the late eighteenth and early nineteenth centuries, however, that much advancement in the knowledge of the topic took place.

John Leake, influenced by William Harvey's historic description of the circulatory system, made one of the first reasonable attempts to explain the etiology of the menopause in his 1777 book *Medical Instructions Towards the Prevention and Cure of Chronic or Slow Diseases Peculiar to Women*. He believed that as long as the "prime of life" continues, along with the circulating force of the blood being more than equal to the resistance of the uterine vessels, the menses will continue to flow. When these vessels become firm from the effect of age, however, the diminished current of blood is insufficient to force the uterine vessels open, and then periodic discharge will cease.

A later development in the history of menstruation studies was to link menstruation with all sorts of other problems, both emotional and organic. In Leake's work he comments that at the time of cessation of menses, women are often afflicted by various chronic diseases. He adds that some women are prone to pain and light-headedness, others are plagued by an intolerable itching at the neck of the bladder, and some are affected by low spirits and melancholy. Leake thought, because it seemed extraordinary that so many disorders should result from such a natural occurrence in a woman's life, that these symptoms can be explained away by indulgence in excesses, luxury, and an "irregularity" in the passions. Laying the blame for complications with the menopause on societal (in particular, female) excesses continued for some time.

Specific disease associations were also made; in 1814, John Burns announced that the cessation of menses seems to cause cancer of the breast in some women. Edward John Tilt, a British physician, wrote one of the first full-length books on *The Change of Life in Health and Disease* (1857). Some of his views were that women should adhere to a strict code of hygiene during menstruation because they are often afflicted with cancer, gout, rheumatism, and nervous disorders.

These beliefs reflect a tendency from the mid-nineteenth century onward for medical literature to associate the menopause with many negative sociological features. For example, Colombat de l'Isère, in his book *Traité des maladies des femmes et de l'hygiène spéciale de leur sexe* (1838; *A Treatise on the Diseases and Special Hygiene of Females*, 1845), expresses his belief that during the menopause women cease to live for the species and live only for themselves. He thought it prudent for men to avoid having erotic thoughts about women in whom these feelings ought to be extinct; he believed that after the menopause sexual enjoyment for women is ended forever.

Not all physicians, however, took such a negative attitude. Some believed that examining this phase in a woman's life presents a challenge. They believed that the boundaries between the physiological and the pathological in this field of study are ill-defined and that it is in the interest of the male gender to conduct more research into this stage of a woman's life. The narrow boundary between normal physiology and pathology was still not fully defined nearly a hundred years later, nor did the many negative and unsubstantiated theories cease. Well into the 1960s, the menopause was still considered "abnormal" and a "negative" state by some physicians.

Three major milestones exist in the history of menopause research in the twentieth century. The first event was the achievement of Adolf Butenandt, who won the Nobel Prize in Chemistry. He succeeded in 1929 in isolating and obtaining, in pure form, a hormone from the urine of pregnant women that was eventually called estrone. The second development was the publication of *Feminine Forever* in 1966, which became an instant best seller. As a result of the book's publication, physicians were prompted to take sides in a heated and continuing debate. The third landmark was the publication of an editorial and two original articles in *The New England Journal of Medicine* of December 4, 1975, claiming an association between exogenous estrogens and endometrial cancer. This claim brought about legal action by initiating, at least in the United States, a series of health administration inquiries.

—*Genevieve Slomski, Ph.D.;*
updated by Karen E. Kalumuck, Ph.D.

See also Aging; Arteriosclerosis; Breast cancer; Cervical, ovarian, and uterine cancers; Endocrinology; Endometrial cancer; Gynecology; Heart disease; Herbal medicine; Hormone therapy; Hormones; Hot flashes; Hysterectomy; Infertility, female; Menstruation; Midlife crisis; Obesity; Osteoporosis; Ovarian cysts; Ovaries; Sterilization; Women's health.

For Further Information:

Corio, Laura E., and Linda G. Kahn. *The Change Before the Change: Everything You Need to Know to Stay Healthy in the Decade Before Menopause.* 2d ed. London: Piatkus Books, 2005.

Doress-Worters, Paula B., and Diana Laskin Siegal. *The New Ourselves, Growing Older: Women Aging with Knowledge and Power.* New York: Simon & Schuster, 1994.

Edelman, Julia Schlam. *Menopause Matters: Your Guide to a Long and Healthy Life.* Baltimore, Maryland: Johns Hopkins University Press, 2010.

"FAQs: Menopause Basics." *North American Menopause Society,* 2013.

Greenwood, Sadja. *Menopause, Naturally: Preparing for the Second Half of Life.* Updated ed. Volcano, Calif.: Volcano Press, 1996.

"Hormone Replacement Therapy." *MedlinePlus,* June 27, 2013.

Love, Susan, and Karen Lindsey. *Dr. Susan Love's Menopause and Hormone Book: Making Informed Choices.* Rev. ed. New York: Three Rivers Press, 2003.

Maas, Paula, Susan E. Brown, and Nancy Bruning. *The Mend Clinic Guide to Natural Medicine for Menopause and Beyond.* New York: Dell, 1997.

"Menopause." *MedlinePlus,* July 1, 2013.

"Osteoporosis." *MedlinePlus,* June 4, 2013.

Sheehy, Gail. *The Silent Passage: Menopause.* Rev. ed. New York: Pocket Books, 1998.

Stoppard, Miriam. *Menopause.* 2d ed. London: DK, 2002.

MENORRHAGIA

Disease/Disorder

Anatomy or system affected: Blood, reproductive system, uterus

Specialties and related fields: Gynecology

Definition: Excessively heavy or prolonged menstrual flow.

Causes and Symptoms

Menorrhagia can be caused by many disorders: anatomic abnormalities of the uterus, hormonal imbalances, certain medical conditions, medications, and malignancy. Common anatomic causes are uterine fibroids and adenomyosis. Irregular menstrual cycles resulting from hormonal imbalances can be associated with menorrhagia. Medical conditions such as blood clotting disorders and liver or thyroid disease contribute to menorrhagia. Medications that prevent blood clotting, such as coumadin or heparin, can lead to increased menstrual flow. Uterine and other reproductive tract cancers can result in unusually heavy menstrual flow.

Symptoms of menorrhagia are uterine bleeding that is excessive (more than 80 milliliters) and/or bleeding that lasts for more than seven days. Unlike metrorrhagia, bleeding occurs at regular intervals. The patient can become anemic and exhibit symptoms of either acute or chronic blood loss. Symptoms and signs which suggest the cause of menorrhagia may be present, such as large palpable fibroids, or evidence of hypothyroidism or liver disease.

Information on Menorrhagia

Causes: Uterine abnormalities (fibroids, adenomyosis); hormonal imbalances; blood clotting disorders; liver or thyroid disease; blood thinners (coumadin, heparin); uterine and other reproductive tract cancers

Symptoms: Excessive uterine bleeding, sometimes anemia

Duration: Chronic

Treatments: Depends on cause and severity; may include iron supplements, oral contraceptives or medroxyprogesterone, hormone injections to induce menopause, high-dose estrogens, dilation and curettage (D & C), thermal ablation, endometrial polyp or fibroid resection, placement of progesterone-impregnated IUD, myomectomy, hysterectomy

Treatment and Therapy

Menorrhagia can be treated via a medical or a surgical approach. The selection of treatment often depends on the cause and severity of the menorrhagia. If menorrhagia is the result of conditions amenable to medical treatment (such as a thyroid disorder), then control of these conditions may decrease the bleeding. If the patient has irregular cycles (for example, because of lack of ovulation), then hormones such as oral contraceptive pills or medroxyprogesterone may be used to regulate the cycles and decrease menstrual flow. A patient who is nearing the menopause can receive hormone injections that place her into an earlier artificial menopause, and hence eliminate menstrual bleeding altogether. If the patient encounters acute and profuse bleeding, then high-dose estrogens may be given.

If menorrhagia is resistent to medical management, then surgical treatment may be necessary. Examples of procedural treatments for menorrhagia are dilation and curettage (D & C), for acute, profuse bleeding; thermal ablation of the endometrial lining; hysteroscopic resection of endometrial polyps or fibroids; and placement of a progesterone-impregnated intrauterine device (IUD). Hysterectomy is the definitive surgery for menorrhagia, no matter what the cause, since menstrual bleeding cannot occur without the uterus. Patients with large fibroids or adenomyosis often are not responsive to medical management. These patients would be candidates for hysterectomy. In patients with large fibroids and menorrhagia who wish to retain childbearing potential, a myomectomy may be performed instead of hysterectomy. If a patient is suspected or known to have a malignancy of the reproductive tract that is causing menorrhagia, then surgical management is the appropriate treatment.

Finally, patients can become severely anemic from menorrhagia, and blood transfusion may be necessary. Mild anemia can be treated with iron supplementation.

—*Anne Lynn S. Chang, M.D.*

See also Anemia; Bleeding; Cervical, ovarian, and uterine cancers; Dysmenorrhea; Endometriosis; Genital disorders, female; Hysterectomy; Menstruation; Myomectomy; Polyps; Reproductive system; Uterus; Women's health.

For Further Information:

Badash, Michelle. "Heavy Menstrual Bleeding." *Health Library*, September 27, 2012.

Golub, Sharon. *Periods: From Menarche to Menopause*. Newbury Park, Calif.: Sage, 1992.

"Heavy Menstrual Bleeding." *Centers for Disease Control and Prevention*, December 12, 2011.

Icon Health. *Menorrhagia: A Medical Dictionary, Bibliography, and Annotated Research Guide to Internet References*. San Diego, Calif.: Author, 2004.

Kasper, Dennis L., et al., eds. *Harrison's Principles of Internal Medicine*. 16th ed. New York: McGraw-Hill, 2005.

"Menorrhagia (Heavy Menstrual Bleeding)." *Mayo Clinic*, June 25, 2011.

O'Donovan, Peter, Paul McGurgan, and Walter Prendiville, eds. *Conservative Surgery for Menorrhagia*. San Francisco: Greenwich Medical Media, 2003.

Stenchever, Morton A., et al. *Comprehensive Gynecology*. 4th ed. St. Louis, Mo.: Mosby/Elsevier, 2006.

Tierney, Lawrence M., Stephen J. McPhee, and Maxine A. Papadakis, eds. *Current Medical Diagnosis and Treatment 2006*. New York: McGraw-Hill Medical, 2006.

MEN'S HEALTH

Anatomy or system affected: All
Specialties and related fields: All
Definition: Issues related to the health and well-being of men.
Key terms:

colonoscopy: examination of the colon using an endoscope inserted into the rectum

digital rectal exam: examination in which a gloved finger is placed in the rectum to feel the prostate gland for lumps, enlargement, or irregularities

endoscope: a flexible tube with a camera device that is inserted into the body

epididymis: the coiled tube behind the testicles that stores and transports sperm

high-risk behaviors: behaviors that increase the chance of injury, disease, or harm

Klinefelter syndrome: a disease in which an extra X chromosome in males causes abnormal development of the testicles

prostate diseases: diseases that affect the prostate gland

prostate-specific antigen (PSA): a glycoprotein produced by the prostate gland; its levels in the blood can indicate the presence of cancer

screening: tests to detect health problems and diseases

sexually transmitted diseases (STDs): contagious diseases that can be spread through sexual contact

sigmoidoscopy: examination of the lower portion of the colon (sigmoid) using an endoscope inserted in the rectum

Major Health Concerns

Men in the United States have a lower life expectancy than do women. Generally, men smoke, drink, and participate in more activities that may result in physical trauma. According to the Centers for Disease Control and Prevention (CDC), the ten leading causes of death among men are accidents, cancer, diabetes, heart disease, lung disease, liver disease, suicide, and homicide.

Accidents or unintentional injuries are the fifth leading cause of death in the United States. The risk of death as a result of a motor vehicle accident is twice as high among men and is highest within the age range of fifteen to twenty-four.

Cancer can occur in anyone at any age, but 76 percent of all cancers are diagnosed in those age fifteen and older. Nonmelanoma skin cancer is the most common cancer. Lung cancer is the leading cause of death among both men and women. Other cancers that affect men include prostate cancer, colon cancer, and testicular cancer.

Skin cancer may be identified as melanoma or nonmelanoma skin cancer. Skin cancers are more common in people with fair skin, hair, and eyes. The most important cause and risk factor for developing skin cancer is excessive sun exposure. Symptoms of skin cancer include skin areas that are crusty, scaly and rough, firm and red, shiny, or waxy, as well as nonhealing sores. The borders of cancerous areas are asymmetrical (uneven). The color is uneven, and the abnormal area is usually larger than six millimeters.

Lung cancer develops from abnormal cell growth in the lining of the lungs. Survival rates of lung cancer are poor. The earlier lung cancer is found, the better the chance for survival. Approximately one in ten survive five years after being diagnosed. Smoking is the number-one cause of lung cancer. Other risk factors include environmental pollution; exposure to radon, asbestos, and gases in closed areas, as in mining; and a family history of lung cancer. At first, one may have no symptoms, but as cancer grows, wheezing, shortness of breath, a persistent cough that worsens over time, coughing blood, chest pain, hoarseness, fatigue, decreased appetite, and neck and face swelling occur.

Colon cancer (colorectal cancer) develops from abnormal cell growth in the lining of the colon. It is the fourth most common cancer in men. About 90 percent of all colorectal cancers are diagnosed after age fifty. Risk factors and causes of colon cancer include a high-fat and low-fiber diet, alcohol abuse, smoking, lack of exercise, diabetes, colitis, irritable bowel, family history of colon cancer, and rectal polyps (growths on the lining of the colon). Polyps are common among those aged fifty and older. In the early stages, there may be no symptoms, but as the cancer grows, symptoms may include a change in bowel movements (diarrhea, constipation, bloody stools that are bright red or very dark, a feeling that the bowel does not empty completely, thin stools), abdominal discomfort (gas pains, cramping, bloating, sense of fullness), vomiting, weight loss, and fatigue.

Prostate cancer is caused by the growth of cancer cells in the prostate gland. Prostate cancer is the third most common cause of death from cancer in men, and it is the most common cause of death from cancer in men over age seventy-five. A definitive cause of prostate cancer is still under investigation. It has been linked to a high-fat diet and elevated testosterone levels. African American men older than age sixty, farmers, tire plant workers, painters, and those exposed to cadmium are at high risk for prostate cancer. Symptoms result from the blocking of urine flow because of prostate enlargement and include frequent urge to urinate (micturia), dribbling urine, painful or burning urination (dysuria), difficulty or inability to urinate, bloody urine or semen, painful ejaculation, and pain or stiffness in the thighs, hips, or lower back.

Testicular cancer is caused by the growth of cancer cells in one or both testicles. It is the most common cancer in men between ages fifteen and thirty-four and is most common in Caucasians. Approximately eight thousand men are diagnosed with testicular cancer annually in the United States. The causes of testicular cancer are still under investigation, but risks include cryptorchidism (undescended testicles) and a family history of testicular cancer. Symptoms of testicular cancer include a dull ache in the groin or low abdomen, pulling or heaviness in the scrotum, testicular or scrotal pain, and testicular enlargement.

Diabetes mellitus is a metabolic disorder in which the pancreas does not produce enough insulin to process and maintain proper blood sugar levels. Over time, poorly controlled diabetes can cause eye, heart, kidney, and nerve damage. About two-thirds of those with diabetes die of heart disease. There are two main types of diabetes. In type 1 diabetes, the body produces no insulin. It affects 10 percent of those with diabetes and is most often seen in males under age thirty. Type 1 diabetes is more prevalent among North Europeans, African Americans, and Hispanics, respectively. The causes of type 1 diabetes are not completely understood, but it is thought to be linked to an inherited, genetic predisposition that is activated by an environmental trigger from exposure to environmental chemicals or viruses that attack the immune system.

In type 2 diabetes, the body either does not produce enough insulin or does not use insulin efficiently. Approximately 90 percent of those with diabetes have type 2 diabetes. The risk of developing this type increases with age and most often affects those over age forty. One-third of men with type 2 diabetes are unaware of it until problems such as erectile dysfunction (impotence), vision loss, or kidney disease develop. Causes and risk factors for developing type 2 diabetes include a family history of diabetes, lack of exercise, a high-fat diet, elevated cholesterol levels, obesity, advancing age, high blood pressure, and being of African American, Hispanic, American Indian, Asian American, or Pacific Islander descent. Symptoms of both types of diabetes include blurred vision, headache, excessive thirst and hunger, unexplained weight loss, dry and itchy skin, slow-healing cuts and bruises, frequent urination, recurring infections, tingling in the hands and feet, mood swings, irritability, depression, and fatigue.

Cardiovascular disease refers to problems that affect the heart (heart disease) and circulation (vascular disease). Heart disease is the number-one killer of men. Being male increases the risk of developing heart disease. The mortality rate for African American men with heart disease is twice as high as for Caucasian men. Causes and risk factors include advancing age, family history, diabetes, elevated cholesterol, high blood pressure, a high-fat diet, lack of regular exercise, obesity, and smoking. Common cardiovascular diseases include coronary artery disease, cardiomyopathy, heart valve disease, heart failure, hyperlipidemia, high blood pressure, and stroke.

Coronary artery disease is the leading cause of heart attacks. In this condition, blood flow through the arteries of the heart is blocked. The most common cause is the buildup of fatty deposits (plaque) in the lining of an artery, called arteriosclerosis. Symptoms include shortness of breath, chest pain (angina), and/or a heart attack (myocardial infarction). Risk factors include smoking, elevated cholesterol, diabetes, high blood pressure, obesity, physical inactivity, and stress.

Cardiomyopathy involves conditions that enlarge the heart and weaken the heart muscle so that it does not pump efficiently. Causes and risk factors for developing cardiomyopathy are aging, alcoholism, high blood pressure, obesity, and smoking. Symptoms include chest pain, shortness of breath, irregular heartbeat, abdominal distention, swelling in the lower legs, fatigue, dizziness, and fainting.

Heart valve disease refers to conditions that damage the heart valves that may result in inadequate closure (prolapse), leaking (regurgitation), or narrowing (stenosis) of the valves so that blood does not circulate adequately. Causes and risk factors for the development of heart valve disease include rheumatic fever, heart attack (myocardial infarction), infections of connective tissue such as systemic lupus erthyematosus (SLE), poliomyelitis, rheumatoid arthritis, aging, congenital birth defects, medications, or radiation treatment. Symptoms of heart valve disease include shortness of breath, chest pain, irregular heart beat, high or low blood pressure, fatigue, and dizziness or faintness upon physical activity.

Heart failure is a condition in which the heart is unable to pump blood to organs and tissues efficiently. Heart failure may develop suddenly or gradually. Congestive heart failure is a condition in which the inability of the heart to pump blood to organs and tissues efficiently leads to a buildup of fluid in the body. Causes and risk factors for heart failure include coronary artery disease, heart valve disease, or cardiomyopathy. Symptoms of heart failure include shortness of breath, chest pain, heart palpitations, fluid retention that causes swelling in the lower legs and abdomen, weight gain (from fluid retention), weakness, dizziness, and fatigue.

Hyperlipidemia refers to elevated fats (lipids) in the blood that eventually form fatty deposits (plaque) on the walls of arteries that lead to coronary artery disease. The most common lipids include high-density lipoprotein (HDL) cholesterol, low-density lipoprotein (LDL) cholesterol, and triglycerides. Hypercholesterolemia refers to elevated blood cholesterol levels (higher than 200 milligrams) and is the leading risk factor for heart disease. High levels of HDL (higher than 60 milligrams) protect against heart disease. High levels of LDL (higher than 100 milligrams) can lead to heart disease. Hypertriglyceridemia refers to elevated triglyceride blood levels (higher than 150 milligrams). Hyperlipidemia increases the risk for heart attack, stroke, and diabetes. Causes and risk factors for hyperlipidemia include diabetes, high blood pressure, hypothyroidism, kidney or liver disease, aging, sex (men have a higher risk for elevated lipids), smoking, a high-fat diet, alcohol abuse, obesity, lack of exercise, hered-

ity, stress, and medications such as corticosteroids, diuretics, and some blood pressure pills.

High blood pressure (hypertension) occurs when the pressure of the blood in the arteries is too high. High blood pressure is referred to as the silent killer because it often creates no symptoms. It is a major risk factor for heart disease. Untreated hypertension can lead to heart failure, heart attack, stroke, and kidney failure. A normal blood pressure is 120/80 or below. Blood pressure above 140/90 is considered high blood pressure. Prehypertension refers to blood pressures between 120/80 and 140/90. In those with diabetes and kidney disease, a blood pressure of 130/80 or higher is too high, and if it is not decreased, then high blood pressure is likely to develop. Causes and risk factors for high blood pressure include aging; race; sex (higher incidence in men); heredity; alcohol or drug abuse; obesity; stress; socioeconomic status; kidney, thyroid, or adrenal gland diseases; diabetes; sensitivity to salt; lack of exercise; and some medications, such as cold, allergy, and migraine medications.

Stroke (also called a brain attack or cerebral vascular accident) can be either ischemic or hemorrhagic. Both prevent oxygen and nutrients from reaching the brain. Ischemic strokes are caused by blockage or narrowing of blood vessels leading to the brain, while hemorrhagic strokes are broken blood vessels that bleed into the brain. Causes and risk factors for a stroke include aging, arteriosclerosis, family history, race (higher incidence in African Americans), sex (higher incidence in men), diabetes, heart disease, high blood pressure, elevated blood lipids, a high-fat diet, lack of regular exercise, obesity, and smoking. Symptoms of a stroke include weakness or numbness of the face, arm, or leg on one side of the body; loss of vision; loss of speech; inability to understand what is being said; headache; dizziness; and walking problems or falling.

Pulmonary or lung diseases affect the health of the lungs. Common lung diseases are chronic obstructive pulmonary disease (COPD), bronchitis, emphysema, asthma, influenza, pneumonia, and lung cancer. Men are vulnerable to these diseases because they are more likely to smoke and to have jobs that involve exposure to hazardous materials.

COPD is the fourth leading cause of death in the United States. There is a strong link between COPD and lung cancer. Causes and risk factors for COPD include smoking; a history of childhood respiratory infections; asbestos, radon, and other air pollutants; and heredity. Symptoms of COPD include coughing, shortness of breath, chest tightness, and wheezing.

Chronic bronchitis occurs when the lining of the lungs become inflamed and swollen so that the airways become small and clogged with excess mucus and oxygen cannot be absorbed. Smoking and exposure to secondhand smoke are the main causes of bronchitis. Allergies, air pollution, infections, and pollutants from mining, farming, and working with textiles are also factors. Symptoms of chronic bronchitis include shortness of breath, coughing, and increased mucus that occurs most days for three months in a year over two consecutive years.

Emphysema occurs when the air sacs (alveoli) that exchange oxygen and carbon dioxide become damaged. Fifty-five percent of those with emphysema are men. Emphysema develops slowly over time, so symptoms do not become evident until it is well established. Smoking and exposure to secondhand smoke are the main causes of emphysema. Allergies, aging, heredity, air pollution, and pollutants from mining, farming, and working with textiles are also factors. Symptoms include a chronic cough with or without mucus production, fatigue, and loss of appetite.

Asthma results in inflammation and swelling in the airways that causes narrowing, preventing air from passing through them. Causes and risk factors for developing asthma include smoking, gastric reflux disease, lung infections, exercise, heredity, allergies, pollution, cold air, and environmental triggers. Symptoms of asthma include wheezing, chest tightness, coughing, and shortness of breath.

Influenza is a contagious viral infection caused by the influenza virus that can be deadly. The elderly, young children, and those with weakened immune systems are at highest risk for serious complications. Symptoms include headache, fever, sore throat, dry cough, nausea, vomiting, diarrhea, fatigue, and muscle weakness and aching. Pneumonia is a deadly infection and/or inflammation of the lungs in which the airways become blocked by pus or fluid so that oxygen cannot be passed to and from the lungs. Individuals affected by heart disease, diabetes, age, or weakened immune systems are at a higher risk of dying from pneumonia. Risk factors and causes of pneumonia include chemicals, bacteria, viruses, and other microbes. Symptoms of pneumonia include fever, chills, sweating, shaking, cough, chest pain, and shortness of breath.

Chronic liver disease is the gradual failure of the liver to function effectively. Cirrhosis of the liver results from scar tissue that replaces healthy liver tissue and hinders the blood flow through the liver so that nutrients, hormones, and drugs are not processed normally. It is the eighth leading cause of death in the United States. Fibrosis of the liver is the overgrowth of scar tissue in the liver (usually from cirrhosis) that results from an infection, inflammation, or injury that prevents the liver from storing vitamins and minerals, regulating blood clotting, producing proteins and enzymes, maintaining hormone balance, and metabolizing or detoxifying substances. Risk factors for chronic liver disease include alcoholism, obesity, a low-fiber and high-fat diet, high blood pressure, elevated blood lipids, family history, and some medications. Symptoms include weakness, fatigue, confusion, loss of appetite, abdominal pain, excessive bruising, swelling in abdomen and legs, gastric bleeding, and yellow skin coloring (jaundice).

Suicide is the eighth leading cause of death among men in the United States. Men are four times more likely to commit suicide than are women. Suicide risk is related to depression, chronic illness, living alone, history of physical or sexual abuse, unemployment, age (highest among men in their twenties, sixties, and seventies), and marital status (higher among the never married, divorced, or recently widowed). Many men do not readily identify their depression and so do not seek treatment. It is estimated that each year more than six million men are affected with depression. Risk factors and causes of depression include loss of a loved one, stress, financial problems, relationship problems, positive or negative life changes, and heredity. Symptoms of depression include feelings of hopelessness, guilt, worthlessness, or helplessness; persistent sadness or anxiety; loss of interest in daily life activities and hobbies; difficulty concentrating; memory loss; indecisiveness; irritability; increased or decreased sleep; loss of energy; fatigue; weight loss or gain; physical ailments; and thoughts of death or suicide.

Men face unique diseases and disorders of the reproductive system. Testicular trauma is most often related to injuries acquired from contact sports or accidents. Symptoms of testicular trauma include pain, swelling, and bruising of one or both testes. Testicular rupture is rare, but it can cause blood to leak into the scrotum and requires surgical repair. Testicular torsion occurs when the spermatic cord twists and cuts the blood supply to the testicle. Adolescent males are often affected as a result of injuries sustained from strenuous activities. Symptoms of testicular torsion are sudden and severe testicular pain, tenderness, and testicular swelling.

Epididymitis is an inflammation of the epididymis. Males ages nineteen to forty are most often affected. Epididymitis is usually caused by an infection and can be the result of a sexually transmitted disease. Symptoms include scrotal pain and swelling, abscess (collection of pus), dysuria, frequent urination, urgency to urinate, abdominal pain, fever, and chills.

Hypogonadism occurs when the testicles do not produce enough testosterone. There are two types. Primary hypogonadism results from an abnormality in the testicles. Secondary hypogonadism results from a problem with the pituitary gland. Causes and risk factors of hypogonadism include undescended testicles, testicular trauma, hemochromatosis (excess iron in the blood), pituitary disorders from a head injury or pituitary tumor, mumps infection, Klinefelter syndrome, aging, chemotherapy or radiation therapy, and medications. Symptoms of hypogonadism include impaired growth of the penis and testicles, decreased muscle mass and body hair, enlarged breasts, infertility, erectile dysfunction, decreased sex drive, fatigue, difficulty concentrating, hot flashes, and depression.

Prostatitis is an inflammation in the prostate gland that is usually caused by a bacterial infection. Risk factors include urinary tract infections, medical procedures requiring insertion of objects into the penis, anal intercourse, benign prostatic hyperplasia (BPH), or prostate enlargement. Symptoms of prostatitis include a tender and swollen prostate, fever; chills; low back, joint, and muscle pain; urinary frequency; dysuria; bloody urine (hematuria); difficulty starting the stream of urine (hesitancy); frequent urination at night (nocturia); and painful ejaculation.

BPH is an enlargement of the prostate gland. It naturally occurs with age and affects 50 percent of men after age sixty and 70 percent of men in their seventies and eighties. When an enlarged prostate presses against the urethra, it blocks the flow of urine. Symptoms of BPH include hesitant urination, frequent urination, urgency to pass urine, weak stream of urine, dribbling urine, dysuria, nocturia, straining to urinate, inability to pass urine (retention), and/or feeling that the bladder is not completely emptied.

Sexually transmitted diseases (STDs) are infections that are transferred through sexual acts such as intercourse, oral sex, sharing sexual objects such as vibrators, and intimate skin-to-skin contact. The United States has the highest number of STDs in the world, with more than 15 million cases reported each year. Almost two-thirds of all STDS occur in adults younger than age twenty-five. STDs include hepatitis B, genital herpes, human papilloma virus (HPV), chlamydia, gonorrhea, and syphilis. STDs can cause infertility and damage to the heart, kidneys, and brain, as well as an increased chance of contracting acquired immunodeficiency syndrome (AIDS). AIDS, the most serious STD, has no cure and can be fatal. STD symptoms may include discharge from the penis; painful sex; dysuria; sore throat from oral sex; pain in the anus from anal intercourse; chancres (painless red sores) on the genitals, tongue, throat, and anus; blisters or warts around the genitals; dark urine; light-colored bowel movements; and yellow skin (jaundice).

Prevention and Treatment Options

The best way for men to manage these health concerns is prevention through education, healthy living, and screenings to identify diseases in their early stages, when they are most treatable.

Skin cancer can be prevented by minimizing sun exposure, wearing protective clothing that covers exposed skin, avoiding the sun during midday, and using sunscreen with SPF 15 or stronger year-round. Men should apply sunscreen at least one-half hour before going into the sun and then reapply it frequently. The American Academy of Dermatology recommends annual screening for skin cancer by a dermatologist. Treatment for skin cancer includes surgery to remove cancerous cells, radiation to shrink and kill cancerous cells, chemotherapy, and photodynamic therapy, in which a light-activated drug that targets cancerous cells is injected and then activated by lasers to destroy cancer cells.

Lung cancer is treated through the surgical removal of tumors, radiation therapy to shrink tumors, chemotherapy, photodynamic therapy, electrosurgery (which concentrates high-energy electromagnetic radiation to destroy tissue), and cryotherapy (which destroys cancerous tissue using extreme cold).

Colon cancer screening includes a rectal examination and stool test for blood every year, sigmoidoscopy every five years, barium enema every five years, and colonoscopy every ten years. Colon cancer screening should begin at age fifty, or sooner if there is a personal or family history of colon cancer or bowel disease. Treatment for colon cancer includes surgical removal of cancerous tissue, chemotherapy, and radiation therapy.

Prostate cancer screening recommendations are annual screenings after age fifty. For high-risk men, annual screenings should begin at age forty. Screenings include a digital rectal exam (DRE) and a prostate-specific antigen (PSA) test. The level of PSA is elevated when there are problems in the prostate. A biopsy may also show abnormal cells in the prostate. Treatment for prostate cancer includes prostatectomy (surgical removal of the prostate), radiation therapy, monthly hormone injections to shrink the prostate cancer cells, or "watchful waiting" until the tumor becomes larger.

Testicular self-examination (TSE) can help identify testicular cancer early. The American Cancer Society recommends that men over the age of fifteen perform monthly TSEs. These examinations are best done after a warm shower. Using both hands, the testicles should be rolled between thumbs and fingers to feel for any lumps. Abnormalities should be reported to a doctor. Treatment for testicular cancer includes orchiectomy (surgical removal of the testes), radiation therapy, and chemotherapy.

Diabetes is screened by a fasting blood glucose test, which measures blood glucose (sugar) after not eating for at least eight hours; a glucose tolerance test, which measures blood glucose two hours after drinking a concentrated sugar beverage; or a random blood glucose test, which checks the level of blood sugar without fasting. It is recommended that men over age forty-five be tested for diabetes every three years and those at high risk for diabetes be tested at age thirty. Treatment of diabetes may require taking hypoglycemic (low blood sugar) medications or insulin injections in addition to following a diabetic diet, monitoring blood glucose, and getting regular exercise.

Coronary artery disease is treated with lifestyle changes such as smoking cessation, exercise, medications, weight control, and a low-fat, high-fiber diet. Angioplasty (the opening of coronary arteries) or coronary artery bypass surgery may be needed. Cardiomyopathy and heart failure are treated with a low-salt, low-fat diet and medications to regulate and strengthen the heartbeat and decrease fluid retention. A cardiac pacemaker can improve the heart rhythm, while an implantable cardiac device (ICD) monitors heart rhythms and gives an electrical shock when a deadly heart rhythm occurs. Heart transplantation is a last resort when heart failure cannot be controlled. Heart valve disease can be treated with medication to regulate heart rhythm and strengthen the heartbeat, relax blood vessels (vasodilators), control blood pressure (antihypertensives), and reduce fluid retention (diuretics). A balloon valvuloplasty introduces an uninflated balloon into the heart valve that is inflated to open the valve and then removed. If symptoms cannot be controlled, surgery may be necessary to repair or replace the affected valve.

Hyperlipidemia treatment includes lifestyle changes to reduce dietary fats and increase fiber in the diet, weight control, and regular exercise. Lipid-reducing medications may be used if lifestyle changes are not effective. If blood lipids are normal, then screening should be done at least every five years starting at age thirty-five. Screening should be done annually for elevated levels. Men who smoke, who have diabetes, or who have heart disease in their family should have their lipids checked starting at age twenty.

Blood pressure screenings should be done at each health

care visit for men aged eighteen and older. Treatment for high blood pressure begins with lifestyle changes such as weight control, smoking cessation, limited alcohol consumption, regular exercise, and a low-fat, high-fiber diet. Antihypertensive medications are generally used if lifestyle changes are not effective.

Stroke can be treated with medications, surgical intervention and rehabilitation to restore optimum function. A carotid endarterectomy removes fatty deposits (plaque) in the artery that leads to the brain. Cerebral angioplasty opens the carotid artery by inflating a balloon into it to compress plaque, remove plaque with a rotating blade, or implant coils (stents) to keep the vessel open. Tissue plasminogen activator (TPA or tPA) is effective in treating strokes caused by blood clots by dissolving the clot and restoring circulation to the brain, but there is only a three-hour window of time in which it will be effective.

Bronchitis treatment is focused on reducing its symptoms, including avoiding smokers and air pollution, increasing fluids to keep mucus thin, humidifying the air to keep the airways open, deep breathing at least every hour to clear airways, and taking medications to open the airways, encourage coughing, and reduce inflammation, swelling, and mucus. If bronchitis worsens, then oxygen may be required to relieve shortness of breath and maintain adequate oxygen levels.

Emphysema treatment includes stopping smoking, avoiding smokers and air pollution, exercising to strengthen the lungs and diaphragm, maintaining a constant comfortable temperature in the home, increasing fluids to keep mucus thin, taking medications to open the airways and thin mucus, and pursed lip breathing (lips partially closed while slowly breathing out to keep airways open). As emphysema worsens, supplemental oxygen may be required.

Asthma treatment begins with controlling the environment. Wearing a mask while cleaning; avoiding fur, feathers, and materials known to cause an attack; humidifying the air; and using an air conditioner in hot weather are some methods of avoiding an asthma attack. Medications for treating asthma include those that open the airways for quick relief; daily medications to control symptoms of inflammation, open airways, and block release of chemicals that cause inflammation; and those that decrease the reaction to irritants. Desensitization is helpful in allergy-induced asthma, in which small amounts of substances that cause an allergic reaction are injected weekly over several months to develop immunity to them. Finally, anti-IgE monoclonal antibody medications help block antibodies that cause asthma attacks.

Men can lower the chances of developing influenza by getting a flu shot every year. Treatment for the flu is based on treating the symptoms and includes drinking adequate fluids, bed rest, and taking medications for fever, aches, cough, congestion, and nausea. Over-the-counter medications can minimize the discomfort of flu symptoms but do not treat the virus. Antiviral medications are helpful in preventing and treating the flu, but they must be given as soon as symptoms begin in order to be effective. Pneumonia can be prevented by having a pneumonia vaccination. It is 90 percent effective,

and one dose prevents infection for five to ten years. Treatment for pneumonia includes drinking adequate fluids, bed rest, taking antibiotics for bacterial pneumonia, and taking medications to relieve fever, aches, cough, and congestion.

Liver disease treatment depends on the problem. Alcohol abuse is the primary cause of liver disease in men. Those at risk for exposure to hepatitis can be vaccinated against hepatitis B and hepatitis A. Treatment may include high blood pressure medication (antihypertensives), chemotherapy, radiation therapy, bile duct drainage, placing coils (stents) in the bile duct or blood vessels in the liver to keep them open, and liver transplantation.

Depression is most often treated by psychological counseling, cognitive behavioral therapy, interpersonal therapies, and antidepressant medications, with generally good results. Other treatments may include exercise, meditation, and light therapy. Treating depression in men can help to prevent suicide.

Testicular trauma can be evaluated by ultrasound or Doppler to identify the extent of injury. Treatment includes ice packs, scrotal support, anti-inflammatory medications, and bed rest for twenty-four hours. Surgical exploration may be warranted if the injury is severe. Testicular torsion is an emergency situation and should be evaluated by a urologist as soon after the injury as possible to prevent irreversible damage to the testicles. Treatment includes pain relief and manual rotation of the testicle to untwist the cord. This procedure is successful 70 percent of the time. If manual rotation does not work, then surgical intervention is necessary.

Treatment for epididymitis includes ice for swelling, a scrotal supporter, antibiotics, bed rest, and anti-inflammatory medicines (ibuprofen, naprosyn). Untreated epididymitis can cause scarring resulting in infertility. If the cause is related to a sexually transmitted disease, then any partners should be checked and provided treatment as well. Using condoms during sex can help to prevent infections.

Treatment for hypogonadism depends on its cause. Testosterone replacement helps in sexual function, increases muscle strength, and prevents bone loss. Pituitary hormones may help increase testosterone levels and sperm production. Surgical removal of a pituitary tumor may help restore testosterone levels as well.

Benign prostatic hypertrophy is treated with medications to lower the tension in the valve under the bladder to allow urine to pass, or to decrease the amount of testosterone so that the prostate shrinks. Surgical removal of the prostate and radiation therapy to shrink the prostate are also optional treatments. There are no screening guidelines for BPH, and digital rectal examination is the only tool.

Prostatitis is not an easy diagnosis to make because symptoms are usually vague. Bacterial cultures of the urine and prostate secretions may or may not show an infection, but antibiotics are usually prescribed, along with medications to relax the prostate and relieve discomfort. Men are encouraged to increase their fluid intake for adequate hydration.

The only way to prevent STDs is through abstinence. Alternative means include education about STDs and their effects and using latex condoms during vaginal, anal, and oral sex. Polyurethane condoms are not as effective as latex, but they are the only alternative for those with latex allergies. Being with one partner (monogamy) who has tested negative for STDs is another way to prevent STDs. Regular screening for STDs are essential for those with multiple sexual partners. When diagnosed early, most STDs can be treated effectively.

Perspective and Prospects

Men's health as a discrete subject within medicine began in the twenty-first century, modeled on the women's health movement. The *Journal of Men's Health and Gender* was founded in 2004. Its goals are to provide information and education about treatment and preventive care specifically for men. The Men's Health Act of 2005 established the Office of Men's Health in the Department of Health and Human Services.

Current men's health issues are in part attributable to the fact that men still tend to participate in risky activities, smoke, drink more alcohol, and be less likely to seek medical attention or participate in health screenings than are women. African American men are twice as likely to develop heart disease than the general population, one-third of men with Type II diabetes are not aware of it, suicide rates among men are four times higher than for women, and almost 69 percent of American men are overweight or obese.

In 2006, the National Center for Health Statistics reported that male life expectancy was seventy-five, about five years less than for women. Lifestyle changes play a large role in improving the life expectancy of men. Eating healthy, staying physically active, having regular medical checkups, and avoiding behaviors that are more prone to end in injury, illness, and death can increase men's life expectancy beyond the present average. Education and program development to engage more men in developing healthy lifestyles are essential for preventing disease and improving quality of life.

—*Sharon W. Stark, R.N., A.P.R.N., D.N.Sc.*

See also Accidents; Alcoholism; Asbestos exposure; Cancer; Cholesterol; Chronic obstructive pulmonary disease (COPD); Circumcision, male; Cirrhosis; Colon cancer; Color blindness; Concussion; Depression; Diabetes mellitus; Erectile dysfunction; Exercise physiology; Gender reassignment surgery; Genital disorders, male; Gulf War syndrome; Gynecomastia; Hair loss and baldness; Hair transplantation; Heart attack; Heart disease; Heart valve replacement; Hemophilia; Hermaphroditism and pseudohermaphroditism; Hormones; Hydroceles; Hypercholesterolemia; Hyperlipidemia; Hypertension; Hypertrophy; Hypospadias repair and urethroplasty; Incontinence; Infertility, male; Klinefelter syndrome; Lung cancer; Mumps; Occupational health; Orchitis; Penile implant surgery; Posttraumatic stress disorder; Proctology; Prostate cancer; Prostate enlargement; Prostate gland; Prostate gland removal; Puberty and adolescence; Pulmonary diseases; Screening; Semen; Sexuality; Sexually transmitted diseases (STDs); Skin cancer; Smoking; Sperm banks; Sports medicine; Steroid abuse; Suicide; Testicles, undescended; Testicular cancer; Testicular surgery; Testicular torsion; Vas deferens; Vasectomy; Women's health.

For Further Information:

Donatelle, Rebecca J. *Health: The Basics.* 7th ed. San Francisco: Benjamin Cummings, 2006. Provides information for lifestyle changes based in current health promotion and disease prevention trends for specific health issues.

Kasper, Dennis L., et al., eds. *Harrison's Principles of Internal Medicine.* 16th ed. New York: McGraw-Hill, 2005. Offers a comprehensive and detailed discussion of most diseases, symptoms, causes, diagnosis, treatment, and expected outcomes.

Litin, Scott C., ed. *Mayo Clinic Family Health Book.* 4th ed. New York: HarperResource, 2009. This handbook provides information regarding healthy living, diseases, and medical care from birth to old age.

Lunenfeld, Bruno, and Louis Gooren, eds. *Textbook of Men's Health.* Boca Raton, Fla.: Parthenon, 2007. Discusses the effects of hormone decline on aging and disease in men.

MedlinePlus. "Men's Health Issues." http://www.nlm.nih.gov/medlineplus/menshealthissues.html#over views. This Web site provides links to news, overviews, and research into conditions affecting men.

National Institutes of Health. "Men's Health." http://health.nih.gov/category/menshealth. This site provides links to other Web sites with information and resources on a variety of issues related to men's health.

Simon, Harvey B. *The Harvard Medical School Guide to Men's Health.* New York: Free Press, 2004. Offers a comprehensive guide based on research for men to improve their health through healthy living and lifestyle changes.

U.S. Department of Health and Human Services. *Healthy People 2010: Understanding and Improving Health.* Rev. ed. Boston: Jones and Bartlett, 2001. A guide for reaching national goals to improve health in the United States. Specific areas of concern are identified, with discussions of physical, social, and psychological factors in disease and the means to address them.

MENSTRUATION

Biology

Anatomy or system affected: Reproductive system, uterus

Specialties and related fields: Endocrinology, gynecology, pediatrics

Definition: The monthly discharge of blood and tissue (menses) by women of childbearing age, caused by changes in hormonal levels.

Key terms:

endometrium: the layer of cells lining the inner cavity of the uterus; the source of menstrual discharge

feedback: a system in which two parts of the body communicate and control each other, often through hormones; can be either negative (inhibitory) or positive (stimulatory)

follicle: a spherical structure within the ovary that contains a developing ovum and that produces hormones; each ovary contains thousands of follicles

hormone: a chemical signal produced in some part of the body that is carried in the blood to another body part, where it has some observable effect

menstrual cycle: the cycle of hormone production, ovulation, menstruation, and other changes that occurs on an approximately monthly schedule in women

ovary: the organ that produces ova and hormones; the two ovaries lie on either side of the uterus, within the abdominal cavity

ovulation: the process by which an ovum is released from its follicle in the ovary; occurs in the middle of each menstrual cycle *ovum (*pl. *ova):* the egg or reproductive cell produced by the female, which when fertilized by a sperm from the male will develop into an embryo

prostaglandins: chemical signals that have local effects on the organ that produces them

uterus: the organ that nourishes and supports the developing embryo; also called the womb

Process and Effects

Menstruation is the monthly discharge of bloody fluid from the uterus. It occurs in humans and in other primates (apes and monkeys), but not in all mammals; for example, horses, cats, and dogs do not menstruate. The menstrual fluid consists of blood, cells, and debris from the endometrial lining of the uterus, and mucus and other fluids. The color of the discharge varies from dark brown to bright red during the period of flow. The menstrual discharge does not normally clot after leaving the uterus, but it may contain endometrial debris that resembles blood clots. The flow lasts from four to five days in most women, with spotting (the discharge of scant fluid) possibly continuing for another day or two. The volume of fluid lost ranges from ten to eighty milliliters, with a median of about forty milliliters. The blood in the menstrual discharge amounts to only a small fraction of the body's total blood volume of about five thousand milliliters, so normal physiological functioning is not usually impaired by the blood loss that occurs during menstruation.

The first menstruation (menarche) typically begins between the ages of eleven and fourteen, when a girl goes through puberty; the last episodes of menstruation occur some forty years later at the time of menopause. Menstruation does not occur during the months of pregnancy or for the

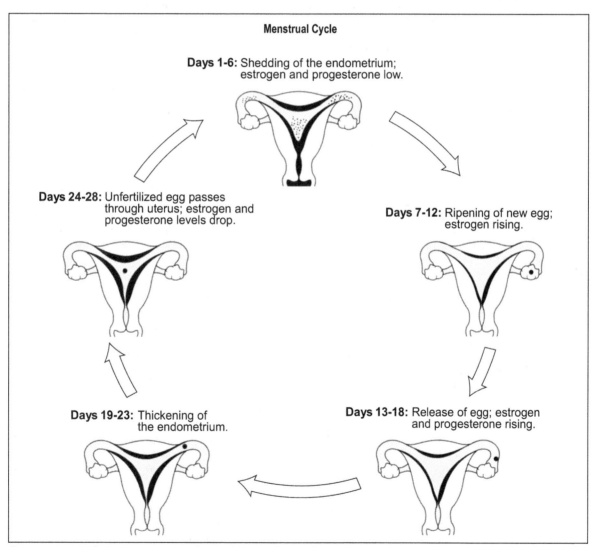

Menstrual Cycle

Days 1-6: Shedding of the endometrium; estrogen and progesterone low.

Days 24-28: Unfertilized egg passes through uterus; estrogen and progesterone levels drop.

Days 7-12: Ripening of new egg; estrogen rising.

Days 19-23: Thickening of the endometrium.

Days 13-18: Release of egg; estrogen and progesterone rising.

Exact timing varies from woman to woman; day 1 is defined as the day of onset of menstrual flow; ovulation occurs in mid-cycle (around day 14). Hormonal levels are rising and falling throughout the cycle.

first few months after a woman has given birth.

Menstruation is the most visible event of the woman's monthly menstrual cycle. The average length of the menstrual cycle in the population is about 29.1 days, but it may vary from sixteen to thirty-five days, with variation occurring between different individuals and in one individual from month to month. Girls who have just gone through puberty and women who are approaching the menopause tend to have more variation in their cycles than do women in the middle of their reproductive years. There is also an age-related change in cycle length: Cycles tend to be relatively long in teenagers, then decrease in length until a woman is about forty years old, after which cycles tend to lengthen and become irregular.

Hormones cause menstruation to be coordinated with other events in the menstrual cycle. Uterine function is regulated by two hormones, estrogen and progesterone, which are produced in the ovaries. In turn, the production of estrogen and progesterone is controlled by follicle-stimulating hormone (FSH) and luteinizing hormone (LH), both of which are produced in the pituitary gland. The hormones from the ovaries and from the pituitary have mutual control over each other: they participate in a feedback relationship. The fact that females produce ova only once a month, in a cycle rather than continuously, is the result of a change in the feedback relationships between the ovarian and pituitary hormones as the menstrual cycle proceeds.

In the first half of the cycle, the follicular phase, a predominant negative feedback effect keeps pituitary hormone levels low while allowing estrogen to increase. Day one of the menstrual cycle is defined as the day of the onset of the menstrual flow. During the days of menstrual bleeding, levels of estrogen and progesterone are low, but FSH levels are high enough to cause the growth of follicles in the ovary. As the follicles start to grow, they secrete estrogen, and increasing amounts are secreted as the follicles continue to enlarge over the next five to ten days. The estrogen exerts negative feedback control over the pituitary: FSH and LH production is inhibited by estrogen, so levels of these hormones remain low during the follicular phase. Besides producing estrogen, the growing follicles contain ova that are maturing and preparing for ovulation. Meanwhile, estrogen acts on the uterus to cause the growth of the endometrial lining. The lining becomes thicker and its blood supply increases; glands located in the lining also grow and mature. These uterine changes are known as endometrial proliferation.

As the woman nears the middle of her cycle, a dramatic change in hormonal feedback occurs. The increasing secretion of estrogen shifts the hormonal system into a positive feedback mode, whereby an increase in estrogen stimulates the release of LH and FSH from the pituitary instead of inhibiting it. Thus, at the middle of the cycle (around day fourteen), simultaneous peaks in levels of estrogen, LH, and FSH occur. The peak in LH triggers ovulation by causing changes in the wall of the follicle, allowing it to break open to release its ovum. Although a group of follicles has matured up to this point, usually only the largest one ovulates, and the remainder in the group die and cease hormone production.

Following ovulation, negative feedback is reestablished. The follicle that just ovulated remains as a functional part of the ovary; it becomes transformed into the corpus luteum, a structure that produces estrogen and progesterone throughout most of the second half of the cycle, the luteal phase. During this phase, the combined presence of estrogen and progesterone reestablishes negative feedback over the pituitary, and LH and FSH levels decline. A second ovulation is prevented because an LH peak is not possible at this time. The combined action of estrogen and progesterone causes the uterus to enter its secretory phase during the second half of the cycle: The glands in the thickened endometrium secrete nutrients that will support an embryo if the woman becomes pregnant, and the ample blood supply to the endometrium can supply the embryo with other nutrients and oxygen. If the woman does in fact become pregnant, the embryo will secrete a hormone that will ensure the continued production of estrogen and progesterone, and because of these hormones, the uterus will remain in the secretory condition throughout pregnancy. Menstruation does not occur during pregnancy because of the high levels of estrogen and progesterone, which continually support the uterus.

If the woman does not become pregnant, the corpus luteum automatically degenerates, starting at about the twenty-fourth day of the menstrual cycle. As the corpus luteum dies, it fails to produce estrogen and progesterone, so levels of these hormones decrease. As the amounts of estrogen and progesterone drop, the uterus begins to produce prostaglandins, chemicals that act as local signals within the uterus. The prostaglandins cause a number of changes in uterine function: blood flow to the endometrium is temporarily cut off, causing the endometrial tissue to die, and the uterine muscle begins to contract, causing further changes in blood flow. The decreased blood flow and the muscle contractions contribute to the cramping pain that many women feel just before and at the time of menstrual bleeding. Menstrual bleeding starts when the blood flow to the endometrium is reestablished and the dead tissue is sloughed off and washed out of the uterus. This event signals the start of a new menstrual cycle.

Complications and Disorders

Many disorders involving menstruation exist. Toxic shock syndrome is a disease that, while not caused directly by menstruation, sometimes occurs during menstruation in women who use tampons to absorb the menstrual flow. The symptoms of toxic shock syndrome—fever, rash, a drop in blood pressure, diarrhea, vomiting, and fainting—are caused by toxins produced by the bacterium *Staphylococcus aureus*. This bacterium is normally present in limited numbers within the vagina, but the use of high-absorbency tampons is associated with a higher-than-normal bacterial growth and toxin production. Toxic shock syndrome requires immediate medical attention, since it may be fatal if left untreated. Women can reduce the risk of toxic shock syndrome by changing tampons often, using lower-absorbency types, and alternating the use of tampons and sanitary napkins.

Amenorrhea is defined as the absence of menstruation. It is usually, but not always, coincident with a lack of ovulation. Amenorrhea may be primary (the woman has never menstruated) or secondary (menstrual cycles that were once normal have stopped). The condition is usually associated with abnormal patterns of hormone secretion, but the problem in hormone secretion may itself be merely the symptom of some other underlying disorder. One of the most common situations leading to both primary and secondary amenorrhea is low body weight, caused by malnutrition, eating disorders, or sustained exercise. Body fat has two roles in reproduction: it provides energy needed for tissue growth and cell functions, and it contributes to circulating estrogen levels. Loss of body fat may create a situation in which the reproductive system ceases to function because of low estrogen levels and because of lack of needed energy. The result is seen as amenorrhea. Emotional or physical stress may also cause amenorrhea, because stress results in the release of hormones that interfere with the reproductive hormones. Ideally, amenorrhea is treated by removing its cause; for example, a special diet or a change in an exercise program can bring about an increase in body fat stores, or stress levels can be reduced through changes in lifestyle or with counseling. Ironically, sometimes birth control pills are prescribed for women with amenorrhea. The pills do not cure the amenorrhea, but they can counteract some of the long-term problems associated with it, such as changes in the endometrial lining and loss of bone density.

Dysmenorrhea refers to abnormally intense uterine pain associated with menstruation. It is estimated that 5 to 10 percent of women experience pain intense enough to interfere with their school or work schedules. Dysmenorrhea may be primary (occurring in women with no known disease) or secondary (caused by a disease condition such as a tumor or infection). Studies have shown uterine prostaglandin levels to be correlated with the degree of pain perceived in primary dysmenorrhea, and drugs that interfere with prostaglandins offer an effective treatment for this condition. These drugs include aspirin, acetaminophen, ibuprofen, and naproxen; some formulas are available without a doctor's prescription, but the stronger drugs require one. Secondary dysmenorrhea is best managed by removing the underlying cause; if this is not possible, the antiprostaglandin drugs may be useful in controlling the pain.

Menorrhagia is excessive menstrual blood loss, usually defined as more than eighty milliliters of fluid lost per cycle. This condition can have serious health consequences because of the loss of red blood cells, which are essential for carrying oxygen to tissues. Women who have given birth to several children are more likely to suffer from menorrhagia, possibly because of enlargement of the uterine cavity and interference with the mechanisms that limit menstrual blood flow. Women who have diseases that interfere with blood clotting may also have menorrhagia. Although the menstrual discharge itself does not usually form clots after it leaves the uterus, clots do form within the uterine endometrium; these clots normally prevent excessive blood loss. Treatment for menorrhagia may begin with iron and vitamin supplements to induce increased red blood cell production, or transfusions may be used to replace the lost red blood cells. If this is unsuccessful, treatment with birth control pills, destruction of the endometrium by laser surgery, or a hysterectomy (surgical removal of the uterus) may be necessary.

Endometriosis is a condition in which endometrial cells from the uterus become misplaced within the abdominal cavity, adhering to and growing on the surface of internal organs. The outside of the uterus, the oviducts (fallopian tubes), the surface of the ovaries, and the outer surface of the intestines can all support the growth of endometrial tissue. Endometriosis is thought to arise during menstruation, when endometrial tissue enters the oviducts instead of being carried outward through the cervix and vagina. Through the oviducts, the endometrial tissue has access to the abdominal cavity. Since the misplaced endometrial tissue responds to hormones in the same way that the normal endometrium does, it undergoes cyclic changes in thickness and attempts to shed at the time of menstruation. Endometriosis results in intense pain during menstruation and can cause infertility because of interference with ovulation, ovum or sperm transport, or uterine function. Endometriosis is treated with birth control pills or with drugs that suppress menstrual cycles, or the endometrial tissue may be removed surgically.

Premenstrual syndrome (PMS) is a set of symptoms that occurs in some women in the week before the start of menstruation, with the symptoms disappearing once menstruation begins. Researchers and physicians who study PMS have struggled to devise a standard definition for the disorder, but the list of possible symptoms is lengthy and varies from woman to woman and even within one woman from month to month. The possible symptoms include both psychological and physical changes: irritability, nervous tension, anxiety, moodiness, depression, lethargy, insomnia, confusion, crying, food cravings, fatigue, weight gain, swelling and bloating, breast tenderness, backache, headache, dizziness, muscle stiffness, and abdominal cramps. A diagnosis of PMS requires that the symptoms show a clear relation to the timing of menstruation and that they recur during most menstrual cycles. Researchers estimate that 3 to 5 percent of women have PMS symptoms that are so severe that they are incapacitating, but that milder symptoms occur in about 50 percent of all women.

Because of the variability in symptoms between women, some researchers believe that there are several subtypes of PMS, each with its own cluster of symptoms. It is possible that each subtype has a unique cause. Suggested causes of PMS include an imbalance in the ratio of estrogen to progesterone following ovulation; changes in the hormones that control salt and water balance (the renin-angiotensin-aldosterone system); increased levels of prolactin (a hormone that acts on the breast); changes in amounts of brain chemicals; altered functioning of the biological clock that determines daily rhythms; poor diet or sensitivity to certain foods; and psychological factors such as attitude toward menstruation, stresses of family or professional life, and underlying personality disorders. Studies evaluating these theories have yielded contradictory results, so that no one cause of PMS has yet been found. Current treatments for PMS include dietary therapy, hormone administration, and psychological counseling, but no treatment has been found effective in all PMS patients.

An interesting phenomenon associated with menstruation is menstrual synchrony, also known as the "dormitory effect." Among women who live together, menstrual cycles gradually become synchronized, so that the women begin to menstruate within a few days of one another. Researchers have found that this phenomenon probably occurs because of pheromones, chemical signals that are produced by an individual and that have an effect on another individual. Pheromones act on the brain through the sense of smell, even though there may not be an odor that is consciously perceived.

Perspective and Prospects

Early beliefs about menstruation were based on folk magic and superstition rather than on scientific evidence. Even today, some cultures persist in believing that menstruating women possess deleterious powers: that the presence of a menstruating woman can cause crops to fail, farm animals to die, or beer, bread, jam, and other foods to be spoiled. Some people believe that these incidents will occur even if the menstruating woman has no evil intention. Because of the possibility of these events, some cultures prohibit menstruating women from interacting with others. In the most rigorous example of such a taboo, some societies require that menstruating women live in special huts for the duration of the bleeding period.

Folk beliefs about menstruating women have been bolstered by religious views of menstruating women as "unclean" and in need of purification. In Orthodox Judaism, there are detailed proscriptions to be observed by a menstruating woman, including the avoidance of sexual intercourse. Seven days after her menstrual flow has stopped, the Orthodox Jewish woman undergoes a ritual purification, after which she may resume sexual relations with her husband. Early Christians absorbed the Jewish belief in the uncleanliness of a menstruating woman and prohibited her from entering church or receiving the sacraments. These injunctions were lifted by the seventh century, but the view of women as spiritually and bodily impure persists in some Christian groups to this day.

Many couples abstain from intercourse during the woman's menstrual period. There is no medical justification for this behavior; in fact, research has demonstrated that intercourse can alleviate menstrual cramping, at least temporarily. Still, surveys have shown that a majority of both men and women think that it is wrong for a woman to have intercourse while menstruating.

There are also persistent beliefs that women's physical and mental abilities suffer during menstruation. In fact, this was the predominant medical opinion up through the nineteenth and early twentieth centuries. Medical writings from this time are filled with injunctions for women to rest and to refrain from exercise and intellectual strain while menstruat-

ing. It was a common belief that education could actually cause physical harm to women. Some men used this advice as justification for excluding women from equal opportunities in education and employment. Starting in the late nineteenth century, however, scientific studies clearly demonstrated that education has no harmful effects and that there is no diminution of intellectual or physical performance during menstruation. Nevertheless, the latter finding has been one that the general population finds difficult to accept.

The latest view of menstruation is that, far from being harmful, menstrual bleeding is directly beneficial to a woman's health. Margie Profet, an evolutionary biologist at the University of California, theorized that menstruation evolved as a means of periodically removing disease-causing bacteria and viruses from the woman's uterus. These organisms might enter the uterus along with sperm after sexual activity. In Profet's view, the energetic cost of replacing the blood and tissue lost through menstruation is more than outweighed by the protective benefits of menstruation. Her theory implies that treatments that suppress menstruation, as birth control drugs sometimes do, are not always advantageous.

The suppression of menstruation through extended or continuous cycling with combined hormonal contraception has recently been reexamined for various benefits, including increased contraceptive efficacy. Some clinicians and consumers have embraced this concept, which can be done with any continuous (no placebo or no-pill interval) use of a monophasic combined oral contraceptive pill, the Ortho Evra patch, or NuvaRing. New formulations of combined oral contraceptives include Seasonale and Seasonique, both of which result in menstrual bleeding every three months, and Lybrel, which eliminates cycles for one year. Other formulations have shortened the one week pill-free interval, resulting in shorter and lighter menses.

—Marcia Watson-Whitmyre, Ph.D.

See also Amenorrhea; Cervical, ovarian, and uterine cancers; Childbirth; Conception; Contraception; Dysmenorrhea; Endocrinology; Endometriosis; Genital disorders, female; Gynecology; Hormones; Hot flashes; Infertility, female; Menopause; Menorrhagia; Ovarian cysts; Ovaries; Pregnancy and gestation; Premenstrual syndrome (PMS); Puberty and adolescence; Reproductive system; Toxic shock syndrome; Uterus; Women's health.

For Further Information:

Ammer, Christine. *The Encyclopedia of Women's Health.* 6th ed. New York: Facts on File, 2009.

Berek, Jonathan S., and Emil Novak, eds. *Berek and Novak's Gynecology.* 15th ed. Philadelphia: Lippincott Williams & Wilkins, 2012.

Covington, Timothy R., and J. Frank McClendon. *Sex Care: The Complete Guide to Safe and Healthy Sex.* New York: Pocket Books, 1987.

Golub, Sharon. *Periods: From Menarche to Menopause.* Newbury Park, Calif.: Sage, 1992.

Loulan, JoAnne, and Bonnie Worthen. *Period: A Girl's Guide to Menstruation.* Rev. ed. Minnetonka, Minn.: Book Peddlers, 2001.

"Menopause." *MedlinePlus*, July 1, 2013.

"Menstruation." *MedlinePlus*, May 28, 2013.

"Premenstrual Syndrome." *MedlinePlus*, April 29, 2013.

Quilligan, Edward J., and Frederick P. Zuspan, eds. *Current Therapy in Obstetrics and Gynecology.* 5th ed. Philadelphia: W. B. Saunders, 2000.

Rako, Susan. *No More Periods? The Risks of Menstrual Suppression and Other Cutting-Edge Issues in Women's Reproductive Health.* New York: Harmony Books, 2003.

Weschler, Toni. *Taking Charge of Your Fertility.* Rev. ed. New York: Collins, 2006.

MENTAL RETARDATION

Disease/Disorder

Anatomy or system affected: Brain, nervous system, psychic-emotional system

Specialties and related fields: Genetics, psychiatry, psychology

Definition: Significant subaverage intellectual development and deficient adaptive behavior often accompanied by physical abnormalities.

Key terms:

educable mentally retarded (EMR): individuals with mild-to-moderate retardation; they can be educated with some modifications of the regular education program and can achieve a minimal level of success

inborn metabolic disorder: an abnormality caused by a gene mutation that interferes with normal metabolism and often results in mental retardation

mental handicap: the condition of an individual classified as "educable mentally retarded"

mental impairment: the condition of an individual classified as "trainable mentally retarded" and typically distinguished from mentally ill

neural tube defects: birth defects resulting from the failure of the embryonic neural tube to close; usually results in some degree of mental retardation

trainable mentally retarded (TMR): individuals with moderate-to-severe retardation; only low levels of achievement may be reached by such persons

Causes and Symptoms

Mental retardation is a condition in which a person demonstrates significant subaverage development of intellectual function, along with poor adaptive behavior. Diagnosis can be made at birth if physical abnormalities also accompany mental retardation. An infant with mild mental retardation, however, may not be diagnosed until problems arise in school. Estimates of the prevalence of mental retardation vary from 1 to 3 percent of the world's total population.

Diagnosis of mental retardation takes into consideration three factors: subaverage intellectual function, deficiency in adaptive behavior, and early-age onset (before the age of eighteen). Intellectual function is a measure of one's intelligence quotient (IQ). Four levels of retardation based on IQ are described by the American Psychiatric Association. An individual with an IQ between 50 and 70 is considered mildly retarded, one with an IQ between 35 and 49 is moderately retarded, one with an IQ between 21 and 34 is severely retarded, and an individual with an IQ of less than 20 is termed profoundly retarded.

A person's level of adaptive behavior is not as easily determined as an IQ, but it is generally defined as the ability to meet social expectations in the individual's own environment. Assessment is based on development of certain skills: sensorimotor, speech and language, self-help, and socialization skills. Tests have been developed to aid in these measurements.

To identify possible mental retardation in infants, the use of language milestones is a helpful tool. For example, parents and pediatricians will observe whether children begin to smile, coo, babble, and use words during the appropriate age ranges. Once children reach school age, poor school achievement may identify those who are mentally impaired. Psychometric tests appropriate to the age of the children will help with diagnosis.

Classification of the degree of mental retardation is never absolutely clear, and dividing lines are often somewhat arbitrary. There has been debate about the value of classifying or labeling persons in categories of mental deficiency. On one hand, it is important for professionals to understand the amount of deficiency and to determine what kind of education and treatment would be appropriate and helpful to each individual. On the other hand, such classification can lead to low self-esteem, rejection by peers, and low expectations from teachers and parents.

There has been a marked change in the terminology used in classifying mental retardation from the early days of its study. In the early twentieth century, the terms used for moderate, severe, and profound retardation were "moron," "imbecile," and "idiot." In Great Britain, the term "feeble-minded" was used to indicate moderate retardation. These terms are no longer used by professionals working with the mentally retarded. "Idiot" was the classification given to the most profoundly retarded until the middle of the twentieth century. Historically, the word has changed in meaning, from William Shakespeare's day when the court jester was called an idiot, to an indication of psychosis, and later to define the lowest grade of mental deficiency. The term "idiocy" has been replaced with the expression "profound mental retardation."

Determining the cause of mental retardation is much more difficult than might be expected. More than a thousand different disorders that can cause mental retardation have been reported. Some cases seem to be entirely hereditary, others to be caused by environmental stress, and others the result of a combination of the two. In a large number of cases, however, the cause cannot be established. The mildly retarded make up the largest proportion of the mentally retarded population, and their condition seems to be a recessive genetic trait with no accompanying physical abnormalities. From a medical standpoint, mental retardation is considered to be a result of disease or biological defect and is classified according to its cause. Some of these causes are infections, poisons, environmental trauma, metabolic and nutritional abnormalities, and brain malformation.

Infections are especially harmful to brain development if they occur in the first trimester of pregnancy. Rubella is a vi-

Information on Mental Retardation

Causes: Often unknown; may include genetic factors, disease, infections, poisons, environmental trauma, metabolic and nutritional abnormalities, brain malformation

Symptoms: Physical abnormalities, subaverage intellectual function, deficiency in adaptive behavior

Duration: Lifelong

Treatments: None; supportive therapy may include special education, physical therapy, family counseling

ral infection that often results in mental retardation. Syphilis is a sexually transmitted disease that affects adults and infants born to them, resulting in progressive mental degeneration.

Poisons such as mercury, lead, and alcohol have a very damaging effect on the developing brain. More recent concerns about mercury in the diets of those who frequently consume fish and other seafood have encouraged some individuals, such as pregnant women, to change their dietary behavior in an effort to avoid potential harm to fetal development. Lead-based paints linger in older houses and are even on toys, causing poisoning in children or otherwise affecting the mental functioning of all persons in the home. Children may mouth or suck on these lead-painted toys, or they may eat chipped house paint and plaster or put them in their mouths; all of these actions possibly cause mental retardation, cerebral palsy, and convulsive and behavioral disorders as a result of lead exposure.

Traumatic environmental effects that can cause mental retardation include prenatal exposure to X rays, lack of oxygen to the brain, or a mother's fall during pregnancy. During birth itself, the use of forceps can cause brain damage, and labor that is too brief or too long can cause mental impairment. After the birth process, head trauma or high temperature can affect brain function.

Poor nutrition and inborn metabolic disorders may cause defective mental development because vital body processes are hindered. One of these conditions, for which every newborn is tested, is phenylketonuria (PKU), in which the body cannot process the amino acid phenylalanine. If PKU is detected in infancy, subsequent mental retardation can be avoided by placing the child on a carefully controlled diet, thus preventing buildup of toxic compounds that would be harmful to the brain.

The failure of the neural tube to close in the early development of an embryo may result in anencephaly (an incomplete brain or none at all), hydrocephalus (an excessive amount of cerebrospinal fluid), or spina bifida (an incomplete vertebra, which leaves the spinal cord exposed). Anencephalic infants will live only a few hours. About half of those with other neural tube disorders will survive, usually with some degree of mental retardation. Research has shown that if a mother's diet has sufficient quantities of folic acid, neural tube closure disorders will be rare or nonexistent.

Microcephaly is another physical defect associated with mental retardation. In this condition, the head is abnormally small because of inadequate brain growth. Microcephaly may be inherited or caused by maternal infection, drugs, irradiation, or lack of oxygen at birth.

Abnormal chromosome numbers are not uncommon in developing embryos and will cause spontaneous abortions in most cases. Those babies that survive usually demonstrate varying degrees of mental retardation, and incidence increases with maternal age. A well-known example of a chromosome disorder is Down syndrome (formerly called mongolism), in which there is an extra copy of the twenty-first chromosome. Gene products caused by the extra chromosome cause mental retardation and other physical problems. Other well-studied chromosomal abnormalities involve the sex chromosomes. Both males and females may be born with too many or too few sex chromosomes, which often results in mental retardation.

Mild retardation with no other noticeable problems has been found to run in certain families. It occurs more often in the lower economic strata of society and probably reflects only the lower end of the normal distribution of intelligence in a population. The condition is probably a result of genetic factors interacting with environmental ones. It has been found that culturally deprived children have a lower level of intellectual function because of decreased stimuli as the infant brain develops.

Treatment and Therapy

Diagnosis of the level of mental retardation is important in meeting the needs of the intellectually handicapped. It can open the way for effective measures to be taken to help these persons achieve the highest quality of life possible for them.

Individuals with an IQ of 50 to 70 have mild-to-moderate retardation and are classified as "educable mentally retarded" (EMR). They can profit from the regular education program when it is somewhat modified. The general purposes of all education are to allow for the development of knowledge, to provide a basis for vocational competence, and to allow opportunity for self-realization. The EMR can achieve some success in academic subjects, make satisfactory social adjustment, and achieve minimal occupational adequacy if given proper training. In Great Britain, these individuals are referred to as "educationally subnormal" (ESN).

Persons with moderate-to-severe retardation generally have IQs between 21 and 49 and are classified as "trainable mentally retarded" (TMR). These individuals are not educable in the traditional sense, but many can be trained in self-help skills, socialization into the family, and some degree of economic independence with supervision. They need a developmental curriculum which promotes personal development, independence, and social skills.

The profoundly retarded are classified as "totally dependent" and have IQs of 20 or less. They cannot be trained to care for themselves, to socialize, or to be independent to any degree. They will need almost complete care and supervision throughout life. They may learn to understand a few simple commands, but they will be able to speak only a few words.

Meaningful speech is not characteristic of this group.

EMR individuals need a modified curriculum, along with appropriately qualified and experienced teachers. Activities should include some within their special class and some in which they interact with students of other classes. The amount of time spent in regular classes and in special classes should be determined by individual needs in order to achieve the goals and objectives planned for each. Individual development must be the primary concern.

For TMR individuals, the differences will be in the areas of emphasis, level of attainment projected, and methods used. The programs should consist of small classes that may be held within the public schools or outside with the help of parents and other concerned groups. Persons trained in special education are needed to guide the physical, social, and emotional development experiences effectively.

A systematic approach in special education has proven to be the best teaching method to make clear to students what behaviors will result in the successful completion of goals. This approach has been designed so that children work with only one concept at a time. There are appropriate remedies planned for misconceptions along the way. Progress is charted for academic skills, home-living skills, and prevocational training. Decisions on the type of academic training appropriate for a TMR individual are not based on classification or labels, but on demonstrated ability.

One of the most important features of successful special education is the involvement of parents. Parents faced with rearing a retarded child may find the task overwhelming and have a great need of caring support and information about their child and the implications for their future. Parental involvement gives the parents the opportunity to learn by observing how the professionals facilitate effective learning experiences for their children at school.

Counselors help parents identify problems and implement plans of action. They can also help them determine whether goals are being reached. Counselors must know about the community resources that are available to families. They can help parents find emotional reconciliation with the problems presented by their special children. It is important for parents to be able to accept the child's limitations. They should not lavish special or different treatment on the retarded child, but rather treat this child like the other children.

Placing a child outside the home is indicated only when educational, behavioral, or medical controls are needed that cannot be provided in the home. Physicians and social workers should be able to do some counseling to supplement that of the trained counselors. Those who offer counseling should have basic counseling skills and relevant knowledge about the mentally retarded individual and the family.

EMR individuals will usually marry, may have children, and often become self-supporting. The TMR will live in an institution or at home or in foster homes for their entire lives. They will probably never become self-sufficient. The presence of a TMR child has a great impact on families and may weaken family closeness. It creates additional expenses and limits family activities. Counseling for these families is very important.

Sheltered employment provides highly controlled working conditions, helping the mentally retarded to become contributing members of society. This arrangement benefits the individual, the family, and society as the individual experiences the satisfaction and dignity of work. The mildly retarded may need only a short period of time in the sheltered workshop. The greater the degree of mental retardation, the more likely shelter will be required on a permanent basis. For the workshop to be successful, those in charge of it must consider both the personal development of the disabled worker and the business production and profit of the workshop. Failure to consider the business success of these ventures has led to failures of the programs.

There has been a trend toward deinstitutionalizing the mentally retarded, to relocate as many residents as possible into appropriate community homes. Success will depend on a suitable match between the individual and the type of home provided. This approach is most effective for the mentally retarded if the staff of a facility is well trained and there is a fair amount of satisfactory interaction between staff and residents. It is important that residents not be ignored, and they must be monitored for proper evaluation at each step along the way. Top priority must be given to preparation of the staff to work closely with the mentally impaired and handicapped.

In the past, there was no way to know before a child's birth if there would be abnormalities. With advances in technology, however, a variety of prenatal tests can be done, and many fetal abnormalities can be detected. Genetic counseling is important for persons who have these tests conducted. Some may have previously had a retarded child, or have retarded family members. Others may have something in their backgrounds that would indicate a higher-than-average risk for physical and/or mental abnormalities. Some come for testing before a child is conceived; others do not come until afterward. Tests can be done on the fetal blood and tissues that will reveal chromosomal abnormalities or inborn metabolic errors.

Many parents do not seek testing or genetic counseling because of the stress and anxiety that may result. Though most prenatal tests result in normal findings, if problems are indicated the parents are faced with what may be a difficult decision: whether to continue the pregnancy. It is often impossible to predict the extent of an abnormality, and weighing the sanctity of life in relation to the quality of life may present an ethical and religious dilemma. Others prefer to know what problems lie ahead and what their options are.

Finally, it is important to realize that problems such as mental retardation may not occur in isolation from other problems. Concurrent physical and mental illnesses may add complexity to managing treatment and services for individuals with more than one condition. Assessment to rule out other conditions remains an important step in ongoing and evolving care for individuals with mental retardation and similar conditions.

Perspective and Prospects

Throughout history, the mentally retarded were first ignored, and then subjected to ridicule. The first attempts to educate the mentally retarded were initiated in France in the mid-nineteenth century. Shortly afterward, institutions for them began to spring up in Europe and the United States. These were often in remote rural areas, separated from the communities nearby, and were usually ill-equipped and understaffed. The institutions were quite regimented, and harsh discipline was kept. Meaningful interactions usually did not occur between the patients and the staff.

The medical approach of the institutions was to treat the outward condition of the mentally retarded and ignore them as people. No concern for their social and emotional needs was shown. There were no provisions for children to play, nor was there concern for the needs of the family of those with mental handicaps.

Not until the end of the nineteenth century were the first classes set up in some U.S. public schools for education of the mentally retarded. The first half of the twentieth century brought about the expansion of the public school programs for individuals with both mild and moderate mental retardation. After World War II, perhaps in response to the slaughter of mentally handicapped persons in Nazi Germany, strong efforts were made to provide educational, medical, and recreational services for the mentally retarded.

Groundbreaking research in the 1950s led to the normalization of society's attitude about the mentally retarded in the United States. Plans to help these individuals live as normal a life as possible were made. The National Association for Retarded Citizens was founded in 1950 and had a very strong influence on public opinion. In 1961, U.S. president John F. Kennedy appointed the Panel on Mental Retardation and instructed it to prepare a plan for the United States to help meet the complex problems of the mentally retarded. The panel presented ninety recommendations in the areas of research, prevention, medical services, education, law, and local and national organization. Further presidential commissions on the topic were appointed and have had far-reaching effects for the well-being of the mentally retarded.

A "Declaration of the Rights of Mentally Retarded Persons" was adopted by the General Assembly of the United Nations in 1971, and the Education for All Handicapped Children Act was passed in the United States in 1975, providing for the development of educational programs appropriate for all handicapped and disabled children and youth. These pieces of legislation were milestones in the struggle to improve learning opportunities for the mentally retarded.

Changes continue to take place in attitudes toward greater integration of the retarded into schools and the community, leading to significant improvements. The role of the family has increased in emphasis, for it has often been the families themselves that have worked to change old, outdated policies. The cooperation of the family is very important in improving the social and intellectual development of the mentally retarded child. Because so many new and innovative techniques have been used, it is very important that programs be evaluated and compared to one another to determine which methods provide the best training and education for the mentally retarded.

—Katherine H. Houp, Ph.D.;
updated by Nancy A. Piotrowski, Ph.D.

See also Batten's disease; Birth defects; Brain; Brain damage; Congenital hypothyroidism; Cornelia de Lange syndrome; Developmental disorders; Down syndrome; Endocrine disorders; Fetal alcohol syndrome; Fragile X syndrome; Genetic diseases; Genetics and inheritance; Learning disabilities; Phenylketonuria (PKU); Prader-Willi syndrome; Pregnancy and gestation; Psychiatry; Psychiatry, child and adolescent; Rubinstein-Taybi syndrome.

For Further Information:

American Association of Intellectual and Developmental Disabilities. http://www.aaidd.org. Formerly the American Association of Mental Retardation, this group for professionals in the mental health field promotes progressive policies, research, effective practices, and universal human rights for the mentally retarded, or for people with intellectual and developmental disabilities, a term preferred by this organization.

Beirne-Smith, Mary, James R. Patton, and Shannon H. Kim, eds. *Mental Retardation*. 7th ed. Upper Saddle River, N.J.: Prentice Hall, 2006. Covers the causes and characteristics of individuals with mental retardation across the life span, explores the benefits of assistive technology, and surveys related legislation and policy issues.

Best Buddies International. http://www.bestbuddies .org. Facilitates support among people with mental retardation and involving them in their communities.

Drew, Clifford J., ed. *Mental Retardation: A Lifespan Approach to People with Intellectual Disabilities*. 8th ed. Boston: Allyn & Bacon, 2004. An introductory and interdisciplinary text that examines all aspects of diagnosis and intervention and discusses multicultural issues related to assessment bias, language differences, and mental retardation in all stages of life.

Dudley, James R. *Confronting the Stigma in Their Lives: Helping People with a Mental Retardation Label*. Springfield, Ill.: Charles C Thomas, 1997. This book is written for those concerned with combating the negative effects of being labeled as having a mental disorder.

Glidden, Laraine Masters. *International Review of Research in Mental Retardation*. New York: Elsevier, 2006. An interdisciplinary text, updated regularly, that surveys recent research into the causes, effects, classification systems, and syndromes of mental retardation. Contributions from nutrition, genetics, psychology, education, and other health and behavioral sciences are included.

Matson, Johnny L., and Rowland P. Barrett, eds. *Psychopathology in the Mentally Retarded*. 2d ed. Boston: Allyn & Bacon, 1993. This book addresses an often-neglected topic: the psychological problems that may be found in those with mental retardation. Discusses special emotional problems based on the causation of deficiencies.

Schalock, Robert, et al. *Intellectual Disability: Definition, Classification, and Systems of Supports*. 11th ed. Washington, D.C.: American Association on Intellectual and Developmental Disabilities, 2010. Written by a committee of experts, this work provides updated, authoritative information on mental retardation, "including best practice guidelines on diagnosing and classifying intellectual disability [mental retardation] and developing a system of supports for people living with an intellectual disability."

MENTAL ILLNESS. See PSYCHIATRIC DISORDERS; SPECIFIC DISEASES.

MENTAL STATUS EXAM
Procedure
Anatomy or system affected: Brain, nervous system, psychoemotional system

Specialties and related fields: Primary care medicine, psychiatry, psychology, emergency medicine

Definition: A clinical tool used for a systematic assessment of cognitive and emotional functioning of an individual.

Overview
Mental Status Exam (MSE) is a clinical tool used for a systematic assessment of cognitive and emotional functioning of an individual. MSE is often incorporated into a health history interview but can be also performed separately. It is very useful for determining an individual's general mental health and eliciting possible problems such as a mood disorder, psychiatric illness, or a physical condition that affects mental status. It is important to remember that certain factors may influence a patient's performance and a clinician's interpretation of the MSE. They include chronic diseases, some medications, educational level, individual behavioral pattern, stress, sleep habits, and the use of alcohol or drugs.

Components
The components of the Mental Status Exam can be divided into four main categories with the acronym A-B-C-T: Appearance, Behavior, Cognition and Thought. These categories and their components are described below.

Appearance. An individual's appearance can provide a wealth of information. It is a broad term that includes elements such as posture, position, hygiene, grooming, and dress. Normal posture is usually erect while position is relaxed. Abnormal findings may include uneven standing position, sitting slumped in a chair, visible facial or general muscle tension, sitting on edge of a chair, or lying curled in bed. Hygiene and grooming should also be considered. Some patients with a history of a stroke may present with unilateral neglect, a condition characterized by complete inattention to one side of the body.

Poor hygiene and inappropriate dress may be indicative of depression, dementia, frontal lobe dysfunction, delirium, or schizophrenia. On the other hand, excessive makeup or flamboyant attire may indicate a manic state or schizophrenia, while meticulous or fastidious grooming may suggest obsessive-compulsive disorder. General appearance such as cachexia or obesity may occur in conjunction with a systemic disease or a mental health disorder such as anorexia nervosa or binge eating disorder.

Behavior. The most important components of behavior include level of consciousness, emotional state, body movements, speech, facial expressions, and general manner of behavior. Level of consciousness (LOC) is one of the most important components of the MSE. A person with a normal LOC is awake, alert, aware of internal and external stimuli, and shows appropriate responses to such stimuli. Impaired consciousness expressed by somnolence, lethargy, stupor, or coma may indicate a neurologic or medical emergency.

Emotional state is expressed by an individual's mood and affect. Mood is a subjective and internal emotional state whereas affect is a clinician's objective evaluation of such. Mood can be assessed by asking a person about the way they feel at this time and most recently. Body language, vocal tone, and facial expressions may assist in determining a patient's affect. Affect can be characterized by emotional range (broad or restricted), intensity (blunted, flat or normal), and stability. It may be congruent with mood or may be different.

Evaluation of body movements is another key element of the MSE. General slowing of physical and emotional reactions and signs of apathy are present in depression, schizophrenia, or organic brain disease. Increased agitation, restlessness, and squirmy movements can occur with bipolar disorder or anxiety. Dragging of feet may be seen in depression or organic brain disease while unusual posturing and odd gestures may be signs of schizophrenia. Changes in body movements over a period of time can occur due to progression of an illness or caused by side effects of certain medications.

When examining speech, it is important to note its overall quality, spontaneity, pace, word choice, sentence structure, and articulation. The manner in which a person speaks is more important than the actual content in this part of the MSE. Speech that is slow and monotonous can occur in conjunction with depression or Parkinsonism. Loud, pressured, or rapid speech is common in manic syndrome. Absence of speech may indicate selective mutism, vegetative state, locked-in syndrome, or a brain lesion.

Facial expressions of a healthy person are proper to the situation and change appropriately with the topic. The eye contact is comfortable. Flat and mask-like facial expression is common in patients with depression or Parkinson's. Frowning and vigilant or darting eyes is a common observation in patients with anxiety or hyperthyroidism.

Cognition. Cognitive assessment includes orientation, attention span, recent memory, remote memory, language, new learning ability, visual spatial skills, judgment, and executive function. Orientation to time, place, person, and situation are often tested during MSE by asking a question such as "Do you know what is today's date?" Disorientation may take place in disorders of organic origin such as dementia or delirium. It is most common for disorientation to occur in the following sequence-first to time, then to place and finally to person.

Attention span is an individual's ability to focus and complete thoughts without digression. Problems with attention are manifested by irrelevant responses to questions as well as quick distractibility by new stimuli. One test of attention span is to provide a series of simple directions and ask to follow them. For example: "Please open the table drawer, take out the red key with your right hand, shift it to your left hand, and put the key in your pocket." Confusional states, fatigue, anxiety, and drug intoxication may impair attention.

Memory is assessed in terms of recent and remote memory as well as the ability to form new memories. Recent memory can be evaluated by asking the patient to describe their life events in the past 24 hours. Remote memory is assessed by inquiring about important historical or patient's own life events. New learning and recall can be tested by asking a patient to remember three to four unrelated words (such as apple, yellow, grass, and winter). During the interview, the examiner asks the patient to repeat the words at 10 and 30 minutes. Deficits in recent memory take place mostly in disorders of organic origin, such as dementia, delirium, amnestic syndrome, or Korsakoff's syndrome in patients with chronic alcoholism. Remote memory shortage can occur due to cerebral cortex damage, which is present in dementia and other diseases.

The most commonly used tests of visual spatial skills are constructional and copying tasks. They include drawing a clock and reproducing figures such as a circle, intersecting circle, and triangle or other figures. Patients with executive dysfunction exhibit poor planning skills. Often times a clock face is too small to contain all the necessary numbers. Those with unilateral neglect ignore half of the clock face. Disturbances in drawing of the figures are often encountered in patients with degenerative disorders, focal brain damages, or toxic and metabolic encephalopathy.

Judgment is an ability to compare alternatives and identify the consequences of actions. It can be evaluated by offering hypothetical daily situations pertinent to a particular patient, and asking for possible solutions. For example, "What would you do if you realized that you lost the keys for your house?" Impaired judgment is often manifested by impulsive or unrealistic decisions and is common in neurologic conditions, schizophrenia, organic brain diseases, and mental retardation.

Executive function is a set of capabilities such as volition, planning, problem solving, reasoning, and effective performance of tasks. The overall executive functioning can be extrapolated from the interview and by asking about everyday functioning. Eliciting the tasks that require assistance or direction can be helpful. Impairment of judgment or insight (patient's awareness of his/her condition and need for treatment) can serve as an early indication of executive dysfunction.

Thought. The main areas of thought processes found on the MSE are thought content, perceptions, and screen for suicidality. Thought content describes particular thoughts that an individual experiences. Healthy thought content is consistent, logical, and realistic. Abnormal findings include obsessions, compulsions, delusions, and thoughts about suicide or homicide. Delusions are common in patients with Lewy body and vascular dementia, Alzheimer's disease, Huntington's disease, and schizophrenia. Delusions that are acute in nature can occur in alcohol or drug intoxication.

Also, it is important to assess for the presence of any perceptual disturbances such as hallucinations or illusions. Hallucinations can involve any of the senses and either have a specific form or be formless. Visual and auditory hallucinations arise with organic brain disease, schizophrenia, bipolar disorder, severe unipolar depression, psychedelic drugs, or alcohol withdrawal.

Screening patients for suicidal ideation is an integral aspect of the MSE. It is usually performed when the patient expresses or portrays feelings of sadness, loneliness, helplessness, hopelessness, grief, or despair. This part of the exam is particularly important in patients with chronic diseases, mental health disorders, or history of prior suicide attempts. A good approach is to begin by asking general questions about the person's feelings and overall outlook on life.

If a clinician remains concerned, then it is important to ask more direct questions such as "Have you ever felt so sad that you wanted to hurt yourself?" or "Do you have a plan and the means (gun, pills etc.) to hurt yourself?" Even if the patient says that he/she will not commit suicide but has suicidal thoughts and a specific plan using a lethal method, it is considered to be high risk.

—*Ilia Jbankov*

For Further Information:

Hazzard, William R., et al. *Principles of Geriatric Medicine and Gerontology.* 5th ed. New York: McGraw-Hill, 2003.

Jarvis, Carolyn. *Physical Examination and Health Assessment.* 5th ed. St. Louis: Saunders/Elsevier, 2008.

Lezak, Muriel D., et al. *Neuropsychological Assessment.* 4th ed. New York: Oxford University Press, 2004.

Snyderman, D., and B.W. Rovner. "Mental Status Examination in Primary Care: A Review." *American Family Physician* 80, no. 8 (2009): 809-814.

Strub, Richard L., and R. William Black. *The Mental Status Examination in Neurology.* 4th ed. Philadelphia: F.A. Davis, 2000.

Mercury poisoning

Disease/Disorder

Anatomy or system affected: Nervous system

Specialties and related fields: Environmental health, epidemiology, neurology, occupational health, pediatrics

Definition: Mercury is a naturally occurring element that can cause neurological damage in humans exposed to it.

Key terms:

methylmercury: a neurotoxin that is the form of mercury that accumulates most easily in biological tissues

neuropathy: any disease of the nervous system

Causes and Symptoms

Mercury is a metallic element once used in a wide variety of applications, ranging from industrial use in processing ore to serving as the indicator fluid in thermometers. In its pure form, mercury is a soft silver-colored metal with a melting point of a frigid -40 degrees Celsius. Consequently, mercury is liquid at room temperature. Mercury and mercury compounds such as methylmercury are known neurotoxins. Prolonged exposure to mercury, either through inhaling mercury vapors or through ingesting it as a contaminant in foodstuffs, will lead to permanent neurological damage. Ingested mercury can also irritate the gastrointestinal tract and has been known to damage kidneys.

Occupational neuropathy has long been anecdotally associated with mercury exposure. The phrase "mad as a hatter," for example, became common in the nineteenth century when workers in the hat industry developed tremors, slurred speech, and problems thinking clearly following exposure to fumes produced by the felting process. A mercury nitrate compound was used to remove animal hair from hides in hat factories. In some cases of long-term exposure, neuropathy progressed to the point where the sufferers experienced hallucinations.

Despite the widespread prevalence of occupational illness among hatters, the nineteenth century medical community did not recognize the dangers of mercury exposure. Mercury was, in fact, used for a variety of medical applications, ranging from treating syphilis to being applied as a topical antiseptic in the form of Mercurochrome. Mercurochrome continued to be used as late as the 1990s, although the Food and Drug Administration (FDA) ruled in 1998 that it would be treated as a "new drug," meaning that any company wishing to manufacture it for nationwide distribution had to submit it for FDA review first.

The mining industry also used mercury extensively. Mercury amalgamates readily with gold dust, making it heavier and causing it to sink into the bottom of rocker boxes as ore is washed as part of placer mining. During the California gold rush, at least 7,600 tons of mercury were deposited into Sierra Nevada streams. Similar amounts were used elsewhere globally, leading to large quantities of mercury being deposited on streambeds and ocean floors. That mercury is now making its way back into the environment in the form of methylmercury, the organic form of mercury that causes most concern among health care professionals today.

Methylmercury is formed when mercury forms a mercury-carbon compound through bacterial action. Manufactured methylmercury and dimethylmercury were common fungicides until the 1970s, when they were banned due to their toxicity.

Treatment and Therapy

With mercury poisoning, prevention is the best form of treatment. Occupational exposure to mercury rarely takes place, and the biggest risk of mercury poisoning today comes from its ingestion within the food chain. Methylmercury bioaccumulates readily and has been found in large concentrations in seafood such as tuna, swordfish, and shark. Numerous studies have shown that when pregnant women consume fish containing high levels of methylmercury the resulting mercury poisoning can cause permanent neurological damage to the developing fetus. Young children are also at risk of developing neuropathy if they eat fish with high mercury levels. This problem was first recognized in the 1970s, but did not become widely publicized until the early twenty-first century. Pregnant women, nursing mothers, and young children are all now advised to avoid some varieties of fish completely, while limiting their consumption of others.

Perspective and Prospects

Although the use of mercury for many applications was discontinued as evidence mounted regarding the dangers of mercury exposure, thimerosal, a mercury compound, continued to be used as a preservative in vaccines used in human medicine into the twenty-first century. In the 1990s, many parents became convinced that thimerosal, which metabolizes readily to ethylmercury, was responsible for the rising rate of autism in American children. Some health activists argued that the increase in autism in the late twentieth century correlated with the increase in the number of vaccines that young children received in the first few years of life. The use of thimerosal as a preservative was discontinued by manufacturers for most vaccines, with the exception of influenza, but research showed that vaccines were not the cause of autism.

One use of mercury that does continue despite several decades of debate over its safety is the application of mercury amalgam tooth fillings in dentistry. The typical "silver" tooth filling is actually 50 percent mercury. Health activists argue that the practice should be stopped, as mercury leaching from the filling into the body could lead to mercury poisoning. In 2002, the FDA concluded that research to date had shown no evidence of ill effects other than rare cases of allergic reactions.

Given the widespread dispersion of mercury into the environment through pollution from numerous industries, mercury exposure will continue to be a health issue for many generations to come. Marine estuaries and ocean floors, as well as inland lakes and rivers, remain contaminated, and methylmercury will continue to work its way up the food chain.

—Nancy Farm Mannikko, Ph.D.

See also Autism; Cavities; Dentistry; Dentistry, pediatric; Environmental diseases; Environmental health; Food poisoning; Immunization and vaccination; Lead poisoning; Nervous system; Neurology; Neurology, pediatric; Occupational health; Poisoning; Toxicology.

For Further Information:

Agency for Toxic Substances and Disease Registry. "Toxic Substances Portal—Mercury." *ATSDR*, February 12, 2013.

Booth, Shawn. "Mercury, Food Webs, and Marine Animals: Implications of Diet and Climate Change for Human Health." *Environmental Health Perspectives* 113, no. 5 (May, 2005): 521–526.

Clampet, Andrew P. "Methylmercury: Formation, Sources, and Health Effects." In *Environmental Health—Physical, Chemical and Biological Factors.* New York: Nova Science Publishers, 2011.

Davidson, Philip W., Gary J. Myers, and Bernard Weiss, eds. *Neurotoxicity and Developmental Disabilities.* New York: Elsevier, 2006.

Friberg, Lars. *Inorganic Mercury.* Geneva: World Health Organization, 1991.

McCoy, Krisha. "Mercury Toxicity." *Health Library*, April, 2013.

MedlinePlus. "Mercury." *MedlinePlus*, July 24, 2013.

US Environmental Protection Agency. "Mercury." *EPA*, July 9, 2013.

WHO Task Group on Environmental Health Criteria for Mercury. *Mercury: Environmental Aspects.* Geneva: World Health Organization, 1989.

MESENCHYMAL STEM CELLS

Treatment

Also known as: Bone marrow stromal stem cells, multipotent stromal cells

Anatomy or system affected: Arms, bones, cells, circulatory system, feet, hands, immune system, joints, knees, legs, ligaments, muscles, musculoskeletal system, spine, tendons

Specialties and related fields: Anesthesiology, biotechnology, orthopedics, plastic surgery, rheumatology, sports medicine

Definition: A self-renewing population of multipotent stem cells present in bone marrow and many other adult tissues.

Key terms:

bone marrow: the soft, highly vascular, fatty tissue inside most bone cavities, which is the source of red and white blood cells

bone marrow aspirate: the removal of a small quantity of bone marrow through a needle

cytokines: small proteins secreted by immune cells that affect cell activity and inflammation

fluoroscope: an instrument that can visualize the form and motion of the deep structures of the body by means of X-ray shadows projected on a fluorescent screen

meniscus: the crescent-shaped cartilage pads between the bottom of the thighbone (femur) and the top of the shinbone (tibia)

multipotent: the ability of particular progenitor cells to differentiate into multiple, but limited cell types

stem cells: undifferentiated cells from a multicellular organism that can self-renew and whose progeny can differentiate into other cell types

Indications and Procedures

Mesenchymal stem cells (MSCs) are multipotent stem cells that have the ability to differentiate into bone-making cells (osteoblasts), cartilage-making cells (chondrocytes), and fat-making cells (adipocytes). They are found in bone marrow (although MSCs constitute only 0.001-0.01 percent of total cells), fat, umbilical cord, muscle, connective tissue skin, and several other tissues. When grown in culture, MSCs adhere to plastic, are spindle-shaped, and express specific cell-surface proteins (CD73, CD90, and CD105).

Because of the ability of MSCs to make cartilage and bone, physicians have used them to treat joint problems that affect the knee, hip, shoulder, back, hand, and ankle, and nonunion

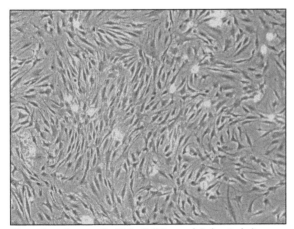

Mesenchymal stem cells. (ScienCell Research Laboratories)

fractures. MSC-based treatments begin with the isolation of bone marrow cells from a bone marrow aspirate. This aspirate is collected from the crest of the ilium of the pelvis with an elongated hollow alignment needle, after which the bone marrow stem cells are concentrated in the laboratory through centrifugation. After concentration, these stem cells are re-injected into the injured area in combination with growth factors from blood platelets taken from peripheral blood. The stem cell injections are not done blindly. Magnetic resonance images (MRIs) of the joint show exactly where the stem cells should go and the injections themselves are guided by means of real-time fluoroscopy or musculoskeletal ultrasound. By placing MSCs directly at the site of the injury, the MSCs can replace damaged cartilage or heal partially torn tendons.

Fat-derived MSCs and associated fat cells (adipocytes) are also being used in plastic surgery to treat facial, breast, and body contour deformities for both reconstructive and aesthetic purposes. Fat for plastic surgery is harvested by means of liposuction and processed by centrifugation. The processed fat is then injected into the desired space.

Uses and Complications

For orthopedic purposes, MSCs can be used to treat osteoarthritis of the knees, hips, shoulders, ankles, and hands. They can also be used to treat partially, but not completely, torn, ligaments, meniscus tears of the knee, and labrum tears and rotator cuff injuries of the shoulder. Generally, MSC administration causes few side effects. Swelling and pain at the site of injection and discomfort from the bone marrow aspiration are some of the most common side effects. Also, if MSCs donated by someone else are injected, there is the possibility that the patient's immune system might reject them. Tumor formation as a result of MSC treatment has not been observed in humans.

Fat-based MSCs and adipocytes for plastic surgery are used to reestablish body contours after injury, surgery, or disease, or to reconstruct the face after an accident or corrective surgery or the breasts after mastectomies. For aesthetic treatments, fat transplantations can remove wrinkles, augment the size of the breast or buttocks, or create new body contours. Complications associated with fat transplantation include infections, and if the fat-based MSCs are mixed with the wrong materials, they can form ectopic bone. Fat transplantation into the breast can cause lumps that calcify. Also, the death of transplanted fat cells (fat necrosis) can produce small calcifications and palpable lumps, which can increase the opacity of the breast and interfere with mammographic scans. No evidence exists to support the concern that transplanting fat into the breast increases the risk of breast cancer, but animal experiments suggest that MSCs can augment the growth of preexisting tumors.

Because MSCs have the ability to suppress the function of immune cells and inflammation through the secretion of cytokines, they have been used to treat autoimmune diseases on an experimental basis. Autoimmune diseases result from an inappropriate immune response against normal cells. Such diseases as Crohn's disease, multiple sclerosis, systemic lupus erythematosis, scleroderma, and graft-versus-host disease have all been treated experimentally with MSCs administered either intravenously or injected directly into damaged tissues. The rationale behind the use of MSCs to treat these diseases, which are characterized by chronic inflammation, is to suppress inflammation so that the damaged tissues and organs can heal and regain their normal level of function.

Perspective and Prospects

Experiments that demonstrated the bone-making capacity of bone-free bone marrow date from the nineteenth century; Tavassoli and Crosby in 1968 and Friedenstein and others in the 1960s and '70s confirmed these results and showed that a bone marrow stem cell population distinct from blood-making stem cells synthesized bone.

Many clinical trials to evaluate the safety and efficacy of MSC treatments are underway. In such trials, MSCs have been used to treat liver disease, fragile bone disease (osteogenesis imperfecta), heart disease, and several other maladies. Genetically engineered MSCs have also been successfully tested in animal models and show remarkable healing potential. MSCs presently represent one of the most fruitful areas of medical research.

—*Michael A Buratovich, Ph.D.*

See also Genetic engineering; Inflammation; Orthopedics; Systemic eclerosis

For Further Information:

Buratovich, Michael A. *The Stem Cell Epistles: Letters to My Students about Bioethics, Stem Cells, and Fertility Treatments.* Eugene, OR: Cascade Books, 2013.

Centeno, Christopher J., *The Stem Cells They Don't Want You to Have: How the New Stem Cell Debate Will Shape the Future of Medicine.* Seattle: Amazon Digital Services, Inc., 2012.

Centeno, Christopher J., and Stephen J. Faulkner. "The Use of Mesenchymal Stem Cells in Orthopedics." *Stem Cells and Cancer Stem Cells.* Vol. 1, edited by M.A. Hayat. New York: Springer, 2012.

Rosing, James H., Granger Wong, Michael S. Wong, David Sahar, Thomas R. Stevenson, and Lee L. Q. Pu. "Autologous Fat Grafting for Primary Breast Augmentation: A Systematic Review." *Aesthetic Plastic Surgery* 35 (2011): 882-890.

MESOTHELIOMA

Disease/Disorder

Anatomy or system affected: Abdomen, lungs, respiratory system

Specialties and related fields: General surgery, occupational health, oncology, pathology, pharmacology, preventive medicine, pulmonary medicine, radiology

Definition: A malignancy originating from the mesothelial surfaces (the lining cells) of the pleural and peritoneal cavities, the pericardium, or the tunica vaginalis. The distribution of mesothelioma may be unifocal or multifocal or may involve the lining cells in a continuous manner. Approximately 80 to 90 percent of all cases have a pleural origin (malignant pleural mesothelioma).

Key terms:

asbestos: a term for a group of naturally occurring silicate minerals with long, thin fibers

ascites: accumulation of fluid in the peritoneal cavity

chemotherapy: treatment of disease by chemicals; usually, systemic therapy of some types of cancer

dyspnea: difficulty or shortness of breathing

pericardium: a fluid-filled conical sac of fibrous tissue that surrounds the heart and the roots of the great blood vessels

peritoneum: a serous membrane that forms the lining of the abdominal cavity

pleura: a serous membrane that covers and protects the lungs

Causes and Symptoms

Mesothelioma is directly attributable to occupational asbestos exposure, with a history of exposure in more than 90 percent of cases. Para-occupational exposure (for example, women whose husbands work in an asbestos environment) has also been suggested. Idiopathic or spontaneous mesothelioma has been reported to occur in the absence of any exposure to asbestos. Other types of mineral fibers, such as erionite or tremolite, have also been shown to induce mesothelioma. The causative role of radiation, genetic factors, and Simian virus 40 is under investigation.

Mesothelioma usually occurs in the fifth to seventh decades of life, and 70 to 80 percent of cases occur in men. Rarely, it can be diagnosed between the ages of twenty and forty; these individuals usually have a history of childhood exposure to asbestos. In industrial countries, the incidence of mesothelioma is 2 in 1 million per year among women and 10 to 30 in 1 million per year among men.

The primary sites of mesothelioma include the pleura (about 90 percent), the peritoneum (about 5 percent), and the pericardium (0.4 percent). Pleural mesothelioma spreads via the fissures of the pleura to encase the lung surfaces. Peritoneal mesothelioma rapidly spreads within the confines of the abdominal cavity to involve most accessible peritoneal and omental surfaces.

Chest pain and/or dyspnea are the typical presenting features of pleural mesothelioma. Pleuritic-type pain can occur in the presence of pleural effusions. Involvement of the mediastinal structures, hoarseness of the voice, and superior vena caval obstruction is possible. Dysphagia (difficulty swallowing) is usually a late finding. Hemoptysis (coughing up blood), lymphadenopathy, and metastatic symptoms are rare. Additional features include chest wall mass, fatigue, fever, sweats, and weight loss. Very rarely, patients may be asymptomatic.

Peritoneal involvement may be found in up to one-third of mesothelioma cases at autopsy. Peritoneal mesothelioma presents with nonspecific symptoms such as loss of appetite, nausea and vomiting, diarrhea or constipation, and, occasionally, ascites (fluid build-up between the abdominal lining and organs). Small bowel obstruction is a late feature.

Physical examination is usually unremarkable except for signs of pleural effusion and pleural thickening as a result of tumor infiltration. Infiltration of the pericardium can result in

---

Information on Mesothelioma

Causes: Primarily occupational asbestos exposure; role played by radiation, genetic factors, possibly simian virus 40

Symptoms: Chest pain, dyspnea, fatigue, fever, sweats, dysphagia and weight loss (pleural mesothelioma); loss of appetite, nausea, vomiting, diarrhea or constipation, ascites (peritoneal mesothelioma)

Duration: Fatal in four to eight months if untreated; survival of sixteen to nineteenth months with treatment

Treatments: Surgery, radiotherapy, chemotherapy

---

signs of cardiac tamponade, compression of the heart because of fluid buildup. Blood tests can reveal an elevated erythrocyte sedimentation rate. Immunohistochemical markers calretinin, WT-1, and cytokeratin are established diagnostic markers. Osteopontin and mesothelin have recently been introduced as new markers for mesothelioma.

Diagnosis is based on the combination of accurate history, examination, radiology, and laboratory testing. Radiological imaging is essential for the diagnosis, staging, and management of mesothelioma. x-rays, computed tomography (CT), magnetic resonance imaging (MRI), and positron emission tomography (PET) can be used to evaluate the disease. In most cases, mesothelioma is readily identified or strongly suspected on routine hematoxylin-eosin histology. The three major histological patterns are sarcomatous, epithelial, and mixed (biphasic).

Treatment and Therapy

Management under a multidisciplinary team consisting of respiratory physicians, oncologists, radiologists, palliative care physicians, and lung cancer specialist nurses should be offered to all patients with mesothelioma. It generally includes multimodality treatment options that combine surgery, chemotherapy, and radiation.

Surgical resection and radiotherapy represent the standard treatment in a patient with resectable malignant pleural mesothelioma. The three most common surgical procedures used are pleurodesis, debulking surgery (cytoreductive surgery or pleurectomy/decortication) and extrapleural pneumonectomy. Radiation therapy can be used to control local tumor growth or as a prophylaxis to reduce the incidence of recurrence and pain at sites of diagnostic or therapeutic instrument insertion, or as part of multimodal definitive treatment. In some cases, it may lead to regression of the disease. Chemotherapy is used to reduce the incidence of distant metastases, to lengthen survival, to improve quality of life, and to provide symptomatic relief. Drugs with single-agent activity include pemetrexed, raltitrexed, vinorelbine, and vinflunine. The addition of pemetrexed or raltitrexed to cisplatin has been shown to prolong survival. For patients with unresectable mesothelioma, the combination of cisplatin and pemetrexed or ralitrexed is the standard treatment.

Most patients need palliation of symptoms early on in the course of the disease and recognition of this by the patient, family, and primary care physician, together with end-of-life care, are essential in the management of patients with mesothelioma.

Life expectancy is poor, with median survival between eight and fourteen months after diagnosis. Identified and verified indicators of poor prognosis include nonepithelioid histology, poor performance status, chest pain, age older than seventy-five, male gender, white blood cell count of 8.3 × 109/liters or greater, platelets greater than 400,000 microliters (μL), and a lactate dehydrogenase (LDH) test of 500 international units per liter (IU/L). With surgery, radiotherapy, and chemotherapy, the survival may be sixteen to nineteen months. In general, the prognosis of peritoneal mesothelioma is worse than that for pleural mesothelioma, with a mean survival time of about seven months.

Perspective and Prospects

Asbestos is considered the main cause of mesothelioma in the Western world. The link between asbestos exposure and mesothelioma was not recognized until 1960, when the disease was first described in South African asbestos miners. The insulating properties of asbestos, however, have been known long before. The pathogenetic role of asbestos has been linked to its ability to cause the release of tumor necrosis factor alpha and other cytokines and growth factors, and to generate mutagenic oxygen radicals from exposed mesothelial cells and nearby macrophages. As of 2009, approximately two thousand to three thousand cases of mesothelioma occur in the United States annually. In 2011, the World Health Organization released results of a study of mesothelioma deaths recorded in the WHO mortality database between 1994 and 2008. During this period, a total of 92,253 deaths from the disease were reported in 83 countries. The incidence of mesothelioma is expected to peak between 2010 and 2020 due to the long latency period (thirty-five to forty-five years after asbestos exposure). Cases of mesothelioma are also expected in those exposed to dust created by the collapse of the Twin Towers in New York following the terrorist attacks of September 11, 2001, particularly among first responders.

Over the past decade, significant advances have been made toward an improved ability to diagnose and stage the disease, define the prognosis, and treat mesothelioma. Novel treatment modalities such as intrapleural chemotherapy, photodynamic therapy, and hyperthermic perfusion have already been used with some success. Immunomodulating, cytokine-targeted treatments (antigrowth factor drugs), and gene therapy are currently under investigation worldwide. These experimental treatments may in the future be combined with standard therapy in multimodality protocols.

—Katia Marazova, M.D., Ph.D.

See also Asbestos exposure; Cancer; Chronic obstructive pulmonary disease (COPD); Environmental diseases; Environmental health; Interstitial pulmonary fibrosis (IPF); Lung cancer; Lungs; Occupational health; Pulmonary diseases; Pulmonary medicine; Pulmonary medicine, pediatric.

For Further Information:

Belli, C., et al. "Malignant Pleural Mesothelioma: Current Treatments and Emerging Drugs." *Expert Opinion on Emerging Drugs* 14, no. 3 (September, 2009): 423–437.

Delgermaa, Vanya, et. al. "Global Mesothelioma Deaths Reported to the World Health Organization between 1994 and 2008." *Bulletin of the World Health Organization*, June 13, 2011.

Hesdorffer, M. E., et al. "Peritoneal Mesothelioma." *Current Treatment Options in Oncology* 9, nos. 2/3 (June, 2008): 180–190.

MedlinePlus. "Mesothelioma." *MedlinePlus*, April 10, 2013.

Ray, M., and H. L. Kindler. "Malignant Pleural Mesothelioma: An Update on Biomarkers and Treatment." *Chest* 136, no. 3 (September, 2009): 888–896.

Smith, Natalie. "Pleural Mesothelioma." *Health Library*, September 1, 2011.

Tsao, A. S., et al. "Malignant Pleural Mesothelioma." *Journal of Clinical Oncology* 27, no. 12 (April, 2009): 2081–2090.

Yang, H., J. R. Testa, and M. Carbone. "Mesothelioma Epidemiology, Carcinogenesis, and Pathogenesis." *Current Treatment Options in Oncology* 9, nos. 2-3 (June, 2008): 147–157.

Zervos, M. D., C. Bizekis, and H. I. Pass. "Malignant Mesothelioma 2008." *Current Opinion in Pulmonary Medicine* 14, no. 4 (July, 2008): 303–309.

METABOLIC DISORDERS

Disease/Disorder

Anatomy or system affected: All

Specialties and related fields: Biochemistry, endocrinology, genetics, nutrition, pediatrics, perinatology

Definition: Disorders resulting from alterations in the pathways by which the body derives energy and synthesizes other molecules from carbohydrates, lipids, and proteins in food; usually caused by genetic defects that result in a missing or faulty enzyme.

Key terms:

anabolic: the metabolic processes by which small molecules are combined to produce larger molecules; used for energy storage or growth of the organism

catabolic: the metabolic processes by which food and stored products are broken down to release energy for use by the cell

enzyme: a protein whose job is to enable chemical reactions to occur in the cell in a timely manner; a biological catalyst

essential: referring to an amino acid, lipid, or vitamin that is necessary for proper cell functioning, but which the human body is ordinarily unable to produce on its own; must be supplied through the diet

metabolism: the process of extracting energy that can be used to power the cells of the body; includes both anabolic and catabolic processes

prenatal/neonatal screening: a tool whereby small volume fluid samples (prenatal) or blood samples (neonatal) are drawn and studied to determine the genetic traits carried by the child; neonatal screening is often mandated by law and used to find metabolic diseases as early in life as possible

Causes and Symptoms

Metabolic disorders of all types are usually inherited from one or both parents who carry a defective gene; the gene is one that codes for an enzyme responsible for a part of the metabolic pathway (either anabolic or catabolic). Much like an assembly line that takes raw material and produces a final product through multiple steps, the metabolism of proteins, lipids, and carbohydrates in the human body requires multiple steps, each with its own enzyme. In some cases, there are multiple pathways to metabolize a particular starting product. In this case, lack of one enzyme may not have a dramatic effect. Other pathways are exclusive, however, and any disruption of an enzyme will lead to disease. In addition to loss of a particular product, some enzyme defects lead to the accumulation of precursor molecules that may be toxic or may interfere with normal function of the cell.

When the deoxyribonucleic acid (DNA) coding for a particular gene is altered, one of three outcomes may be seen: no change (silent mutation), partial loss of ability of the enzyme to do its job (mild disease), or complete loss of enzyme function (mild to severe disease). Diseases in the human are not known for all enzymes that could potentially be lost; this is most likely because disruption of an enzyme that is absolutely necessary in early development of the fetus will lead to early (and undetected) loss of the fetus.

Disorders of metabolism may be classified according to the pathways that are disrupted. Disorders associated with protein/amino acid metabolism may be seen when amino acids cannot be effectively broken down or when they cannot be transported into the cells of the body for use in building new proteins. Most of these disorders are seen early in life, since many proteins are essential for growth and development of the body. Examples of amino acid metabolism disorders are phenylketonuria (PKU) and maple syrup urine disease (MSUD). Other amino acid/protein disorders are homocystinuria, citrullinemia, alkaptonuria, and tyrosinemia.

Phenylalanine is an essential amino acid involved in the production of tyrosine, which in turn is converted to dopamine and serotonin. In PKU, the absence of this conversion means that phenylalanine accumulates in the body, causing toxic reactions within the brain and other organs. Mental retardation is the most obvious effect of this toxicity; other symptoms may include seizures, skin rashes, nausea and vomiting, and aggressive behavior. Phenylacetate (a byproduct of excess phenylalanine) is secreted in sweat and urine, giving a distinctive odor to the child.

Leucine, isoleucine, and valine are amino acids that have a branched side chain. As a result of the presence of this special shape, an enzyme that can convert these enzymes is needed in order to metabolize food containing them. In MSUD, that enzyme is absent or deficient and these amino acids accumulate in the urine, giving a distinctive smell for which the disorder is named. If left untreated, this can lead to vomiting, staggering, confusion, coma, and eventual death from degeneration of the developing nerves early in life. A total of six different genes are responsible for production of the branched-chain alpha-ketoacid dehydrogenase enzyme complex, thus leading to some variation in the severity of the disease. While this disease is rare in the general population, the Mennonite com-

---

Information on Metabolic Disorders

Causes: Missing or faulty enzymes
Symptoms: Depends on enzyme affected; may include mental retardation, seizures, rashes, nausea, vomiting, coma, delayed development, organ damage, paralysis, dementia, blindness
Duration: Chronic and often fatal
Treatments: Ranges from none to dietary restrictions to enzyme therapy

---

munity of Pennsylvania has a high rate of carriers for these mutations and thus is particularly affected.

Lipids (fats) are used in numerous ways in the human body, including for energy, temperature regulation, cell membrane structure, and nerve function. A variety of enzymes are responsible for breaking down and processing both stored and dietary lipids. In the absence of efficient processing of lipids, accumulations occur that can be extremely harmful to the organs of the body. Examples of lipid metabolism disorders are fatty acid oxidation disorders and Tay-Sachs disease. Other lipid metabolism disorders include Gaucher's disease, Refsum disease, Niemann-Pick disease, Tangier disease, carnitine uptake defect, and trifunctional protein deficiency.

Several enzymes are involved in pathways that help stored lipids to be broken down and turned into energy. In the most common fatty acid oxidation disorder the enzyme deficient in this pathway is medium-chain acyl-coenzyme A dehydrogenase (MCAD). This is one of the most common errors of metabolism among people of northern European descent. A buildup of acyl-coenzyme A leads to delayed development, heart muscle weakness, and enlarged liver; death may occur. Symptoms develop shortly after birth and are most severe if the child goes without food for a prolonged period of time, or following exercise and the need for more energy to the cells (thus triggering the lipid breakdown pathways).

Perhaps the best known of the lipid metabolism disorders, Tay-Sachs disease results from errors in the enzyme β-hexosaminidase, which is responsible for breaking down the lipid GM2 ganglioside. The gene for this enzyme is known to reside on chromosome 15, and the absence of this enzyme allows large amounts of the ganglioside to accumulate in neurons. This accumulation leads to neurodegeneration that often results in floppy muscle tone, then paralysis, dementia, blindness, and death by age three or four. Less severe forms lead to long-term problems in the nervous system that progress throughout life. Tay-Sachs disease is most commonly seen in the Ashkenazi Jewish community but is also seen in the French Canadian population of Quebec and the Cajun population of Louisiana.

Carbohydrates (especially glucose) are the principal fuels for the body on a daily basis. Carbohydrate metabolism requires a variety of intracellular enzymes, as well as those responsible for transport and entry into the cell. Diseases or disorders of carbohydrate metabolism can be quite severe. Examples of carbohydrate metabolism disorders are type 1 diabetes mellitus and glycogen storage diseases.

The ability to get glucose (the primary carbohydrate) into the cells of the body requires the hormone insulin. A lack in the production of insulin in the pancreas (type 1 diabetes) leads to hyperglycemia (high blood levels of glucose) and a lack of glucose for energy within the cells. In addition to lack of cellular energy, this can lead to increased risk of blindness, heart disease, kidney failure, neurological diseases, and problems with circulation in the extremities. Type 1 diabetes may result from any one of several known mutations in DNA, the most common of which has been tracked to chromosome 6. In some forms of type 1 diabetes, the body attacks either the insulin or the pancreatic cells that produce it, making this an autoimmune disease.

Glycogen is the branched-chain storage form of glucose in the liver and muscles of the body. Glycogen storage diseases are actually a group of eleven similar diseases that result in the inability of the body to produce sufficient glucose for the bloodstream to be used by cells of the body to produce energy. In addition to low blood sugar levels, children with these diseases often have enlarged livers, swollen abdomens, and weak muscles. Elevated levels of lipids in the blood (taking the place of glucose as an energy source), may lead to acidosis and stress on the heart and kidneys.

In addition to the transport, storage, and breakdown of proteins, lipids, and carbohydrates, metabolism involves alterations in the use of elements such as iron and copper and the synthesis, storage, and use of the components of DNA and ribonucleic acid (RNA). Diseases and disorders in each of these areas are known as well. Examples include Wilson disease, Menkes disease, hereditary hemochromatosis, and Lesch-Nyhan syndrome.

Copper is necessary in cells for energy metabolism, bone production, and nerve maturation. Wilson disease and Menkes disease are disorders of copper transport and absorption that lead to a buildup of copper to toxic levels in the liver and the brain. Both liver disease and neurological damage can be present if they are not diagnosed early on; eventually, toxicity can be seen in many other organs as well. Menkes disease is usually fatal during infancy. Both diseases have been mapped to chromosome 13 and appear to be the result of proteins that are part of a transmembrane pump system. Menkes disease is transmitted as an X-linked recessive trait, while Wilson's disease is autosomal recessive.

Hereditary hemochromatosis is a disorder of iron metabolism seen predominantly in those of Northern European, Caucasian descent and traceable to a mutation on chromosome 6. Because iron is not adequately metabolized, the levels stored in the body grow over time, leading to symptoms that include cirrhosis of the liver, cardiomyopathy (heart muscle disease), alterations in skin pigmentation, joint damage, and decreased functioning of the gonads. Because men generally retain iron better than women do, symptoms often occur earlier in men. Symptoms also occur early in alcoholics, as alcohol consumption affects uptake of dietary iron.

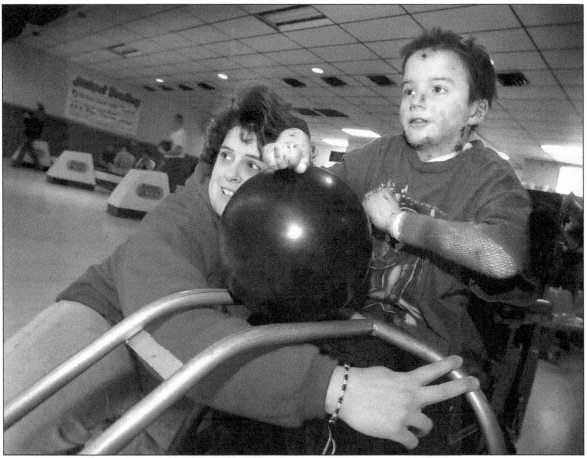

This child suffers from an incurable inborn metabolic error known as epidermolysis bullosa, which makes his skin blister at the touch. (AP/ Wide World Photos)

Both DNA and RNA are constructed in part from nitrogen-containing bases; these bases are chemically grouped as purines and pyrimidines. The body can both make and recycle these bases. One of the genes involved in the recycling of purines (HPRT1) is located on the X chromosome. In Lesch-Nyhan syndrome, several known mutations result in low levels of the enzyme, and thus a lack of purine recycling. The resulting disease is seen almost exclusively in males and causes accumulation of uric acid (the starting point in purine synthesis). Uric acid leads to gout (painful deposits in the skin and joints) and kidney stones. For unknown reasons, this enzyme deficiency also leads to self-mutilation (biting of the fingers and tongue). Severe muscle weakness and mental retardation generally occur.

Treatment and Therapy

The most important diagnostic tool available for metabolic disorders is routine neonatal genetic screening. In 2005, a report by the American College of Medical Genetics recommended a core panel of twenty-eight metabolic disorders that should be screened for in all newborn children. This list includes disorders of protein metabolism, carbohydrate metabolism, and lipid metabolism, as well as a few multisystem disorders. Such screening does not prevent disorders but does allow early detection and therefore early intervention with diet, drugs, and other regimens that allow extended life spans for those afflicted. As of 2013, newborn screening in the United States varies from state to state, with most states testing for more than thirty disorders.

Once detected, treatment of metabolic disorders is quite varied and is related to the underlying cause of the disorder. For protein/amino acid disorders, dietary restrictions are a key element in treatment. For instance, in PKU, phenylalanine intake must be restricted starting in the first few weeks of life. This means elimination of most forms of natural protein and substitution with phenylalanine-free foods. Patients with homocysteinuria often improve with vitamin B_6 (pyridoxine) or vitamin B_{12} (cobalamin). In maple syrup urine disease, restricting the dietary intake of the three branched-chain amino acids to the minimal amount required for growth and development allows for the best improvement. Vitamin B_1 (thiamine) is helpful in those with mild disease; dialysis is used in those with severe disease. Gene therapy is a possibility in the future.

In lipid disorders, control of diet is also essential. With fatty acid oxidation disorders it is important that patients eat often, never skip meals, and consume a diet high in carbohydrates and low in lipids. Treatment with intravenous glucose is helpful during attacks. The long-term outcome is very good in those who follow a strict dietary regimen. Likewise, in Refsum disease, a diet with little or no phytanic acid (carefully controlled plant products that contain no chlorophyll) is the key; plasmapheresis may be also be helpful. Other lipid disorders, including Gaucher's and Tay-Sachs, require drug intervention. Gaucher's type I patients (especially those without nervous system damage) can be treated with enzyme replacement therapy; the modified enzyme is given intravenously every two weeks. Enzyme therapy has been shown to stop, and even reverse, many of the symptoms of this disease. The late-onset (less severe) form of Tay-Sachs has seen some promise from treatment with a ganglioside synthesis inhibitor. Treatment of the infantile form has shown little promise, since much of the neurological damage occurs prior to birth and reversing neurological damage that has already occurred has proven to be extremely difficult.

Type 1 diabetes can usually be controlled well with daily insulin (artificial) and control of diet (to match the amount of energy needed for daily activities). Although islet cell transplantation or immunosuppression has been on the drawing board for several years, no real success has yet been obtained.

Other metabolic disorders run the gamut from easy to impossible to treat. Hereditary hemochromatosis, for instance, is easy to control, with therapeutic phlebotomy (blood-letting) to remove excess iron that has built up. Early diagnosis and treatment leads to a normal life span. By contrast, there is no cure for Niemann-Pick disease, and these children generally die of infection or degeneration of the central nervous system. For Menkes disease, administration of copper histidinate has shown promise, but it increases the patient's life span only by a few years (less than ten). In Lesch-Nyhan syndrome, medications are used to decrease the levels of uric acid; restraint against self-mutilation is commonly needed. Advances in gene therapy look promising for several of these conditions as well.

Perspective and Prospects

Metabolic disorders have existed since the earliest humans roamed the earth, but it was not until the early twentieth century that the mechanism for these disorders was recognized. The term "inborn error of metabolism" was coined by Archibold Garrod, a British physician who published a classic text on the subject in 1923, following a study of children with alkaptonuria. This was the first such treatise to explain how symptoms often seen in sickly children could be explained on the basis of enzyme defects. Many of these diseases, such as diabetes, had been well established and named years before but not yet understood in terms of their biochemistry. The genetic basis for these disorders was not determined until much later—the 1970s and beyond.

Another early pioneer in this field was the German pediatrician Albert Niemann, who in 1914 described in detail a child with nervous system impairment. This condition later became known as Niemann-Pick disease, when Luddwick Pick took tissue samples from several such children after their deaths and provided chemical evidence of a distinct lipid storage problem.

The discovery of insulin in the 1920s provided the first opportunity to treat a metabolic disease in a standardized way, as insulin could be extracted and purified in a controlled laboratory setting. The availability of insulin has saved millions of lives since its discovery.

The hope for the future is gene therapy. The first gene therapy successes were recorded in children with enzyme deficiencies, and there are many trials throughout the world aimed at improving the chances of survival and healthy lives of those with similar metabolic disorders through correction of the genetic defect. In the future, such therapy might even be available in utero.

—*Kerry L. Cheesman, Ph.D.*

See also Arthritis; Diabetes mellitus; Digestion; Endocrinology; Endocrinology, pediatric; Enzyme therapy; Enzymes; Fatty acid oxidation disorders; Food biochemistry; Fructosemia; Gastroenterology; Gastroenterology, pediatric; Gastrointestinal system; Gaucher's disease; Genetic diseases; Glands; Glycogen storage diseases; Glycolysis; Gout; Hemochromatosis; Hormones; Kidney disorders; Lipids; Maple syrup urine disease (MSUD); Mental retardation; Metabolic syndrome; Metabolism; Mucopolysaccharidosis (MPS); Niemann-Pick disease; Nonalcoholic steatohepatitis (NASH); Obesity; Obesity, childhood; Phenylketonuria (PKU); Tay-Sachs disease; Wilson's disease.

For Further Information:

Gilbert, Hiram F. *Basic Concepts in Biochemistry.* 2d ed. New York: McGraw-Hill, 2002.

National Institute of General Medical Sciences (US). *The Structures of Life.* Bethesda, Md.: US Department of Health and Human Services, Public Health Service, National Institutes of Health, National Institute of General Medical Sciences, 2007. NIH publication no. 07-2778.

MedlinePlus. "Metabolic Disorders." *MedlinePlus*, May 21, 2013.

National Newborn Screening and Global Resource Center. "Families: Newborn Screening." *NNSGRC: National Newborn Screening & Global Resource Center*, April 22, 2013.

Nussbaum, Robert L., et. al.. *Thompson and Thompson Genetics in Medicine.* 7th ed. Philadelphia: Saunders/Elsevier, 2007.

Scriver, Charles R., et al., eds. *The Metabolic and Molecular Bases of Inherited Disease.* 8th ed. New York: McGraw-Hill, 2002.

Wheeler, Patricia G. "Newborn Screening Tests." *KidsHealth from Nemours*, September 2012.

METABOLIC SYNDROME

Disease/Disorder

Also known as: Insulin resistance syndrome, Syndrome X, Deadly Quartet

Anatomy or system affected: All

Specialties and related fields: Cardiology, endocrinology, internal medicine, nutrition

Definition: A constellation of metabolic changes that affect most major organ systems and may impinge on practically all systems of the body, often beginning with excess weight or obesity.

Key terms:

atherosclerosis: fat deposition and pathologic changes in the arterial surface and walls of major blood vessels of the body

diabetes mellitus type 2: peripheral resistance to insulin and increases in serum glucose and insulin concentrations, with damage to arteries in various organs

dyslipidemia: abnormal blood lipid levels, especially characterized by high serum triglycerides and very low-density lipoproteins (VLDLs) and depressed serum high-density lipoprotein (HDL) cholesterol

hyperinsulinemia: an abnormally high serum insulin concentration

obese: having a body mass index (BMI), calculated as weight in kilograms divided by height in meters squared, that is greater than 30

overweight: having a BMI that is between 25 and 29.9

steatohepatitis: an increased fat content in the liver independent of alcohol consumption

Causes and Symptoms

Metabolic syndrome is a complex medical disorder. According to guidelines issued by the National Cholesterol Education Program/Adult Treatment Panel III (NCEP/ATP III), diagnosis of metabolic syndrome is made when an individual displays at least three of the following risk factors: abdominal obesity, elevated triglycerides, low levels of the high-density lipoprotein (HDL) type of cholesterol, high blood pressure, and the presence of more than 100 milligrams per deciliter (mg/dL) of glucose in the blood after fasting.

The National Heart, Lung, and Blood Institute (NHLBI) estimates that as many as forty-seven million adults in the United States suffer from metabolic syndrome, which is around 25 percent of the total adult population. A study published in *National Health Statistics Reports* in May 2009 reported that 34 percent of the study's 3,423 adults aged twenty and older met the criteria for metabolic syndrome. Age plays a large role in metabolic syndrome, with the likelihood of being diagnosed increasing as an individual gets older. Total body weight is also an indicator of the likelihood of the metabolic syndrome criteria being met. Males who are overweight are six times as likely as normal-weight males to be diagnosed with metabolic syndrome, and those who are obese are thirty-two times as likely.

In females, being overweight leads to a fivefold increase in the chances of being diagnosed with metabolic syndrome and obesity a seventeen-fold increase, compared to women of normal weight. Disturbingly, metabolic syndrome is now being recognized in children and adolescents; this is probably related to the increase in obesity and type 2 diabetes mellitus seen in this age group over recent years. There is also evidence to demonstrate a genetic component to metabolic syndrome; further research will clarify this.

Key aspects of the metabolic syndrome are an energy imbalance and resultant altered metabolic pathways. The abnor-

---

Information on Metabolic Syndrome

Causes: Unknown; possibly poor utilization of glucose and abnormal cellular metabolism

Symptoms: Lipid abnormalities, insulin resistance, abdominal obesity, high blood pressure; may result in diabetes, heart disease, stroke, colon cancer, nonalcoholic steatohepatitis (NASH), polycystic ovary disease, chronic renal failure

Duration: Chronic

Treatments: Weight loss, diet modification, drug therapy

---

mal metabolic reactions seen in metabolic syndrome confer an increased risk for type 2 diabetes mellitus and cardiovascular disease (CVD). Several other diseases—colon cancer, nonalcoholic steatohepatitis (NASH), polycystic ovary disease, and chronic renal failure—can also be a consequence of this syndrome.

The National Health and Nutrition Examination Survey determined that the most prevalent risk factor displayed by individuals with metabolic syndrome is abdominal obesity. This is when fat is stored in the abdominal region of the body as opposed to in the buttocks and thighs. People with abdominally stored fat are often said to have "apple" type bodies; those with fat stored lower, in the buttocks and thighs, are said to be "pear" shaped. Men are typically apples and women are pears. Cortisol is a stress response hormone that promotes fat deposition in the abdominal area in individuals with chronic stress. Nearly all cases of overweight and obesity, including abdominal obesity, are due to excess calorific intake (overeating) combined with a sedentary lifestyle. In the United States, around one-third of the adult population is obese. Obesity greatly increases the risk for type 2 diabetes and cardiovascular disease.

Abnormal levels of fats in the blood is called dyslipidemia. In people who are overweight or obese, the levels of lipids in the body are so high that the pathways involved in fat synthesis and breakdown cannot keep up, and chronically high blood lipids are seen.

In addition, due to impaired insulin action and incorrect handling of glucose by their cells, individuals with type 2 diabetes tend to have high levels of blood triglyceride and low HDL cholesterol levels. This puts type 2 diabetics and obese individuals at high risk for CVD.

The second most prevalent factor seen in patients diagnosed with metabolic syndrome is hypertension, or high blood pressure. One in four Americans suffers from hypertension. If untreated, it can lead to CVD and kidney failure. The atherosclerotic process is accelerated in the metabolic syndrome and in type 2 diabetes because of the presence of multiple metabolic abnormalities. In insulin resistance, plaque formation may be enhanced because of the increased expression of adhesion molecules on endothelial cells and an increased rate of monocyte adhesion to endothelial cells. Circulating plasminogen is also more likely activated, which typically leads to increased clotting. In addition, hypertension may contribute to an increased risk of stroke in those with the metabolic syndrome.

The third most prevalent factor is hyperglycemia, or impaired fasting glucose. To satisfy the criterion for metabolic syndrome the glucose level in the blood after fasting must be over 100 mg/dl. A person with 100 to 125 mg/dl would be considered prediabetic, and diabetes is diagnosed when the fasting level of glucose is 126 mg/dl or above. Increases in blood glucose are indicative of a phenomenon called insulin resistance. Here, the cells of the body do not respond properly to insulin, and as a result glucose cannot enter the cells for use or storage so it remains in the circulating blood. Chronically elevated blood glucose concentration permits glucose molecules to combine with diverse proteins in the body, including hemoglobin within red blood cells, by a process known as glycation or glycosylation. Glycation also leads to blood vessels becoming rigid, a factor that contributes to CVD.

Any one of the risk factors listed on the NCEP/ATP III guidelines can cause chronic health problems, specifically type 2 diabetes mellitus and CVD. Diagnosis of metabolic syndrome requires that at least three out of the five criteria are met. This translates into a vastly increased risk for these chronic health problems; the reason why the life span of individuals diagnosed with metabolic syndrome is an average of fourteen years shorter than those without the disease.

Treatment and Therapy

Treatment strategies for the metabolic syndrome focus on weight loss through a comprehensive program utilizing behavioral changes, including improved nutrition and an increase in physical activities. The long-term goal of therapy is a better balance between the intake of food energy sources and energy expenditure, so that a healthier body weight can be achieved. Dietary treatment typically requires the involvement of nutritionists and registered dieticians to provide educational information and institute changes in food selection.

Physicians provide overall care, and concomitant with lifestyle changes use the prescription of medications for one or more of the components of metabolic syndrome. Metformin is a drug used to treat type 2 diabetes mellitus; it works by improving insulin action, and has also been shown to stop the development of impaired fasting glucose to type 2 diabetes in patients with metabolic syndrome. Angiotensin-converting enzyme (ACE) inhibitors are used in the treatment of hypertension. They are successful in treating hypertension and, in addition, have a beneficial effect on insulin resistance in metabolic syndrome. Another class of drugs is the statins, which are used to improve cholesterol levels in people with metabolic syndrome. Statins also appear to cause a reduction in inflammation seen in metabolic syndrome, leading to a reduction in CVD.

Since the emerging epidemic of the metabolic syndrome is expected to continue, both preventive and treatment strategies are needed. Prevention aimed toward reducing the development of this syndrome in children and adolescents should involve schools and community agencies.

Perspective and Prospects

Recognition of the metabolic syndrome essentially paralleled the increases in overweight and obesity in the United States in the early 1990s. Physicians were diagnosing many overweight and obese patients with the major components of the metabolic syndrome without linking them to a major health trend. Other countries of affluence were also reporting cases.

The metabolic syndrome was first defined in 1998 by the World Health Organization (WHO). The WHO criteria included a BMI of more than thirty; a blood triglyceride level greater than or equal to 150 mg/dl; HDL cholesterol level under 35 mg/dl in men and 39 mg/dl in women; blood pressure over 140/90 mm Hg; impaired glucose tolerance, insulin tolerance or type 2 diabetes; insulin resistance; and microalbuminuria (protein in the urine). In 2001 the NCEP/ATP III released their guidelines for the diagnosis of metabolic syndrome, which quickly became the most widely accepted. These differed from the WHO guidelines in several ways. Firstly, BMI measurement was replaced with waist circumference measurement when it became clear that it was not necessarily the total body fat content, but the way in which it is deposited in the body that is important to pathogenesis. A waist circumference of over forty inches for men and over thirty-five inches for women is considered a risk factor for metabolic syndrome. Secondly, the HDL values were changed to less than 40 mg/dl for men and 50 mg/dl for women, and blood pressure limit was lowered to 130/85 mm Hg. A fasting glucose level of over 110 mg/dl was defined as a risk for metabolic syndrome. Finally, insulin resistance and microalbumiuria were removed from the criteria. In 2005 the guidelines were updated by American Heart Association (AHA) and NHLBI; the fasting blood glucose level was lowered to 100 mg/dl. These are the currently used criteria for the diagnosis of metabolic syndrome.

The metabolic syndrome has deadly consequences because of the nature of the chronic diseases that it spawns. This problem will worsen in the future in the United States because excessive calorific intake, eating the wrong kinds of food (for example highly processed food containing high fructose corn syrup, trans fats, or too much salt), and too little physical activity continue to dominate society. The epidemic nature of this syndrome requires that new public health measures be initiated and implemented as soon as possible. Preventive strategies need to be instituted to reduce the enormous impact of this syndrome anticipated in the United States in the coming decades. The overall cost of treatment will be enormous.

—*Claire L. Standen, Ph.D.; additional material by John J. B. Anderson, Ph.D.*

See also Arteriosclerosis; Diabetes mellitus; Endocrine disorders; Endocrinology; Endocrinology, pediatric; Hormones; Hyperlipidemia; Hypertension; Metabolic disorders; Obesity; Obesity, childhood; Weight loss and gain.

For Further Information:

Byrne, Christopher D., and Sarah H. Wild, eds. *The Metabolic Syndrome*. 2d ed. Hoboken, N.J.: John Wiley & Sons, 2011.
Chrousos, George P., and Constantine Tsigos, eds. *Stress, Obesity,*

and Metabolic Syndrome. Boston: Blackwell/New York Academy of Sciences, 2006.

Codario, Ronald A. *Type 2 Diabetes, Pre-diabetes, and the Metabolic Syndrome*. 2d ed. Totowa, N.J.: Humana Press, 2011.

Ervin, R. Bethene. "Prevalence of Metabolic Syndrome Among Adults 20 Years of Age and Over, by Sex, Age, Race and Ethnicity, and Body Mass Index: United States, 2003–2006." *National Health Statistics Reports* no. 13 (May 5, 2009): 1–7.

Hansen, Barbara C., and George A. Bray, eds. *The Metabolic Syndrome: Epidemiology, Clinical Treatment, and Underlying Mechanisms*. Totowa, N.J.: Humana Press, 2008.

Houston, Mark C. *The Handbook of Hypertension*. Hoboken, N.J.: Wiley-Blackwell, 2009.

Levine, T. Barry, and Arlene Bradley Levine. *Metabolic Syndrome and Cardiovascular Disease*. 2d ed. Hoboken, N.J.: Wiley-Blackwell, 2013.

MedlinePlus. "Metabolic Syndrome." *MedlinePlus*, May 20, 2013.

Scholten, Amy. "Metabolic Syndrome." *Health Library*, May 14, 2013.

METABOLISM

Biology

Anatomy or system affected: Gastrointestinal system, intestines, kidneys, liver, pancreas, spleen, stomach

Specialties and related fields: Biochemistry, cytology, exercise physiology, gastroenterology, nutrition, pharmacology

Definition: The processes by which the substance of plants and animals incidental to life is built up and broken down.

Key terms:

adipose tissue: tissue that stores fat; occurs in humans beneath the skin, usually in the abdomen or in the buttocks

anabolism: the metabolic activity through which complex substances are synthesized from simpler substances

basal metabolic rate (BMR): the standardized measure of metabolism in warm-blooded organisms

calorie: a measurement of heat, particularly in measuring the value of foods for producing energy and heat in an organism

catabolism: the complete breaking down of molecules by an organism for the purpose of obtaining chemical building blocks

essential nutrients: molecules that an organism needs for survival but cannot manufacture itself

standard metabolic rate (SMR): the standardized measure of metabolism in cold-blooded organisms

storage compounds: areas in the body that store nutrients not immediately required by an organism

Structure and Functions

Metabolism is an ongoing process in living organisms. It is fundamentally concerned with the chemistry of life. An organism's metabolic rate is the rate at which it consumes the energy it derives from the nutrients that sustain it. Organisms consume energy by converting chemical energy to heat and external work; most of the latter is converted to heat also, as external work, such as walking or moving in any way, overcomes friction. A workable measure of metabolic rate, therefore, is the rate at which an organism produces heat. The food that organisms ingest is measured in calories, each calorie being the measure of what is required to raise the temperature of one kilogram of water by one degree Celsius.

Metabolism consists of two essential underlying processes, anabolism and catabolism. In vertebrates, the food ingested is immediately mixed with digestive enzymes in the mouth. These enzymes are produced by the salivary glands. As a ball of food, a bolus, passes through the digestive system, additional enzymes found in the stomach, the pancreas, and the small intestine work upon it, accelerating the digestive process.

Some nonenzymes are also vital to the digestive process. Most notable are hydrochloric acid, which, in the stomach, is a necessary ingredient for the efficient use of the stomach's pepsin, and bile salts in the small intestine, nonenzymes essential to the digestive process. The action of the digestive apparatus results in catabolism, or the breaking down of the components of food, notably lipids, carbohydrates, and proteins, into small molecules used to build and repair cells. Such molecules, through absorption, traverse the wall of the small intestine to enter the blood or the lymph so that they can be distributed throughout the body to meet its immediate requirements.

Amino acids break down protein, permitting it to enter the bloodstream, whereas glucose and other enzymes act to break down the large carbohydrates into small molecules that are absorbed into the bloodstream. After they are catabolized into smaller molecules, the lipids or fats, unlike proteins and carbohydrates, enter the lymphatic system rather than the bloodstream, which they can enter only after they have passed through the lymphatic system.

Organisms typically cannot digest all the types of nutrients they ingest. Most vertebrates, for example, are incapable of digesting cellulose, the major carbohydrate component of most plants. This material, therefore, simply passes through the digestive system and is excreted. Fiber, which passes through the digestive tract essentially undigested, performs a valuable function in keeping the colon clear and, over the long term, in preventing colon cancer.

A remarkably complex biochemical process occurs when the circulatory system delivers its absorbed sugars, lipids, and amino acids to the parts of the body where they are needed to build new cells and repair existing cells. Sometimes, this process requires the conversion of sugar molecules to fat molecules or animo acids. For a cell to construct a protein, it must connect in a specific, complex order the many animo acid molecules that the process requires. While some of the requisite amino acids result directly from ingesting nutrients, others are not available in this way and must be obtained through the synthesis of sugar molecules.

Molecules that an organism need for survival but that it cannot manufacture itself are obtained through ingestion. Such molecules are called essential nutrients. It takes twenty different kinds of amino acids, for example, to manufacture protein, but the body is capable of producing only half of these. Because green plants can synthesize all twenty forms of amino acids, they are a major and ready source of the es-

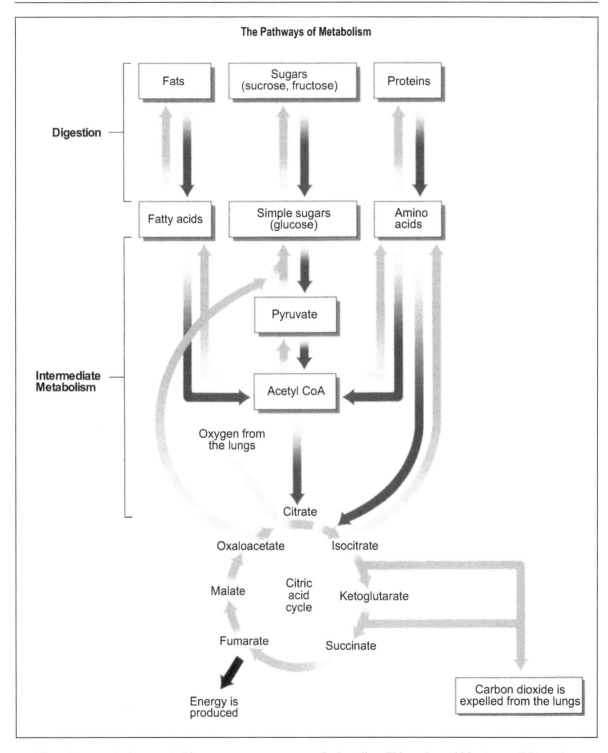

The Pathways of Metabolism

sential nutrients required to sustain life.

Also, as part of a nutritional chain, one can note that although neither humans nor chickens can synthesize valine, a vital amino acid, chickens obtain valine by eating grain that is rich in it. Humans, in turn, eat chickens, through which they obtain valine. This amino acid is also available to humans through the green vegetables they eat.

The food that organisms ingest is used both to provide the necessary building blocks for the synthesis of membranes, enzymes, and other parts of cells and to provide energy. If the nutrients ingested are greater than the body's requirements for such synthesis and for the production of energy, then food molecules may be husbanded for future use in storage compounds within the organism. The excess stored in this way is usually in the form of lipids. In humans, such excesses are stored essentially around the abdomen and buttocks, where they can accumulate in considerable quantity.

If a human's food supply is severely reduced or completely cut off, the body draws on these reserves, using the stored fat cells until they have been completely depleted. Afterward, nutrients, mostly proteins, will be drawn from muscle mass, the sudden reduction of which can quickly eventuate in death.

The survival of organisms is usually dependent upon the work that they perform. Energy to carry out this work is derived through the splitting of the chemical bonds of adenosine triphosphate (ATP) and the splitting of the bonds of food molecules. Highly sophisticated and refined series of biochemical reactions called cellular respiration and aerobic catabolism permit most animals to transfer energy from the chemical bonds of nutrient molecules to the bonds of ATP.

Every cell in the body has the enzymes and cellular equipment to carry out aerobic catabolism and to manufacture its own ATP. Oxygen, carried through the blood, is the essential ingredient in aerobic catabolism, which results in the oxidization of nutrient molecules and their being broken up into small molecules composed largely of carbon dioxide and water. In this process, energy is released, some of it lost as heat and some of it conserved in the bonds of ATP.

As amino acids, lipids, and carbohydrates are catabolized in humans, the lipids and carbohydrates are used by the muscles, whereas the brain gains its energy almost exclusively through the glucose that catabolized carbohydrates produce. Excess amino acids are converted by the liver and, to a smaller extent, by the kidneys to carbohydrates or lipids.

In a process called anaerobic glycolysis, which involves the creation of ATP without the presence of oxygen, energy is produced by converting glucose or glycogen into lactic acid. The body cannot excrete lactic acid, thereby making impossible its accumulation in its original form in the body. Lactic acid is released into the bloodstream after exercise and, subjected to oxygen, is metabolized by the liver and either converted to glucose or oxidized aerobically in order to release additional energy.

As vertebrates age, their metabolic rate often decreases. In humans, a decreased metabolic rate, reduced activity in old age, and a failure to reduce caloric intake can result in substantial weight gain. Therefore, as humans age, their physicians usually encourage them to engage in physical activity and to reduce the overall number of calories that they consume. Physical activity generally helps to sustain the basal metabolism at levels higher than those found among the sedentary.

Disorders and Diseases

All metabolic disorders stem either from genetic or environmental origins, or from a combination of the two. For example, a person with a predisposition for diabetes, an inherited genetic disorder, may exacerbate this predisposition by indulging in a diet high in fats and carbohydrates, by overindulging in alcoholic beverages, and by engaging in little physical activity.

Environmental factors such as diet and exercise can hasten the onset of a disease that lurks in one's genes. People with this predisposition who control diet and alcohol consumption and who make strenuous exercise regular parts of their daily activity, however, may forestall the onset of the disease, possibly keeping it at bay for their entire lifetimes.

Significant advances were first made in the 1960s in tracing the genetic origins of diseases. The discovery that deoxyribonucleic acid (DNA), the molecular basis of heredity, exists in the nucleus of every cell of living organisms was a major biochemical discovery. It has led to vastly increased insights into heredity and into metabolic disorders of genetic origin, certainly the overwhelming majority of all such disorders. Among the many metabolic disorders attributable to inheritance are diabetes, arthritis, gout, phenylketonuria (PKU), Tay-Sachs disease, Niemann-Pick disease, and hemochromatosis.

Microbiologists can detect a number of abnormalities in fetuses by analyzing the amniotic fluid that surrounds them in the womb. This process, known as amniocentesis, can identify more than twenty inherited metabolic disorders before an infant is born. Genetic manipulation in utero can alter some metabolic disorders, thereby bypassing or modifying faulty or abnormal genes. The genes of a person carrying a predisposition for a metabolic defect usually do not carry the information required for the synthesizing of a particular protein, usually an enzyme. This deficiency inhibits catalytic activity and blocks a metabolic pathway, resulting in a genetic abnormality.

In a minority of cases, the protein serves a role in transport or acts as a cell-surface receptor. Whatever role the protein in question serves, a delicate balance exists within the cells. When this balance is disturbed, metabolic problems ensue. For example, a gene may be responsible for producing an enzyme that converts one substance to another substance. If this gene is defective, the enzyme derived from it may be deficient and may fail to carry out the conversion or carry it out so slowly as to result in an inefficient conversion. While the first substance, a protein, accumulates in the cell, causing a surplus, it will be in short supply in the cell involved in the conversion, resulting in a deficiency. The surplus or the shortage may eventuate in a metabolic disorder, the genetic disbalance often revealing itself in overt symptoms.

Evidence of metabolic disorders can occur at any time in a person's life. They sometimes are detectable prenatally, but they may occur in early childhood, adolescence, adult life, or old age. In some cases, the onset of a serious metabolic disorder will be followed quickly by death. Many people suffering from such disorders, however, live long, active, full lives, many of them exceeding the average life span. Some metabolic disorders, such as diabetes, are manageable over long periods through diet and medication.

Some types of metabolic disorders can be treated successfully with massive doses of vitamins. At least twenty fairly common disorders respond favorably to such treatment. For example, Wilson disease, which results in excessive amounts of copper being accumulated in the tissues, is generally treated successfully with D-penicillamine, a compound that removes copper from the tissues and deposits it into the urinary system for excretion as urine.

Certain nutrients trigger metabolic disorders in some organisms. The avoidance of these nutrients can prevent the triggering of the disorder on a permanent basis. Also, where the disorder results from a deficiency of an end product in a reaction, the disorder may be forestalled by replacing the end product.

Perspective and Prospects

Metabolism was scarcely understood until the 1770s, when Joseph Priestley discovered oxygen and set other researchers on the path to understanding its role in the biochemical aspects of all life. In the next decade, Antoine-Laurent Lavoisier and Adair Crawford were the first researchers to measure the heat produced by animals and to suggest convincingly that animal catabolism is a form of combustion.

These early, tentative steps toward understanding how organisms derive energy and how they expend it led to further research that, in 1828, resulted in Friedrich Wohler's synthesis of an organic compound, urea, from inorganic substances, demonstrating that the compounds that living organisms produce can be converted from inorganic to organic through metabolism.

It was not until 1842 that Justus von Liebig categorized foods as falling into three essential types: carbohydrates, lipids, and proteins. He measured the caloric values of nutrients and advanced considerably what was known about nutrition and its role in metabolism. At about the same time, Julius Robert von Mayer and James Joule discovered that motion, heat, and electricity are all forms of the same thing, energy. It was not until the 1890s, however, that Max Rubner and Wilbur Atwater demonstrated conclusively through empirical data that animals release energy according to thermodynamic and biochemical principles established through studies of inanimate systems.

Landmark discoveries about metabolism proceeded into the twentieth century. In 1907, Walter Fletcher and Frederick Gowland Hopkins discovered that lactic acid results when glucose is subjected to the anaerobic contraction of muscles. Five years later, Hopkins discovered substances that are now recognized as vitamins, a term invented in 1912 by Casimir Funk. Ten years later, Frederick Banting and others pinpointed insulin as a substance that could be synthesized and used to reduce levels of blood sugar in humans, thereby making diabetes a manageable rather than a clearly fatal disorder.

A turning point in the understanding of metabolism and especially of metabolic disorders came in 1926 when James B. Sumner purified the first enzyme, showing it to be a protein, clearly leading to the realization that metabolic disorders result from a faulty protein in the genes. In 1941, Fritz Lipmann established the central role of ATP as a carrier of energy in living organisms, and the following year, Rudolf Schoenheimer demonstrated that the adult body's chemical constituents are in constant flux, suggesting that normal, healthy organisms are constantly renewing themselves.

As one surveys the future in terms of the rapidly increasing knowledge of metabolism and genetics, it is clear that genetic engineering offers daunting biological challenges. Birth defects can be detected well before birth, and many of them, through genetic manipulation, can be prevented. It is now within the capability of genetic engineering to predetermine the sex of a fetus and to control matters of gender. Amniocentesis can reveal abnormalities by the second trimester of pregnancy, revealing such conditions as metabolic disorders.

The capabilities that currently lie within reach pose substantial ethical problems and challenges. For example, if a fetus clearly shows evidence of being afflicted with a metabolic disorder, what use should be made of this information? Some parents would elect to terminate the pregnancy, given the challenges of raising such a child.

—*R. Baird Shuman, Ph.D.*

See also Acid-base chemistry; Arthritis; Caffeine; Carbohydrates; Cholesterol; Diabetes mellitus; Digestion; Endocrinology; Endocrinology, pediatric; Enzyme therapy; Enzymes; Exercise physiology; Fatty acid oxidation disorders; Food biochemistry; Fructosemia; Gastroenterology; Gastroenterology, pediatric; Gastrointestinal system; Gaucher's disease; Genetic diseases; Glands; Glycogen storage diseases; Glycolysis; Gout; Hemochromatosis; Hormones; Kidney disorders; Lipids; Macronutrients; Maple syrup urine disease (MSUD); Metabolic disorders; Metabolic syndrome; Mucopolysaccharidosis (MPS); Niemann-Pick disease; Nonalcoholic steatohepatitis (NASH); Obesity; Obesity, childhood; Phenylketonuria (PKU); Protein; Tay-Sachs disease; Wilson's disease.

For Further Information:

Appleton Amber, Olivia Van Bergen, and Ming Yeong Lim. *Metabolism and Nutrition*. New York: Mosby/Elsevier, 2013.

Barasi, Mary E. *Human Nutrition: A Health Perspective*. 2d ed. New York: Oxford University Press, 2003.

Becker, Kenneth L., et al., eds. *Principles and Practice of Endocrinology and Metabolism*. 3d ed. Philadelphia: Lippincott Williams and Wilkins, 2001.

Devlin, Thomas M., ed. *Textbook of Biochemistry: With Clinical Correlations*. 7th ed. Hoboken, N.J.: Wiley-Liss, 2011.

Edwards, Christopher R., and Dennis W. Lincoln, eds. *Recent Advances in Endocrinology and Metabolism*. 4th ed. New York: Churchill Livingstone, 1992.

Feek, Colin, and Christopher Edwards. *Endocrine and Metabolic Disease*. New York: Springer, 1988.

Gropper, Sareen S., and Jack L. Smith. *Advanced Nutrition and Human Metabolism*. 6th ed. Belmont, Calif.: Cengage Learning, 2013.

Hoffmann, Georg F., et al. *Inherited Metabolic Diseases*. Philadelphia: Lippincott Williams & Wilkins, 2002.

Isaacs, Scott, and Neil Shulman. *The Hormonal Balance: Understanding Hormones, Weight, and Your Metabolism*. Boulder, Colo.: Bull, 2007.

Karsenty, Gerard. *Translational Endocrinology of Bone: Reproduction, Metabolism, and the Central Nervous System*. Oxford: Elsevier/Academic, 2013.

King, Richard A., Jerome I. Rotter, and Arno G. Motulsky, eds. *The Genetic Basis of Common Diseases*. 2d ed. New York: Oxford

University Press, 2002.

Kronenberg, Henry M., et al., eds. *Williams Textbook of Endocrinology*. 12th ed. Philadelphia: Saunders/Elsevier, 2011.

Whitehead, Roger G. *New Techniques in Nutritional Research*. San Diego, Calif.: Academic Press, 1991.

METASTASIS. *See* CANCER; MALIGNANCY AND METASTASIS.

METHICILLIN-RESISTANT STAPHYLOCOCCUS AUREUS (MRSA) INFECTIONS

Disease/Disorder

Also known as: Methicillin-resistant staph infections

Anatomy or system affected: Blood, blood vessels, bones, circulatory system, feet, hands, heart, joints, kidneys, legs, liver, muscles, musculoskeletal system, nose, respiratory system, skin, spine, spleen

Specialties and related fields: Bacteriology, cardiology, critical care, dermatology, epidemiology, family medicine, general surgery, internal medicine, microbiology, nursing, orthopedics, pediatrics, pharmacology, podiatry, public health, pulmonary medicine, radiology, rheumatology, sports medicine

Definition: An infection caused by a virulent and destructive bacteria that is resistant to common antibiotics and difficult to treat. It may be localized to one area of the body or may become systemic (spread throughout the body).

Key terms:

abscess: a collection of pus

bacteremia: bacterial infection of the blood

bacterial endocarditis: bacterial infection of the heart valves

cellulitis: infection of the skin and underlying tissue

culture: growth of bacteria in laboratory conditions

osteomyelitis: infection of bone

septic arthritis: infection of a joint

surgical debridement: removal of diseased tissue

surgical drainage: removal of pus

Causes and Symptoms

Staphylococcus aureus is a bacterium commonly found on skin, especially in the nose, axilla (underarm), groin, and rectal areas. Methicillin resistance is the genetically acquired ability of some strains to withstand exposure to a class of antibiotics designed to treat staphylococci. Methicillin-resistant *Staphylococcus aureus* (MRSA) infections occur when a visible or microscopic break in the skin allows these bacterial organisms to enter the body. Such points of entry may be the result of injury, such as an abrasion sustained wrestling or playing football, or surgical, as in a cesarean section or a joint replacement. Needles used to inject medication or illicit drugs can also introduce these bacteria. Sometimes the source is as innocuous as a hair follicle, and occasionally the source of a bloodstream infection is never identified.

Many strains of MRSA are virulent and destructive. Infections are characterized by fever and by pain, redness, and swelling at the site. Pus may drain from the area or may build up as an abscess within infected tissue. MRSA may be invasive, meaning that it spreads deep into tissues and into the bloodstream, traveling through the body and infecting other sites. The most common site of infection is the skin, where MRSA may cause cellulitis (infection of the skin layers), folliculitis (infection of hair follicles), or boils (abscesses complicating folliculitis). It is a common cause of foot and leg infections in patients with diabetes. Osteomyelitis (bone infection) can occur by direct invasion from an overlying skin infection or through trauma (fracture or foreign body such as shrapnel). When bacteria enter the bloodstream, they may find a focus in any organ or tissue and infect that area, sometimes even forming abscesses in these secondary sites. The spine, spleen, and kidneys are common secondary sites. Bacterial endocarditis, or infection of the heart valves and linings, is a particularly dangerous form of MRSA infection and is very difficult to treat. MRSA infections can complicate surgical procedures, causing infection of the incision and sometimes invading deeper tissues or spreading systemically. MRSA infection of surgically placed foreign bodies (artificial joints, bone plates and pins, heart valves) sometimes occurs. MRSA pneumonia can occur in hospitalized patients who require respirators and is a rare but sometimes fatal complication of influenza.

Treatment and Therapy

Treatment of MRSA infections is challenging both because of the organism's resistance to antibiotics and because of its aggressive and persistent nature. When possible, laboratory testing of the infecting organism can help guide the selection of antibiotics most likely to be effective. Specimens from the infected site (pus, infected tissue, blood) can be cultured for bacterial growth and the bacteria subjected to testing for susceptibility to a variety of antibiotics. Those shown in the laboratory to kill or inhibit growth of the cultured bacteria are those most likely to be effective in treating infection.

The antibiotics most commonly used for treating MRSA infections are vancomycin, linezolid, daptomycin, quinupristin/dalfopristin, clindamycin, and various forms of sulfa drugs and tetracyclines. Intravenous (IV) treatment is necessary for severe infections. Some infections, such as bacterial endocarditis and osteomyelitis, require antibiotics for six weeks or more, and relapse is not unusual. Surgical debridement to remove diseased or dead tissue or surgical drainage of an abscess may be necessary in addition to antibiotics. MRSA infection involving a foreign body (for example, a prosthetic joint) is particularly difficult to eradicate; removal of the foreign body is often recommended in addition to antibiotics.

Perspective and Prospects

Since the discovery of microorganisms as a cause of disease, *Staphylococcus aureus*, a common inhabitant of normal skin, has been shown capable of causing severe, life-threatening infection under some conditions. The introduction of antibiotics proved it able to adapt rapidly through mutation, as some strains became resistant first to penicillin and later to

---

Information on MRSA Infections

Causes: Bacteria entering through break in skin from trauma, surgery, injection; point of entry may be unidentifiable

Symptoms: Fever, pain, redness, swelling, pus if localized

Duration: days to weeks; can be fatal if systemic

Treatments: Antibiotics, surgery

---

the semi-synthetic penicillins (such as methicillin) designed to treat penicillin-resistant staphylococci. Initially, these antibiotic-resistant strains were found almost entirely in hospitals and nursing homes, where exposure to antibiotics and evolutionary pressure favored their development. Since the 1990s, MRSA has become widespread outside these settings. Some of these "community-acquired" strains, or CA-MRSA (as distinguished from hospital-acquired or HA-MRSA), have caused severe infections and even death in young, otherwise healthy people who became infected through minor sports injuries or following influenza. Public health authorities have instituted more stringent guidelines for cleaning athletic equipment, immediate showering after practices and competitions, excluding infected athletes from participation, covering open wounds with bandages, and so on. Education and public awareness of appropriate hygiene and infection control measures are important in reducing spread of the infection through communities. Efforts to reduce unnecessary or inappropriate antibiotic use (overprescription, or premature discontinuation of a prescription) may help to prevent the further development of antibiotic-resistant bacteria. Research and development of more effective antibiotics are essential for improving cure rates for severe MRSA infections.

—*Margaret Trexler Hessen, M.D.*

See also Antibiotics; Bacterial infections; Bacteriology; Drug resistance; Epidemiology; Hospitals; Iatrogenic disorders; Infection; Staphylococcal infections.

For Further Information:
Bowman, M. C., D. A. Wohl, and A. H. Kaplan. "Staphylococcal Infections." In *Netter's Internal Medicine*, edited by M. S. Runge and M. A. Greganti. 2d ed. Philadelphia: Saunders/Elsevier, 2009.

Brooks, G. F., et al., eds. *Jawetz, Melnick, and Adelberg's Medical Microbiology*. 25th ed. New York: McGraw-Hill, 2010.

McCoy, Krisha. "Methicillin-Resistant Staph Infection." *Health Library*, September 30, 2012.

"Methicillin-Resistant Staphylococcus Aureus (MRSA)." *National Institute of Allergy and Infectious Diseases*, April 3, 2012.

"Methicillin-Resistant Staphylococcus Aureus (MRSA) Infections." *Centers for Disease Control and Prevention*, April 15, 2011.

Yok, Q. al-, and P. Moreillon. "*Staphylococcus aureus* (Including Staphylococcal Toxic Shock)." In *Mandell, Douglas, and Bennett's Principles and Practice of Infectious Diseases*, edited by G. L. Mandell, J. E. Bennett, and R. Dolin. 7th ed. Philadelphia: Churchill Livingstone/Elsevier, 2010.

MICROBIOLOGY
Specialty

Anatomy or system affected: Cells, immune system

Specialties and related fields: Bacteriology, environmental health, epidemiology, immunology, pathology, public health, virology

Definition: The study of organisms too small to be seen by the unaided human eye, especially the identification, transmission, and control of microorganisms that cause disease.

Key terms:

deoxyribonucleic acid (DNA): the genetic material of a cell that directs the synthesis of proteins; ribonucleic acid (RNA) is the intermediary needed to complete protein synthesis

flora: the microorganisms that are commonly found on or in the human body; also called microflora

infectious disease: an illness caused by a microorganism or its products, in contrast to diseases caused by factors such as heredity or poor nutrition

microorganism: an organism that is too small to be seen without a magnifying lens; also known as a microbe

pathogen: an organism that causes an infectious disease

Science and Profession

Microbiology is the field of science that focuses on microorganisms, living things that can be studied only by using microscopes and other special equipment. Microorganisms have an important place in the ecology of the planet. They form a basis for food chains and, as decomposers, recycle many materials in the environment. Because microbes are everywhere, humans come in contact with a wide variety every day; many live on or in the human body. Most of these organisms either are harmless or are prevented from multiplying by the immune system and other defenses. Others are able to penetrate these defenses and cause an illness. Medical microbiologists study microorganisms that cause these diseases. These pathogens come primarily from four groups: bacteria, fungi, protozoans, and viruses.

Bacteria, along with blue-green algae, belong to the Monera kingdom and are the simplest organisms that exist in cellular form. The bacterial chromosome consists of a loop of deoxyribonucleic acid (DNA) containing several hundred genes. Because it is unprotected by a nuclear membrane, bacterial DNA can be manipulated more easily than can DNA in plants and animals. Several traits are used to identify bacterial species. There are three basic shapes: coccus (round), bacillus (rod), and spirillum (spiral). The gram stain procedure divides bacteria into two main groups based on their cell wall content. Other staining procedures can identify the presence of such structures as flagella, capsules, and endospores, which may have implications for control measures. For example, endospores are resistant to many common disinfectants, and boiling them for up to four hours may not destroy them. In addition to staining, chemical and metabolic tests are used to differentiate bacterial species.

Although the fungi kingdom includes larger organisms

such as mushrooms, the ones of interest to medical microbiology are the yeasts, molds, and related microorganisms. Like plants, they have cell walls. They cannot manufacture their own food by photosynthesis, however, and must either be saprophytes, living on dead organic material, or parasites, obtaining nutrients from another living organism. Fungi reproduce by means of spores that are released and carried by the air to a suitable medium. They thrive in a warm, moist environment with a carbohydrate source of food.

Protozoa, members of the Protista kingdom, are often referred to as one-celled animals. They have no cell walls and must ingest or absorb their food. Their ability to move enables them to spread more quickly than can nonmotile microbes. Four main categories exist. The amoebas move by means of projections called pseudopodia. The flagellates move by means of long hairlike structures (flagella) that whip back and forth. Ciliates are covered with short hairlike structures (cilia) that beat in a synchronized way to cause movement. Sporozoans must move by means of the circulation of blood and tissue fluids within a host. Of all the microorganisms, protozoa are the ones that most resemble human cells. Treatment for a protozoal disease must be monitored closely; most chemicals that are effective against protozoa are also toxic to humans.

Viruses are on the borderline between living and nonliving things. They are not cellular in form, unlike all other forms of life. Each virus particle, called a virion, is made up of a protein coat and a nucleic acid core of either DNA or RNA. Viruses are classified by size, shape, type of nucleic acid in their core, and type of cell they invade or disease they cause.

To reproduce, a virion attaches itself to a living cell and injects its core into the cell. The nucleic acid then takes over the cell's protein-manufacturing apparatus to make new virus particles. The host cell ruptures as these viruses are released to infect other cells. Some viral DNA can incorporate itself into the host DNA and remain dormant until some factor triggers a new reproductive cycle. Viruses usually can attack only one type of cell or species; however, mutations can occur that allow them to infect other species. For example, human immunodeficiency virus (HIV), the cause of acquired immunodeficiency syndrome (AIDS), is believed to have mutated from simian immunodeficiency virus (SIV) in monkeys.

Diagnostic and Treatment Techniques

When the type of microorganism causing an infectious disease is unknown, a medical microbiologist follows a series of procedures known as Koch's postulates. Named for Robert Koch, who proposed them, these procedures identify and confirm that a particular microorganism is the cause of the disease. First, the microorganism must be present in the tissues of all individuals who have the disease. This means that all the microorganisms in a sample of diseased tissue must be identified and classified so that a possible pathogen may be differentiated from the normal flora. Second, the suspected pathogen must be isolated and grown in a pure culture. Many microorganisms can be grown on a simple medium called

nutrient agar. Some microorganisms may need specific nutrients added to the medium or may be obligate parasites—that is, they can grow only on or in living cells. Anaerobic organisms cannot grow at all if oxygen is present. Since these special needs are not known in advance, the detection of some pathogens may be difficult.

The third step the researcher takes is to inoculate an animal with the organism in an effort to duplicate the disease. In the case of human diseases, mammals—such as rabbits, guinea pigs, and mice—are used. Finding the right animal subject may also pose a problem, since not all animals are susceptible to human diseases. For example, armadillos must be used to study leprosy, because the more common laboratory animals are not susceptible to it. In the last of Koch's procedures, the organism must be reisolated from the diseased animal. This step verifies the identity of the pathogen and confirms that it is the same as the original form. If the organism has been identified correctly as the cause of the disease, researchers can then proceed to learn more about the microorganism and its role in the disease process.

The identification of a pathogen as the cause of a specific disease and knowledge of its biological characteristics aid medical researchers in finding prevention and treatment strategies. To cause illness, a microorganism must meet several criteria. First, it must survive transfer to the new host. Some pathogens can form protective structures, such as endospores, that will keep them alive outside a host for a long period of time. A pathogen that cannot survive outside a host must be passed directly in some way from an infected person to a healthy one. Second, a pathogen must overcome the host's defenses. Some may enter through a wound, bypassing the skin barrier that protects the human body from many infections. Some produce chemicals that damage cells and weaken the body. Still others may be able to cause illness only if the person's defenses are weakened by some factor such as age, malnutrition, or another existing illness. Finally, the organism must cause some damage to the host, resulting in the symptoms and signs associated with that illness. The disease process can best be understood by examining several examples of pathogens, the diseases they cause, and the strategies used against them.

The members of the genus *Clostridium* are all anaerobic, form endospores, and produce toxins. Among the bacteria in this group are the pathogens that cause gangrene, tetanus, and botulism. Gangrene usually occurs when a wound has cut off the blood supply to an area of the body. *Clostridium perfringens* enters the body and is able to survive because the lack of blood has created an anaerobic condition. It produces a toxin that destroys surrounding tissue, allowing it to spread. Antibiotics may be effective in preventing the bacteria from spreading to healthy tissue but, because drugs are transported in the blood, may not be able to reach the infected site. Placing the patient in a chamber containing oxygen under high pressure is one strategy used to destroy anaerobic bacteria. *Clostridium tetani* also enters the body through a wound—sometimes a very small one. Since this organism is common and a small wound may go unnoticed, regular immunizations with tetanus vaccine are recommended. Once *C. tetani* bacteria enter the body, they produce a neurotoxin. This nerve poison causes the muscles to stiffen, resulting in a condition called tetanus, or lockjaw. In addition to antibiotics, an antitoxin must be given to neutralize the poison. *Clostridium botulinum* causes botulism, a type of food poisoning. If proper canning techniques are not used, the endospores will germinate. The food then provides a medium on which they can grow, and the sealed can provides the perfect anaerobic conditions. *C. botulinum* produces a neurotoxin that, if it is not destroyed by adequate cooking, will produce neurological symptoms such as double vision and dizziness. This disease must be treated by an appropriate antitoxin or death from respiratory failure can occur in a matter of days.

The human intestine contains large numbers of microorganisms. Some of them provide benefits to their host by producing vitamins and inhibiting the growth of other, potentially harmful, microorganisms. Disease can result if the balance is changed. *Escherichia coli*, part of the normal intestinal flora, can cause infections when it is transferred to another part of the body, such as the urinary bladder. In developing countries, *E. coli* bacteria contaminate drinking water in such large numbers that they result in infantile diarrhea, a common cause of death in those countries. A 1993 epidemic in the United States involved a particularly virulent strain of *E. coli* that had been ingested in improperly cooked ground beef. The characteristics of the strain, combined with the large number of bacteria in the meat, disrupted the intestinal balance of those who ingested it, caused hundreds of people to become ill, and resulted in the deaths of three young children.

The use of antibiotics can disrupt the natural balance by destroying beneficial bacteria as well as pathogens. *Candida albicans*, a yeastlike fungus, is part of the normal human flora. Its growth in the intestine is controlled by certain kinds of bacteria. When antibiotics are used, these beneficial bacteria are destroyed, and the *Candida* begins to multiply. This may not only result in intestinal yeast infections but also contribute to yeast infections in the vagina and other areas where *Candida* can be found. Strategies used to restore the balance may involve eating yogurt or capsules containing *Acidophilus*, one of the beneficial bacteria. Sugars, an important source of food for yeast, should be eliminated from the diet. If these measures do not work, antifungal medication may have to be used.

Fungi that cause skin infections such as athlete's foot are called dermatophytes. When an infected person takes a shower, dermatophyte spores are left in the shower stall. The warm, moist environment then allows the spores to survive until a potential new host comes. Since feet are usually enclosed in shoes and socks, the dermatophytes are again provided with an ideal warm, moist environment. Prevention strategies involve using fungicidal disinfectants to kill the spores and wearing sandals in the shower to avoid coming in contact with the spores. Treatment includes antifungal medication and making the environment less suitable for fungi by keeping the feet dry.

Protozoa are also vulnerable to dry conditions. *Entamoeba histolytica*, the cause of amebic dysentery, is usually ingested in contaminated water. It can, however, form cysts, which allows it to resist drying and freezing. An individual can become ill after eating food rinsed in contaminated water or drinking a "safe" beverage that contained ice made from contaminated water.

Plasmodium species are responsible for malaria, which kills two million people in the world each year. Because this protozoan cannot live outside a host, it is dependent on the female *Anopheles* mosquito to transmit it from one person to another. When a mosquito "bites," it actually pierces the skin with a hypodermic-like mouth and injects a local anesthetic to prevent the host from feeling its presence. At the same time, if it is infected with *Plasmodium*, it will inject malarial parasites into the bloodstream. These parasites spend most of their life cycle inside red blood cells, where they are protected from normal immune defenses. When they have multiplied, they rupture the cells as they leave. Treatment involves maintaining sufficiently high levels of medicine, such as quinine, in the plasma that the parasites die. The most important public health strategy is to control the mosquito population and prevent transmission.

Other than bacteria, viruses are the most common pathogens. The mode of transmission of viruses from one host to another depends on the type of virus. Some can survive for a long period of time outside a host, others must be transferred quickly through the air or by contact, and others can survive only when passed directly into the host by body fluids or insect bites. The damage done to the host depends on the type of tissue that is infected by the virus. For example, the Epstein-Barr virus invades the lymphatic system. It causes the enlarged lymph nodes and abnormal lymphocytes that are characteristic of mononucleosis. It is also associated with Burkitt lymphoma and Hodgkin's disease, both of which are cancers of the lymphatic system. The human immunodeficiency virus (HIV) invades the T lymphocytes, the white blood cells that are crucial to the functioning of the immune system. Damage to the immune system not only makes the individual vulnerable to disease organisms coming from outside the body but also disrupts the balance between the host and normal human flora. This allows other viruses, bacteria, protozoa, and fungi such as *Candida* to multiply and cause potentially fatal secondary infections.

Perspective and Prospects

Infectious diseases have had devastating effects on human populations and societies. For example, during the eighty-year period starting in 1347, recurrent plague epidemics resulted in the deaths of 75 percent of the European population. For many centuries, some physicians and others hypothesized that invisible creatures were the cause of disease. In 1546, Girolamo Fracastoro suggested the presence of germs (seeds) of disease that could be passed from person to person. Because these creatures could not be seen, this "germ" theory was not widely accepted. Then, in 1673, Antoni van Leeuwenhoek began sending descriptions and pictures of what he called "animalcules" to the Royal Society of London. An amateur scientist, Leeuwenhoek made simple microscopes and systematically studied the objects and materials around him. His discoveries of what are now known to be protozoa and bacteria were verified, and they opened the field of microbiology as a science. Using their new knowledge of the microbial world, nineteenth-century researchers began to reexamine the germ theory of disease. In 1857, Louis Pasteur, a chemist, discovered that certain bacteria caused wine to spoil. A few years later, he isolated a protozoan as a cause of a silkworm disease and predicted that microbes could cause human illness. In 1875, Robert Koch, a German physician, devised a procedure by which he demonstrated that anthrax was caused by a specific type of bacterium, *Bacillus anthracis*. His experiments led to widespread acceptance of the germ theory of disease, and his procedures provided a systematic method by which researchers could identify those germs. The twenty-five years that followed are referred to as the golden age of microbiology; one by one, nearly all the major bacterial pathogens were identified.

During this intense period of discovery, researchers soon found that although fine porcelain filters were used to trap microorganisms, in some cases the liquid filtrate was capable of causing disease. The term "virus," meaning poison, was used because it was thought at first that the liquid contained a toxic substance. Pasteur hypothesized that there might be an organism too small to be seen using the light microscope. Later, this was verified, when researchers were able to remove the water from the filtrate, leaving crystals. After the invention of the electron microscope in 1933, individual virions could be seen.

The discovery of pathogens quickly led to research aimed at finding ways to prevent and treat infectious diseases. The contagious nature of disease was known in ancient times. This is illustrated by the practices of Greek physicians and Jewish hygiene laws. Prior to Koch's work, Ignaz Phillipp Semmelweis in the 1840s and Joseph Lister in the 1860s showed that antiseptic techniques could control transmission of diseases. In 1849, John Snow traced the source of a cholera epidemic to a water pump in London. The knowledge that a specific pathogen was involved made it possible for more specific means of prevention to be applied. Within ten years of Koch's report, Pasteur developed vaccines for anthrax and rabies. Immunizations for many infectious diseases were developed, public sanitation measures were taken to reduce the contamination of food and water, and surgeons adopted techniques to control surgical and wound infection.

Although progress in disease prevention was being made, once a person became ill, treatment was still primarily a matter of keeping the patient alive until the disease ran its course. In the early twentieth century, a German physician named Paul Ehrlich began to search for what he called a "magic bullet"—a chemical that would specifically treat a disease by killing the pathogens that caused it. After several years of work, compound 606, an arsenic derivative, was made available to treat syphilis. Sulfa drugs were developed in the 1920s. In 1929, Alexander Fleming discovered penicillin, a substance produced by the mold *Penicillium* that could destroy bacteria in cultures. In 1939, Ernst Chain and Howard Florey used penicillin successfully to treat bacterial infections. In 1944, Selman Waksman discovered streptomycin and used the term "antibiotic" to refer to a substance manufactured by a living organism that kills or inhibits the growth of a pathogen.

By the 1970s, it seemed that the end of infectious disease as a major medical problem was in sight. Several developments brought an end to this complacency. Strains of *Staphylococcus* appeared that were resistant to common antibiotics and caused an increase in postsurgical infections. Antibiotic-resistant strains of gonorrhea and syphilis also became widespread. Childhood diseases, once thought to be under control, reappeared as a result of neglected vaccination programs. Increased world travel also facilitated the spread of disease from country to country. Then, in 1981, AIDS was first described; within a few years, it became a worldwide health problem. As people with AIDS began to succumb to previously uncommon secondary diseases, these diseases had to be studied. A new antibiotic-resistant strain of tuberculosis also appeared as a direct result of the AIDS epidemic. These developments have reemphasized the study of microbiology and demonstrated its importance to human health.

—Edith K. Wallace, Ph.D.

See also Antibiotics; Bacterial infections; Bacteriology; Bionics and biotechnology; Cells; Cytology; Cytopathology; Diagnosis; DNA and RNA; Drug resistance; Epidemiology; Fungal infections; Gastroenterology; Gastroenterology, pediatric; Gastrointestinal disorders; Gastrointestinal system; Genetic engineering; Gram staining; Immune system; Immunization and vaccination; Immunology; Laboratory tests; Microscopy; Mutation; Pathology; Pharmacology; Pharmacy; Prion diseases; Protozoan diseases; Serology; Toxicology; Tropical medicine; Urinalysis; Urinary system; Urology; Urology, pediatric; Viral infections.

For Further Information:

Alcamo, I. Edward. *Microbes and Society: An Introduction to Microbiology.* 2d ed. Sudbury, Mass.: Jones and Bartlett, 2008.

Biddle, Wayne. *A Field Guide to Germs.* 2d ed. New York: Anchor Books, 2002.

Gallo, Robert. *Virus Hunting.* New York: Basic Books, 1991.

Gladwin, Mark, and Bill Trattler. *Clinical Microbiology Made Ridiculously Simple.* 4th ed. Miami: MedMaster, 2009.

Hogg, Stuart. *Essential Microbiology.* 2d ed. Malden: Wiley-Blackwell, 2013.

Jensen, Marcus M., and Donald N. Wright. *Introduction to Microbiology for the Health Sciences.* 4th ed. Englewood Cliffs, N.J.: Prentice Hall, 1997.

Madigan, Michael T., and John M. Martinko. *Brock Biology of Microorganisms.* 12th ed. San Francisco: Pearson/Benjamin Cummings, 2009.

Mishra, Saroj K., and Dipti Agrawal. *A Concise Manual of Pathogenic Microbiology.* Malden: Wiley-Blackwell, 2012.

Murray, Patrick R., Ken S. Rosenthal, and Michael A. Pfaller. *Medical Microbiology.* 6th ed. Philadelphia: Mosby/Elsevier, 2009.

Slonczewski, Joan, and John W. Foster. *Microbiology: An Evolving Science.* New York: Norton, 2013.

MICROSCOPY

Procedure

Anatomy or system affected: Cells

Specialties and related fields: Bacteriology, cytology, histology, microbiology, pathology, virology

Definition: The use of a microscope to make extremely small objects appear larger in order to make them visible.

Indications and Procedures

Conventional microscopy uses a beam of light to illuminate a thin slice of material to be viewed. The material may be stained to provide contrast among its components. The visible light is aimed through the material and collected in a lens. Additional lenses magnify the image until it is visible to the eye of the viewer.

Electron microscopy is a procedure in which a beam of electrons, rather than visible light, is projected toward an object to be viewed. The object is prepared by coating it with a fine layer of metal, frequently gold, that is one or two atoms thick. The electrons reflect off the coated object and hit a screen. The image on the screen is magnified and becomes visible to the human eye. An alternative procedure involves a very thin section of material that is dried and put into a vacuum chamber. A beam of electrons is directed through the prepared specimen. A coated screen receives the electron beam and transforms the image into one visible to the human eye.

Fluorescence microscopy is a procedure that is based on the fact that fluorescent materials emit visible light when they are irradiated with ultraviolet light, which is outside the spectrum visible to the human eye. Some materials manifest this property naturally; others may have to be treated with fluorescent solutions in a process similar to staining. When the absorption of the specimen is in the relatively long ultraviolet range, two filters are also used. The first is placed over the light source to eliminate all but the desired long ultraviolet rays. The second is placed over the eyepiece. The result is a field that becomes dark and allows any red or yellow fluorescence to be visible.

Uses and Complications

Microscopy has extended the range of understanding for physical objects. Intracellular organelles are routinely made visible. Microscopy has made possible the science of microbiology. Fluorescence allows immunoglobulins to be routinely assayed. Viruses are too small to be seen with a light microscope, but electron microscopy has enabled virologists to view and classify viruses.

The drawbacks of current microscopy techniques are primarily that only small samples of material can be viewed at a time. Usually, the material must be destroyed while it is being prepared. Living tissue may be viewed, but only at levels of magnification below those possible at the limits of normal microscopy and far below those possible with electron microscopy.

Electron microscopy allows the greatest amount of magnification for objects. Because the wavelength of electrons is thousands of times shorter than that of visible light, the result-

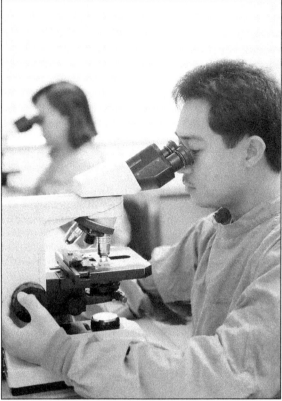

Microscopes are essential in the analysis of laboratory specimens. (PhotoDisc)

ing magnification is several thousand times greater than that possible with visible light. The use of subatomic particles theoretically increases the potential of magnification, but a continuous source of subatomic particles is difficult and quite expensive to supply.

—*L. Fleming Fallon, Jr., M.D., Ph.D., M.P.H.*

See also Antibiotics; Bacteriology; Cells; Cytology; Cytopathology; Diagnosis; Gram staining; Laboratory tests; Microbiology; Microscopy, slitlamp; Pathology.

For Further Information:

Black, Jacquelyn G., and Laura J. Black. *Microbiology*. Hoboken, N.J.: Wiley, 2013.

Hawkes, Peter W., and John C. H. Spence, eds. *Science of Microscopy*. New York: Springer, 2007.

Madigan, Michael T., and John M. Martinko. *Brock Biology of Microorganisms*. 13th ed. San Francisco: Pearson/Benjamin Cummings, 2012.

Murray, Patrick R., Ken S. Rosenthal, and Michael A. Pfaller. *Medical Microbiology*. 6th ed. Philadelphia: Mosby/Elsevier, 2009.

Singleton, Paul, and Diana Sainsbury. *Dictionary of Microbiology and Molecular Biology*. Rev. 3d ed. Hoboken, N.J.: John Wiley & Sons, 2007.

Spector, David L., and Robert D. Goldman, eds. *Basic Methods in Microscopy: Protocols and Concepts from Cells—A Laboratory Manual*. Cold Spring Harbor, N.Y.: Cold Spring Harbor Laboratory Press, 2006.

MICROSCOPY, SLITLAMP
Procedure
Also known as: Biomicroscope
Anatomy or system affected: Eyes
Specialties and related fields: Ophthalmology
Definition: The use of a special instrument to examine the tissues of the eye.

Indications and Procedures
The slit-lamp microscope, or biomicroscope, is used to examine and evaluate tissues of the eye with both stereopsis and multiple values of optical magnification. The anterior segment of the eye is observed with several types of illumination: diffuse, direct (both broad and narrow beam, the latter allowing an almost slidelike examination of the clear corneal layers), indirect (side illumination), retroillumination (in which abnormalities are back-illuminated with light reflected from more internal structures), specular (in which light is reflected off various layers to show the detail of each surface), and sclerotic scatter (internal illumination). Various dyes (such as fluorescein or rose bengal) may be employed to help differentiate normal from abnormal tissues.

The instrument has two coaxial rotating arms controlled by a joystick level; one arm carries the adjustable slit-lamp illumination system, with attendant filters and optical stops, and the other arm carries the observation optics (a binocular microscope). An adjustable chin and forehead rest positions the subject's head.

Auxiliary devices allow the measurement of intraocular pressure (tonometer) and corneal thickness (pacometer) and the evaluation of the angle between the cornea and iris (gonioscope lens). Cameras, both still and video, may be attached at various sites. High-powered auxiliary optical lenses have also been developed, which allow the clinician to use the slit-lamp microscope to observe the posterior pole of the eye (through the pharmacologically dilated pupil), including the optic nerve and most of the retina. Ophthalmic lasers can also be attached to this system in order to treat the various structures of the eye as they are observed directly through the same optics, using the principle of the reversibility of the path of light.

Allvar Gullstrand received a Nobel Prize in 1911 for his contributions to optics, and the same year he introduced his refinement of the slit-lamp microscope. Modern instruments and techniques are largely based on his work.
—*Barry A. Weissman, O.D., Ph.D.*

See also Eye infections and disorders; Eye surgery; Eyes; Laser use in surgery; Microscopy; Ophthalmology; Optometry; Vision; Vision disorders.

For Further Information:
A.D.A.M. Medical Encyclopedia [Internet]. Atlanta (GA): A.D.A.M., Inc.; ©2005. Slit-lamp exam; [updated 2013 Feb 7; cited 2013 June 26]; [about 4 p.]. Available from: http://www.nlm.nih.gov/medlineplus/ency/article/003880.htm.
Duane, Thomas David, William Tasman, and Edward A. Jaeger. *Duane's Ophthalmology*. Rev. ed. Philadelphia: Lippincott Williams & Wilkins, 2011.

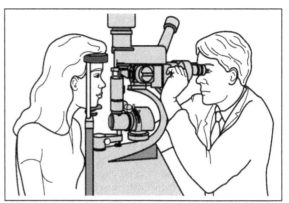
The slitlamp microscope, or biomicroscope, is used by ophthalmologists to examine the health of the eye.

Kaufman, Paul L., and Albert Alm. *Adler's Physiology of the Eye: Clinical Application*. 10th ed. St. Louis, Mo.: Mosby, 2003.
Ledford, Janice K., and Valerie N. Sanders. *The Slit Lamp Primer*. 2d ed. Thorofare, N.J.: SLACK, 2006.
Newell, Frank W. *Ophthalmology: Principles and Concepts*. 8th ed. St. Louis, Mo.: Mosby, 1996.
Riordan-Eva, Paul, and John P. Whitcher. *Vaughan and Asbury's General Ophthalmology*. 18th ed. New York: Lange Medical Books/McGraw-Hill, 2011.
Sutton, Amy L., ed. *Eye Care Sourcebook: Basic Consumer Health Information About Eye Care and Eye Disorders*. 3d ed. Detroit, Mich.: Omnigraphics, 2008.
Wenzel, Martin. *Specular Microscopy of Intraocular Lenses: Atlas and Textbook for Slit-Lamp and the Specular Microscopic Examinations*. New York: Thieme Medical, 1993.

MINIMALLY CONSCIOUS STATE
Disease/Disorder
Anatomy or system affected: Central nervous system
Specialties and related fields: Neurology, neuropsychology, neurosurgery, nursing, occupational therapy, physiatry, physical therapy, speech language pathology
Definition: A condition of severely altered consciousness in which minimal, but definite, behavioral evidence of self or environmental awareness is demonstrated.
Key terms:
arousal: the degree of wakefulness
awareness: the perception of one's self and the environment
brain connectivity: a pattern of structural and functional interactions within and between cortical and subcortical structures
disorder of consciousness (DoC): a medical condition caused by acquired brain injury (traumatic or nontraumatic) and characterized by impairments in arousal and awareness of self and environment

Causes and Symptoms
Minimally conscious state (MCS) is one of several disorder of consciousness (DoC) syndromes associated with alteration in arousal, impaired self and environmental awareness, and disruption of brain connectivity necessary for supporting

conscious awareness. The most severe disorder, coma, is characterized by complete loss of arousal and no behavioral signs of awareness. In the vegetative state (VS), the arousal system recovers and sleep-wake cycles return, but behavioral signs of awareness remain absent. In coma and VS, subcortical functions are partially preserved, but interactions between cortical and subcortical structures are severely diminished or completely lost. Conversely, MCS is characterized by near-normal to normal wakefulness and at least one definitive behavioral sign of awareness. The hallmark feature of MCS is inconsistency in volitional responses. The transition from coma and VS to MCS is coupled to the recovery of cortico-cortical and cortico-subcortical connectivity.

The diagnostic criteria for MCS are based on reproducible or sustained behavioral evidence of one or more of the following:

- simple command-following
- gestural or verbal yes/no responses (regardless of accuracy)
- intelligible verbalization
- purposeful behavior, including movements or affective behaviors that occur in contingent relation to relevant environmental stimuli and are not due to reflexive activity (e.g., visually tracking a moving object)

While most people progress through MCS in less than three months, others may remain in MCS permanently. Clear evidence of either of the following behaviors mark emergence from MCS:

- functional interactive communication (i.e., consistent and accurate yes-no responses to personal or situational orientation questions)

OR

- functional object use (i.e., appropriate demonstration of the use of at least two common objects)

Observational assessment of behavior remains the "gold standard" for differential diagnosis among DoC. This method may lead to misdiagnosis as the evaluation of level of consciousness may be confounded by fluctuations in arousal level, sensory deficits, motor limitations, cognitive dysfunction, language impairment, diminished behavioral drive, and other factors. Use of standardized assessments, such as the Coma Recovery Scale-Revised (CRS-R), has been shown to decrease the rate of misdiagnosis.

Treatment and Therapy

Currently, there are no standards of care for treatment of persons in MCS. Prevention of common medical complications associated with severe brain injury, avoidance of prolonged immobilization, and management of environmental stimulation are typically the primary goals of rehabilitation. Common complications include, but are not limited to, spasticity, autonomic dysfunction, pneumonia, urinary tract infection, and sleep disturbance.

Pharmacologic agents are often used to promote arousal, increase behavioral initiation, decrease agitation, and regulate sleep in patients in MCS. However, amantadine hydro-chloride is the only therapeutic agent shown to be effective in increasing the rate of recovery in patients in traumatic VS and MCS. There is also growing interest in the sleep medication, zolpidem, as a few case studies have reported dramatic increases in arousal, speech, and volitional behavior within 30 minutes of administration. A broad range of other treatment interventions, including other drug therapies, invasive and noninvasive brain stimulation procedures and cognitive rehabilitation, have been used to promote recovery, although their effectiveness remains largely unproven.

Science and Profession

While there is no consensus on the best method of treatment for MCS, a collaborative, multidisciplinary approach that engages the expertise of multiple clinical specialties is essential for effective management of the wide-ranging and long-term needs of this population.

During the acute hospitalization, stabilization, and management of the primary and secondary effects of the injury necessitate the collective expertise of neurologists, neurosurgeons, and physiatrists. Once the critical medical issues have been stabilized, the patient may be evaluated and treated by a rehabilitation team consisting of physical and occupational therapists, speech language pathologists, and clinical neuropsychologists. When implementing a multidisciplinary approach, clinicians across specialties collaborate on common assessment strategies and treatment goals.

Perspective and Prospects

MCS was originally referred to as the minimally responsive state; however, this term was abandoned to avoid conflating reflexive and automatic behavioral responses with those that are volitional. The diagnosis of MCS was formally established by the Aspen Neurobehavioral Workgroup in 2002. A major impetus for differentiating patients in MCS from those in VS was a growing body of research showing that the outcome from MCS was significantly more favorable relative to VS. Many subsequent studies have validated these findings and suggest that people who reach MCS within the first three months of injury have a lower mortality rate and are more likely to have a lower degree of functional disability by 12 months postinjury. Current efforts are underway to improve detection of MCS early after injury, better define the upper boundary of MCS, and identify factors that influence outcome.

—*Matthew Doiron, B.A., Yelena Guller, Ph.D., and Joseph T. Giacino, Ph.D.*

See also Concussion; Glasgow coma scale; Neuropsychology; Neuroscience traumatic brain injury

For Further Information:

Fins J.J., M. McMaster, L. Gerber, and J.T. Giacino. "The Minimally Conscious State: A Diagnosis in Search of an Epidemiology." *Archives of Neurology* 64 (2007): 1400-1405.

Giacino, Joseph. "The Minimally Conscious State: Defining the Borders of Consciousness." *Progress in Brain Research, The Boundaries of Consciousness: Neurobiology and Neuropathology,* edited by Steven Laureys. Amsterdam: Elsevier, 2005.

Giacino, J.T., et al., "Placebo-Controlled Trial of Amanatadine for Severe Traumatic Brain Injury." *New England Journal of Medicine* 366, no. 9 (2012):819-826.

Giacino, J.T., et al. "The Minimally Conscious State: Definition and Diagnostic Criteria." *Neurology* 58, no. 3 (2002): 349-353.

Giacino, J.T., and K.A. Kalmar. "The Vegetative and Minimally Conscious States: A Comparison of Clinical Features and Functional Outcome during the First Year Post-Injury." *Journal of Head Trauma Rehabilitation* 12 (1997): 36-51.

Giacino, J., J.J. Fins, A. Machado, and N.D. Schiff. "Central Thalamic Deep Brain Stimulation to Promote Recovery from Chronic Posttraumatic Minimally Conscious State: Challenges and Opportunities." *Neuromodulation: Journal of the International Neuromodulation Society* 15, no. 4 (2012): 339-349.

Nakase-Richardson, W.J., and J.T. Giacino. "Longitudinal Outcome of Patients with Disordered Consciousness in the NIDRR TBI Model Systems Programs." *Journal of Neurotrauma* 29, no. 1 (2011): 59-65.

Schiff, N.D., et al. "Fmri Reveals Large-Scale Network Activation in Minimally Conscious Patient." *Neurology* 64, no. 3 (2005): 514-523.

Schnakers, C., A. Vanhaudenhuyse, J. Giacino, M. Ventura, M. Boly, S. Majerus, and S. Laureys. (2009). "Diagnostic Accuracy of the Vegetative and Minimally Conscious State: Clinical Consensus versus Standardized Neurobehavioral Assessment." *BMC Neurology* 9, no. 1 (2009): 35.

MIRROR NEURONS

Anatomy

Anatomy or system affected: Brain

Specialties and related fields: Neuroscience, psychology

Definition: Neurons within the brain that fire during both the execution and observation of an action.

Key terms:

autism: a spectrum of disorders characterized by poor social interactions, deficits in communication, and stereotypical motor behaviors

theory of mind: the ability to infer the mental states of others

Structure and Functions

Mirror neurons were first discovered in the early 1990s in the premotor cortex and inferior parietal lobe of primates. These neurons fired when a monkey made a particular motor movement, such as reaching out to grasp an object, as well as when he observed another monkey make the same movement. Thus, these neurons were coined "mirror neurons" because they fire during both the execution and observation of the same movement. Mirror neurons can also respond to some nonmotor-based information. For example, some mirror neurons respond to sounds associated with particular actions, such as shells cracking when eating peanuts.

Whether or not mirror neurons fire is greatly dependent on the goal or intention of a motor action. An interesting phenomenon is that mirror neurons respond to goal-directed movements even when part of the motor sequence is hidden from view, e.g., seeing an object hidden behind a screen and then seeing a hand reach behind the screen as if to grasp the object. However, these same neurons do not respond to the same sequence when it is not goal-directed, e.g., a hand mimicking grasping a nonexistent object. Likewise, mirror neurons can differentiate between the same motor movement with two different end goals. For example, mirror neurons will fire differently for the action of grasping a piece of food when followed by eating the food compared to when followed by placing the food in a container.

Differences Between Humans and Primates

Thus far, mirror neurons have only been directly observed in nonhuman primates. There is a variety of evidence from neuroimaging techniques such as functional magnetic resonance imaging (fMRI) that suggest there is mirror-like activity in humans. However, there are several differences between these systems in humans and primates. Imaging studies have found regions of mirror-like behavior in human brains that are outside the activity zones found in primates. Additionally, supposed human mirror neurons respond to a wider array of actions and stimuli such as meaningless movements, gestures, emotion, and pain.

These differences in humans and primates have caused debate regarding the classification of mirror neurons. In primates, mirror neurons are considered to be a sub-category of motor neurons. However, human studies tend to define mirror neurons more broadly as neurons which fire for a given state or behavior within an individual and when that same state or behavior is observed in another individual. These mirrored states may not be motor-related, e.g., neurons that fire when one feels disgusted and when observing someone else with an expression of disgust.

Disorders and Diseases

It has been proposed that a "broken" mirror neuron system in humans could underlie the symptoms of autism, which include poor social cognition, deficits in communication, and stereotyped motor behaviors such as flapping hands. Autistics are thought to have a poor theory of mind, which is the ability to infer the mental states of others. This leads to an inability to understand the intentions of others or empathize with others. Mirror neurons have been proposed as a neural mechanism for a theory of mind because their firing links the observed motor actions of others onto one's own motor repertoire. Likewise, mirror neurons may provide a neural mechanism for imitation, which may be a stepping stone to develop broader social skills. Autistic children are poor imitators, and their inability to imitate gestures may contribute to their underdeveloped communication skills. It is difficult to infer a direct relationship between these deficits and faulty mirror neurons, but this discussion has stimulated a new area of research in autism.

The neuroimaging data on mirror neurons and autism is mixed. Neuroanatomically, autistics have less brain tissue in mirror neurons regions. Some studies report a correlation between social impairment and abnormal mirror neuron activity. However, autistics also have reduced brain tissue in regions that process emotion and social cues but are not mirror neuron areas. Thus, a mirror neuron explanation may be too simplistic and dysfunction in these additional areas may better explain symptoms of autism.

Despite the inconclusive evidence, some proponents are proposing therapeutic techniques via sensorimotor training to improve mirror neuron function. It has been shown in primates that training can alter mirror neuron activity. Whether training will prove successful in autistic individuals is still to be seen.

Perspective and Prospects

It is important to consider that mirror neurons were only discovered a mere two decades ago. The function and ontology of these neurons is still not known and is widely debated. One theory of mirror neuron function is that they contribute to understanding the actions and intentions of others, which has led to the implication that mirror neurons may be involved in social cognition. However, as discussed, the data on mirror neurons and disorders such as autism is mixed.

It is also not clear if these neurons are hardwired from birth, and thus perhaps serve a function such as social cognition, or if they are learned from experience. If the latter is true, mirror neurons may simply reflect behavior rather than contribute to it. This may be a more accurate picture of mirror neurons as they are only a small percentage of all motor neurons (by one estimate in primates, approximately 6 percent).

Lastly, the differences between humans and primates raise questions on the definition of mirror neurons. In primates, mirror neurons are a subset or a particular firing pattern of motor neurons. However, in humans, mirror-like activity has been found in more regions of the brain and in response to a wider array of stimuli than in primates. This could be due to a more advanced system in humans. However, more research is necessary to further understand the function and ontology of these neurons.

—*Joyce W. Lacy, Ph.D.*

See also Autism; Neuroscience; Premotor cortex

For Further Information:

Casile, A. "Mirror Neurons (and Beyond) in the Macaque Brain: An Overview of 20 Years of Research." *Neuroscience Letters* 540 (2013): 3-14.

Chong, T. T-J., R. Cunnington, M. A. Williams, N. Kanwisher, and J. B. Mattingley. "fMRI Adaptation Reveals Mirror Neurons in Human Inferior Parietal Cortex." *Current Biology* 18 (2008): 1576-1580.

Gallese, V., M. J. Rochat, and C. Berchio. "The Mirror Mechanism and Its Potential Role in Autism Spectrum Disorder." *Developmental Medicine & Child Neurology* 55 (2012): 15-22.

Hamilton, A. F. "Reflecting on the Mirror Neuron System in Autism: A Systematic Review of Current Theories." *Developmental Cognitive Neuroscience* 3 (2013): 91-105.

Umilta, M. A., E. Kohler, V. Gallese, L. Fogassi, L. Fadiga, C. Keysers, and G. Rizzolatti, G. "I Know What You Are Doing: A Neurophysiological Study." *Neuron* 31 (2001): 155-165.

Singer, T., B. Seymour, J. O'Doherty, H. Kaube, R. J. Dolan, and C. D. Frith. "Empathy for Pain Involves the Affective But Not Sensor Components of Pain." *Science* 303 (2004): 1157-1162.

Wicker, B., C. Keysers, J. Plailly, J-P. Royet, V. Gallese, and G. Rizzolatti, "Both of Us Disgusted in my Insula: The Common Neural Basis of Seeing and Feeling Disgust." *Neuron* 40 (2003): 655-664.

MISCARRIAGE

Disease/Disorder

Also known as: Spontaneous abortion

Anatomy or system affected: Psychic-emotional system, reproductive system, uterus

Specialties and related fields: Embryology, gynecology, obstetrics, perinatology, psychology

Definition: A pregnancy that self-terminates within the first twenty weeks of gestation; the same condition occurring after twenty weeks is termed a stillbirth.

Key terms:

abortion: the medical term for intended and unintended pregnancy loss

blighted ovum: a condition in which the gestational sac and placenta grow without a developing child inside

ectopic pregnancy: a pregnancy in which the implantation of the fertilized egg occurs anywhere outside the uterus, usually in the Fallopian tube

human chorionic gonadotropin (hCG): the hormone, produced only in pregnancy, that makes the uterine lining receptive for the developing embryo or fetus; pregnancy tests determine its presence

molar pregnancy: abnormal, cystlike placental tissue that grows either in place of the developing child (complete mole) or in addition to the developing child (partial mole)

recurrent miscarriage: a condition in which a woman experiences three consecutive miscarriages

threatened abortion: when the symptoms of a miscarriage first occur

Causes and Symptoms

Approximately 15 to 20 percent of all known pregnancies will end in miscarriage. Furthermore, it is estimated that 50 to 75 percent of all fertilized eggs fail to implant in the uterus—a situation generally unknown to the woman. The likelihood of a miscarriage drops during the pregnancy's duration: approximately 10 percent in the first four weeks after implantation, 5 percent for the next six weeks, and 3 percent for the following eight weeks. (The stillbirth rate is approximately 1 percent.)

The symptoms of a threatened abortion may include spotting of blood, which may turn into heavier bleeding; cramping, possibly accompanied by lower back pain and vaginal discharge of tissue, clots, or pinkish fluid. A completed miscarriage may also demonstrate changes in pregnancy signs, such as nausea and breast sensitivity. A hormonal sign of a threatened abortion is the failure of human chorionic gonadotropin (hCG) levels to double every two days.

There are three conditions where a woman experiences a miscarriage and the developing child is missing in the sac. About 30 percent of miscarriages before the eighth gestational week are blighted ova, as an embryo has failed to develop. Complete molar pregnancies arise when a sperm (or two) fertilize an egg that has lost its genes. The resulting development of pregnancy tissues—absent the developing child—usually leads to the symptoms of a miscarriage in the

Information on Miscarriage

Causes: Genetic abnormalities, uterine or cervical defects, hormonal or immune disorders; risks increase with poor health, history of reproductive tract disease or miscarriage, age over forty-five, certain substances (caffeine, cocaine, nicotine), radiation exposure, STDs

Symptoms: Spotting that turns into heavier bleeding; cramping and lower back pain; vaginal discharge (tissue, clots, pinkish fluid); nausea; loss of pregnancy signs

Duration: Acute

Treatments: None in first two months of pregnancy; later, magnesium sulfate for preeclampsia or premature contractions, cervical stitch for incompetent cervix

first several gestational weeks, but expulsion of the placenta may not occur. Because of the higher likelihood of residual disease (including cancer) in the abnormal tissue if any is left behind, surgical removal of the molar tissue is often warranted. Women who have aborted a molar pregnancy are advised to not get pregnant again for a year, and then they must be closely monitored for subsequent pregnancies, as they are at increased risk for further abnormalities that can become malignant. Finally, a woman may have a recognized pregnancy yet not realize that she was actually pregnant with twins and that one died. This "vanishing twin syndrome" occurs in an estimated 3.5 percent of all twin pregnancies.

Analyses reveal the probability of the most common causes of miscarriages: 50 to 60 percent, genetic abnormalities; 10 to 15 percent, defects in the uterus (such as double or septal uterus) or the cervix (such as incomplete closure); and 10 to 15 percent, hormonal (such as low progesterone or thyroxin) and/or immune disorders (such as lupus or antiphosphid antibody syndrome). A woman's poor health, history of disease (such as endometriosis), history of miscarriages, and advanced age (a 75 percent miscarriage rate for women forty-five and older) also increase the probability of a miscarriage. Recent studies have indicated that the presence of bacterial vaginosis is associated with late-onset miscarriages and preterm deliveries. The presence of the bacteria known as beta strep in the mother's birth canal is tied to preterm labor when it goes untreated. Lifestyle choices that can compromise a successful pregnancy may involve the abuse of substances such as caffeine, cocaine, or nicotine; the contraction of sexually transmitted diseases (STDs), such as chlamydia, human immunodeficiency virus (HIV), or human papillomavirus (HPV); or exposure to harmful agents, such as radiation.

Treatment and Therapy

Little can be done to stop a miscarriage in the first two months of pregnancy, though some effective interventions are possible in later gestational periods. Magnesium sulfate is effective in combating preeclampsia (high blood pressure during pregnancy) and premature labor contractions. A cervical stitch (cerclage) can rectify an incompetent cervix (premature dilation). Most medical efforts, however, are directed toward the prevention of future miscarriages—the treatment of disease, lifestyle changes, RhO shots for Rh problems—and recovery from the present miscarriage. For example, medications to reduce the risk of miscarriage include antibiotics, which treat or prevent infections, and aspirin and similar medications that treat blood-clotting issues. Surgical procedures are also used to prevent miscarriages by treating certain uterine problems, such as uterine fibroids and a weakened cervix.

There are two aspects of recovery from a miscarriage. The physical part involves the natural or artificial removal of pregnancy tissue—either chemically, as with pitocin, or surgically, as with dilation and curettage (D & C)—and the establishment of a new menstrual cycle. A typical physical recovery ranges from a few days to a few weeks for the miscarriage itself and one to two months after the miscarriage for the next period. Women are usually advised to wait one to two normal periods before trying to conceive again. Approximately 60 percent of women trying to conceive will be successful within six months of the miscarriage.

The psychological recovery may take longer than the physical recovery. Social support, good mental health prior to the miscarriage, deeper religious faith, and successful grieving (mourning, not denying, the loss and then moving forward in life) are some of the factors correlated with a better psychological recovery. Support groups exist for individuals who have suffered miscarriage, stillbirth, or infant death. Similar groups exist to provide support to individuals who are pregnant after the loss of an earlier pregnancy. Such support is essential in decreasing anxiety.

Perspective and Prospects

Until the latter half of the twentieth century, miscarrying women received little satisfaction from the medical community. In fact, many of the drugs introduced in the mid-twentieth century, such as diethylstilbestrol (DES) and its numerous estrogenic cousins, caused more harm than good. However, by the latter part of the twentieth century significant progress was made in diagnosing and preventing miscarriages.

In the early twenty-first century, three avenues of research appear to be promising. Studies are revealing certain genetic predispositions for miscarriages, such as the low production of nitric oxide, resulting in less blood to the uterus. Miscarriages are also being linked to autoimmune disorders and hormonal deficiencies. Use of hormone injections to women who are found to have a hormonal imbalance can help to prevent miscarriage. Finally, assisted reproductive technologies offer intriguing possibilities, such as the ethically controversial opportunity to screen preimplantation embryos for chromosomal abnormalities. In these and other areas of research, new hopes are being raised for old griefs.

—Paul J. Chara, Jr., Ph.D.,
and Kathleen A. Chara, M.S.;
updated by Robin Kamienny Montvilo, R.N., Ph.D.

See also Abortion; Addiction; Assisted reproductive technologies; Ectopic pregnancy; Fetal alcohol syndrome; Genetic diseases; Genetics and inheritance; Obstetrics; Placenta; Pregnancy and gestation; Premature birth; Stillbirth; Teratogens; Uterus; Women's health.

For Further Information:

Eisenberg, Arlene, Heidi E. Murkoff, and Sandee E. Hathaway. *What to Expect When You're Expecting.* 4th ed. New York: Workman, 2009.

Friedman, Lynn, and Irene Daria. *A Woman Doctor's Guide: Miscarriage—The Support and Facts You Need to Get Through Pregnancy Loss.* New York: Kensington, 2001.

Jutel, A. "What's in a Name? Death Before Birth." *Perspectives in Biology and Medicine* 49, no. 3 (2006): 425–434.

Lanham, Carol Cirruli. *Pregnancy After a Loss: A Guide to Pregnancy After a Miscarriage, Stillbirth, or Infant Death.* New York: Berkley, 1999.

Larsen, E. C. "New Insights into Mechanisms behind Miscarriage." *BMC Medicine* 11, no. 1 (June, 2013): 154.

Tranquilli, A. L. "Miscarriages: Causes, Symptoms and Prevention." *Obstetrics and Gynecology Advances.* New York: Nova, 2012.

Ugwumadu, A. H., and P. Hay. "Bacterial Vaginosis: Sequelae and Management." *Current Opinions in Infectious Disease* 12, no. 1 (1999): 53–59.

Wood, Deborah. "Miscarriage." *Health Library*, September 10, 2012.

MITES. *See* BITES AND STINGS; LICE, MITES, AND TICKS; PARASITIC DISEASES.

MITRAL VALVE PROLAPSE
Disease/Disorder

Anatomy or system affected: Circulatory system, heart

Specialties and related fields: Cardiology, family medicine, internal medicine, vascular medicine

Definition: The inability of the mitral valve in the heart to close properly.

Causes and Symptoms

The mitral valve connects the heart's left ventricle and left atrium. The oxygenated blood, having already passed through the right heart chambers and the lungs, arrives in the left atrium through the pulmonary veins and then passes through the mitral valve into the left ventricle. Compression of the left ventricle pumps the blood into the aorta and on to the rest of the body. A properly functioning mitral valve closes and prevents regurgitation or backflow into the left atrium. Mitral valve prolapse occurs when the two leaves of

---

Information on Mitral Valve Prolapse

Causes: Rheumatic fever, inflammation of heart lining (endocarditis), cardiac tumors, genetic error

Symptoms: Undue fatigue after exercise, shortness of breath, chest pain

Duration: Chronic

Treatments: Regular exercise; good eating habits; occasionally, surgery

---

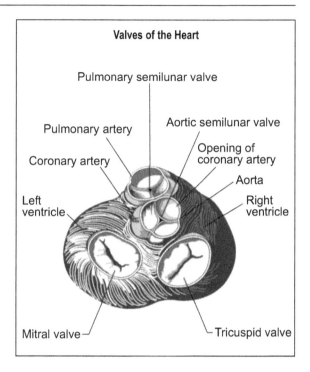

Valves of the Heart

Pulmonary semilunar valve

Pulmonary artery

Aortic semilunar valve

Coronary artery

Opening of coronary artery

Aorta

Left ventricle

Right ventricle

Mitral valve

Tricuspid valve

---

the mitral valve close imperfectly, allowing leakage. This condition, known also as mitral valve insufficiency prolapse, is the most common cardiac syndrome. Found in all segments of society, it is most common in young adult women.

Mitral valve prolapse has several possible causes including rheumatic fever, inflammation of the heart lining (endocarditis), cardiac tumors, or most often, genetic error. Its symptoms are undue fatigue after exercise, shortness of breath, and chest pain. Other common complaints are anxiety, depression, and panic, all related to stress. The number of diagnosed cases in Western countries is rising markedly and may be the result of more sophisticated diagnostic techniques or the increasing stress in modern society.

Perspective and Prospects

Until the 1960s, the detection of mitral valve prolapse was through a characteristic "click" heard by the physician when the mitral leaves attempted to close. Now the use of echocardiograms, allowing ultrasound images of the beating heart and blood flow, is standard practice.

People with mitral valve prolapse lead a normal life, and many are unaware that they have the condition. Repeated irregularity in breathing or an inexplicable shortness of breath is a sign to see one's physician. Regular exercise and good eating habits are recommended for this mild condition. Only in severe cases is mitral valve prolapse treated surgically or considered life-threatening.

—*K. Thomas Finley, Ph.D.*

See also Anxiety; Cardiac surgery; Cardiology; Cardiology, pediatric; Circulation; Congenital heart disease; Echocardiography; Endocarditis; Fatigue; Heart; Heart disease; Rheumatic fever; Stress.

For Further Information:

Alpert, Joseph S., James E. Dalen, and Shahbudin H. Rahimtoola, eds. *Valvular Heart Disease*. 3d ed. Philadelphia: Lippincott Williams & Wilkins, 2000.

Badash, Michelle. "Mitral Valve Prolapse." *Health Library*, May 9, 2013.

Boudoulas, Harisios, and Charles F. Wooley, eds. *Mitral Valve: Floppy Mitral Valve, Mitral Valve Prolapse, Mitral Valvular Regurgitation*. 2d ed. Armonk, N.Y.: Futura, 2000.

Crawford, Michael, ed. *Current Diagnosis and Treatment—Cardiology*. 3rd ed. New York: McGraw-Hill Medical, 2009.

Eagle, Kim A., and Ragavendra R. Baliga, eds. *Practical Cardiology: Evaluation and Treatment of Common Cardiovascular Disorders*. 3rd ed. Philadelphia: Lippincott Williams & Wilkins, 2009.

Frederickson, Lyn. *Confronting Mitral Valve Prolapse Syndrome*. New York: Warner Books, 1992.

Gersh, Bernard J., ed. *The Mayo Clinic Heart Book*. 2d ed. New York: William Morrow, 2000.

"Mitral Valve Prolapse." *Mayo Clinic*, April 21, 2011.

"What Is Mitral Valve Prolapse?" *National Heart, Lung, and Blood Institute*, July 1, 2011.

MOLD AND MILDEW
Biology, Disease/Disorder

Anatomy or system affected: Immune system, lungs, nose, respiratory system, skin

Specialties and related fields: Environmental health, microbiology, pediatrics, pulmonary medicine, toxicology

Definition: Mold is a generalized term describing nonfruiting fungi, often microscopic and living in moist areas both outdoors and inside buildings, which consume nutrients and produce spores. Mold, which thrives in humid and closed spaces, has contributed to the development of effective pharmaceuticals but has also been blamed for various health problems and diseases.

Key terms:

conidiophore: a spore-creating area on hyphae in fungi

conidium: spores

hyphae: thin tubes in fungi that secure food and grow, expanding mold size

mycelium: mold colonies consisting of numerous meshed hyphae

mycologists: scientists who study the biological field specializing in fungi and similar spore producers that do not undergo photosynthesis

mycotoxins: poisons released by fungi

Structure and Functions

Mold grows in wet environments where abundant food, primarily organic materials such as cellulose, provides nourishment. Although mycologists consider mildew to be an outdoor fungal plant disease, that term is popularly used to designate mold found indoors on cloth and wooden objects. Thousands of mold species and millions of strains exists. Scientists have found molds both on Earth and in space. Mold spores are always present in air, moving with currents and surrounding humans. They cannot totally be eliminated inside buildings.

Information on Mold and Mildew

Causes: Exposure to parasitic fungi

Symptoms: Allergies, runny nose, sinus problems, coughing, rashes, asthma attacks, headaches, nausea, memory loss

Duration: Acute to chronic

Treatments: Frequent household cleaning, allowing air to circulate, keeping moisture levels in check

---

Fungi release enzymes to digest food in hyphae to create cells and energy. Mold eats dust, paper, and leather products, living in basements and cooling and heating systems. It can be found in walls, in insulation, and on ceilings. Flooding intensifies mold growth. Mold perishes if food sources are completely devoured or if mites that eat mold spores are present.

Mold hyphae have conidiophores that make conidium. Shaped as spirals, ovals, or spheres, mold spores can be barbed or smooth. If spores have access to nutrients, moisture, air, and sufficiently warm temperatures, then germination starts within twelve to forty-eight hours of being discharged from the conidiophore, and an initial hyphae emerges from the spore. As the hyphae consumes food, a mycelium forms in a period ranging from several days to almost two weeks later for *Stachybotrys chartarum*, also called black mold.

Although some molds such as penicillin are helpful, many molds are toxic. In their spores usually, but sometimes in hyphae, molds create mycotoxins, which protect them from bacteria and can cause sickness in other organisms. The access of molds to food and water affects their production of mycotoxins, which are not created by every mold. Molds do not discharge mycotoxins every place that they grow, nor do they always create toxic quantities of mycotoxins. Molds are mostly benign when outdoors because mycotoxins frequently scatter in the air. Inside, however, mycotoxins can accumulate in dangerous amounts.

Disorders and Diseases

Scientists have proven that outdoor molds can cause many human, plant, and animal illnesses. Some researchers have considered inside molds to be detrimental to human health, associating them with weakened immune systems and various ailments because people have suspected that exposure to indoor molds intensified their allergies and asthma. Some have blamed contact with molds in their homes and other buildings for triggering headaches, skin rashes, nosebleeds, and fevers.

Based on animal testing and cases of humans exposed to moldy agricultural products, medical researchers recognize known mold dangers. For example, black mold produces satratoxin, which can attack and destroy brain cells, particularly neurons, impeding the ability to smell and detect odors. *Trichothecenes* mycotoxins created by *Stachybotrys* and *Fusarium* molds can cause sore throats, blistered skin, and excessive bleeding. *Aspergillus flavus* produces aflatoxins, which can be carcinogenic. Aspergillosis, a disease affecting the lungs, is triggered by mycotoxins created by *Aspergillus* molds. *Claviceps purpurea*, referred to as ergot, produces mycotoxins that can be hallucinogenic. Some forms of that mycotoxin are useful, however, in soothing migraines or inducing childbirth.

Although individual mold mycotoxins might be harmless, mixtures of mycotoxins can be potentially damaging as their adverse effects combine. The degree to which molds might cause health problems depends on the concentration of mycotoxins and how they invade body systems, specifically whether humans breathe or ingest spores and where the spores settle within their bodies. The size of spores influences their impact on people's health. Researchers hypothesize that some mycotoxins might reach vulnerable lung tissues because they are too tiny to be stopped by nasal defenses that block other harmful microorganisms.

Perspective and Prospects

In 1837, scientists initially became aware that black mold existed when it was found in wallpaper in a Prague, Czechoslovakia, residence. By 1986, William Croft, B. B. Jarvis, and C. S. Yatawara presented the first scientific paper, published in *Atmospheric Environment*, discussing the toxicity of indoor mold. They suggested that black mold spores located in a Chicago house, which later proved lethal to laboratory animals, might be linked to health issues that the residents experienced.

During 1993 and 1994, physicians treated infants whose lungs bled at a Cleveland, Ohio, children's hospital. An investigation by hospital physicians and Centers for Disease Control and Prevention (CDC) personnel revealed that the infants lived in homes containing black mold spores. The media printed stories blaming black mold for the infants' sickness, while hospital officials emphasized the complexity of the situation and the need for a thorough investigation to verify if mold had caused the medical conditions.

The possible dangers of indoor molds again became news in 1999, when *USA Weekend* magazine warned of health hazards allegedly attributed to black mold. Lawsuits resulting in several million dollars in damages increased public awareness of the mold health issue as the media sensationalized the topic. Litigation and mold-related services escalated; con artists took advantage of people's fears of toxic mold. Some legislation relevant to mold and health concerns required house sellers to reveal whether mold had ever existed in structures for sale.

In 2004, the Institute of Medicine of the National Academies in the United States published a consensus report on damp indoor spaces and health. The report concluded that an association exists between damp indoor environments and problems such as upper respiratory-tract symptoms, coughing, wheezing, and asthma symptoms in some human populations. Research in this area continues to lead to healthier work and home environments. Reductions in dampness in indoor spaces improve health and also address known problems such as mold, bacteria, and dust.

—*Elizabeth D. Schafer, Ph.D.*

See also Allergies; Aspergillosis; Asthma; Blisters; Coughing; Environmental diseases; Environmental health; Fungal infections; Headaches; Immune system; Immunology; Lungs; Microbiology; Multiple chemical sensitivity syndrome; Nasopharyngeal disorders; Pulmonary diseases; Pulmonary medicine; Rashes; Respiration; Sinusitis; Skin; Skin disorders; Sore throat; Wheezing.

For Further Information:

Lankarge, Vicki. *What Every Home Owner Needs to Know About Mold (And What to Do About It)*. New York: McGraw-Hill, 2003.

May, Jeffrey C., and Connie L. May. *Mold Survival Guide for Your Home and for Your Health*. Baltimore: Johns Hopkins University Press, 2004.

Money, Nicholas P. *Carpet Monsters and Killer Spores: A Natural History of Toxic Mold*. New York: Oxford University Press, 2004.

Shoemaker, Ritchie C. *Mold Warriors: Fighting America's Hidden Health Threat*. Baltimore: Gateway Press, 2007.

MOLES

Disease/Disorder
Also known as: Nevi pigmentosa
Anatomy or system affected: Skin
Specialties and related fields: Dermatology, family medicine, plastic surgery
Definition: Nonmalignant marks, pigmented spots, or growths on the skin.

Causes and Symptoms

The common mole, also known as a nevus pigmentosus, is a mark, spot, or growth found on the skin that is generally benign and may be either congenital (present at birth) or developmental. Moles may be various colors, shapes, and sizes, and they can be flat or raised. Caucasian adults usually have approximately twenty pigmented nevi, the majority of which are less than 0.5 inch in diameter, with fewer pigmented ones evident at birth.

A mole is primarily the result of an accumulation of melanocytes, cells that form the skin pigment melanin. The greater the number of melanocytes, the darker the brown color of the mole. When the melanocytes are located deep below the skin surface, the mole appears dark bluish in color. Melanocytes also form the relatively larger vascular nevi (birthmarks) that derive from abnormal vascular construction in the skin. Types of birthmarks include the strawberry hemangioma and the port-wine stain, which arise from poorly developed blood vessels, and the nevus anemicus, which is attributed to a reduced blood flow.

Treatment and Therapy

In most cases, moles are benign, but occasionally they develop into malignant melanoma, a form of skin cancer. This transformation may be indicated by the development of a flat, pigmented zone around the base of a mole or the progressive enlargement of an existing mole. Other evidence of skin cancer involves a sudden increase in size, color, texture, shape, or sensation; irregular edges; loss of the hair surrounding a mole; and ulceration and bleeding. If cancer is suspected, a doctor can test for cancer cells by performing a biopsy to remove all or part of the mole.

Information on Moles

Causes: Congenital and environmental factors, aging
Symptoms: Flat or raised mark, spot, or growth on skin
Duration: Short-term to chronic
Treatments: Removal through cauterization, laser treatment

A newly formed mole is usually flat. If it arises between the dermis and the epidermis, then the mole is called a junction nevus, which may become malignant. A dermatologist's care in a timely manner is usually recommended. The main treatment involves removal of the mole by cauterization or laser treatment.

Moles occasionally disappear with age. Generally, however, more nevi form with aging, such as freckles, and they are usually permanent. The growth of new moles and darkening or other changes in existing ones should be monitored. Moles that are unsightly or irritated may be surgically removed. New moles are usually dome-shaped and elevated slightly above the surrounding skin. Plucking the hair associated with moles is not recommended, as this may damage the skin and lead to ulceration and bleeding.

—*Soraya Ghayourmanesh, Ph.D.*

See also Birthmarks; Dermatology; Dermatology, pediatric; Melanoma; Skin; Skin cancer; Skin disorders; Warts.

For Further Information:

Alan, Rick. "Moles." *Health Library*, May 11, 2013.
Burns, Tony, et al., eds. *Rook's Textbook of Dermatology.* 7th ed. Malden, Mass: Blackwell Science, 2004.
Lacouture, Mario E. *Dermatology and the Cancer Patient: Conditions of the Skin, Hair, and Nails During Cancer Treatment and Survivors.* Hoboken: Wiley-Blackwell, 2013.
McClay, Edward F., and Jodie Smith. *One Hundred Questions and Answers About Melanoma and Other Skin Cancers.* Boston: Jones and Bartlett, 2004.
Mackie, Rona M. *Clinical Dermatology.* 5th ed. New York: Oxford University Press, 2003.
Marks, James G., Jr., and Jeffrey J. Miller. *Lookingbill and Marks" Principles of Dermatology.* 4th ed. Philadelphia: Saunders/Elsevier, 2006.
Schofield, Jill R., and William A. Robinson. *What You Really Need to Know about Moles and Melanoma.* Baltimore: Johns Hopkins University Press, 2000.
Shenenberger, DW. "Cutaneous Malignant Melanoma: A Primary Care Perspective." *American Family Physician* 85, no. 2 (2012): 161–168.
Turkington, Carol, and Jeffrey S. Dover. *The Encyclopedia of Skin and Skin Disorders.* 3d ed. New York: Facts On File, 2007.
Weedon, David. *Skin Pathology.* 3d ed. New York: Churchill Livingstone/Elsevier, 2010.

MONKEYPOX
Disease/Disorder

Anatomy or system affected: Immune system, respiratory system, skin
Specialties and related fields: Dermatology, emergency medicine, internal medicine, public health, virology

Definition: A rare disease, originating in the rain forests of Central and West Africa, that affects animals and humans and is caused by a virus.

Causes and Symptoms

Monkeypox is a poxvirus in the *Orthopoxvirus* genus, which contains three other species affecting humans: variola (smallpox), vaccinia (the current smallpox vaccine), and cowpox (the original smallpox vaccine). The virion is large and brick-shaped, containing double-stranded deoxyribonucleic acid (DNA) that has been decoded and comprises 196,858 base pairs. Since smallpox was declared eradicated in 1979, monkeypox is regarded as the most serious naturally occurring poxvirus infection.

Bites or direct contact with an infected animal may result in transmission. Person-to-person spread also occurs through respiratory droplets, requiring close contact with an infected host. Direct contact with body fluids or skin lesions may also transmit the virus. Less commonly, virus-contaminated objects from infected humans, pets, or laboratory animals may spread the disease indirectly.

The disease can affect persons of any age, but children are more common. The incubation period varies from about six to sixteen days, and the illness commences with a fever that may be accompanied by headache and enlarged lymph nodes. One to three days later, a maculopapular rash develops. The rash primarily involves the periphery (head and extremities) and resembles smallpox more than chickenpox, which is more centrally (trunk) located. However, lymphadenopathy is not usually seen in smallpox. The rash of monkeypox may involve the palms and soles. The skin lesions progress through a vesiculopustular stage before finally crusting. Secondary infection and scarring may occur. Lesions may also be seen in the mouth and upper respiratory tract, producing a cough and occasionally respiratory distress. Spread of the infection to the brain, causing encephalitis, is a rare but serious complication. The illness typically lasts two to four weeks, and while mortality rates as high as 10 percent have been reported from Africa, fatal cases are rare with modern health care.

Treatment and Therapy

Smallpox vaccine is about 85 percent protective against monkeypox infection, and individuals at risk should receive the vaccine. Exposed individuals should receive the vaccine within four days of exposure but may benefit up to two weeks after exposure. Vaccinia immunoglobulin may be considered for treatment or prophylaxis, although its effectiveness is unproven. The antiviral agent cidofovir is active against monkeypox in vitro and in animals. Unfortunately, the efficacy of cidofovir for human cases is unknown. Because cidofovir is a toxic drug, it should be considered for treatment only in severe cases and should not be used for prophylaxis.

Perspective and Prospects

In 1958, monkeypox was first described in captive *Cynomolgous* monkeys in Copenhagen, Denmark. The first

---

Information on Monkeypox

Causes: Viral infection transmitted by bite or direct contact with infected animal (primarily African rodents); also transmitted person-to-person through respiratory droplets, direct contact with body fluids or skin lesions

Symptoms: Rash, fever, headache, lymph node enlargement, coughing; may spread to brain, causing encephalitis

Duration: Two to four weeks

Treatments: Protection with smallpox vaccine before or after exposure; antiviral drug cidofovir only in severe cases

---

human case was identified in 1970 in the Democratic Republic of Congo. African squirrels are the main reservoir of monkeypox, but the virus has been found in a number of other African rodents.

A shipment of eight hundred African rodents from Ghana to an animal distributor in Texas during April 2003, resulted in the infection of coinhabiting captive prairie dogs. Many of these animals were sold as pets, and the result was eighty-one human cases of monkeypox in six states. All patients survived, but 25 percent required hospitalization and two children had severe disease.

Low herd immunity, along with repeated introduction of monkeypox from the African wild reservoir, will likely produce more human illness, both in Africa and at distant sites. The use of smallpox vaccine in high-risk and exposed persons, along with antiviral agents such as cidofovir for severe cases, should limit disease and improve outcomes.

—*H. Bradford Hawley, M.D.*

See also Immunization and vaccination; Rashes; Smallpox; Viral infections; Zoonoses.

For Further Information:

Beltz, Lisa A. *Emerging Infectious Diseases: A Guide to Diseases, Causative Agents, and Surveillance*. San Francisco: Jossey-Bass, 2011.

Bernard, Susan M. "Qualitative Assessment of Risk for Monkeypox Associated with Domestic Trade in Certain Animal Species, United States." *Emerging Infectious Diseases* 12, no. 12 (December 1, 2006): 1827.

Centers for Disease Control and Prevention. "Multistate Outbreak of Monkeypox—Illinois, Indiana, and Wisconsin, 2003." *Morbidity and Mortality Weekly Report* 52 (June 13, 2003): 537–540.

Centers for Disease Control and Prevention. "Update: Multistate Outbreak of Monkeypox—Illinois, Indiana, Kansas, Missouri, Ohio, and Wisconsin, 2003." *Morbidity and Mortality Weekly Report* 52 (July 2, 2003): 1–3.

Hutlin, Yvan J. F., et al. "Outbreak of Human Monkeypox, Democratic Republic of Congo, 1996-1997." *Emerging Infectious Diseases* 7 (May/June, 2001): 434–438.

JeÅ3/4ek, ZdenÄªk, and Frank Fenner, eds. *Human Monkeypox*. New York: S. Karger, 1988.

"Monkeypox." *Centers for Diesease Control and Prevention*, Sept. 5, 2008.

"Monkeypox." *World Health Organization*, Feb. 2011.

"Monkeypox Virus Infections." *MedlinePlus*, Jan. 14, 2013.

MONONUCLEOSIS

Disease/Disorder

Also known as: Infectious mononucleosis, the kissing disease

Anatomy or system affected: Heart, lymphatic system, spleen, throat

Specialties and related fields: Family medicine, pediatrics, virology

Definition: An acute viral infectious disease that produces lymph node enlargement (hyperplasia).

Key terms:

anorexia: loss of appetite

dysphagia: difficulty in swallowing

lymph nodes: glandlike masses or knots of lymphatic tissue that are distributed along the lymphatic vessels to filter bacteria or foreign bodies from the body

periorbital: referring to the region around the eyes

spleen: a large lymphatic organ in the abdominal cavity that forms lymphocytes and other blood cells and stores blood

splenomegaly: enlargement of the spleen

Causes and Symptoms

Mononucleosis is caused by the Epstein-Barr virus, which is transmitted through infected saliva or by blood transfusions. It has an incubation period of four to six weeks. The saliva may remain infective for as long as eighteen months, and after the primary infection, the virus may be present in the nasal secretions and shed periodically for the rest of the host's life. Many cases occur in adolescents—hence the popular name "the kissing disease." The virus can be cultured from the throat of 10 to 20 percent of most healthy adults. The incidence of mononucleosis varies seasonally among high school and college students but does not vary among the general population. The disease is fairly common in the United States, Canada, and Europe and occurs in both sexes.

Mononucleosis is characterized by fever, fatigue, anorexia, a sore throat, chills, a skin rash, bleeding gums, red spots on the tonsils, malaise, and periorbital edema. Lymph nodes in the neck enlarge, and splenomegaly develops in about half of patients. In a small number of patients, liver involvement with mild jaundice occurs.

The diagnosis is made by several different tests, such as the differential white blood count. In mononucleosis, lymphocytes and monocytes make up greater than 50 percent of the blood cells, with a figure of more than 10 percent being atypical. The leukocyte count is normal early in the disease but rises during the second week. Serology studies show an increase in the heterophile antibody titer, although the monospot test is more rapid and can detect the infection earlier and is widely used. Children under four years of age often test negative for heterophil antibodies, but the test will identify 90 percent of cases in older children, adolescents, and adults.

Treatment and Therapy

The treatment of mononucleosis is mainly supportive, since the disease is self-limiting. The patient is usually placed on

Information on Mononucleosis

Causes: Viral infection

Symptoms: Fever, malaise, lymph node enlargement, sore throat, chills, rash, bleeding gums, red spots on tonsils

Duration: Four to six weeks

Treatments: Supportive therapy, including bed rest, limited activity, acetaminophen (Tylenol), increased fluid intake

bed rest during the acute stage of the disease, and activity is limited to prevent rupture of the enlarged spleen, usually for at least two months. Acetaminophen (such as the brand Tylenol) is given for the fever, and saline gargles or lozenges may be used for the sore throat. Patients need to increase their fluid intake. Many doctors use corticosteriods such as prednisone during the course of the disease to lessen the severity of the symptoms. If rupture of the spleen occurs, emergency surgery is necessary to remove the organ.

Complications are uncommon but may include rupture of the spleen, secondary pneumonia, heart involvement, neurologic manifestations such as Guillain-Barré syndrome, meningitis, encephalitis, hemolytic anemia, and orchitis (inflammation of the testes).

Perspective and Prospects

Viruses, such as the one responsible for mononucleosis, were first studied in the 1930s, and they remain a challenge to laboratory investigators. Most information about viruses has come from studying their effects, rather than the viruses themselves. The majority of methods for destroying or controlling viruses are ineffective. There is no prevention for many of the diseases caused by viruses, such as infectious mononucleosis. It may be reassuring to know that the disease seldom causes severe complications if the symptoms are treated and medical care is given to those infected with the Epstein-Barr virus.

—Mitzie L. Bryant, B.S.N., M.Ed.

See also Childhood infectious diseases; Chronic fatigue syndrome; Epstein-Barr virus; Fatigue; Fever; Hodgkin's disease; Immune system; Jaundice; Lymphadenopathy and lymphoma; Lymphatic system; Otorhinolaryngology; Sore throat; Viral infections.

For Further Information:

Alan, Rick. "Mononucleosis." *Health Library*, March 25, 2013.

Beers, Mark H., et al., eds. *The Merck Manual of Diagnosis and Therapy*. 19th ed. Whitehouse Station, N.J.: Merck Research Laboratories, 2011.

Dreher, Nancy. "What You Need to Know About Mono." *Current Health 2* 23, no. 7 (March, 1997): 28–29.

Harkness, Gail, ed. *Medical-Surgical Nursing: Total Patient Care*. 10th ed. St. Louis, Mo.: Mosby, 1999.

Kimball, Chad T. *Colds, Flu, and Other Common Ailments Sourcebook*. Detroit, Mich.: Omnigraphics, 2001.

Litin, Scott C., ed. *Mayo Clinic Family Health Book*. 4th ed. New York: HarperResource, 2009.

"Mononucleosis." *Mayo Clinic*, December 19, 2012.

"Mononucleosis." *MedlinePlus*, May 15, 2012.

Shrader, Laurel, and John Zonderman. *Mononucleosis and Other Infectious Diseases*. Rev. ed. New York: Chelsea House, 2000.

Sompayrac, Lauren. *How Pathogenic Viruses Work*. Boston: Jones and Bartlett, 2002.

Woolf, Alan D., et al., eds. *The Children's Hospital Guide to Your Child's Health and Development*. Cambridge, Mass.: Perseus, 2002.

MORGELLONS DISEASE

Disease/Disorder

Anatomy or system affected: Psychic-emotional system, skin

Specialties and related fields: Dermatology, neurology, psychiatry

Definition: A skin disorder characterized by a pattern of dermatologic symptoms described as insectlike sensations, with skin lesions varying from very minor to disfiguring, and associated with disabling fatigue, joint pain, and various neuropsychiatric symptoms. In the first decade of the twenty-first century, the cause, transmission, and treatment remained under investigation.

Key terms:

obsession: a recurrent and persistent thought or impulse associated with continuous and involuntary preoccupation that cannot be expunged by logic or reasoning

psychosomatic illness: a disorder in which physical symptoms are caused or aggravated by psychological factors

skin biopsy: a removal of a piece of skin for the purpose of further microscopic examination

skin lesion: superficial growth or patch of the skin that differs from the surrounding area surrounding

Causes and Symptoms

Morgellons disease is a pattern of dermatologic symptoms first described several centuries ago. Patients typically complain of insectlike sensations, such as persisting itching, stinging, biting, pricking, burning, and crawling. They often have skin lesions that can vary from very minor to disfiguring. Some patients, however, have no visible changes in the skin. In some cases, fiberlike material can be obtained from the skin lesions; patients describe this material as "fibers," "fiber balls," and "fuzz balls." In other cases, "granules" can be removed from the skin, described by the patients as "seeds," "eggs," and "sands." The majority of patients report disabling fatigue, reduced capacity to exercise, joint pain, and sleep disturbances. Additional symptoms may include hair loss, neurological symptoms, weight gain, recurrent fever, orthostatic intolerance, tachycardia, decline in vision, memory loss, and endocrine abnormalities (such as diabetes type 2, Hashimoto's thyroiditis, hyperparathyroidism, or adrenal hypofunction).

The disease may occur at any age and has a large geographic distribution. It occurs in both males and females. Cases of elderly women living alone seem more frequently reported. Physical stress was reported to be a common precursor. Rural residence and exposure to unhygienic conditions (contact with soil or waste products) are often described. Results from routine laboratory tests are often

---

Information on Morgellons Disease

Causes: Unknown; under investigation
Symptoms: Insectlike skin sensations of stinging, persisting itching, biting, pricking, burning, and crawling; minor to disfiguring skin lesions; disabling fatigue; joint pain; psychosomatic and neurological symptoms
Duration: Chronic
Treatments: Symptomatic and supportive skin care, antipsychotic medications

---

variable and inconsistent.

The vast majority of these patients have been diagnosed with psychosomatic illness. Prior psychiatric diagnosis (such as bipolar disorder, paranoia, schizophrenia, depression, and drug abuse) has been recorded in more than 50 percent of patients . Patients are obsessively focused on the skin symptoms in terms of complaints and measures to eradicate the disease and to prevent contagion. They usually seek help from between ten and forty physicians and complain of being not understood or taken seriously. Usually, patients are intensely anxious and not open to the idea that they may have a psychological or neurological pathology. They often experience extreme frustration.

Morgellons disease has also been reported in association with conditions that are characterized by itching, such as renal disease, malignant lymphoma, or hepatic disease.

The etiology of Morgellons disease remains under investigation. So far, no examinations, biopsies, and tests have been able to provide evidence supporting any possible cause. Skin biopsies from patients with Morgellons disease typically reveal nonspecific pathology or inflammatory process/reaction with no observable pathogen. In a 2012 study from the US Centers for Disease Control and Prevention (CDC) researchers did not find any evidence that Morgellons is caused by either an environment substance or an infectious agent.

Treatment and Therapy

The management of patients with Morgellons disease is symptomatic and supportive. It can include skin care with baths, topical ointments, and emollients. It is important for the treating physician (in most cases, a dermatologist) to refer the patient to a psychiatrist or to prescribe appropriate psychoactive medication. Long-term treatment with pimozid (0.5 to 2 milligrams once daily) has been suggested. Risperidone and aripiprazone have also been reported to be efficient. Patients should be convinced that the medication may be needed for months or years.

Perspective and Prospects

Morgellons disease was initially described in France, in 1674, by Sir Thomas Browne. "The Morgellons" was the term used to describe dermal complaints such as hairlike extrusions and sensations of movement beneath the skin reported by children. By the early seventeenth century, this condition was thought to be caused by the parasite *Dranculus*

(later called *Dracontia*), and the suggested treatment consisted of filament removal from the skin. Michel Ettmuller produced the only known drawing dating from 1682 of "The Morgellons," the objects associated with what was then believed to be a parasitic infestation in children.

The name "Morgellons disease" was created in 2002 to describe patients presenting with this clinical set of symptoms and to provide an alternative to "delusion of parasitosis." Although the condition was first described many centuries ago, much attention has recently been given to the disease because of the Internet, mass media, and the online support group Morgellons Research Foundation at www.morgellons.com. There is still a discussion whether Morgellons disease is very similar, if not identical, to "delusion of parasitosis." Thus, whether Morgellons disease is a delusional disorder or even a disease has been a mystery for more than three hundred years. So far, research about Morgellons is sparse and limited. General practitioners, mental health professionals, and the general public need to be aware of the signs and symptoms of this mysterious condition. Some authors suggest the term "syndrome" instead of "disease."

—Katia Marazova, M.D., Ph.D.

See also Antidepressants; Anxiety; Bipolar disorders; Body dysmorphic disorder; Delusions; Dermatology; Factitious disorders; Hallucinations; Hypochondriasis; Itching; Neurology; Neurology, pediatric; Neurosis; Psychiatric disorders; Psychiatry; Psychosis; Psychosomatic disorders; Skin; Skin disorders; Stress.

For Further Information:

"CDC Study of an Unexplained Dermopathy." *Centers for Disease Control and Prevention*, January 25, 2012.
Harvey, William T., et al. "Morgellons Disease: Illuminating an Undefined Illness—A Case Series." *Journal of Medical Case Reports* no. 3 (2009): 8243.
Fair, Brian. "Morgellons: Contested Illness, Diagnostic Compromise and Medicalisation." *Sociology of Health & Illness* 32, no. 4 (May 2010): 597–612.
Koblenezer, Caroline S. "The Challenge of Morgellons Disease." *Journal of the American Academy of Dermatology* 55 (2006): 920–22.
"Morgellons Disease: Managing a Mysterious Skin Condition." *Mayo Clinic*, April 11, 2012.
Savely, Virginia R., Mary M. Leitao, and Raphael B. Stricker. "The Mystery of Morgellons Disease: Infection or Delusion?" *American Journal of Clinical Dermatology* 7, no. 1 (2006): 1–5.

MOSQUITO BITES. *See* BITES AND STINGS; INSECT-BORNE DISEASES

MOTION SICKNESS
Disease/Disorder
Also known as: Carsickness, airsickness, seasickness
Anatomy or system affected: Ears, gastrointestinal system, head, nervous system, stomach
Specialties and related fields: Family medicine, neurology, otorhinolaryngology
Definition: A disorder characterized by nausea, vomiting, and vertigo and caused by a combination of repetitive back-and-forth and up-and-down movements.

Key terms:

cranial: pertaining to the bones of the head

medulla oblongata: a continuation of the spinal cord that forms the lower portion of the brain stem; the site of many regulatory centers, as for cardiac rhythm, breathing, and the diameter of blood vessels

transdermal patch: a drug delivery system in which medication is slowly released from a patch and absorbed through the skin over a period of days

vertigo: a specific type of dizziness in which people feel as though either they themselves are spinning around or the room is spinning around them

Causes and Symptoms

Motion sickness appears to be caused by overstimulation of the balance centers of the inner ears by repeated back-and-forth and up-and-down movements. Messages are carried from this area of the inner ear, known as the vestibular apparatus, to the medulla oblongata in the brain, which is responsible for the vomiting reaction. The nerve pathways for this journey are not entirely known, but certainly the cranial nerve, which is responsible for hearing and balance, is involved. Responses in the medulla oblongata set into motion automatic motor reactions in the upper gastrointestinal tract, diaphragm, and abdominal muscles that lead to vomiting.

Individuals vary considerably in their susceptibility to motion sickness, and experts believe that there may be an inherited tendency toward the problem. Shifting visual input (such as watching waves on the horizon), a poorly ventilated environment, and fear and anxiety all seem to play a role in the development and severity of motion sickness.

The diagnosis of motion sickness is usually self-evident. Vertigo, nausea, and vomiting follow exposure to a repetitive and usually irregular rocking motion while in a moving vehicle or on an amusement park ride. The first indication of motion sickness may be yawning, excessive salivation, pale skin, and sweating. The person may begin to breathe deeply or complain of sleepiness. The patient may also develop a need for air, dizziness, or a headache. In most cases, nausea and vomiting occur sooner or later. On an extended trip, patients with motion sickness may eventually develop a tolerance to the motion and feel better, or they may continue to feel sick. If severe rocking motions develop once again, however, patients may also become sick again. Repeated vomiting may lead to dehydration and low blood pressure. Depression is another feature of prolonged motion sickness.

Treatment and Therapy

This malady is far easier to prevent than to treat. People who suffer from motion sickness should avoid drinking liquids just before and during short trips. On longer trips, they should limit liquids and have only small, easy-to-digest foods at regular intervals. Plenty of fresh air may also help prevent sickness. Those prone to motion sickness should not read in a car or other moving vehicle. Focusing the eyes well above the horizon while riding in a car or on a boat may help. People who are susceptible to motion sickness should also avoid

> ### Information on Motion Sickness
>
> **Causes:** Overstimulation of balance centers of inner ears, shifting visual input, poorly ventilated environment, fear and anxiety
>
> **Symptoms:** Yawning, excessive salivation, pale skin, sweating, nausea, vomiting, vertigo
>
> **Duration:** Acute
>
> **Treatments:** Over-the-counter or prescription medications; preventive measures

amusement park rides that involve swinging and rocking.

Sufferers of motion sickness may be treated with over-the-counter or prescription medications an hour before travel begins. Medications used for this purpose include diphenhydramine, promethazine, prcochlorperazine, chlorpromazine, scopolamine, dimenhydrinate, cyclizine, buclizine, and meclizine. They are available in a variety of forms, including tablets, rectal suppositories, and transdermal patches. Many of these drugs cause sleepiness, which may be helpful during a trip but cause drowsiness or lack of alertness on arrival. Another common side effect of some of these drugs is dry mouth. In most cases, these medications are more effective when given before vomiting begins. An extract of ginger root has been recommended as a treatment using a natural substance, and so having fewer side effects. Some objective studies, however, have failed to demonstrate its efficacy.

If the person has already begun vomiting, medications must be given by injection, rectal suppository, or a transdermal patch. In cases of prolonged vomiting, where dehydration is a concern, the patient may require intravenous fluids. Of particular concern is the individual who is already ill with another disease and also suffers from motion sickness. Such patients may have serious complications related to the vomiting and resulting dehydration.

Nonpharmacologic treatments for motion sickness abound. The best known are acupressure wristbands. The autogenic-feedback training (AFT) exercise, designed by the National Aeronautics and Space Administration (NASA), is a self-regulation and biofeedback training scheme that has shown promise in studies of space motion sickness in astronauts. It requires a minimum of six hours of training and so is not the quick fix that drugs promise. NASA scientists have also explored devices for holding the astronaut's head steady, since head movement appears to exacerbate motion sickness. Such an apparatus might be applicable to the civilian population as well.

Perspective and Prospects

Motion sickness is a common problem in children and some adults. New drugs to treat the problem are being explored. A number of chemicals showing promise are related to or interact with serotonin, a chemical that participates in a number of regulatory systems in the body. Drug companies are working on new drug delivery systems to make antinausea medications easier to take. Other advances include drug regimens that will provide antinausea effects without sleepiness.

—Rebecca Lovell Scott, Ph.D., PA-C;
updated by Carl W. Hoagstrom, Ph.D.

See also Acupressure; Acupuncture; Audiology; Balance disorders; Biofeedback; Dehydration; Dizziness and fainting; Ear infections and disorders; Ears; Gastrointestinal system; Nausea and vomiting; Nervous system; Neurology; Neurology, pediatric; Over-the-counter medications.

For Further Information:

Canalis, Rinaldo, and Paul R. Lambert, eds. *The Ear: Comprehensive Otology.* Philadelphia: Lippincott Williams & Wilkins, 2000.

Chang, Chih-Hui, et al. "Console Video Games, Postural Activity, and Motion Sickness During Passive Restraint." *Experimental Brain Research* 229, no. 2 (August, 2013): 235–242

Crampton, George H., ed. *Motion and Space Sickness.* Boca Raton, Fla.: CRC Press, 1990.

Diels, C., and P. A. Howarth. "Frequency Characteristics of Visually Induced Motion Sickness." *Human Factors* 55, no. 3 (June, 2013): 595–604.

Ferrari, Mario. *PDxMD Ear, Nose, and Throat Disorders.* Philadelphia: PDxMD, 2003.

Litin, Scott C., ed. *Mayo Clinic Family Health Book.* 4th ed. New York: HarperResource, 2009.

Mendel, Lisa Lucks, Jeffrey L. Danhauer, and Sadanand Singh. *Singular's Illustrated Dictionary of Audiology.* San Diego, Calif.: Singular, 1999.

Spock, Benjamin, and Robert Needlman. *Dr. Spock's Baby and Child Care.* 8th ed. New York: Pocket Books, 2004.

Thorton, W. E., and R. Bonato. "Space Motion Sickness and Motion Sickness: Symptoms and Etiology." *Aviation, Space, and Environmental Medicine* 84, no. 7 (July, 2013): 716–721.

Zajonc, Timothy P., and Peter S. Roland. "Vertigo and Motion Sickness, Part 1: Vestibular Anatomy and Physiology." *Ear, Nose, and Throat Journal* 84 (September, 2005): 581–584.

Zajonc, Timothy P., and Peter S. Roland. "Vertigo and Motion Sickness, Part 2: Pharmacological Treatment." *Ear, Nose, and Throat Journal* 85 (January, 2006): 25–35.

MOTOR NEURON DISEASES
Disease/Disorder

Anatomy or system affected: Muscles, musculoskeletal system, nerves, nervous system, spine

Specialties and related fields: Neurology

Definition: Progressive, debilitating, and eventually fatal diseases affecting nerve cells in muscles.

Key terms:

Babinski's sign: an abnormal response to a neurological test involving a brisk stroke with a sharp object on the bottom of the foot; the normal response is for the toes to bunch together and curve downward, while the abnormal response is for the big toe to pull upward and not in unison with the other toes

corticospinal tracts: neurological pathways descending from the brain to the spinal cord that control and allow voluntary movement

fasciculations: spontaneous electrical impulses from neurons that result in irregular, involuntary muscular contractions; in motor neuron disease, these contractions indicate nerve death

lower motor neuron: a nerve cell whose cell body resides either in the brain stem (to form a cranial nerve) or in the spinal cord (to form a spinal motor neuron)

motor neuron: a nerve that functions either directly or indirectly to control a target organ

muscular atrophy: a wasting of muscle mass; a greatly reduced size of muscle cells caused by the lost innervation (neuron death) or disuse of muscles

spasticity: an abnormal condition in which the limbs demonstrate resistance to passive movement as a result of damage to the corticospinal tracts; the reflexes are hyperactive

tropic factors: chemicals released from nerve cells that have a vital influence on muscle health; in the absence of tropic factors, muscles atrophy

upper motor neuron: a nerve whose cell body resides within the brain but whose axon descends the brain stem and spinal cord to form a corticospinal tract

Causes and Symptoms

In motor neuron diseases, certain nerves die, specifically those that allow any and all body movement. The actual cause of spontaneous motor neuron death is unknown, but genetic defects, neurotoxins, viruses, autoimmune disruptions, and metabolic disorders are contributing factors.

The predominant features of motor neuron disorders are muscular weakness, muscular wasting, and the presence of fasciculations. As a nerve dies, it can no longer effectively innervate its target muscle, but neighboring nerves may sprout to keep the muscle active. A consequence of nerve sprouting is the onset of brief, spontaneous contractions, or twitches. These visible twitches are called fasciculations. Eventually, as increasing numbers of nerves die, fewer healthy nerves are left to sprout until, finally, all muscles are denervated. Dead nerves cannot prompt muscle movement, nor can they release tropic factors as they do in health. This loss of tropic input from the neuron causes muscular atrophy and renders the muscle useless.

Motor neuron diseases are usually first noticed in the hands or upper limbs, where muscle weakness and decreased ability to use arms or hands cause problems. Unlike some disorders, motor neuron diseases fail to show stages of exacerbation or remission. Rather they progress—either rapidly or slowly, but relentlessly—until death, usually as a result of respiratory complications.

Although there are childhood forms, motor neuron diseases are more likely to strike between the ages of fifty and fifty-five, and they are seen in males more than females by a ratio of 1.5 to 1. Motor neuron diseases seem to occur rarely in the obese person and tend to afflict otherwise healthy, thin, and perhaps athletic persons. A famed person afflicted by the debilitating motor neuron disease amyotrophic lateral sclerosis (ALS) was baseball player Lou Gehrig, in whose memory it is often called Lou Gehrig's disease.

Motor neuron diseases are often subgrouped into three categories: ALS, progressive spinal muscular atrophy, and progressive bulbar (brain-stem) palsy. In the plural form, motor neuron diseases refer to all forms of the affliction, whereas the singular form, motor neuron disease, is synonymous with ALS.

Amyotrophic lateral sclerosis is the most familiar of the motor neuron diseases primarily because it accounts for a full 60 percent of all such disorders. The name has clinical meaning: "Amyotrophy" refers to the loss of muscle bulk as a result of missing tropic factors from dying or dead neurons, "lateral" refers to the locations within the spinal cord that are affected, and "sclerosis" refers to the hardened quality of the lateral regions of the diseased spinal cord, which otherwise would be soft tissue. The brain stem may also be sclerotic (hardened). ALS has an incidence of 1 or 2 persons per 100,000, although some Pacific islands, such as Guam, seem to have a higher incidence attributable to undetermined genetic factors. In addition, some populations show an autosomal dominant genetic component. ALS is fatal, and death generally occurs as a result of respiratory failure within three to five years after the onset of symptoms.

ALS is characterized by upper and lower motor neuron signs of neural death; thus the presence of both fasciculations and spasticity is required for a diagnosis. Spasticity is a medical term that describes a certain kind of muscular resistance (stiffness) to movement. In particular, spastic means a resistance that increases the more rapidly a muscle is extended; tendon reflexes are also hyperactive and Babinski's sign (abnormal reflexes of the toes) must be present. Babinski's sign reveals the death of neurons in the corticospinal tracts, which signals the occurrence of upper motor neuron death. The presence of fasciculations reveals lower motor neuron death.

Progressive spinal muscular atrophy (SMA) will show only lower motor neuron signs—namely, muscular weakness, fasciculations, and atrophy. Babinski's sign or spasticity is not found. The early symptoms may include increased clumsiness in using the fingers for fine movements (including writing or using kitchen utensils), stiffness of the fingers and hands, and cramping of the upper and lower limbs. Once the brain-stem nerves become involved, difficulty in speaking and swallowing occur. Of all persons afflicted with one of the motor neuron diseases, 7 to 15 percent will have lower motor neuron signs only and are presumed to have the progressive spinal muscular atrophy form.

Progressive bulbar palsy literally means progressive brain-stem paralysis. This form of motor neuron disease accounts for 20 to 25 percent of all cases. The tongue is usually the first place to show muscular wasting and fasciculations. As the nerves controlling the tongue die, the tongue shrivels and shrinks so that speaking, chewing, and moving solids or liquids to the back of the mouth for swallowing become difficult or impossible.

Children can be afflicted with spinal muscular atrophy. This disease is believed by many experts to be completely unique from the adult form. The childhood form seems to be more associated with environmental and genetic factors. (This concept is greatly debated, however, since the actual cause of any of the motor neuron diseases is unknown.) Three forms of childhood SMA have been identified: type 1, or acute infantile SMA (also known as Werdnig-Hoffman disease); type 2, or intermediate SMA; and type 3, or juvenile

---

Information on Motor Neuron Diseases

Causes: Unknown; possibly genetic defects, neurotoxins, viruses, autoimmune disruptions, metabolic disorders
Symptoms: Muscle weakness or wasting, twitching or spasticity, decreased ability to use arms or hands, increased clumsiness
Duration: Chronic, sometimes progressive
Treatments: None; management of symptoms and palliative care

SMA (also known as Kugelberg-Welander disease).

Of children afflicted with SMA, 25 percent have type 1. This form of the disease is an autosomal recessive genetic disorder that occurs in 1 of 15,000 to 25,000 births. In an experienced mother, there may be awareness of minimal fetal movement in the last trimester of pregnancy; the fetus tends to stay still as a result of muscular weakness. Upon birth, the newborn may be a "floppy" baby of great weakness and may immediately have trouble with nursing and breathing. In other cases, it may take three to six months before symptoms begin. Because of the eventual weakening of the muscles of respiration, the child becomes prone to respiratory infections that cannot be cleared because of a lost cough reflex. Death usually occurs at two to three years of age.

When a child fails to stand or walk between six to twelve months of age, the physician considers the possibility that the child has type 2 SMA. An abnormal curvature of the spine to the forward and sideways position (kyphoscoliosis) is often seen, but rarely is there any problem with feeding or breathing. It is generally the case that very fine tremors of the child's hands can be noticed, and sometimes contractures of the hips and knees can occur. There is no delay in terms of mental health or intellect for these children.

Type 3 SMA is most often seen in the adolescent, but this disease can be observed in some children as early as five years of age. The predominant feature is weakness of the hip muscles. Since these children have been walking for some time, a change in their walking gait to a waddle can be seen over the course of years. Most people with type 3 SMA must use wheelchairs in their mid-thirties, but some may lose their ability to walk earlier. Type 3 SMA has been shown to be an autosomal recessive disorder in many cases, but there are also reported cases of sporadic occurrences within families that have previously been unaffected. Clearly, there are unanswered questions about this disease.

It should be noted that controversy abounds on the assigned classifications of motor neuron diseases. This controversy arises from the fact that the origins of the diseases are not known. Since cause has not been established for any form of motor neuron disease, physicians must use clusters of symptoms to sort the differences in disease manifestation. This sorting is used to plan the best possible treatment programs for the circumstances; nevertheless, these distinctions may seem arbitrary once more is known about the causes of motor neuron death.

Treatment and Therapy

Perhaps one of the most frustrating attributes of motor neuron diseases is that neither prevention nor effective treatment and cures are available. For a person living with motor neuron disease, physicians and health care professionals must work as a team to manage the symptoms of the diseases and offer palliative care.

In general, patients are encouraged to use and exercise their muscles cautiously in order to avoid disuse atrophy, but activity to the point of fatigue is forbidden since it is believed to aggravate the progression of muscular wasting. In addition, exposure to cold may worsen muscular contractures. Physical therapy facilitates a delay in the total loss of willed body movement by allowing the use of braces, walkers, and wheelchairs as modes of locomotion. Adults are encouraged to continue nonexertive work for as long as possible; it aids both the body and the mind to maintain independence and a sense of wholeness, well-being, and dignity.

As muscular control of the voice wanes, sketch pads, word boards, and computers can aid the ill person in communicating with loved ones, doctors, nurses, and colleagues. In addition, respiratory therapy aids in maintaining healthy breathing in spite of ever-weakening respiratory muscles. Prophylactic immunizations for influenza and pneumococci are given, especially to those who are wheelchair-dependent or bedridden. Forced deep breathing and coughing are needed at least once every four hours to bring up any congestion that may otherwise lead to grave consequences. Almost all persons with motor neuron diseases die from respiratory insufficiency. For this reason, it is imperative that the patient and physician discuss respiratory care early after diagnosis to determine whether the patient wants to be placed on mechanical ventilators in the later stages of the disease. Other issues such as tube feedings should be discussed while the patient is still able to voice an opinion and express any concerns about the dying process associated with the disease .

The past decade has seen a significant increase in the offering of fake treatments for motor neuron diseases by unaccredited organizations and physicians online. Many of these treatements offer patients relief from symptoms using human or animal stem cells. There remains no credible scientific evidence that stem cells of any kind are beneficial in the treatment of motor neuron disease. Reputable medical organization and law enforcement officials in the United States have stepped up efforts to combat scams and hoaxes offering false promises to patients and their familes.

Perspective and Prospects

Life can be socially difficult for people with motor neuron diseases. Others tend to assume that persons who must use wheelchairs and are unable to control mouth movements (so that speech and swallowing are lost and drooling may occur) are not intelligent, thinking, or aware. This is a sad misperception.

Many persons suffering from a motor neuron disease rise above its physical challenges to conquer in spirit that which the body cannot. For example, former United States senator Jacob Javits labored hard to improve the awareness of and funding for ALS in spite of being on a ventilator and completely immobile because of his battle with the disease. Another example of how well the intellect is preserved in this physically tragic disease can be seen in the life and work of the world-renowned astrophysicist Stephen Hawking.

Until there is an established cause or causes for these diseases, effective treatments or cures are likely to remain hidden. The research continues in the hope of pinning down the ever-elusive motor neuron diseases.

—Mary C. Fields, M.D.

See also Amyotrophic lateral sclerosis; Aphasia and dysphasia; Hospice; Huntington's disease; Muscle sprains, spasms, and disorders; Muscles; Nervous system; Neuralgia, neuritis, and neuropathy; Neurology; Neurology, pediatric; Palliative medicine; Palsy; Paralysis; Spinal cord disorders; Spine, vertebrae, and disks; Terminally ill: Extended care.

For Further Information:

Bear, Mark F., Barry W. Connors, and Michael A. Paradiso. *Neuroscience: Exploring the Brain*. 3d ed. Philadelphia: Lippincott Williams & Wilkins, 2007.

Bloom, Floyd E., M. Flint Beal, and David J. Kupfer, eds. *The Dana Guide to Brain Health*. New York: Dana Press, 2006.

Heilman, Kenneth M. *Matter of Mind: A Neurologist's View of Brain-Behavior Relationships*. New York: Oxford University Press, 2002.

Kuncl, Ralph W. *Motor Neuron Disease*. 1st ed. Philadelphia: Saunders Ltd., 2002. Print.

National Institute of Neurological Disorders and Stroke (NINDS). *Motor Neuron Diseases Information Page*. http://www.ninds. nih.gov/disorders/motor_neuron_diseases.

Parker, James N., and Philip M. Parker, eds. *Official Patient's Sourcebook on Amyotrophic Lateral Sclerosis*. San Diego, Calif.: Icon Health, 2003.

Parsons, Malcolm, and Michael Johnson. *Diagnosis in Color: Neurology*. New York: Mosby, 2001.

Talbot, Kevin. *Motor Neuron Disease (The Facts)*. Oxford UP, 2008. Print.

Thompson, Charlotte E. *Raising a Child with a Neuromuscular Disorder: A Guide for Parents, Grandparents, Friends, and Professionals*. New York: Oxford University Press, 2000.

Turner, Bradley J., and Julie B. Atkin, eds. *Motor Neuron Diseases: Causes, Classification and Treatments (Neurology - Laboratory and Clinical Research Developments)*. Hauppauge, New York: Nova Biomedical Books, 2012. Print.

MOTOR SKILL DEVELOPMENT

Development

Anatomy or system affected: Bones, circulatory system, eyes, joints, muscles, musculoskeletal system, nerves, nervous system, psychic-emotional system

Specialties and related fields: Exercise physiology, genetics, neonatology, neurology, orthopedics, pathology, pediatrics, perinatology, physical therapy, psychology, sports medicine

Definition: The process of change in motor behavior with advancing age and the numerous physiological and psychological processes that underlie these changes, which describe the adjustments in posture, movement, and skillful manipulation of objects achieved through the coordination of several neurologic control structures.

Key terms:

central nervous system: the brain and spinal cord, which process incoming information from the peripheral nervous system and form the main network of coordination and control in advanced organisms

motor control: the nature and cause of movement, which focuses on stability and movement of the body, and the manipulation of objects, which is achieved through the coordination of many structures organized both hierarchically and in a parallel manner

motor learning: the acquisition and modification of movement as a result of practice and experience, which leads to relatively permanent intrinsic changes in the ability to perform skilled activities; not directly measurable, but inferred from measures of motor performance

motor performance: the directly measurable extent to which the objective of a motor task is met, the scientific study of which originated as a branch of experimental psychology

motor skills: skills in which both movement and the outcome of actions are emphasized

peripheral nervous system: the system of nerves that link the central nervous system to the rest of the body; consists of twelve pairs of cranial nerves, thirty-one pairs of spinal nerves, and the autonomic nervous system

skeletal muscle: striated muscle that contracts voluntarily and involuntarily to carry out the functions of body support, posture, and locomotion

somatosensory system: the system by which muscle, joint, and cutaneous sensory receptors contribute to the perception and control of movement through ascending pathways

Physical and Psychological Factors

Motor skill development, the process of change in motor behavior with increasing age, focuses on adjustments in posture, movement, and the skillful manipulation of objects. Early researchers attributed essentially all developmental changes to modifications occurring within the central nervous system, with increasing motor abilities reflecting increasing neural maturation. Modern researchers have determined that the central nervous system works in combination with other body systems (such as the musculoskeletal, cardiovascular, and respiratory systems) and the environment to influence motor development, with all systems interacting in an extremely complex fashion as the individual ages.

Prenatal development of motor behavior takes place between approximately seven weeks after conception and birth, as was first determined during the 1970s using technology to visualize the fetus in utero. Following approximately eight weeks of gestation, the fetus is able to exert reflex and reaction actions, as well as active spontaneous movement. It is currently believed that the ability to self-initiate movements within the womb is an integral part of development, as compared to the traditional view that the fetus is passive and reflexive.

Infancy, the period from birth until the child is able to stand and walk, lasts approximately twelve months. The neonate begins life essentially helpless against the force of gravity and gradually develops the ability to align body segments with respect both to other body segments and to the environment. The Bayley Scales of Infant Development measure the following milestones of motor skill development for the first year of life (with the average age of accomplishment listed in parentheses): erect and steady head holding (0.8 months), side to back turning (1.8 months), supported sitting (2.3 months), back to side turning (4.4 months), momentary independent sitting (5.3 months), rolling from back to stomach (6.4 months), steady independent sitting (6.6 months), early supported stepping movements (7.4 months), arm pull to standing position (8.1 months), assisted walking (9.6 months), independent standing (11.0 months), and independent walking (11.7 months). The transition from helplessness to physical independence during the first twelve months creates many changes for growing children and their caregivers. New areas of exploration open up for the baby as greater body control is gained, the force of gravity is conquered, and less dependence on holding and carrying by caregivers is required.

During the first three months after birth, the infant's motor skill development focuses on getting the head aligned from the predominating posture of flexion. Flexor tone, the tendency to maintain a flexed posture and to rebound back into flexion when the limbs are extended and released, probably results from a combination of the elasticity of soft tissues that were confined to a flexed position while in the womb and of central nervous system activity. As antigravity activity progresses, the infant develops the ability to lift the head. Movements during this period involve brief periods of stretching, kicking, and thrusting of the limbs, in addition to turning and twisting of the trunk and head. Infants tend to be the most active prior to feeding and more quiet and sleepy after feeding.

The third to sixth months after birth are marked by great strides in overcoming the force of gravity by both flexion and extension movements. The infant becomes more competent in head control with respect to symmetry and midline orientation with the rest of the body, is able to sit independently for brief periods, and can push up onto hands and knees. These major milestones enable considerably more independence and permit a much greater ability to interact with the rest of the world.

During the sixth to ninth months after birth, the infant is constantly moving and exploring the surrounding environment. As nine months is approached, most babies are able to pull themselves into a standing position using a support such as furniture. The child expends a great deal of energy to stand and often bounces up and down once standing is achieved. The up-and-down bouncing eventually leads to the shifting of body weight from side to side and the taking of first steps, with a caregiver assisting alongside the furniture; this is often called cruising.

The ninth to twelfth months involve forward creeping on hands and knees. This locomotor pattern requires more complicated alternating movements of the opposite arms and legs. Some infants have a preference for creeping even after they are able to walk independently, with many preferring plantigrade creeping (on extended arms and legs) to walking. The ease to which the child moves from sitting to creeping, kneeling, or standing is greatly improved and balance is developed to the point where the child can pivot around in circles while sitting, using the hands and feet for propulsion. The child begins to move efficiently from standing to floor sitting and can initiate rolling from the supine position using flexed legs. Unsupported sitting is accomplished with ease, and weight while sitting can be transferred easily from buttocks to hands.

The early childhood period lasts from infancy until about six years. It involves the child attaining new skills but not necessarily new patterns of movement, with the learning patterns that were acquired during the first year of life being put to use in more meaningful activities. The locomotor pattern of walking is refined, and new motor skills that require increased balance and control of force—such as running, hopping, jumping, and skipping—are mastered.

Running is usually begun between years two and four, as the child learns to master the flight phase and the anticipatory strategies necessary when there is temporarily no body contact with the ground. It is not until about age five or six that control during running with respect to starting, stopping, and changing directions is effectively mastered. Jumping develops at about age 2.5, as the ability and confidence to land after jumping from a height such as a stair is achieved. The ability to jump to reach an overhead object then emerges, with early jumpers revealing a shallow preparatory crouch that progresses to a deeper crouch. Hopping, an extension of the ability to balance while standing on one leg, begins at about age 2.5 but is not performed well until about age six, when a series of about ten hops can be performed consecutively and are incorporated into games such as hopscotch. Skipping, a step and a hop on one leg followed by a step and hop of the other leg, is generally not achieved until about six years, with the opportunity and encouragement for practice being a primary determining factor, as with other locomotor skills.

Throwing is typically acquired during the first year, but advanced throwing, striking (such as with a plastic baseball and bat), kicking (such as with a soccer ball), and catching are not developed until early childhood. Catching develops at approximately age three, with the child initially holding the arms in front of the body and later making anticipatory adjustments to account for the direction, speed, and size of the thrown object. Kicking, which requires balancing on one foot while transferring force to an object with the other foot, begins with little preparatory backswing and eventually develops to involve the knee, hip, and lean of the trunk at about age six.

Fine motor manipulation skills in the upper extremity that are important to normal activities of daily living such as feeding, dressing, grooming, and handwriting are greatly improved in early childhood. The key components include locating a target, which requires the coordination of eye-head movement; reaching, which requires the transportation of the hand and arm in space; and manipulation, which includes grip formation, grasp, and release.

During later childhood (the period from seven years to about eleven years), adolescence, and adult life throughout the remainder of the life span, changes in movement are influenced predominantly by age. Adolescence begins with the onset of the physical changes of puberty, at approximately eleven to twelve years of age in girls and twelve to thirteen years of age in boys, and ends when physical growth is curtailed. Most authorities believe that the growth spurt of adolescence leads to the emergence of new patterns of movement within the skills that have already been acquired. Most adolescents have strong drives to develop self-esteem and become socially acceptable with their peers in school and various recreational activities. Cooperation and competition become strong components of motor skill development, whereby many skills are stabilized prior to adolescence and preferences for various sports activities emerge. Boys typically demonstrate increased speed and strength as compared to girls, despite recent dramatic changes in available opportunities for girls in recreational and competitive sports activities. Even though age-related changes in motor behavior continue throughout adulthood, the physical skills that permit independence are primarily acquired during the first year of life.

Psychological factors that influence motor skill development include attention level, stimulus-response compatibility, arousal level, and motivation. The level of attention when attempting a motor task is critical, with humans displaying a relatively fixed capacity for concentration during different stages of development. Stimulus identification, response selection, and response programming stages—whereby an individual remembers or determines how to perform a task—affect skill development because the central nervous system takes longer to synthesize and respond to more complex skills. Also important are stimulus-response compatibility—the better the stimulus matches the response, the shorter the reaction time—and arousal, which is described as an "inverted U" by the Yerkes-Dodson model. The inverted U hypothesis implies that there exists an optimal level of psychological arousal to learn or perform a motor skill efficiently, with performance declining when the arousal level at a given moment in time is too great or too small. At a low level of arousal, the scope of perception is broad, and all stimuli (including irrelevant information) are being processed. As arousal level increases, perception narrows so that when the optimal level of arousal is reached and attention is sufficiently focused, concentration on only the stimuli relevant to successful skill learning and performance is enabled. If arousal level surpasses this optimal level, perception narrows to the point of tunnel vision, some relevant stimuli are missed, and learning and skill performance are reduced. The influence of personal motivation during motor skill development encompasses the child's perceived relevance of the activity and also the child's individual ability to recognize the goal of the activity and desire to achieve it.

Three main factors that affect motor skill development in

early and later childhood include feedback, amount of practice, and practice conditions. Feedback can be intrinsic, arising from the somatosensory system and senses such as vision and hearing, as information is gathered about a movement and its consequences rather then the actual achievement of the goal. In pathological conditions such as cerebral palsy, intrinsic feedback is often greatly impaired. Feedback can also be extrinsic and is often divided by researchers into knowledge of results, or information about the success of the movement in accomplishing the goal that is available after the skill is completed, and knowledge of performance, or information about skill performance technique or strategy. Knowledge of results provides information about errors as well as successes. True learning occurs by a process of trial and error, with the nervous system serving to detect and correct inappropriate or inefficient movements.

Disorders and Effects

Physical therapists, psychologists, teachers, and other professionals who work with pediatric patients often plan their treatment interventions and instructional lessons based on the normal age-related progression of motor skill development. Motor skill development is often significantly decreased as a consequence of a neurological impairment, however, with the child's resulting movement patterns revealing primary impairments such as inadequate activation of muscle, secondary impairments such as contractures, and compensatory strategies that are adopted to overcome the impairment and achieve mobility. The categories for impairments that have an impact on motor development can generally be divided into musculoskeletal, neuromuscular, sensory, perceptual, and cognitive.

Damage to various nervous system structures somewhat predictably reduces the motor control of movement via both positive symptoms (the presence of abnormal behavior) and negative symptoms (the loss of normal behavior). Positive symptoms include the presence of exaggerated reflexes and abnormalities of muscle tone. Negative symptoms include the loss of muscular strength and the inappropriate selection of muscles during task performance. The broad spectrum of muscle tone abnormalities ranges from flaccidity to rigidity, with muscle spasticity defined as the velocity-dependent increase in tonic stretch reflexes (also called muscle tone), with exaggerated tendon jerks resulting from changes in the threshold of the stretch reflex.

Secondary effects of central nervous system lesions are not directly caused by the lesions themselves but develop as a consequence of the lesions. For example, children with cerebral palsy often exhibit the primary problem of spasticity in muscles of the lower extremities, which causes the secondary problem of muscular and tendon tightness in the ankles, knees, and hips. The secondary problem of limited range of motion in these important areas for movement often impairs motor skills more than the primary problem of spasticity, with the resulting movement strategies reflecting the growing child's best attempt to compensate.

Another common compensatory strategy seen in children

with a motor development dysfunction involves standing with the knee hyperextended because of an inability to generate enough muscular force to keep the knee from collapsing. Standing with the knee in hyperextension keeps the line of gravity in front of the knee joint. Contractures of joints are frequent consequences of disordered postural and movement patterns. For example, a habitual crouched sitting posture results in chronic shortening of the hamstring, calf, and hip flexor muscles, and a backward-tipped pelvis accommodates the shortened hamstrings. Chronic shortening of the calf muscles often results in toe walking (in which the heel does not strike the ground) and a reduced walking speed and stride length, because of decreased balance and leg muscle strength. Changes in the availability of sensory information and cognitive factors such as fear of falling and inattention may also contribute strongly to motor skill development in some pediatric patients.

Perspective and Prospects

Interest in the scientific study of motor development was greatly enhanced by Myrtle B. McGraw's *The Neuromuscular Maturation of the Human Infant* (1945). It described four stages of neural maturation: a period in which movement is governed by reflexes as a result of the dominance of lower centers within the central nervous system; a period in which reflex expression declines as a result of maturation of the cerebral cortex and the inhibitory effect of the cortex over lower centers; a period in which an increase in the voluntary quality of activity as a result of increased cortical control produces deliberate or voluntary movement; and a period in which integrative activity of the neural centers takes place, as shown by smooth and coordinated movements.

Arnold Gesell then used cinematography to conduct extensive observations of infants during various stages of growth. He described the maturation of infants based on four behavior categories: motor behavior, adaptive behavior, language development, and personal-social development. Gesell identified six principles of development. The principle of motor priority and fore-reference states that the neuromotor system is laid down before it is voluntarily utilized. The principle of developmental direction states that development proceeds in head-to-foot and proximal-to-distal directions. The principle of reciprocal interweaving states that opposing movements such as extension and flexion show a temporary dominance over one another until they become integrated into mature motor patterns. The principle of functional asymmetry states that humans have a preferred hand, a dominant eye, and a lead foot, with this unilateral dominance being subject to change during development. The principle of self-regulation states that periods of stability and instability culminate into more stable responses as maturity proceeds. The principle of optimal realization states that the human action system has strong growth potential toward normal development if environmental and cultural conditions are favorable and if compensatory and regeneration mechanisms come into play when damage occurs to facilitate attainment of the maximum possible growth.

Esther Thelen suggested the dynamic systems theory. This theory argues that the maturing nervous system interacts with other biomechanical, psychological, and social environment factors to create a dimensional system whereby behavior represents a compression of the degrees of freedom.

A more refined systems theory of motor control developed by Anne Shumway-Cook and Marjorie Woollacott claims that the three main factors that interact in the development of efficient locomotion are progression (ability to generate rhythmic muscular patterns to move the body in the desired direction), stability (the control of balance), and adaptation (the ability to adapt to changing task and environmental requirements). These three factors generally appear sequentially, with muscular patterns appearing first, followed by equilibrium control, and finally adaptive capabilities. Although research on the emergence of human motor skills has primarily concentrated on the developmental milestones of infants and children, it appears that important changes in motor behavior continue throughout the human life span.

—*Daniel G. Graetzer, Ph.D.*

See also Cerebral palsy; Cognitive development; Developmental stages; Growth; Muscular dystrophy; Muscle sprains, spasms, and disorders; Muscles; Nervous system; Physical examination; Reflexes, primitive; Speech disorders; Well-baby examinations.

For Further Information:

Berk, Laura E. *Child Development*. 9th ed. Boston: Pearson/Allyn & Bacon, 2013.

Feldman, Robert S. *Development Across the Life Span*. 6th ed. Upper Saddle River, N.J.: Pearson/Prentice Hall, 2011.

Haywood, Kathleen, Mary Ann Roberton, and Nancy Getchell. *Advanced Analysis of Motor Development*. Champaign, Ill.: Human Kinetics, 2012.

Kail, Robert V., and John C. Cavanaugh. *Human Development: A Life-Span View*. 6th ed. Belmont, Calif.: Wadsworth Cengage Learning, 2013.

Kalverboer, Alex F., Brian Hopkins, and Reint Geuze, eds. *Motor Development in Early and Later Childhood: Longitudinal Approaches*. New York: Cambridge University Press, 1993.

Ludlow, Ruth, and Mike Phillips. *The Little Book of Gross Motor Skills*. London: Featherstone Education, 2012.

Nathanson, Laura Walther. *The Portable Pediatrician: A Practicing Pediatrician's Guide to Your Child's Growth, Development, Health, and Behavior from Birth to Age Five*. 2d ed. New York: HarperCollins, 2002.

Newell, K. M. "Motor Skill Acquisition." *Annual Review of Psychology* 42 (1991): 213–37.

Shumway-Cook, Anne, and Marjorie Woollacott. *Motor Control: Translating Research into Clinical Practice*. 4th ed. Philadelphia: Lippincott Williams & Wilkins, 2012.

Sugden, David, and Michael G. Wade. *Typical and Atypical Motor Development*. London: Mac Keith Press, 2013.

Thelen, Esther, and Linda B. Smith. *A Dynamic Systems Approach to the Development of Cognition and Action*. 5th ed. Cambridge, Mass.: MIT Press, 2002.

MOUTH AND THROAT CANCER
Disease/Disorder

Anatomy or system affected: Gums, mouth, neck, teeth, throat
Specialties and related fields: Dentistry, general surgery, oncology, radiology

Definition: A malignancy of the lips, tongue, gums, salivary glands, or pharynx.

Key terms:

biopsy: the removal and examination of body tissue to determine whether it is cancerous

esophagus: a muscular tube connecting the pharynx and the stomach

pharynx: the area connecting the back of the throat to the esophagus

squamous cells: flat ephithelial cells that resemble scales

Causes and Symptoms

Often, dentists detect cancers of the mouth and throat during routine dental examinations. People who visit their dentists regularly, preferably twice a year, will likely have such cancers detected and diagnosed in their earliest stages when treatment is effective and the cure rate high.

Valid generalizations can be made about the causes of mouth and throat cancers. The most significant cause is the regular use of tobacco products. Cigarette smoking over long periods often results in these cancers or in lung cancer. Males, especially those over forty, have a higher rate of mouth and throat cancer than do females. Pipe and cigar smokers are at greater risk of cancer than are cigarette smokers, and a correlation also exists between the use of chewing tobacco and snuff and the development of mouth cancer. About 90 percent of people suffering from mouth and/or throat cancer have been consistent users of tobacco.

A second causal factor is the regular consumption of substantial quantities of alcoholic beverages, usually over four drinks a day. Some 80 percent of people suffering from mouth and/or throat cancer have used alcohol regularly and in substantial quantities. They are particularly subject to cancers on the floor of the mouth, the tonsils, the lower pharynx, and the tongue.

People who smoke two packs of cigarettes a day and consume over four drinks a day increase the likelihood that they will develop mouth and/or throat cancers by forty times. Other factors in such cancers are poor dental hygiene, ill-fitting dentures, or irregular teeth that cause irritations in the mouth. Those whose work brings them into direct contact with certain toxic chemicals are also at risk.

The most common symptom of lip cancer is the formation of a small, whitish patch (leukoplakia), usually painless, on the lip. It frequently consists of squamous cells. As it develops, it may become ulcerous, causing bleeding and compromising surrounding tissue. If the tongue becomes involved, then it may stiffen. As the malignancy advances, the tongue often becomes painful. Speech, chewing, and swallowing become progressively difficult.

Cancer of the oropharynx, the mid-section of the pharynx, is often accompanied by difficulty in swallowing and hoarseness. Such cancers may also cause patients to expectorate blood-stained sputum. A sore throat frequently accompanies this form of cancer, and earache may also occur, although both of these symptoms frequently result from other causes.

Information on Mouth And Throat Cancer

Causes: Tobacco, alcohol, dental problems, toxins, severe acid reflux disease
Symptoms: May include whitish patches on lips, stiff tongue, bloody sputum, sore throat, earache
Duration: Chronic
Treatments: Surgery, radiation therapy, chemotherapy, plastic surgery

People with severe and consistent stomach acid reflux are vulnerable to throat cancer.

Treatment and Therapy

The usual treatment of mouth and throat cancer is surgery to remove the affected tissue. Such surgery is almost always followed by a course of radiation, which may also precede such surgery to shrink any tumors that might be present. Sometimes, removal of the tongue is indicated, although this is a very drastic treatment because of the problems that it causes for the patient, whose ability to speak and to chew and swallow food will be drastically compromised. Cancer of the tongue is the most aggressive form of mouth cancer, which is justification for using drastic measures to deal with it. Facial disfiguration may also be involved in treating cancers of this sort, so extensive plastic surgery may be necessary following it.

Throat cancers usually require the surgical removal of cancerous tissue followed by radiation, but treatment with anticancer medications may also be involved in the management of such cancers. Often, a biopsy is performed in the operating room prior to surgery, usually in conjunction with invasive procedures that permit surgeons and oncologists to view the pharynx, the lungs, and the esophagus using laryngoscopes, bronchoscopes, or esophagoscopes.

Perspective and Prospects

Cancer of the mouth and throat constitute about 8 percent of all the cancers diagnosed in the United States annually. The American Cancer Society estimates that, in 2013, approximately 36,000 people in the United States will develop oral cavity or oropharyngeal cancer and that about 6,850 people will die of these cancers. When an early diagnosis is made and is followed by prompt treatment, a cure results in 75 percent of cases. More than half the people diagnosed with mouth cancer, even those for whom late diagnoses are made, survive for at least five years following treatment. As in all cancers, early detection is the key to effective management and desirable outcomes.

Perhaps the most important factor in reducing the incidence of mouth and throat cancer is to convince young people not to develop the habit of using tobacco products and not to abuse alcohol. People who are already smokers and drinkers are well advised to stop smoking and to limit their alcohol intake to two drinks a day or less.

No conclusive correlation has been made between mouth and throat cancer and secondhand smoke. As an increasing number of public venues and workplaces have become smoke-free, however, people who patronize or work in such places have been smoking less.

Most inveterate smokers want to overcome the habit, but nicotine addiction is so powerful that giving it up is difficult. Various methods have proved helpful in enabling people to control their habits, among them hypnosis, acupuncture, laser treatment, psychotherapy, and nicotine replacement through patches or nicotine chewing gum.

In 2013, researchers from Penn State reported the results of their study of about two thousand smokers who took part in the US National Health and Nutrition Examination Survey. They found that people who smoked a cigarette within five minutes of waking up in the morning were more likely to develop lung and oral cancer than other smokers. The research team published their findings in the March 29, 2013, issue of *Cancer Epidemiology, Biomarkers and Prevention.*

—*R. Baird Shuman, Ph.D.*

See also Addiction; Alcoholism; Biopsy; Cancer; Carcinogens; Carcinoma; Cells; Chemotherapy; Dental diseases; Dentistry; Dermatology; Dermatopathology; Esophagus; Glands; Laryngectomy; Malignancy and metastasis; Nasopharyngeal disorders; Oncology; Oral and maxillofacial surgery; Pharyngitis; Pharynx; Plastic surgery; Radiation therapy; Skin cancer; Skin lesion removal; Smoking; Sore throat; Tumor removal; Tumors.

For Further Information:

American Cancer Society. "Oral Cavity and Oropharyngeal Cancer." *American Cancer Society*, February 26, 2013.

DeConno, Franco, et al. "Mouth Care." In *Oxford Textbook of Palliative Medicine*, edited by Derek Doyle et al. 3d ed. New York: Oxford University Press, 2006.

Dougherty, Lisa, and Sara E. Lister, eds. *The Royal Marsden Hospital Manual of Clinical Nursing Procedures*. 8th ed. Oxford: Wiley-Blackwell, 2011.

Hahn, Michael J., and Anne Jones. *Head and Neck Nursing*. Edinburgh, N.Y.: Churchill Livingstone, 2000.

Hellwig, Jennifer. "Throat Cancer." *Health Library*, May 1, 2013.

Lydiatt, William M., and Perry J. Johnson. *Cancers of the Mouth and Throat: A Patient's Guide to Treatment*. Omaha, Nebr.: Addicus Books, 2012.

MedlinePlus. "Oral Cancer." *MedlinePlus*, April 12, 2013.

Preidt, Robert. "HealthDay: 'Wake-Up Cigarette May Raise Risk for Lung, Mouth Cancers." *MedlinePlus*, April 5, 2013.

MRI. *See* MAGNETIC RESONANCE IMAGING (MRI).

MUCOPOLYSACCHARIDOSIS (MPS)
Disease/Disorder

Also known as: Diferrante syndrome, Hunter syndrome, Hurler's syndrome, Morquio syndrome
Anatomy or system affected: All
Specialties and related fields: Cardiology, embryology, genetics, pediatrics
Definition: A genetic disorder characterized by accumulations of mucopolysaccharides in tissues.

Causes and Symptoms

Six distinct classes of mucopolysaccharidosis (MPS) have been described, with a number of subclasses. The basis for all mucopolysaccharidosis categories is found in recessive genetic defects of gene products associated with the metabolism of mucopolysaccharides, long chains of sugar molecule that are used to build connective tissue in the body. Specific symptoms are associated with each type, which is a function of which gene locus is at fault. All involve the degradation of specific mucopolysaccharides: dermatan sulfate, heparan sulfate, or keratan sulfate. At least ten enzymes are involved in these metabolic pathways.

The specific syndrome depends upon which enzyme, or which combination, is at fault. For example, MPS I, also called Hurler's syndrome, results from a deficiency of the enzyme alpha-L-iduronidase (IDUA) and is associated with early childhood defects in disparate sites such as the aorta or cornea. Other common symptoms include physical distortion of the face, dwarfism, organ enlargement, mental deficiencies, and shortened life span. MPS IV, also known as Morquio syndrome, is related to reduced activity of galactosamine-6-sulfatase and causes symptoms similar to those in other forms of the disorder.

Diagnosis has generally been based upon laboratory testing for the decreased presence of enzymes involved in the metabolic pathway, as well as the observed accumulation of intermediate polysaccharides such as heparan sulfate in cell lysosomes, reflecting the lack of breakdown. Recent procedures have taken advantage of more accurate laboratory tests, as in use of polymerase chain reaction (PCR) or deoxyribonucleic acid (DNA) blotting techniques for the analysis of specific genes. Fetal cells obtained by means of amniocentesis or chorionic villus sampling and grown in culture can also be tested for defects in the suspected pathways. Generally, symptoms begin to develop after the age of two.

The same tests can be useful for the detection of carriers who do not express the defective traits. The frequency of diagnosis in various populations has ranged from 1 in 25,000 to 1 in 125,000, with significant variation in the specific type.

Treatment and Therapy

All forms of MPS are progressive, resulting in physical or structural abnormalities of varying severity. Death usually occurs before the age of twenty, though in the most severe types, the child rarely reaches the teenage years. Treatment is primarily symptomatic. Bone marrow transplants have been attempted as a means to replace defective enzymes, with little success. Prospects are currently poor. Most advances have involved improved diagnosis as well as the detection of carriers for the various traits.

—Richard Adler, Ph.D.

See also Enzyme therapy; Enzymes; Gaucher's disease; Genetic counseling; Genetic diseases; Glycogen storage diseases; Lipids; Metabolic disorders; Metabolism; Neonatology; Niemann-Pick disease; Screening; Tay-Sachs disease.

Information on Mucopolysaccharidosis (MPS)

Causes: Genetic enzyme defects
Symptoms: Depends on type; may include defects in aorta or corneas, facial distortion, dwarfism, organ enlargement, mental deficiencies, shortened life span
Duration: Progressive and fatal
Treatments: None; alleviation of symptoms

For Further Information:

Bach, G., et al. "The Defect in the Hunter Syndrome: Deficiency of Sulfoiduronate Sulfatase." *Proceedings of the National Academy of Sciences* 70 (1973): 2134–38.

Booth, C., and H. Nadler. "Demonstration of the Heterozygous State in Hunter's Syndrome." *Pediatrics* 53 (1974): 396–99.

Guarany, Nicole Ruas, et al. "Functional Capacity Evaluation of Patients with Mucopolysaccharidosis." *Journal of Pediatric Rehabilitation Medicine* 5, no. 1 (2012): 37–46.

Icon Health. *Hunter Syndrome: A Medical Dictionary, Bibliography, and Annotated Research Guide to Internet References.* San Diego, Calif.: Author, 2004.

Icon Health. *Hurler Syndrome: A Medical Dictionary, Bibliography, and Annotated Research Guide to Internet References.* San Diego, Calif.: Author, 2004.

"Mucopolysaccharidoses Fact Sheet." *National Institute of Neurological Disorders and Stroke*, April 29, 2013.

Muenzer, Joseph. "Overview of Mucopolysaccharidoses." *Rheumtology* 50, no. 5 (December 2011): pv4–v12.

Porter, Robert S., et al., eds. *The Merck Manual Home Health Handbook.* Whitehouse Station, N.J.: Merck Research Laboratories, 2009.

Scriver, Charles, et al., eds. *The Metabolic and Molecular Basis of Inherited Disease.* 8th ed. New York: McGraw-Hill, 2001.

MULTIPLE BIRTHS

Biology
Anatomy or system affected: All
Specialties and related fields: Embryology, genetics, neonatology, obstetrics, pediatrics
Definition: The presence of two or more fetuses in the womb.
Key terms:

chromosomes: the rod-shaped structures in the nucleus of a cell that carry genes

concordance: the condition among twins of having the same physical or psychological trait

dizygotes: fraternal twins; born from two ova separately fertilized by two sperm

embryo: the cells growing after conception until the eighth week of pregnancy

monozygotes: identical twins; born of a single ovum that divides after a single sperm fertilizes it

ovum: the egg cell released from the ovaries during ovulation

placenta: the membrane sac developed from the uterine wall that passes nutrients to the fetus through interconnected blood vessels

ultrasonography: an imaging technique that uses high-frequency sound waves to view fetuses in the womb, as well as other internal structures *zygote:* a fertilized ovum before multicellular development begins

Introduction

Multiple births have historically been rare events, but the incidence is increasing with assisted reproductive technologies. The most common multiple births are twins; this occurs in approximately one of every eighty complete pregnancies. Twins can come from a single egg or from two different eggs. Triplets occur in approximately one in every eight hundred completed pregnancies. Quadruplets occur in one in every eight thousand completed pregnancies. Quintuplets occur naturally in approximately one of every eighty thousand completed pregnancies.

As the number of fetuses increases, the chances that all will survive decreases. Multiple births are most commonly combinations of twins and single eggs. By reviewing the mechanics of twin formation, greater multiples can be understood.

The Different Types of Twins

Two types of twins are well known: fraternal twins and

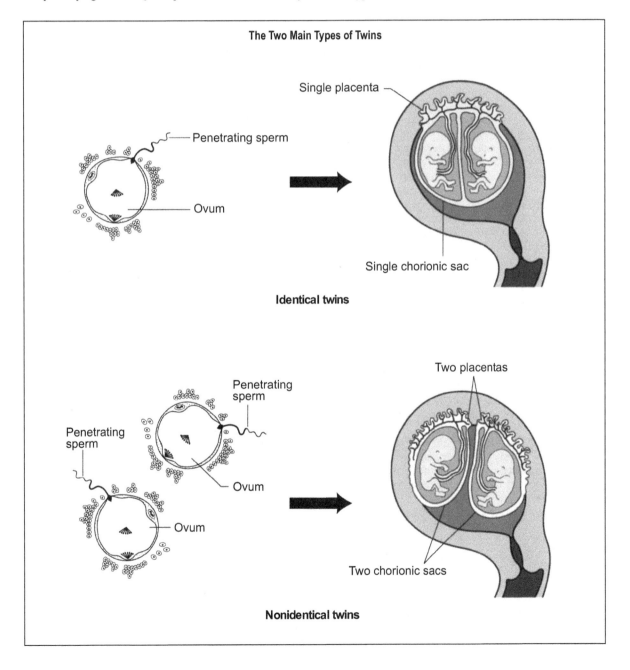

The Two Main Types of Twins

Single placenta

Penetrating sperm

Ovum

Single chorionic sac

Identical twins

Penetrating sperm

Penetrating sperm

Ovum

Ovum

Two placentas

Two chorionic sacs

Nonidentical twins

identical twins. Behind these general terms, however, lies considerable variation. This variation is based on the many changes that a human ovum can undergo after it is released by the ovary, is fertilized, travels along the Fallopian tube to the uterus, and implants there to develop into an embryo.

Fraternal twins are also known as dizygotic or binovular twins. In a normal menstrual cycle, only a single egg is released. When a sperm penetrates an ovum, the fertilized egg releases a chemical that prevents other sperm from penetrating the same egg. If a second egg has been released, however, it can also be fertilized. A newly fertilized egg is called a zygote. If both zygotes succeed in attaching to the uterine walls, a twin pregnancy begins. Usually, this dual insemination occurs during a single release of semen in a single copulation, so that the embryos have the same father. Occasionally, the two eggs may be fertilized in separate copulations during the same ovulation, a phenomenon called superfecundation. It is then possible for dizygotic twins to have different fathers. This possibility seems to have long been recognized. The Greek myth of Leda and the Swan derives from such a pregnancy.

Fraternal twins have separate placentas and membranes in the womb. The placenta comprises maternal and fetal tissues interconnected by blood vessels. Nutrients pass from the mother to the fetus through the placenta. Waste products are removed from the fetus by a reverse process. Sometimes, the placentas press against each other in the womb and fuse. Having had separate placentas or one fused together, however, does not affect the nature of the twins after birth. Fraternal twins, even though they share the same birthday, are no more similar in appearance or manner than two siblings from separate births.

Identical twins are the result of different initial events. They are also called monozygotic or monovular twins. Identical or look-alike twins originate when a single egg spontaneously divides after penetration by a sperm cell. Each half develops separately. The reason for this division is not known. One theory holds that sometimes the fertilized ovum does not implant in the uterus right away as is normally the case. During the delay, the chromosomes double and the zygote halves, with each half then implanting and becoming a separate embryo.

Another theory suggests that early in the pregnancy, a genetic mutation occurs in one of the cells. Later, while the embryo is still no more than a few hundred cells, the normal cells recognize the genetic difference and reject the mutant cells, much as the immune system rejects substances foreign to it. The rejected group of cells develops separately. If this theory proves to be true, identical twins must not be completely identical after all. Cases in which one identical twin has a genetic disease and the other remains healthy appear to support this theory, although mutation in one twin may occur after splitting rather than causing the splitting.

Variation sometimes appears after birth in monozygotic siblings. Twins can vary in birth weight greatly (one may weigh twice as much), develop at different rates, and die from unrelated natural causes. As a rule, however, identical twins share an overwhelming majority of traits. When two (or more) siblings share a trait, they are considered to be concordant for that trait. Typically, body structures and coloration will be strikingly concordant. Features such as facial shape, hair texture and color, eye color, and height are typical examples of concordance. "Mirror" twins are an uncommon phenomenon. They show mirror-image symmetry in some traits. For example, one may be left-handed while the other is right-handed. Whorls on the scalp may also occur as mirror images. In very rare cases, one mirror twin will have situs inversus: the placement of all internal organs is reversed. An individual with situs inversus will have the liver and appendix on the left side of the abdomen and the spleen on the right.

Genetic variation may account for the subtle variations in even the most concordant of twins. The internal environment of the womb also has an effect. Most identical twin fetuses share the same placenta but have different inner or chorionic sacs. They may have separate placentas (and separate chorions) depending on when the initial splitting of the zygote took place. Usually, those sharing a single placenta have separate chorions. In the rarest variation, the fetuses also share the same amnion. The degree of separation or number of barriers can influence the amount of oxygen or nutrients that each twin receives. Relatively minor differences can affect development.

A third type of twin is theoretically possible. During maturation and before becoming fertilized, the mature ovum could divide into a secondary oocyte (the cell to be fertilized) and a much smaller polar body. It is possible for the ovum to divide into roughly equal portions, both of which are viable and contain the same genetic material. If separate sperm then fertilize these ova, they would become two zygotes. Such twins would have exactly the same maternal genes, but a portion of the paternal genes would differ. They would be less identical than monozygotes but more so than dizygotes. Although this type of twinning has been described in rats and mice, no human case has been indisputably identified and reported.

A fourth variant of twinning is conjoined twins, popularly called Siamese twins. Conjoined twins share some tissue. This can range from simple joining of skin on the head or shoulders to having one heart or kidney or two torsos and a single pair of legs. Conjoined twins are identical (or monozygotic) twins created by incomplete cell division during early fetal life. The portions of cells that divide normally continue to develop in a normal fashion. The cells that did not divide completely also develop normally. The result is a portion of the body that is duplicated and a portion that is not. If the incomplete division occurred early in fetal development, the amount of shared tissue is likely to be greater than with an incomplete division that occurred later in fetal development.

About one-third of all twin births result in identical twins. The proportion of males and females is approximately equal. The incidence of identical twins remains constant throughout the world's diverse ethnic populations. Fraternal twins, however, show different proportions and distributions. About half the pairs have the same gender (with a nearly equal number of male-male and female-female pairs); about half are male-female pairs. Fraternal twin births occur most frequently among rural Nigerians (45 pairs per 1,000 births) and least frequently among Chinese and Japanese parents (4 pairs per 1,000 births). European and American rates, for both blacks and whites, are approximately halfway between these extremes.

Evidence suggests that women inherit a tendency to conceive fraternal twins from their mothers. There is little scientific evidence to support the belief that fathers possess a gene for monozygotic twins. Physiological factors can increase the likelihood of a woman having fraternal twins. Women who are tall and heavy and who have previously given birth to children have more twins than small women or those who have not been pregnant before. Women between thirty-five and forty years of age are the most likely to have twins, but the chances decrease thereafter.

Naturally occurring multiple pregnancies (triplets and more) are usually combinations of twins. Identical triplets do rarely occur, but triplets consisting of two identical and one fraternal sibling are the norm. Naturally occurring multiple births of four or more infants are almost always combinations of twins. Physicians can ascertain the status of multiple birth siblings by examining placentas and chorionic sacs.

Possible Complications

Multiple births create special problems for mothers. Specifically, they are more difficult to carry in the womb and to nurture through infancy than singletons. Multiples are smaller, so that vaginal deliveries are easier. Many physicians, however, recommend birth by cesarean section to manage complications better. Most twins are born healthy, but they must be monitored carefully. As the number of fetuses increases, their size decreases. Because they are not fully mature, this increases the chances for medical problems.

Positively identifying multiple fetuses in the womb is not always an easy task, even though medical science has developed a variety of techniques. The traditional signs of considerable fetal movement, multiple heartbeats, and a large weight gain by the mother can be inaccurate and contradictory. Tests for the human chorionic gonadotropin hormone in the mother's blood or urine or alpha-fetoprotein in the blood may suggest the presence of multiple fetuses if the hormone or protein levels are unusually elevated. Nevertheless, imaging technologies provide the most reliable test. Ultrasonography has supplanted X-rays, which declined in use because of the radiation hazard to fetuses. The images produced by ultrasonography can usually resolve multiple fetuses early in the pregnancy.

A multiple pregnancy itself strains the mother's body and is particularly subject to medical complications. Typically, a mother carrying multiple fetuses gains from 30 to 80 pounds, about twice the weight of a single pregnancy. The added weight can cause skeletal and muscular problems. The fetuses' demands on the mother's body may also worsen preexisting medical conditions, such as heart or kidney disease. As the multiple fetuses develop, their size stretches the uterus, which can initiate early labor. For this reason, the premature

birth rate is higher for multiple fetuses than for single fetuses. Twins occasionally reach full term; triplets and greater multiples do not.

Similarly, multiple pregnancies miscarry at more than three times the rate of singletons. Occasionally, one fetus will develop at the expense of the other by drawing a disproportionate amount of nutrients from the mother, a condition called twin transfusion syndrome. In cases of identical (monozygotic) twins who share a single placenta, a phenomenon known as a twin-twin transfusion can occur. When this occurs, one twin receives most of the blood, nutrients, and oxygen, in turn becoming much larger than the other twin. In some instances, the smaller twin (the donor) perishes due to lack of these vital substances. In other cases, the larger twin (the recipient) succumbs to heart failure as a result of having to pump the increased blood flow. A new surgical technique (ablation) is currently being used in the third trimester to sever the connection, stopping the twin-twin transfusion. If one fetus dies for any reason, then the mother's body may reabsorb it partially or completely, a phenomenon known as the vanishing twin. Some doctors believe that because of unobserved vanishing twins, miscarriages, and induced abortions, the number of twin conceptions has been underestimated.

Doctors carefully monitor the fetal development of multiple fetuses to ensure their health and, especially, to prepare for delivering them. Amniocentesis and genetic tests detect potential biochemical defects, genetic anomalies, and diseases. Ultrasonography allows doctors to identify defects in shape and the relative position of the fetuses in the womb. Their position is important during labor. Normally, babies are born head-first. In multiples, one of the fetuses frequently lies crosswise or feet-first. These positions greatly lengthen and complicate delivery, so that the second fetus runs a higher risk of dying during labor. Moreover, the mother's over distended uterus, unable to contract properly after delivery, might begin to bleed. If labor lasts too long it could result in dangerous maternal exhaustion. Because of such problems, many obstetricians recommend delivery by cesarean section-that is, by cutting a passage through the abdomen into the uterus-at the first sign of trouble to either mother or fetuses.

The prematurity and low birth weight common in multiple infants means that many are placed on life support. Studies have found that multiple infants suffer congenital defects as much as three times more often than singletons. Identical siblings are the most likely of all to have abnormalities. Heart malformations are most common. According to some studies, closed esophagus, clubfeet, excess fingers or toes, and forms of mental retardation such as Down syndrome occur at a slightly higher rate.

Conjoined twins are relatively rare, appearing approximately once in a hundred thousand pregnancies. Most are attached at the back, or at the back of the head or neck. In an extreme rarity, one identical twin has a full set of chromosomes while the other has only the X chromosome from the mother; in this case the twin will be a female with a condition called Turner Syndrome. Therefore, identical twins will be of opposite gender if the first twin has the XY chromosomes that define a male and the other is a female with Turner Syndrome.

That multiple birth siblings develop in the same environment and from a common origin allows researchers to trace the genetic and environmental influences on human development in general. Most of this research has been conducted on twins because of the relative rarity of triplets or larger groups of siblings. The reasoning is straightforward. In the case of identical twins, either their genetic heritage (nature) or the environment (nurture) dominates in determining how they grow mentally and physically. Researchers have tested the idea by tracking down identical twins that were separated while young, usually at birth, and reared separately. If genetics control development, then the separated twins should still look and behave similarly. If environment predominates, then separated twins should show variations in appearance and temperament.

The reported research results have been mixed. Some separated twins do not look or act any more alike than siblings born separately. Others show an uncanny degree of similarity throughout their lives-dressing the same way, marrying in the same year, having the same number of children, and dying nearly at the same time of the same disease. Their intelligence, which many scientists believe is heavily influenced by environment, nevertheless shows high concordance.

Perspective and Prospects

Worldwide, superstitions and a strong moral overtone have traditionally accompanied multiple births. Some societies view one twin as automatically good and the other evil and treat them accordingly as they mature. Others believe twins are shameful, a sign of corruption or promiscuity in the mother. These babies might be killed at birth or separated because of it. An African curse reflects the deep suspicion that some societies have held for twins: "May you be the mother of twins." On the other hand, some nations believed that twins have divine origin or power over the elements or special talents for prophecy and telepathy.

Multiple siblings enjoy a special advantage: They are rarely lonely. Some twins even share their own private language, a phenomenon known as idioglossa. Their common development means increased requirements of time and money for their families. It also provides continuous opportunities for sharing and relying on each other. The many national and international organizations created by and for twins and other multiple birth siblings reflect their pride in their status.

Triplets have historically had a reasonable chance for survival. Before the advent of support equipment for premature babies, lung immaturity was the factor that usually determined life or death. Surfactant is a chemical that is secreted in the seventh month of pregnancy. Without surfactant, lung tissues stick together and infants cannot breathe. Because of the combined size of all fetuses, many multiple infants are born before the seventh month of gestation. The Dionne quintuplets, who were born in the 1930s, were unusual in that for the first time in history, all five survived into adulthood. Modern support technology has helped several sets of sextuplets (six

infants) to survive. In 1997, the same technology permitted all the McCaughey sextuplets (seven infants) to survive. This was the first time such an event had occurred. (The chances of naturally conceiving sextuplets are one in eight to ten million conceptions.) In 2009, controversy erupted when Nadya Suleman gave birth to octuplets (eight infants), all of whom survived. A fertility doctor had implanted eight embryos into Suleman, a single mother who already had six children conceived through artificial insemination.

Advances in the field of assisted reproduction have increased the odds of multiple pregnancies. Women who have difficulty conceiving are initially treated with drugs that cause more than one egg to be released during ovulation. This increases the chance of pregnancy but also increases the chance of carrying multiple fetuses. Couples who seek medical assistance to achieve pregnancy routinely use fertility drugs. A woman will have several eggs or zygotes implanted to improve the odds of successfully initiating a pregnancy. The result of this approach is an increased number of multiple births. In 1988, twelve fetuses, which were miscarried, resulted from a fertility drug. Artificially induced pregnancies have posed ethical dilemmas for many who believe that scientists should not manipulate human biological processes.

Multiple births raise other moral and ethical questions as well. Genetic tests can now identify potential fetal defects in the womb early enough that surgeons can remove a defective fetus without harming the healthy fetus, a procedure called selective birth, selective abortion, or selective feticide. Those who hold abortions to be immoral have reservations about selective feticide even when the defective fetus has little chance of surviving and may threaten the lives of the remaining healthy fetuses. That selective feticide may be used simply because a mother does not want to rear more than one child has caused far greater concern. Since the procedure is tricky to perform and can result in the death of all fetuses, most doctors find selective feticide for nonmedical reasons to be ethically indefensible.

Twin births bear witness to the successes of modern health care. In the United States, incidents of multiple births, both fraternal and identical, have increased since the 1970s, and more multiples are surviving to adulthood. Fertility drugs may account for part of the increase, as does the trend among American women to delay childbearing until their thirties or forties. Nevertheless, prenatal care, better diet, improvements in neonatal intensive care, and education about pregnancy and birth are as important.

—Roger Smith, Ph.D., and
L. Fleming Fallon, Jr., M.D., Ph.D., M.P.H.;
updated by Samar Aslam, M.D.

See also Abortion; Amniocentesis; Assisted reproductive technologies; Birth defects; Cesarean section; Childbirth; Childbirth complications; Chorionic villus sampling; Conception; Embryology; Ethics; Gamete intrafallopian transfer (GIFT); Genetics and inheritance; In vitro fertilization; Miscarriage; Neonatology; Obstetrics; Pregnancy and gestation; Premature birth; Reproductive system; Sibling rivalry; Ultrasonography; Uterus

For Further Information:

Bowers, Nancy A. *The Multiple Pregnancy Sourcebook*. Chicago: Contemporary Books, 2001. The author, a perinatal nurse specializing in multiple-birth education, provides an excellent guide on topics such as infertility technology, prenatal testing, prenatal development, risk factors and complications, the birth of multiples, and adapting one's life to raise multiples.

Cunningham, F. Gary, et al., eds. *Williams Obstetrics*. 24th ed. New York: McGraw-Hill, 2014. This standard textbook in obstetrics would complement a similar text in gynecology. Provides wide coverage of events related to pregnancy and childbirth. A well-written text for the serious reader who wants detailed information.

Luke, Barbara, and Tamara Eberliein. *What to Expect When You're Expecting Twins, Triplets, or Quads: A Complete Resource*. 3rd ed. New York: HarperCollins, 2013. Two authors, a professor of obstetrics and gynecology and a health journalist, have written what is perhaps the best received book on the topic by expectant mothers and their families. Focuses on the practical preparations, including nutritional and lifestyles planning, how to find the right specialist, and reduce the risk of prenatal harm to the babies.

Malmstrom, Patricia Maxwell, and Janet Poland. *The Art of Parenting Twins*. New York: Random House International, 2000. Malmstrom and Poland cover the biology and causes of twinning; the emotional terrain of parenting multiples; the differences between twin and single pregnancies; twin development in babyhood, toddlers, the preschool and school-age years, and adolescence; and twins' relationships with each other from babyhood to adulthood.

Malone, J.A., S.P. Margevicius, and E.G. Damato. "Multiple Gestation: Side Effects of Antepartum Bed Rest." *Biological Research in Nursing* 8, no. 2 (2006): 115-128. An overview of problems encountered by pregnant women as a result of the bed rest that is often required to deal with multiples.

Mann, Denise. "11 Things You Didn't Know about Twin Pregnancies." WebMD Feature Article. WebMD, 2013. www.webmd. com/baby/features. A clearly written and straightforward overview of the less commonly known and under-appreciated aspects of twin pregnancies. The online version of the article also has additional links that will be of interest to expectant mothers and their families.

Moore, Keith L., and T.V.N. Persaud. *The Developing Human*. 8th ed. Philadelphia: Saunders/Elsevier, 2011. An outstanding textbook on human embryonic development, with information about the development of multiple embryos.

Noble, Elizabeth. *Having Twins and More: A Parent's Guide to Pregnancy, Birth, and Early Childhood*. 3rd ed. New York: Houghton-Mifflin, 2003. This book is well written and easy to understand. The author is a professional with many years of experience with multiple births.

Novotny, Pamela P. *The Joy of Twins and Other Multiple Births: Having, Raising, and Loving Babies Who Arrive in Groups*. Avenel, NJ: Crown Books, 1994. The author provides interesting information for parents of multiple infants.

Rand, L., K.A. Eddleman, and J. Stone. "Long-Term Outcomes in Multiple Gestations." *Clinical Perinatology* 32, no. 2 (2005): 495-513. An in-depth look at problems for which multiples are at high risk and their likelihood of occurring.

Rothbart, Betty. *Multiple Blessings: From Pregnancy Through Childhood-A Guide for Parents of Twins, Triplets, or More*. San Francisco: Hearst Books, 1994. In a clear presentation of all the facts, the author helps parents through all stages of pregnancy, providing advice on feeding, home care, juggling hectic schedules, and other critical issues related to the raising of twins and triplets.

MULTIPLE CHEMICAL SENSITIVITY SYNDROME
Disease/Disorder

Anatomy or system affected: Eyes, immune system, lungs, muscles, nerves, nervous system, respiratory system, skin

Specialties and related fields: Dermatology, environmental health, epidemiology, immunology, neurology, occupational health, public health, toxicology

Definition: An increasing intolerance to commonly encountered chemicals at concentrations well tolerated by other people.

Causes and Symptoms

Multiple chemical sensitivity (MCS) syndrome, idiopathic environmental intolerance (IEI), reactive airway disease, and sick building syndrome are overlapping disorders caused by intolerance of environmental chemicals. Exactly how many people are affected by MCS is unknown. The onset is often associated with initial acute chemical exposure; patients may report the onset of MCS after moving into a new house, being exposed to chemicals in the workplace, or using pesticides in the home. Patients often describe an increasing intolerance to commonly encountered chemicals at concentrations well tolerated by other people. Diagnosis is made when the following six criteria are met: repeated exposure reproduces symptoms, the condition is chronic, low chemical exposure levels cause symptoms, symptoms improve with the removal of offending chemicals, responses are triggered by multiple unrelated chemicals, and multiple systems are affected.

Symptoms usually wax and wane with exposure and are more likely to occur in patients with preexisting histories of migraine or classical allergies. Idiosyncratic medication reactions (especially to preservative chemicals) are common in MCS patients, as are dysautonomic symptoms (such as vascular instability), poor temperature regulation, and food intolerance. It is thought that patients with MCS have organ abnormalities involving the liver, the nervous system (including the brain and the limbic, peripheral, and autonomic systems), the immune system, and perhaps porphyrin metabolism, probably reflecting chemical injury to these systems. There is often a substantial overlap of MCS symptoms with fibromyalgia and chronic fatigue syndrome.

The common clinical symptoms may include headaches (often migraine), chronic fatigue, musculoskeletal aching, chronic respiratory inflammation (rhinitis, sinusitis, laryngitis, asthma), attention-deficit disorder, and hyperactivity in younger children. Less common complaints include tremor, seizure, and mitral valve prolapse. Agents associated with the onset of MCS include gasoline, kerosene, natural gas, pesticides (especially chlordane and chlorpyrifos), organic solvents, new carpet and other renovation materials, adhesives and glues, fiberglass, carbonless copy paper, fabric softener, formaldehyde and glutaraldehyde, carpet shampoo (lauryl sulfate) and other cleaning agents, isocyanates, combustion products (poorly vented gas heaters, overheated batteries), and medications (dinitrochlorobenzene for warts,

---

> ### Information on
> ### Multiple Chemical Sensitivity Syndrome
>
> **Causes:** Environmental exposure to chemicals
> **Symptoms:** Headaches (often migraine); chronic fatigue, musculoskeletal aching; chronic respiratory inflammation (rhinitis, sinusitis, laryngitis, asthma); attention-deficit disorder; hyperactivity (affecting younger children); food intolerance
> **Duration:** Acute to chronic
> **Treatments:** Alleviation of symptoms, supportive therapy

intranasally packed neosynephrine, prolonged antibiotics, and general anesthesia with petrochemicals).

It is believed that the mechanisms that lead to MCS may be multifactorial and include neurogenic inflammation (respiratory, gastrointestinal, and genitourinary symptoms), kindling and time-dependent sensitization (neurologic symptoms), and immune activation or impaired porphyrin metabolism (multiple-organ symptoms). Pathological findings of MCS have rarely been examined. A preliminary study of nasal pathology in these patients indicates that they are characterized by defects in the junctions between cells, desquamation of the respiratory epithelium, glandular hyperplasia, lymphocytic infiltrates, and peripheral nerve fiber proliferation. A consistent physiologic abnormality in these patients has not been established.

Psychiatric, personality, cognitive/neurologic, immunologic, and olfactory studies have been conducted comparing MCS subjects with various control groups. Thus far, the most consistent finding is that patients with MCS have a higher rate of psychiatric disorders across studies and relative to diverse comparison groups. Since these studies are cross-sectional, however, causality cannot be implied. Various working groups have proposed several research questions addressing the relationship between neurogenic inflammation and toxicant-induced loss of tolerance with the development of MCS.

Treatment and Therapy

The management of patients with MCS at present involves symptomatic and supportive therapy. There is a general consensus among researchers and clinicians that in order to treat patients with MCS effectively, a double-blind, placebo-controlled study performed in an environmentally controlled facility, with rigorous documentation of both objective and subjective responses, is needed to help elucidate the nature and origin of MCS.

—Shih-Wen Huang, M.D.; updated by
Sharon W. Stark, R.N., A.P.R.N., D.N.Sc.

See also Allergies; Antihistamines; Asthma; Autoimmune disorders; Chronic fatigue syndrome; Dermatitis; Dermatology; Dizziness and fainting; Environmental diseases; Fatigue; Fibromyalgia; Hay fever; Headaches; Host-defense mechanisms; Immune system; Immunology; Laryngitis; Lungs; Migraine headaches; Mold and mildew; Nasopharyngeal disorders; Nausea and vomiting; Occupational health; Pulmonary medicine; Rashes; Seizures; Sinusitis; Skin; Skin disorders; Sore throat; Wheezing.

For Further Information:

Baron-Faust, Rita, and Jill P. Buyon. *The Autoimmune Connection: Essential Information for Women on Diagnosis, Treatment, and Getting on with Your Life.* Chicago: Contemporary Books, 2003.

Barrett, Stephen J., and Ronald E. Gots. *Chemical Sensitivity: The Truth About Environmental Illness.* Amherst, N.Y.: Prometheus Books, 1998.

Delves, Peter J., et al. *Roitt's Essential Immunology.* 12th ed. Hoboken, N.J.: John Wiley & Sons, 2011.

Dwyer, John M. *The Body at War: The Story of Our Immune System.* 2d ed. New York: J. M. Dent, 1993.

McCormick, Gail. *Living with Multiple Chemical Sensitivity: Narratives of Coping.* Jefferson, N.C.: McFarland, 2000.

MCS Referral and Resources. http://www.mcsrr.org.

Morgan, Monroe T. *Environmental Health.* 3d ed. Belmont, Calif.: Thomson/Wadsworth, 2003.

Owen, Judy, Jenni Punt, and Sharon Stranford. *Kuby Immunology.* 7th ed. New York: W. H. Freeman, 2013.

MULTIPLE SCLEROSIS
Disease/Disorder

Anatomy or system affected: Muscles, musculoskeletal system, nerves, nervous system, spine
Specialties and related fields: Immunology, internal medicine, neurology, pediatrics
Definition: A debilitating chronic inflammatory disease affecting the central nervous system.

Key terms:

autoimmunity: a condition in which the immune system fails to recognize its own tissues as "self" and mounts an immune response against its own cells

demyelination: the destruction of myelin

disseminated sclerosis: another name for multiple sclerosis (MS)

myelin: a fatty substance wrapping nerves as a sheath that accelerates electric impulse propagation

primary progressive MS: the most aggressive form of MS, characterized by the absence of remissions and continual decline

relapsing-remitting MS: the most common form of MS, characterized by unpredictable attacks (relapses) followed by periods free of symptoms (remission)

remyelination: the repair of myelin

sclerosis: a process of hardening of tissues

secondary progressive MS: a form that occurs in patients who initially had relapsing-remitting MS and transition to a more aggressive MS

Causes and Symptoms

Multiple sclerosis (MS) is a chronic and disabling disease of the nervous system. Symptoms can be mild, such as limb numbness, or severe, such as paralysis and loss of vision. How the disease will progress and its severity in specific individuals are difficult to predict because it progresses differently in each of its victims.

Multiple sclerosis is caused by degeneration of the ner-

Information on Multiple Sclerosis

Causes: Genetic and environmental factors; possibly viral infection
Symptoms: Tingling, numbness, slurring of speech, blurred or double vision, loss of coordination, muscle weakness and/or tightness, fatigue, bowel and bladder control difficulties, sexual dysfunction, paralysis, impaired cognitive functions
Duration: Chronic with recurrent episodes
Treatments: Steroids, human interferons, regular exercise

vous system. A fatty substance called myelin surrounds and protects many nerve fibers of the brain and spinal cord. Myelin is important because it speeds up signals that move along the nerve fibers. In MS, the body attacks its own tissues, termed an autoimmune reaction, and a breakdown in the myelin layer along the nerves occurs. When any part of the myelin sheathing is destroyed, nerve impulses to and from the brain are slowed, distorted, or interrupted. The disease is called "multiple" because it affects many areas of the brain. Scleroids are hardened, scarred patches that form over the damaged areas of myelin.

The initial symptoms of MS may include tingling, numbness, slurred speech, blurred or double vision, loss of coordination, and muscle weakness. Later manifestations include unusual fatigue, muscle tightness, bowel and bladder control difficulties, sexual dysfunction, and paralysis. The most common cognitive functions influenced are short-term memory, abstract reasoning, verbal fluency, and speed of information processing. All the mental and physical symptoms listed may come or go in any combination. The symptoms may also vary from mild to severe in intensity throughout the course of the disease.

The symptoms of MS not only vary from person to person but also may periodically vary within the same person. This makes the prognosis of the disease difficult to foresee. Although the general course of the disease may be anticipated, the symptoms and their severity seem to be quite unpredictable in most individuals. In the "classic" course of MS, as time progresses, chronic problems gradually accumulate over many years, slowly worsening the sufferer's quality of life. The total level of disability will vary from patient to patient.

The typical pattern of MS is marked by active periods of the disease during which the nerves are being ravaged by the immune system. These periods are called attacks, relapses, or exacerbations. The active periods of the disease are followed by calm periods called remissions. The cycle of attack and remission will differ from sufferer to sufferer. Some people have few attacks, and their MS disabilities slowly accumulate over time; in these sufferers, it takes decades to become truly debilitated. Most people with MS have what is known as the relapsing-remitting form of the disease. They suffer many attacks over time, and these attacks occur unpredictably; the attacks are then followed by complete remission which may

last months or years. Again, the injuries may take many years to accumulate to complete disability.

The most aggressive form of the disease is primary progressive MS. In this type of MS, the disease follows a rapid course that steadily worsens from its first onset. Although there are still attacks and partial remission, the attacks are quite severe and occur more regularly in time. Full paralysis may develop in primary progressive MS in three to five years. Secondary progressive MS occurs in patients who initially have the relapsing-remitting type and later develop the more aggressive form.

Both genetic and environmental factors have been implicated in inducing the onset of MS. Viral infection has been suggested as a cause, but no single virus has ever been shown to be associated with MS. Although infections such as the common cold, flu, and gastroenteritis increase the risk of relapse, flu vaccination is safe in patients with MS. Risk may be conferred by exposure to a specific environment during adolescence, but that environment and the genetic risk factors have not yet been characterized. The support for the genetic component comes from examining identical twins. The likelihood of MS in the second identical twin, when the first twin has MS, is 30 percent.

Researchers Sharon Lynch and John Rose suggested that certain racial and geographic populations are less susceptible than others to the disease. MS is uncommon in Japanese people as well as among American Indians. The disease is more common among Northern European Caucasians as well as among North Americans of higher latitudes. There is an additional sexual dimorphism in the epidemiology of MS; the disease is found more frequently in women, by a ratio of 2:1.

The disease usually begins its first manifestations in late adolescence (around age eighteen) to early middle age (around age thirty-five). It is not clear how the interaction between the genetics of the sufferer and the environment may trigger onset. The progressive type of MS is more common over the age of forty, so those with late-onset MS often have the quickest deterioration of motor function. The reason that an older age predisposes someone to primary chronic progressive MS is still not clear.

Studies by Swiss researcher Avinoam Safran have shown that occasionally MS manifests after the age of fifty. This condition has been named late-onset multiple sclerosis. Late-onset MS is not rare. Nearly 10 percent of MS patients demonstrate their first symptom after the age of fifty. This type of MS is often not recognized by physicians, who do not expect it in the aged.

Treatment and Therapy

Scientists have been encouraged by advancements in MS diagnosis using the MRI brain scan. In 2002 they announced that these scans appear to detect damage around nerve fibers in patients with possible early signs of MS. This detection helps doctors predict those who will eventually develop MS and how severe one's experience with the disease might be. In turn, this allows a drug regimen to begin earlier. In the past, doctors did not officially diagnose MS or start treatment until patients had two episodes of nerve problems in different areas of the body—reoccurrences that could come years apart while damage nonetheless continued silently. New research has found that putting patients on MS drugs at the first sign of nerve inflammation drastically slows the chances of developing MS within a few years, although most will eventually still develop the disease.

While there is no cure for MS, there are many effective treatments. In most cases, steroidal drugs are used to treat relapses or attacks of the disease. Corticotropin was the first steroidal immunosuppressant to be used widely in MS treatment. The primary effect of the drug is to shorten the duration of an attack, although it does not appear to reduce the severity of the attack. Although it is still used with patients who respond well to it, corticotropin has been supplanted by other drugs. Methylprednisolone is an immunosuppressant and steroid that has replaced corticotropin. It has been shown to control the inflammation that accompanies demyelination. These steroids seem to work by sealing leaking blood vessels in the brain and reducing the responsiveness of the white blood

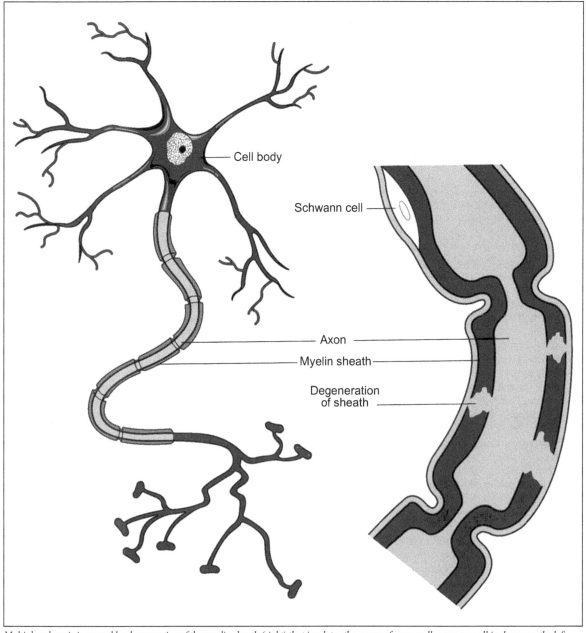

Cell body

Schwann cell

Axon

Myelin sheath

Degeneration of sheath

Multiple sclerosis is caused by degeneration of the myelin sheath (right) that insulates the axons of nerve cells; a nerve cell is shown on the left.

In the News: New Drug Treatments for Multiple Sclerosis

The neurodegeneration that characterizes multiple sclerosis (MS) results from the destruction of myelin that surrounds and protects nerves by the immune system. Myelin-specific T cells are required for this attack. Corticosteroids have been used as therapy because of their known immunosuppressive properties. They have proved to be effective against the symptoms of MS episodes, but they have serious side effects and can be taken only for short times. Because they suppress the immune system in a general, nonspecific way, they inhibit not only the destruction of myelin but also the body's ability to fight infection. This problem has led to the deaths of some MS patients. In addition, corticosteroids do not delay the long-term progression of MS. More recently, interferon-β has been used to treat MS. Although interferon-β therapy can be given for long periods and has been shown to reduce the frequency of relapses and to slow the progression of the disease, why it works is not known. One theory is that it reduces inflammation.

New drugs on the horizon aim to stop the progression of MS and eliminate all relapses. The theory behind them is that a drug should targeted to inhibit only the components of the immune system that destroy myelin. Such drugs, unlike the drugs currently available, would be attacking the underlying cause of MS, rather than its symptoms, and would be expected to cause few or no side effects.

Two of these new drugs, Tovaxin from Opexa Therapeutics and a not-yet named candidate, now called RTL1000, from Artielle Immuno-Therapeutics, act by specifically inactivating the patient's own myelin-specific T cells, while not interacting with other immune system cells. Myelin-specific T cells are required for the destruction of myelin, and when a large number of them are inactivated, myelin destruction slows down.

Another approach is being developed by Immune Response. Their drug NeuroVax acts by specifically stimulating patients' cells that down-regulate myelin-specific T cells. Clinical trials of NeuroVax are underway.

—*Lorraine Lica, Ph.D.*

Zocor—part of the statin class—showed early positive signs of similar anti-inflammatory effects in humans. Another strategy using a monoclonal antibody, Natalizumab, was approved in 2006 for the treatment of the relapsing form of MS. In 2010, the Food and Drug Administration (FDA) approved fingolimod, the first oral drug for MS treatment.

During the 1990s, in a study supported by the National Institutes of Health and conducted at the Mayo Clinic, plasma exchange, also called plasmapheresis, was proven to be an effective treatment for certain patients suffering from severe symptoms of multiple sclerosis who were not responsive to conventional methods of treatment. Plasma exchange involves the removal of the patient's blood; the elimination of the plasma-containing antibodies that target myelin, which is then replaced by a fluid with similar properties, usually containing albumin; and its subsequent return to the patient. This procedure has been used for treatment of other

cells of the immune system so that they cannot attack the myelin as easily.

Several federally approved drugs can slow the rate of attacks: Avonex, Rebif, and Betaseron are preparations of interferon (proteins regulating the immune system), and Copaxone is a mixture of small peptides that protects myelin. Although these drugs do not stop MS entirely, they actually limit the level of myelin destruction, as observed in magnetic resonance imaging (MRI) scans of the brain. Avonex slows down the rate of progression to disability, and all four slow down the natural course of MS. University of Western Ontario researcher George Ebers was the first to perform experimental treatments on MS patients with interferons. The myelin sheath is actually produced by a special nerve cell called an oligodendrocyte; presumably the oligodendrocytes are stimulated to protect themselves by exposure to interferons. Patients treated with human interferons demonstrated a 34 percent reduction in frequency of attacks; that reduction was sustained over five years of treatment. More impressive was the 80 percent reduction of MS activity detected in their brains. Steroid treatment was rarely required in these patients.

In 2002, researchers announced that preliminary studies using mice and a class of statin drugs used to lower cholesterol in heart patients showed an improvement and some reversal of the debilitating symptoms of MS. The animal data was encouraging because of their demonstration that the statin drugs appear to reprogram the immune cells that attack myelin so they instead protect nerve coatings. Also in 2002, another parallel study using MS patients and the drug sold as

autoimmune diseases such as myasthenia gravis and Guillain-Barré syndrome in the past.

Investigators concluded that plasma exchange might contribute to recovery from an acute attack in people with MS who have not responded to standard steroid treatment. Therefore, they recommended that this treatment only be considered for individuals experiencing a severe, acute attack that is not responding to high-dose steroids. Since the vast majority (90 percent) of people experiencing acute attacks respond well to the standard steroid treatment, plasma exchange would be considered a treatment alternative only for the approximately 10 percent who do not. For those 10 percent, however, plasma exchange may offer an important and beneficial treatment option. Because the exact reasons for the effectiveness of plasmapheresis are not known, researchers feel that further studies are warranted based on the idea that some people may have antibodies in their plasma that are instrumental in certain disease activities that allow disabilities to occur.

As additional therapy, patients with MS should participate in a regular exercise program. Exercise is vital to the maintenance of functional ability in MS sufferers. It strengthens muscles, benefits gait, and generally improves coordination. The best type of exercise is aquatic in nature. Sufferers are often heat-intolerant, and participation in a regular aerobic program would be unpleasant. Also, aquatic exercise is a low-impact activity that puts less stress on chronically sore muscles. Exercise programs also encourage socialization of patients and engender peer support.

Perspective and Prospects

The first written report of MS was published in 1400 when the famed Dutch skater Lydwina of Schieden was diagnosed. It was recognized initially as a wasting disease of unknown origin. The disease was described clinically by Jean-Martin Charcot in 1877. Charcot initially characterized the clinical signs and symptoms of MS. He recognized that the disease affects the nervous system and tried many remedies, without success. In 1890, the cause of MS was thought to be suppression of sweat; the treatment was electrical stimulation and bed rest. At the time, life expectancy for a sufferer was five years after diagnosis. By 1910, MS was thought to be caused by toxins in the blood, and purgatives were alleged the best treatment. In the 1930s, poor circulation was believed to cause MS, and blood-thinning agents became the treatment of choice. In the 1950s through the 1970s, MS was thought to be caused by severe allergies; treatments included antihistamines. Not until the 1980s was the basis of MS understood and effective treatment developed.

By the early twenty-first century, it was estimated that thousands of peopel had this disorder of the brain and spinal cord, which causes disruption in the smooth flow of electrical messages from brain and nerves to the body. The progress of the disease is slow and may take decades to achieve complete nerve degeneration and paralysis. Although often considered a disease of youth, MS has the potential to become an increasing problem in aging populations. More cases of late-onset MS have come to light in individuals over forty years of age, including such celebrities as comedian Richard Pryor, entertainer Annette Funicello, and talk-show host Montel Williams.

Several novel therapies that have been under investigation are sphingosine receptor modulator (fingolimod), vitamin D, inosine (Axosine), and antimicrobial agents. Various combinations of drugs are also being examined and include mitoxantrone (an immunosuppressant) and Copaxone. Current clinical trials are likely to reveal treatment strategies that will further facilitate controlling of the symptoms and progression of MS.

—James J. Campanella, Ph.D.;
updated by W. Michael Zawada, Ph.D.

See also Amyotrophic lateral sclerosis; Muscle sprains, spasms, and disorders; Muscles; Nervous system; Neuralgia, neuritis, and neuropathy; Neuroimaging; Neurology; Paralysis; Spinal cord disorders; Spine, vertebrae, and disks.

For Further Information:

"About MS." *National Multiple Sclerosis Society*, 2013.
Alan, Rick, and Rimas Lukas. "Multiple Sclerosis—Adult." *Health Library*, Sept. 30, 2012.
Alan, Rick, Rebecca Stahl, and Kari Kassir. "Multiple Sclerosis—Child." *Health Library*, June 6, 2012.
Blackstone, Margaret. *The First Year—Multiple Sclerosis: An Essential Guide for the Newly Diagnosed*. 2d ed. New York: Avalon, 2007.
Halbreich, Uriel. *Multiple Sclerosis: A Neuropsychiatric Disorder*. Boston: American Psychiatric Press, 1993.
Iams, Betty. *From MS to Wellness*. Chicago: Iams House, 1998.
Kalb, Rosalind, ed. *Multiple Sclerosis: The Questions You Have, the Answers You Need*. 5th ed. New York: Demos Vermande, 2012.
Litin, Scott C., ed. "Multiple Sclerosis." In *Mayo Clinic Family Health Book*. 4th ed. New York: HarperResource, 2009.
Matthews, Bryan. *Multiple Sclerosis: The Facts*. 4th ed. New York: Oxford University Press, 2001.
"Multiple Sclerosis." *MedlinePlus*, May 7, 2013.
"NINDS Multiple Sclerosis Information Page." *National Institute of Neurological Disorders and Stroke*, Aug. 14, 2012.
Polman, Chris H., et al. *Multiple Sclerosis: The Guide to Treatment and Management*. 6th ed. New York: Demos Vermande, 2006.
Russell, Margot. *When the Road Turns: Inspirational Stories About People with MS*. Deerfield Beach, Fla.: Health Communications, 2001.
Salter, Robert Bruce. *Textbook of Disorders and Injuries of the Musculoskeletal System*. 3d ed. Baltimore: Williams & Wilkins, 1999.

Mumps

Disease/Disorder

Also known as: Epidemic parotitis

Anatomy or system affected: Genitals, glands, nervous system, pancreas

Specialties and related fields: Family medicine, pediatrics

Definition: An acute, contagious childhood disease caused by a virus and characterized by swollen salivary glands.

Key terms:

encephalitis: infection and inflammation of the brain

meningitis: infection and inflammation of the covering of the brain

orchitis: infection, inflammation, and swelling of a testicle or ovary; usually occurs only on one side and usually only in adults with mumps infection

parotitis: infection, inflammation, and swelling of the parotid gland, the major salivary gland located near the angle of the jaw; this swelling will often push out the earlobe

Causes and Symptoms

Mumps infection is acquired after contact with infected respiratory secretions. An infected person can spread the disease from twelve to twenty-two days after infection. One case in a family generally means that every family member has been infected. Mumps is most commonly transmitted in the winter and early spring. During the sixteen- to eighteen-day incubation period, the virus grows first in the nose and throat, moves to the regional lymph nodes and then into the bloodstream, and spreads to multiple organs and the central nervous system.

One-third of patients with mumps infection do not have symptoms or have very mild symptoms. Mumps is more se-

---

Information on Mumps

Causes: Viral infection

Symptoms: Swollen salivary glands, fever, headache, stomach upset, loss of appetite, mildly congested nose, red rash; occasionally organ infection or joint inflammation

Duration: Sixteen to eighteen days

Treatments: Alleviation of symptoms with mild pain medications, adequate fluid and nutritional intake

vere after puberty. The first symptoms include fever, headache, stomach upset, loss of appetite, and a mildly congested nose. The most common finding is swelling of the salivary glands. This swelling usually starts on one side and then moves to both sides in three-quarters of cases. Salivary gland pain is most pronounced during the first few days and is associated with discomfort when eating or drinking acidic foods such as orange juice. Rarely, a thin red rash can occur. The fever usually resolves in three to five days, and the salivary gland swelling subsides within seven to ten days.

Between 1 and 10 percent of patients have clinical evidence of central nervous system infection, most commonly meningitis but very rarely encephalitis. Infection of the central nervous system is more common in males than in females. Central nervous system disease typically occurs one to three weeks after the onset of salivary gland swelling, but it can also precede or follow this swelling. Symptoms include headache, fever, lethargy, stiff neck, and vomiting. Seizures occur in 20 percent of hospitalized patients. Central nervous system infection is almost always limited, without any lasting effect or complications. Hearing loss occurs during mumps illness in 4 percent of patients but is not higher in those with central nervous system involvement. Higher-tone deficits are noted most frequently. Recovery from hearing loss usually occurs within a few weeks following onset. Persistent hearing loss is usually only one-sided.

Orchitis, an infection of the testicles or ovaries, can also occur with mumps. The highest risk for this disease occurs after puberty, usually in males from fifteen to twenty-nine years of age. Between 14 and 35 percent of males with mumps infection develop orchitis. Fever, malaise, vomiting, and stomach pain are common symptoms. Testicular pain, swelling, and tenderness generally last for three to seven days. Involvement is one-sided in most cases. Symptoms usually began four to eight days following the onset of salivary gland swelling, but they can occur in the absence of gland swelling.

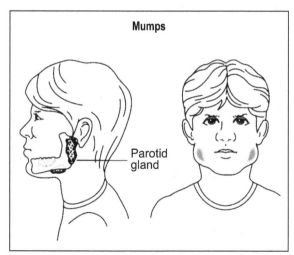

Mumps

Parotid gland

Mumps causes a characteristic swelling of the parotid (salivary) glands.

Mumps infection can cause other, less common complications. Infection of the kidney is almost always limited, but rare reports of kidney failure with mumps do exist. Multiple joint migratory arthritis with joint fluid has been described and is usually of short duration. Joint complaints are more common in males in their twenties. The usual signs of joint disease occur one to three weeks after the onset of salivary gland swelling. The large joints are more commonly affected.

Inflammation of the heart occurs in 4 to 15 percent of patients with mumps. It is most common in adults and generally resolves itself within two to four weeks. Infection and inflammation of the pancreas can occasionally occur. Pancreatitis can lead to fatty diarrhea and, very rarely, diabetes. Women who have mumps infection during pregnancy do not have an increased risk of delivering an infant with congenital malformation.

Very rarely, mumps will cause death. It is unclear why, prior to the advent of vaccination, mumps infection killed people each year. More than 50 percent of deaths are of adults.

Not all patients with salivary gland swelling have mumps. Swelling in this area of the face may be attributable to another disease of the salivary gland or another disease affecting other tissues in the face such as lymph nodes or bones. Persistent or recurrent swelling of the parotid gland should be evaluated by a physician.

Treatment and Therapy

Conservative therapy is indicated for mumps infection. No antiviral therapy is available. Adequate fluids and nutrition are important. A patient's diet should avoid acidic foods and should be light and generous in fluids. Occasionally, mild pain medications may be necessary for severe headaches or salivary gland discomfort. Stronger pain medications may be needed with testicular involvement. In unusual cases where vomiting is severe, intravenous fluids may be required. A spinal tap (lumbar puncture) is rarely indicated, but patients who have this procedure frequently find that it relieves their headaches.

Exposure to mumps infection may cause anxiety in adult family members or day care employees. A child with mumps should be isolated for nine days after the start of salivary gland swelling. Vaccine administration will probably not prevent infection after exposure, and a history of family exposure to mumps probably indicates past infection. The physician will reassure any adult exposed family members and indicate that it is unlikely that the vaccine will prevent this disease. Nevertheless, exposure may dictate the need to administer the vaccine, as determining immune status is generally not practicable.

Mumps is a self-limited illness and does not require the administration of antiviral medications, antibiotics, or antibody preparations. Mumps vaccine should be given to children to prevent this disease. The combined vaccine containing measles, mumps, and rubella (MMR) vaccines should be given to children first when they are twelve months to fifteen months of age; a second dose should be given before the child first starts school (four through six years of age). About 98 percent

---

In the News:
Mumps Outbreak in the United States

In December, 2005, several students at an unnamed college in eastern Iowa displayed symptoms of illness that included glandular swelling in the salivary region. Antibody testing indicated that the students had active cases of mumps. Several weeks later, an additional case was diagnosed. In the following months, additional cases were reported in the surrounding states of Illinois, Kansas, Minnesota, and Nebraska; serotyping of isolated viruses indicated that all cases originated from a similar or identical strain. Since not all the cases were directly linked with each other—that is, involved known contact—the suspicion among health workers is that portions of the outbreak were maintained through inapparent infections.

The source of the illness remains unclear, but the initial case may have been contracted in Great Britain. During 2005, some 56,000 cases were diagnosed there, and the strain that first appeared in Iowa appears to be identical. It is likely that a student had either traveled to Great Britain during the period of the outbreak or had contact with someone who had.

By the time that the illness had run its course in the summer of 2006, more than 4,700 persons had been diagnosed with mumps, with cases reported as far away as California. Approximately 25 percent were college students. Mumps is generally a benign infection, and while there were no fatalities, pregnant women and persons with compromised immune systems, such as those who are HIV-positive, may be at risk for severe illness. An unusual feature of the outbreak was that more than two-thirds of the patients had already received the recommended two doses of the mumps vaccine in the form of the MMR (measles, mumps, rubella) vaccine, calling into question the long-term effectiveness of current immunization practices. In the light of the outbreak, health authorities recommended that all students be sure of prior immunization against mumps, or that they receive an additional two doses of the vaccine.

—*Richard Adler, Ph.D.*

---

cine in its present form or in another form should be considered for administration both to decrease adverse reactions and to decrease its cost and improve its applicability to a broader population.

—*Peter D. Reuman, M.D., M.P.H.*

See also Childhood infectious diseases; Encephalitis; Fever; Glands; Immunization and vaccination; Infertility, male; Meningitis; Orchitis; Viral infections.

For Further Information:

American Medical Association. *American Medical Association Family Medical Guide.* 4th rev. ed. Hoboken, N.J.: John Wiley & Sons, 2004.

Badash, Michelle, and Kari Kassir. "Mumps." *Health Library*, Sept. 27, 2012.

Beers, Mark H., et al., eds. *The Merck Manual of Diagnosis and Therapy.* 18th ed. Whitehouse Station, N.J.: Merck Research Laboratories, 2006.

Bellenir, Karen, and Peter D. Dresser, eds. *Contagious and Noncontagious Infectious Diseases Sourcebook.* Detroit, Mich.: Omnigraphics, 1996.

"Fast Facts about Mumps." *Centers for Disease Control and Prevention*, Mar. 24, 2010.

Gorbach, Sherwood L., John G. Bartlett, and Neil R. Blacklow, eds. *Infectious Diseases.* 3d ed. Philadelphia: W. B. Saunders, 2004.

Litin, Scott C., ed. *Mayo Clinic Family Health Book.* 4th ed. New York: HarperResource, 2009.

"Mumps." *Centers for Disease Control and Prevention*, Oct. 6, 2010.

"Mumps." *MedlinePlus*, May 2, 2013.

"Mumps Vaccination: Who Needs It?" *Centers for Disease Control and Prevention*, Jan. 12, 2012.

Sompayrac, Lauren. *How Pathogenic Viruses Work.* Boston: Jones and Bartlett, 2002.

Woolf, Alan D., et al., eds. *The Children's Hospital Guide to Your Child's Health and Development.* Cambridge, Mass.: Perseus, 2002.

MÜNCHAUSEN SYNDROME BY PROXY
Disease/Disorder

Anatomy or system affected: All

Specialties and related fields: Ethics, family medicine, pediatrics, psychiatry, psychology

Definition: A disorder in which a parent fabricates, simulates, or induces a medical condition in a child in order to receive attention and acknowledgment as the source of information about the child's health.

Key terms:

covert video surveillance: the monitoring of a child using video equipment in which the parent is unaware of the taping

narcissistic personality disorder: a disorder characterized by maladaptive patterns of behavior that are used to deal with common life situations

Causes and Symptoms

Münchausen syndrome by proxy may occur in different forms. In its least invasive form, this syndrome involves lying about a child's medical problems. For example, a father may claim that his child stopped breathing or had a seizure. The harm to the child comes from the medical studies that are

---

of children will respond to this vaccine and not acquire mumps infection.

Perspective and Prospects

The term "mumps" is derived from an English dialect meaning "grimace," attributed to the painful parotid gland swelling. The virus was first described in 1934, and a live vaccine was first licensed in 1967. Prior to 1980, the age-group most affected by mumps was five- to nine-year-olds. In the 1980s, this group shifted to children and adolescents aged ten to nineteen. In the 1990s, most cases occurred in adults over twenty. This change was caused by the increased use of the mumps vaccine in children but not in adults.

Vaccination has been very successful, especially when combined with measles and rubella vaccine, given in the second year of life, and repeated prior to school. Side effects from mumps vaccine are extremely rare and can include anything that is seen in mumps infection. Recent research in the area has been directed toward determining whether the vac-

---

Information on Münchausen Syndrome by Proxy

Causes: Psychological disorder
Symptoms: Lying about or inducing a child's medical problems
Duration: Chronic
Treatments: Psychotherapy

---

ordered by the physician in an attempt to evaluate and diagnose the condition. A second situation involves the simulation of symptoms in the child. For example, a mother may maintain that her child is experiencing hematuria, and examination of the urine reveals the presence of blood. The blood comes not from the child but from some external source, such as the mother's menstrual blood or animal blood from packaged meat. Again, the child is subjected to needless diagnostic tests, some of which can be invasive.

The most injurious form of Münchausen syndrome by proxy comes when a parent induces the symptoms in the child. This can be done in many ways: The parent can administer syrup of ipecac to induce vomiting, administer substances such as diphtheria-tetanus-pertussis (DTaP) vaccine to cause a fever, or inject fecal materials into already existing intravenous lines to induce a bacterial bloodstream infection. Parental induction of an apparent life-threatening event (ALTE) has been documented through the use of covert video surveillance. Parents have been observed placing their hands or other objects over the infant's face. Many of these children demonstrated bleeding from the mouth or gums, a finding not reported in any of the control infants who were experiencing an ALTE.

In addition to being subjected to multiple and invasive diagnostic procedures, some children die as a direct result of their parents" actions. Some families have a history of sudden or unexplained deaths of siblings that may be attributable to Münchausen syndrome by proxy or other types of child abuse.

Treatment and Therapy

A physician should become concerned about the possibility of Münchausen syndrome by proxy in a child with multiple health care visits in whom an explanation for the problems is elusive. The most common complaints include bleeding, vomiting, apnea, seizures, and fever. In each case, the chronic nature of the problems and the constant switching of health care providers should be clues. Statements by experienced physicians such as "I've never seen anything like this" should also signal that the child may be the victim of Münchausen syndrome by proxy. Some physicians become trapped in the process of ordering multiple studies for fear of missing an exotic disease.

On the other hand, some parents represent the "worried well." These people bring their children in for many minor complaints: every runny nose, low-grade temperature, or nonapparent skin rash. Their motivation is not personal attention. Rather, they are fearful and view their children as vulnerable.

The psychologic profile of the parent helps to distinguish the overly concerned mother from the one with Münchausen syndrome by proxy. The usual perpetrator is the child's mother. The father is often detached, distant, and not involved in the child's care, although cases in which the father is the perpetrator have been documented. Most perpetrators are believed to have borderline personalities and narcissistic personality disorders. They enjoy the attention that they receive in a medical setting. Medical staff members often characterize these individuals as excellent parents because they are knowledgeable about their child's health, attentive to his or her needs, and cooperative with the staff. Many of the mothers have some type of medical or science background, which facilitates their understanding of medical conditions. Some have worked in physicians" offices, making them knowledgeable about medical terminology or procedures. Psychological assessment is needed to help define parental pathology. Members of the medical staff may be disbelieving of the diagnosis, since they often find the parent to be nice and helpful. Many parents deny the accusations and are resistant to psychiatric intervention.

The task of the medical team is to entertain the diagnosis, obtain evidence, and protect the child. In some institutions, covert video surveillance is used to catch the parent in the act of inflicting the symptoms. Although there is concern about issues of privacy, legal counsel at most institutions has supported the use of covert video surveillance because it assesses the situation of the child.

Perspective and Prospects

Münchausen syndrome by proxy was initially described by Roy Meadow in 1977. In the twenty years after his initial report, more than three hundred cases were reported in the literature. The diversity of ways in which this syndrome is inflicted on children has expanded with each case report. In many cases, the prognosis for affected children is somewhat guarded because of the complexity of establishing the diagnosis on a legal level.

Once the child and the parent are separated, the symptoms resolve. Cases may be difficult to substantiate in court, without the presence of concrete evidence. Some children suffer from long-term sequelae, sometimes behaving like invalids because of the role in which they have been cast since childhood. There are reports of self-destructive behavior and Münchausen syndrome in some survivors. Psychological counseling is critical to ensure the well-being of these children. In most cases, the children cannot be returned to the parental perpetrator because of the intractable nature of the parent's problem.

—*Carol D. Berkowitz, M.D.*

See also Bacterial infections; Critical care; Critical care, pediatric; Domestic violence; Emergency medicine; Emergency medicine, pediatric; Fever; Hypochondriasis; Nausea and vomiting; Physical examination; Psychiatric disorders; Psychiatry; Psychiatry, child and adolescent; Psychosomatic illness.

For Further Information:

American Psychiatric Association. *Diagnostic and Statistical Manual of Mental Disorders: DSM-5.* 5th ed. Arlington, Va.: Author, 2013.

Eminson, Mary, and R. J. Postlethwaite, eds. *Münchausen Syndrome by Proxy Abuse: A Practical Approach.* Boston: Butterworth-Heinemann, 2000.

Feldman, Marc D. *Playing Sick? Untangling the Web of Munchausen Syndrome, Munchausen by Proxy, Malingering, and Factitious Disorder.* New York: Brunner-Routledge, 2004.

Gregory, Julie. *Sickened: The Memoir of a Münchausen by Proxy Childhood.* New York: Bantam, 2003.

Kaneshiro, Neil K., David C. Dugdale III, and David Zieve. "Munchausen Syndrome by Proxy." *MedlinePlus*, Feb. 21, 2011.

McCoy, Krisha, Rebecca J. Stahl, and Brian Randall. "Factitious Disorder." *Health Library*, Mar. 15, 2013.

New, Michelle. "Munchausen by Proxy Syndrome." *KidsHealth.* Nemours Foundation, Mar. 2012.

Rosenberg, D. A. "Münchausen Syndrome by Proxy." In *Child Abuse: Medical Diagnosis and Management*, edited by Robert M. Reece, et al. 3d ed. Elk Grove, Ill.: American Academy of Pediatrics, 2009.

Southall, D. P., M. C. Plunkett, and M. W. Banks, et al. "Covert Video Recordings of Life-Threatening Child Abuse: Lessons for Child Protection." *Pediatrics* 100, no. 5 (November, 1997): 735–760.

Zangwill, Monica, and Brian Randall. "Smothered by Something that Looks Like Love, but Isn't: Munchausen Syndrome by Proxy." *Health Library*, July 10, 2012.

MUSCLE SPRAINS, SPASMS, AND DISORDERS

Disease/Disorder

Also known as: Myopathies

Anatomy or system affected: Legs, ligaments, muscles, musculoskeletal system

Specialties and related fields: Exercise physiology, family medicine, osteopathic medicine, physical therapy, sports medicine

Definition: Injuries, defects, or disorders of the muscles of the body.

Causes and Symptoms

There are three kinds of muscle tissue in the human body: smooth muscle, cardiac muscle, and striated muscle. Smooth muscle tissue is found around the intestines, blood vessels, and bronchioles in the lung, among other areas. These muscles are controlled by the autonomic nervous system, which means that their movement is not subject to voluntary action. They have many functions: They maintain the airway in the lungs, regulate the tone of blood vessels, and move foods and other substances through the digestive tract. Cardiac muscle is found only in the heart. Striated muscles are those that move body parts. They are also called voluntary muscles because they must receive a conscious command from the brain in order to work. They supply the force for physical activity, and they also prevent movement and stabilize body parts.

Muscles are subject to many disorders: Muscle sprains, strains, and spasms are common events in everyone's life and, for the most part, are harmless, if painful, results of overexercise, accidents, falls, bumps, or countless other events. Yet these symptoms can also signal serious myopathies, or disorders within muscle tissue.

Myopathies constitute a wide range of diseases. They are classified as inflammatory myopathies or metabolic myopathies. Inflammatory myopathies include infections by bacteria, viruses, or other microorganisms, as well as other diseases that are possibly autoimmune in origin (that is, resulting from and directed against the body's own tissues). In metabolic myopathies, there is some failure or disturbance in the body's ability to maintain a proper metabolic balance or electrolyte distribution. These conditions include glycogen storage diseases, in which there are errors in glucose processing; disorders of fatty acid metabolism, in which there are derangements in fatty acid oxidation; mitochondrial myopathies, in which there are biochemical and other abnormalities in the mitochondria of muscle cells; endocrine myopathies, in which an endocrine disorder underlies muscular symptoms; and the periodic paralyses, which can be the result of inherited or acquired illnesses. This is only a partial list of the myopathies, the symptoms of which include weakness and pain.

Muscular dystrophies are a group of inherited disorders in which muscle tissue fails to receive nourishment. The results are progressive muscular weakness and the degeneration and destruction of muscle fibers. The symptoms include weakness, loss of coordination, impaired gait, and impaired muscle extensibility. Over the years, muscle mass decreases and the arms, legs, and spine become deformed.

Neuromuscular disorders include a wide variety of conditions in which muscle function is impaired by faulty transmission of nerve impulses to muscle tissue. These conditions may be inherited; they may be attributable to toxins, such as in food poisoning (for example, botulism) or by pesticide poisoning; or they may be side effects of certain drugs. The most commonly seen neuromuscular disorder is myasthenia gravis.

The muscular disorders most often seen are those that result from overexertion, exercise, athletics, accidents, and trauma. Injuries sustained during sports and games have become so significant that sports medicine has become a recognized medical subspecialty. Besides the muscles, the parts of the body involved in these disorders include tendons (tough, stringy tissue that attaches muscles to bones), ligaments (tissue that attaches bone to bone), synovia (membranes enclosing a joint or other bony structure), and cartilage (soft, resilient tissue between bones). A sprain is an injury in which ligaments are stretched or torn. In a strain, muscles or tendons are stretched or torn. A contusion is a bruise that occurs when the body is subjected to trauma; the skin is not broken, but the capillaries underneath are, causing discoloration. A spasm is a short, abnormal contraction in a muscle or group of muscles. A cramp is a prolonged, painful contraction of one or more muscles.

Sprains can be caused by twisting the joint violently or by forcing it beyond its range of movement. The ligaments that connect the bones of the joint stretch or tear. Sprains occur most often in the knees, ankles, and arches of the feet. There is pain and swelling, and at least some immobilization of the joint.

A strain is also called a pulled muscle. When too great a demand is placed on a muscle, it and the surrounding tendons can stretch and/or tear. The main symptom is pain; swelling and muscle spasm may also occur.

Muscle spasms and cramps are common. Sometimes they occur spontaneously, such as the calf muscle cramps that occur at night. Sometimes they are attributable to muscle strain (the charley horse that tightens thigh muscles in runners and other athletes). Muscles that are used often will go into spasm, such as those in the thumb and fingers of writers (writer's cramp), as can muscles that have remained in one position for too long. Muscle spasms and cramps can also occur as direct consequences of dehydration; they are common in athletes who perspire excessively during hot weather.

Some injuries to muscles and joints occur so regularly that they are named for the activities associated with them. A good example is tennis elbow, a condition that results from repeated, vigorous movement of the arm, such as swinging a tennis racket, using a paintbrush, or pitching a baseball. Runners" knee can afflict joggers and other athletes. It is usually caused by sprains in the knee ligaments; there is pain and there may be partial or total immobilization of the knee. Achilles tendinitis, as the name suggests, is inflammation of the Achilles tendon in the heel. It is usually the result of excessive physical activity that causes small tears in the tendon. Pain and immobility are symptoms. Tendinitis can occur in other joints as well; elbows and shoulders are common sites. Tenosynovitis is inflammation of the synovial membrane that sheathes the tendons in the hand. It may be caused by bacterial infection or may be attributable to overexertion.

Tumors and cancerous growths in muscle tissue are rare. If a lump appears in muscle, it is usually a lipoma, a fatty deposit that is benign. One tumor, called rhabdomyosarcoma, however, is malignant and can be fatal.

Treatment and Therapy

The myopathies are a wide group of diseases, and treatment varies considerably among them. The muscular dystrophies also vary in their treatment methods. Physical therapy is recommended to prevent contractures, the permanent, disfiguring muscular contractions that are a feature of the disease. Orthopedic appliances and surgery are also used. Because these diseases are genetic, it is sometimes recommended that people with a familial history of muscular dystrophy be tested for certain genetic markers that would suggest the possibility of disease in their children.

Myasthenia gravis is treated with drugs that increase the number of neurotransmitters available where nerves and muscles come together. The drugs help improve the transmission of information from the brain to the muscle tissue. In some cases, a procedure called plasmapheresis is used to eliminate blood-borne substances that may contribute to the disease. Surgical removal of the thymus gland is helpful in alleviating symptoms in some patients.

In treating the many muscle disorders that are caused by athletic activity and excessive wear and tear on the muscle, the R-I-C-E formula is recommended. The acronym stands for rest-ice-compression-elevation: The patient must rest and not use or exercise the limb or muscle involved; an ice pack is applied to the injury; compression is supplied by wrapping a moist bandage snugly over the ice, reducing the flow of fluids to the injured area; and the injured limb is elevated. If there is a fracture involved, the limb must be properly splinted or otherwise immobilized before elevation. The ice pack is held in place for twenty minutes and removed, but the bandage is held in place. Ice therapy can be resumed every twenty minutes.

Heat is also part of the therapy for strains and sprains, but it is not applied until after the initial swelling has gone down, usually after forty-eight to seventy-two hours. Heat raises the metabolic rate in the affected tissue. This brings more blood to the area, carrying nutrients that are needed for tissue repair. Moist heat is preferred, and it can be supplied by an electrical heating pad, a chemical gel in a plastic bag, or hot baths and whirlpools. In using pads and chemical gels, there should be a layer of toweling or other material between the heat source and the body. The temperature for a whirlpool or hot bath should be about 106 degrees Fahrenheit. Only the injured part should be immersed, if possible. As in the ice treatments, heat should be applied for twenty minutes and can be repeated after twenty minutes of rest.

Analgesics are given for pain. Over-the-counter preparations such as aspirin, acetaminophen, or ibuprofen are used most often. Sometimes, when pain is severe, more potent medications are required. Steroids are sometimes prescribed to reduce inflammation, and nonsteroidal anti-inflammatory drugs (NSAIDs) can alleviate both pain and inflammation. If a strained muscle or tendon is seriously torn or otherwise damaged, surgery may be required. Similarly, if a sprain involves torn or detached ligaments, they may have to be surgically repaired.

Muscle spasms and cramps may require both manipulation and the application of heat or cold. The affected limb is gently extended to stretch the contracted muscle. Massage and immersion in a hot bath are useful, as are cold packs.

Tennis elbow, runners" knee, and tendinitis respond to R-I-C-E therapy. Ice is applied to the injured site, and the limb is elevated and allowed to rest. When tenosynovitis is caused by bacterial infection, prompt antibiotic therapy may be necessary to avoid permanent damage. When it is attributable to overexertion, analgesics may help relieve pain and inflammation. Rarely, a corticosteroid is used when other drugs fail.

Often, the injured site requires physical therapy for the full range of motion to be restored. The physical therapist analyzes the patient's capability and develops a regimen to restore strength and mobility to the affected muscles and joints. Physical therapy may involve massage, hot baths, whirlpools, weight training, and/or isometric exercise. Orthotic devices may be required to help the injured area heal.

An important aspect of sports medicine and the treatment of sports-related muscle disorders is prevention. Many painful, debilitating, and immobilizing episodes can be avoided by proper training and conditioning, intelligent exercise practice, and restriction of exertion. Before undertaking any sport or strenuous physical activity, the individual is advised to warm up by gentle stretching, jogging, jumping, and other mild muscular activities. Arms can be rotated in front of the body, over the head, and in circles perpendicular to the ground. Knees can be lifted and pulled up to the chest. Shoulders should be gently rotated to relax upper-back muscles. Neck muscles are toned by gently and slowly moving the head from side to side and in circles. Back muscles are loosened by bending forward and continuing around in slow circles.

If a joint has been injured, it is important to protect it from further damage. Physicians and physical therapists often recommend that athletes tape, brace, or wrap susceptible joints, such as knees, ankles, elbows, or wrists. Sometimes a simple commercial elastic bandage, available in various configurations specific to parts of the body, is all that is required. Neck braces and back braces are used to support these structures.

Benign muscle tumors require no treatment, or may be surgically removed. Malignant tumors may require surgery, radiation, and chemotherapy.

Perspective and Prospects

With the increased interest in physical exercise in the United States has come increasing awareness of the dangers of muscular damage that can arise from improper exercise, as well as of the cardiovascular risks that lie in wait for weekend athletes. Warm-up procedures are universally recommended. Individual exercisers, those in gym classes, professional athletes, and schoolchildren are routinely taken through procedures to stretch and loosen muscles before they start strenuous activity.

Greater attention is being paid to the special needs of young athletes, such as gymnasts. Over the years, new athletic toys and devices have constantly been developed for the young: Skateboards, skates, scooters, and bicycles expose children to a wide range of bumps, falls, bruises, strains, and sprains. Protective equipment and devices have been designed especially for them: Helmets, padding, and special uniforms give children more security in accidents. Similarly, adults should take the time and trouble to outfit themselves correctly for the sports and athletics in which they engage: Joggers should tape, wrap, and brace their joints; and cyclists

should wear helmets.

Nevertheless, the incidence of sports- and athletics-related muscular damage is relatively high, pointing to the necessity for increased attention to prevention. The growth of sports medicine as a medical specialty helps considerably in this endeavor. Physicians and nurses in this area are trained to deal with the various problems that arise, and they are often expert commentators on the best means to prevent problems.

—C. Richard Falcon

See also Amyotrophic lateral sclerosis; Ataxia; Back pain; Bell's palsy; Beriberi; Botox; Cerebral palsy; Chronic fatigue syndrome; Electromyography; Exercise physiology; Fibromyalgia; First aid; Guillain-Barré syndrome; Hemiplegia; Hypertrophy; Kinesiology; Motor neuron diseases; Multiple sclerosis; Muscles; Muscular dystrophy; Myasthenia gravis; Neurology; Neurology, pediatric; Numbness and tingling; Osteopathic medicine; Overtraining syndrome; Palsy; Paralysis; Paraplegia; Parkinson's disease; Physical rehabilitation; Poliomyelitis; Ptosis; Quadriplegia; Rabies; Rheumatoid arthritis; Rotator cuff surgery; Seizures; Speech disorders; Sphincterectomy; Sports medicine; Tendon disorders; Tendon repair; Tetanus; Tics; Torticollis; Weight loss and gain; Whiplash.

For Further Information:

Brukner, Peter, and Karim Khan. *Brukner & Khan's Clinical Sports Medicine*. 4th ed. New York: McGraw-Hill , 2010. Print.

Kirkaldy-Willis, William H., and Thomas N. Bernard, Jr., eds. *Managing Low Back Pain*. 4th ed. New York: Churchill Livingstone, 1999.

Litin, Scott C., ed. *Mayo Clinic Family Health Book*. 4th ed. New York: HarperResource, 2009.

McArdle, William, Frank I. Katch, and Victor L. Katch. *Exercise Physiology: Energy, Nutrition, and Human Performance*. 7th ed. Boston: Lippincott Williams & Wilkins, 2010.

Marieb, Elaine N., and Katja Hoehn. *Human Anatomy and Physiology*. 9th ed. San Francisco: Pearson/Benjamin Cummings, 2010.

MacAuley, Domhnall. *Oxford Handbook of Sport and Exercise Medicine*. 2nd ed. Oxford UP, 2012. Print.

Rouzier, Pierre A. *The Sports Medicine Patient Advisor*. 3rd ed. Valley Stream, New York: SportsMed Press, Print.

Salter, Robert Bruce. *Textbook of Disorders and Injuries of the Musculoskeletal System*. 3d ed. Baltimore: Williams & Wilkins, 1999.

MUSCLES

Anatomy

Anatomy or system affected: Arms, gastrointestinal system, legs, ligaments, musculoskeletal system

Specialties and related fields: Cardiology, exercise physiology, orthopedics, osteopathic medicine, physical therapy, sports medicine

Definition: Cardiac muscle, skeletal muscle, and smooth muscle—all of which have the ability to contract, making possible body movement, peristalsis (the movement of food through the gastrointestinal system), and the circulation of blood throughout the body.

Key terms:

cardiac muscle: a type of muscle, found only in the heart, that makes up the major portion of the heart; involved in the movement of blood through the body

muscle contraction: the shortening of a muscle, which may

result in the movement of a particular body part

muscle fibers: elongated muscle cells that make up skeletal, cardiac, and smooth muscles

musculature: the arrangement of skeletal muscles in the body

skeletal muscle: a type of muscle that attaches to bone and causes movement of body parts; the only type that is under conscious, voluntary control

smooth muscle: a type of muscle found in the walls of internal organs such as the stomach, intestines, and urinary bladder; involved in the movement of food through the digestive tract

Structure and Functions

More than half of the body weight of humans is made up of muscle. Three types of muscles are found in the body: skeletal muscle, cardiac muscle, and smooth muscle. These muscles are composed of different types of muscle cells and perform different functions within the body. The characteristics and functions of each of these three muscle types will be discussed separately, starting with skeletal muscle.

Skeletal muscles attach to and cover bones. This type of muscle is often referred to as voluntary muscle because it is the only muscle type that can be controlled or made to move by consciously thinking about it. Skeletal muscles perform four important functions: bringing about body movement, helping to maintain posture, helping to stabilize joints such as the knee, and generating body heat.

Nearly all body movement is dependent upon skeletal muscle. Skeletal muscle is needed not only to be able to run and jump but also to speak, to write, and to move and blink the eyes. These movements are brought about by the contraction or shortening of skeletal muscles. These muscles are attached to two bones or other structures by tough thin strips or cords of tissue known as tendons. When a muscle contracts or shortens, it pulls the tendons, which then pull on the bones or other structures to which they are connected. In this way, the desired movement is brought about.

Skeletal muscles also aid in the maintenance of posture. Posture is defined as the ability to maintain a position of the body or body parts: for example, the ability to stand or to sit erect. The constant force of gravity must be overcome in order to maintain a standing or seated posture. Small adjustments to the force of gravity are constantly being made through slight contractions of skeletal muscle.

Skeletal muscles—or, more appropriately, their tendons—help to maintain joint stability. Many of the tendons that connect muscles to bones cross movable joints such as the knee and the shoulder. These tendons are kept taut by the constant contraction of the muscles to which they are attached. As a result, they act as walls to prevent the joints from dislocating or shifting out of the normal positions.

More than 40 percent of the human body is composed of skeletal muscle. Skeletal muscles generate heat as they contract. As a result, skeletal muscles are of extreme importance in maintaining normal body temperature. When the body is exposed to cold temperatures, it begins to shiver. This shivering is the result of muscle contractions, which serve to gener-

ate body heat and maintain the body's normal temperature.

Skeletal muscles are made up of skeletal muscle cells. These cells are long and tube-shaped and therefore are referred to as skeletal muscle fibers. In some instances, these muscle fibers may be a foot long. When individual skeletal muscle fibers are viewed under a microscope, they display bands that are referred to as striations. For this reason, skeletal muscle is often called striated muscle.

Each skeletal muscle, depending upon its size, is made up of hundreds or thousands of skeletal muscle fibers. These muscle fibers are surrounded by a tough connective tissue that holds the muscle fibers together. These muscle fibers and their surrounding connective tissue form a skeletal muscle. In the human body, there are more than six hundred skeletal muscles. It is the arrangement of these muscles in the body that is referred to as the musculature, or muscle system.

Smooth muscles are often referred to as involuntary muscles because they cannot be made to contract by conscious effort. Smooth muscles are typically found in the walls of internal organs such as the esophagus, stomach, intestines, and urinary bladder. The primary function of smooth muscles in these organs is to enable the passage of material through a tube or tract. For example, the contraction of smooth muscles in the intestines helps to move digested materials through the digestive system.

Smooth muscle is composed of smooth muscle cells. These cells differ from skeletal muscle fibers in that they are short and spindle-shaped. They also differ from skeletal muscle cells in that they are not striated. Furthermore, smooth muscle cells usually are not surrounded by a tough connective tissue to form a muscle; instead, they are arranged in layers.

Cardiac muscle is found only in the heart. Like smooth muscle, cardiac muscle cannot be made to contract by means of conscious effort. Like skeletal muscle, however, cardiac muscle is striated. The contraction of cardiac muscle results in the contraction of the heart. This, in turn, results in the pumping of blood throughout the body.

Although many differences exist among skeletal, smooth, and cardiac muscle, all have one thing in common—their ability to contract. The methods by which this contraction is brought about in skeletal muscle, however, are different from those used by smooth muscle and cardiac muscle.

In order for skeletal muscles to contract, they must first be electrically stimulated. This electrical stimulation is brought about by nerves that are closely associated with the muscle fibers. Each muscle fiber has a branch of a nerve, known as an axon terminal, that lies very close to it. This axon terminal does not touch the muscle fiber, but is separated from it by a tiny space known as the synaptic cleft (or gap). An electrical impulse from the nerve causes the release of a chemical called a neurotransmitter into the synaptic cleft. The specific type of neurotransmitter for skeletal muscle is known as acetylcholine. The neurotransmitter will then pass through the synaptic cleft to the muscle fiber membrane, where it will bind to a special site known as a receptor. When the neurotransmitter binds to the receptor, it causes an electrical impulse to travel down the muscle fiber. This, in turn, causes the contraction of the muscle fiber. When most or all of the muscle fibers contract, the result is the contraction of the entire muscle.

The muscle fibers and muscle will remain in a contracted state as long as the neurotransmitter is bound to the receptor on the muscle fiber membrane. In order for the muscle fiber to relax, the neurotransmitter must be released from the receptor to which it is bound. This is accomplished by the destruction of the neurotransmitter. Another chemical, known as an enzyme, is released into the synaptic cleft. This enzyme destroys the neurotransmitter; thus, the neurotransmitter is no longer bound to the receptor. In skeletal muscle, this enzyme is called acetylcholinesterase, because it destroys the neurotransmitter acetylcholine.

The contraction of cardiac muscle differs from that of skeletal muscle in that each cardiac muscle fiber does not have an axon terminal associated with it. Cardiac muscle is capable of making its own electrical impulse; it does not need a nerve to initiate the electrical impulse for every cardiac muscle fiber. An impulse is started in a particular place in the heart, called the atrioventricular (A-V) node. This impulse spreads from muscle fiber to muscle fiber. Thus, each cardiac muscle fiber stimulates those fibers next to it. The electrical impulse spreads so fast that nearly all the cardiac muscle fibers contract at the same time. As a result, the single impulse that began in the A-V node causes the entire heart to contract.

Disorders and Diseases

Any type of muscle disorder has the ability to disrupt the normal functions performed by muscles. Skeletal muscle disorders can disrupt body movement and the ability to maintain posture. If these disorders affect the diaphragm, the principal breathing muscle, they can also be fatal.

Perhaps the most common and least detrimental muscle disorder is disuse atrophy. When muscles are not used, the muscle fibers will become smaller, a process called atrophy. As a result of the decrease in the diameter of the muscle fibers, the entire muscle also becomes smaller and therefore weaker.

Disuse atrophy occurs in such circumstances as when an individual is sick or injured and must remain in bed for prolonged periods of time. As a result, the muscles are not used and begin to atrophy. Disuse atrophy is also fairly common in astronauts. This occurs as a result of the lack of gravity against which the muscles must work. If a muscle does not work against a load or force, such as gravity, it will tend to decrease in size.

In general, disuse muscle atrophy is easily treated. The primary treatment is to exercise the unused muscle. Physical activity, particularly those activities in which the muscle must work to lift or pull a weight, will result in an enlargement in the diameter of the skeletal muscle fibers, and thus of the entire muscle. The increase in the diameter of the muscle fibers and muscle is referred to as hypertrophy.

Another common muscle disorder is a muscle cramp. A muscle cramp is a spasm in which the muscle undergoes

strong involuntary contractions. These involuntary contractions, which may last for as short a time as a few seconds or as long as a few hours, are extremely painful. Muscle cramps appear to occur more frequently at night or after exercise. Treatment for cramps involves rubbing and massaging the affected muscle.

Muscles are often overused or overstretched. When this is the case, it is possible for the muscle fibers to tear. When the muscle fibers are torn, the result is a muscle strain, more often referred to as a pulled muscle. Although pulled muscles may be painful, they are usually not serious. Treatment for pulled muscles most often involves the resting of the affected muscle. If the muscle fibers are torn completely apart, surgery may be required to reattach the muscle fibers.

Among the more serious skeletal muscle disorders is muscular dystrophy. The term "muscular dystrophy" is used to define those muscle disorders that are genetic or inherited. These diseases most often begin in childhood, but a few cases have been reported to begin during adult life. Muscular dystrophy results in progressive muscle weakness and muscle atrophy. The most common form of muscular dystrophy is known as Duchenne muscular dystrophy. This form of muscular dystrophy primarily affects males. In those affected with Duchenne muscular dystrophy, muscular weakness and atrophy begin to appear at three to five years of age. There is a progressive loss of muscle strength and muscle mass such that, by the age of twelve, those individuals afflicted with the disorder are confined to a wheelchair. Usually between the ages of fourteen and eighteen, the patients develop serious and sometimes fatal respiratory diseases as a result of the impairment of the diaphragm, the primary breathing muscle. The progressive deterioration of the muscles cannot be stopped, but it may be slowed with exercise of the affected muscles.

Myasthenia gravis is also a severe muscle disorder. This disease results in excessive weakness of skeletal muscles, a condition known as muscle fatigue. Those with myasthenia gravis complain of fatigue even after performing normal everyday body movements. Although severe, myasthenia gravis is usually not fatal unless the diaphragm is affected.

Myasthenia results from a decrease in the availability of the receptors for acetylcholine. If fewer acetylcholine receptors are available on the muscle fibers, less acetylcholine binds to the muscle fiber receptors; this binding is needed for contraction to occur. As a result, fewer muscle fibers within the muscle contract. The fewer muscle fibers within the entire muscle that contract, the weaker the muscle.

Myasthenia gravis affects about one in every ten thousand individuals. Unlike Duchenne muscular dystrophy, myasthenia gravis may affect any group, and, overall, women are affected more frequently than men. Myasthenia gravis is usually first detected in the facial muscles, particularly those of the eyes and eyelids. Those afflicted have droopy eyelids and experience difficulty in keeping the eyes open. Other symptoms are weakness in those muscles involved in chewing and difficulty swallowing as a result of weakening of the tongue muscles. In most patients, there is also some weakening of the muscles of the legs and arms.

The prognosis for the treatment of myasthenia gravis is very good. The most important treatment for the disorder is the use of anticholinesterase drugs. These drugs inhibit the breakdown of acetylcholine. As a result, there is a large amount of acetylcholine in the neuromuscular junction to bind with the limited number of acetylcholine receptors. This, in turn, increases the ability and number of the muscle fibers that are able to contract, resulting in an increase in muscle strength and the ability to use the muscles without fatigue.

Also of interest is the effect of pesticides and the way in which they affect muscle function. Some pesticides are classified as organic pesticides that inhibit the enzyme acetylcholinesterase. If acetylcholinesterase is inhibited, it will no longer break down the acetylcholine that is bound to the receptor on the skeletal muscle membrane. If the acetylcholine is not removed from the receptor, the muscle cannot relax and is therefore in a constant state of contraction. As a result, the respiratory muscles are unable to contract and relax, a process required for breathing. Thus, organic pesticides function to prevent the respiratory muscles from working, and an affected animal will die as a result of not being able to breathe.

Muscle fibers also require a blood supply in order to keep them alive. If the blood supply to the muscle fibers is inhibited, death of the muscle fibers can result. If enough muscle fibers are affected, death of the muscle can result. This most commonly occurs in cardiac muscle. If the blood supply to the cardiac muscle making up the heart is reduced or cut off, the result is a decrease in the ability of the cardiac muscle to contract. This, in turn, leads to heart failure.

Perspective and Prospects

The study of muscles and musculature is as old as the study of anatomy itself. The first well-documented study of muscles was done by Galen of Pergamum in the first century. Galen made drawings of muscles and described their functions. In all, Galen described more than three hundred muscles in the human body, almost half of all the muscles now known.

The first refined drawings and descriptions of the skeletal muscles of the body were made in the late fifteenth century. Among those who stood out as muscle anatomists during this period was Leonardo da Vinci, whose drawings of the skeletal muscles of the body were magnificent. His chief interest in the muscles of the body, like Galen's, was their function. He accurately described, among many other muscles, the muscles involved in the movement of the lips and cheeks.

A major step to the understanding of muscle physiology did not occur until the late eighteenth century. Luigi Galvani in 1791 discovered the relationship between muscle contraction and electricity when he found that an electrical current could cause the contraction of a frog leg. The use of electrical stimulation to study muscle contraction and function was fully utilized in the mid-nineteenth century by Duchenne de Boulogne. The actual measurement of the electrical activity in a muscle came about in 1929, with the invention by Edgar Douglas Adrian and Detlev Wulf Bronk of the needle electrode, which could be placed into the muscle to record the muscle's electrical activity. This recording of the electrical activity of the muscle is known as an electromyogram, or EMG. Electromyograms are important in the evaluation of the electrical activity of resting and contracting muscles. Since the discovery of EMGs, they have been used by anatomists, muscle physiologists, exercise physiologists, and orthopedic surgeons to study and diagnose muscle diseases. Furthermore, the knowledge gained from EMGs has led to the making of artificial limbs that can be controlled by the electrical impulses of the existing muscles.

Knowledge of muscle names, muscle anatomy, and movement, as well as muscle physiology, is needed for many medical fields. These fields include kinesiology, the study of movement; physical and occupational therapy; the treatment and rehabilitation of those who are disabled by injury; exercise physiology and sports medicine, in which the effects of exercise on muscle and the damage of muscle as a result of sports injuries are studied; and, finally, orthopedic surgery, which is the surgical repair of damaged bones, joints, and muscles.

—David K. Saunders, Ph.D.

See also Acupressure; Amyotrophic lateral sclerosis; Anesthesia; Anesthesiology; Ataxia; Bed-wetting; Bell's palsy; Botox; Breasts, female; Cells; Cerebral palsy; Chronic fatigue syndrome; Diaphragm; Electromyography; Exercise physiology; Fibromyalgia; Glycolysis; Guillain-Barré syndrome; Head and neck disorders; Hemiplegia; Kinesiology; Lower extremities; Mastectomy and lumpectomy; Motor neuron diseases; Multiple sclerosis; Muscle sprains, spasms, and disorders; Muscular dystrophy; Myasthenia gravis; Myomectomy; Orthopedic surgery; Orthopedics; Orthopedics, pediatric; Osteopathic medicine; Overtraining syndrome; Palsy; Paralysis; Paraplegia; Parkinson's disease; Physical rehabilitation; Poisoning; Poliomyelitis; Ptosis; Quadriplegia; Rabies; Respiration; Rotator cuff surgery; Seizures; Speech disorders; Sphincterectomy; Sports medicine; Steroid abuse; Tendon disorders; Tendon repair; Tetanus; Tics; Torticollis; Tremors; Upper extremities; Weight loss and gain; Whiplash.

For Further Information:
Blakey, Paul. *The Muscle Book*. Honesdale, Pa.: Himalayan Institute, 2000.
Burke, Edmund. *Optimal Muscle Performance and Recovery*. Rev. ed. New York: Putnam, 2003.
Cash, Mel. *Pocket Atlas of the Moving Body*. New York: Crown, 2000.
Clarkson, Hazel M. *Musculoskeletal Assessment: Joint Motion and Muscle Testing*. Philadelphia: Wolters Kluwer Health/Lippincott Williams & Wilkins, 2013.
Guyton, Arthur C., and John E. Hall. *Guyton and Hall Textbook of Medical Physiology*. 12th ed. Philadelphia: Saunders/Elsevier, 2011.
Marieb, Elaine N. *Essentials of Human Anatomy and Physiology*. 10th ed. San Francisco: Pearson/Benjamin Cummings, 2012.
Shier, David N., Jackie L. Butler, and Ricki Lewis. *Hole's Essentials of Human Anatomy and Physiology*. 11th ed. Boston: McGraw-Hill, 2012.
Pocock, Gillian, Christopher D. Richards, and Dave A. Richards. *Human Physiology*. New York: Oxford University Press, 2013.
Tortora, Gerard J., and Bryan Derrickson. *Principles of Anatomy and Physiology*. 13th ed. Hoboken, N.J.: John Wiley & Sons, 2012.
Willems, Mark. *Skeletal Muscle: Physiology, Classification, and Disease*. New York: Nova Biomedical, 2013.

MUSCULAR DYSTROPHY
Disease/Disorder

Anatomy or system affected: Legs, muscles, musculoskeletal system

Specialties and related fields: Genetics, pediatrics, physical therapy

Definition: A group of related diseases that attack different muscle groups, are progressive and genetically determined, and have no known cure.

Key terms:

disease: an interruption, cessation, or disorder of a body function or system, usually identifiable by a group of signs and symptoms and characterized by consistent anatomical alterations

distal: situated away from the center of the body; the farthest part from the midline of the body

DNA (deoxyribonucleic acid): a type of protein found in the nucleus of a cell comprising chromosomes that contain the genetic instructions of an organism

dystrophin: both the gene and the protein that are defective in Duchenne muscular dystrophy

dystrophy: an improper form of a tissue or group of cells (literally, "bad nourishment")

enzyme: a protein secreted by a cell that acts as a catalyst to induce chemical changes in other substances, remaining apparently unchanged itself in the process

fiber: a slender thread or filament; the elongated, threadlike cells that collectively constitute a muscle

genetic: imparted at conception and incorporated into every cell of an organism

muscle: a bundle of contractile cells that is responsible for the movement of organs and body parts

muscle group: a collection of muscles that work together to accomplish a particular movement

Causes and Symptoms

Muscles, attached to bones through tendons, are responsible for movement in the human body. In muscular dystrophy, muscles become progressively weaker. As individual muscle fibers become so weak that they die, they are replaced by connective tissue, which is fibrous and fatty rather than muscular. These replacement fibers are commonly found in skin and scar tissue and are not capable of movement, and the muscles become progressively weaker. There are several different recognized types of muscular dystrophy. These have in common degeneration of muscle fibers and their replacement with connective tissue. They are distinguished from one another on the basis of the muscle group or groups involved and the age at which individuals are affected.

The most common type is Duchenne muscular dystrophy. In this disease, the muscles involved are in the upper thigh and pelvis. The disease strikes in early childhood, usually between the ages of four and seven. It is known to be genetic and occurs only in boys. Two-thirds of affected individuals are born to mothers who are known to carry a defective gene; one-third are simply new cases whose mothers are geneti-

cally normal. Individuals afflicted with Duchenne muscular dystrophy suffer from weakness in their hips and upper thighs. Initially, they may experience difficulty in sitting up or standing. The disease progresses to involve muscle groups in the shoulder and trunk. Patients lose the ability to walk during their early teens. As the disease progresses, portions of the brain become affected, and intelligence is reduced. Muscle fibers in the heart are also affected, and most individuals die by the age of twenty.

The dystrophin gene normally produces a very large protein called dystrophin that is an integral part of the muscle cell membrane. In Duchenne muscular dystrophy, a defect in the dystrophin gene causes no dystrophin or defective dystrophin to be produced, and the protein will be absent from the cell membrane. As a result, the muscle fiber membrane breaks down and leaks, allowing fluid from outside the cell to enter the muscle cell. In turn, the contents of affected cells are broken down by other chemicals called proteases that are normally stored in the muscle cell. The dead pieces of muscle fiber are removed by scavenging cells called macrophages. The result of this process is a virtually empty and greatly weakened muscle cell.

A second type is Becker's muscular dystrophy, which is similar to the Duchenne form of the disease. Approximately three in two hundred thousand people are affected, and it too is found only among males. The major clinical difference is the age of onset. Becker's muscular dystrophy typically first appears in the early teenage years. The muscles involved are similar to those of Duchenne muscular dystrophy, but the course of the disease is slower. Most individuals require the use of a wheelchair in their early thirties and eventually die in their forties.

Myotonic dystrophy is a form of muscular dystrophy that strikes approximately five out of one hundred thousand people in a population. Myotonia is the inability of a muscle group to relax after contracting. Individuals with myotonic dystrophy experience this difficulty in their hands and feet. On average, the disease first appears at the age of nineteen. The condition is benign, in that it does not shorten an affected person's life span. Rather, it causes inconveniences to the victim. Affected persons also experience a variety of other problems, including baldness at the front of the head and malfunction of the ovaries and testes. The muscles of the stomach and intestines can become involved, leading to a slowing down of intestinal functions and diarrhea.

Another type is limb girdle muscular dystrophy. The muscles of both upper and lower limbs—the shoulders and the pelvis—are involved. The onset of this dystrophy form is variable, from childhood to middle age. While the disorder is not usually fatal, it does progress, and victims experience severe disability about twenty years after the disease first appears. While this variant is also genetically transmitted, men and women are about equally affected.

One type of muscular dystrophy found almost exclusively among individuals of Scandinavian descent is called distal dystrophy. It first appears relatively early in adult life, between the thirties and fifties. The muscles of the forearm and hand be-

---

Information on Muscular Dystrophy

Causes: Genetic defect
Symptoms: Ranges widely; may include progressive muscle weakness, loss of coordination, impaired gait, reduced intelligence, malfunction of ovaries or testes, slowed intestinal functions, impaired swallowing, impaired eye movement
Duration: Chronic
Treatments: None; supportive care (physical therapy, braces, orthopedic surgery, drug therapy)

---

come progressively weaker and decrease in size. Eventually, the muscles of the lower leg and foot also become involved. This form of muscular dystrophy is not usually fatal.

Oculopharyngeal muscular dystrophy is a particularly serious form that involves the muscles of the eyes and throat. In this disease, victims are affected in their forties and fifties. There is progressive loss of control of the muscles that move the eyes and loss of the ability to swallow. Death usually results from starvation or from pneumonia acquired when the affected individual accidentally inhales food or drink.

A type of muscular dystrophy for which the location of the genetic abnormality is known is facioscapulohumeral muscular dystrophy; the defect is confined to the tip of the fourth chromosome. This disease initially involves the muscles of the face and later spreads to the muscles of the posterior or back of the shoulder. Eventually, muscles in the upper thigh are involved. The affected person loses the ability to make facial expressions and assumes a permanent pout as a result of loss of muscle function. As the condition advances, the shoulder blades protrude when the arms are raised. Weakness and difficulty walking are eventually experienced. As with other forms of muscular dystrophy, there is some variability in the degree to which individuals are affected. Occasionally, a variety of deafness occurs involving the nerves that connect the inner ear and the brain. Less commonly, victims become blind.

There are other variants of muscular dystrophy that have been recognized and described. These forms of the disease, however, are rare. The main problem facing physicians is differentiating accurately the variety of muscular dystrophy seen in a particular patient so as to arrive at a correct diagnosis.

Treatment and Therapy

The diagnosis of muscular dystrophy is initially made through observation. Typically, parents notice changes in their affected children and bring these concerns to the attention of a physician. The physician takes a careful family history and then examines a suspected victim to make a tentative or working diagnosis. Frequently, knowledge of other family members with the condition and observations are sufficient to establish a firm diagnosis. Occasionally, a physician may elect to order physiological or genetic tests to confirm the tentative diagnosis. As Duchenne muscular dystrophy is the most common form of muscular dystrophy, it provides a convenient example of this process.

A diagnosis of Duchenne or any other form of muscular dystrophy is rarely made before the age of three. This form of the disease almost always occurs in boys. (Variants, rather than true Duchenne muscular dystrophy, are seen in girls, but this situation is extremely rare.) The reason for this finding is that the genetic defect occurs on the X chromosome, of which males only possess one. Approximately two-thirds of all victims inherit the defective chromosome from their mothers, who are asymptomatic carriers; thus, the condition is recessive and said to be X-linked. The disease occurs in the remaining one-third of victims as a result of a fresh mutation, in which there is no family history of the disease and the parents are not carriers.

Victims usually begin to sit, walk, and run at an older age than normally would be expected. Parents describe walking as waddling rather than the usual upright posture. Victims have difficulty climbing stairs. They also have apparently enlarged calf muscles, a finding called muscular hypertrophy. While the muscles are initially strong, they lose their strength when connective and fatty tissues replace muscle fibers. The weakness of muscles in the pelvis is responsible for difficulties in sitting and the unusual way of walking. Normal chil-

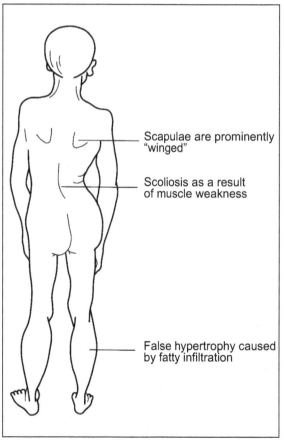

Scapulae are prominently "winged"

Scoliosis as a result of muscle weakness

False hypertrophy caused by fatty infiltration

Duchenne muscular dystrophy, the most common type, is characterized by prominently "winged" scapulae, scoliosis, false hypertrophy of the calves, and other less visible effects; children are the victims, usually not surviving beyond age twenty.

In the News: The Path Toward Gene Therapy for Muscular Dystrophy

Gene therapy in the treatment of Duchenne muscular dystrophy (DMD), the gravest and most common form of muscular dystrophy, has been a subject of intensive research. The goal of such therapy is to introduce the normal gene for dystrophin, which is defective in DMD, into diseased muscle cells so that their ability to withstand the wear and tear of contractile activity is restored. Significant progress in this effort was reported in the October, 2002, issue of the *Proceedings of the National Academy of Science of the United States of America* by collaborating groups at the University of Washington in Seattle and the University of Michigan in Ann Arbor.

The researchers used as their model system the transgenic *mdx* mouse, which carries a truncated dystrophin gene and therefore produces virtually no dystrophin protein. The leg muscles of such mice are susceptible to contraction-induced injury and subsequent deterioration, much as in human DMD.

To deliver functionally effective levels of normal full-length dystrophin, the gene was engineered into an adenovirus, which was then injected directly into the *mdx* leg muscles. This viral vector, which is related to the family of viruses that cause the common cold, is an excellent choice as a genetic vehicle because of its efficiency at infecting muscle cells. However, the researchers needed to make significant changes to the adenoviral deoxyribonucleic acid (DNA) in order to overcome two major problems. First, the dystrophin gene is extremely large and therefore is not amenable to being inserted into a viral DNA sequence. Second, the immune systems of the mice tend to reject the adenoviral DNA. To solve both of these problems, the viral vector was stripped of all unnecessary DNA ("gutted") so that it would accommodate the entire cDNA sequence of dystrophin while not being rejected.

The gutted adenoviral vector made it possible for the first time to introduce full-length dystrophin into adult *mdx* leg muscles without eliciting an immune response. One month later, the muscle tissue near the injection sites was making 25 to 30 percent of normal dystrophin levels; furthermore, there was a 40 percent improvement in contraction-induced injury. These findings constitute an important step toward the use of adenoviral vector-based gene therapy to treat DMD. For the therapy to be truly effective, it will be necessary to develop systemic techniques for delivering the normal gene to all muscles.

—Mary A. Nastuk, Ph.D.

dren are able to go directly from a sitting position to standing erect. Victims of Duchenne muscular dystrophy first roll onto their stomachs, then kneel and raise themselves up by pushing their hands against their shins, knees, and thighs; they literally climb up themselves in order to stand. These children also have a pronounced curvature of their lower backs, an attempt by the body to compensate for the weakness in the muscles of the hips and pelvis.

There is frequently some weakness in the muscles of the shoulder. This finding can be demonstrated by a physician, but it is not usually seen by parents and is not an early problem for the victim. A physician tests for this weakness by lifting the child under the armpits. Normal children will be able to support themselves using the muscles of the shoulder. Individuals with Duchenne muscular dystrophy are unable to hold themselves up and will slip through the physician's hands. Eventually, these children will be unable to lift their arms over their heads. Most victims of Duchenne muscular dystrophy are unable to walk by their teen years. The majority die before the age of twenty, although about one-quarter live for a few more years. Most victims also have an abnormality in the muscles of the heart that leads to decreased efficiency of the heart and decreased ability to be physically active; in some cases, it also causes sudden death. Most victims of Duchenne muscular dystrophy suffer mental impairment.

As their muscles deteriorate, their measured intelligence quotient (IQ) drops approximately twenty points below the level that it was at the onset of the disease. Serious mental handicaps are experienced by about one-quarter of victims.

Other forms of muscular dystrophy are similar to Duchenne muscular dystrophy. Their clinical courses are also similar, as are the methods of diagnosis. The critical differences are the muscles involved and the age of onset.

Laboratory procedures used to confirm the diagnosis of muscular dystrophy include microscopic analysis of muscle tissue, measurement of enzymes found in the blood, and measurement of the speed and efficiency of nerve conduction, a process called electromyography. Some cases have been diagnosed at birth by measuring a particular enzyme called creatinine kinase. It is possible to diagnose some types of muscular dystrophy before birth with chorionic villus sampling or amniocentesis.

There is no specific treatment for any of the muscular dystrophies. Physical therapy is frequently ordered and used to prevent the remaining unaffected muscles from losing their tone and mass. In some stages of the disease, braces, appliances, and orthopedic surgery may be used. These measures do not reverse the underlying pathology, but they may improve the quality of life for a victim. The cardiac difficulties associated with myotonic dystrophy may require treatment with a pacemaker. For victims of myotonic dystrophy, some relief is obtained by using drugs; the most commonly used pharmaceuticals are phenytoin and quinine. The inability to relax muscles once they are contracted does not usually present a major problem for sufferers of myotonic dystrophy.

More useful and successful is prevention, which involves screening individuals in families or kinship groups who are potential carriers. Carriers are persons who have some genetic material for a disease or condition but lack sufficient genes to cause an apparent case of a disease or condition; in short, they appear normal. When an individual who is a carrier conceives a child, however, there is an increased risk of the offspring having the disease. Genetic counseling should be provided after screening, so that individuals who have the gene for a disease can make more informed decisions about having children.

Chemical tests are available for use in diagnosing some forms of muscular dystrophy. Carriers of the gene for Duchenne muscular dystrophy can be detected by staining a muscle sample for dystrophin; a cell that is positive for Duchenne muscular dystrophy will have no stained dystrophin molecules. The dystrophin stain test is also used to diagnose Becker's muscular dystrophy, but the results are not quite as consistent or reliable. Approximately two-thirds of carriers and fetuses at risk for both forms of muscular dystrophy can be identified by analyzing DNA. Among individuals at risk for myotonic dystrophy, nine out of ten who carry the gene can be identified with DNA analysis before they experience actual symptoms of the disease.

Perspective and Prospects

Muscular dystrophy has been recognized as a medical entity for several centuries. Initially, it was considered to be a degenerative disease only of adults, and it was not until the nineteenth century that the disease was addressed in children with Guillaume-Benjamin-Amand Duchenne's description of progressive weakness of the hips and upper thighs. An accurate classification of the various forms of muscular dystrophy depended on accurate observation and on the collection of sets of cases. Correct diagnosis had to wait for the development of accurate laboratory methods for staining muscle fibers. The interpretation of laboratory findings depended on the development of biochemical knowledge. Thus, much of the integration of knowledge concerning muscular dystrophy is relatively recent.

Genes play an important role in the understanding of muscular dystrophy. All forms of muscular dystrophy are hereditary, although different chromosomes are involved in different forms of the disease. The development of techniques for routine testing and diagnosis has also occurred relatively recently. Specific chromosomes for all forms of muscular dystrophy have not yet been discovered. Considering initial successes of the Human Genome Project, an effort to identify all human genes, it seems likely that more precise genetic information related to muscular dystrophy will emerge.

There still are no cures for muscular dystrophies, and many forms are relentlessly fatal. Cures for many communicable diseases caused by bacteria or viruses have been discovered, and advances have been made in the treatment of cancer and other degenerative diseases by identifying chemicals that cause the conditions or by persuading people to change their lifestyles. Muscular dystrophy, however, is a group of purely genetic conditions. Many of the particular chromosomes involved are known, but no techniques are yet available to cure the disease once it is identified.

The availability of both a mouse model and a dog model of Duchenne muscular dystrophy, however, has facilitated the testing of gene therapy for this disease. Dystrophic mouse early embryos have been cured by injection of a functional copy of the dystrophin gene; however, this technique must be performed in embryos and is not useful for human therapy. Two avenues of research under way in these animal models are the introduction of normal muscle-precursor cells into dystrophic muscle cells and the direct delivery of a functional dystrophin gene into dystrophic muscle cells. It is hoped that these studies lead to a cure for the disease.

In the meantime, muscular dystrophy continues to cause human suffering and to cost victims, their families, and society large sums of money. The disease is publicized on an annual basis via efforts to raise money for research and treatment, but there is little publicity on an ongoing basis. For these reasons, muscular dystrophy remains an important medical problem in contemporary society.

—L. Fleming Fallon, Jr., M.D., Ph.D., M.P.H.;
updated by Karen E. Kalumuck, Ph.D.

See also Connective tissue; Genetic counseling; Genetic diseases; Genetics and inheritance; Hypertrophy; Muscle sprains, spasms, and disorders; Muscles; Pediatrics; Physical rehabilitation; Screening.

For Further Information:

Alan, Rick. "Muscular Dystrophy." *Health Library*, September 20, 2011.

Beers, Mark H., et al., eds. *The Merck Manual of Diagnosis and Therapy*. 19th ed. Whitehouse Station, N.J.: Merck Research Laboratories, 2011.

Behrman, Richard E., Robert M. Kliegman, and Hal B. Jenson, eds. *Nelson Textbook of Pediatrics*. 18th ed. Philadelphia: Saunders/Elsevier, 2007.

Brown, Susan S., and Jack A. Lucy, eds. *Dystrophin: Gene, Protein, and Cell Biology*. New York: Cambridge University Press, 1997.

Emery, Alan E. H. *Muscular Dystrophy: The Facts*. 3rd ed. New York: Oxford University Press, 2008.

"Facts about Muscular Dystrophy." *Centers for Disease Control and Prevention*, April 6, 2012.

Goldman, Lee, and Dennis Ausiello, eds. *Cecil Textbook of Medicine*. 23d ed. Philadelphia: Saunders/Elsevier, 2007.

Kumar, Vinay, Abul K. Abbas, and Nelson Fausto, eds. *Robbins and Cotran Pathologic Basis of Disease*. 8th ed. Philadelphia: Saunders/Elsevier, 2010.

"Muscular Dystrophy: Hope Through Research." *National Institute of Neurological Disorders and Stroke*. February 14, 2013.

Tierney, Lawrence M., Stephen J. McPhee, and Maxine A. Papadakis, eds. *Current Medical Diagnosis and Treatment 2007*. New York: McGraw-Hill Medical, 2006.

Wolfson, Penny. *Moonrise: One Family, Genetic Identity, and Muscular Dystrophy*. New York: St. Martin's Press, 2003.

MUTATION

Biology

Anatomy or system affected: Cells, immune system

Specialties and related fields: Cytology, genetics, pathology

Definition: An error in the process that copies genetic information for each new generation, resulting in an alteration in the organism that can be beneficial, harmful, or neutral.

Key terms:

alleles: alternate forms of a gene; each person has two alleles of each gene, and these alleles may be the same or different; a person inherits one allele from each parent

chromosomes: the parts of a cell that contain genetic information, made of DNA covered with protein; each human cell has twenty-three pairs of chromosomes

deoxyribonucleic acid (DNA): a long, spiral-shaped molecule that makes up the bulk of chromosomes; the sequence of subunits contains the genetic information of the cell and organism

gene: the basic unit of inheritance; at the molecular level, a gene consists of a segment of DNA that codes for a particular protein

genotype: the genetic makeup of an individual; it is usually expressed as a list of alleles

heterozygous: having two different alleles for a particular gene

homozygous: having two identical alleles of a particular gene

meiosis: a special kind of cell division whereby four cells are produced; each cell has only half of the original number of chromosomes; meiosis produces the sex cells (eggs and sperm)

nucleotides: the subunits from which DNA is made

The Function of Genes

An individual is not a random assortment of characteristics. The way individuals look, their physiological makeup, their susceptibility to disease, and even how long they may live are determined by information received from their parents. The smallest unit of information for inherited characteristics is the gene. For each characteristic, an individual has two copies of the gene controlling that characteristic. The gene can have two forms, called alleles. For example, the alleles for eye color can be designated using the letters B and b, with the B allele carrying the information for brown eyes and the b allele specifying blue eyes. Thus the genotype, or genetic makeup, of an individual can be one of three types: BB, bb, or Bb. A BB individual will have brown eyes. A bb person will have blue eyes. A Bb individual will have brown eyes since the brown allele is dominant over the blue one. The dominant allele will always be expressed, whether present as two copies or only one. For a recessive allele to be expressed, an individual must have two recessive alleles (bb).

When a person reproduces, he or she passes on one allele for each gene to the child. Therefore, the child also has two alleles for each gene, one from each parent. A person with two identical alleles for a given gene is said to be homozygous for that trait and can pass on only one kind of allele. Someone with two different alleles for a particular gene is said to be heterozygous. A heterozygous person will pass on the dominant allele to 50 percent of his or her children, on average; the other 50 percent will receive the recessive allele. Alleles are passed on in the sex cells—the eggs and sperm. Eggs and sperm are produced by a special type of cell division, meiosis, that reduces by half the amount of genetic information carried by the cell. When an egg is fertilized by a sperm cell, the amount of genetic information is once again doubled. In "normal" cell division, called mitosis, the amount of genetic material in each cell is kept constant. After fertilization, the egg cell divides repeatedly by mitosis to produce the millions of cells that make up the embryo and later the adult organism.

If the genetic makeup of a couple for a given trait is known, the probable characteristics of their children for this trait can be predicted. For example, one can predict the eye color for children of a brown-eyed husband and blue-eyed wife. Assuming that the husband comes from a family of only brown-eyed people, one can be fairly certain that he is homozygous for this trait (BB). Since his wife has blue eyes, and blue is recessive, she must be homozygous for the other allele (bb).

Their children will each have a brown allele from their father and a blue allele from their mother; they will all be heterozygous (Bb). Since brown is dominant, they will all have brown eyes.

One can take this example a step further and predict the outcome for the next generation. If one of this couple's brown-eyed sons marries a blue-eyed woman, then one can predict the eye colors of their children using a simple diagram called a Punnett square. (Reginald Crundall Punnett contributed much to the early study of genetics.)

Using this simple tool, with the possible alleles in the sperm cells along the top and those from the eggs down the side, one can show all the possible combinations of inherited alleles (see figure 1). These boxes represent the genotypes of

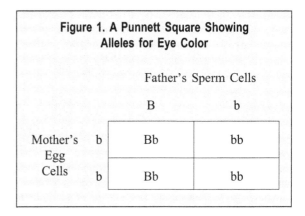

Figure 1. A Punnett Square Showing Alleles for Eye Color

Father's Sperm Cells

		B	b
Mother's Egg Cells	b	Bb	bb
	b	Bb	bb

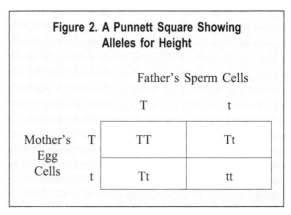

Figure 2. A Punnett Square Showing Alleles for Height

Father's Sperm Cells

		T	t
Mother's Egg Cells	T	TT	Tt
	t	Tt	tt

the fertilized eggs. In this case, one would expect about half of their children to have brown eyes (the Bb boxes) and half to have blue eyes (the bb boxes). Since chance determines exactly which sperm actually fertilizes the egg in every conception event, however, such a prediction is not always accurate. Nevertheless, the more children they have, the closer the actual percentage of brown-eyed or blue-eyed children will be to half.

Actually, the inheritance of eye color is somewhat more complicated than it is described above. Several genes contribute to eye color. Depending on the mix of dominant and

The Relationship Between Genotype and Blood Type		
Genotype	Blood Type	Comments
AA AO	A A	These two genotypes produce identical blood types.
BB BO	B B	These two genotypes produce identical blood types.
AB	AB	Both dominant alleles are expressed.
OO	O	With no dominant alleles, the recessive allele is expressed.

recessive alleles for each gene involved, eye color can range from pale blue to dark brown. Other combinations produce green eyes.

In addition, many genes do not show complete dominance. For example, evidence shows that height is controlled by several genes that exhibit incomplete dominance. One homozygous individual (TT) will be tall, the other (tt) will be short, and the heterozygous individual(Tt) will be of medium height. The laws that determine how the alleles may be passed on from generation to generation, however, are exactly the same. One can use a simplified example of two people who are heterozygous for a hypothetical height gene. If both parents are heterozygous, each will be able to produce two kinds of sex cells, those with "tall" alleles and those with "short" alleles. From all the possible outcomes shown in the boxes of the Punnett square, one would predict 25 percent tall (TT), 25 percent short (tt), and 50 percent medium-height (Tt) children.

If several genes are involved, a wide range of heights is possible. A person who is homozygous for the "tall" alleles in most of the height genes will be very tall. Someone homozygous for most of the "short" alleles will be short. Someone who is heterozygous in most of these genes will be of medium height. Since even relatively short people will have some "tall" alleles, and since chance determines which sex cells are actually used, it is possible for two short people to have a tall child: By chance, the egg and sperm that united had more than the usual share of "tall" alleles.

The preceding examples have used genes that have only two alleles: brown or blue, tall or short. There are genes, however, for which more than two alleles are possible—although any one individual may have only two alleles in his or her genetic makeup. A good example of such a gene is the one that controls human blood type. There are three blood type alleles: A, B, and O. The A and B alleles are dominant, while the O allele is recessive. This allows for the various types of blood.

A person with an A allele produces a particular chemical in the blood. Similarly, the B allele causes the production of a

different chemical. The O allele produces no chemical at all. If a chemical not already present in the blood is introduced, such as in a blood transfusion, the body will react against it, destroying the new blood. Since people with type O blood produce neither chemical, they are sometimes referred to as "universal donors." Their blood can be given safely to anyone. Similarly, people with AB blood can receive any other blood type because their bodies already contain both types of chemical.

One can also use a blood type example to show how parents can produce children who are genetically unlike both parents. The mother has type A blood and is heterozygous (AO), while the father has type B blood and is also heterozygous (BO). Their child could have any of the four blood types.

Although blood type is not an obvious visible feature, many genes that express themselves in an individual's appearance behave in a similar manner. Therefore, one should not be surprised to see two parents with a child who resembles neither of them.

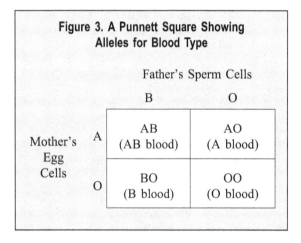

Figure 3. A Punnett Square Showing Alleles for Blood Type

The genes that control heredity actually consist of strands of deoxyribonucleic acid (DNA) that make up the chromosomes. Humans have twenty-three pairs of chromosomes in each cell. This explains how an individual can have two alleles for each gene, one on each chromosome of a pair. The exception is the sex chromosomes, which are different in males and females. Sex chromosomes come in two kinds, a relatively large X and a small Y. The X chromosomes can carry many more genes than the Y. Females have two X chromosomes and thus have two alleles for every gene found on the X chromosome. Males have only one X chromosome; therefore, they only have one allele for those genes carried on the X. The Y chromosome of the male has been shown to carry very little, although important, genetic information. Genes carried on the X chromosome are called sex-linked, since they typically are expressed in only one sex—the male. Females may be merely carriers of a sex-linked trait.

One sex-linked trait is the disorder called hemophilia. A hemophiliac fails to produce a chemical that allows the blood to clot. This disorder is usually fatal if the hemophiliac is not constantly supplied with the clotting factor. Such an individual would simply bleed to death following even the slightest injury. Suppose that a woman who carries the trait for hemophilia marries a man who does not have the disorder. Hemophilia is a recessive condition; therefore, the woman has one normal X chromosome and one bearing the recessive allele (denoted by Xh). Since the normal allele directs the production of the clotting factor, her blood can clot and she is perfectly normal. Since her husband is not a hemophiliac, his one X chromosome must bear the normal allele. One can use a Punnett square to predict the likelihood of their children inheriting the disease. About half of them will be carriers for the trait, but there is no way of knowing which ones they are. Of the sons, one half will be normal and the other half will suffer from hemophilia.

How Mutations Occur

There is a variety of genetic information in the human population, leading to a diversity of internal and external features. The process of sexual reproduction randomly selects among that variety for each new individual who is born. Mutation is the process that created the variety originally, and it can continue to add to it today.

A human being begins as a single fertilized cell. That cell contains two copies of the genetic information in its twenty-three pairs of chromosomes. The cell divides constantly during growth and development to produce the millions of cells that make up an adult. Each one of those cells, with very few exceptions, also has twenty-three pairs of chromosomes. In order for each cell to have its own double copy of information, the DNA that makes up the chromosomes must replicate, once for each cell division. This process of replication must ensure that the information contained in the DNA is copied exactly, and for the most part, it is.

To understand how a mistake can occur, one must look at the structure of DNA, the genetic blueprint. The DNA molecule resembles a spiral staircase. The outside rails are strings of sugar molecules hooked together by phosphate groups. The steps are made of bases that project from each sugar-phosphate backbone toward the middle. The information is contained in the sequence of base pairs that make up the steps of the staircase. The bases that can form such a pair are determined by their shape and bonding properties. Of the four bases, only two pairs are possible. Adenine (A) always pairs with thymine (T), leaving cytosine (C) and guanine (G) to form the other pair. This structure explains the accuracy with which DNA replicates. During replication, the original molecule unwinds from its spiral structure. The two strands separate, and a new complementary strand forms on each of the original strands. The order of bases on the new strand is determined by the original strand and the base-pairing rules. Where there is an A in the old strand, there must be a T in the new one. The other bases will not fit because they do not have the correct shape or bonding properties. Similarly, where the old strand has a C, the new one must have a G. Each base is attached to a deoxyribose sugar and a phosphate group, all three forming a nucleotide. Once all

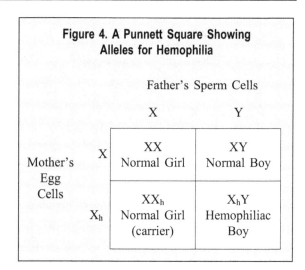

Figure 4. A Punnett Square Showing Alleles for Hemophilia

		Father's Sperm Cells	
		X	Y
Mother's Egg Cells	X	XX Normal Girl	XY Normal Boy
	Xh	XX$_h$ Normal Girl (carrier)	X$_h$Y Hemophiliac Boy

proper nucleotides are linked together, the new strand is complete, the original DNA is rewound, and there are two molecules where there once was one.

The accuracy with which the DNA template is copied is impressive. It has been estimated that an error occurs only once for every 100,000 nucleotides copied. The replication of DNA is a chemical process that relies on random movements of molecules to put the correct ones together. There are enzymatic systems to make sure that only the correct nucleotides end up as part of the new DNA strand. There are also error detection and correction mechanisms that can remove an incorrect nucleotide and replace it with the correct one. This correction process reduces the error rate to one in 10 billion. Nevertheless, with the amount of DNA that has to be copied, mistakes do occur. If a mistake is made in a gamete (sperm or egg cell), the mutated DNA can be passed on to future generations.

The mistake will not be detected until the section of DNA that contains it is actually used by the cell to make a specific protein molecule. At the molecular level, a gene is a section of DNA that has the information necessary to make a particular protein molecule. Proteins are the working molecules of the body: They make up flesh and bone and the enzymes that speed up chemical reactions. The sequence of bases on a DNA molecule codes for the sequence of amino acids that makes up a protein molecule. Since there are twenty commonly used amino acids, and a protein can contain thousands of amino acids, there is an almost infinite number of different protein molecules. A mutation on a DNA molecule will usually mean that one amino acid in the protein for which it codes is changed.

Changing one unit in a thousand may not seem very significant, and usually it is not. Such a small change in a protein molecule generally has very little effect on the functioning of that molecule. Perhaps this mutation will make the molecule able to withstand a slightly higher temperature before breaking down. If the protein is an enzyme, the change may speed or slow its reaction time by a little bit. During human evolution, an individual may have been able to live slightly longer if the mutated protein was slightly improved in function. The longer that he or she lived, the greater was the chance that the individual could produce offspring—who would also have the mutated gene. In this way, positive, useful mutations became more common in the population. A change that made the protein less functional was less likely to be reproduced since the individual possessing the mutation may not have lived long enough to have children.

A slight change in a protein can make a very big difference. The hemoglobin (the oxygen-carrying protein in red blood cells) of a person with sickle cell disease differs from normal hemoglobin by one amino acid. The amino acid, however, is in a critical position. With the changed amino acid, the hemoglobin clumps uselessly in the cell and does not carry oxygen. This is a lethal mutation, as a person afflicted with sickle cell disease cannot live very long. One would assume that this mutation would not survive in the human population. Yet, in some parts of Africa, the mutant allele is carried by as much as 20 percent of the black population. To understand how this can be, one must consider the heterozygous individual. With one normal allele and one mutant one, such an individual makes both kinds of hemoglobin, including enough normal hemoglobin to be able to live comfortably under normal conditions. Moreover, the presence of the altered hemoglobin confers significant resistance to malaria. Because the heterozygous individual has a selective advantage over the other two genotypes, this mutant allele not only has been maintained but even has increased in the black population in Africa.

Perspective and Prospects

The modern study of genetics is conducted mostly at the molecular level. One project has identified every human gene and its location on a specific chromosome. Dubbed the Human Genome Project, it was a cooperative venture among scientists worldwide. This map tells researchers where each gene is located, and it is hoped that the defective copies in people with genetic diseases can be repaired using this knowledge. Genetic engineering techniques have already isolated many genes. For example, the gene for the production of insulin has been identified and extracted from human cells in culture. The gene has been inserted into the chromosomes of bacteria, and the bacteria are then grown in large quantities in commercial cultures. The insulin that they produce is harvested, purified, and made available to diabetics. This genuine human insulin is more potent than the insulin extracted from animals. In addition, such a process is essential for diabetics who suffer adverse reactions to the inevitable impurities that are found in insulin extracted from animals.

Ultimately, it should be possible to insert a functioning gene, like the one for insulin, directly into an afflicted person's chromosomes—thus curing the genetic disease. The cured individual, however, would still be able to pass the defective allele on to his or her children. The possibility of splicing genes into the chromosomes of sex cells does not seem likely in the near future.

More traditional genetics is also of value to prospective parents. A woman with a history of hemophilia in her family would want to know the chances that her children could inherit the disease. A genetic counselor would analyze the family tree of the woman and calculate a statistical probability. Some other genetic diseases can be detected in a fetus still in the womb. For example, a condition called phenylketonuria (PKU) can cause severe mental retardation and other medical problems. A genetic analysis of prospective parents with a family history of the condition could indicate the likelihood of PKU occurring in their children. If the chances are high, cells of the couple's child can be extracted and tested early in pregnancy. In the case of PKU, early detection can be used to prevent the effects of the disease. If the diet of the mother and then the newborn are carefully regulated, the toxic chemical that causes the disease will not accumulate in the fetus or newborn.

Genetic mutations have not stopped occurring in modern society. In fact, they are more likely. Many environmental factors have been shown to increase the mutation rate in animals. Several types of radiation and many chemicals can increase the mutation rate. This is why an x-ray technician will place a lead apron over the abdomen of a patient being x-rayed. Lead prevents the x-rays from penetrating to the genital organs, where actively dividing DNA is particularly sensitive to the radiation. Such care should always be taken to protect the genetic makeup of future generations.

—*James Waddell, Ph.D.*

See also Bacteriology; Biostatistics; Cancer; Carcinogens; DNA and RNA; Embryology; Environmental diseases; Environmental health; Genetic counseling; Genetic diseases; Genetic engineering; Genetics and inheritance; Genomics; Microbiology; Oncology; Pathology; Radiation sickness; Screening.

For Further Information:

Campbell, Neil A., et al. *Biology: Concepts and Connections*. 6th ed. San Francisco: Pearson/Benjamin Cummings, 2009.

Klug William S., et al., eds. *Essentials of Genetics*. Boston: Pearson, 2013.

Lewin, Benjamin. *Lewin's Genes X*. 10th rev. ed. Sudbury, Mass.: Jones and Bartlett, 2011.

Lewis, Ricki. *Human Genetics: Concepts and Applications*. 10th ed. Dubuque, Iowa: McGraw-Hill, 2012.

Pierce, Benjamin A. *Genetics Essentials: Concepts and Connections*. New York: W. H. Freeman, 2013.

Radman, Mirislav, and Robert Wagner. "The High Fidelity of DNA Duplication." *Scientific American* 259 (August, 1988): 40–46.

Rusting, Ricki L. "Why Do We Age?" *Scientific American* 267 (December, 1992): 130–35.

Sanders, Mark Frederick, and John L. Bowman. *Genetic Analysis: An Integrated Approach*. Boston: Benjamin Cummings, 2012.

Stahl, Franklin W. "Genetic Recombination." *Scientific American* 256 (February, 1987): 90–101.

MYASTHENIA GRAVIS
Disease/Disorder

Anatomy or system affected: Immune system, musculoskeletal system, nervous system

Specialties and related fields: Immunology, neurology

Definition: A disorder characterized by selective muscle fatigue following repeated use; it is caused by an abnormal immune reaction to specific receptors on the muscle surface.

Key terms:

acetylcholine: a chemical released by motor neuron terminals; it causes muscle contraction

acetylcholine receptor: a protein on the surface of muscle cells; binding of acetylcholine to this receptor causes muscle cells to contract

acetylcholinesterase: an enzyme that degrades acetylcholine

antibody: a protein produced by the immune system to inactivate substances detected as foreign

autoimmune disease: a disorder in which the immune system targets proteins that are normal components of body tissues

thymus: a gland located at the base of the neck; part of the immune system

---

Information on Myasthenia Gravis

Causes: Autoimmune disorder in which immune system fails to recognize muscle receptors as "self"

Symptoms: Weakness of muscles following repeated use, resulting in visual disorders, difficulty chewing and swallowing, slurred speech, limb weakness, breathing difficulties; in most cases, abnormal thymus gland

Duration: Chronic, usually progressive

Treatments: Alleviation of symptoms; may include medications (neostigmine, prednisone, azathioprine), surgery (removal of thymus), plasma exchange

---

Causes and Symptoms

Myasthenia gravis is a neuromuscular disorder characterized by weakness of skeletal muscles following repeated use. The prevalence of the disease in the United States is approximately 14 in 100,000. It occurs in both genders of all ethnic groups, and the average age of onset is under forty for women and over sixty for men.

Normally, body movements result from the contraction of skeletal muscles, which are voluntary muscles attached to bone. These muscles are stimulated to contract by motor neurons in the brain and spinal cord. Nerve impulses travel down the motor neurons to their terminals, where a small amount of a substance known as a neurotransmitter is released onto the muscle's surface. In this case, the neurotransmitter is the chemical acetylcholine. When acetylcholine binds to specific receptors on the muscle surface, contraction results.

In myasthenia gravis, an autoimmune disease, the patient's immune system fails to recognize the acetylcholine receptors on skeletal muscle as part of "self"; thus, antibodies are erroneously produced against these receptors. Antibody binding to acetylcholine receptors causes the total number of functional receptors to be reduced because they are internalized and degraded by the muscle cells. With fewer remaining receptors, the muscle's contractile response is weakened.

The root cause of this aberrant immune response remains unknown. The thymus, a gland involved in immune function, is abnormal in about 75 percent of patients with the disease. Two distinct thymic anomalies may occur in myasthenia gravis: One of these is thymic hyperplasia (an increase in the number of certain immune cells in the thymus) or thymoma (a thymic tumor). In some late-onset cases of myasthenia gravis, however, the thymus appears normal or even shrunken—yet these cases are also accompanied by elevated levels of antibodies recognizing acetylcholine receptors. Such inconsistencies are part of the reason that the relationship between the thymus and myasthenia gravis is not fully understood.

Skeletal muscle weakness is a symptom common to all forms of myasthenia gravis. Because this weakness is exacerbated with muscle use, it is not surprising that the first muscles to be affected are those used most often. Thus, the earliest signs of the disease often involve the muscles of the eye, including drooping of the eyelids and double vision. As other muscle groups become affected, advancing symptoms may include difficulty in chewing and swallowing, slurred speech, limb weakness, and breathing difficulties. Although symptoms are highly variable from patient to patient, they often fluctuate in severity with a similar daily pattern: Weakness is usually more pronounced in the evening than in the morning. Factors other than exertion that can provoke symptoms include viral illness, excitement, elevated temperature, menses, and pregnancy.

Although the long-term course of the disease can vary, it is usually progressive. In a minority of patients, weakness affects only the eye muscles. In other cases, progression is often most rapid within the first three years and may be punctuated with spontaneous temporary remissions. Treatment can help keep the symptoms under control.

Early symptoms are not always recognized as being linked to myasthenia gravis. A definitive diagnosis includes testing for the presence of antibodies that bind acetylcholine receptors. In addition, impaired nerve-muscle communication should be demonstrated in the form of specific muscle weakness elicited by repetitive nerve stimulation. Finally, it should be shown that muscle weakness is briefly relieved following the administration of edrophonium. This drug blocks the breakdown of acetylcholine, temporarily increasing the amount of the neurotransmitter available to act on muscle receptors.

Treatment and Therapy

Several treatment options have been developed with the goal of symptomatic control of myasthenia gravis. Treatment must be individually tailored depending on disease history and severity. Therapies include medications, surgery, and plasma exchange.

To improve neuromuscular transmission, drugs can be given to inhibit the action of acetylcholinesterase, the naturally occurring enzyme that degrades acetylcholine, thus prolonging the availability of acetylcholine so that its contractile effect is enhanced. Such drugs include neostigmine. Another pharmacological approach is to suppress the immune system with drugs such as prednisone and azathioprine; as a result, the production of abnormal antibodies is reduced.

Thymectomy, the surgical removal of the thymus, is commonly recommended as a treatment for myasthenia gravis. In general, this procedure is considered the most effective approach for obtaining sustained relief or remission. Maximum postsurgical improvement may take several years to occur, and results are usually best in younger patients early in their disease.

Plasma exchange is used as an immediate intervention to combat the sudden onset of severe symptoms such as respiratory failure, or in cases where the patient has not responded to other treatments. In this procedure, abnormal antibodies are removed from the blood plasma.

Perspective and Prospects

Myasthenia gravis was first described by the British physician Thomas Willis in 1685. Although relatively rare, it was the first neurological disease to be identified as having an autoimmune basis. The understanding of the disease was aided by converging research among neurophysiologists, neurologists, and immunologists; as such, these combined approaches have helped to elucidate other autoimmune diseases.

Although patients undergoing treatment for myasthenia gravis can expect a normal life span marked by significant improvement of their symptoms, as of 2013 there was no cure for the disease. Research is aimed at gaining a better understanding of the factors triggering the autoimmune response in myasthenia gravis, elucidating the relationship between the thymus and the disease, and fully understanding the molecular basis of normal and aberrant nerve-muscle transmission. This research should guide developments in treatment strategy, with a key goal being to cure the immune abnormality that underlies the disease.

—*Mary A. Nastuk, Ph.D.*

See also Autoimuune disorders; Electromyography; Glands; Immune system; Immunology; Immunopathology; Muscle sprains, spasms, and disorders; Muscles; Muscular dystrophy; Thymus gland.

For Further Information:

Carson-DeWitt, Rosalyn. "Myasthenia Gravis (MG)." *Health Library*, September 10, 2012.

Kaminski, Henry J., ed. *Myasthenia Gravis and Related Disorders.* 2d ed. New York: Humana Press, 2010.

Kasper, Dennis L., et al., eds. *Harrison's Principles of Internal Medicine.* 16th ed. New York: McGraw-Hill, 2005.

MedlinePlus. "Myasthenia Gravis." *MedlinePlus*, April 19, 2013.

National Institute of Neurological Disorders and Stroke. "NINDS Myasthenia Gravis Information Page." *NINDS*, December 4, 2012.

Parker, James N. and Philip M. Parker. *Myasthenia Gravis: A Medical Dictionary, Bibliography, and Annotated Research Guide to Internet References.* San Diego, Calif.: ICON Health Publications, 2004.

Vincent, Angela. "Unravelling the Pathogenesis of Myasthenia Gravis." *Nature Reviews Immunology* 2 (October, 2002): 797 804.

MYOCARDIAL INFARCTION. *See* HEART ATTACK.

MYOMECTOMY

Procedure

Anatomy or system affected: Reproductive system, uterus
Specialties and related fields: Gynecology
Definition: The removal of a uterine myoma, also known as a fibroid or leiomyoma.

Indications and Procedures

The most common indication for a myomectomy is the need to remove a symptomatic fibroid. In many cases, these fibroids are large (greater than 8 centimeters). A myomectomy is chosen over a hysterectomy (removal of the uterus) if the patient desires future childbearing and if there is no evidence of malignancy of the uterus. A myomectomy can be performed using abdominal, laparoscopic, vaginal, or hysteroscopic approaches. The choice of approach depends on the location and size of the fibroids, as well as on the experience of the surgeon.

The most common type is abdominal myomectomy. This procedure is performed in the operating room with the patient under general anesthesia. The abdomen is incised and entry into the pelvic cavity is obtained. The uterus is then identified and inspected for fibroids. Some surgeons apply a tourniquet to the uterine arteries for hemostasis. A vasocontrictive agent is injected into the myometrium surrounding the fibroid to minimize blood loss. The myometrium over the fibroid is then incised, and the fibroid is dissected out. Finally, the myometrial defect is closed with a suture to stop blood flow. In patients desiring fertility, care is taken to minimize entry into the endometrial cavity, as the procedure may increase the risk of uterine rupture with pregnancy.

In laparoscopic and vaginal myomectomies, access to the fibroids is obtained using endoscopic instruments and through an incision in the vagina, respectively. In hysteroscopic myomectomies, access to fibroids in the endometrial cavity is obtained using a hysteroscope inserted through the cervical canal. The hysteroscope holds an instrument that shaves away fibroids in the endometrial cavity.

Uses and Complications

The primary use of myomectomy is the relief of symptoms caused by fibroids. These symptoms can be any of the following: pressure sensation, pelvic pain, dyspareunia (painful intercourse), menorrhagia (excessive menstruation), dysmenorrhea (painful menstruation), urinary urgency or frequency, urinary incontinence, and constipation.

The short-term risks of abdominal myomectomies are the same as those for most pelvic surgeries. These risks are small but include infection, damage to internal organs such as the bowel or bladder, blood loss requiring transfusion, and complications from anesthesia. Long-term consequences include an increased risk of uterine rupture with future pregnancy, the recurrence of fibroid growth, and pelvic adhesion (scar tissue) formation. Laparoscopic myomectomies are less invasive than abdominal myomectomies, but the same short-term and long-term risks are present. Hysteroscopic myomectomies carry less risks than abdominal procedures, since no incision is made on the abdomen and there is no entry into the pelvic cavity, but the risks unique to hysteroscopy exist, such as uterine perforation and fluid overload.

—Anne Lynn S. Chang, M.D.

See also Dysmenorrhea; Genital disorders, female; Gynecology; Hysterectomy; Menorrhagia; Menstruation; Muscles; Reproductive system; Tumor removal; Tumors; Uterus; Women's health.

For Further Information:

Bieber, Eric J., and Victoria M. Maclin, eds. *Myomectomy*. Malden, Mass.: Blackwell Science, 1998.

DeCherney, Alan H., et al. *Current Diagnosis and Treatment: Obstetrics and Gynecology*. New York: McGraw-Hill Medical, 2013.

Falcone, T., and M. A. Bedaiwy. "Minimally Invasive Management of Uterine Fibroids." *Current Opinion in Obstetrics and Gynecology* 14, no. 4 (August, 2002): 401–07.

Hoffman, Barbara L., et al. *Williams Gynecology*. New York: McGraw-Hill Medical, 2012.

Rock, John A., and Howard W. Jones III, eds. *Te Linde's Operative Gynecology*. 10th ed. Philadelphia: Wolters Kluwer/Lippincott Williams & Wilkins, 2008.

Stenchever, Morton A., et al. *Comprehensive Gynecology*. 4th ed. St. Louis, Mo.: Mosby/Elsevier, 2006.

Tulandi, Togas, ed. *Uterine Fibroids: Embolization and Other Treatments*. New York: Cambridge University Press, 2003.

Youngkin, Ellis Quinn, et al. *Women's Health: A Primary Care Clinical Guide*. Boston: Pearson, 2013.

MYOPIA
Disease/Disorder
Also known as: Nearsightedness
Anatomy or system affected: Eyes
Specialties and related fields: Ophthalmology, optometry
Definition: A visual defect that impairs the perception of distant objects.

Causes and Symptoms

Nearsightedness (myopia) occurs when light from distant objects reaches a focal point in front of the retina, the photoreceptive tissue of the eye. Consequently, vision of distant objects is blurred on the retina. The primary cause of myopia is an eyeball that is too long from front to back. People whose parents have myopia are more likely to have it, indicating a genetic cause; a few studies have also shown correlations between higher testosterone levels in the womb and later incidence of myopia. Research has also found that prolonged eyestrain, especially from long periods of reading or other close work, can distort the shape of the eye. This may be one reason why more highly educated people manifest higher

---

Information on Myopia

Causes: Unknown; possibly higher testosterone levels in womb, genetic predisposition, prolonged eyestrain
Symptoms: Impaired perception of distant objects
Duration: Varies
Treatments: Wearing concave lenses, correction through laser surgery

---

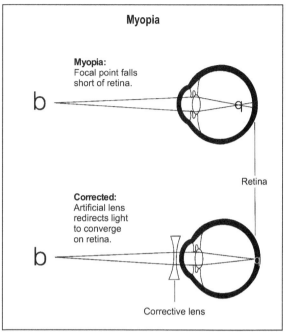

Myopia is commonly termed "nearsightedness" because most light rays entering the eye will not resolve, or focus, on the retina unless they are coming from a very near distance; corrective lenses or surgery can solve this problem.

rates of nearsightedness than individuals with less formal education.

All children are born nearsighted; by the age of six months, however, vision begins to improve. Myopia is an uncommon problem in younger school-age children but begins to increase in prevalence as children move into their teenage years. From the twenties until the forties, the rate of visual deterioration tends to slow down. As people enter middle and old age, however, the rate of visual decline accelerates again. People past the age of seventy are fourteen times as likely to experience myopia resulting in legal blindness as those in their twenties.

Treatment and Therapy

For several centuries, nearsightedness has been corrected by the use of a concave lens, which moves the focal point of light in myopic eyes closer to the retina. The first eyeglasses, invented in late-thirteenth-century Italy, had convex lenses that corrected for farsightedness; not until the fifteenth century did glasses with concave lenses appear. As the twentieth century drew to a close, innovative surgical approaches were developed to correct for myopia. Most of these procedures, such as laser surgery, move the focal point of light closer to the retina by changing the shape of the cornea.

—Paul J. Chara, Jr., Ph.D.

See also Aging; Blurred vision; Cataracts; Glaucoma; Eye infections and disorders; Eye surgery; Eyes; Laser use in surgery; Ophthalmology; Optometry; Optometry, pediatric; Sense organs; Vision; Vision disorders.

For Further Information:

Buettner, Helmut, ed. *Mayo Clinic on Vision and Eye Health: Practical Answers on Glaucoma, Cataracts, Macular Degeneration, and Other Conditions*. Rochester, Minn.: Mayo Foundation for Medical Education and Research, 2002.

"Facts About Myopia." *National Eye Institute*, October, 2010.

Icon Health. *Myopia: A Medical Dictionary, Bibliography, and Annotated Research Guide to Internet References*. San Diego, Calif.: Author, 2004.

National Foundation for Eye Research. http://www .nfer.org.

"Nearsightedness." *MedlinePlus*, September 3, 2012.

Riordan-Eva, Paul, and John P. Whitcher. *Vaughan and Asbury's General Ophthalmology*. 18th ed. New York: Lange Medical Books/McGraw-Hill, 2011.

Sutton, Amy L., ed. *Eye Care Sourcebook: Basic Consumer Health Information About Eye Care and Eye Disorders*. 3d ed. Detroit, Mich.: Omnigraphics, 2008.

MYRINGOTOMY

Procedure

Anatomy or system affected: Ears

Specialties and related fields: Family medicine, otorhinolaryngology

Definition: The creation of an opening in the eardrum (tympanic membrane) to allow drainage of accumulated fluid in the middle ear.

Indications and Procedures

Fluid can collect in the middle ear as a result of infection or allergy; this fluid consists of blood, pus, water, and debris. An ear, nose, and throat specialist may surgically insert small tubes into the middle ear to facilitate drainage. Usually, local anesthesia is administered, particularly if the patient is a young child.

This procedure, called myringotomy, is used to relieve pain caused by pressure and to prevent temporary or permanent hearing loss. Physiologically, the problem involves blockage of the Eustachian tube, a narrow canal that connects the middle ear to the back of the nasal cavity. This tube regulates air pressure in the middle-ear cavity, allowing the hearing mechanism to function properly and helping to maintain a sense of balance.

Prior to performing a myringotomy, medical treatment may involve the prescription of antihistamines, decongestants, and perhaps steroids, which usually reduce the swelling of the Eustachian tube and sometimes preclude a myringotomy. After the procedure, improvement in hearing is usually immediate, and the middle-ear infection should heal. Antibiotic eardrops may be prescribed; three or four drops should be placed in each ear twice a day for five days. In approximately six to twelve months, the myringotomy tube will be expelled into the outer ear canal automatically and can be removed by a physician. Treatment may include follow-up visits every two months.

Uses and Complications

Postoperatively, it is not unusual for the patient to experience a certain amount of pulsation, popping, clicking, and other sounds in the ear. It is important during the postoperative period to make certain that the patient does not get water in his or her ear, especially when the tube is in place. When washing the hair or face, cotton covered with petroleum jelly may be placed in the outer part of the ear. For long-term protection, earplugs may be used during showering, bathing, and swimming. Diving, deep swimming, and any other activities that may place pressure on the eardrum are not recommended.

—*John Alan Ross, Ph.D.*

See also Deafness; Ear infections and disorders; Ear surgery; Ears; Hearing; Hearing loss; Otorhinolaryngology; Surgery, pediatric.

For Further Information:

A.D.A.M. Medical Encyclopedia [Internet]. Atlanta (GA): A.D.A.M., Inc.; ©2005. Ear tube insertion; [updated 2012 July 30; cited 2013 June 27]; [about 2 p.]. Available from: http://www.nlm.nih.gov/medlineplus/ency/article/003015.htm.

American Medical Association. *American Medical Association Family Medical Guide*. 4th rev. ed. Hoboken, N.J.: John Wiley & Sons, 2004.

Bluestone, Charles D. *Pediatric Otolaryngology*. New York: McGraw-Hill, 2013.

Canalis, Rinaldo, and Paul R. Lambert, eds. *The Ear: Comprehensive Otology*. Philadelphia: Lippincott Williams & Wilkins, 2000.

Ferrari, Mario. *PDxMD Ear, Nose, and Throat Disorders*. Philadelphia: PDxMD, 2003.

Johnson, Jonas T., Clark A. Rosen, and Byron J Bailey, eds. *Bailey's Head and Neck Surgery—Otolaryngology*. Philadelphia: Wolters Kluwer Health/Lippincott Williams & Wilkins, 2013.

Pender, Daniel J. *Practical Otology*. Philadelphia: J. B. Lippincott, 1992.

Sataloff, Robert T., and Joseph Sataloff. *Hearing Loss*. 4th ed. New York: Taylor & Francis, 2005.

Turkington, Carol, and Allen E. Sussman. *The Encyclopedia of Deafness and Hearing Disorders*. Rev. 2d ed. New York: Facts On File, 2004.

Woolf, Alan D., et al., eds. *The Children's Hospital Guide to Your Child's Health and Development*. Cambridge, Mass.: Perseus, 2002.

NAIL REMOVAL
Procedure

Anatomy or system affected: Feet, hands, nails

Specialties and related fields: Emergency medicine, family medicine, internal medicine, pediatrics, podiatry, sports medicine

Definition: The partial or total removal of either fingernails or toenails.

Indications and Procedures

Nail removal is one of the most common office procedures seen in primary care. Nail disorders leading to removal occur most often in toenails, but they can also occur in fingernails. Common reasons for removal are infection, ingrown nails, or trauma. Patients usually experience pain and inability to function in their normal activities. Rarely are there any systemic signs or symptoms, such as fever, chills, or nausea, unless the cause is a serious infection.

The patient's foot or hand is first cleansed and draped. Sterile techniques are used throughout the procedure. Patients undergoing partial or total nail removal require adequate anesthesia, which is usually done through a digital block. This procedure is performed at the base of the digit with lidocaine or a similar anesthetic to numb the entire finger or toe. The provider should wait five minutes for the anesthesia to become effective. A tourniquet may be applied to minimize bleeding and enhance anesthesia. An instrument is then used to separate the nail from the nail bed with the least trauma possible. In a complete removal, the nail is gently pulled away from the nail bed. In a partial removal, scissors are used to cut the desired amount of nail away from the intact nail. Some providers will also chemically destroy the nail matrix in the area of the partial removal to prevent recurrent ingrown nails, if clinically indicated.

Compression for a few minutes may be needed to slow any bleeding from the nail removal. Topical antibiotic ointment may be applied with gauze and a compression dressing. When a toenail is removed, patients may walk immediately after the procedure and resume any activity as tolerated. Local wound care instructions are given, and if the procedure is performed secondary to an infected digit, oral antibiotics may be ordered. The procedure usually takes approximately fifteen minutes to complete.

Uses and Complications

Partial nail removal or trimming may also be performed in diabetic patients or those unable to perform routine nail care. Fungal infections cannot be cured with nail removal alone, though in severe or painful cases, the procedure may be performed in conjunction with the administration of antifungal agents.

Nail removal has few complications if performed properly. Pain is one of the most common complications of the procedure, especially if the digit was already infected. Bacterial infection may also occur after the procedure without proper wound care management. Bleeding may occur, as epinephrine is not used in digital blocks. Adequate compression or cautery usually stops any continued bleeding after the procedure. Patients must also be warned that the nail may not grow back with the same shape prior to removal. Nails should be cut straight across without curvature to prevent any ingrown nail recurrence.

—Jeffrey R. Bytomski, D.O.

See also Bacterial infections; Diabetes mellitus; Feet; Lower extremities; Nails; Podiatry; Upper extremities; Wounds.

For Further Information:

Clark, Robert E., and Whitney D. Tope. "Nail Surgery." In *Cutaneous Surgery*, edited by Roland G. Wheeland. Philadelphia: W. B. Saunders, 1994.

"Nail Diseases." *MedlinePlus*, April 11, 2013.

Woods, Michael, et al. "Ingrown Toenail Removal." *Health Library*, May 2, 2013.

Zuber, Thomas J. "Ingrown Toenail Removal." *American Family Physician* 65, no. 12 (June 15, 2002): 2547–2554.

NAILS
Anatomy

Anatomy or system affected: Hands, feet, skin

Specialties and related fields: Dermatology, histology

Definition: The thin, horny plates covering the dorsal ends of the fingers or toes.

Key terms:

cuticle: cutaneous or skin tissue that surrounds the nail plate on its proximal sides and provides a protective barrier to the nail bed; it is attached to the proximal nail fold and to the nail plate

hyponychium: cutaneous tissue underlying the free nail at its point of separation from the nail bed; structurally similar to the cuticle

keratinocytes: matrix basal epithelial cells that differentiate, fill with keratin, and form the dead horny substance making up the nail plate

lunula: a whitish, crescent-shaped area at the end of the proximal nail fold that marks the end of the nail matrix and is the site of mitosis and nail growth

onychomycosis: common nail disorder in which fungal organisms invade the nail bed causing progressive changes in the color, texture, and structure of the nail

Structure and Functions

Nails function to protect fingers and toes against bumps and trauma. Fine touch is amplified and skillful manipulation of small objects with the fingers is enabled by the presence of nails. Nails also provide the ability to scratch, both as a temporary relief of an itch and in personal defense. Nails are important social communicators of beauty and sexuality and hence are the focus of a major cosmetic industry.

Biologically, nails are characterized as plates of tightly packed, hard epidermis cells filled with a protein called keratin. Nails are normally seen on the dorsal side (the side opposite the palm or sole) of all fingers and toes. The anatomy of the normal nail consists of a nail plate, proximal nail fold, nail bed, matrix, and hyponychium. These components are epithelial-derived structures, like skin and hair, which emerge from the live germinative zone of the epidermis. In nails, these cells differentiate and form the horny layer, which is considered to be dead.

The nail plate is a relatively hard and flat, transparent, horny structure that is rectangular in shape. It rests on the underlying nail bed but typically extends beyond the bed as an unattached, free-growing edge reaching toward or beyond the tip of the finger or toe. On the fingers, the thickness of the plate in adults increases from about 0.7 millimeters at the proximal edge to about 1.6 millimeters at the distal edge. The terminal tip thickness varies considerably between persons.

Normally, a pinkish nail bed is seen through the transparent nail plate. Frequently in the thumbnail and sometimes in the other fingernails, a whitish, semi-moon-shaped structure called the lunula is seen that extends under the proximal nail fold. The borders of the nail plate are covered by skin structures: two lateral folds and a single proximal fold.

The proximal nail fold is the cutaneous or skin structure that is in continuity with the visible proximal border of the nail but overlies part of the nail root. The ventral side (underside) of the proximal nail fold provides physical protection to the germinative zone of the nail and aids in the physical attachment of the nail plate. About a fourth of the total surface area of the nail plate is located under the proximal fold. The cuticle is a layer of epidermis extending from the proximal nail fold and attached to the dorsal side of the nail. The cuticle functions to provide a physical seal against microbes and chemical irritants, which may otherwise enter the matrix and affect nail production.

The nail bed is the portion of the digit upon which the nail rests. The nail bed is highly vascular, with numerous capillaries. It consists of epithelial tissue and extends from the lunula

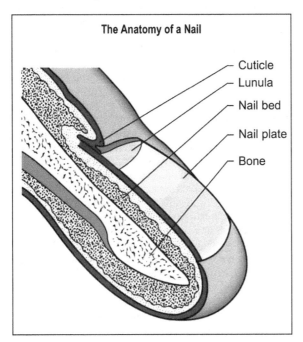

The Anatomy of a Nail

- Cuticle
- Lunula
- Nail bed
- Nail plate
- Bone

to the point where the bed separates from the nail. A series of fine longitudinal folds in the nail bed corresponds to the undersurface structure of the nail. This arrangement enhances the adherence of the nail plate to the nail bed.

The nail matrix is generally considered the most proximal part of the nail bed and is bordered by the proximal nail fold. On the distal end it is bordered by the distal margin of the lunula. The nail matrix epithelium cells consist predominantly of keratinocytes in both a basal and a spinous layer. Melanocytes and Langerhans cells are intermingled with keratinocytes. It is within the matrix that the germinating center of nail growth is found. Basal epithelial cells increase in number through mitosis, or division, and then differentiate into keratinocytes, which are epithelial cells filled with keratin protein. These keratinocytes condense their cytoplasm, lose their nucleus, and form flat, horny-looking dead cells. As further cell division occurs in the nail matrix, more distal keratinocytes are pushed out to form the nail plate.

The hyponychium consists of epidermis tissue that underlies the edge of the nail plate and extends from the nail bed to the distal groove. It functions to provide a defense against entry of bacteria under the free edge of the nail plate. Excessively vigorous cleaning may damage the hyponychium and allow for bacteria to enter more readily under the nail plate.

The turnover rate of matrix cells determines the growth rate of the nail. This rate varies with age, environmental conditions, nutritional status, and the specific digit. The growth rate proportionately increases with the length of the digit; thus the middle finger nail grows the fastest while the growth rate in the little finger is the slowest. Fingernails grow three times as rapidly as toenails. The growth rate is more rapid in the winter than in the summer. Furthermore, nails grow faster in young children than in older adults. It takes about six months for a fingernail to completely grow in. Male nails grow faster than female nails. Nails on the dominant hand grow faster than those on the other hand.

If nails are protected and untrimmed, they can grow to considerable lengths. Such long nails were prized by the wealthy classes in imperial Chinese culture as an indication of status. The practice of painting toenails red may have originated in the Ottoman seraglio, where it was a signal of menstrual status.

Nails continue to grow throughout life without a resting phase. Contrary to folk belief, nails cease growing when an individual dies. The matrix cells stop producing deoxyribonucleic acid (DNA) and dividing soon after death, and thus the nail bed cannot grow longer. The appearance of nail growth after death is due to a retraction or shrinkage of nail matrix tissue, resulting in the apparent lengthening of the nail plate.

Professional grooming of the nails for both men and women is termed a manicure. Manicure procedures include cutting the nails according to fashion standards to improve their cosmetic appearance. A pedicure is the term applied to grooming the toenails. Typically, the nails are first soaked in a soapy solution to soften the nail plate and to remove dirt and debris. It is often fashionable to trim the nails to a delicate arc at the middle of the fingertip. The corners of the nail are typically filed. While this shape is attractive in creating the illusion of longer, slender fingers, it heightens the probability of nail plate fractures, hangnails, or ingrown nails. The cuticle, considered to be unattractive by manicurists, is typically minimized, partially removed, or traumatized. This may increase the incidence of fungal invasion and disease. Most of the problems associated with a manicure arise from excessive manipulation of the cuticle.

Nail polish typically consists of pigments suspended in a volatile solvent that also contains a film-forming agent. When the polish is applied to the finger, a covering film develops over the nail. The film is permeable to oxygen, which allows gas exchange to occur between the atmosphere and the nail plate. Resins and plasticizers are added to the polish to increase the flexibility of the film and to minimize chipping. The variety in nail polish color is due to the addition of coloring agents. Deep red nail polishes can cause a temporary yellowish staining of the nail plate.

Nail adornments are sometimes used. Frequently, small nail jewels or ribbons are applied to the fingernails immediately before the nail polish dries, allowing the decoration to adhere to the nail plate. Since some people frequently develop contact dermatitis in reaction to nickel, gold or nickel-free jewels should be selected. Artificial nail tips made of plastic also are glued to the nail tip to create the illusion of an elongated natural nail tip. The gluing may cause nail problems, since a portion of the natural nail is occluded by the glue. This occlusion inhibits oxygen transfer and stresses the nail plate. Frequently, the nail may thin and be unable to support its own weight after the plastic tip is removed. Removal of the plastic tip may result in nail pitting.

Disorders and Diseases

Nails are useful indicators of skin disease and internal disorders. An abnormally pigmented band in the nail may indicate a malignant melanoma. A yellow nail may indicate psoriasis or a fungal infection. Pulmonary disease or smoking may also cause yellow or brownish nails. Antimalarial drugs may cause the nail to darken in appearance. Frequently, psoriasis causes pitting of nails and an acceleration in their growth rate. Chronic chest disease or a cyanotic congenital heart disorder is frequently associated with club-shaped deformity of the nail plate. Beau's lines, which are transverse depressions in the nail plates, are associated with illnesses such as coronary thrombosis, pneumonia, and severe injuries. Drug treatment may cause nail breakdown or destruction or complete shedding of the nail plate.

An unexplained aspect of nail physiology is its relationship to lung physiology. Hippocrates first described a connection between lung parenchymal disorders and an edema in the connective tissue beneath the lunula that results in clubbing. The relationship has long been recognized, but the causal link is still unknown.

An ingrown nail results when a deformed nail grows improperly into the skin or when the skin around the nails engulfs part of the nail. Wearing narrow, tight shoes can cause or worsen this pathology. Initially, symptoms may be slight or mild, but with time may come increasing pain. The affected area becomes reddish and, if not treated, may become infected. If infected, the area becomes swollen, inflamed, and painful. Blisters may develop. Treatment involves trimming away the nail from the infected area, allowing the inflammation to decline and the area to heal.

Clubbing is a disorder characterized by a bulblike enlargement of the nail with increased horizontal and longitudinal curvatures. Clubbing involves both fingers and toes and commonly begins at puberty. The disorder may be genetically inherited or acquired. Clubbed nails often have a spongy feel when pressure is placed on the proximal nail fold. This is due to the expanded soft tissue that underlies the nail. Acquired clubbing is often associated with another clinical pathology, most commonly pulmonary or cardiovascular disease. However, at times it is also associated with gastrointestinal inflammatory disease or cystic fibrosis.

A fungal infection is the cause of onychomycosis, which is the most common nail disorder. About half of all nail problems can be linked to this disease, which affects as many as 15 to 20 percent of people in North America. It is uncommon in children and more frequently seen in aged adults.

Several fungi may cause onychomycosis, although most belong to the group called dermatophytes. The fungi are present in soil, and indirect transmission to humans frequently occurs through public swimming pools and shower floors. Some yeasts and molds are also thought to cause this clinical condition. Alternatively, this infection is associated with athlete's foot infection. Typically this condition is found in toenails more frequently than fingernails. The presence of the fungus is further evidenced by scaling on the plantar surface of the foot, where it is often harbored.

In onychomycosis, the fungal organism invades the nail bed, causing a progressive change in the color, texture, and structure of the nail. The nail may turn white, thicken, and even detach from the nail bed. Debris from the infected nail often collects under its free edge. If untreated, the pathology may involve the entire nail plate, and rarely will the nail unit spontaneously heal itself.

Since several organisms may induce the pathology, effective treatment depends on matching the curative with the causal agent. Topically applied antifungals are seldom effective because most cannot penetrate the nail-plate barrier to reach the causal organism. Systemically (orally) administered antifungal therapy frequently uses one of several drugs such as griseofulvin, thiabendazole, or ketoconazole. These drugs are generally effective in halting further invasion of the fungus. While treatment continues, the new nail growth is usually normal, so treatment typically continues until the old nail is replaced by new nail and is then discontinued.

More than seventy tumors have been associated with parts of the nail. They may originate from the epidermis, dermis, subcutaneous tissues, or bone and may be found in the nail bed, nail matrix, hyponychium, or nail fold. The tumors may take various forms, including warts, erosion or ulceration of the nail bed, malignant neoplasms from underlying melanocytes, benign fibromas of the connective tissue, or squamous cell carcinomas. Diagnosis usually is made by taking a biopsy of the affected area. Treatment typically involves surgical removal of the tumor.

Perspective and Prospects

The earliest cellular growth leading to nail formation can be seen histologically at eight weeks of human development, the end of the embryonic period. Microscopically, the cells forming the proximal edge of the nail field and the future matrix can be distinguished at this time. The earliest gross anatomical appearance of nails is seen on the finger digit surface at about nine weeks of development, the very early fetal stage. By eleven weeks of age, the nail field is seen clearly on the hand digits of the fetus. By twenty weeks of age, the fetus shows a nail plate and bed and a proximal cuticle. By thirty-two weeks, the third trimester of pregnancy, adult-type nail structures are visible in the fetus, including a nail plate, matrix, and bed and a forming hyponychium.

Aging results in changes and disorders in nails. When people get older, the color, contour, growth rate, surface texture, and thickness of the nail plate change. Some disorders are more prevalent with aging, such as brittle nails, splitting or fissuring of the nail plate, and increased infections. Aged nails appear dull and opaque, with their color varying from yellow to gray. Frequently in older persons, the lunula is decreased in size or is absent. The growth rate of nails decreases with aging. The most rapid period of growth is during the first thirty years, after which the rate steadily declines. Nail plate thickness frequently increases with advanced age, in combination with discoloration and loss of translucency of the nail plate.

For many years, blood and urine specimens have been used to detect and measure body concentrations of therapeutic drugs or drugs of abuse. During the past decade, alternative biological specimens such as nails and hair have been frequently used as the basis for drug detection. The basis for drug detection in nail clippings is that the dividing epidermal cells that form the nail plate also incorporate drugs from the systemic circulation. The subsequent cornification of these cells traps the drug within the forming nail plate. Drug-detection methods involve taking a sample of nail clippings and extracting and identifying drug molecules via immunochemical or chromatographic techniques. These techniques are extremely sensitive and capable of detecting minute quantities of drug in the samples; as little as ten milligrams of nail clippings is required to detect the presence of drugs. Twenty-first-century drug-screening methods have detected amphetamines and cocaine in nail clippings. Using nail clippings for drug analysis and screening provides a long-term measure of drug exposure that may potentially represent months of drug use. Furthermore, nail clippings are relatively easy to collect and involve a noninvasive procedure; samples are easily stored, and once incorporated in the nail tissue, most of the drugs are presumably stable.

Modern medicine in the early twenty-first century still lacks adequate descriptive science as well as understanding of the molecular mechanisms that control nail development and growth. To date, the specific genes or gene products that initiate nail growth have not been identified. The molecular basis for brittle nails, clubbing, and other nail pathologies is not known. Is onychomycosis affected by a systemic immune deficit? What causes yellow nail syndrome? Answers to these questions as well as additional information about the molecular control of nail physiology will greatly increase understanding and lead to better treatments for nail disorders.

—*Roman J. Miller, Ph.D.*

See also Feet; Fungal infections; Lower extremities; Nail removal; Pulmonary diseases; Skin; Skin disorders; Upper extremities.

For Further Information:

Baran, R., et al., eds. *Baran and Dawber's Diseases of the Nails and Their Management*. 3d ed. Malden, Mass.: Blackwell Science, 2001.

Du Vivier, Anthony. *Atlas of Clinical Dermatology*. 4th ed. Edinburgh: Churchill Livingstone, 2012.

"Fingernails: Dos and Don'ts for Healthy Nails." *Mayo Clinic*, December 8, 2011.

Hordinsky, Maria K., Marty E. Sawaya, and Richard K. Scher, eds. *Atlas of Hair and Nails*. Philadelphia: Churchill Livingstone, 2000.

Mix, Godfrey F. *The Salon Professional's Guide to Foot Care*. Albany: Milday SalonOvations, 1999. .

"Nail Diseases." *MedlinePlus*, July 9, 2013.

Porter, Robert S., et al., eds. *The Merck Manual Home Health Handbook*. Whitehouse Station, N.J.: Merck Research Laboratories, 2009.

Standring, Susan, et al., eds. *Gray's Anatomy*. 40th ed. New York: Churchill Livingstone/Elsevier, 2008.

Zaias, Nardo. *The Nail in Health and Disease*. 2d ed. Norwalk, Conn.: Appleton & Lange, 1992.

NARCOLEPSY

Disease/Disorder

Anatomy or system affected: Brain, nervous system, psychic-emotional system

Specialties and related fields: Neurology

Definition: An apparently inherited disorder of the nervous system characterized by brief, numerous, and overwhelming attacks of sleepiness throughout the day.

Key terms:

cataplexy: brief periods of partial or total loss of skeletal muscle tone, usually triggered by emotional stimuli, which can cause the person to collapse

electroencephalogram (EEG): a recording of brain wave activity using electrodes attached to the scalp

excessive daytime sleepiness: a strong tendency to fall asleep, accompanied by reduced energy and lack of alertness during the entire day

hypnogogic hallucination: a bizarre, sometimes frightening, dreamlike occurrence just as one is falling asleep or just after waking

maintenance of wakefulness test: a polysomnographic technique to measure a person's ability to remain awake during repeated trials throughout the day

multiple sleep latency test: a polysomnographic technique to measure how quickly one falls asleep during repeated trials throughout the day

polysomnography: the continuous recording of brain waves, eye movements, skeletal muscle movements, and other body functions to determine bodily changes during the stages of sleep

REM sleep: a period of intense brain activity, often associated with dreams; named for the rapid eye movements that typically occur during this time

sleep paralysis: an inability to move voluntarily, occurring just at the beginning of sleep or upon awakening

---

Information on Narcolepsy

Causes: Genetic factors

Symptoms: Attacks of irresistible sleepiness in daytime, episodes of cataplexy, hypnogogic hallucinations, sleep paralysis, memory difficulties, eye fatigue, sleep apnea

Duration: Chronic with acute episodes

Treatments: Stimulant medications (dextroamphetamine, pemoline, Ritalin), tricyclic antidepressants, supportive counseling

---

Causes and Symptoms

Narcolepsy (*narco* meaning "numbness" and *lepsy* meaning "seizure") consists primarily of attacks of irresistible sleepiness in the daytime. The sleepiness is extreme; it has been described as the feeling that most people would experience if they tried to add columns of numbers in the middle of the night after forty-eight hours without sleep.

The narcoleptic's day is broken up by a series of brief and repetitive sleep attacks, perhaps even two hundred attacks in a single day. These transient, overpowering attacks of sleepiness may last from a few seconds to thirty minutes, with an average spell lasting two minutes. It is excruciatingly difficult, and frequently impossible, to ignore the urge to sleep, no matter how inconvenient or inappropriate. Narcoleptics typically fall asleep suddenly, on the job, in conversation, standing up, and even while eating, driving, or making love.

These sleep attacks result from an abrupt failure in resisting sleep, as opposed to a sudden surge in sleepiness, because narcoleptics are actually sleepy all day. The misconception that their daytime sleepiness is caused by insufficient nighttime sleep prompts undiagnosed patients to spend inordinately long hours in bed. Narcoleptics will be sleepy during the day regardless of how much sleep they get at night.

One of the most prominent and troubling features of narcolepsy is cataplexy, a sudden loss of muscle tone that causes the person to collapse. Cataplexy, the second most common symptom of narcolepsy, is experienced by approximately 70 percent of those diagnosed with the disorder. It occurs during the daytime while the person is awake. It may involve all the muscles at once or only a select few, so the severity may range from total collapse to the ground to partial collapse of a limb or the jaw. The cataplectic sometimes remains conscious, able to think, hear, and see, although vision may be blurred. At other times, there is a brief loss of consciousness, associated with an experience of dreaming. Although most attacks of cataplexy last less than a minute, occasionally they go on for several minutes or more. Cataplexy is often triggered by enjoyable feelings, laughter, or excitement during which the person suddenly crumples into a heap. For other patients, a strong negative emotion, such as fear or anger, precipitates an attack.

Many narcoleptics notice the symptom of excessive daytime sleepiness (EDS) for as much as a year before the onset of cataplexy. After many years of experiencing cataplexy, some patients find that less emotional stimulus is required to induce the muscle collapse and that increasingly more muscles are involved. Others find that this symptom diminishes, possibly because they have become adept at anticipating and avoiding the situations that trigger attacks. It has been noted that other hypersomnias—that is, other diseases of excessive sleepiness—do not include cataplexy; only narcoleptics suffer from this embarrassing and troubling symptom of muscle collapse.

Many narcoleptics also experience hypnogogic hallucinations, dreams that intrude into the waking state. In normal sleep, dreaming generally occurs approximately ninety minutes after falling asleep; narcoleptics begin their sleeping episodes with vivid dreams. These hallucinations are extremely realistic and often violent. The patient sees someone else in the room or hears someone calling his or her name, for the hallucinations are nearly always visual and are usually auditory. The vivid sights, sounds, and feelings characteristic of hypnogogic hallucinations are thought to occur while the person is awake, both during the day and just at the edges of nighttime sleep. Since narcoleptics typically fall asleep dozens if not hundreds of times a day, they can experience these disturbing hallucinations with great frequency.

Narcoleptics may suffer from another frightening symptom: sleep paralysis. This condition occurs at the beginning or end of sleep and renders immobile virtually every voluntary muscle, except those around the eyes. During sleep paralysis, the mind is awake and one is aware of the external surroundings, but the muscles refuse to move. The paralysis usually lasts only a few seconds, but it may continue for as long as twenty minutes. Sleep researchers find that almost everyone has an episode of sleep paralysis that lasts a few seconds some time during his or her lifetime. When the paralysis continues for more than a few seconds, however, it is usually a sign of narcolepsy. Although either sleep paralysis or hypnogogic hallucinations alone are distressing enough, they may happen simultaneously. However, it is estimated that only 10 to 25 percent of narcoleptics experience all four major symptoms of this sleep disorder.

Because of their frequent, irresistible sleep attacks, narcoleptics often wobble back and forth between sleep and wakefulness in a state that has been likened to sleepwalking and is termed automatic behavior. When in this state, the person seems to behave normally but later does not remember extended periods of time. For example, narcoleptics might find themselves in a different building or several exits farther down a highway than they last remembered. Obviously, automatic behavior is very anxiety-producing; it is very troubling to narcoleptics to be unable to remember what they have done in the minutes or hours that have just passed.

In addition to these memory difficulties, some narcoleptics experience constant eye fatigue, difficulty focusing, and double vision. They also have a higher incidence of the heart abnormality called mitral valve prolapse, which affects blood flow to the left ventricle.

Although narcolepsy is an illness of excessive daytime sleepiness, the nighttime sleep of those afflicted is far from normal as well. It is often troubled by restlessness and frequent awakenings, which are brief or may last for hours. Patients also experience many nightmares. Many narcoleptics talk, cry out, or thrash about periodically during the night.

One narcoleptic in ten has the added complication of suffering from sleep apnea. This sleep disorder consists of recurrent interruptions in breathing during sleep. This further disturbance of nighttime sleep aggravates the narcoleptic's tendency to excessive daytime sleepiness.

Narcolepsy was once thought to be extremely rare. By the late twentieth century, however, it became one of the most diagnosed sleep disorders, behind insomnia, obstructive sleep apnea, and restless legs syndrome. Nevertheless, many medical officials consider narcolepsy to be an underdiagnosed condition.

Males and females are equally affected by narcolepsy. Although the disorder has been diagnosed in a five-year-old, its symptoms most frequently appear for the first time during adolescence. In about 75 percent of cases, the attacks begin between the ages of fifteen and twenty-five; only 5 percent of cases begin before the age of ten. Onset is rare after the age of forty; if narcolepsy seems to appear in an older person, it has probably existed undiagnosed for years. Sleep researchers believe that the extra need for sleep characteristic of adolescence may make this stage of development particularly vulnerable for the onset of narcolepsy. Thus, this disorder may typically begin in adolescence because it is somehow triggered by the brain changes associated with sexual maturation.

While many members of the general population have scattered episodes of excessive daytime sleepiness, they are not considered narcoleptics. It is not until a person has one to several attacks each day that narcolepsy is suspected.

Treatment and Therapy

Narcolepsy is a disease of the nervous system. Although incurable, it can be successfully treated with various medications once it has been diagnosed. The diagnosis of narcolepsy, however, is often slow to occur. The average interval between the first appearance of symptoms and diagnosis is often as long as thirteen years. Because early symptoms are usually mild, narcoleptics typically spend years wondering whether they are sick or whether they merely lack initiative. They are often called lazy because they repeatedly nap during the day and are lethargic even when awake. Diagnosis is made more difficult by the wide range of severity of symptoms. For example, excessive daytime sleepiness may trouble a person for ten or twenty years before cataplexy appears. Patients may even occasionally experience a temporary or partial remission in their condition. Narcoleptics often fight off their sleep attacks by ingesting large amounts of caffeine and never realize that they have an actual disease until years later.

If narcolepsy is suspected, a polysomnographic study is done at a sleep disorders center to confirm the diagnosis. The most reliable confirmation of narcolepsy can be obtained by what is called the multiple sleep latency test (MSLT). The MSLT is easy, convenient, inexpensive, and very informative. The person is given four or five opportunities to lie down and fall asleep during the daytime. Normal individuals take fifteen to thirty minutes to fall asleep. In the MSLT, falling asleep in less than five minutes is considered abnormal. Those afflicted with narcolepsy always fall asleep in less than five minutes and often within a minute. The maintenance of wakefulness test (MOWT) is also used in the confirmation of narcolepsy. In the MOWT, the person is kept all day in a comfortable reclining position. Polysomnography is used to measure the patient's ability to stay awake and how many times he or she falls asleep.

Along with the MSLT and the MOWT, a thorough physical examination is needed to discover if the person has some other disorder that can mimic narcolepsy; an underactive thyroid gland, diabetes, chronic low blood sugar, anemia, and a malfunctioning liver can each cause excessive daytime sleepiness. Similarly, drug use, poor nutrition, emotional frustration, dissatisfaction, or poor motivation can also result in the type of sleepiness that a narcoleptic experiences.

When the diagnosis of narcolepsy is confirmed, treatment usually consists of stimulant medications such as dextroamphetamine, pemoline, or methylphenidate (Ritalin) during the daytime. These stimulant drugs can increase alertness and cut down the number of sleep attacks from perhaps several per day to several per month. Unfortunately, patients can quickly develop tolerance to these medications.

Even on low doses, some patients become irritable, aggressive, or nervous, or they may develop obesity and sexual problems. It is very important, therefore, to monitor a narcoleptic carefully, determining the lowest effective dose and the best times of day to take it. It may be months before the positive effects of drug therapy are fully experienced. The MSLT will often be given on a day that one takes the medication and on another when it is not taken, in order to evaluate the success of a given treatment.

Because specific drug and dosage schedules may have to be altered frequently, patients may repeatedly have to face drug withdrawal symptoms such as intensified sleepiness and disturbing dreams. To prevent adverse reactions, narcoleptics must often avoid certain foods and common medications. Their use of stimulant drugs may even be viewed as morally wrong, in these days of widespread drug abuse, by neighbors or coworkers who do not comprehend that narcolepsy is a disabling disease.

If cataplexy is present, medications other than amphetamines or Ritalin are required and useful. The class of drugs called tricyclic antidepressants, including protriptyline and imipramine, or the class of drugs called monoamine oxidase inhibitors may alleviate cataplexy. These medicines can often reduce attacks—for example, from three a day to three a month. In addition, effective treatment for cataplexy usually also relieves sleep paralysis and hypnogogic hallucinations.

Since the development of tolerance is common and these drugs can aggravate the symptom of sleepiness, determining the best timing and dose is critical. Another side effect of cataplexy drugs is impaired sexual function in males. Some men even discontinue these medications periodically for a day or two in order to sustain sexual relations. In addition, none of the drugs used for any symptoms of narcolepsy are safe to take during pregnancy.

In some cases, narcoleptics can be treated without medication if they carefully space naps during the day to relieve excessive sleepiness. Patients keep nap diaries to rate their alertness at regular intervals during the day. They then schedule short, strategically timed naps during those daytime periods when their sleep attacks are most likely to occur.

Naps are particularly valuable in treating children with narcolepsy because the consequences of a lifetime of medication on their development or on the course of their illness is unknown. Some children who show hyperactive behavior actually have narcolepsy; they are working frantically to overcome their persistent sleepiness and to keep themselves awake. Children with narcolepsy may also justifiably fear falling asleep, day or night, because of hallucinations and sleep paralysis.

It is evident that supportive counseling must be a strong component of treatment, whatever the patient's age. Sensitive medical monitoring can offer narcoleptics a measure of satisfactory daily living, but the use of stimulants to improve alertness may also make them more aware of their limitations and, therefore, more frustrated. Depression is not the cause of narcolepsy but may result primarily from the disruption in their lives and the feeling that they are denied the right to a "normal" life. Their constant sleepiness engenders feelings of inferiority and inadequacy. Narcoleptics usually refrain from mentioning their hallucinations and try to hide their automatic behavior for fear of being labeled insane. Loss of work, broken marriages, and social isolation are often witnesses to the crippling effects of narcolepsy.

Of all the people with narcolepsy seen at major sleep disorders centers, more than one-half have been completely disabled with respect to regular employment by the age of forty. With part-time, homebound, or self-employment, however, most narcoleptics can gain self-respect and help support themselves through work that is safe and tailored to their needs. They must be given tasks that can be divided into parts performed in relatively short time periods.

Drug and nap therapy can do little for narcoleptics without education of their families, friends, acquaintances, employers, and coworkers about the reality of this neurological disease. Most people find it hard to accept the notion that sleepiness cannot be controlled and insist that narcoleptics could be more alert if they tried harder. Narcoleptics are often stigmatized as slackers or incompetents, or assumed to be drug abusers or closet drinkers. It is most important that patients and all the people in their lives comprehend that excessive daytime sleepiness is not the patients" "fault."

Further help for narcoleptics seems to lie in animal studies, which may fill in many important pieces of the narcolepsy puzzle. The effects of the disease on behavior, the way in which it is inherited, and the benefits and risks of specific drugs continue to be evaluated in narcoleptic dogs.

Perspective and Prospects

Once viewed as "all in the mind," narcolepsy is now recognized as a neurological disorder. Its origin is unknown, but research has already discovered evidence of possible causes. An understanding of narcolepsy both depended on and advanced the understanding of normal sleep and of other sleep disorders. Scientists define sleep as a reduction in awareness of and interaction with the environment, lowered movement and muscle activity, and partial or complete suspension of voluntary behavior and consciousness.

Although narcolepsy was named and described in 1880, it could not be genuinely studied until the 1930s, when the electroencephalograph (EEG) was developed to record brain activity during the various stages of sleep. By the 1940s, this advancement led to a description of the narcoleptic tetrad, the four usual symptoms of narcolepsy: excessive daytime sleepiness, cataplexy, sleep paralysis, and hypnogogic hallucinations.

In the 1950s, narcolepsy still only rated a paragraph in one neurology textbook, which mistakenly called it a rare variety of epilepsy. A major discovery occurred in 1960: Narcoleptics bypass the normal stages of light and deep sleep and fall directly into rapid eye movement (REM) sleep. Thus, sudden-onset REM period (or SOREMP) became the major distinguishing feature of this brain disorder.

It was soon noted that relatives of narcoleptics are sixty times more likely to have the disease than members of the general population. Clearly, there is a hereditary factor involved, and geneticists have joined the hunt for narcolepsy's cause. The hereditary aspects of the disease are particularly important to counselors because parents with narcolepsy may feel guilty if their child develops it. (Indeed, some patients abandon plans to have children.) Geneticists have found a gene that may be responsible for narcolepsy. Since the gene produces an antigen called DR2 on patients" white blood cells, which is not found in nonnarcoleptics, immunologists have also begun to search for the origins of narcolepsy.

Rapid advances have been made in the last few years in determining the cause of narcolepsy. The disease is thought to arise from a biochemical imbalance in the brain that disturbs the mechanism that activates the on/off cycle of sleep. Biochemists are studying the possible relationship of various brain chemicals called neurotransmitters to narcolepsy. A defect in the way in which the body produces or uses dopamine, acetylcholine, or some other neurotransmitter is suspected to precipitate narcolepsy, which never spontaneously disappears once it is developed. The newest discovery has been the finding of abnormalities in the structure and function of a particular group of nerve cells, called hypocretin neurons, in the brains of patients with narcolepsy. The molecules implicated in narcolepsy are neuropeptides known as orexins (originally described as hypocretins). Researchers discovered that changes in the hypocretin receptor 2 and preprohypocretin genes are able to produce narcolepsy in animals. In one study involving nine human subjects, hypocretin could not be detected in seven of the subjects. Other studies have produced hypocretin knockout mice, which have symptoms that are quite similar to those found in human narcoleptics. Hypocretins have been found to occur normally in the regions of the central nervous system that appear to be involved in the regulation of sleep. An autosomal recessive mutation has been discovered in narcoleptic dogs that alters the hypocretin receptor 2 gene. In humans, a similar disruption or deficiency in hypocretin is associated with most cases of narcolepsy, although it is still unclear as to what underlies the exact genetic predisposition to the disease. Scientists speculate that they one day may cure narcolepsy or reduce its effects with drugs mimicking secretions of the missing nerve cells or even with brain-cell transplants.

Two interesting discoveries may help in the diagnosis of narcolepsy even before the classical clinical symptoms develop. There is some evidence that REM sleep is entered with abnormal rapidity years before the disorder develops. The drug physostigmine salicylate has no effect on normal dogs but elicits cataplexy in puppies with narcolepsy. Both these discoveries may be useful in screening the children of narcoleptics.

Because narcolepsy involves the fundamental processes of sleep, the combined efforts of neuroscientists, geneticists, biochemists, immunologists, and other scientists to unravel its mysteries will continue to yield important information about the basic mechanism of sleep—that state in which humans spend almost one-third of their lives.

—Grace D. Matzen

See also Apnea; Brain; Electroencephalography (EEG); Hallucinations; Memory loss; Nervous system; Neurology; Neurology, pediatric; Paralysis; Sleep; Sleep disorders; Sleeping sickness; Unconsciousness.

For Further Information:

Bassetti, Claudio L., Michel Billiard, and Emmanuel Mignot, eds. *Narcolepsy and Hypersomnia.* New York: Informa Healthcare, 2007.

Caldwell, J. Paul. *Sleep: The Complete Guide to Sleep Disorders and a Better Night's Sleep.* Rev. ed. Toronto, Ont.: Firefly Books, 2003.

Dement, William C. *The Sleepwatchers.* 2d ed. Menlo Park, Calif.: Stanford Alumni Association, 1996.

Hartmann, Ernest. *The Sleep Book: Understanding and Preventing Sleep Problems in People over Fifty.* Glenview, Ill.: Scott, Foresman, 1987.

Hollenstein, Jenna, and Rimas Lukas. "Narcolepsy." *Health Library,* Sept. 30, 2012.

Jasmin, Luc, David C. Dugdale III, and David Zieve. "Narcolepsy." *MedlinePlus,* Sept. 26, 2011.

Kryger, Meir H., Thomas Roth, and William C. Dement, eds. *Principles and Practices of Sleep Medicine.* 5th ed. Philadelphia: Saunders/Elsevier, 2011.

"Sleep Disorders." *MedlinePlus,* May 14, 2013.

"Narcolepsy Fact Sheet." *National Institute of Neurological Disorders and Stroke,* Dec. 28, 2011.

"About Narcolepsy." *Narcolepsy Network,* 2013.

Poceta, J. Steven, and Merrill Mitler, eds. *Sleep Disorders: Diagnosis and Treatment.* Totowa, N.J.: Humana Press, 1998.

Reite, Martin, John Ruddy, and Kim E. Nagel. *Concise Guide to Evaluation and Management of Sleep Disorders.* 3d ed. Washington, D.C.: American Psychiatric Press, 2002.

Walsleben, Joyce A., and Rita Baron-Faust. *A Woman's Guide to Sleep: Guaranteed Solutions for a Good Night's Rest.* New York: Crown, 2001.

"What Is Narcolepsy?" *National Heart, Lung, and Blood Institute,* Nov. 1, 2010.

NARCOTICS
Treatment
Anatomy or system affected: Brain, spinal cord and peripheral nerves

Specialties and related fields: Pharmacology

Definition: Narcotics are drugs, which mimic the action of the body's own painkilling substances, to treat pain, anxiety, coughing, diarrhea, and insomnia.

Key terms:

agonist: a drug that mimics the effects of a hormone or neurotransmitter normally found in the body

analgesia: relief of pain; analgesics are compounds that stop the neurotransmission of pain messages

antagonist: a drug that acts to block the effects of a hormone or neurotransmitter normally found in the body

brainstem: the region between the brain and spinal cord that controls vital functions such as breathing and heart rate

central nervous system: the brain and spinal cord

dependence: a craving for a drug

endogenous: something naturally found in the body, such as neurotransmitters

exogenous: something originating outside the body and administered orally or by injection

neurotransmitter: a chemical substance released by one nerve cell to stimulate or inhibit the function of an adjacent nerve cell; a chemical message released from a neuron

opioids: endogenous or exogenous substances (opiates) that relieve pain and cause euphoria

opiates: drugs made from the opium flower, such as opium, morphine, and codeine

synthetically made neuron: a nerve cell that can conduct electrical impulses from one region of the body to another; it is capable of releasing neurotransmitters

tolerance: diminished effect of a drug over time due to its chronic use

withdrawal: the body's response, both physical and mental, when an addictive substance is reduced or not given to the body

The Effects of Narcotics

Narcotics are drugs commonly used to treat pain (analgesics), suppress coughing, control diarrhea, and aid in anesthesia. These drugs are some of the oldest and most commonly used agents in medicine. They have psychoactive effects on the body which either block (an antagonist) or mimic (an agonist) the effects of naturally occurring chemicals. Researchers have studied the many effects of opiates, such as morphine, codeine, and heroin in comparison to the body's own endogenous opioids. Naturally occurring opioids, such as endorphins, dynorphins, and enkephalins, act as neurotransmitters, which send chemical signals throughout the human nervous system to relieve pain and increase euphoria.

To understand how opioids affect the body's response to pain, one must first understand the physiology of pain. When tissues are damaged, they release chemical substances into the space outside of the damaged cell, known as the extracellular space. Sensory neurons that have the ability to detect these chemicals are known as pain neurons. Once the chemicals bind to receptors on a pain neuron, the neuron is stimulated to send an ascending electrical message from the peripheral nerve, to the spinal cord and eventually to the brain. One type of neurotransmitter that transfers this message is called substance P. Once released and transmitted, two actions occur when the message arrives to the brain. The first is an immediate initiation of a reflex, which attempts to remove the tissue from the source of injury. For example, when one accidentally places an arm on a hot stove, a neural reflex causes the muscles of the limb to retract the arm from the burner. This is accomplished when the pain neuron releases a descending chemical message (neurotransmitter) from the brain to the spinal cord which then stimulates peripheral neurons that control the muscles of the affected limb. The second action of sensory pain occurs in terms of memory where appropriate behavioral modification can take place. For example, one may become more cautious around the kitchen after burning one's arm on the stove.

Regulation of pain occurs via neurotransmitters such as 5-hydroxytryptamine (5-HT) receptors, glycine, gamma-aminobutyric acid (GABA), and opioids. Morphine acts as an exogenous opioid, dampening the transmission of pain messages at various sites in the nervous system. One of the most clinically important places is within the spinal cord at the region where the pain neurons release substance P. Opioids are known to reduce the amount of substance P that is released and thereby decreasing the stimulatory message in the neural pathway to the brain. If the pain impulses traveling to the brain are reduced, so is one's perception of pain. The second area of the nervous system known to be involved in regulating the perception of pain is a dense area of neurons located between the brain and spinal cord referred to as the brainstem. When researchers stimulated a particular region of the brainstem, pain impulses traveling to the brain were reduced by the modulation of endogenous opioids.

Considering exogenous opioids mimic endogenous opioids, one may wonder why there is a need for narcotic drugs if the body already produces opioids such as endorphins and enkephalins. The answer is that every individual has a different degree of pain tolerance. How much pain one can endure also changes with certain circumstances. For example, one hardly notices the pain of a cut when participating in an exciting outdoor game. If the same wound occurs while one's attention is focused on it, however, the cut becomes noticeably painful. Perhaps the best explanation for the differing interpretation of pain during these activities and among different people is the endogenous opioid system. It is postulated that the analgesic effects of acupuncture are a result of stimulating neurons to release endorphins, enkephalins, and dynorphins. In the same way, with the administration of narcotics, one artificially increases the amount of opioids in the body in order to block pain impulses.

Opioids also act on the brainstem to modulate other pathways not associated with pain. They suppress coughing in a way that is similar to their effect on neural signals to decrease pain messages to the brain. Narcotics appear to inhibit the release of neurotransmitters responsible for the cough reflex. Unfortunately, opiates can simultaneously activate other areas of the brainstem responsible for nausea and vomiting. This unwanted side effect is related to the dose and type of drug used. Therefore, physicians can usually diminish the vomiting response with appropriate treatment selections. Perhaps the most dangerous problem with opioid usage is the effect on the brainstem's regulation of respiration. When the brainstem senses that the level of carbon dioxide is too high, breathing is increased to rid the body of this excess gas. Narcotics decrease the responsiveness of the brainstem to carbon dioxide. Therefore, breathing rates tend to be inappropriately low, causing a buildup of carbon dioxide.

Constriction of the pupils of the eyes is a very common side effect of opiates on the visual system. In fact, this constriction serves as an important diagnostic clue in examining a patient who has taken an overdose of a narcotic.

Opiates have a constipating effect, indirectly through the central nervous system and directly through their influence on the intestines. Opiates cause a decrease in peristalsis, concerted muscular contractions of the intestinal wall that would normally move food toward the anus.

Most opiate analgesics have no direct effect on the heart and blood vessels. Thus, they do not alter heart rate or blood pressure to any significant degree. The only noticeable effect on the cardiovascular system is a flushing and warming of the skin because of a slight increase in blood flow. Occasionally, this is accompanied by sweating. Kidney function tends to be depressed by opiates, which may be attributable to a decrease in the amount of blood that is filtered through the kidneys. There is also a decrease in the ability to urinate, as these drugs increase contraction of the muscle that prevents urine from leaving the bladder.

Uses and Complications

Medical personnel utilize narcotics to alter the body for the patient's advantage. Narcotics such as opiates are used for the relief of pain and anxiety, adjuncts for anesthesia, reduction of coughing, and control of diarrhea.

Opiate analgesics are among the most effective and valuable medications for the treatment of acute and chronic pain.

They are often used to treat pain in the postoperative period, in which they effectively reduce or eliminate the short-term pain from tissue trauma that is caused by surgery. When pain is reduced, patients tend to eat, sleep, and recover much more rapidly. Physicians often prescribe narcotics such as morphine or codeine for an as-needed basis ("PRN"). By doing so, the patient, who knows firsthand the effectiveness of the drug, can control the frequency of analgesic administration. In fact, patients are usually advised to administer a small dose before the pain becomes too intense, thus decreasing the pain message before it reaches a higher level, requiring a higher dosage for relief.

A painful sensation consists of the neural response to the tissue damage and the patient's reaction to the stimulus. The analgesic properties of narcotics are related to their ability to diminish both pain perception and the reaction of the patient to pain. These drugs effectively raise the threshold for pain, perhaps because of the euphoria experienced by patients given opioids. For example, a patient in pain who is given morphine experiences a pleasant floating sensation with a great reduction in distress and anxiety. It is interesting to note, however, that some subjects do not experience euphoria when given morphine. In fact, they tend to have an unpleasant response known as dysphoria, which often includes restlessness and a feeling of general discomfort.

Physicians and other health care workers must achieve a delicate balance between alleviating pain from known causes and masking pain as a warning signal from unexpected sources. For example, a patient having abdominal surgery would likely require relatively high doses of analgesics to reduce the postoperative pain. Yet the administration of an analgesic could mask the pain from an unexpected abdominal infection. Therefore, if used excessively, narcotics may prevent the early recognition of complications.

In addition to their analgesic effects, opiates tend to have a sedative effect and are often used as an adjunct to anesthesia. Potent opiates are used in relatively large doses to achieve general anesthesia, particularly in patients undergoing heart surgery. These narcotics are also commonly used during other surgeries in which it is important that heart function be affected only minimally. Examples of narcotic agents used in anesthesia include fentanyl (Sublimaze), sufentanil, alfentanil, and propofol.

Suppression of the cough reflex is a clinically useful effect of opiates. Therapeutic doses needed to reduce coughing are much lower than doses to achieve analgesia. The opioid derivatives most commonly used to suppress the cough reflex are codeine, dextromethorphan, and noscapine. The exact mechanism of action is unknown; however, it is thought to act on the brainstem.

Diarrhea from almost any cause can be controlled with opiates. Diphenoxylate (Lomotil) and loperamide (Imodium) are commonly used to treat diarrhea and do not possess analgesic properties. These drugs appear to act on the nerves within the intestinal tract to decrease muscular activity.

Like all drugs, narcotics have both beneficial and undesired effects. The toxic effects of an opioid depend on the dosage, the agent used, the clinical condition in which it is used, and an individual patient's response to the drug. Some of the more common unwanted side effects include restlessness and hyperactivity instead of sedation, respiratory depression, nausea and vomiting, increased pressure within the brain, low blood pressure, constipation, urinary retention, and itching around the nose. Most of these conditions are of short duration and resolve after the drug has been discontinued.

Patients on chronic opiate therapy may develop tolerance and become physically and mentally dependent upon these agents. Many people abuse narcotics in high dosages in order to experience euphoric effects. With chronic use, the euphoric effects diminish and the user eventually requires higher doses to achieve the same euphoria. Physiological adaptation to the long-term use of opioids (two to three weeks) causes the development of tolerance towards these drugs.

Exogenous opioids take the place of endogenous ones. Therefore, the nervous system and other physiological systems attempt to bring the levels of these neurotransmitters back to normal. First, the liver speeds up its metabolism of the drugs to eliminate them from the system more rapidly. Second, the regions of the nervous system that respond to opioids become desensitized by reducing the number of neural receptors that are available. Finally, after a few weeks of high levels of opiates, changes in other areas of the brain attempt to compensate for the rising opioid levels. Individuals who abruptly stop taking the drugs enter a period of withdrawal in which they experience symptoms similar to a bad case of influenza. Morphine and heroine withdrawal symptoms usually start within twelve hours of the last dose. Peak symptoms of narcotic withdrawal occur after one to two days. Most symptoms gradually subside and resolve after one week. It should be emphasized that, under a physician's direction, the abuse potential of narcotics is very low.

There are certain clinical conditions in which opiates should not be used or should be used with extreme caution. Because of the potential for respiratory depression with opiate treatment, these drugs should not be administered to patients with head injuries or impaired lung function. Most opioid drugs can cross the placenta and therefore should be avoided during pregnancy; with long-term use, the infant can be born addicted to narcotics.

Fortunately, some drugs can reverse the effects of narcotics when required. Three commonly used opioid antagonists are nalmefene, naloxone (Narcan), and naltrexone (Trexan). When these agents are given in the absence of an opioid agonist, they have no noticeable effect. When administered to a morphine-treated patient, however, they completely reverse the opioid effects almost immediately. These narcotic antagonists are particularly useful in treating patients who have taken an overdose of opiates. Such patients often arrive in the hospital emergency room with severe respiratory depression or in a coma. These antagonists will normalize respiration, restore consciousness, and counteract other opioid effects. Interestingly, individuals who have become tolerant to and dependent upon opioids will immediately experience withdrawal symptoms when given naloxone or naltrexone.

Perspective and Prospects

Narcotic drugs were originally found in the opium poppy five thousand years ago. Opium is obtained from the milky fluid of the unripe seed capsules of the poppy plant. The juice is dried in the air and forms a brown, sticky substance. With continued drying, the mass can be pulverized into powder. It is this powder that opiates are derived from. Morphine, codeine, and papaverine are the natural opiates that are used clinically. Most other narcotics are chemically derived.

The opium poppy, Papaver somniferum, was named after the Roman god of sleep, Somnis. Ancient Egyptian medical texts listed opium as a cure for illness and as a poison. Although opium was used extensively, the abuse potential was low because the poppy has a very bitter taste. Smoking opium became popular in eighteenth century China as a treatment for severe diarrhea and was also a socially acceptable drug used mainly for its euphoric effects.

The opium poppy contains more than twenty distinct agents with a variety of potencies and unwanted side effects. In 1806, a pharmacist refined opium into one active substance, morphine, which was found to be ten times as potent. Morphine was named after Morpheus, the Greek god of dreams, because of its powerful sedative effects. The discovery of other medically active agents quickly followed. Codeine and papaverine were identified next and found to be slightly less potent than morphine. At this time, clinicians used these purified products rather than the crude opium juice.

Shortly after purified narcotics became available, so did the widespread use of hypodermic needles. This allowed physicians to administer narcotics directly into the bloodstream. The injected opioids would rapidly travel via the blood to the brain and exert its effects. In the United States, morphine found widespread use as an analgesic for wounded soldiers during the Civil War. It was one of the most powerful painkillers available to physicians, but its unrestricted availability created great potential for addiction with long-term use.

Opioid derivations became so popular that hundreds of medications became available to the public in many different forms. Tonics promised to cure everything from "tired blood" to common aches and pains. Their widespread unregulated usage allowed for potential addiction. At the beginning of the twentieth century, the U.S. government attempted to address this issue by making it illegal to buy any opiate-containing compound without a prescription. Chemists then tried to synthesize compounds with morphine-like characteristics but without the addictive effects.

Physicians now have a vast selection of narcotics with different pharmacological properties to choose from. For example, there are drugs without addictive, euphoric, or sedative properties that can treat coughing or diarrhea. Narcotic analgesics can only be prescribed and administered under the direction of a physician. With proper medical supervision, the benefit of narcotics can be maximized and the side effects, including addiction, can be minimized. Morphine is still used as a potent pain reliever, and when used appropriately, there is less potential for addiction. With further research into opioids and pain pathways, the potential for further medical usage remains an endless possibility.

—*Matthew Berria, Ph.D.;*
updated by Cristina Cesaro, D.O.,
and Jimmy Bajaj, D.O.

See also Addiction; Anesthesia; Anesthesiology; Coughing; Diarrhea and dysentery; Marijuana; Over-the-counter medications; Pain; Pain management; Pharmacology; Prescription drug abuse; Self-medication; Substance abuse

For Further Information:

Acker, Caroline Jean. *Creating the American Junkie: Addiction Research in the Classic Era of Narcotic Control.* Baltimore: Johns Hopkins University Press, 2002. A fascinating examination of how the construction of addiction in the early twentieth century was influenced by a nexus of actors and events: psychiatrists, pharmacologists, and the American Medical Association's campaign to reduce prescriptions of opiates.

Davenport-Hines, Richard. *The Pursuit of Oblivion: A Global History of Narcotics.* New York: W.W. Norton, 2002. Blends social, political, and cultural history to trace the evolution of drugs, their role in society, and addiction.

Griffith, H. Winter. *Complete Guide to Prescription and Nonprescription Drugs.* Revised and updated by Stephen Moore. New York: Penguin Group, 2010. A complete guide to both prescription and nonprescription drugs, including major uses, unwanted effects, precautions, and interactions with other drugs. A highly organized, useful tool for the nonscientist.

Inaba, Darryl S., William E. Cohen, and Michael E. Holstein. *Uppers, Downers, All Arounders: Physical and Mental Effects of Psychoactive Drugs.* 6th ed. Ashland, OR: CNS, 2007. Mainly covers drug abuse, but also contains brief descriptions of the history and medical uses for drugs with abuse potential. A reader-friendly book that offers numerous statements from drug addicts regarding their addiction and, in some cases, their recovery.

Ling, W., and D.R. Wesson. "Drugs of Abuse: Opiates." *Western Journal of Medicine* 152 (May, 1990): 565-572. This article reviews the ways that addiction can be treated. Also addresses the use of narcotic antagonists in the treatment of drug overdose.

Liska, Ken. *Drugs and the Human Body, with Implications for Society.* 8th ed. Upper Saddle River, NJ: Pearson/Prentice Hall, 2009. Examines the use of drugs in the North American culture by discussing such topics as what constitutes a drug and where drugs come from, federal laws, drug metabolism, and the different classifications of drugs.

Voth, Eric A., Robert L. Dupont, and Harold M. Voth. "Responsible Prescribing of Controlled Substances." *American Family Physician* 44 (November, 1991): 1673-1680. This article details some of the important problems in prescribing narcotics. Gives a description of characteristics that both health care workers and nonprofessionals can watch for in their attempts to identify drug abusers.

NASAL POLYP REMOVAL

Procedure

Anatomy or system affected: Head, nose

Specialties and related fields: Family medicine, general surgery, otorhinolaryngology

Definition: The excision of benign growths that project from the mucous membrane lining the nasal cavity.

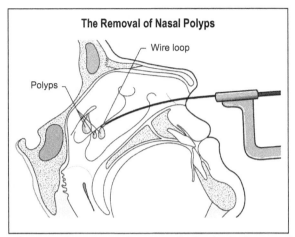

The Removal of Nasal Polyps

Wire loop

Polyps

Allergies or chronic sinus infections can lead to the development of nasal polyps, distended areas of the nasal lining. If they interfere with breathing or the sense of smell or if they cause frequent nosebleeds, the polyps may be removed with a wire loop.

Indications and Procedures

Nasal polyps are swollen masses that project from the nasal wall. These benign structures are commonly found in patients with allergies. They may cause chronic nasal obstruction, which results in diminished air flow through the nasal cavity.

Once a polyp is detected, the physician may prescribe a nasal spray to reduce its size, such as the corticosteroids beclometasone or flunisolide. This treatment is usually effective for small nasal polyps that cause only minor symptoms. When pharmacological management is not successful, the polyps should be removed surgically.

Surgical removal of nasal polyps (nasal polypectomy) is typically done as an outpatient procedure. It requires either general anesthesia or local anesthesia with sedation. After the patient is asleep or sedated, the lining of the nasal cavity is injected with a combination of local anesthesia and epinephrine to control pain and bleeding. The surgeon (usually an otorhinolaryngologist) visualizes the polyps with a headlight, and the polyps are removed with specialized long surgical instruments inserted into the nasal cavity. After the polyps are removed, the nasal passages are packed with ointment-coated gauze to help control bleeding and aid in the healing of the nasal mucosa. The gauze is removed in the physician's office a few days after the surgery. Once the packing is removed, the patient enjoys improved breathing through the nasal passages.

Uses and Complications

There are relatively few complications associated with nasal polyp removal. Some of the more common complications include bleeding from the surgical site, nasal and ear discomfort or anxiety as a result of the packing, and nausea from the anesthesia. The recurrence of nasal polyps after polypectomy is not unusual. Patients with cystic fibrosis have a high rate of occurrence of nasal polyps and often have recurrent problems.

—*Matthew Berria, Ph.D. and Douglas Reinhart, M.D.*

See also Allergies; Nasopharyngeal disorders; Oral and maxillofacial surgery; Otorhinolaryngology; Polyps; Sense organs; Sinusitis; Smell.

For Further Information:

Adelman, Daniel C., Thomas B. Casale, and Jonathan Corren, eds. *Manual of Allergy and Immunology.* 5th ed. Philadelphia: Wolters Kluwer Health/Lippincott Williams & Wilkins, 2012.

Benjamin, Bruce, et al. *A Colour Atlas of Otorhinolaryngology.* Edited by Michael Hawke. Philadelphia: J. B. Lippincott, 1995.

Bull, P. D. *Lecture Notes: Diseases of the Ear, Nose and Throat.* 10th ed. Malden, Mass.: Blackwell Science, 2007.

PDxMD. *PDxMD Ear, Nose, and Throat Disorders.* Philadelphia: Author, 2003.

Icon Health. *Nasal Polyps: A Medical Dictionary, Bibliography, and Annotated Research Guide to Internet References.* San Diego, Calif.: Author, 2004.

Kimball, Chad T. *Colds, Flu, and Other Common Ailments Sourcebook.* Detroit, Mich.: Omnigraphics, 2001.

Lewy, Jennifer, and Marcin Chwistek. "Nasal Polyp." *Health Library,* March 15, 2013.

Morelock, Michael, and J. B. Vap. *Your Guide to Problems of the Ear, Nose, and Throat.* Philadelphia: Lippincott Williams & Wilkins, 1985.

"Nasal Polyps." *Mayo Clinic,* February 19, 2011.

Settipane, Guy A., et al., eds. *Nasal Polyps: Epidemiology, Pathogenesis and Treatment.* Providence, R.I.: OceanSide, 1997.

Vorvick, Linda J., Seth Schwartz, and David Zieve. "Nasal Polyps." *MedlinePlus,* August 31, 2011.

NASOPHARYNGEAL DISORDERS
Disease/Disorder

Anatomy or system affected: Nose, respiratory system, throat

Specialties and related fields: Family medicine, occupational health, otorhinolaryngology

Definition: Disorders of the nose, nasal passages (sinuses), and pharynx (mouth, throat, and esophagus).

Key terms:

acute disease: a short and sharp disease process

chronic disease: a lingering illness

esophagus: the tube that leads from the pharynx to the stomach

larynx: the organ that produces the voice, which lies between the pharynx and the trachea; commonly called the voice box

nasopharyngeal: referring to the nose and pharynx (the upper part of the throat that leads from the mouth to the esophagus)

trachea: a tube that leads from the throat to the lungs; commonly called the windpipe

Causes and Symptoms

Nasopharyngeal disorders are all the diseases that can be present in the nasal cavity and the pharynx. These include the common cold, pharyngitis (sore throat), laryngitis (inflammation of the larynx), epiglottitis (inflammation of the lid over the larynx), tonsillitis (inflammation of the lymph nodes at the rear of the mouth), sinusitis (inflammation of the sinus cavities that surround the nose), otitis media (earache that is often associated with nasopharyngeal infection), nosebleed,

Information on Nasopharyngeal Disorders

Causes: May include bacterial or viral infection, nasal obstruction (polyps), environmental allergens or toxins

Symptoms: Sore throat; inflamed lymph nodes, larynx, and sinus cavities; earache or ear infection; nosebleeds; nasal obstruction; fever; difficulty breathing or swallowing; general malaise; bad breath

Duration: Acute to chronic

Treatments: Antibiotics, over-the-counter medications, surgery; if severe, emergency intubation

nasal obstruction, halitosis (bad breath), and various other disorders.

The common cold is one of the most prevalent diseases that afflict humankind. Pharyngitis, or sore throat, often accompanies the common cold, or it may appear by itself. Acute infections can be caused by viruses or bacteria, often by certain streptococcus strains—hence the common term for the disorder, strep throat. Acute pharyngitis can also be caused by chemicals or radiation. As a chronic disorder, pharyngitis can be caused by lingering infection in other organs such as the lungs and sinuses, or it can be attributable to constant irritation from smoking, drinking alcohol, or breathing polluted air. The usual symptoms of pharyngitis include sore throat, difficulty swallowing, and fever. The infected area appears red and swollen.

Ordinarily, pharyngitis is not serious. If certain strains of streptococcus are the cause, however, then the infection may progress to rheumatic fever. This disease appears to be the result of an immune system reaction to some streptococcus bacteria. It can have painful effects in many parts of the body, including the joints, and can do permanent damage to parts of the heart. In rare cases, rheumatic fever can be fatal.

Acute laryngitis is usually caused by a viral infection, but bacteria, outside irritants, or misuse of the voice are other causes. Ordinarily, the vocal cords produce sounds by vibrating in response to the air passing over them. When inflamed or irritated, they swell, causing distortion in the sounds produced. The affected person's voice becomes hoarse and raspy and may even diminish to a soft whisper. This distortion of sound is the main symptom of laryngitis; other possible symptoms include a sore throat and congestion that causes constant coughing. The condition generally resolves itself and requires no treatment. Chronic laryngitis has the same symptoms but does not go away spontaneously. It may be caused by an infectious agent but more likely is attributable to some irritant activity, such as constantly misusing one's voice, smoking, drinking alcohol, or breathing contaminated air.

The epiglottis is a waferlike tissue covered by a mucous membrane that sits on top of the larynx. It can become infected by such microorganisms as the bacteria *Haemophilus influenzae* type b, causing a condition called epiglottitis. Although the symptoms of epiglottitis can resemble those of pharyngitis, the infection can quickly progress to a very serious, life-threatening disorder. Epiglottitis usually afflicts children from two to four years of age, but adults can also be affected. The infection can begin rapidly, causing the epiglottis to swell and obstruct the airway to the lungs, creating a major medical emergency. Within twelve hours of the onset of symptoms, 50 percent of patients require hospitalization and intubation (insertion of a breathing tube into the trachea). The symptoms are high fever, severe sore throat, difficulty breathing, difficulty swallowing, and general malaise. As the airway becomes more and more occluded, the patient begins to gasp for air. The lack of oxygen may cause cyanosis (blue color in the lips, fingers, and skin), exhaustion, and shock.

Another disease associated with the larynx is croup, or laryngotracheobronchitis. As the medical name indicates, croup involves the larynx, the trachea, and the bronchi (the large branches of the lung). It is usually caused by a virus, but some cases are attributable to bacterial infection. Children from three to five years of age are the usual victims. This disease causes the airways to narrow due to inflammation of the inner mucosal surfaces. Inflammation causes coughing, but the narrowed airway causes the cough to be sharp and brassy, like the barking of a seal. Croup is usually relatively benign, but sometimes it progresses to a severe disease requiring hospitalization.

Various other disorders can afflict the larynx, such as damage to the vocal cords because of infection by bacteria, fungi, or other microorganisms. The vocal cords can also be damaged by misusing one's voice, smoking, or breathing contaminated air. Polyps (masses of tissue growing on the surface), nodes (little knots of tissue), or so-called singer's nodules may develop. Sores called contact ulcers may form on the vocal cords.

Tonsillitis is an inflammation of the tonsils, two large lymph nodes located at the back of the throat. It may also involve the adenoids, lymph nodes located at the top of the throat. The function of these lymph nodes is to remove harmful pathogens (disease-causing organisms) from the nasopharyngeal cavity. At times, the load of microorganisms that they absorb becomes more than they can handle, and they become infected. The tonsils and adenoids may then become enlarged. A sore throat develops, along with a headache, fever, and chills. Glands of the neck and throat feel sore and may become enlarged. Young adults can also suffer from quinsy, or peritonsillar abscess. In this condition, one of the tonsils becomes infected and pus forms between the tonsil and the soft tissue surrounding it. Quinsy is characterized by pain in the throat or the soft palate, pain on swallowing, fever, and a tendency to lean one's head toward the affected side.

The nasal sinuses are four pairs of cavities in the bone around the nose. There are two maxillary sinuses, so called because they are found in the maxilla, or upper jaw. Slightly above and behind them are the ethmoid sinuses, and behind them are the sphenoid sinuses. Sitting over the nose in the lower part of the forehead are the two frontal sinuses. All these sinuses are lined with a mucous membrane and have small openings that lead into the nasal passages. Air moves in and out of the sinuses and allows mucus to drain into the nose.

In acute sinusitis, infection builds up in the mucous membrane of any or all of the sinuses. The membrane lining the sinus swells and shuts the opening into the nasal passages. At the same time, membranes of the nose swell and become congested. Mucus and pus build up inside the sinuses, causing pain and pressure. Most often, sinusitis accompanies the common cold: the mucous membrane that lines the nose extends into the sinuses, so the infection of a cold can readily spread into the sinuses. The various viruses responsible for the common cold may be involved, as well as a wide group of bacteria. Chronic sinusitis can be caused by repeated infections that have allowed scar tissue to build up, closing the sinus openings and impeding mucus drainage, or it may be the result of allergies.

According to the Centers for Disease Control and Prevention, chronic sinusitis is the most common long-term illness in the United States, surpassing the rates for asthma, arthritis, and congestive heart disease and causing nearly fourteen million doctor's office visits per year. For reasons that are not yet understood, sinusitis sufferers are often beset with inflammation of the ducts, trapping mucus, bacteria, and viruses inside and allowing nasal polyps to develop. Researchers have been very interested in finding causes and effective treatments for

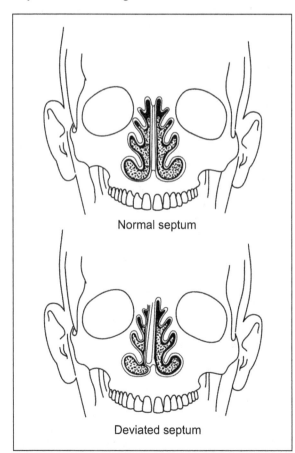

Normal septum

Deviated septum

A deviated septum is a malformation in the cartilage between the nostrils, either present at birth or caused by a blow to the nose.

sinusitis. In the late twentieth century, most chronic cases of sinusitis were treated with fiber-optic surgery that allowed access to the cramped sinus passageways. However, patients often returned within weeks or months with ongoing problems. This fact has recently prompted a reconsideration of the problem and its underlying causes as well as a struggle to redefine sinusitis. Some medical experts suspect that inflammation or the responses of the immune system are the culprit but note that additional research must be completed before any definitive answers are found.

Tissues in the nasopharyngeal cavity may be affected by conditions occurring in other parts of the body. For example, vocal cord paralysis may be caused by vascular accidents, certain cancers, tissue trauma, and other events.

Some infections in the nasopharyngeal cavity can spread to the ear through the eustachian tubes that connect the two areas. Chief among the diseases of the ear that can be associated with nasopharyngeal disorders are the various forms of acute otitis media, an earache occurring in the central part of the ear. There are four basic types of otitis media. In the first type, serous otitis media, there is usually no infection, but fluid accumulates inside the middle ear because of the blockage of the eustachian tube or the overproduction of fluid; the condition is usually mild, with some pain and temporary loss of hearing. The second type is otitis media with effusion; with this condition comes both infection and accumulation of fluid. The third form is acute purulent otitis media, the most serious type. Pus builds up inside the middle ear, and its pressure may rupture the eardrum, allowing discharge of blood and pus. The fourth type is secretory otitis media, which usually occurs after several bouts of otitis media. Cells within the middle ear start producing a fluid that is thicker than normal and produced in greater amounts.

Chronic otitis media is bacterial in origin. It is characterized by a perforation of the eardrum and chronic pus discharge. The eardrum is a flat, pliable disk of tissue that vibrates to conduct sounds from the outside to the inner-ear structures. The perforation that occurs in chronic otitis media can be one of two types: a relatively benign perforation occurring in the central part of the eardrum or a potentially dangerous perforation occurring near the edges of the eardrum. The latter perforation can be associated with loss of hearing, increased discharge of pus and other fluids, facial paralysis, and the spread of infection to other tissues. When the perforation of chronic otitis media is near the edges of the eardrum, something called a cholesteatoma develops. This accumulation of matter grows in the inner ear and can be destructive to bone and other tissue.

The same organisms that cause otitis media can be responsible for a condition called mastoiditis. The mastoid process is a bone structure lined with a mucous membrane. Infection from otitis media can spread to this area and in severe cases can destroy the bone. Mastoiditis used to be a leading cause of death in children.

Nosebleeds are common and most often result from a blow to the nose, but they can also be caused by colds, sinusitis, and breathing dry air. The septum (the cartilaginous tissue that separates the nostrils) and the surrounding intranasal mucous membrane contain many tiny blood vessels that are easily ruptured. If an individual receives a blow to the nose, these vessels can break and bleed. They can also rupture due to irritation from a cold or other condition. Breathing very dry air sometimes causes the nasal mucous membrane to crust over, and bleeding can follow. Nosebleeds are not usually serious, but sometimes they are indicative of an underlying condition, such as hypertension (high blood pressure), a tumor, or another disease.

Nasal obstruction is common during colds and allergy attacks, but it can also be caused by a deviated septum, a malformation in the cartilage between the nostrils that can be congenital or caused by a blow to the nose. Nasal obstruction can also be attributable to nasal polyps, nasal tumors, or swollen adenoids. A common source of nasal obstruction is overuse of nasal decongestants. These agents relieve nasal congestion by reducing intranasal inflammation and swelling. If used too often or for too long, however, they can cause the very problem that they were intended to cure: intranasal blood vessels dilate, the area swells, secretions increase, and the nose becomes blocked. This is known as rebound congestion or, in medical terminology, rhinitis medicamentosa (nasal inflammation that is caused by a medication).

Halitosis, or bad breath, can be considered a nasopharyngeal disorder in the sense that it can originate in the mouth. It can be caused by diseases of the teeth or gums, but the most common causes are smoking or eating aromatic foods such as onions and garlic. Bad breath may also be a sign of disease conditions in other parts of the body, such as certain lung disorders or cancer of the esophagus. Hepatic failure, a liver dysfunction, may be accompanied by a fishy odor on the breath. Azotemia, the retention of nitrogen in the blood, may give rise to an ammonia-like odor. A sweet, fruity odor on the breath of diabetic patients may accompany ketoacidosis, a condition that occurs when there are high levels of glucose in the blood. Sometimes, young children stick foreign objects or other materials into their noses; it has been reported that these materials can fester, causing severe halitosis. Bad breath is rarely apparent to the individual who has it, however offensive it may be to others. A good way to check one's breath is to lick the back of one's hand and smell the spot; malodor, if it exists, will usually be apparent.

Treatment and Therapy

Nasopharyngeal disorders are most often mild illnesses that can be treated at home. For example, acute pharyngitis, or sore throat, is easily managed most of the time. The patient is advised to rest, gargle with warm salt water several times a day, and soothe the pain with lozenges or anesthetic gargles. If the infection is caused by a virus, it usually will clear without further treatment. If the physician suspects that the infection is bacterial in origin, throat smears may be taken so that the organism can be identified. If bacteria are discovered, antibiotic therapy will be undertaken to eradicate the pathogens. This is particularly important if the infection is caused by certain strains of streptococcus bacteria. In this case, it is vital to

destroy the organism in order to avoid the development of rheumatic fever.

In cases of acute laryngitis caused by viral infection, the patient is advised to rest his or her voice, inhale steam, and drink warm liquids. If bacteria are the cause of the laryngitis, antibiotic therapy is undertaken. In treating chronic laryngitis, the physician must discover the cause and remove it. If allergy is the cause, antihistamine therapy could help. If the cause is bacterial, antibiotic therapy is used. If smoking or drinking alcohol is the problem, the patient should be counseled to stop. The simple palliative measures used for acute laryngitis—resting the voice, drinking warm liquids, and breathing steam—are also useful for chronic laryngitis.

Symptoms of epiglottitis are often similar to those of sore throat. If there is any evidence of difficulty in breathing, however, the patient should be seen by a physician quickly, as an emergency situation may be developing. If epiglottitis is obstructing the airway, the patient should be treated in an intensive care setting. Antibiotics must be given to the patient to treat the infection. It is important to make an airway for the patient, and it may be necessary to insert a tube into the trachea to allow the patient to breathe.

Before the age of antibiotics, tonsillitis was often treated surgically, with both tonsils and adenoids removed. This procedure is now rare, as the infection usually responds to antibiotic therapy. Similarly, in the case of peritonsillar abscess or quinsy, antibiotics usually clear the condition satisfactorily. In some cases, accumulations of pus may be removed surgically. If the abscesses return, it may be advisable to remove the tonsils.

As a rule, a child with croup is treated at home. Because the disease is usually caused by viruses, antibiotics are not used unless bacteria are known to be involved. Steam is often used to help liquefy mucus deposits on the interior walls of the trachea, the larynx, and the bronchi. The patient is given warm liquids to drink and is closely watched so that any signs that the condition is getting worse will be detected. The following symptoms should alert the caregiver to the possibility that an emergency situation is developing and that medical help is needed quickly: drooling, difficulty breathing or swallowing, inability to bend the neck forward, blue or dark color in the lips, high-pitched sounds when inhaling, rapid heartbeat, and loss of consciousness.

The main goals of therapy for sinusitis are to control infection, relieve the blockage of the sinus openings to permit drainage, and relieve pain. When sinusitis is known to be of bacterial origin, an appropriate antibiotic will be used to eradicate the organism. Often, however, sinusitis is attributable to viral infection, and other procedures are used to treat it. Inhaling steam is useful for thinning secretions and promoting drainage, as are mucolytic agents such as guaifenesin. Decongestant sprays and oral decongestants reduce swelling and open passages. Analgesics can be given for pain. In certain circumstances, the sinuses are drained surgically.

Acute otitis media is most often diagnosed with the aid of an otoscope, an instrument that the doctor uses to look at the eardrum and surrounding tissues. The eardrum will be a dull red color, bulging, and perhaps perforated. While a viral infection may precede otitis media, the causative microorganisms for this and related ear infections, such as mastoiditis, are usually bacteria. Antibiotics are used both to treat the infections and to prevent the spread of disease to other areas. The drugs are usually taken orally. Penicillin and its derivatives are used, as are erythromycin and sulfisoxazole. Antibiotic therapy for acute otitis media is usually continued for ten days to two weeks. Sometimes pus and other fluids and solid matter build up in the inner ear, and it may be necessary to pierce the eardrum in order to remove these deposits. To help relieve blockage of the eustachian tubes, a topical vasoconstrictor may be used in the nose to reduce the swelling of blood vessels. Antihistamines could be helpful to patients with allergies but are otherwise not indicated.

For chronic otitis media, it is necessary to clean both the outer ear canal and the middle ear thoroughly. A mild acetic acid solution with a corticosteroid is used for a week to ten days. Meanwhile, aggressive oral antibiotic therapy is undertaken to eradicate the pathogen. The perforated eardrum associated with chronic otitis media can usually be repaired surgically with little or no loss of function, and the cholesteatoma must be surgically removed.

Simple nosebleeds can be treated by pinching the nose with the fingers and breathing through the mouth for five or ten minutes to allow the blood to clot. Also, a plug of absorbent paper or cloth can be inserted into the bleeding nostril. A nosebleed that does not stop easily should be seen by a physician.

Nasal obstruction resulting from colds or allergies is treated by appropriate medications, decongestants for colds and antihistamines for allergies. A deviated septum may require surgery. The only therapy for rhinitis medicamentosa, or rebound congestion caused by overuse of nasal decongestants, is to stop the medication and endure the congestion for as long as it takes the condition to clear. Sometimes it is necessary to consult a physician.

For simple halitosis caused by smoking or food, breath fresheners (with or without "odor-fighting" chemicals) are often used, even though they usually simply replace a "bad" odor with a "good" one. Some people believe that chewing parsley or other leaves rich in chlorophyll will counteract the smell of garlic. When halitosis is attributable to tooth or gum disease, it will persist until the condition is cured. Halitosis may be of diagnostic value in certain situations where a characteristic odor could alert the physician to the possibility of a disease condition.

Perspective and Prospects

Diseases and infections of the nasal cavity and throat have always been common among human populations, as have therapies to deal with them. Until the advent of antibiotics, some of these disorders were quite serious, especially in young children, but modern medications and surgeries, where appropriate, have greatly lessened the danger. The widespread use of a vaccine against *Haemophilus influenzae* type b, the most common causative organism of epiglottitis, has made this life-threatening disease a rarity. Many over-the-counter drugs are used to combat sore throats, sinus congestion, and other nasopharyngeal symptoms of the common cold, although colds themselves remain incurable because of the hundreds or thousands of different microorganisms that may be responsible.

Despite the numerous medications that can be taken, however, more serious infections or diseases, such as chronic tonsillitis or laryngitis, require a doctor's care, with more potent prescription drugs and surgery if needed. The treatments available to physicians and patients for the symptoms of nasopharyngeal disorders are many, but the search continues for better drugs and perhaps preventive measures such as vaccinations to address the causes of these conditions.

—C. Richard Falcon

See also Allergies; Antihistamines; Choking; Common cold; Decongestants; Ear infections and disorders; Ears; Earwax; Esophagus; Halitosis; Hearing; Hearing loss; Laryngectomy; Laryngitis; Mouth and throat cancer; Multiple chemical sensitivity syndrome; Nasal polyp removal; Nosebleeds; Oral and maxillofacial surgery; Otorhinolaryngology; Pharyngitis; Pharynx; Plastic surgery; Respiration; Rhinitis; Rhinoplasty and submucous resection; Sinusitis; Smell; Sore throat; Strep throat; Taste; Tonsillectomy and adenoid removal; Tonsillitis; Tonsils; Voice and vocal cord disorders.

For Further Information:

Friedman, Ellen M., and James P. Barassi. *My Ear Hurts! A Complete Guide to Understanding and Treating Your Child's Ear Infections.* Darby, Pa.: Diane, 2004.

Greene, Alan R. *The Parent's Complete Guide to Ear Infections.* Allentown, Pa.: People's Medical Society, 1999.

Kimball, Chad T. *Colds, Flu, and Other Common Ailments Sourcebook.* Detroit: Omnigraphics, 2001.

Litin, Scott C., ed. *Mayo Clinic Family Health Book.* 4th ed. New York: HarperResource, 2009.

PDxMD. *PDxMD Ear, Nose, and Throat Disorders.* Philadelphia: Author, 2003.

Wagman, Richard J., ed. *The New Complete Medical and Health Encyclopedia.* 4 vols. Chicago: J. G. Ferguson, 2002.

NATIONAL CANCER INSTITUTE (NCI)

Organization

Definition: A federal agency devoted to the study of cancer, as well as communication and education about this condition.

Key terms:

carcinogenesis: the biological process of the initiation, promotion, and progression of cancer

epidemiology: the study of the relationships between a host, an agent, and an environment that lead to a condition or disease

Overview

The US Department of Health and Human Services (HHS) is the federal agency responsible for public health. The HHS includes eleven divisions, one of which is the National Institutes of Health (NIH). The National Cancer Institute (NCI) is one of twenty-seven institutes and centers within the NIH. The institute was established in 1937 under the National

Cancer Institute Act and in 1944 was made part of the National Institutes of Health under the Public Health Service Act. NCI is the principal federal agency for cancer research and training. Following special legislation in 1971 that amended the Public Health Service Act and created the National Cancer Act, the scope of the NCI has continued to broaden through new initiatives and legislation.

The purpose of the NCI is to eliminate cancer as far as possible and to discover treatment for those cancers which cannot be eradicated. The NCI approaches these goals by supporting research, coordinating efforts in prevention and treatment, facilitating the movement of research findings into medicine, and providing education and resources for patients and their families, health educators, and scientists. The NCI conducts research in its own laboratories and clinics in Bethesda, Maryland, but also supports and coordinates research projects conducted by universities, hospitals, research foundations, and businesses throughout the United States and many other countries.

The Organization and Focus of the NCI

The NCI is organized by the Office of the Director into nearly thirty centers, offices, and divisions. Each of the intiatives specializes in a different aspect of cancer research, although there is overlap among them. The Office of Cancer Centers, for example, supports cancer research at academic and research institutions across the United States, while the Office of Cancer Genomics specifically supports research programs that focus on the molecular components of cancer.

Another group, the Office of Cancer Nanotechnology Research, is in charge of the NCI Alliance for Nanotechnology in Cancer Program, which works to develop nanotechnology-based tools for research, detection, treatment, monitoring, and prevention. The Center to Reduce Cancer Health Disparities works through research, training, and partnerships to reduce cancer disparities among diverse populations. The Center for Global Health fosters international collaboration and sharing of research resources among government agencies, nongovernment organizations, biotechnology companies, and pharmaceutical companies. In 1998, the Office of Cancer Complementary and Alternative Medicine was established to coordinate research and communication activities in the arena of complementary and alternative medicine, both within the NCI and with other agencies.

The main purpose of the NCI's basic, clinical intramural research program, the Center for Cancer Research, is to improve the lives of those affected by cancer as well as by HIV/AIDS. The NCI's other intramural initiative is the Division of Cancer Epidemiology and Genetics, whose goal is prevention. This division focuses on the factors that could lead to cancer growth, namely genetic predisposition, lifestyle factors, environmental contaminants, occupational exposures, medications, radiation, and infectious agents; the group also works on epidemiological methods development.

Research in cancer cell biology, such as carcinogenesis and cancer immunology, falls within the realm of the extramural Division of Cancer Biology. This division also examines the biological and health effects of exposures to ionizing and nonionizing radiation. The efforts of the Division of Cancer Prevention center on early detection methods and the efficacy of nutritional or lifestyle changes on cancer prevention. The results of research in this area led to the 5 a Day for Better Health program. Initiated in 1991, this program is a collaborative effort between the food industry and the NCI, which encourages Americans to eat five or more servings of vegetables and fruits each day as part of a low-fat, high-fiber diet. The goal of this type of diet is to prevent the risk of cancer, heart disease, diabetes, and stroke. The Division of Cancer Treatment and Diagnosis includes programs in biomedical imaging, cancer diagnosis, cancer therapy evaluation, developmental therapeutics, and radiation research. The Division of Cancer Control and Population Sciences supports a wide array of research in the areas of surveillance, genetics, epidemiology, and behavior.

The mission of the Coordinating Center for Clinical Trials (CCCT), established in 2006, is to facilitate the bringing of new scientific discoveries and tools to the medical clinic. Research areas supported by the CCCT include cancer genetics, cancer vaccines and immunotherapy, molecular therapeutics, experimental transplantation, and advanced technology. The clinical cancer genetics program integrates all aspects of clinical and laboratory medicine, particularly in studies of breast, colon, renal, and prostate cancer. Processes include molecular diagnostics, novel imaging techniques, and the molecular assessment of normal tissues in at-risk populations. The cancer vaccines and immunotherapy program investigates the clinical feasibility of using vaccines against known conditions associated with cancer, such as the human papillomavirus (HPV vaccines Cervarix and Gardasil) and human immunodeficiency virus (HIV), as well as with cancer-specific products, such as in melanoma and in lymphomas. The molecular therapeutics program is concerned with most clinical trial experiments. Important discoveries include the development of paclitaxel (Taxol) as an effective anticancer agent, the development of zidovudine (AZT, Retrovir) as an important anti-HIV drug, and the use of adoptive immunotherapy in the treatment of malignant melanoma. The scientific thrust of the molecular therapeutics program is the belief that the analysis of the molecular profile of individual cancers will help determine the most effective chemotherapeutic approaches. The experimental transplantation program examines bone marrow biology in order to advance transplantation techniques and the effectiveness of this approach.

Integrating many programs and divisions is the advanced technology initiative. New technology is an essential key to identifying genetic elements involved in cancer initiation and progression, as well as in drug efficacy and drug resistance. Although many drugs have been discovered that inhibit the growth of cancer cells successfully, they also affect healthy cells. This causes side effects that have a negative impact on patients" health and quality of life. New therapeutics and technology have been investigated to minimize or eliminate these side effects and enhance the effectiveness of therapy.

Another division of the NCI is the Division of Extramural Activities, which is responsible for handling all applications for funding and for monitoring research that has received funding from the NCI. Extramural activities also include the oversight of scientific communications. To enhance communication, the NCI has a number of advisory boards and groups that provide the institute with input from the public, medical, and research communities.

The NCI has helped strengthen the information base for cancer care decision making. Researchers, medical providers, and patients seek to better understand what constitutes quality cancer care. The Cancer Information Service, established in 1975, is the section of the NCI that is the link to the public, attempting to explain research findings in a clear, timely, and understandable manner. To this end, the Cancer Information Service helps develop education efforts that target minority audiences and people with limited access to health care information or services.

Perspective and Prospects

To be successful in managing this range of responsibilities and breadth of mission, the NCI has a budget in the billions of dollars. Although cancer is the second leading cause of death in the United States and is a leading cause of death worldwide, through the years, the work of the NCI has led to a decline in the number of deaths due to this disease. Creative and dedicated scientists at the NCI are committed to lowering its numbers even further.

—*Karen Chapman-Novakofski, R.D., L.D.N., Ph.D.*

See also Cancer; Chemotherapy; Clinical trials; Department of Health and Human Services; Environmental diseases; Environmental health; Epidemiology; Genetics and inheritance; National Institutes of Health (NIH); Nutrition; Oncology; Preventive medicine; Radiation therapy.

For Further Information:

"About NCI." *National Cancer Institute,* 2013.

"Cancer." *World Health Organization,* Jan. 2013.

"Cancer: Addressing the Cancer Burden at a Glance." *Centers for Disease Control and Prevention,* 30 Aug. 2012.

Hewitt, Maria Elizabeth, et al., eds. *Ensuring Quality Cancer Care.* Washington, DC: National Academy Press, 1999.

Lerner, Barron H. *The Breast Cancer Wars: Fear, Hope, and the Pursuit of a Cure in Twentieth-Century America.* New York: Oxford University Press, 2003.

National Cancer Institute. *The Cancer Information Service: A Fifteen-Year History of Service and Research.* Bethesda, Md.: Author, 1993.

National Cancer Institute. *National Cancer Institute's Research Programs: Pursuing the Central Questions of Cancer Research.* Bethesda, Md.: Author, 1999.

National Cancer Institute. *NCI Fact Book.* Bethesda, Md.: Author, 1979.

"NCI Mission Statement." National Cancer Institute, 2013.

"NCI Organization." *National Cancer Institute,* 2013.

Reuben, Suzanne H. *Assessing Progress, Advancing Change: 2005–2006 Annual Report.* Bethesda, Md.: National Institutes of Health, National Cancer Institute, 2006.

Varmus, Harold. "Professional Judgment Budget 2013." *National Cancer Institute,* 2013.

NATIONAL INSTITUTES OF HEALTH (NIH)
Organization

Definition: The National Institutes of Health (NIH), composed of more than twenty-five separate institutes, centers, and offices, is one of eight agencies constituting the U.S. Department of Health and Human Services.

Key terms:

AIDSLINE: a database that is part of the National Library of Medicine (NLM) and is devoted to the topic of research on acquired immunodeficiency syndrome (AIDS)

CATLINE: the online catalog of books and manuscripts in the NLM

grant proposals: research plans that outline scientific methods to pursue new knowledge, the required budget, and the resulting products and significance of that work

institute: a specific subagency of the NIH that has the charge of advancing scientific discovery and clinical practice in a specific area of medical science

MEDLINE: a database that is available via the Internet featuring current and historical medical literature, research articles, monographs, presentations, and abstracts

History and Mission

The National Institutes of Health (NIH) is a US federal agency that occupies a multibuilding campus in Bethesda, Maryland. It consists of a variety of offices, institutes focused on specific medical problems, research laboratories and centers, a center for scientific review, and a national medical library. Its main goal is to discover knowledge that will improve the state of public health for all persons, especially those in the United States. This goal extends to all medical conditions afflicting men, women, and children of all ethnic backgrounds. It also extends to seeking knowledge in areas of basic biological research, clinical research, and research on policy and practice in health care.

The National Institute of Health (precursor to the NIH) was formally established by the Ransdell Act of 1930, which bestowed the name on what was formerly called the Hygienic Laboratory (HL) of the Marine Hospital Service (MHS) in New York. The Ransdell Act also allowed for the establishment of fellowships for basic medical and biological research. The very beginnings of the NIH extend back to 1887, however, when basic laboratory work into medical problems was pursued by the MHS, the founding body of the United States Public Health Service (PHS). The MHS was formed in 1798 to provide hospital care for seamen, but by the 1880s it had shifted its focus to screening ship passengers for infectious diseases capable of starting epidemics.

New European research in the 1880s suggesting that microorganisms caused such diseases spurred American interest in medical research and helped form the original HL. Work by the HL continued, with the laboratory eventually moving from the MHS to its own Washington, DC, campus. The study of microorganisms continued, extending from study of individual persons to studying the effects of bacteria on water and air pollution. Progress for such work was rewarded in 1901 with governmental money for the construction of a building (completed in 1904) to house the HL and further foster work focused on advancing the public health. Because the value of such work was not well established, however, no permanent funding was provided, leaving the organization subject to ongoing evaluation and supplemental funding.

In 1902 the MHS was reorganized and renamed the Public Health and Marine Hospital Service (PH-MHS); in 1912 it adopted the shortened name of the Public Health Service (PHS). During the intervening time, the HL continued its work and expanded to work in chemistry, pharmacology, zoology, immunology, and the regulation and production of vaccines and antitoxins. Additionally, new scientific staff were added to the staff of medical doctors already on board. Changes in the mission of the organization in 1912 also opened the door for the pursuit of research on noncontagious diseases and water pollution. This work continued during World War I in the form of examining sanitation, anthrax outbreaks, smallpox, tetanus, influenza, and other combat-related conditions. The success of the PHS's work in these areas caught the attention of legislators and resulted in the Ransdell Act of 1930, which established both the National Institute of Health and the practice of setting aside public monies for funding medical research. In 1937, the National Cancer Institute (NCI) was created. In 1944, the PHS formally designated the NCI as a component of the NIH, setting the pattern of a problem-focused structure within the NIH that continues to the present.

World War II led the NIH to focus almost exclusively on war-related problems. This involved examinations of fitness for military service and issues such as dental problems and syphilis. The effects of hazardous substances and conditions on workers in war industries; risks armed service professionals faced from lack of oxygen, cold temperatures, and blood clots while flying; burns, shock, bacterial infections, and fever; and the development of vaccines and therapies for tropical diseases such as malaria also composed much of its work during this time.

Successes established during the wars by such medical research led the PHS to take the 1944 Public Health Service Act to Congress. This act led to grant-funding mechanisms being extended from the NCI alone to the entire National Institute of Health. Additionally, an increasing public interest in health organizations caused Congress to create additional institutes for research on mental health, dental diseases, and heart disease between 1946 and 1949. In 1948, the National Heart Act allowed for the formal pluralization of the National Institutes of Health, rather than a singular institute with the NCI as a subinstitute. The Public Health Service Act of 1944 also provided funding for the Warren Grant Magnuson Clinical Center, which opened in 1953 to focus exclusively on clinical research on health.

From this point forward, each of the individual institutes now composing the NIH came into being. By 1960 there were ten institutes, and by 2013 there were twenty-seven institutes and centers. As different health interests develop and ad-

vances in medical knowledge are needed, the NIH has responded by allocating its resources to pursue goals in those areas. This has been done both by developing institutes and also by creating specialized offices to pursue contemporary medical problems.

Illness and medicine know no boundaries, however, so the NIH has also maintained an interest in global public health issues. Such interest was formally shown in 1947, when grants were first awarded to investigators abroad. Similarly, in 1968, the John E. Fogarty International Center (FIC) was created to coordinate international research efforts, involving liaisons with the World Health Organization and a variety of international research organizations. The FIC also supports language translation, documentation, and reviews of new health findings. It facilitates biomedical communications through its maintenance of the National Library of Medicine (NLM), MEDLINE, CATLINE, AIDSLINE, and numerous other databases for researchers, physicians, and the public at large. Similarly, focused consensus development conferences, where investigators and clinicians from around the world can meet to evaluate new and existing therapies, are another way in which international interests are pursued.

In keeping with its practical focus, the NIH has strived to seek out knowledge that yields new drugs, devices, and procedures that are useful not just for the government but for the public at large as well. In 1986, the Technology Transfer Act allowed for a partnership between NIH-funded research and the private sector. Encouraging researchers to examine possible commercial and practical applications of basic medical research to wide-reaching clinical or research use benefits overall scientific and health progress. Partnering with business allows private industries to take over the process of marketing and developing products in a manner more affordable to them than to the government, allowing the government to focus on development while benefiting through the use of the eventual marketed products.

Organizational Structure and Method

The NIH is organized to accomplish its goals by using its offices, institutes, and research centers. Research is conducted on the NIH campus in its own funded laboratories as well as in the labs of scientists supported by NIH funding, who are stationed in institutes of higher education, teaching hospitals, and research institutions in the United States and other countries. In addition to supporting ongoing research, the NIH also supports research infrastructure by maintaining a library and a variety of printed and electronic resources to facilitate communication among its researchers, the larger scientific community, policymakers, and the public. Scientific research also is supported through development of one of the most valuable resources known to medicine: new researchers. The NIH sponsors a variety of training programs focusing on medical training and research in order to keep a large body of high-quality scholars and investigators in development. Such programs extend from career development for postdoctoral researchers and predoctoral training, to high school level learning in the sponsoring of internships and other learning experiences for teenagers interested in medical science careers.

Funding for research and training programs outside the NIH campus and research centers is facilitated through grant proposal programs that distribute federal tax monies devoted to such endeavors. Applicants to such programs are able to submit independent proposals for work related to the goals of the NIH that they believe is demanded by the state of science and knowledge. They are also able to submit proposals in response to program announcements and calls for proposals on specific topics as outlined by the institutes and offices of the NIH. Many different grant mechanisms exist for such proposals, including grants supporting the work of individual trainees, training programs for cohorts of researchers at different stages of career development, the ongoing work of career scientists, small grants for new or experimental work, focused projects, and even centers of research excellence where many researchers focus on the same topic of study. In addition, grant support is offered to sponsor conferences and academic meetings on special topics in health research and training.

To receive this funding, those wishing to be considered must submit proposals for confidential peer review through the Center for Scientific Review (CSR), which is part of the NIH structure. Proposals are reviewed by panels of experts who evaluate the research plans, goals, staff, environment, and overall innovation and merit of the work proposed. In addition, ethical considerations about the proposed research are reviewed and considered for both animal welfare and the welfare of human research participants. Emphasis on ethical issues has been a long-standing issue for medical research. It was, however, highlighted in the 1960s, when grantees receiving NIH grant monies were required to state the ethical principles guiding their research on humans, and in 1979, when written guidelines for research on human subjects were established. Once through peer review, proposals are reviewed again by a national advisory council to determine the priority of the work in addressing the goals of the NIH and its institutes and offices. After the proposals are approved by this council for advancement, the individual institutes (sometimes cooperating with specific NIH offices) work to fund them with the monies allotted. Unfortunately, not all proposals can be funded. It should be noted that even after funding, the work of the NIH continues so as to ensure that proper research ethics are followed through the life of the research.

Research funded by the NIH is facilitated by the various institutions and research offices that fall under its organizational umbrella, each focusing on a discrete area of health interest. Some of the institutions involved include the NCI; the National Eye Institute; the National Heart, Lung, and Blood Institute; and the National Human Genome Research Institute. Also included are the National Institutes on Aging, Alcohol Abuse and Alcoholism, Allergy and Infectious Diseases, Arthritis and Musculoskeletal and Skin Diseases, Child Health and Human Development, Deafness and Other Communication Disorders, Dental and Craniofacial Research, Diabetes and Digestive and Kidney Diseases, Drug Abuse, Environmental Health Sciences, Mental Health, Minority Health and Health Disparities, and Neurological Disorders and Stroke.

In addition to these institutes, the NIH has numerous offices focusing on specific issues or populations that need to be addressed in health research. These offices focus on contemporary issues of importance for research and include the Offices of Technology Transfer, AIDS Research, Research on Women's Health, Behavioral and Social Sciences Research, Dietary Supplements, Rare Diseases, Science Policy, Biotechnology Activities, Science Education, and Information Technology. There are also offices that focus on the management of research, specific organizational issues at the NIH, or the communication of information from the NIH to members of the public. These include the Offices of Intramural Research, Extramural Research, Evaluation, Human Resources, Financial Management, Acquisition and Logistics Management, Management Assessment, and Communications and Public Liaison as well as the NIH Legal Advisor and the Freedom of Information Act Office.

Perspective and Prospects

The NIH has been responsible for supporting some very influential research for more than one hundred years, garnering more than eighty Nobel Prizes for NIH-supported work. More vaccines against infectious diseases are available than ever before. The successful mapping of the human genome has set the stage for enhanced genetic testing and the development of gene therapies. Substantial decreases in mortality rates have been achieved for heart disease and strokes. Survival rates for individuals afflicted by cancer have increased, as have survival rates for infants with respiratory distress syndrome. Recovery from spinal cord injuries has been enhanced so as to lessen the probability of long-term disability. Advances in the pharmacological and behavioral treatment of mental health problems such as depression, anxiety, bipolar disorders, and schizophrenia have been achieved. Preventive approaches in dentistry have been highly successful in stopping and slowing dental problems.

Given such successes, billions of dollars of federal tax monies continue to be devoted to the NIH budget to foster continued scientific advances. New work focused on improving prevention, screening, assessment, diagnosis, and treatment for conditions such as AIDS, alcoholism and drug dependence, Alzheimer's disease, arthritis, blindness, communication disorders, diabetes, heart disease, kidney disease, lung cancer, lupus, mental illnesses, Parkinson's disease, stroke, and other persisting conditions continues on a daily basis. While great successes have been achieved to date, new research is needed that will focus on specialized approaches that may enhance health for women, minorities, youth, and the elderly. The combination of these needs, past successes, and governmental commitment to improving the state of the public health ensures that the NIH will continue onward with its mission for the foreseeable future.

—*Nancy A. Piotrowski, Ph.D.*

See also Childhood infectious diseases; Department of Health and Human Services; Disease; Environmental diseases; Environmental health; Epidemics and pandemics; Epidemiology; Health Canada; Immunization and vaccination; National Cancer Institute (NCI); Occupational health; World Health Organization.

For Further Information:

Desalle, Rob. *Epidemic! The World of Infectious Disease.* New York: New Press, 1999.

Eberhart-Philips, Jason. *Outbreak Alert: Responding to the Increasing Threat of Infectious Diseases.* Oakland, Calif.: New Harbinger, 2000.

Garrett, Laurie. *Betrayal of Trust: The Collapse of Global Public Health.* New York: Hyperion, 2001.

Guest, Charles, et al. Oxford Handbook of Public Health Practice. 3d ed. Oxford: Oxford University Press, 2013.

Institute of Medicine. *Scientific Opportunities and Public Needs: Improving Priority Setting and Public Input at the National Institutes of Health.* Washington, D.C.: National Academy Press, 1998.

Lee, Philip R., and Carroll L. Estes, eds. *The Nation's Health.* 7th ed. Sudbury, Mass.: Jones and Bartlett, 2003.

National Institutes of Health. "About NIH." US Department of Health and Human Services, June 6, 2013.

National Institutes of Health. "Institutes, Centers, and Offices." US Department of Health and Human Services, August 1, 2013.

Shnayerson, Michael, and Mark J. Plotkin. *The Killers Within: The Deadly Rise of Drug Resistant Bacteria.* Boston: Little, Brown, 2003.

Tulchinsky, Theodore H., and Elena A. Varavikova. *The New Public Health: An Introduction for the Twenty-first Century.* San Diego, Calif.: Academic Press, 2000.

Nausea and Vomiting

Disease/Disorder

Anatomy or system affected: Brain, gastrointestinal system, nervous system, stomach

Specialties and related fields: Gastroenterology, otorhinolaryngology

Definition: Nausea is an unpleasant subjective sensation, accompanied by epigastric and duodenal discomfort, which often culminates in vomiting, the regurgitation of the contents of the stomach.

Key terms:

affect: the emotional reactions associated with experience

antiemetics: drugs that prevent or relieve the symptoms of nausea and/or vomiting

chemoreceptor trigger zone: a sensory nerve ending in the brain that is stimulated by and reacts to certain chemical stimulation localized outside the central nervous system

emesis: the act of vomiting

psychogenic: of mental origin

psychotropics: drugs that affect psychic function, behavior, or experience

Causes and Symptoms

Nausea is defined as a subjectively unpleasant sensation associated with awareness of the urge to vomit. It is usually felt in the back of the throat and epigastrium and is accompanied by the loss of gastric tone, duodenal contractions, and reflux of the intestinal contents into the stomach. Retching is

defined as labored, spasmodic, rhythmic contractions of the respiratory muscles (including the diaphragm, chest wall, and abdominal wall muscles) without the expulsion of gastric contents. Vomiting, or emesis, is the forceful expulsion of gastric contents from the mouth and is brought about by the powerful sustained contraction of the abdominal muscles, the descent of the diaphragm, and the opening of the gastric cardia (the cardiac orifice of the stomach).

Nausea and vomiting are important defense mechanisms against the ingestion of toxins. The act of emesis involves a sequence of events that can be divided into three phases: preejection, ejection, and postejection. The preejection phase includes the symptoms of nausea, along with salivation, swallowing, pallor, and tachycardia (an abnormally fast heartbeat). The ejection phase comprises retching and vomiting. Retching is characterized by rhythmic, synchronous, inspiratory movements of the diaphragm, abdominal, and external intercostal muscles, while the mouth and the glottis are kept closed. As the antral (cavity) portion of the stomach contracts, the proximal (nearest the center) portion relaxes and the gastric contents oscillate between the stomach and the esophagus. During retching, the hiatal portion of the diaphragm does not relax, and intra-abdominal pressure increases are associated with a decrease in intrathoracic pressure.

In contrast, relaxation of the hiatal portion of the diaphragm (near the esophagus) permits a transfer of intra-abdominal pressure to the thorax during the act of vomiting. Contraction of the muscles of the anterior abdominal wall, relaxation of the esophageal sphincter, an increase in intrathoracic and intragastric pressure, reverse peristalsis (movement of the contents of the alimentary canal), and an open glottis and mouth result in the expulsion of gastric contents. The postejection phase consists of autonomic and visceral responses that return the body to a quiescent phase, with or without residual nausea.

The complex act of vomiting, involving coordination of the respiratory, gastrointestinal, and abdominal musculature, is controlled by what researchers label the emetic center. This center in the brain stem has access to the motor pathways responsible for the visceral and somatic output involved in vomiting, and stimuli from several areas within the central nervous system can affect this center. These include afferent (inward-directed) nerves from the pharynx and gastrointestinal tract, as well as afferents from the higher cortical centers (including the visual center) and the chemoreceptor trigger zone (CTZ) in the area postrema (a highly vascularized area of the brain stem). The CTZ can be activated by chemical stimuli received through the blood or the cerebrospinal fluid. Direct electrical stimulation of the CTZ, however, does not result in emesis.

Clinical assessment of nausea and vomiting usually focuses on the occurrence of vomiting, that is, the frequency and number of episodes. Nausea, however, is a subjective phenomenon unobservable by another. Few data collection instruments that measure separately the patient's experience of nausea and vomiting and his or her symptom distress have been reported in the literature. In fact, the Rhodes Index of Nausea and Vomiting (INV) Form 2 is the only available tool that measures the individual components of nausea, vomiting, and retching. This index measures the patient's perception of the duration, frequency, and distress from nausea. The frequency, amount, and distress from vomiting; and the frequency, amount, and distress from retching (dry heaves). The INV score provides a measurement of the total symptom experience of the patient.

While the causes of nausea and vomiting are numerous—they include gastrointestinal diseases, infections, intracranial disease, toxins, radiation sickness, psychological trauma, migraines, and circulatory syncope—three of the most common causes are motion sickness (air, sea, land, or space), pregnancy, and anesthesia administered during operative procedures.

The sequence of symptoms and signs that constitute motion sickness is fairly characteristic. Premonitory symptoms often include yawning or sighing, lethargy, somnolence, and a loss of enthusiasm and concern for the task at hand. Increasing malaise is directed toward the epigastrium, a sensation best described as "stomach awareness," which progresses to nausea. Diversion of the blood flow from the skin toward the muscles results in pallor. A feeling of warmth and a desire for cool air is often accompanied by sweating. Frontal headache and a sensation of disorientation, dizziness, or light-headedness may also occur. As symptoms progress, vomiting occurs early in the sequence of symptoms for some; in others, malaise is severe and prolonged and vomiting is delayed. After vomiting, there is often a temporary improvement in well-being; however, with continued provocative motion, symptoms build again and vomiting recurs. The symptoms may last for minutes, hours, or even days.

The most coherent explanation for the development of motion sickness is provided by sensory conflict theory. Motion sickness is generally thought to occur as the result of a "sensory conflict" between information arising from the semicircular canals and organs of the vestibular system, visual and other sensory input, and the input that is expected on the basis of past experience or exposure history. It is argued that conflicts between current sensory inputs are by themselves insufficient to produce motion sickness since adaptation occurs

even though the conflicting inputs continue to be present. Visual input alone, however, can produce symptoms of motion sickness, such as watching motion pictures shot from a moving vehicle or looking out of the side window (as opposed to the front window) of a moving vehicle.

Nausea and/or vomiting in the early morning during pregnancy, so-called morning sickness, is so common that it is accepted as a symptom of normal pregnancy. Occurring soon after waking, it is often retching rather than actual vomiting and usually does not disturb the woman's health or her pregnancy. The symptoms nearly always cease before the fourteenth week of pregnancy. In a much smaller proportion of cases, approximately one in one thousand births, the vomiting becomes more serious and persistent, occurring throughout the day and even during the night. The term "hyperemesis gravidarum" is given to this serious form of vomiting. Theories on the etiology of morning sickness have tended to be grouped under four main areas: endocrine (caused by estrogen and progesterone levels), psychosomatic (a conscious or unconscious wish not to be pregnant), allergic (a histamine reaction), and metabolic (a lack of potassium).

Nausea and vomiting occur frequently as unpleasant side effects of the administration of anesthesia in many clinical procedures. Most postoperative vomiting is mild, and only in a few cases will the problem persist so as to cause electrolyte disturbances and dehydration. The factors affecting postoperative nausea and vomiting may be divided into two categories: by the type of patient and surgery, and by the anesthetic and preoperative and postoperative medication uses. Patients with a history of motion sickness have a predisposition to postoperative vomiting. Nearly 43 percent of patients who vomited following previous surgery vomited again, whereas slightly more than 14 percent of those who did not vomit previously had an emetic episode at their next operation. Patients undergoing their first anesthetic procedure had an incidence of vomiting of approximately 30 percent.

No direct association between vomiting and age has been found. That vomiting may be hormonally related, however, is suggested by the higher incidence of nausea and vomiting in the latter half of the menstrual cycle. Other factors that may affect nausea and vomiting associated with anesthesia include patient weight (female obese patients being particularly more vulnerable), amount of hydration, metabolic status, and psychological state.

With regard to the type of surgery performed, the highest incidence of nausea and vomiting appears to be associated with abdominal surgery, as well as ear, nose, and throat surgery, with middle-ear surgery being the major category. The length of surgery, and therefore the duration of anesthesia, also has a direct effect on nausea and vomiting. Short (thirty-minute to sixty-minute) operations using cyclopropane had an emetic incidence of 17.5 percent, while operations lasting one and a half to three and a half hours had an incidence of 46.4 percent.

Most of the causes of vomiting associated with general anesthesia are expected to be eliminated with regional or spinal anesthesia. The type of anesthesia used also has an effect on nausea and vomiting. Research indicates that cyclopropane, ether, and nitrous oxide are potent emetics.

Treatment and Therapy

Since the generation of sensory conflict underlies all motion environments that give rise to motion sickness, practical measures that reduce conflict are likely to reduce motion sickness incidence. Motion sickness can be minimized if the subject has the widest possible view of a visual reference in which the earth is stable. Passengers aboard ships are less likely to be seasick if they remain on deck at midship, where vertical motion is minimized, and view the horizon. In a car or bus, individuals should be in a position to see the road directly ahead, since the movement of this visual scene will correlate with the changes in the direction of the vehicle. While head movements in a rotating environment are known to precipitate motion sickness, there is no clear experimental evidence that they elicit nausea in mild linear oscillation. Thus, some nonpharmacologic remedies for motion sickness are restricting head movements, lying in a supine position, or closing the eyes. In addition, the use of acupressure wrist bands has proven effective in combating motion sickness.

Pharmacologically, the drug hyoscine hydrobromide (also called hyoscine or scopolamine) emerged as a valuable prophylactic drug following extensive research during World War II into the problems of motion sickness in troops transported in aircraft, ships, and landing craft. It remains one of the most effective drugs for short-duration exposures to provocative motion. Doses in excess of 0.6 milligram, however, are very likely to lead to drowsiness, and there is much experimental evidence that hyoscine impairs short-term memory. Hyoscine can be absorbed transdermally, and in order to extend the duration of action, a controlled-release patch was developed to deliver 1.2 milligrams on application and 0.01 milligram hourly thereafter. There is substantial evidence of its sustained effectiveness, but, perhaps as a result of variable absorption rates, there is an increased risk of blurred vision after more than twenty-four hours of use.

Amphetamines, ephedrine, and a number of antihistamines (such as dimenhydrinate) have been found to be clinically useful in motion sickness. Following oral administration, these drugs are generally slower than hyoscine in reaching their peak efficacy, but they have a longer duration of action.

For most susceptible subjects whose exposure to motion sickness-inducing stimuli is infrequent, prophylactic drugs offer the only useful treatment. When exposure to provocative stimuli is more frequent, as for example in professional aircraft pilots, spontaneous adaption occurs during training and an initially high incidence of motion sickness decreases with time.

In medical conditions in which the cause is relatively unknown, it is usual to find a wide variety of suggested therapies; nausea and vomiting during pregnancy and hyperemesis gravidarum (the serious, persistent form of vomiting in pregnancy) are no exception. Prior to 1968, treatments numbered approximately thirty. In subsequent years,

however, suggested therapy has been mainly drugs of the antiemetic variety. Yet since the thalidomide tragedy (in which severe deformities occurred in the children of women who took this drug), there has been a reluctance to use drugs of any kind during early pregnancy. Probably the only value of drug therapy is at the stage of morning sickness, when antiemetics or mild sedatives may counter the feeling of nausea and prevent women from experiencing excessive vomiting and entering the vicious cycle of dehydration, starvation, and electrolyte imbalance. Once the patient has reached the stage of hyperemesis gravidarum, much more basic therapy is required, and the regimen calls for correction of dehydration, carbohydrate deficiency, and ionic deficiencies. This program is best managed by intravenous therapy, with or without the addition of vitamin supplements and sedative agents.

Nonpharmacologic self-care actions for morning sickness fall into the three broad categories of manipulating diet, adjusting behavior, and seeking emotional support. Some of the most effective self-care actions are getting rest, eating several small meals rather than three large ones, avoiding bad smells, avoiding greasy or fried foods, avoiding cooking, and receiving extra attention and support.

In terms of postoperative nausea and vomiting caused by anesthesia, it has been found that routine antiemetic prophylaxis of patients undergoing elective surgical procedures is not indicated, since fewer than 30 percent of patients experience postoperative nausea and vomiting. Of those who develop these symptoms, many have transient nausea or only one or two bouts of emesis and do not require antiemetic therapy. In addition, commonly used antiemetic drugs can produce significant side effects, such as sedation. Nevertheless, antiemetic prophylaxis may be justified in those patients who are at greater risk for developing postoperative nausea and/or vomiting. Such therapy is often given to patients with a history of motion sickness or to those undergoing gynecologic procedures, inner-ear procedures, oral surgery (in which the jaws are occluded by wires, causing a high risk of breathing in vomitus), and operations on the ear or eye and plastic surgery operations (in order to avoid disruption of delicate surgical work).

Many different antiemetic drugs are available for the treatment of postoperative nausea and vomiting. Researchers have found it difficult to interpret the results of antiemetic drug studies because the severity of postoperative vomiting and the response to therapeutic agents can be influenced by many variables in addition to the antiemetic drug being studied. Even with the use of the same drugs in a homogeneous population undergoing the same procedure, the severity of emesis varies from individual to individual.

Because antiemetic drugs have differing sites of action, better results can be obtained by using a multidrug approach. If a combination of drugs with a similar site of action is used, however, the incidence of side effects may be increased. There are few data regarding combination antiemetic prophylaxis or therapy for postoperative nausea and emesis. Drug combinations have been avoided in postsurgical patients because of concerns about additive central nervous system toxicity. An exception is the combination of low-dose droperidol and metoclopramide, which appears to be more effective than droperidol alone for outpatient gynecologic procedures.

Although a full stomach is best avoided before any operative procedure, with situations such as emergencies, in which danger from vomiting is acute, a rapid sequence of administering anesthesia (induction) and clearing the air passage (intubation) remains the method of choice to avoid nausea and vomiting in patients with a full stomach. After the procedure, it is recommended that the patient minimize movement in order to avoid nausea and vomiting. Also, it has been found that avoiding eating solid food for at least eight hours after a surgical procedure is helpful in preventing postoperative nausea and vomiting.

Perspective and Prospects

Though it has existed for as long as there have been human beings, the symptom of nausea has never received much attention in health care practice or research. In fact, until the early 1970s the sensation of nausea was frequently dismissed as merely a passing phenomenon. The rationale for this dismissal was most likely the understanding that nausea is self-limiting (it always passes with time), is never life-threatening in itself, is probably psychogenic in nature (at least to some degree), and, being subjective, is very difficult to measure. In addition, in the past the most predictable nausea was related to pregnancy, which may also explain the lack of attention given to nausea.

Until the late 1980s, there was still little research being conducted on the nausea associated with pregnancy, although it is a common symptom. The historical lack of interest in nausea and vomiting during pregnancy may be traced to the fact that, since the symptoms generally persist only through the first trimester, health care professionals have viewed the problem as relatively insignificant. As more pregnant women work outside the home in demanding positions, however, these women have exhibited less tolerance for illness. Demands upon the health care industry and upon personal physicians for more research and effective treatment have become more widespread.

While it is surprising that nausea has received scant attention in the history of clinical research, it is even more astonishing that vomiting, an observable behavior, has received so little attention as well. Although vomiting is a primitive neurologic process that has remained almost unchanged in the evolution of animals, the mechanisms that regulate the behavior remain virtually unknown.

One reason for the paucity of information on the subject of nausea in particular stems from the lack of a reliable animal model. This fact has hampered research aimed at establishing the etiological basis for nausea and its relationship to vomiting. While some species of lower animals, for example rats, cannot vomit, it is not known whether rats experience the phenomenon of nausea. Thus no effective means of measuring nausea in lower animals has been devised.

Since the early 1970s, there has been a noticeable increase in research on nausea as a drug side effect because it was so frequently seen in cancer chemotherapy clinical trials sponsored by the National Cancer Institute and the American Cancer Society. As more powerful chemotherapy agents and aggressive combinations were clinically investigated, patients began to experience severe, potentially life-threatening nausea and vomiting. Older drugs such as antihistamines, phenothiazines, and benzodiazepines are still used for their antiemetic characteristics, but they are augmented by newer agents such as benzamides, neurokinin-1-receptor antagonists, and serotonin antagonists.

Aside from the pharmacological investigations of new drugs and drug combinations in the treatment of nausea and vomiting, an interesting branch of scientific investigation has begun the process of exploring alternative ways of managing these symptoms. Behavioral interventions, such as progressive muscle relaxation, biofeedback, imagery, or music therapy, have been used to alleviate postchemotherapy anxiety. These methods may also be used to treat other patients suffering from the symptoms of nausea and vomiting, such as pregnant women.

Another noninvasive, nonpharmacologic measure that has been considered in the relief of nausea and vomiting is transcutaneous electrical nerve stimulation (TENS). Several research studies indicate that TENS may be useful in alleviating chemotherapy-related nausea and vomiting, including delayed nausea and vomiting. Side effects from using TENS units are negligible, and with further study they may prove to be an acceptable, helpful relief measure.

—*Genevieve Slomski, Ph.D.*

See also Acid reflux disease; Anesthesia; Appetite loss; Botulism; Bulimia; Chemotherapy; Colitis; Crohn's disease; Diaphragm; Digestion; Eating disorders; Esophagus; Food biochemistry; Food poisoning; Gastroenteritis; Gastroenterology; Gastroenterology, pediatric; Gastrointestinal disorders; Gastrointestinal system; Heartburn; Indigestion; Influenza; Lactose intolerance; Motion sickness; Multiple chemical sensitivity syndrome; Noroviruses; Poisoning; Poisonous plants; Pregnancy and gestation; Radiation sickness; Rotavirus; Salmonella infection; Stomach, intestinal, and pancreatic cancers; Ulcer surgery; Ulcers; Vagotomy.

For Further Information:

Blum, Richard H., and W. LeRoy Heinrichs. *Nausea and Vomiting: Overview, Challenges, Practical Treatments, and New Perspectives*. Philadelphia: Whurr, 2000.

Casey, Georgina. "Treating Nausea and Vomiting." *Kai Tiaki Nursing New Zealand* 18, no. 11 (December, 2012): 20–24.

Edmundowicz, Steven A., ed. *Twenty Common Problems in Gastroenterology*. New York: McGraw-Hill, 2002.

Funk, Sandra G., et al., eds. *Key Aspects of Comfort: Management of Pain, Fatigue, and Nausea*. New York: Springer, 1989.

Hesketh, Paul J., ed. *Management of Nausea and Vomiting in Cancer and Cancer Treatment*. Sudbury, Mass.: Jones and Bartlett, 2005.

Kucharczyk, John, David J. Stewart, and Alan D. Miller, eds. *Nausea and Vomiting: Recent Research and Clinical Advances*. Boca Raton, Fla.: CRC Press, 1991.

Litin, Scott C., ed. *Mayo Clinic Family Health Book*. 4th ed. New York: HarperResource, 2009.

Palatty, Princy Lous, et al. "Ginger in the Prevention of Nausea and

Vomiting." *Critical Reviews in Food Science and Nutrition* 53, no. 7 (2013): 659.

Rao, Kamakshi V., and Aimee Faso. "Chemotherapy-Induced Nausea and Vomiting: Optimizing Prevention and Management." *American Health and Drug Benefits* 5, no. 4 (July, 2012): 232–240.

Sleisenger, Marvin H., ed. *The Handbook of Nausea and Vomiting*. New York: Caduceus Medical/Parthenon, 1993.

NECK INJURIES AND DISORDERS. *See* HEAD AND NECK DISORDERS.

NECROSIS
Disease/Disorder
Also known as: Gangrene, mortification
Anatomy or system affected: Bones, cells
Specialties and related fields: Oncology, orthopedics
Definition: Tissue damage occurring as a result of cell death.

Causes and Symptoms

"Necrosis" refers to the degeneration of cells or tissues after cell death occurs for any reason, generally in localized regions of the body. Thus, necrosis is tissue degeneration, which occurs secondary to cell death from any cause. Necrosis is most commonly the result of ischemia, traumatic injury, bacterial infection, or toxins (including excessive steroids or alcohol).

In its earliest stage, there are often no symptoms of necrosis. Tissue damage begins to occur within twelve hours of cell death. When symptoms do begin to occur, they range from atrophy to decreased range of motion and pain to the development of gangrenous tissue.

Treatment and Therapy

The damage done to the tissue resulting from cell death is permanent. Any treatment of necrosis is aimed at minimizing further cell death and tissue injury. In the case of heart disease, treatment of the underlying condition to alleviate hypoxia prevents further cell death from ischemia. In the case of bacterial infection, antibiotics are used to treat the infection and prevent cell death and tissue damage. In the case of necrosis of bone tissue from decreased blood supply, the aim of treatment is to minimize further bone loss. This type of necrosis, known as "avascular necrosis" or "osteonecrosis," is treated with nonsteroidal anti-inflammatory drugs (NSAIDs) to relieve pain, exercise to improve range of motion, electrical treatment to stimulate bone growth, or surgery to reshape or graft bone or to replace joints.

Perspective and Prospects

The term "necrosis" was used nearly two thousand years ago in ancient Greek textbooks to refer to changes within tissue, long after cell death had occurred, that were visible to the naked eye. With the advent of light microscopy, the tissue damage following cell death became visible within twelve to twenty-four hours.

In 1859, Rudolf Virchow, in his renowned text *Cellular*

Information on Necrosis

Causes: Cell death leading to degeneration of tissue over time
Symptoms: Pain, tissue decay
Duration: Permanent, irreversible
Treatments: Pain relievers (NSAIDs), surgery

Pathology as Based upon Physiological and Pathological Histology, discussed degeneration, necrosis, mortification, and gangrene, using these terms more or less synonymously. It should be noted that he used the term "necrosis" to refer to an advanced stage of tissue breakdown. At this point, the breakdown had to be visible to the naked eye, since light microscopy had not yet been developed. Today, using the microscope, tissue damage resulting from cell death is obvious and often identical whether caused by ischemia, traumatic injury, bacteria, or toxins.

—*Robin Kamienny Montvilo, R.N., Ph.D.*

See also Cells; Circulation; Gangrene; Ischemia; Necrotizing fasciitis; Osteonecrosis; Pathology; Vascular medicine; Vascular system.

For Further Information:

A.D.A.M. Medical Encyclopedia. "Necrosis." *MedlinePlus*, March 23, 2013.

"Cell Death." In *Pathology: Clinicopathologic Foundations of Medicine*, edited by Raphael Rubin, David Sheldon Strayer, and Emanuel Rubin. 6th ed. Baltimore: Lippincott, 2012.

Majno, G., and I. Joris. "Apoptosis, Oncosis, and Necrosis: An Overview of Cell Death." *American Journal of Pathology* 146, no. 1 (1995): 3–15.

"Necrosis." In *Taber's Cyclopedic Medical Dictionary*, edited by Donald Venes. 21st ed. Philadelphia: F. A. Davis, 2010.

Parker, J. N., and P. M. Parker. *The Official Patient's Sourcebook on Avascular Necrosis*. San Diego, Calif.: Icon Health, 2002.

NECROTIZING FASCIITIS
Disease/Disorder
Anatomy or system affected: Blood vessels, muscles, skin
Specialties and related fields: Bacteriology, critical care, dermatology, emergency medicine, epidemiology, histology, plastic surgery, vascular medicine
Definition: An invasive bacterial infection that occurs in the connective tissue between the skin and muscle known as the fascia, cutting off blood flow; it must be urgently treated surgically and, even in the best circumstances, has a high mortality rate.

Causes and Symptoms

Although it had been identified in the past, in 1994 there were numerous headline newspaper reports describing a new "flesh-eating bacteria." These articles detailed the devastating effect of seemingly minor wounds infected with streptococcal bacteria. Patients quickly become very sick, with a rapidly progressive downward course, even from trauma resulting in a deep muscle bruise or muscle strain or in "minor"

Information on Necrotizing Fasciitis

Causes: Bacterial infection
Symptoms: Fever, inflammation, severe pain, blistering at site of infection, tissue death
Duration: Acute
Treatments: Emergency care, extensive surgical debridement, antibiotics

---

cuts and scrapes.

In the former nonpenetrating injuries, it is likely that the bacteria were already present in the blood and then seeded the site of damage. Most of these patients, however, did not recall any prior recent infection that may have made them susceptible. Penetrating injuries, where the normally protective barrier of the skin has been broken, were often minor and not originally treated as contaminated or infected. Other cases of necrotizing fasciitis are caused by surgical infections and bowel contamination. These cases are more rare and often found to have a mixture of bacteria, such as staphylococci or *Escherichia coli* (*E. coli*).

Patients with necrotizing fasciitis have fever, inflammation, severe pain, and blistering at the site of infection. If this cellulitis is not recognized and urgently treated, the infection will quickly spread in the layers of connective tissue just under the skin known as the fascia. As the bacteria multiply, they cause blood vessels supplying the skin to form clots and thus cut off blood flow to the skin. Without nutrients, oxygen, and the ability to remove waste products, the skin dies. Once this occurs, the nerves are destroyed and the patient no longer has the excruciating pain. The skin at this point appears to be "eaten away." The possibility exists that the underlying muscle adjacent to the fascia will become infected. Thus, the potential for muscle death as well as skin death is of great concern, particularly if the infection begins in the arms, legs, abdomen, or back, as these areas have large muscle groups directly underlying the skin. In necrotizing fasciitis, the extremities and the area around the genitals and anus (perineum) are most commonly and extensively involved. Multiplication and movement of these streptococcal bacteria and their toxins into the bloodstream produces a shock-like state.

Treatment and Therapy

The patient with necrotizing fasciitis must be stabilized quickly in an intensive care unit, where fluids can be administered and heart and lung condition can be closely monitored. The only lifesaving treatment available is extensive surgical debridement to remove the necrotic (dead) tissue and slow the spread of the bacteria. Antibiotics including penicillins, clindamycin, and gentamicin are given to help eradicate the pathogen. Because the infection spreads so rapidly, death often results even with heroic surgical and drug therapy unless the condition is diagnosed and treated early. Fortunately, these infections remain relatively rare.

—*Matthew Berria, Ph.D.*

See also Antibiotics; Bacterial infections; Bacteriology; Connective tissue; Dermatology; Epidemiology; Fascia; Necrosis; Shock; Skin; Skin disorders; Streptococcal infections; Toxic shock syndrome; Wounds.

For Further Information:
Berman, Kevin. "Necrotizing Soft Tissue Infection." *MedlinePlus*, November 22, 2011.
Biddle, Wayne. *A Field Guide to Germs*. 3d ed. New York: Anchor Books, 2010.
Forbes, Betty A., Daniel F. Sahm, and Alice S. Weissfeld. *Bailey and Scott's Diagnostic Microbiology*. 12th ed. St. Louis, Mo.: Mosby/Elsevier, 2007.
MedlinePlus. "Streptococcal Infections." *MedlinePlus*, May 7, 2013.
Roemmele, Jacqueline A., and Donna Batdorff. *Surviving the Flesh-Eating Bacteria: Understanding, Preventing, Treating, and Living with the Effects of Necrotizing Fasciitis*. Garden City Park, N.Y.: Avery, 2000.
Snyder, Larry, et al. *Molecular Genetics of Bacteria*. 4th ed. Washington, D.C.: ASM Press, 2013.
Wilson, Brenda A., Abigail A. Salyers, et al. *Bacterial Pathogenesis: A Molecular Approach*. 3d ed. Washington, D.C.: ASM Press, 2011.
Wilson, Michael, Brian Henderson, and Rod McNab. *Bacterial Disease Mechanisms: An Introduction to Cellular Microbiology*. New York: Cambridge University Press, 2002.

NEONATAL BRACHIAL PLEXUS PALSY
Disease/Disorder

Also known as: Erb's palsy, obstetric brachial plexus palsy, birth brachial plexus palsy
Anatomy or system affected: Arms, nerves
Specialties and related fields: Neonatology, neurology, obstetrics, organizations and programs, orthopedics, pediatrics, perinatology, physical therapy, plastic surgery, psychology, radiology
Definition: A motor disability evident early in life that manifests as weakness of the affected arm due to stretching or compression of the nerves of the brachial plexus during the perinatal period, with passive range of motion greater than active.

Key terms:

brachial plexus: complex of nerves that carry motor and sensory function to the arm

contractures: permanent shorting of muscles or joints

Erb's palsy: stereotyped clinical presentation of neonatal brachial plexus palsy resulting from injury to the C5, C6, and sometimes C7 spinal nerve roots

Horner's syndrome: ptosis (eyelid drooping), miosis (abnormal constriction of the pupil of the eye), and anhydrosis (decreased sweating on the face)

incidence: the rate at which a certain event occurs or the number of new cases of a specific disorder occurring during a certain period in a population at risk

pan-plexopathy: a form of neonatal brachial plexus palsy comprising of injury to all of the spinal nerve roots manifesting as a flaccid arm

perinatal period: the period immediately before and after birth, commencing at 20 weeks of gestation and ending at 28 weeks after birth (140 days total) *range of motion:* movement of a joint from full flexion to full extension

shoulder dystocia: diagnosed when the delivery of the fetal head is not followed by the emergence of the shoulder due to impaction of the fetus' shoulder in the birth canal

Causes and Symptoms

Children with neonatal brachial plexus palsy (NBPP) have a weak or paralyzed arm, and their passive range of motion is greater than their active range of motion. NBPP becomes evident early in life and usually results from stretching or compression of the nerves of the brachial plexus during the perinatal period. NBPP occurs with an incidence of 1.5 cases per 1000 live births, with or without shoulder dystocia at the time of both vaginal and cesarean delivery. Risk factors for NBPP include abnormal positioning of the fetus, labor abnormalities, artificial labor induction, large fetus, and shoulder dystocia. However, except for shoulder dystocia, none of these risk factors are statistically significant clinical predictors for the occurrence of NBPP.

Compression or stretching of the nerves of the brachial plexus can occur during development in the uterus or during the descent and emergence of the fetus from the uterus and pelvis with maternal pushing and naturally expulsive forces. Biomechanically, nerve injury can result from forces applied by clinicians, or natural physical events that move the fetus

> ### Information on Neonatal Brachial Plexus Palsy
>
> **Causes:** Damage to the nerves of the brachial plexus during or after birth
> **Symptoms:** One of the arms does not move normally
> **Duration:** Depends on the severity; some children recover completely, others only partially, while some are permanently affected
> **Treatments:** Physical and occupational therapy, exercises, orthopedic or neural surgery

from the uterus through the birth canal and out of the mother's pelvis. No one force or factor seems to be responsible for the cause of NBPP, but the available data do suggest that the occurrence of NBPP may be a multifactorial event.

The brachial plexus is a very complex structure that connects the spinal nerves in the neck to their terminal branches in the arm and is divided into 5 zones: (1) C5 through T1 spinal nerve roots; (2) upper, middle, and lower trunks; (3) anterior and posterior divisions of each trunk; (4) lateral, posterior, and medial cords; and (5) terminal branches. These nerves carry the signals necessary for the normal movement and sensation in the entire arm. The brachial plexus is analogous to a set of intersecting highways with overpasses, underpasses, and multiple merging traffic intersections, with several roads leading into (analogous to the spinal nerve roots)

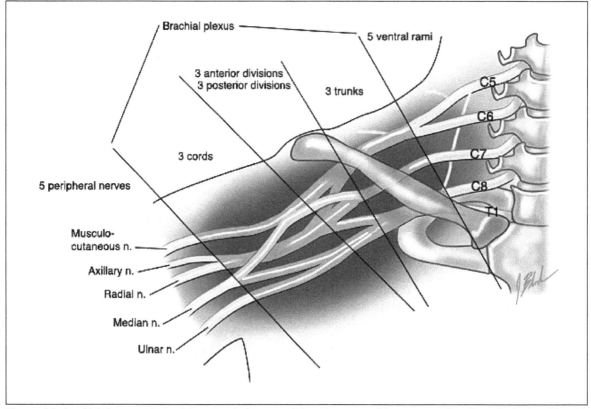

Nerves of the brachial plexus, cervical and thoracic spinal nerves and the major nerves of the upper arm. (http://www.backpain-guide.com)

and out of (analogous to the terminal branches) the intersections. However, for simplicity, the nerve roots can be indexed to the muscles in the following fashion: C5-shoulder movement, C6-elbow flexion, C7-elbow extension, C8/T1-hand and finger movement.

Not all cases of NBPP are the same, and the symptoms may be radically different depending on which parts of the brachial plexus are injured. The intricate intersecting nature of the brachial plexus implies that thousands of potentially different palsies can ensue, but in reality, only a few variations actually occur. The most useful classification scheme for clinical presentation of NBPP is the Narakas Grade system that represents the extent of the spinal nerve root injury: only C5 and C6 nerve roots are injured in Grade 1, C5, C6, C7 nerve roots in Grade 2, and C5 through T1 injured in Grade 3 (without Horner's syndrome) and Grade 4 (with Horner's syndrome). When this classification system is used in 2-4 week old affected babies, it may guide the prognosis for spontaneous recovery, since up to 90 percent of the patients with Grade 1 NBPP regain functional use of the affected arm, but less than 5 percent of the patients with Grade 4 NBPP regain functional use without medical and/or surgical intervention.

Other classification systems are based on the clinical manifestations of NBPP. Erb's palsy, the most common type of NBPP, is synonymous with an "upper" plexus palsy that specifically results from damage to C5, C6, and sometimes C7 spinal nerve roots. Patients with Erb's palsy present a "waiter's tip" posture when their affected arm is pulled toward the midline of the body, an internally rotated shoulder, flexed wrist, extended fingers that result from loss of both shoulder control and elbow bending. Contrastingly, the extremely rare Klumpke's palsy is synonymous with a "lower" plexus palsy characterized by a flaccid hand attached to an otherwise active arm. Total plexus palsy or pan-plexopathy is equivalent to Narakas Grade 3 and 4 and is recognized by loss of total function of the arm.

Treatment and Therapy

Lack of normal arm movement observed during the perinatal period warrants confirmation of the diagnosis of NBPP by a specialist. Possible skeletal injuries or fractures should be confirmed by clinical and radiographic evaluation since these injuries may preclude early occupational/physical therapy. Immobilization of the arm is not recommended except in the case of skeletal injuries.

With regard to the specific motor function of the affected arm, the treating physician assesses the passive and active range of motion of the affected arm. Available assessment scales of motor function in NBPP are used to determine the extent and severity of nerve injury, to prognosticate potential functional recovery, and to guide and assess the outcomes from further treatment. Traditional scales focus only upon the affected arm, but more recently, assessment methods are focusing upon the overall function of the child. Supplementing the physical examination with electrodiagnostic / electromyographic (EMG) and radiographic (magnetic resonance imaging, MRI) findings are helpful to decide whether

surgical nerve reconstruction will be beneficial.

Early referral of those babies with severe or extensive NBPP to interdisciplinary specialty clinics can improve overall functional outcomes as the baby grows. Regardless of the need for surgical intervention, rehabilitation management is critical. Occupational/physical therapy to maintain the normal passive range of motion in all upper extremity joints (especially shoulder external rotation and forearm rotation) facilitates successful functional recovery. Parents and caregivers should consider themselves to be the patient's primary therapist by performing range of motion exercises regularly, with multimedia assistance if available (e.g., during every diaper change). Reinforced use of the affected arm while constraining the normal arm (similar to patching a lazy eye) can aid the child's recognition of the arm and strengthen the arm through increased arm use during age-appropriate activities. Normal childhood developmental milestones must be encouraged, including crawling. Splinting may be used during sleep to avoid contractures or to protect floppy joints. As the child grows, recreational activities like swimming, dance, sports, and potentially therapist-designed video game platforms can help to sustain the goals of formal occupational/physical therapy.

For NBPP patients who do not recover with conservative management, surgical nerve reconstruction may be an option, usually occurring between 3-9 months of age. Although the indications and timing for nerve reconstruction have not been absolutely established, most practitioners agree that babies with the extensive total brachial plexus palsy and those with the severe Erb's palsy will benefit from nerve surgery. The goal of nerve reconstruction is not to regain a normal arm, but surgical intervention is a step towards a functional arm with adequate movement, if not power. Nerve repair using autologous nerve graft and/or nerve transfer (using a good nerve to re-innervate an injured one) constitute the primary options for reconstructing the function of the brachial plexus. As nerve repair and transfer rely upon regrowth of the normal portions of the nerve through the residual pathways after injured nerve is cleared away (Wallerian degeneration), and as this nerve regeneration is very slow, the ultimate functional outcome from nerve reconstruction surgery may not be apparent for 1-3 years.

Toddlers and older children with incomplete recovery following neurosurgical or conservative treatment may have functional limitations because of residual muscle weakness and soft tissue contractures, especially around the shoulder and elbow. MRI imaging can guide the decision to pursue orthopedic intervention. Internal rotation contracture of the shoulder is most common and can be associated with progressive shoulder joint deformity and instability. Indications for surgical intervention include persistent internal rotation contracture despite aggressive nonsurgical therapy, progressive joint deformity, and obvious joint dislocation. Surgical options include muscle lengthening combined with tendon transfers, corrective bone surgery (osteotomies), and open or arthroscopic reduction of the shoulder joint.

For children with residual elbow, forearm, and hand problems, secondary procedures by a hand surgeon may be appropriate. These procedures include soft tissue releases, joint fusions, muscle transfers, and corrective osteotomies. The usual age for secondary reconstruction of the elbow/forearm function is 4-6 years of age, and for wrist/hand function is 6-13 years of age.

For all surgical interventions, the most important factor in producing the optimal result is a cooperative child with intense investment from assertive parents/caretakers. The parents must understand the objectives of the surgical procedure and work hard with their children in postoperative rehabilitation-and maintenance of function by being their children's primary therapists. Surgery alone without subsequent rehabilitation management and therapy is unlikely to yield the desired outcome.

Perspective and Prospects

Overall, the majority of infants with NBPP have a good prognosis for recovering adequate functional use of the affected arm-with rehabilitation management and therapy, supplemented with surgical intervention when and where appropriate and desired by the patient and parents/caretakers. Early occupational/physical therapy can support the spontaneous recovery of function and minimize consequent musculoskeletal comorbidities along with more efficient recovery of function after surgery. Despite the similar incidence of NBPP to cerebral palsy, public awareness of this perinatal disorder and its lifelong implications (medical and psychosocial) for the more extensively/severely affected children are significantly lacking. Similarly, published research studies regarding NBPP number only a fraction of that regarding cerebral palsy. Therefore, current efforts exist not only to find new medical treatment techniques but also to increase awareness, to address and improve the quality of life for patients with NBPP via traditional and recent technology-assisted modalities. Early referral to an interdisciplinary specialty brachial plexus clinic can avail the patient of the most current treatment paradigms to achieve the optimal outcome.

—*Lynda J.-S. Yang, M.D., P.D., F.A.A.N.S.*

See also Neonatology; Neurology; Neurology, pediatric; Obstetrics; Occupational health; Orthopedics; Physical rehabilitation

For Further Information:

Bowerson, M., V.S. Nelson, and L.J. Yang. "Diaphragmatic Paralysis Associated with Neonatal Brachial Plexus Palsy." *Pediatric Neurology* 42, no. 3 (March 2010) 234-236. Case study of a NBPP baby whose diaphragm was also paralyzed.

Chung, Kevin C., Lynda J.-S.Yang, and John E. McGillicuddy, eds. *Practical Management of Pediatric and Adult Brachial Plexus Palsies.* London: Elsevier, 2011. Extensive overview of the medical and surgical techniques for managing disorders of the brachial plexus. Presents a multidisciplinary approach to pediatric brachial plexus palsy treatment and rehabilitation, obstetric considerations, and other timely topics in the field (includes DVD).

Mehta, S.H., and B. Gonik. "Neonatal Brachial Plexus Injury: Obstetrical Factors and Neonatal Management." *Journal of Pediatric Rehabilitation Medicine* 4, no. 2 (2011) 113-118. A review of the potential causes of and risk factors for NBPP.

Murphy, K.M., L. Rasmussen, S.L. Hervey-Jumper, D. Justice, V.S.
Nelson, and L.J. Yang. "An Assessment of the Compliance and Utility of a Home Exercise DVD for Caregivers of Children and Adolescents with Brachial Plexus Palsy: A Pilot Study." *PM & R* 4, no. 3 (March 2012) 190-197. Small, initial study of the efficacy of home exercises for NBPP children.

Piatt, J.H., Jr. "Birth Injuries of the Brachial Plexus." *Clinical Perinatology* 32, no. 1 (March 2005) 39-59. Excellent summary of the classification of various types of NBPP.

Squitieri, L.. B.P. Larson, K.W. Chang, L.J. Yang, and K.C. Chung. "Medical Decision-Making among Adolescents with Neonatal Brachial Plexus Palsy and Their Families: A Qualitative Study." *Plastic and Reconstructive Surgery* 131, no. 6 (June, 2013): 880e-887e. A study that examines why patients make particular treatment choices and stresses the need for proper patient education.

NEONATOLOGY

Specialty

Anatomy or system affected: All

Specialties and related fields: Cardiology, critical care, embryology, genetics, obstetrics, pediatrics, perinatology

Definition: A subspecialty of pediatrics that involves the care of newborn infants from birth through the first month of life, especially those infants with life-threatening conditions such as prematurity, genetic defects, and serious illnesses.

Key terms:

congenital disorders: abnormalities present at birth that occurred during fetal development as a result of genetic errors, exposure to toxins and microorganisms, or maternal illness

incubator: in the nursery, a plexiglass unit that encloses the premature or sick infant to allow strict temperature regulation

intrauterine growth retardation: the condition of infants who are born significantly smaller than the standard for the number of weeks that they have spent in the uterus

neonatal intensive care unit: a hospital nursery with advanced equipment and specially trained staff to maintain the vital functions of sick newborns and to monitor their progress closely

neonatal period: the first month of life; derived from the Greek *neo* (meaning "new") and the Latin *natum* (meaning "birth")

prematurity: strictly defined, birth before a full-term pregnancy (thirty-eight weeks); more commonly associated with birth before thirty-five weeks

respirator: a machine that inflates and deflates the lungs, imitating normal breathing; connected to the patient through a tube placed into the windpipe (endotracheal tube)

respiratory distress syndrome: a life-threatening illness primarily of premature infants; immature lungs lack surfactant, a vital substance that keeps the tiny air sacs (alveoli) from collapsing upon exhalation

Science and Profession

Neonatology has grown dramatically since its beginnings in the late 1960s, and neonatologists have become an integral part of the obstetric-pediatric team at major medical centers throughout the world. In addition to being cared for by physicians who specialize in neonatology, some neonatal infants, in particular those who are critically ill or premature, are cared for by nurse practitioners with the specialty certification of neonatal nurse practitioner (NNP). In large part because of an ever-expanding technological base and marked advances in scientific research, these health care professionals have changed the outlook for premature and sick newborns.

As a subspecialty of pediatrics, neonatology is concerned with the most critical time of transition and adjustment—the first four weeks of life, or the neonatal period—whether the infant is healthy (a normal birth) or sick (as a result of genetic problems, obstetric complications, or medical illness). By the early 1970s, it became increasingly clear to health administrators that hospitals throughout the United States had varying abilities to care for medical and pediatric cases requiring the most sophisticated staff and equipment. Consequently, they developed a system that designated hospitals as either level I (small, community hospitals), level II (larger hospitals), or level III (major regional medical centers, also called tertiary care centers). It was in the last group that the most advanced neonatal care could be delivered. In these major centers, there are two types of nurseries, separating the normal healthy infant from the sick or high-risk infant: the routine nursery and the neonatal intensive care unit (NICU).

Routine nurseries are the temporary home of the vast majority of newborns. The services of the neonatologist are rarely needed here, and the general pediatrician or family practitioner observes and examines the infant for twenty-four to forty-eight hours to be sure that it has made a smooth transition from intrauterine to extrauterine life. These babies soon leave the hospital for their homes. Those neonates with minor problems arising from multiple births, difficult deliveries, mild prematurity, and minor illness are easily managed by a primary care physician in consultation with a neonatologist, perhaps at another hospital. It is in the neonatal intensive care unit, however, that the most difficult situations present themselves. Here several teams of pediatric subspecialists—surgeons, cardiologists, anesthesiologists, and highly trained nurses, along with many other health professionals—are led by a neonatologist, who coordinates the team's efforts. These newborns have life-threatening conditions, often as a result of extreme prematurity (more than six weeks earlier than the expected date of delivery), major birth defects (genetic or developmental), severe illness (such as overwhelming infections), or being born to drug- or alcohol-addicted mothers. They require the most advanced technological and medical interventions, often to sustain life artificially until the underlying problem is corrected. It is in this setting that the most dramatic successes of neonatology are found.

After hours of being inside a forcefully contracting uterus and sustaining the stress of passing through a narrow birth canal, the newborn emerges into a dry, cold, and hostile environment. The umbilical cord, which has provided oxygen and nutrients, is clamped and cut; the fluid-filled lungs must now exchange air instead, and the respiratory center of the infant's brain begins a lifetime of spontaneous breathing, usually her-

alded by crying. The vast majority of neonates make this extraordinary adjustment to extrauterine life without difficulty. At one minute and again at five minutes, the newborn is evaluated and scored on five physical signs: heart rate, breathing, muscle tone, reflexes, and skin tone. The healthy infant is vigorously moving, crying, and pink regardless of race. These Apgar scores, named for neonatology pioneer Virginia Apgar, evaluate the need for immediate resuscitation. A brief physical examination follows, which can identify other life-threatening abnormalities.

It is essential to remember that the medical history of a neonate is in fact the medical and obstetric history of its mother, and seemingly normal infants may develop problems shortly after birth. Risk factors include very young or middle-aged mothers; difficult deliveries; babies with Rh-negative blood types; mothers with diabetes mellitus, kidney disease, or heart disease; and concurrent infections in either the mother or the baby. Anticipating these problems of the healthy newborn by using the Apgar scores and the results of the physical examination allows the proper assignment of the infant to the nursery or NICU.

The NICU is a daunting place containing high-tech equipment, a tangle of wires and tubes, the sounds of beeps and alarms, and tiny, fragile infants. All this technology serves two simple purposes: to monitor vital functions and to sustain malfunctioning or nonfunctioning organ systems. Looked at individually, however, the machines and attachments become much more understandable. The incubator, perhaps the most common device, maintains a warm, moist environment of constant temperature at 37 degrees Celsius (98.6 degrees Fahrenheit). Small portholes with rubber gloves allow people to touch the child safely. Generally, the infants will have small electrodes taped on their chests, connected to video monitors that record the heart and breathing rates and that will sound alarms if significant deviations occur. These monitors will also record blood pressure through an arm or thigh cuff. To ensure immediate access to the blood, for delivering medications and taking blood for testing, catheters (plastic tubes) are placed into larger arteries or veins near the umbilicus, neck, or thigh (in adults, intravenous access is found in the arms).

The remaining equipment is used for the very serious business of life support, in particular the support of the respiratory system. Maintaining adequate oxygenation is critical and can be accomplished in several ways, depending on the baby's needs. The least stressful are tubes placed in the nostrils or a face mask, but these methods require that breathing be spontaneous although inadequate. More often, unfortunately, neonates with the types of problems that bring them to an intensive care unit cannot breathe on their own. In these cases, a tube must be connected from the artificial respirator into the windpipe (the endotracheal tube). Warm, moistened, oxygen-rich air is delivered under pressure and removed from the lungs rhythmically to simulate breathing. Tranquilizers and paralytic agents are used to calm and immobilize the infant. Sick or premature infants are also generally unable to feed or nurse naturally, by mouth. Again, several methods of feeding

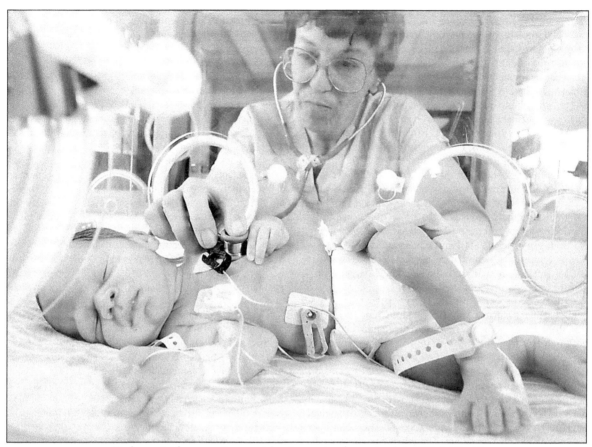

Newborns at risk may require a special environment such as an incubator. (Digital Stock)

can be employed, depending on the problems and the length of time that such feedings will be needed. For the first few days, simple solutions of water, sugar, and protein can be given through the intravenous catheters. These lines, because of the very small, fragile blood vessels of the newborn, are seldom able to carry more complex solutions. A second method, known as gavage feeding, employs tubing that is inserted through the nose directly into the stomach. Through that tube, infant formula (water, sugar, protein, fat, vitamins, and minerals) and, if available, breast milk can be given.

As the underlying problems are resolved, the infant is slowly weaned, first feeding orally and then breathing naturally. Next, the infant will be placed in an open crib, and gradually the tangled web of tubes and wires will clear. With approval from the neonatologist, the baby is transferred to the routine nursery, a transitional home until discharge from the hospital is advisable.

Diagnostic and Treatment Techniques

Neonatology has amassed an enormous body of knowledge about normal neonatal anatomy and physiology, disease processes, and, most important, how to manage the wide variety of complications that can occur. Specific treatment protocols have been developed that are practiced uniformly in all neonatal intensive care units. Short-term stays (twenty-four to forty-eight hours) are meant to observe and monitor the infant with respiratory distress at birth that required immediate intervention. Long-term stays, lasting from several weeks to months, are the case for the sickest newborns, most commonly those with severe prematurity and low birth weight (less than 1,500 grams), respiratory distress syndrome (also known as hyaline membrane disease), congenital defects, and drug or alcohol addictions.

Infants born prematurely make up the major proportion of all infants at high risk for disability and death, and each passing decade has seen younger and younger babies being kept alive. While many maternal factors can lead to preterm delivery, often no explanation can be found. The main problem of prematurity lies in the functional and structural immaturity of vital organs. Weak sucking, swallowing, and coughing reflexes lead to an inability to feed and to the danger of choking. Lungs that lack surfactant, a substance that coats the millions of tiny air sacs (alveoli) in each lung to keep them from collapsing and sticking together after air is exhaled, cause severe breathing difficulty as the infant struggles to reinflate the lungs. When premature delivery is inevitable but not immediate, lung maturity can be increased by administration of steroids to the mother. An immature immune system cannot protect the newborn from the many viruses, bacteria, and other microorganisms that exist. Inadequate metabolism causes low body temperature and inadequate use of food or medications. Neurological immaturity can lead to mental retardation, blindness, and deafness.

Aggressive management of the preterm baby begins in the delivery room, with close cooperation between the obstetrician and the neonatologist. Severely preterm infants, some born after only twenty weeks of pregnancy, require immediate respiratory and cardiac support. Placement of the endotracheal tube, assisted ventilation with a handheld bag, and delicate chest compressions similar to the cardiopulmonary resuscitation (CPR) performed on adults to stimulate the heartbeat are each accomplished quickly. Once the respiratory and circulatory systems have been stabilized, excess fluid will be suctioned, while a brief physical examination is performed to note any abnormalities that require immediate attention. As soon as transport is considered safe, the newborn is sent to the NICU. If the infant has been delivered at a small community hospital, this may involve ambulance or even helicopter transport to the nearest tertiary care center.

Once in the unit, the neonate will be placed in an incubator and attached to video monitors that record heart rate, breathing, and blood pressure. The endotracheal tube can now be attached to the respirator machine, and intravenous or intra-arterial catheters will be placed to allow the fluid and medication infusions and the blood drawing for the battery of tests that the neonatologist requires. Feeding methods can be set up as soon as the infant has stabilized. Within a short time after delivery, the premature newborn has had a flurry of activity about it and is surrounded by the most sophisticated

equipment and staff available. Supporting the immature organs becomes the first priority, although the ethical issues of saving very sick infants must soon be addressed as complications begin to occur. Nearly 15 percent of surviving preterm infants whose birth weights were less than 2,000 grams have serious physical and mental disabilities after discharge. The majority, however, grow to lead normal, healthy lives.

Congenital defects are common, and it is estimated that the majority of miscarriages are a direct result of congenital defects that are incompatible with life. Many infants that do survive development and delivery die shortly after birth despite the most sophisticated and heroic attempts to intervene. The causes of such defects are arbitrarily assigned to two broad categories, although a combination of these factors is the most likely explanation: genetic errors (such as breaks, doubling, and mutations) and environmental insults (such as chemicals, drugs, viruses, radiation, and malnutrition). In the United States, among the most common birth defects that require immediate intervention are heart problems, spina bifida (an open spine), and tracheoesophageal fistulas and esophageal atresias (wrongly connected or incomplete wind and food pipes).

The birth of a malformed infant is rarely expected, and the neonatologist's team plays a key role in its survival. Congenital heart disease is the most prevalent life-threatening defect. During development in utero, the umbilical cord supplies the necessary oxygen; it is not until birth, when that lifeline is cut, that the neonate's circulatory and respiratory systems acquire full responsibility. At delivery, all may appear normal, and the one-minute Apgar score may be high. Several minutes later, however, the pink skin color may begin to darken to a purplish

Number of Infant Deaths in the United States, 2004

Cause of Death	
Congenital malformations, deformations, and chromosomal abnormalities	5,622
Disorders related to short gestation and low birth weight	4,642
Sudden infant death syndrome (SIDS)	2,246
Newborn affected by maternal complications of pregnancy	1,715
Accidents (unintentional injuries)	1,052
Newborn affected by complications of placenta, cord, and membranes	1,042
Respiratory distress	875
Bacterial sepsis	827
Neonatal hemorrhage	616
Diseases of the circulatory system	593
All other causes	8,706
Total	27,936

Source: National Center for Health Statistics.

blue (cyanosis), indicating that insufficient oxygen is being extracted from the air. Immediately, the infant receives rescue breathing from the bag mask. Upon admission to the neonatal unit, the source of the cyanosis must be determined. A chest x-ray may provide significant information about the anatomy of the heart and lungs, but special tests are usually needed to pinpoint the problem. Catheters that are threaded from neck or leg vessels into the heart can reveal the pressure and oxygen content of each chamber in the heart and across its four valves. Echocardiograms, video pictures similar to sonograms generated by sound waves passing through the chest, enhance the data provided by the x-rays and catheterizations, and a diagnosis is made. Based on the physical signs and symptoms of the newborn, a treatment plan is devised.

Because of the nature of congenital defects and structural abnormalities, their correction generally requires surgery. Openings between the heart's chambers (septal defects), valves that are too narrow or do not close properly, and blood vessels that leave or enter the heart incorrectly are all common defects treated by the pediatric heart surgeon. Because of the delicacy of the operation and the vulnerability of the newborn, surgery may be postponed until the baby is larger and stronger while it is provided with supplemental oxygen and nutrients. The risk of such operations is high, and depending on the degree of abnormality, several operations may be required.

Another group of infants who have benefited from advances in neonatology are those born to drug-addicted women. The lives of these infants are often complicated by congenital defects and life-threatening withdrawal symptoms. For example, heroin-addicted babies are quite small, are extremely irritable and hyperactive, and develop tremors, vomiting, diarrhea, and seizures. The newborn must be carefully monitored in the unit, and sedatives and antiseizure medications are given, sometimes for as long as six weeks. Cocaine and its derivatives frequently cause premature labor, fetal death, and maternal hemorrhaging during delivery. Infants that do survive often have serious congenital defects and suffer withdrawal symptoms. The risk of acquired immunodeficiency syndrome (AIDS) adds another dimension to an already complicated picture.

Perspective and Prospects

Throughout human history, maternal and neonatal deaths have been staggering in number. Ignorance and unsanitary conditions frequently resulted in uterine hemorrhaging and overwhelming infection, killing both mother and baby. Highly inaccurate records at the beginning of the twentieth century in New York City show maternal death averaging 2 percent; in fact, the rate was probably greater, since most births occurred at home. Neonatal deaths from respiratory failure, congenital defects, prematurity, and infection loom large in these medical records. The expansion of medical, obstetric, and pediatric knowledge and technology that began after World War II has dramatically lowered maternal and infant mortality. It should not be forgotten, however, that nonindustrialized nations, the majority in the world, remain devastated by the neonatal problems that have plagued

civilization for thousands of years.

Ironically, the problems associated with neonatology in Western nations are now at the other end of the spectrum: saving and prolonging life beyond what is natural or "reasonable." As neonatology advanced scientifically and technically, saving life took precedence over ethical issues. The famous and poignant story of Baby Doe in the early 1980s illustrates the dilemmas that occur daily in neonatal intensive care units. Baby Doe was a six-pound, full-term male born with Down syndrome and severe congenital defects of the heart, trachea, and esophagus. These malformations were deemed surgically correctable, although the underlying problem of Down syndrome, a disease characterized by intellectual disabilities and particular facial and body features, would remain. The parents did not agree to any operations and requested that all treatment be withheld. Baby Doe was given only medication for sedation and died within a few days. The case was later related by the attending physician in a letter to *The New England Journal of Medicine*, sparking enormous controversy. On July 5, 1983, a law was passed in effect stating that all newborns with disabilities, no matter how seriously afflicted, should receive all possible life-sustaining treatment, unless it is unequivocally clear that imminent death is inevitable or that the risks of treatment cannot be justified by its benefit. The legislators believed that Baby Doe had been allowed to die because of his underlying condition of Down syndrome.

Since then, attorneys, ethicists, juries, and courts have used the example of Baby Doe, and the law that grew from it, to interpret many cases that have come to light. Life-and-death decisions are made on a daily basis in the neonatal care unit. They are always difficult, but they usually remain a private matter between the parents and the neonatologist. These cases become public matters, however, when the family disagrees with the medical staff. Then the question of what is in the best interest of the child is compounded by who will pay for the treatments and who will care for the baby after it is discharged.

Such ethical dilemmas will continue as expertise and technology grow. A multitude of questions, previously relegated to philosophy and religion, will arise, and the benefits of saving a life will have to be weighed against its quality and the resources necessary to maintain it.

—*Connie Rizzo, M.D., Ph.D.;*
updated by Alexander Sandra, M.D.

See also Apgar score; Birth defects; Blue baby syndrome; Bonding; Cardiology, pediatric; Cesarean section; Childbirth; Childbirth complications; Chlamydia; Circumcision, male; Cleft lip and palate; Cleft lip and palate repair; Cognitive development; Colic; Congenital disorders; Congenital heart disease; Craniosynostosis; Critical care, pediatric; Cystic fibrosis; Developmental disorders; Developmental stages; Down syndrome; Embryology; Endocrinology, pediatric; Failure to thrive; Fetal alcohol syndrome; Fetal surgery; Gastroenterology, pediatric; Genetic diseases; Genetics and inheritance; Hematology, pediatric; Hemolytic disease of the newborn; Hydrocephalus; Intraventricular hemorrhage; Jaundice, neonatal; Metabolic disorders; Motor skill development; Multiple births; Nephrology, pediatric; Neurology, pediatric; Obstetrics; Orthopedics, pediatric; Pediatrics; Perinatology; Phenylketonuria (PKU); Polydactyly and syndactyly; Premature birth; Pulmonary medicine, pediatric; Rh factor; Shunts; Sudden infant death syndrome (SIDS); Surgery, pediatric; Tay-Sachs disease; Teratogens; Toxoplasmosis; Urology, pediatric; Well-baby examinations.

For Further Information:

Behrman, Richard E., Robert M. Kliegman, and Hal B. Jenson, eds. *Nelson Textbook of Pediatrics*. 18th ed. Philadelphia: Saunders/ Elsevier, 2007.

Bradford, Nikki. *Your Premature Baby: The First Five Years*. Toronto, Ont.: Firefly Books, 2003.

Crisp, Stuart, and Jo Rainbow, eds. *Emergencies in Paediatrics and Neonatology*. 2d ed. Oxford: Oxford University Press, 2013.

Cunningham, Nicholas, ed. *Columbia University College of Physicians and Surgeons: Complete Guide to Early Child Care*. New York: Crown, 1990.

Levin, Daniel L., and Frances C. Morriss, eds. *Essentials of Pediatric Intensive Care*. 2d ed. New York: Churchill Livingstone, 1997.

MacDonald, Mhairi G., Mary M. K. Seshia, and Martha D. Mullett, eds. *Avery's Neonatology: Pathophysiology and Management of the Newborn*. 6th ed. Philadelphia: Lippincott Williams & Wilkins, 2005.

Martin, Richard J., Avroy A. Fanaroff, and Michele C. Walsh, eds. *Fanaroff and Martin's Neonatal-Perinatal Medicine: Diseases of the Fetus and Infant*. 2 vols. 8th ed. Philadelphia: Mosby/Elsevier, 2006.

Meeks, Maggie, Maggie Hallsworth, and Helen Yeo, eds. *Nursing the Neonate*. 2d ed. Malden: Wiley-Blackwell, 2013.

Moore, Keith L., and T. V. N. Persaud. *The Developing Human*. 8th ed. Philadelphia: Saunders/Elsevier, 2008.

Ruhlman, Michael. *Walk on Water: Inside an Elite Pediatric Surgery Unit*. New York: Viking-Penguin, 2003.

Sadler, T. W. *Langman's Medical Embryology*. 11th ed. Philadelphia: Lippincott Williams & Wilkins, 2009.

Sinha, Sunil, Lawrence Miall, and Luke Jardine. *Essential Neonatal Medicine*. 5th ed. Malden: Wiley-Blackwell, 2012.

Woolf, Alan D., et al., eds. *The Children's Hospital Guide to Your Child's Health and Development*. Cambridge, Mass.: Perseus, 2002.

NEPHRECTOMY

Procedure

Anatomy or system affected: Abdomen, kidneys, urinary system

Specialties and related fields: General surgery, nephrology, oncology, urology

Definition: The removal of the kidney, which may be performed to treat disorders and disease or for the purpose of transplantation.

Key terms:

adrenal gland: a small hormone-producing gland which is adjacent to the upper pole of the kidney

donor nephrectomy: a procedure in which a kidney is removed for transplantation into another patient; the kidney can be removed from a person who is brain-dead but whose heart is still beating (cadaveric donor nephrectomy) or from a relative of the recipient (a living related donor)

nephroureterectomy: a procedure similar to a radical nephrectomy, with the additional removal of the ureter and a cuff of the bladder; performed to treat transitional cell carcinomas of the ureters and the pelvis of the kidneys

radical nephrectomy: a procedure in which a kidney is removed along with the covering layers of tissue and the adjacent adrenal gland; performed with cancerous conditions

renal cell carcinoma (RCC): cancer of the small tubules of the kidney; generally known as kidney cancer

simple nephrectomy: a procedure in which a kidney is removed but the covering layers of tissue and the adjacent adrenal gland are left intact; usually performed to treat benign (noncancerous) conditions

transitional cell carcinoma (TCC): cancer arising from the lining of the urine-collecting system of the kidneys, ureters, and bladder

ureters: the tubes that drain urine from the kidneys to the bladder

Indications and Procedures

A kidney may be removed for several reasons, including congenital defects, trauma, cancer, inflammation, and transplantation. Congenital problems, or birth defects, associated with the kidneys include abnormal development, nonfunctional cysts, blockage, tumors, and cysts that leave the kidneys functional but which cause difficulty in breathing because of their large size. A kidney may be removed if the organ or its main blood vessels have been damaged beyond repair by trauma, such as a gunshot wound. Cancer is one of the most common reasons for nephrectomy; kidney cancers include renal cell carcinomas, transitional cell carcinomas, and tumors in the capsules of the kidneys or in surrounding layers of tissue. Infections or abscesses in the kidney that are beyond medical treatment and that become life-threatening may also necessitate a nephrectomy. Finally, a kidney may be removed from a donor for transplantation.

Simple nephrectomies involve removal of the kidney only, whereas radical nephrectomies include removal of the kidney and surrounding glands. Depending on the underlying disease and the surgeon's preference and experience, the kidney can be approached from the front, side, or back. The incisions used to reach the kidney are similar for simple, radical, and donor nephrectomies, but the steps that follow differ once the abdomen has been entered. For a nephroureterectomy, in which the kidney, the connecting ureter, and a part of the bladder are removed, the surgeon makes either one long, S-shaped incision starting in the flank and ending near the bladder, or two separate incisions.

In the frontal approach to nephrectomy, the patient lies on his or her back and the abdomen and peritoneal cavity are opened. The intestines near the kidney are pushed to the side, and the kidney is approached from the front. The advantage of this approach includes better evaluation of the liver and the structures surrounding the kidney, better control of the blood vessels, and easy removal of clots from veins if necessary. The disadvantages of this approach are the possibility of adhesions developing in the intestines and lung complications after the surgery. The frontal approach may also be laparoscopic, in which a number of small incisions are made in the abdomen; a camera is fed through one incision, and surgical

Nephrectomy

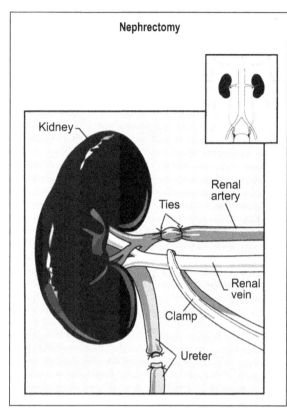

Kidney

Ties

Renal artery

Renal vein

Clamp

Ureter

The removal of a kidney may be necessary because of disease or because the kidney is intended for transplantation into another patient; the inset shows the location of the kidneys.

tools through another; one of the incisions is then made larger for the removal of the kidney. A laparoscopic nephrectomy takes longer to perform but has a shorter recovery period with less postoperative discomfort.

In the side approach, the patient is placed on his or her side and the incision is made through the eleventh or twelfth ribs. The kidney is approached from behind. This type of incision involves cutting into muscle and results in significant postoperative pain. The main advantage is that the peritoneal cavity is not entered.

In the back approach, known as a dorsal lumbotomy, the patient is placed face-down and a muscle-splitting incision is used. The kidney is approached from behind. This method is usually used for a simple nephrectomy. Its primary advantages are less postoperative pain and avoidance of the peritoneal cavity. Its main disadvantage is a limited view of the surgery site.

In a simple nephrectomy, after the kidney has been exposed, Gerota's fascia (the covering envelope of the kidney) is opened, and the fat around the kidney is dissected. The adjacent blood vessels and the connecting ureter are tied and cut, and the kidney is removed. In a radical nephrectomy, the adjacent adrenal gland and surrounding lymph glands are also removed in the one block. For a nephroureterectomy, the ureter is not cut close to the kidney but is removed all the way down to

the bladder. A 2-centimeter cuff of bladder is cut off, the entire specimen is removed, and the hole in the bladder is closed.

The techniques used with kidney transplantation differ for cadaveric (deceased) donor nephrectomy and living related donor (LRD) nephrectomy. For cadaveric donor nephrectomy, the abdominal aorta (the main artery bringing blood to the kidney) and the inferior vena cava (the main vein taking blood away from the kidney) are isolated above and below the kidneys and cannulated with pipes to irrigate both kidneys with cold preservation fluid. Both kidneys and ureters, along with their related blood vessels, are removed. For LRD nephrectomy, the kidney is dissected along with its blood vessels and ureter. Great care is taken to obtain the maximum length of ureter and blood vessels without causing damage to the donor.

Uses and Complications

The major complications of nephrectomy during surgery are bleeding, damage to surrounding structures, and problems related to anesthesia. Therefore, there is significant evaluation of the patient before surgery. A battery of tests may be performed, including blood testing, urinalysis, electrocardiography, and x-rays. A thorough medical examination is done to determine whether the patient can be placed under anesthesia safely. The patient's blood is also typed and cross-matched in the event that a transfusion is required. Good surgical skills, the availability of blood for transfusion, and proper anesthesia techniques usually ensure that any complications that occur are not life-threatening. Nevertheless, the patient may also experience complications during the procedure that are not directly related to the surgery, such as a heart attack.

After a nephrectomy, the patient is at some risk for other problems. These complications may include bleeding, infection, intestinal obstruction, blood clots in the legs or lungs, or a heart attack.

Perspective and Prospects

Significant advances have been made in nephrectomy since the first such procedure was performed by Gustav Simmons in 1869. Thorough preoperative evaluation; improved anesthesia techniques; a greater understanding of anatomy, physiology, and pathology (including the nature of infections and microorganisms); and the discovery of antibiotics have all led to better surgical techniques. As a result, the death rate for nephrectomy operations is only 1 percent.

—*Saeed Akhter, M.D.*

See also Adrenalectomy; Dialysis; Hemolytic uremic syndrome; Kidney cancer; Kidney disorders; Kidney transplantation; Kidneys; Nephritis; Nephrology; Nephrology, pediatric; Transplantation.

For Further Information:
Brenner, Barry M., et al., ed. *Brenner and Rector's The Kidney.* 9th ed. Philadelphia: Saunders/Elsevier, 2012.
Danovitch, Gabriel M., ed. *Handbook of Kidney Transplantation*. 5th ed. Philadelphia: Lippincott Williams & Wilkins, 2010.
Hinman, Frank, Jr. *Atlas of Urologic Surgery.* 2d ed. Philadelphia: W. B. Saunders, 1998.
"Kidney Removal." *MedlinePlus*, October 9, 2012.

Kohnle, Diana. "Nephrectomy." *Health Library*, May 23, 2013.

Marshall, Fray F., ed. *Textbook of Operative Urology*. Philadelphia: W. B. Saunders, 1996.

"Nephrectomy (Kidney Removal)." *Mayo Clinic*, May 23, 2012.

Novick, Andrew C., and Stevan B. Streem. "Surgery of the Kidney." In *Campbell-Walsh Urology*, edited by Patrick Walsh et al. 9th ed. 4 vols. Philadelphia: Saunders/Elsevier, 2007.

Schrier, Robert W., ed. *Diseases of the Kidney and Urinary Tract*. 8th ed. Philadelphia: Wolters Kluwer Health/Lippincott Williams & Wilkins, 2007.

NEPHRITIS

Disease/Disorder

Anatomy or system affected: Blood vessels, immune system, kidneys

Specialties and related fields: Immunology, internal medicine, nephrology

Definition: An inflammatory response of the kidneys, particularly of the glomeruli, to infectious agents or immunological challenges.

Key terms:

albuminuria: excretion in the urine of the protein albumin, usually as a result of changes occurring in the glomeruli

amyloidosis: the deposition of immunoglobulin fibrils in various tissues, including the kidneys

dialysis: the use of artificial membranes to remove metabolites from the blood when the kidneys fail; the peritoneum can also be used (peritoneal dialysis)

filtration rate: the amount of fluid passing per minute from blood across the glomerular capillaries to form glomerular fluid

glomeruli: structures consisting mainly of capillary blood vessels contained in a capsule, across whose walls water and solutes pass (filter) to form glomerular fluid

glomerulonephritis: inflammation of glomeruli

hematuria: the presence of red blood cells or red blood cell casts in the urine

immunoglobulins: proteins associated with immune responses

nephrotic syndrome: a condition involving edema, the retention of water and of sodium and chloride ions, urinary protein losses greater than 3 grams per day, and hypoalbuminemia

proteinuria: the presence of proteins, including globulins, in the urine; usually considered a sign of changes in the glomerular structures

renal blood flow: the amount of whole blood entering the renal arteries per minute; a fraction of water and solutes is removed to form urine

renal failure: severe kidney insufficiency requiring the use of dialysis or transplantation to return and maintain composition of body fluids at or near normal values

renal insufficiency: the inability of the kidneys to maintain a normal internal environment of the body and its fluids

streptococci: bacteria responsible for the development of some cases of acute glomerulonephritis, but without infection of the kidneys

tubules: hollow structures conducting glomerular fluid to the collecting ducts and the renal pelvis; they produce composition and volume changes of glomerular fluid passing through them and may reabsorb some of the protein that crosses the glomerular capillaries

Causes and Symptoms

Nephritis means any inflammatory responses of the kidney, whether the cause is infectious or immunological. Generally, it involves mainly the glomeruli, where the initial formation of urine takes place. The term is therefore equivalent in meaning to glomerulonephritis. Pathological changes may also occur in the interstitium (the extravascular, extracellular domain in which the tubules are embedded) and affect tubular functions. This condition, referred to as tubulointerstitial nephritis, is associated with localized cellular infiltrates and the accumulation of fluid.

The classic cause of acute glomerulonephritis is an infection in the throat or of the skin by a nephritogenic strain of Group A streptococci. The clinical presentation can be dramatic and can be associated not only with a sore throat but also with headaches, shortness of breath, and swelling of the ankles. Physical examination may find hypertension, rales in the lungs, peripheral pitting edema, and changes in the retinal vessels. In the chronic form, the onset is usually insidious; an infection may have been forgotten or ignored, without specific complaints except for some ankle edema, tiredness, and perhaps pallor. The physical findings for chronic glomerulonephritis are similar to but less striking than in the acute form.

The diagnosis in each type of nephritis is presumed on the basis of urinalysis, with a finding of blood (hematuria) in the acute form; proteinuria (actually mainly albuminuria, although globulins may also be present); and a decreased glomerular filtration rate. Diagnosis is established on the basis of renal biopsy with examination by both light and electron microscopy. Throat cultures and streptococcal group determination are appropriate if an infection is suspected.

Both conditions may be followed by the development of nephrotic syndrome, which is characterized by major losses of albumin in the urine, decreased serum albumin concentrations (hypoalbuminemia), the retention of water and of sodium and chloride ions, and massive edema and ascites (fluid leakage from blood vessels into the abdomen). Nephrotic syndrome may also appear without any history or evidence of a preceding episode of acute glomerulonephritis. On renal biopsy, essentially no changes or only minimal changes may be noted on inspection by light microscopy (minimal change disease), although characteristic changes are found with electron microscopy affecting particularly the foot processes (podocytes) of the glomeruli.

Acute glomerulonephritis resolves spontaneously and rapidly in about 95 percent of cases, without detectable residual damage to kidney functions. Apart from control of hypertension, no specific treatment is available. The edema is rarely sufficient to warrant the use of diuretics. Antibiotics are not indicated unless there is evidence of an infection. Patients can be considered to be cured but should nonetheless be followed

Information on Nephritis

Causes: Inflammation of kidney from bacterial infection (often streptococcal) or immune disorder

Symptoms: In acute form, sore throat, headache, shortness of breath, ankle swelling, hypertension, edema; in chronic form, ankle swelling, fatigue, pallor; either may lead to nephrotic syndrome (loss of albumin in urine, decreased serum albumin, water retention, sodium and chloride ion retention, massive edema and ascites)

Duration: Acute or chronic

Treatments: Usually none needed for acute form; for nonresolving or chronic form, dietary control (decreased protein and potassium), steroids, hemodialysis or peritoneal dialysis, kidney transplantation

in the event of a reappearance of symptoms or manifestations.

In nonresolving acute glomerulonephritis and in chronic glomerulonephritis, there can be progression of damage to the glomeruli so that the number of functioning glomeruli (normally, about one million in each kidney) diminishes. This process may be gradual or may occur as a part of acute exacerbations that subside but leave the patient with diminished renal functions. As a result, glomerular filtration is decreased and the accumulation of metabolic end-products, particularly urea, occurs in the blood and tissue fluids. Abnormalities of acid-base regulation appear with decreased blood pH (acidemia), decreased serum bicarbonate concentration, and increased potassium concentration. Generally, a significant anemia exists, and renal blood flow is decreased so that the metabolic activities of the renal tubule cells are affected. Renal insufficiency is established, and dietary control is instituted, with decreased intakes of protein and potassium. Paradoxically, with decreased glomerular function, proteinuria decreases, serum albumin increases, and edema decreases or disappears.

Unfortunately, the progression of glomerular dysfunction continues, and dietary measures provide insufficient control of metabolic abnormalities. Resort is then made to hemodialysis or peritoneal dialysis to control the metabolic abnormalities and lift dietary restrictions to some degree while the patient awaits kidney transplantation. During this waiting period, stimulants of the bone marrow, such as erythropoietin, are administered in the expectation of maintaining the red cell count and the hematocrit at a satisfactory level. Transplants will require the use of immunosuppressive agents to prevent rejection unless an identical twin is the donor.

Other diseases in which glomerular damage can occur include diabetes mellitus, amyloidosis, systemic lupus erythematosus (SLE), Wegener's granulomatosis, Goodpasture's syndrome, syphilis, and human immunodeficiency virus (HIV) infection. Common problems associated with glomerular damage of any etiology are hypertension, strokes, heart failure, pulmonary edema, arteriolar vasoconstriction and sclerosis, impaired vision from exudates, pericarditis, and pericardial effusions.

Treatment and Therapy

Acute glomerulonephritis is characterized by the disappearance of signs and symptoms, or at least their marked reduction, in most patients. In 90 to 95 percent of cases, there is no progression and no recurrence. In some patients, the problems may reappear after apparent complete remission, while in others the disease progresses, often to nephrotic syndrome. This phase, too, disappears as the disease worsens, reaching the stage where hemodialysis or peritoneal dialysis becomes necessary. A renal biopsy can aid in determining the appropriate treatment. For example, if the biopsy confirms that poststreptococcal nephritis is present, then no specific treatment is available. If progressive glomerulonephritis is the diagnosis, then steroids may be indicated.

Hemodialysis depends on an arteriovenous shunt being created, usually in the forearm, so that the patient's blood can pass through a dialysis machine, which functions in a manner similar to glomeruli. Usually, several sessions, two or three times per week for several hours at a time, are required. Peritoneal dialysis involves the introduction of large amounts of fluid into the peritoneal cavity and its withdrawal after adequate exchanges with body fluids across the peritoneal surfaces have occurred. Hemodialysis requires going to a hospital or specialized facility, while pertoneal dialysis can be performed at home. Both procedures require careful and frequent monitoring of the patient's acid-base, electrolyte, and metabolic statuses.

While arrangements can usually be made for local dialysis, patients on dialysis lose a significant degree of mobility and independence. This independence can be regained to a considerable degree through kidney transplantation. Kidneys may be obtained from cadavers, unrelated living donors, and related living donors, such as identical twins. Except with the latter group, rejection phenomena may occur. Infections can occur with the use of immunosuppressive agents. Rarely, malignancies can be introduced with transplanted kidneys.

A low protein intake is recommended in the later stages of glomerulonephritis because too high a protein intake may accelerate the progression of the disease. Lack of control of water intake may lead to edema. Anemia is common in the later stages and may require the administration of erythropoietin.

In the nephrotic phase and in minimal change disease, control of edema is sought through one or more of the following measures: salt restriction, diuretics, intravenous (IV) administration of concentrated human serum albumin, corticosteroids (such as prednisone, which is more likely to be effective in minimal change disease), and other immunosuppressive agents. Nephrotic syndrome may occur in the presence of other underlying diseases, such as lupus, diabetes mellitus, HIV infection, syphilis, amyloidosis, and microvascular angiopathies. Specific treatments should be used when applicable.

Perspective and Prospects

The monograph *Reports of Medical Cases* by Richard Bright, published in 1827, marks the first clear description of nephritis through clinical findings (edema), laboratory assessment (proteinuria), and gross structural changes in the kidneys at postmortem. For many years, nephritis was referred to as Bright's disease. Apart from the measurement of blood constituents such as urea and creatinine, functional assessment was limited until the development, by Donald D. Van Slyke, of the clearance concept, defined as the amount of a given substance excreted in the urine per unit time relative to its concentration in plasma or blood. Van Slyke focused on the clearance of urea, while P. B. Rehberg in Denmark proposed that the clearance of creatinine could be used as a measure of the glomerular filtration rate. Glomerular fluid had been shown by Newton Richards to have the same composition as an ultrafiltrate of plasma. Accordingly, if creatinine was neither secreted nor reabsorbed by the tubules, then its clearance would be equivalent to the glomerular filtration rate.

The assumptions with respect to creatinine were shown to be incorrect, and inulin, a polyfructoside studied by Homer Smith, was found to be a reliable and correct indicator for measuring the glomerular filtration rate. Smith and his collaborators systematized and advanced knowledge of the kidney as a whole organ in a quantitative manner. Detailed understanding of the components of the whole organ progressed rapidly with the discovery of the significance of countercirculation in establishing the solute concentration gradient from cortex to medulla reported by H. Wirz and B. Hargitay. Functions of limited segments of the tubules (and later of individual cells) have provided additional important information on transport and metabolic processes in the kidneys.

On the clinical side, the introduction of renal biopsies and of hemodialysis (and later peritoneal dialysis) by way of an arteriovenous shunt made for more accurate diagnoses and longer life expectancies for patients with chronic renal disease. Further encouragement was provided by the development of techniques for successful renal transplants, first from identical twins, then from living donors and cadavers. Problems of rejection remain. Another major challenge is to find the means of delaying or arresting the progression of chronic renal disease before dialysis and transplants become necessary.

A study published in the *Journal of Epidemiology and Community Health* in May 2013 reported that half of over 1,100 adults treated for stroke in Boston, Massachusetts between 1999 and 2004 lived in close proximity to a major roadway. According to researchers, there is evidence that air pollution caused by traffic can cause harm to the arteries that supply blood to the kidneys.

—Francis P. Chinard, M.D.

See also Bacterial infection; End-stage renal disease; Hemolytic uremic syndrome; Kidney cancer; Kidney disorders; Kidneys; Nephrectomy; Nephrology; Nephrology, pediatric; Proteinuria; Pyelonephritis; Renal failure; Stone removal; Stones; Streptococcal infection; Systemic lupus erythematosus (SLE); Transplantation.

For Further Information:

Brenner, Barry M. "Retarding the Progression of Renal Disease." *Kidney International* 64 (2003): 370-378.

_____, ed. *Brenner and Rector's The Kidney.* 8th ed. Philadelphia: Saunders/Elsevier, 2008.

Cameron, J. Stewart, and Richard J. Glassock, eds. *The Nephrotic Syndrome.* New York: Marcel Dekker, 1988.

D'Amico, G., and C. Bazzi. "Pathophysiology of Proteinuria." *Kidney International* 63 (2003): 809-825.

Eddy, A. A., and J. M. Symons. "Nephrotic Syndrome in Children." *The Lancet* 362 (2003): 629-639.

Hricik, D. E., M. Chung-Park, and J. R. Sedor. "Glomerulonephritis." *New England Journal of Medicine* 339 (1998): 888-899.

Lue, Shih-Ho. "Residential Proximity to Major Roadways and Renal function."Â *Journal of Epidemiology and Community Health.* 10.1136 (2012). Print.

NEPHROLOGY

Specialty

Anatomy or system affected: Abdomen, blood, kidneys, urinary system

Specialties and related fields: Biochemistry, biotechnology, endocrinology, genetics, hematology, internal medicine, urology

Definition: The field of medicine that deals with the anatomy and physiology of the kidneys.

Key terms:

analyte: any chemical substance undergoing measurement; includes charged electrolytes found in the blood, such as sodium or potassium

creatinine: a nitrogen-containing by-product of metabolism; levels of creatinine may be indicative of kidney function

endocrine: referring to a process in which cells from an organ or gland secrete substances into the blood; these substances in turn act on cells elsewhere in the body

glomerulonephritis: inflammation of the glomeruli, the clusters of blood vessels and nerves found throughout the kidney

nephritis: any disease or pathology of the kidney that results in inflammation

nephron: the structural and functional unit of the kidney; composed of the renal corpuscle, the loop of Henle, and renal tubules

nephrotic syndrome: an abnormal condition of the kidneys characterized by a variety of conditions, including edema and proteinuria; often accompanies glomerular dysfunction and diabetes

renal: pertaining to the kidney

urea: a waste product of protein metabolism that represents the form in which nitrogen is eliminated from the body

Science and Profession

Nephrology is the branch of medicine that deals with the function of the kidneys. As a consequence, a nephrologist frequently deals with problems related to homeostasis, that is, the maintenance of the internal environment of the body. The most obvious function of the kidneys is their ability to regulate the excretion of water and minerals from the body, at the same time serving to eliminate nitrogenous wastes in the form of urea. While such waste material, produced as by-products of cell metabolism, is removed from the circulation, essential nutrients from body fluids are retained within the renal apparatus. These nutrients include proteins, carbohydrates, and electrolytes, some of which help maintain the proper acid-base balance within the blood. In addition, cells in the kidneys regulate red blood cell production through the release of the hormone erythropoietin.

The human excretory system includes two kidneys, which lie in the rear of the abdominal cavity on opposite sides of the spinal column. Urine is produced by the kidneys through a filtration network composed of 2 million nephrons, the actual functional units within each kidney. Two ureters, one for each kidney, serve to remove the collected urine and transport this liquid to the urinary bladder. The urethra drains urine from the bladder, voiding the liquid from the body.

Each adult human kidney is approximately 11 centimeters in length, with a shape resembling a bean. When the kidney is sectioned, three anatomical regions are visible: a light-colored outer cortex; a darker inner region, called the medulla; and the renal pelvis, the lowest portion of the kidney. The cortex consists primarily of a network of nephrons and associated blood capillaries. Tubules extending from each nephron pass into the medulla. The medulla, in turn, is visibly divided into about a dozen conical masses, or pyramids, with the base of the pyramid at the junction between the cortex and medulla and the apex of the pyramid extending into the renal pelvis. The loops (such as the loop of Henle) and tubules within the medulla carry out the reabsorption of nutrients and fluids that have passed through the capsular network of the nephron. The tubules extend through the medulla and return to the cortical region.

There are approximately 1 million nephrons in each kidney. Within each nephron, the actual filtration of blood is carried out within a bulb-shaped region, Bowman's capsule, which surrounds a capillary network, the glomerulus. In most individuals, a single renal artery brings the blood supply to the kidney. Since the renal artery originates from a branch of the aorta, the body's largest artery, the blood pressure within this region of the kidney is high. Consequently, hypotension, a significant lowering of blood pressure, may also result in kidney failure.

The renal artery enters the kidney through the renal pelvis, branching into progressively smaller arterioles and capillaries. The capillary network serves both to supply nutrition to the cells that make up the kidney and to collect nutrients or fluids reabsorbed from the loops and tubules of the nephrons. Renal capillaries also enter the Bowman's capsules in the form of balls or coils, the glomeruli. Since blood pressure remains high, the force filtration in a nephron pushes about 20 percent of the fluid volume of the glomerulus into the cavity portion of the capsule. Most small materials dissolved in the blood, including proteins, sugars, electrolytes, and the nitrogenous waste product urea, pass along within the fluid into the capsule. As the filtrate passes through the series of convoluted tubules extending from the Bowman's capsule, most

nutrients and salts are reabsorbed and reenter the capillary network. Approximately 99 percent of the water that has passed through the capsule is also reabsorbed. The material which remains, much of it waste such as urea, is excreted from the body.

Nephrology is the branch of medicine that deals with these functions of the kidney. Loss of kidney function can quickly result in a buildup of waste material in the blood; hence kidney failure, if untreated, can result in serious illness or death. Within the purview of nephrology, however, is more than the function of the kidneys as filters for the excretion of wastes. The kidneys are also endocrine organs, structures that secrete hormones into the bloodstream to act on other, distal organs. The major endocrine functions of the kidneys involve the secretion of the hormones renin and erythropoietin.

Renin functions within the renin-angiotensin system in the regulation of blood pressure. It is produced within the juxtaglomerular complex, the region around Bowman's capsule in which the arteriole enters the structure. Cells within the tubules of the nephron closely monitor the blood pressure within the incoming arterioles. When blood pressure drops, these cells stimulate the release of renin directly into the blood circulation.

Renin does not act directly on the nephrons. Rather, it serves as a proteolytic enzyme that activates another protein, angiotensin, the precursor of which is found in the blood. The activated angiotensin, called angiotensin II, has several effects on kidney function that involve the regulation of blood pressure. First, by decreasing the glomerular filtration rate, it allows more water to be retained. Second, angiotensin II stimulates the release of the steroid hormone aldosterone from the adrenal glands, located in close association with the kidneys. Aldosterone acts to increase sodium retention and transport by cells within the tubules of the nephron, resulting in increased water reabsorption. The result of this complex series of hormone interactions within the kidney is a close monitoring of both salt retention and blood pressure and volume. In this manner, nephrology also relates to the pathophysiology of hypertension—high blood pressure.

The kidneys also regulate the production of erythrocytes, red blood cells, through the production of the hormone erythropoietin. Erythropoietin is secreted by the peritubular cells associated with regions outside the nephrons in response to lowered oxygen levels in the blood, also monitored by cells within the kidney. The hormone serves to stimulate red cell production within the bone marrow. Approximately 85 percent of the erythropoietin in blood fluids is synthesized within the kidneys, the remainder by the liver.

Since proper kidney function is related to a wide variety of body processes, from the regulation of nitrogenous waste disposal to the monitoring and control of blood pressure, nephrology may deal with a number of disparate syndromes. The kidney may represent the primary site of a disease or pathology, an example being the autoimmune phenomenon of glomerulonephritis. Renal failure may also result from the indirect action of a more general systemic syndrome, as is the case with diabetes mellitus. In many cases, the decrease in kidney function may result from any number of disorders, which poses many problems for the nephrologist.

Proper function of the kidney is central to numerous homeostatic processes within the body. Thus nephrology by necessity deals with a variety of pathophysiological disorders. Renal dysfunction may involve disorders of the organ itself or pathology associated with individual structures within the kidneys, the glomeruli or tubules. Likewise, the disorder within the body may be of a more general type, with the kidney being a secondary site of damage. This is particularly true of immune disorders such as lupus (systemic lupus erythematosus) or diabetes. Conditions that affect proper kidney function may result from infection or inflammation, the obstruction of tubules or the vascular system, or neoplastic disorders (cancers).

Immune disorders are among the more common processes that result in kidney disease. They may be of two types: glomerulonephritis or the more general nephrotic syndrome. Glomerulonephritis can result either from a direct attack on basement membrane tissue by host antibodies, such as with Goodpasture's syndrome, or indirectly through deposits of immune (antigen-antibody) complexes, such as with lupus. Nephritis may also be secondary to high blood pressure. In any of these situations, inflammation resulting from the infiltration of immune complexes and/or from the activation of the complement system may result in a decreased ability of the glomeruli to function. Treatment of such disorders often involves the use of corticosteroids or other immunosuppressive drugs to dampen the immune response. Continued recurrence of the disease may result in renal failure, requiring dialysis treatment or even kidney transplantation.

Activation of the complement system as a result of immune complex deposition along the glomeruli is a frequent source of inflammation. Complement consists of a series of some dozen serum proteins, many of which are pharmacologically active. Intermediates in the complement pathway include enzymes that activate subsequent components in a cascade fashion. The terminal proteins in the pathway form a "membrane attack complex," capable of significantly damaging a target (such as the basement membrane of a Bowman's capsule). Activation of the initial steps in the pathway begins with either the deposition of immune complexes along basement membranes or the direct binding of antibodies on glomerular surfaces. The end result can be extensive nephrotic destruction.

Nephrotic syndrome, which can also result in extensive damage to the glomeruli, is often secondary to other disease. Diabetes is a frequent primary disorder in its development; approximately one-third of insulin-dependent diabetics are at risk for significant renal failure. Other causes of nephrotic syndrome may include cancer or infectious agents and toxins.

Diagnostic and Treatment Techniques

Nephrologists can measure glomerular function using a variety of tests. These tests are based on the ability of the basement membranes associated with the glomeruli to act as filters. Blood cells and large materials such as proteins dissolved in the blood are unable to pass through these filters. Plasma, the liquid portion of the blood containing dissolved factors involved in blood-clotting mechanisms, is able to pass through the basement membrane, the driving force for filtration being the hydrostatic pressure of the blood (blood pressure).

The glomerular filtration rate (GFR) is defined as the rate by which the glomeruli filter the plasma during a fixed period of time. Generally, the rate is determined by measuring either the time of clearance of the carbohydrate inulin from the blood or the rate of clearance of creatinine, a nitrogenous byproduct of metabolism. Though the rate may vary with age, it generally is about 125 to 130 milliliters of plasma filtered per minute.

Any significant decrease in the GFR is indicative of renal failure and can result in significant disruptions of acid-base or electrolyte balance in the blood. A decrease in the GFR can sometimes be observed through measurements of urine output. Healthy individuals usually excrete from 1 to 2 liters of urine per day. If the urine output drops to less than 500 milliliters (0.5 liter) per day, a condition known as oliguria, the body suffers a diminished capacity to remove metabolic waste products (urea, creatinine, or acids). Taken to an extreme, in which the filtering capacity is completely shut down and urine formation drops below 100 milliliters per day (anuria), the resulting uremia may cause death in a matter of days.

Anuria may have a variety of causes: kidney failure; hypotension, in which blood pressure is insufficient to maintain glomerular filtration; or a blockage in the urinary tract. As waste products, fluids, and electrolytes (especially sodium and potassium) build up, the person may appear puffy, be feverish, and exhibit muscle weakness. Heart arrhythmia or failure may also occur. Mediation of the problem, in addition to attempts to alleviate the reasons for kidney dysfunction, include regulation of fluid, protein, and electrolyte uptake. Medications are also used to increase the excretion of potassium and tissue fluids, assuming that the cause is not a urinary blockage.

The nephrologist or other physician may also monitor kidney function through measurements of serum analytes or through observation of certain chemicals within the urine. The levels of blood, urea, and nitrogen (BUN), nitrogenous substances in the blood, present a rough measure of kidney function. Generally, BUN levels change significantly only after glomerular filtration has been significantly disrupted. The levels are also dependent on the amount of protein intake in the diet. When changes occur as a result of renal dysfunction, BUN levels can be a useful marker for the progression of the disease. A more specific indicator of renal function can be the creatinine concentration within the blood. Serum creatinine, unlike BUN levels, is not related to the diet. In the event of renal failure, however, changes in BUN levels usually can be detected earlier than those of creatinine.

As the glomeruli lose their ability to distinguish large from small molecules during filtration, protein can begin to appear in the urine, the condition known as proteinuria. Usually, the level of protein in the urine is negligible (less than 250 milligrams per day). A transient proteinuria can result from heavy exercise or minor illness, but persistent levels of more than 1 gram per day may be indicative of renal dysfunction or even complications of hypertension. Generally, if the problem resides in the loss of tubular reabsorption, levels of protein generally are below 1 to 2 grams per day, with that amount usually consisting of small proteins. If the problem is a result of increased glomerular permeability caused by inflammation, levels may reach greater than 2 grams per day. In cases of nephrotic syndrome, excretion of protein in the urine may exceed 5 grams per day.

Measurement of urine protein is a relatively easy process. A urine sample is placed on a plastic stick with an indicator pad capable of turning colors, depending on the protein concentration. Analogous strips may be used for detection of other materials in urine, including acid, blood, or sugars. The presence of either red or white blood cells in urine can be indicative of infection or glomerulonephritis.

In addition to the filtration of blood fluids through the nephrons, the reabsorption of materials within the tubules results in increased urine concentration. A normal GFR within a healthy kidney produces a urine concentration three or four times as great as that found within serum. As kidney failure progresses, the concentration of urine begins to decrease, with the urine becoming more dilute. The kidneys compensate for the decreased concentration by increasing the amount of urine output: The frequency of urination may increase, as well as the volume excreted (polyuria). In time, if renal failure continues, the GFR will decrease, resulting in the retention of both analytes and water.

Determination of urine concentration is carried out following a brief period of dehydration: deprivation of fluids for about fifteen hours prior to the test. This dehydration will result in increased production by the hypothalamus of antidiuretic hormone (ADH), or vasopressin, a chemical that decreases the production of urine through increased renal tubule reabsorption of water. The result is a more concentrated urine. Following the dehydration period, the patient's urine is collected over a period of three hours and assessed for concentration. Significantly low values may be indicative of kidney disease.

A battery of tests in addition to those already described may be utilized in the diagnosis of kidney disease. These may include intravenous pyelography (in which a contrast medium is injected into the blood and followed as it passes through the kidneys), kidney biopsy, and ultrasound examinations. Diagnosis and course of treatment depend on an evaluation of these tests.

Perspective and Prospects

The roots of modern nephrology date from the seventeenth century. In the early decades of that century, the English physician William Harvey demonstrated the principles of blood circulation and the role of the heart in that process. Harvey's theories opened the door for more extensive analysis of organ systems, both in humans and in other animals. As a result, in 1666, Italian anatomist Marcello Malpighi, while exploring organ structure with the newly developed microscope, discovered the presence of glomeruli (what he called Malpighian corpuscles) within the kidneys. Malpighi thought that these structures were in some way connected with collecting ducts in the kidneys that had recently been found by Lorenzo Bellini. Malpighi also suspected that these structures played a role in urine formation.

Sir William Bowman, in 1832, was the first to describe the true relationship of the corpuscles discovered by Malpighi to urine secretion through the tubules. Bowman's capsule, as it is now called, is a filter that allows only the liquid of the blood, as well as dissolved salts and urea within the blood, into the tubules, from which the urine is secreted. It remained for Carl Ludwig, in 1842, to complete the story. Ludwig suggested that the corpuscles function in a passive manner, in that the filtrate is filtered by means of hydrostatic pressure through the capsule into the tubules and from there concentrated as water and solutes that are reabsorbed.

The first definitive work on urine formation, *The Secretion of the Urine*, was published by Arthur Robertson Cushny in 1917. In the monograph, Cushny offered a thorough analysis of the data published on kidney function. Though Cushny was incorrect in some of his conclusions, the work catalyzed intensive research activity on the functions of the kidney. A colleague of Cushny, E. Brice Mayrs, made the first attempt to determine the glomerular filtration rate, measuring the clearance of sulfate in rabbits. In 1926, the Danish physiologist Poul Brandt Rehberg demonstrated the superiority of creatinine as a marker for glomerular filtration; the "guinea pig" for the experiment was Rehberg himself.

A pioneer in renal physiology, Homer William Smith, began his research while serving in the United States Army during World War I. Until he retired in 1961, Smith was involved in much of the research related to renal excretion. It was Smith who developed inulin clearance as a measure of the GFR; his later years dealt with studies on mechanisms of solute excretion.

With the newer technology of the late twentieth century, more accurate methods for analysis became available. These have included ultrasound scanning, intravenous pyelography, and angiography. In addition, better understanding of immediate causes of many kidney problems has served to control or prevent some forms of renal failure.

—*Richard Adler, Ph.D.*

See also Abdomen; Abdominal disorders; Adrenalectomy; Blood and blood disorders; Cysts; Diabetes mellitus; Dialysis; Edema; End-stage renal disease; Hemolytic uremic syndrome; Internal medicine; Kidney cancer; Kidney disorders; Kidney transplantation; Kidneys; Lithotripsy; Nephrectomy; Nephritis; Nephrology, pediatric; Polycystic kidney disease; Pyelonephritis; Renal failure; Stone removal; Stones; Systemic lupus erythematosus (SLE); Terminally ill: Extended care; Transplantation; Urinalysis; Urinary system; Urology; Urology, pediatric.

For Further Information:

Brenner, Barry M., ed. *Brenner and Rector's The Kidney.* 8th ed. Philadelphia: Saunders/Elsevier, 2008.
Cameron, Stewart. *Kidney Disease: The Facts.* 2d ed. New York:

Oxford University Press, 1990.

Floege, Jurgen, Richard J. Johnson, and John Feehally. *Comprehensive Clinical Nephrology: Expert Consult*. St. Louis: Mosby/Elsevier, 2010.

Hricik, Donald E., R. Tyler Miller, and John R. Sedor, eds. *Nephrology Secrets*. 2d ed. Philadelphia: Hanley & Belfus, 2003.

Legrain, Marcel, et al. *Nephrology*. Trans. M. Cavaillé-Coll. New York: Masson, 1987.

Lerma, Edgar, and Allen R. Nissenson. *Nephrology Secrets*. 3d ed. Philadelphia: Elsevier Mosby, 2011.

Marieb, Elaine N. *Essentials of Human Anatomy and Physiology*. 9th ed. San Francisco: Pearson/Benjamin Cummings, 2009.

Mitchell, Rosner H, and Edgar V. Lerma. *Clinical Decisions in Nephrology, Hypertension and Kidney Transplantation*. New York: Springer, 2013.

O'Callaghan, Chris A., and Barry M. Brenner. *The Kidney at a Glance*. Boston: Blackwell Scientific, 2000.

Tanagho, Emil A., and Jack W. McAninch, eds. *Smith's General Urology*. 17th ed. New York: McGraw-Hill, 2008.

Wallace, Robert A., Gerald P. Sanders, and Robert J. Ferl. *Biology: The Science of Life*. 4th ed. New York: HarperCollins, 1996.

Whitworth, Judith A., and J. R. Lawrence, eds. *Textbook of Renal Disease*. 2d ed. New York: Churchill Livingstone, 1994.

NERVOUS SYSTEM

Anatomy

Anatomy or system affected: Ears, nerves, spine

Specialties and related fields: Neurology

Definition: The major control system of the body, which synchronizes physiologic activity by interpreting incoming stimuli and which is responsible for memory and reasoning; it is composed of the central nervous system (the brain and spinal cord) and the peripheral nervous system (nerve processes, sensory receptors, and ganglia).

Key terms:

cerebrospinal fluid (CSF): the extracellular fluid of the central nervous system; it flows through the ventricles of the brain and the central canal of the spinal cord, circulating nutrients and providing a cushion for the brain

effector: a general term referring to skeletal, smooth, and cardiac muscles or glands that respond to impulses produced by the nervous system

glial cells: nonexcitable cells of the nervous system; they include astrocytes, microglial cells, oligodendrocytes, and Schwann cells

receptors: membrane-bound proteins with specific binding sites for neurotransmitters

synapse: a juncture between neurons or between neurons and muscle

Structure and Functions

The nervous system serves as the major control system of the human body. It is responsible for the synchronization of body parts, the integration of physiologic activity, the interpretation of incoming stimuli, and all intellectual activity, including memory and abstract reasoning. The nervous system regulates these activities by communication between various nerve cells; by controlling the actions of skeletal, smooth, and cardiac muscle; and by stimulating the secretion of products from various glands of the body.

Anatomically, the nervous system is divided into the central nervous system, which is composed of the brain and the spinal cord, and the peripheral nervous system, which includes all nervous structures outside the central nervous system—primarily nerve processes, sensory receptors, and a limited number of cells of the nervous system that are located in special structures known as ganglia. Ganglia are found at various locations throughout the body. They are the only locations of neurons outside the central nervous system. Information from incoming cells can be transmitted to the ganglion cells, which in turn can transmit that information to other locations.

Although the brain and the spinal cord contain several different types of cells that are morphologically unique, there is only one type of functional cell present, which by convention is always referred to as the neuron. The neuron is one of the few cells in the body that cannot reproduce; a fixed number of these cells develop in infancy, and the number never increases, though it can decrease in the event of injury or disease.

The neuron consists of a cell body that is similar to that of the typical animal cell familiar to most people. In addition, the neuron has extensions called processes. In the typical neuron, there are two types of processes: dendrites and axons.

Usually a neuron has many dendrites. Dendrites are very short; they receive information from nearby cells and relay that information to the cell body. Each cell has only a single axon, which may be very long, extending up and down the spinal cord or from the spinal cord to the ends of the fingers or toes. The axons conduct information from the cell bodies to the effectors—that is, the muscles and glands—or to other neurons.

Functionally, the nervous system is divided into two areas: the somatic nervous system and the autonomic nervous system. The somatic system controls posture and locomotion by stimulating the skeletal muscles. It is responsible for knowing where the body is in space and for ensuring that there is sufficient muscle contraction (tone) to maintain posture. Responses of the somatic system occur through the motor neurons.

The autonomic nervous system regulates internal activities through the innervation, or nerve stimulation, of the smooth muscles or the glands. It is anatomically different from the somatic nervous system in that the stimulation of body parts always involves two neurons. The cell body of the second neuron in the sequence is located in a ganglion outside the central nervous system.

The autonomic nervous system is broken down further into two divisions: the sympathetic and the parasympathetic. The sympathetic system is also known as the "fight or flight" reaction, since it evolved from the mechanism in lower animals by which an animal would prepare to fight a predator or run from it. More commonly, it is referred to in humans as the adrenaline response, which is active during stressful situations, strenuous physical activity, public performance, or competition.

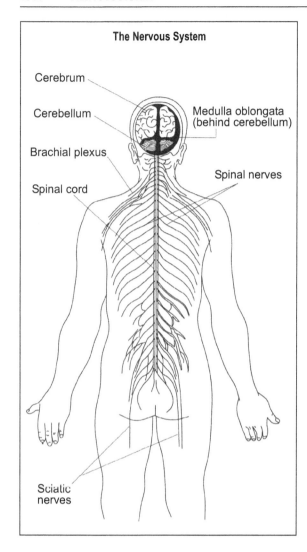

The Nervous System

Cerebrum

Cerebellum

Brachial plexus

Spinal cord

Medulla oblongata
(behind cerebellum)

Spinal nerves

Sciatic
nerves

tors on their dendrites. Neurotransmitters may either stimulate or inhibit the activity of the second cell. If there is significant stimulation of the second cell, it will conduct the information along its axon and release a neurotransmitter from the axon terminal, which will in turn stimulate or inhibit the next neuron or effector. There must be a mechanism for the immediate removal of neurotransmitters from the synaptic cleft if the stimulation of the second neuron is to cease and if other impulses are to be conducted.

Neurotransmitters can influence only those cells that have the appropriate receptors on their surfaces. It is through the neurotransmitter-receptor complex that neurotransmitters are able to influence cells, and any alteration of the number or type of receptors on a cell membrane will lead to an alteration of cellular functioning.

The axons of some neurons are covered with multiple layers of a cell membrane known as myelin. The myelin is produced by specialized cells in the brain known as oligodendrocytes and by cells in the peripheral axons known as Schwann cells. Myelin serves as an insulator for axons and is effective in speeding up the conduction of nerve impulses. It is essential for the normal functioning of the nervous system.

The brain and spinal cord are enclosed by three membranes of dense connective tissue called the meninges, which separate the nervous system from other tissue and from the skull and spinal cord. From the outside inward, they are the dura mater, the arachnoid mater, and the pia mater. Many of the blood vessels of the brain travel through the meninges; therefore, the surface of the brain is very vascular and is subject to bleeding or clotting after trauma.

Disorders and Diseases

Diseases of the nervous system can be arranged into several general categories: infections, congenital diseases, seizure disorders, circulatory diseases, traumatic injury, demyelinating diseases, degenerative diseases, mental diseases, and neoplasms.

Infections of the nervous system are described according to the tissues infected. If the meninges are infected, the disease is known as meningitis; if the brain tissue is infected, the disease is referred to as encephalitis. The development of abscesses in the nervous tissue can also occur. The conditions described can be caused by viruses, bacteria, protozoa, or other parasites.

In most cases, the organism that causes meningitis is spread via the bloodstream. It is also possible for infections to be spread via an infected middle ear or paranasal sinus, a skull fracture, brain surgery, or a lumbar puncture. The infectious agent can usually be determined by analyzing the spinal fluid. Bacterial infections are treated with antibiotics, while viral infections receive only supportive treatment.

An abscess of nervous tissue is usually a complication resulting from an infection at some other anatomical site, particularly from middle-ear infections or sinus infections. Abscesses may also occur following penetrating injuries. The abscess can create pressure inside the skull and, if left un-

The parasympathetic system, which is responsible for the digestive functions of the body, controls stimulation of salivary gland secretions, increased blood flow to digestive organs, and movement of material through the digestive system. The sympathetic and parasympathetic systems usually function in balance; the parasympathetic system predominates after meals, and the sympathetic system predominates during periods of stress or physical activity.

Neurons communicate with other neurons or effectors through the release of chemical messengers known as neurotransmitters. At the termination of the axon, there is a widened area known as the synaptic knob, which produces and stores neurotransmitters. The effects of neurotransmitters are always localized and of short duration. There are many types of neurotransmitters, some of which are well known, such as acetylcholine and norepinephrine.

Neurotransmitters are released in response to an electrical impulse that is conducted along the axon. Once released, a neurotransmitter binds to cells that have appropriate recep-

treated, may rupture and lead to death.

Viral encephalitis is an acute disease that is often spread to humans by arthropods from animal hosts. After a carrier insect bites a human, the virus is spread to the brain of the human via the bloodstream. The specific causative agent often goes undiagnosed. Some well-known forms of encephalitis are herpes simplex encephalitis, poliomyelitis, rabies, and cytomegalovirus encephalitis. In addition, some forms of encephalitis fall into the category of slow virus infections, which have latent periods as long as several years between the time of infection and the development of encephalitis.

Other serious infections include neurosyphilis, which occurs in the late stages of untreated syphilis infections; toxoplasmosis, a protozoan infection that is extremely dangerous to fetuses but rarely causes serious problems in adults; cerebral malaria; and African trypanosomiasis, which is also known as sleeping sickness.

Congenital diseases of the brain vary in the degree of malfunction they produce. Spina bifida is a general term for a group of disorders in which the vertebrae do not develop as they should. As a result, the spinal cord may protrude from the lower back. In some cases, the effects may be so minimal as to produce no symptoms; in other cases, however, these malformations may lead to major neurologic impairment.

Hydrocephalus is another congenital malformation, one that may lead to an increase in the size of the ventricles of the brain. It may be caused by blockage of the flow of spinal fluid in the fetus. In some cases, the spinal fluid produced by the nervous system fills the ventricles and limits the space available for the growing brain and nervous tissue. The result under these conditions is the presence of larger-than-normal ventricles and a smaller-than-normal amount of nervous tissue.

A seizure disorder is any sudden burst of excess electrical activity in the neurons of the brain. Epilepsy is a general term for seizure disorders. The condition may be mild and have only minimal effects, or it may be severe, leading to convulsions. The cause is often unknown, but epilepsy may result from infection, trauma, or neoplasms.

Cerebrovascular accident (CVA) is the term used to describe a variety of malfunctions of blood circulation in the nervous system that are not a result of trauma. More commonly, the term *stroke* is used to describe the condition. Strokes have many causes that generally fall into two categories: ischemic and hemorrhagic.

Ischemic strokes are those in which the nervous tissue is deprived of oxygen as a result of an impairment of blood flow to the area. An ischemic stroke is most commonly the result of a blood clot that blocks the blood vessels leading to the brain or the blood vessels in the brain itself. Since the cells can live for only a few minutes without oxygen, an ischemic stroke can result in neurological impairment or even death.

In hemorrhagic strokes, there is bleeding in the brain itself. It may be caused by hypertension or by the rupture of a weakened blood vessel, which is known as an aneurysm. Both ischemic and hemorrhagic strokes lead to the death of neurons in the affected area. The degree of damage to the brain is determined by the number of cells destroyed by the oxygen deprivation.

Traumatic injury to the brain can generally be classified as penetrating or nonpenetrating. Penetrating injuries produce a risk of infection as well as bleeding at the site of the wound. Since many large blood vessels are located in the meninges, even injuries that penetrate only into the meninges may be sufficient to cause serious injury. Nonpenetrating injuries may also cause bleeding of the meninges, which can limit blood flow to the nervous tissue or put excessive pressure on the tissue.

Injury to the spinal cord may result in severing the spinal cord from the brain. If this should occur, communications between the brain and any structures below the area of the injury are lost, as is all sensory and motor function in those areas. Since neurons are unable to regenerate and axon repair is limited, there is little hope for reversal of this condition, although extensive research is being conducted in this area.

Demyelinating diseases are those that result in changes in the myelin sheaths of neurons. The most common example is multiple sclerosis, which affects myelin in the central nervous system but not in the peripheral nervous system. Although there are varying degrees of severity, the condition causes limb weakness, impaired perception, and optic neuritis, among other things. Some cases present only mild symptoms, while others are degenerative and can lead to death, sometimes within months. Many patients, however, survive for more than twenty years. The cause of these diseases is not yet clear, although viral infections have been associated with some demyelinating diseases.

Degenerative diseases are those in which there is a gradual decline in nervous function. The disease may be hereditary, as in the case of Huntington's disease, or may occur without any apparent genetic basis, as in the case of Parkinson's disease. Parkinson's disease involves the death of certain neurons in the brain and a decreased concentration of neurotransmitters. As the disease progresses, there is a gradual loss of motor ability and, ultimately, a complete loss of motor function. Not much is known about neurotransmitter replacement or mechanisms to stop degenerative diseases.

Little is known about mental diseases such as schizophrenia and manic depression. They appear to involve abnormal levels of neurotransmitters or errors in the membrane receptors associated with those neurotransmitters. Success in localizing the causes of these diseases has been slow in coming; there has been much more success in the development of medications to treat them.

Cancer of the brain can be primary or metastatic. Metastatic tumors, the more common variety, can arise from any source. Of the primary neoplasms, the most common are those derived from glial cells, which are responsible for more than 65 percent of all primary neoplasms. The second most common are neoplasms resulting from transformation of cells of the meninges. Since neurons cannot divide, neuron tumors are almost nonexistent except in children.

Perspective and Prospects

When the control system of the body experiences a malfunction, the effects are wide ranging. Since the nervous system is responsible for regulating so many diverse activities, nervous-system injury or disease must be treated immediately if the patient is to survive. This problem is further complicated by the fact that the brain is a difficult organ to study, because of its location within the skull and because its cells are vital and can be studied only after they have died.

Disease or injury of the cells of the nervous system, especially the brain, creates problems that are unique to that organ for several reasons, including the fact that those cells cannot repair themselves and cannot divide. In addition, the cells of the brain are restricted to a limited area. The cells of the nervous system are unique in that they are so highly specialized that they are not capable of cell division. As a result, humans have the greatest number of neurons during early childhood. Any neural injury or disease that kills cells results in a decreased number of neurons. Furthermore, the space in the skull is tightly packed with cells and cerebrospinal fluid, leaving no room for blood that might result from an injury or fluid accumulation due to tissue infection or tumors. Any of these conditions will increase the pressure within the skull and will also increase the extent of the injury to the nervous tissue.

Although there is no mechanism for replacing cells that have died, the prognosis is not totally bleak. There are cells in the brain that can, in the event of disease or injury, assume the responsibilities of the dead cells. For example, a person who has lost the capacity to speak following a stroke may be retaught to speak using cells that previously did not perform that function.

Among the problems with which the nervous system must cope, there are many things that can go wrong at the synapse of a neuron. The cell may produce too little or too much neurotransmitter. It is possible that the neurotransmitter may not be released on cue or that, if it is released, the postsynaptic cells will not have the appropriate receptors. There also may be no mechanism for removal of the neurotransmitter from the synaptic cleft. These are only a few of the problems that can interfere with communication between different neurons or between neurons and other effectors. As science learns more about the communication system of neurons, efforts to correct these problems will intensify. Already there are many drugs available that can alter activity at the synapse. Correcting these errors can lead to methods for the treatment of mental diseases.

Someday it may be possible to transplant healthy neurons from one person to another. This procedure may permit physicians to prevent total paralysis in a person who has suffered a broken neck or total loss of motor function in an individual who suffers from Parkinson's disease. In 1990, normal neurons were grown in tissue culture for the first time. Such scientific breakthroughs will lead to more and better treatments for individuals who suffer from diseases of the nervous system.

—*Annette O'Connor, Ph.D.*

See also Acupressure; Acupuncture; Alzheimer's disease; Amnesia; Amputation; Anesthesia; Anesthesiology; Aneurysmectomy; Aneurysms; Anxiety; Aphasia and dysphasia; Apnea; Aromatherapy; Ataxia; Autism; Balance disorders; Behçet's disease; Bell's palsy; Biofeedback; Botox; Brain; Brain damage; Brain disorders; Brain tumors; Caffeine; Carpal tunnel syndrome; Cells; Cerebral palsy; Cluster headaches; Coma; Computed tomography (CT) scanning; Concussion; Craniotomy; Cysts; Deafness; Dementias; Disk removal; Dizziness and fainting; Dyslexia; Ear infections and disorders; Ear surgery; Ears; Electrical shock; Electroencephalography (EEG); Electromyography; Encephalitis; Epilepsy; Fetal alcohol syndrome; Fetal tissue transplantation; Ganglion removal; Guillain-Barré syndrome; Hallucinations; Head and neck disorders; Headaches; Hearing loss; Hemiplegia; Huntington's disease; Hydrocephalus; Hypothalamus; Intraventricular hemorrhage; Laminectomy and spinal fusion; Lead poisoning; Learning disabilities; Leprosy; Leukodystrophy; Lower extremities; Lumbar puncture; Memory loss; Meningitis; Mental retardation; Migraine headaches; Motor neuron diseases; Motor skill development; Multiple sclerosis; Narcolepsy; Neuralgia, neuritis, and neuropathy; Neurofibromatosis; Neuroimaging; Neurology; Neurology, pediatric; Neurosurgery; Numbness and tingling; Paget's disease; Palsy; Paralysis; Paraplegia; Parkinson's disease; Physical rehabilitation; Poisoning; Poliomyelitis; Porphyria; Premenstrual syndrome (PMS); Quadriplegia; Rabies; Reflexes, primitive; Restless legs syndrome; Sciatica; Seizures; Sense organs; Shingles; Shock therapy; Skin; Sleep disorders; Snakebites; Spina bifida; Spinal cord disorders; Spine, vertebrae, and disks; Strokes; Sympathectomy; Systems and organs; Tetanus; Tics; Touch; Toxicology; Transient ischemic attacks (TIAs); Tremors; Unconsciousness; Upper extremities; Vagotomy; Vagus nerve.

For Further Information:

Afifi, Adel K., and Ronald A. Bergman. *Functional Neuroanatomy: Text and Atlas*. 2d ed. New York: Lange Medical Books/McGraw-Hill, 2005.

"Autonomic Nervous System Disorders." *MedlinePlus*, April 17, 2013.

Barondes, Samuel H. *Molecules and Mental Illness*. 2d ed. New York: Scientific American, 1999.

Bear, Mark F., Barry W. Connors, and Michael A. Paradiso. *Neuroscience: Exploring the Brain*. 3d ed. Philadelphia: Lippincott Williams & Wilkins, 2007.

Bloom, Floyd E., M. Flint Beal, and David J. Kupfer, eds. *The Dana Guide to Brain Health: A Practical Family Reference from Medical Experts*. New York: Dana Press, 2006.

Goldman, Steven A. "Biology of the Nervous System." *Merck Manual Home Health Handbook*, November 2007.

McCance, Kathryn L., and Sue M. Huether. *Pathophysiology: The Biologic Basis for Disease in Adults and Children*. 6th ed. St. Louis, Mo.: Mosby/Elsevier, 2010.

McLendon, Roger E., Marc K. Rosenblum, and Darell D. Bigner, eds. *Russell and Rubinstein's Pathology of Tumors of the Nervous System*. 7th ed. 2 vols. London: Hodder Arnold, 2006.

"Neurologic Diseases." *MedlinePlus*, July 4, 2013.

Nicholls, John G., et al. *From Neuron to Brain*. 5th ed. Sunderland, Mass.: Sinauer, 2012.

Underwood, J. C. E., and S. S. Cross, eds. *General and Systematic Pathology*. 5th ed. New York: Churchill Livingstone/Elsevier, 2009.

Woolsey, Thomas A., Joseph Hanaway, and Mokhtar H. Gado. *The Brain Atlas: A Visual Guide to the Human Central Nervous System*. 3d ed. Hoboken, N.J.: Wiley, 2007.

SALEM HEALTH

MAGILL'S MEDICAL GUIDE

ENTRIES BY ANATOMY OR SYSTEM AFFECTED

ALL
Abscesses
Abuse of the elderly
Accidents
Acupuncture
Adrenal glands
Aging
Aging: Extended care
Alternative medicine
Anatomy
Antibiotic resistance
Antibiotics
Antihypertensives
Anti-inflammatory drugs
Antioxidants
Autoimmune disorders
Autopsy
Bionics and biotechnology
Birth defects
Burkitt's lymphoma
Cancer
Carcinogens
Carcinoma
Chemotherapy
Chronic granulomatous disease
Clinical trials
Club drugs
Coccidioidomycosis
Cockayne Disease
Collagen
Congenital disorders
Critical care
Cryosurgery
Cysts
Death and dying
Diagnosis
Dietary reference intakes (DRIs)
Disease
Embryology
Emergency medicine
Emergency rooms
Emerging infectious diseases
Environmental diseases
Enzyme therapy
Epidemics and pandemics
Epidemiology
Epidermal nevus syndromes
Family medicine
Fascia
Fatigue
Fever
First aid

First responder
Food guide plate
Forensic pathology
Genetic diseases
Genetic engineering
Genetic Imprinting
Genetics and inheritance
Genomics
Geriatric assessment
Geriatrics and gerontology
Grafts and grafting
Growth
Healing
Herbal medicine
Histology
Homeopathy
Hydrotherapy
Hyperadiposis
Hyperthermia and hypothermia
Hypertrophy
Hypochondriasis
Iatrogenic disorders
Imaging and radiology
Immunopathology
Infection
Inflammation
Insect-borne diseases
Internet medicine
Interpartner violence
Invasive tests
Leptin
Lesions
Longevity
Macronutrients
Magnetic resonance imaging (MRI)
Malignancy and metastasis
Malnutrition
Massage
Medical home
Meditation
Men's health
Metabolic disorders
Metabolic syndrome
Mucopolysaccharidosis (MPS)
Multiple births
Münchausen syndrome by proxy
Neonatology
Noninvasive tests
Nursing
Nutrition
Occupational health
Oncology

Opportunistic infections
Ovaries
Over-the-counter medications
Pain
Pain management
Palliative care
Palliative medicine
Paramedics
Parasitic diseases
Pathology
Pediatrics
Perinatology
Physical examination
Physician assistants
Physiology
Phytochemicals
Plastic surgery
Positron emission tomography (PET)
    scanning
Preventive medicine
Progeria
Prognosis
Prostheses
Protein
Proteomics
Psychiatry
Psychosomatic disorders
Puberty and adolescence
Radiation therapy
Radiopharmaceuticals
Retroviruses
Safety issues for children
Safety issues for the elderly
Screening
Self-medication
Shock
Signs and symptoms
Stem cells
Stress
Stress reduction
Substance abuse
Sudden infant death syndrome (SIDS)
Suicide
Supplements
Surgical procedures
Surgical technologists
Syndrome
Systemic lupus erythematosus (SLE)
Systemic sclerosis
Systems and organs
Teratogens
Terminally ill: Extended care

Toxic shock syndrome
Toxicology
Transitional care
Tumor removal
Tumors
Viral hemorrhagic fevers
Viral infections
Vitamin D deficiency
Vitamins and minerals
Well-baby examinations
Wounds
Xenotransplantation
Zoonoses

ABDOMEN
Abdominal disorders
Adrenalectomy
Amebiasis
Amniocentesis
Aneurysmectomy
Appendectomy
Appendicitis
Back pain
Bariatric surgery
Bladder removal
Bypass surgery
Campylobacter infections
Candidiasis
Cesarean section
Cholecystectomy
Cholecystitis
Colitis
Colon
Colon therapy
Colorectal cancer
Colorectal polyp removal
Colorectal surgery
Constipation
Culdocentesis
Cushing's syndrome
Diabetes mellitus
Dialysis
Diarrhea and dysentery
Digestion
Diverticulitis and diverticulosis
Eating disorders
Endoscopic retrograde
    cholangiopancreatography (ERCP)
Endoscopy
Enemas
Fistula repair
Gallbladder
Gallbladder diseases
Gastrectomy
Gastroenteritis
Gastroenterology
Gastrointestinal disorders

Gastrointestinal system
Gastrostomy
Gaucher's disease
Hernia
Hernia repair
Ileostomy and colostomy
Incontinence
Internal medicine
Intestinal disorders
Intestines
Irritable bowel syndrome (IBS)
Kidney transplantation
Kidneys
Laparoscopy
Liposuction
Lithotripsy
Liver
Liver transplantation
Mesothelioma
Nephrectomy
Nephrology
Obesity
Pancreas
Pancreatitis
Peristalsis
Peritonitis
Polyps
Pregnancy and gestation
Prostate cancer
Reproductive system
Roseola
Shunts
Small intestine
Splenectomy
Stents
Sterilization
Stevens-Johnson syndrome
Stone removal
Stones
Tubal ligation
Tularemia
Ulcerative colitis
Ultrasonography
Urinary disorders
Urinary system
Urology
Vasculitis

ANUS
Amebiasis
Anal cancer
Colon therapy
Colorectal cancer
Colorectal polyp removal
Colorectal surgery
Endoscopy
Enemas

Episiotomy
Fistula repair
Hemorrhoid banding and removal
Hemorrhoids
Hirschsprung's disease
Human papillomavirus (HPV)
Intestinal disorders
Intestines
Irritable bowel syndrome (IBS)
Polyps
Rape and sexual assault
Rectum
Soiling
Sphincterectomy
Syphilis
Ulcerative colitis

ARMS
Amputation
Arthroplasty
Auras
Carpal tunnel syndrome
Casts and splints
Charcot-Marie-Tooth Disease
Cornelia de Lange syndrome
Cutis marmorata telangiectatica
    congenita
Dyskinesia
Fracture and dislocation
Fracture repair
Gigantism
Hemiplegia
Liposuction
Mesenchymal stem cells
Muscles
Neonatal brachial plexus palsy
Phlebotomy
Pityriasis alba
Quadriplegia
Roseola
Rotator cuff surgery
Sarcoma
Skin lesion removal
Slipped disk
Spinocerebellar ataxia
Streptococcal infections
Tendinitis
Thalidomide
Tremors
Upper extremities

BACK
Ankylosing spondylitis
Back pain
Bone disorders
Bone marrow transplantation
Bones and the skeleton

Chiropractic
Cushing's syndrome
Disk removal
Dwarfism
Juvenile rheumatoid arthritis
Kyphosis
Laminectomy and spinal fusion
Neuroimaging
Osteoporosis
Pityriasis alba
Pityriasis rosea
Sarcoma
Sciatica
Scoliosis
Slipped disk
Stevens-Johnson syndrome
Streptococcal infections
Sympathectomy
Tendon disorders

BLADDER
Abdomen
Abdominal disorders
Bed-wetting
Bladder cancer
Bladder removal
Candidiasis
Catheterization
Cystitis
Cystoscopy
Diuretics
Endoscopy
Fetal surgery
Fistula repair
Hematuria
Incontinence
Internal medicine
Lithotripsy
Polyps
Pyelonephritis
Schistosomiasis
Smoking
Sphincterectomy
Stone removal
Stones
Toilet training
Ultrasonography
Uremia
Urethritis
Urinalysis
Urinary disorders
Urinary system
Urology
Williams syndrome

BLOOD
Acquired immunodeficiency

syndrome (AIDS)
Anemia
Angiography
Antibodies
Aspergillosis
Avian influenza
Babesiosis
Biological therapies
Bleeding
Blood pressure
Blood testing
Blood vessels
Bone marrow transplantation
Bulimia
Candidiasis
Carbohydrates
Circulation
Cold agglutinin disease
Connective tissue
Cushing's syndrome
Cyanosis
Cytomegalovirus (CMV)
Deep vein thrombosis
Defibrillation
Dialysis
Disseminated intravascular
   coagulation (DIC)
Diuretics
E. coli infection
Ebola virus
End-stage renal disease
Epstein-Barr virus
Ergogenic aids
Fetal surgery
Fetal tissue transplantation
Fistula repair
Fluids and electrolytes
Glycolysis
Gulf War syndrome
Heart
Hematology
Hematomas
Hematuria
Hemolytic disease of the newborn
Hemolytic uremic syndrome
Hemophilia
Histiocytosis
Host-defense mechanisms
Hyperbaric oxygen therapy
Hypercholesterolemia
Hyperlipidemia
Hypoglycemia
Immune system
Immunization and vaccination
Jaundice
Laboratory tests
Leukemia

Liver
Lymph
Malaria
Menorrhagia
Methicillin-resistant staphylococcus
   aureus (MRSA) infection
Nephrology
Pharmacology
Phenylketonuria (PKU)
Phlebotomy
Plasma
Pulse rate
Rh factor
Salmonella infection
Schistosomiasis
Septicemia
Serology
Sickle cell disease
Single photon emission computed
   tomography (SPECT)
Snakebites
Staphylococcal infections
Sturge-Weber syndrome
Subdural hematoma
Thalassemia
Thrombocytopenia
Thrombolytic therapy and TPA
Thrombosis and thrombus
Thymus gland
Transfusion
Transplantation
Ultrasonography
Uremia
Von Willebrand's disease
Wiskott-Aldrich syndrome
Yellow fever

BLOOD VESSELS
Aneurysms
Angiography
Angioplasty
Arteriosclerosis
Avian influenza
Bedsores
Bile
Bleeding
Blood and blood disorders
Blood pressure
Blood testing
Blood vessels
Bruises
Bypass surgery
Caffeine
Carotid arteries
Catheterization
Cholesterol
Circulation

Claudication
Cluster headaches
Cold agglutinin disease
Cutis marmorata telangiectatica
   congenita
Deep vein thrombosis
Defibrillation
Diabetes mellitus
Disseminated intravascular
   coagulation (DIC)
Diuretics
Dizziness and fainting
Edema
Electrocauterization
Embolism
Embolization
End-stage renal disease
Endarterectomy
Erectile dysfunction
Eye infections and disorders
Facial transplantation
Hammertoe correction
Heart
Heart disease
Heat exhaustion and heatstroke
Hematomas
Hemorrhoid banding and removal
Hemorrhoids
Hormone therapy
Hypercholesterolemia
Hypertension
Hypotension
Infarction
Intravenous (IV) therapy
Ischemia
Kawasaki disease
Klippel-Trenaunay syndrome
Leptospirosis
Methicillin-resistant staphylococcus
   aureus (MRSA) infection
Necrotizing fasciitis
Nephritis
Neuroimaging
Obesity
Phlebitis
Phlebotomy
Plasma
Polycystic kidney disease
Polydactyly and syndactyly
Pulse rate
Raynaud's phenomenon
Rocky Mountain spotted fever
Roundworms
Schistosomiasis
Scleroderma
Scurvy
Single photon emission computed

tomography (SPECT)
Stenosis
Stents
Strokes
Sturge-Weber syndrome
Temporal arteritis
Thalidomide
Thrombolytic therapy and TPA
Thrombosis and thrombus
Toxemia
Transient ischemic attacks (TIAs)
Umbilical cord
Varicose vein removal
Varicose veins
Vascular medicine
Vascular system
Vasculitis
Venous insufficiency
Von Willebrand's disease

BONES
Amputation
Ankylosing spondylitis
Arthritis
Arthroplasty
Aspergillosis
Back pain
Bone cancer
Bone disorders
Bone grafting
Bone marrow transplantation
Bowlegs
Bunions
Cartilage
Casts and splints
Cells
Chiropractic
Cleft lip and palate
Cleft lip and palate repair
Connective tissue
Craniosynostosis
Cushing's syndrome
Dengue fever
Disk removal
Dwarfism
Ear surgery
Ears
Eating disorders
Ewing's sarcoma
Facial transplantation
Failure to thrive
Feet
Foot disorders
Fracture and dislocation
Fracture repair
Gaucher's disease
Gigantism

Hammertoe correction
Head and neck disorders
Hearing
Heel spur removal
Hip fracture repair
Hip replacement
Histiocytosis
Hormone therapy
Jaw wiring
Joints
Kneecap removal
Kyphosis
Laminectomy and spinal fusion
Leishmaniasis
Lower extremities
Marfan syndrome
Mesenchymal stem cells
Methicillin-resistant staphylococcus
   aureus (MRSA) infection
Motor skill development
Necrosis
Neurofibromatosis
Neurosurgery
Niemann-Pick disease
Nuclear medicine
Nuclear radiology
Orthopedic surgery
Orthopedics
Osteochondritis juvenilis
Osteogenesis imperfecta
Osteomyelitis
Osteonecrosis
Osteopathic medicine
Osteoporosis
Paget's disease
Periodontitis
Physical rehabilitation
Pigeon toes
Podiatry
Polydactyly and syndactyly
Prader-Willi syndrome
Rheumatology
Rickets
Rubinstein-Taybi syndrome
Sarcoma
Scoliosis
Spina bifida
Spinal cord disorders
Sports medicine
Syphilis
Teeth
Temporomandibular joint (TMJ)
   syndrome
Tendon disorders
Tendon repair
Upper extremities

BRAIN

Abscess drainage
Acidosis
Acquired immunodeficiency
  syndrome (AIDS)
Addiction
Adrenoleukodystrophy
Agnosia
Alcoholism
Altitude sickness
Alzheimer's disease
Amnesia
Anesthesia
Anesthesiology
Aneurysmectomy
Aneurysms
Angelman syndrome
Angiography
Anorexia nervosa
Anosmia
Antianxiety drugs
Antidepressants
Aortic stenosis
Aphasia and dysphasia
Apnea
Aromatherapy
Aspergillosis
Ataxia
Attention-deficit disorder (ADD)
Auras
Autism
Batten's disease
Biofeedback
Body dysmorphic disorder
Brain damage
Brain disorders
Brain tumors
Brucellosis
Bulimia
Caffeine
Carbohydrates
Carotid arteries
Cerebral palsy
Chiari malformations
Chronic wasting disease (CWD)
Cluster headaches
Cognitive development
Cognitive enhancement
Concussion
Cornelia de Lange syndrome
Craniotomy
Creutzfeldt-Jakob disease (CJD)
Cutis marmorata telangiectatica
  congenita
Cytomegalovirus (CMV)
Defibrillation
Dehydration

Dementias
Depression
Developmental stages
Dizziness and fainting
Down syndrome
Drowning
Dwarfism
Dyskinesia
Dyslexia
Electroencephalography (EEG)
Embolism
Embolization
Encephalitis
Endocrine glands
Endocrinology
Enteroviruses
Epilepsy
Ergogenic aids
Eye infections and disorders
Failure to thrive
Fetal alcohol syndrome
Fetal surgery
Fetal tissue transplantation
Fibromyalgia
Fragile X syndrome
Frontal lobe syndrome
Frontotemporal dementia (FTD)
Gigantism
Glioma
Gulf War syndrome
Head and neck disorders
Headaches
Hearing
Hearing loss
Hemiplegia
Hemolytic disease of the newborn
Hormone therapy
Huntington's disease
Hydrocephalus
Hypertension
Hypnosis
Hypotension
Hypothalamus
Infarction
Intraventricular hemorrhage
Ischemia
Kawasaki disease
Kinesiology
Kluver-Bucy syndrome
Korsakoff's syndrome
Lead poisoning
Learning disabilities
Leptospirosis
Leukodystrophy
Light therapy
Listeria infections
Lumbar puncture

Melatonin
Memory loss
Meningitis
Mental retardation
Mental status exam
Mirror neurons
Narcolepsy
Narcotics
Nausea and vomiting
Neuroimaging
Neurology
Neuropsychology
Neuroscience
Neurosis
Neurosurgery
Niemann-Pick disease
Nuclear radiology
Pharmacology
Phenylketonuria (PKU)
Phrenology
Pick's disease
Pituitary gland
Poliomyelitis
Polycystic kidney disease
Prader-Willi syndrome
Prion diseases
Psychiatric disorders
Rabies
Restless legs syndrome
Resuscitation
Reye's syndrome
Rocky Mountain spotted fever
Roseola
Sarcoidosis
Schizophrenia
Seizures
Shock therapy
Shunts
Single photon emission computed
  tomography (SPECT)
Sleep
Sleep disorders
Sleeping sickness
Sleepwalking
Spina bifida
Spinocerebellar ataxia
Split-brain
Strokes
Sturge-Weber syndrome
Subdural hematoma
Synesthesia
Syphilis
Teeth
Tetanus
Thrombosis and thrombus
Tics
Tinnitus

Tourette's syndrome
Transient ischemic attacks (TIAs)
Traumatic brain injury
Vagus nerve
Vertigo
Weight loss medications
Wernicke's aphasia
West Nile virus
Williams syndrome
Wilson's disease

BREASTS
Abscess drainage
Breast cancer
Breast disorders
Breast-feeding
Breast surgery
Cyst removal
Fibrocystic breast condition
Gender reassignment surgery
Glands
Gynecology
Gynecomastia
Hormone therapy
Klinefelter syndrome
Mammography
Mastectomy and lumpectomy
Mastitis
Premenstrual syndrome (PMS)
Raynaud's phenomenon
Stevens-Johnson syndrome
Tumor removal

CELLS
Acid-base chemistry
Alzheimer's disease
Antibodies
Bacteriology
Batten's disease
Biological therapies
Biopsy
Breast cancer
Cholesterol
Cloning
Conception
Cytology
Cytomegalovirus (CMV)
Cytopathology
Defibrillation
Dehydration
Diuretics
Electrocauterization
Epstein-Barr virus
Erectile dysfunction
Ergogenic aids
Eye infections and disorders
Fluids and electrolytes

Food biochemistry
Gaucher's disease
Gene therapy
Genetic counseling
Glycolysis
Gram staining
Gulf War syndrome
Hearing
Host-defense mechanisms
Hyperplasia
Immune system
Immunization and vaccination
In vitro fertilization
Karyotyping
Kinesiology
Laboratory tests
Lipids
Magnetic field therapy
Mesenchymal stem cells
Microbiology
Microscopy
Mutation
Necrosis
Parkinson's disease
Pharmacology
Phlebotomy
Plasma
Rhinoviruses
Sarcoma
Sickle cell disease
Sleep
Thymus gland
Turner syndrome

CENTRAL NERVOUS SYSTEM
Delirium
Minimally conscious state

CHEST
Achalasia
Aneurysmectomy
Antihistamines
Asthma
Bacillus Calmette-Guérin (BCG)
Bronchiolitis
Bronchitis
Bypass surgery
Cardiac rehabilitation
Cardiology
Choking
Cold agglutinin disease
Common cold
Congenital heart disease
Coughing
Cystic fibrosis
Defibrillation
Diaphragm

Electrocardiography (ECG or EKG)
Emphysema
Gulf War syndrome
Gynecomastia
Heart
Heart transplantation
Heart valve replacement
Heimlich maneuver
Hiccups
Legionnaires' disease
Lung cancer
Lungs
Oxygen therapy
Pacemaker implantation
Palpitations
Pityriasis rosea
Pleurisy
Pneumocystis jirovecii
Pneumothorax
Pulmonary diseases
Pulmonary medicine
Respiration
Resuscitation
Rhinoviruses
Sarcoidosis
Streptococcal infections
Thoracic surgery
Trachea
Tuberculosis
Vasculitis
Whooping cough

CIRCULATORY SYSTEM
Acute respiratory distress syndrome
  (ARDS)
Aneurysms
Angina
Angiography
Angioplasty
Antibodies
Antihistamines
Apgar score
Arteriosclerosis
Avian influenza
Biofeedback
Bleeding
Blood and blood disorders
Blood pressure
Blood testing
Blood vessels
Blue baby syndrome
Bypass surgery
Cardiac arrest
Cardiac rehabilitation
Cardiac surgery
Cardiology
Cardiopulmonary resuscitation (CPR)

Carotid arteries
Catheterization
Chest
Cholera
Cholesterol
Circulation
Claudication
Cold agglutinin disease
Computed tomography (CT) scanning
Congenital heart disease
Coronary artery bypass graft
Cutis marmorata telangiectatica
    congenita
Decongestants
Deep vein thrombosis
Defibrillation
Dehydration
Diabetes mellitus
Dialysis
Disseminated intravascular
    coagulation (DIC)
Diuretics
Dizziness and fainting
Drowning
Ebola virus
Echocardiography
Edema
Electrocardiography (ECG or EKG)
Electrocauterization
Embolism
Encephalitis
End-stage renal disease
Endarterectomy
Endocarditis
Ergogenic aids
Exercise physiology
Facial transplantation
Food allergies
Gigantism
Heart
Heart attack
Heart disease
Heart failure
Heart transplantation
Heart valve replacement
Heat exhaustion and heatstroke
Hematology
Hemolytic uremic syndrome
Hemorrhoid banding and removal
Hemorrhoids
Hormone therapy
Hormones
Hyperbaric oxygen therapy
Hypercholesterolemia
Hypertension
Hypotension
Immune system

Intravenous (IV) therapy
Ischemia
Juvenile rheumatoid arthritis
Kawasaki disease
Kidneys
Kinesiology
Klippel-Trenaunay syndrome
Lead poisoning
Liver
Lymph
Lymphatic system
Mesenchymal stem cells
Methicillin-resistant staphylococcus
    aureus (MRSA) infection
Mitral valve prolapse
Motor skill development
Obesity
Osteochondritis juvenilis
Oxygen therapy
Pacemaker implantation
Palpitations
Phlebitis
Phlebotomy
Placenta
Plasma
Preeclampsia and eclampsia
Pulmonary edema
Pulse rate
Resuscitation
Reye's syndrome
Rocky Mountain spotted fever
Roundworms
Sarcoidosis
Schistosomiasis
Scleroderma
Septicemia
Shunts
Single photon emission computed
    tomography (SPECT)
Smoking
Snakebites
Sports medicine
Staphylococcal infections
Stenosis
Stents
Steroid abuse
Streptococcal infections
Strokes
Sturge-Weber syndrome
Temporal arteritis
Testicular torsion
Thrombocytopenia
Thrombolytic therapy and TPA
Thrombosis and thrombus
Toxemia
Transfusion
Transient ischemic attacks (TIAs)

Transplantation
Typhoid fever
Typhus
Uremia
Varicose vein removal
Varicose veins
Vascular medicine
Vascular system
Vasculitis
Venous insufficiency
Yellow fever

EARS
Adenoids
Adrenoleukodystrophy
Agnosia
Altitude sickness
Antihistamines
Aspergillosis
Audiology
Auras
Bell's palsy
Cartilage
Charcot-Marie-Tooth Disease
Cold agglutinin disease
Cornelia de Lange syndrome
Cytomegalovirus (CMV)
Deafness
Decongestants
Dyslexia
Ear infections and disorders
Ear surgery
Earwax
Facial transplantation
Fetal alcohol syndrome
Fragile X syndrome
Hearing
Hearing aids
Hearing loss
Hearing tests
Histiocytosis
Leukodystrophy
Measles
Ménière's disease
Motion sickness
Myringotomy
Nervous system
Neurology
Osteogenesis imperfecta
Otoplasty
Otorhinolaryngology
Pharynx
Raynaud's phenomenon
Rubinstein-Taybi syndrome
Sense organs
Speech disorders
Streptococcal infections

Tinnitus
Tonsillitis
Vasculitis
Vertigo
Williams syndrome
Wiskott-Aldrich syndrome

ENDOCRINE SYSTEM
Addison's disease
Adrenalectomy
Adrenoleukodystrophy
Amenorrhea
Anorexia nervosa
Assisted reproductive technologies
Bariatric surgery
Biofeedback
Carbohydrates
Computed tomography (CT) scanning
Congenital adrenal hyperplasia
Congenital hypothyroidism
Corticosteroids
Cushing's syndrome
Diabetes mellitus
Dwarfism
End-stage renal disease
Endocrine disorders
Endocrine glands
Endocrinology
Ergogenic aids
Failure to thrive
Fibrocystic breast condition
Gender reassignment surgery
Gestational diabetes
Gigantism
Glands
Goiter
Gynecomastia
Hashimoto's thyroiditis
Hormones
Hyperparathyroidism and
   hypoparathyroidism
Hypoglycemia
Hypothalamus
Klinefelter syndrome
Lead poisoning
Liver
Melatonin
Nonalcoholic steatohepatitis (NASH)
Obesity
Overtraining syndrome
Pancreas
Pancreatitis
Parathyroidectomy
Pituitary gland
Placenta
Plasma
Polycystic ovary syndrome

Postpartum depression
Prader-Willi syndrome
Preeclampsia and eclampsia
Prostate gland
Prostate gland removal
Sexual differentiation
Small intestine
Steroid abuse
Steroids
Testicular cancer
Testicular surgery
Thymus gland
Thyroid disorders
Thyroid gland
Thyroidectomy
Turner syndrome
Weight loss medications
Williams syndrome

EYES
Acquired immunodeficiency
   syndrome (AIDS)
Adenoviruses
Adrenoleukodystrophy
Agnosia
Angelman syndrome
Ankylosing spondylitis
Antihistamines
Aspergillosis
Astigmatism
Auras
Batten's disease
Behçet's disease
Bell's palsy
Blindness
Blurred vision
Botox
Cataract surgery
Cataracts
Chlamydia
Color blindness
Conjunctivitis
Corneal transplantation
Cornelia de Lange syndrome
Cutis marmorata telangiectatica
   congenita
Cytomegalovirus (CMV)
Dengue fever
Diabetes mellitus
Dry eye
Dyslexia
Enteroviruses
Eye infections and disorders
Eye surgery
Face lift and blepharoplasty
Facial transplantation
Fetal alcohol syndrome

Fetal tissue transplantation
Galactosemia
Gigantism
Glaucoma
Gonorrhea
Gulf War syndrome
Hay fever
Juvenile rheumatoid arthritis
Keratitis
Kluver-Bucy syndrome
Laser use in surgery
Leptospirosis
Leukodystrophy
Lyme disease
Macular degeneration
Marfan syndrome
Motor skill development
Multiple chemical sensitivity
   syndrome
Myopia
Ophthalmology
Optometry
Pigmentation
Pterygium/Pinguecula
Ptosis
Refractive eye surgery
Reiter's syndrome
Rubinstein-Taybi syndrome
Sarcoidosis
Scurvy
Sense organs
Sjögren's syndrome
Sphincterectomy
Spinocerebellar ataxia
Stevens-Johnson syndrome
Strabismus
Sturge-Weber syndrome
Styes
Syphilis
Tears and tear ducts
Trachoma
Transplantation
Vasculitis
Vision
Vision disorders
Williams syndrome

FEET
Athlete's foot
Bones and the skeleton
Bowlegs
Bunions
Charcot-Marie-Tooth Disease
Cold agglutinin disease
Cornelia de Lange syndrome
Corns and calluses
Dyskinesia

Flat feet
Foot disorders
Fragile X syndrome
Frostbite
Ganglion removal
Gout
Hammertoe correction
Hammertoes
Heel spur removal
Lower extremities
Mesenchymal stem cells
Methicillin-resistant staphylococcus
    aureus (MRSA) infection
Nail removal
Nails
Orthopedic surgery
Orthopedics
Pigeon toes
Podiatry
Polydactyly and syndactyly
Raynaud's phenomenon
Rubinstein-Taybi syndrome
Spinocerebellar ataxia
Sports medicine
Stevens-Johnson syndrome
Streptococcal infections
Tendinitis
Tendon repair
Thalidomide
Tremors

GALLBLADDER

Abscess drainage
Bariatric surgery
Bile
Cholecystectomy
Cholecystitis
Chyme
Endoscopic retrograde
    cholangiopancreatography (ERCP)
Fistula repair
Gallbladder cancer
Gallbladder diseases
Gastroenterology
Gastrointestinal system
Internal medicine
Laparoscopy
Liver transplantation
Malabsorption
Nuclear medicine
Polyps
Stone removal
Stones
Typhoid fever
Ultrasonography

GASTROINTESTINAL SYSTEM

Abdomen
Abdominal disorders
Achalasia
Acid reflux disease
Acidosis
Acquired immunodeficiency
    syndrome (AIDS)
Adenoviruses
Allergies
Amebiasis
Anal cancer
Angelman syndrome
Ankylosing spondylitis
Anorexia nervosa
Anthrax
Anus
Appendectomy
Appendicitis
Asbestos exposure
Avian influenza
Bacterial infections
Bariatric surgery
Beriberi
Bulimia
Bypass surgery
Campylobacter infections
Candidiasis
Carbohydrates
Childhood infectious diseases
Cholecystectomy
Cholecystitis
Cholera
Cholesterol
Chyme
Clostridium difficile infection
Colic
Colitis
Colon
Colon therapy
Colonoscopy and sigmoidoscopy
Colorectal cancer
Colorectal polyp removal
Colorectal surgery
Computed tomography (CT) scanning
Constipation
Crohn's disease
Cytomegalovirus (CMV)
Diabetes mellitus
Diarrhea and dysentery
Digestion
Diverticulitis and diverticulosis
E. coli infection
Eating disorders
Ebola virus
Embolization
Endoscopic retrograde

cholangiopancreatography (ERCP)
Endoscopy
Enemas
Enterocolitis
Esophagus
Fiber
Fistula repair
Food allergies
Food biochemistry
Food poisoning
Fructosemia
Gallbladder
Gallbladder cancer
Gallbladder diseases
Gastrectomy
Gastroenteritis
Gastroenterology
Gastrointestinal disorders
Gastrostomy
Giardiasis
Glands
Gluten intolerance
Gulf War syndrome
Hand-foot-and-mouth disease
Hemolytic uremic syndrome
Hemorrhoid banding and removal
Hemorrhoids
Hernia
Hernia repair
Histiocytosis
Host-defense mechanisms
Ileostomy and colostomy
Incontinence
Internal medicine
Intestinal disorders
Intestines
Irritable bowel syndrome (IBS)
Klippel-Trenaunay syndrome
Kwashiorkor
Lactose intolerance
Laparoscopy
Lipids
Liver
Malabsorption
Malnutrition
Meckel's diverticulum
Metabolism
Motion sickness
Muscles
Nausea and vomiting
Nonalcoholic steatohepatitis (NASH)
Noroviruses
Obesity
Pancreas
Pancreatitis
Peristalsis
Peritonitis

Pharynx
Pinworms
Poisoning
Polycystic kidney disease
Polyps
Proctology
Protozoan diseases
Pyloric stenosis
Radiation sickness
Rectum
Reiter's syndrome
Rotavirus
Roundworms
Salmonella infection
Scleroderma
Sense organs
Shigellosis
Shunts
Small intestine
Smallpox
Smoking
Soiling
Staphylococcal infections
Stenosis
Stevens-Johnson syndrome
Tapeworms
Taste
Teeth
Toilet training
Toxoplasmosis
Trichinosis
Tumor removal
Typhoid fever
Ulcer surgery
Ulcerative colitis
Ulcers
Vagotomy
Vasculitis
Weaning
Weight loss and gain

GENITALS
Adrenoleukodystrophy
Aphrodisiacs
Assisted reproductive technologies
Behçet's disease
Candidiasis
Catheterization
Cervical procedures
Chlamydia
Congenital adrenal hyperplasia
Contraception
Cyst removal
Embolization
Endometrial biopsy
Episiotomy
Erectile dysfunction

Ergogenic aids
Fragile X syndrome
Gender identity disorder
Gender reassignment surgery
Glands
Gonorrhea
Gynecology
Hemochromatosis
Hermaphroditism and
   pseudohermaphroditism
Herpes
Hormone therapy
Human papillomavirus (HPV)
Hydroceles
Hyperplasia
Hypospadias repair and urethroplasty
Klinefelter syndrome
Kluver-Bucy syndrome
Masturbation
Mumps
Orchitis
Pap test
Pelvic inflammatory disease (PID)
Penile implant surgery
Prader-Willi syndrome
Rape and sexual assault
Reproductive system
Rubinstein-Taybi syndrome
Semen
Sexual differentiation
Sexual dysfunction
Sexuality
Sexually transmitted diseases (STDs)
Sperm banks
Sterilization
Stevens-Johnson syndrome
Streptococcal infections
Syphilis
Testicular cancer
Testicular surgery
Testicular torsion
Toilet training
Trichomoniasis
Urethritis
Urology
Uterus
Vas deferens
Vasectomy

GLANDS
Abscess drainage
Addison's disease
Adrenalectomy
Adrenoleukodystrophy
Assisted reproductive technologies
Biofeedback
Breast cancer

Breast disorders
Breast-feeding
Breast surgery
Cushing's syndrome
Cyst removal
Dengue fever
Diabetes mellitus
DiGeorge syndrome
Dwarfism
Endocrine disorders
Endocrine glands
Endocrinology
Epstein-Barr virus
Ergogenic aids
Eye infections and disorders
Gender reassignment surgery
Goiter
Gynecomastia
Hashimoto's thyroiditis
Hormones
Hyperhidrosis
Hyperparathyroidism and
   hypoparathyroidism
Hypoglycemia
Hypothalamus
Immune system
Internal medicine
Liver
Mastitis
Melatonin
Mumps
Neurosurgery
Nuclear medicine
Nuclear radiology
Pancreas
Parathyroidectomy
Pituitary gland
Prader-Willi syndrome
Prostate gland
Prostate gland removal
Quinsy
Semen
Sexual differentiation
Sleep
Steroids
Sweating
Testicular cancer
Testicular surgery
Thymus gland
Thyroid disorders
Thyroid gland
Thyroidectomy

GUMS
Abscess drainage
Bulimia
Cavities

Cleft lip and palate repair
Dengue fever
Dental diseases
Dentistry
Dentures
Fluoride treatments
Gingivitis
Gulf War syndrome
Gum disease
Jaw wiring
Mouth and throat cancer
Oral and maxillofacial surgery
Orthodontics
Periodontal surgery
Periodontitis
Root canal treatment
Scurvy
Teeth
Teething
Tooth extraction
Wisdom teeth

HAIR
Alopecia
Angelman syndrome
Anorexia nervosa
Collodion baby
Cornelia de Lange syndrome
Cushing's syndrome
Dermatitis
Dermatology
Gigantism
Gulf War syndrome
Hair
Hair transplantation
Klinefelter syndrome
Pigmentation
Radiation sickness

HANDS
Amputation
Arthritis
Arthroplasty
Bursitis
Carpal tunnel syndrome
Casts and splints
Charcot-Marie-Tooth Disease
Cold agglutinin disease
Cornelia de Lange syndrome
Corns and calluses
Dyskinesia
Fetal alcohol syndrome
Fracture and dislocation
Fragile X syndrome
Frostbite
Ganglion removal
Gigantism

Mesenchymal stem cells
Methicillin-resistant staphylococcus
    aureus (MRSA) infection
Nail removal
Nails
Neurology
Orthopedic surgery
Orthopedics
Polydactyly and syndactyly
Raynaud's phenomenon
Rheumatology
Rubinstein-Taybi syndrome
Scleroderma
Skin lesion removal
Spinocerebellar ataxia
Sports medicine
Stevens-Johnson syndrome
Streptococcal infections
Tendinitis
Tendon repair
Thalidomide
Tremors
Upper extremities
Vasculitis

HEAD
Alopecia
Altitude sickness
Aneurysms
Angelman syndrome
Angiography
Antihistamines
Bell's palsy
Botox
Brain
Brain disorders
Brain tumors
Cluster headaches
Concussion
Cornelia de Lange syndrome
Craniosynostosis
Craniotomy
Dengue fever
Dizziness and fainting
Dyskinesia
Electroencephalography (EEG)
Epilepsy
Eye infections and disorders
Facial transplantation
Fetal alcohol syndrome
Fibromyalgia
Hair transplantation
Head and neck disorders
Headaches
Hemiplegia
Hydrocephalus
Meningitis

Motion sickness
Nasal polyp removal
Neuroimaging
Neurology
Neurosurgery
Oral and maxillofacial surgery
Paget's disease
Pharynx
Rubinstein-Taybi syndrome
Seizures
Shunts
Single photon emission computed
    tomography (SPECT)
Spinocerebellar ataxia
Sports medicine
Stevens-Johnson syndrome
Strokes
Sturge-Weber syndrome
Tears and tear ducts
Temporomandibular joint (TMJ)
    syndrome
Thrombosis and thrombus
Tinnitus
Tremors
Whiplash

HEART
Acidosis
Anemia
Aneurysmectomy
Aneurysms
Angina
Angiography
Angioplasty
Anorexia nervosa
Anxiety
Aortic stenosis
Apgar score
Arrhythmias
Arteriosclerosis
Aspergillosis
Atrial fibrillation
Avian influenza
Beriberi
Biofeedback
Bites and stings
Blood pressure
Blood vessels
Blue baby syndrome
Brucellosis
Bulimia
Bypass surgery
Caffeine
Cardiac arrest
Cardiac rehabilitation
Cardiac surgery
Cardiology

Cardiopulmonary resuscitation (CPR)
Carotid arteries
Catheterization
Congenital heart disease
Cornelia de Lange syndrome
Coronary artery bypass graft
Defibrillation
Depression
Diabetes mellitus
DiGeorge syndrome
Diphtheria
Diuretics
Drowning
Echocardiography
Electrical shock
Electrocardiography (ECG or EKG)
End-stage renal disease
Endocarditis
Enteroviruses
Ergogenic aids
Exercise physiology
Fatty acid oxidation disorders
Fetal alcohol syndrome
Gangrene
Glycogen storage diseases
Heart attack
Heart disease
Heart failure
Heart transplantation
Heart valve replacement
Hemochromatosis
Hormone therapy
Hypercholesterolemia
Hypertension
Hypotension
Infarction
Internal medicine
Interstitial pulmonary fibrosis (IPF)
Intravenous (IV) therapy
Juvenile rheumatoid arthritis
Kawasaki disease
Kinesiology
Lyme disease
Marfan syndrome
Methicillin-resistant staphylococcus
   aureus (MRSA) infection
Mitral valve prolapse
Mononucleosis
Obesity
Oxygen therapy
Pacemaker implantation
Palpitations
Plasma
Prader-Willi syndrome
Pulmonary edema
Pulse rate
Renal failure

Respiratory distress syndrome
Resuscitation
Reye's syndrome
Rheumatic fever
Rheumatoid arthritis
Rubinstein-Taybi syndrome
Sarcoidosis
Scleroderma
Single photon emission computed
   tomography (SPECT)
Sleeping sickness
Sports medicine
Stenosis
Stents
Steroid abuse
Streptococcal infections
Strokes
Syphilis
Teeth
Thoracic surgery
Thrombolytic therapy and TPA
Thrombosis and thrombus
Transplantation
Ultrasonography
Uremia
Whooping cough
Williams syndrome

HIPS
Ankylosing spondylitis
Arthritis
Arthroplasty
Arthroscopy
Back pain
Bones and the skeleton
Bowlegs
Chiropractic
Dwarfism
Fracture and dislocation
Fracture repair
Hip fracture repair
Hip replacement
Liposuction
Lower extremities
Orthopedic surgery
Orthopedics
Osteochondritis juvenilis
Osteonecrosis
Osteoporosis
Paget's disease
Physical rehabilitation
Pigeon toes
Rheumatology
Sciatica

IMMUNE SYSTEM
Acquired immunodeficiency

syndrome (AIDS)
Adenoids
Adenoviruses
Allergies
Ankylosing spondylitis
Anorexia nervosa
Anthrax
Antibodies
Antihistamines
Arthritis
Asthma
Bacillus Calmette-Guérin (BCG)
Bacterial infections
Bacteriology
Bedsores
Bile
Biological therapies
Bites and stings
Blood and blood disorders
Bone grafting
Bone marrow transplantation
Candidiasis
Cells
Chagas' disease
Childhood infectious diseases
Chronic fatigue syndrome
Cold agglutinin disease
Conjunctivitis
Cornelia de Lange syndrome
Coronaviruses
Corticosteroids
Coughing
Cytology
Cytomegalovirus (CMV)
Cytopathology
Dermatology
Dermatopathology
DiGeorge syndrome
Disseminated intravascular
   coagulation (DIC)
Ehrlichiosis
Endocrinology
Epstein-Barr virus
Facial transplantation
Fetal tissue transplantation
Food allergies
Fungal infections
Gluten intolerance
Gram staining
Guillain-Barré syndrome
Gulf War syndrome
Hashimoto's thyroiditis
Hay fever
Hematology
Histiocytosis
Hives
Host-defense mechanisms

Juvenile rheumatoid arthritis
Klippel-Trenaunay syndrome
Kneecap removal
Ligaments
Lyme disease
Mesenchymal stem cells
Methicillin-resistant staphylococcus
    aureus (MRSA) infection
Motor skill development
Obesity
Orthopedic surgery
Orthopedics
Osteoarthritis
Osteochondritis juvenilis
Osteomyelitis
Osteonecrosis
Physical rehabilitation
Pigeon toes
Polymyalgia rheumatica
Reiter's syndrome
Rheumatology
Rotator cuff surgery
Rubella
Sarcoidosis
Sarcoma
Scleroderma
Spondylitis
Sports medicine
Streptococcal infections
Syphilis
Temporomandibular joint (TMJ)
    syndrome
Tendinitis
Tendon repair
Tularemia
Von Willebrand's disease

KIDNEYS
Abdomen
Abdominal disorders
Abscess drainage
Addison's disease
Adrenalectomy
Anemia
Anorexia nervosa
Aspergillosis
Avian influenza
Babesiosis
Carbohydrates
Cholera
Diabetes mellitus
Dialysis
Diuretics
Drowning
End-stage renal disease
Ergogenic aids
Fructosemia

Hantavirus
Hematuria
Hemolytic uremic syndrome
Hypertension
Hypotension
Infarction
Internal medicine
Intravenous (IV) therapy
Kidney cancer
Kidney disorders
Kidney transplantation
Laparoscopy
Leptospirosis
Lithotripsy
Metabolism
Methicillin-resistant staphylococcus
    aureus (MRSA) infection
Nephrectomy
Nephritis
Nephrology
Nuclear medicine
Nuclear radiology
Polycystic kidney disease
Polyps
Preeclampsia and eclampsia
Proteinuria
Pyelonephritis
Renal failure
Reye's syndrome
Rocky Mountain spotted fever
Sarcoidosis
Scleroderma
Scurvy
Sickle cell disease
Stone removal
Stones
Syphilis
Toilet training
Transplantation
Typhoid fever
Typhus
Ultrasonography
Uremia
Urinalysis
Urinary disorders
Urinary system
Urology
Vasculitis
Williams syndrome

KNEES
Amputation
Angelman syndrome
Arthritis
Arthroplasty
Arthroscopy
Bowlegs

Bursitis
Cartilage
Casts and splints
Endoscopy
Exercise physiology
Fracture and dislocation
Joints
Kneecap removal
Liposuction
Lower extremities
Lyme disease
Mesenchymal stem cells
Orthopedic surgery
Orthopedics
Osgood-Schlatter disease
Osteonecrosis
Physical rehabilitation
Pigeon toes
Rheumatology
Sports medicine
Stevens-Johnson syndrome
Tendinitis
Tendon repair

LEGS
Amputation
Arthritis
Arthroscopy
Auras
Back pain
Bone disorders
Bones and the skeleton
Bowlegs
Bursitis
Bypass surgery
Casts and splints
Charcot-Marie-Tooth Disease
Claudication
Cornelia de Lange syndrome
Cutis marmorata telangiectatica
    congenita
Deep vein thrombosis
Dwarfism
Dyskinesia
Fracture and dislocation
Fracture repair
Gigantism
Hemiplegia
Hip fracture repair
Kneecap removal
Liposuction
Lower extremities
Mesenchymal stem cells
Methicillin-resistant staphylococcus
    aureus (MRSA) infection
Muscles
Muscular dystrophy

Numbness and tingling
Orthopedic surgery
Orthopedics
Osteoporosis
Paget's disease
Paralysis
Paraplegia
Physical rehabilitation
Pigeon toes
Poliomyelitis
Quadriplegia
Rheumatology
Roseola
Sarcoma
Sciatica
Slipped disk
Spinocerebellar ataxia
Sports medicine
Stevens-Johnson syndrome
Streptococcal infections
Tendinitis
Tendon disorders
Tendon repair
Thalidomide
Tremors
Varicose vein removal
Vascular system
Vasculitis
Venous insufficiency

LIGAMENTS
Ankylosing spondylitis
Back pain
Bowlegs
Casts and splints
Collagen
Connective tissue
Electrocauterization
Eye infections and disorders
Flat feet
Joints
Mesenchymal stem cells
Muscles
Orthopedic surgery
Orthopedics
Osteogenesis imperfecta
Physical rehabilitation
Pigeon toes
Sports medicine
Tendon disorders
Tendon repair
Whiplash

LIVER
Abdomen
Abdominal disorders
Abscess drainage

Acquired immunodeficiency
  syndrome (AIDS)
Alcoholism
Amebiasis
Aspergillosis
Babesiosis
Bile
Blood and blood disorders
Brucellosis
Cholecystitis
Chyme
Circulation
Cirrhosis
Cold agglutinin disease
Cytomegalovirus (CMV)
Edema
Embolization
Endoscopic retrograde
  cholangiopancreatography (ERCP)
Ergogenic aids
Fatty acid oxidation disorders
Fetal surgery
Fructosemia
Galactosemia
Gastroenterology
Gastrointestinal system
Gaucher's disease
Glycogen storage diseases
Hematology
Hemochromatosis
Hemolytic disease of the newborn
Hepatitis
Histiocytosis
Hypercholesterolemia
Immune system
Internal medicine
Jaundice
Kaposi's sarcoma
Leptospirosis
Liver cancer
Liver disorders
Liver transplantation
Malabsorption
Malaria
Metabolism
Methicillin-resistant staphylococcus
  aureus (MRSA) infection
Niemann-Pick disease
Nonalcoholic steatohepatitis (NASH)
Phenylketonuria (PKU)
Polycystic kidney disease
Reye's syndrome
Shunts
Thrombocytopenia
Transplantation
Typhoid fever
Wilson's disease

Yellow fever

LUNGS
Abscess drainage
Acquired immunodeficiency
  syndrome (AIDS)
Acute respiratory distress syndrome
  (ARDS)
Adenoviruses
Allergies
Altitude sickness
Antihistamines
Apgar score
Apnea
Asbestos exposure
Aspergillosis
Asphyxiation
Asthma
Avian influenza
Bacterial infections
Bronchi
Bronchiolitis
Bronchitis
Cardiopulmonary resuscitation (CPR)
Chest
Childhood infectious diseases
Chlamydia
Choking
Chronic obstructive pulmonary
  disease (COPD)
Cold agglutinin disease
Common cold
Coronaviruses
Coughing
Croup
Cystic fibrosis
Cytomegalovirus (CMV)
Diaphragm
Drowning
Edema
Embolism
Emphysema
Endoscopy
Exercise physiology
Fetal surgery
Hantavirus
Hay fever
Heart transplantation
Heimlich maneuver
Hiccups
Histiocytosis
H1N1 influenza
Hyperbaric oxygen therapy
Hyperventilation
Hypoxia
Infarction
Influenza

Internal medicine
Interstitial pulmonary fibrosis (IPF)
Intravenous (IV) therapy
Kaposi's sarcoma
Kinesiology
Legionnaires' disease
Leptospirosis
Lung cancer
Lung surgery
Measles
Mesothelioma
Mold and mildew
Multiple chemical sensitivity
    syndrome
Niemann-Pick disease
Oxygen therapy
Plague
Pleurisy
Pneumocystis jirovecii
Pneumonia
Pneumothorax
Pulmonary diseases
Pulmonary edema
Pulmonary hypertension
Pulmonary medicine
Quinsy
Respiration
Respiratory distress syndrome
Resuscitation
Rhinoviruses
Roundworms
Sarcoidosis
Schistosomiasis
Scleroderma
Severe acute respiratory syndrome
    (SARS)
Sickle cell disease
Stevens-Johnson syndrome
Thoracic surgery
Thrombolytic therapy and TPA
Thrombosis and thrombus
Transplantation
Tuberculosis
Tumor removal
Vasculitis
Wiskott-Aldrich syndrome

LYMPHATIC SYSTEM
Acquired immunodeficiency
    syndrome (AIDS)
Adenoids
Antibodies
Bacillus Calmette-Guérin (BCG)
Bacterial infections
Biological therapies
Blood and blood disorders
Blood vessels

Breast cancer
Breast disorders
Bruises
Chlamydia
Cold agglutinin disease
Colorectal cancer
Coronaviruses
DiGeorge syndrome
Edema
Elephantiasis
Embolism
Epstein-Barr virus
Gaucher's disease
Hay fever
Hodgkin's disease
Immune system
Kawasaki disease
Klippel-Trenaunay syndrome
Leishmaniasis
Leptospirosis
Lower extremities
Lung cancer
Lymph
Lymphadenopathy and lymphoma
Mononucleosis
Overtraining syndrome
Prostate cancer
Roundworms
Rubella
Sarcoidosis
Skin cancer
Sleeping sickness
Small intestine
Splenectomy
Thymus gland
Tonsillectomy and adenoid removal
Tonsillitis
Tonsils
Tularemia
Upper extremities
Vascular medicine

MOUTH
Acid reflux disease
Acquired immunodeficiency
    syndrome (AIDS)
Adenoids
Angelman syndrome
Auras
Behçet's disease
Bell's palsy
Candidiasis
Canker sores
Chickenpox
Cleft lip and palate repair
Cold sores
Cornelia de Lange syndrome

Crowns and bridges
Dengue fever
Dental diseases
Dentistry
Dentures
DiGeorge syndrome
Dyskinesia
Eating disorders
Endodontic disease
Epstein-Barr virus
Esophagus
Facial transplantation
Fetal alcohol syndrome
Fluoride treatments
Gingivitis
Gum disease
Hand-foot-and-mouth disease
Heimlich maneuver
Herpes
Jaw wiring
Kawasaki disease
Lisping
Measles
Mouth and throat cancer
Oral and maxillofacial surgery
Orthodontics
Periodontal surgery
Pharynx
Quinsy
Rape and sexual assault
Raynaud's phenomenon
Reiter's syndrome
Root canal treatment
Rubinstein-Taybi syndrome
Sense organs
Sjögren's syndrome
Taste
Teething
Temporomandibular joint (TMJ)
    syndrome
Thumb sucking
Tooth extraction
Ulcers
Wisdom teeth

MUSCLES
Acidosis
Acupressure
Amputation
Anesthesia
Anesthesiology
Apgar score
Avian influenza
Back pain
Bed-wetting
Bedsores
Bell's palsy

Muscles
Muscular dystrophy
Myasthenia gravis
Neurology
Nuclear medicine
Nuclear radiology
Numbness and tingling
Orthopedic surgery
Orthopedics
Osgood-Schlatter disease
Osteoarthritis
Osteochondritis juvenilis
Osteogenesis imperfecta
Osteomyelitis
Osteonecrosis
Osteopathic medicine
Paget's disease
Palsy
Paralysis
Parkinson's disease
Physical rehabilitation
Poisoning
Poliomyelitis
Prader-Willi syndrome
Precocious puberty
Rabies
Radiculopathy
Respiration
Restless legs syndrome
Rheumatoid arthritis
Rheumatology
Rickets
Scoliosis
Seizures
Sleepwalking
Slipped disk
Speech disorders
Sphincterectomy
Spinal cord disorders
Spinocerebellar ataxia
Sports medicine
Staphylococcal infections
Teeth
Tendinitis
Tendon disorders
Tendon repair
Tetanus
Tics
Tourette's syndrome
Trichinosis
Upper extremities
Weight loss and gain

NAILS
Anorexia nervosa
Athlete's foot
Collodion baby

Dermatology
Fungal infections
Malnutrition
Nail removal
Podiatry

NECK
Botox
Carotid arteries
Casts and splints
Chiari malformations
Choking
Congenital hypothyroidism
Dyskinesia
Encephalitis
Endarterectomy
Facial transplantation
Goiter
Hashimoto's thyroiditis
Head and neck disorders
Heimlich maneuver
Hyperparathyroidism and
    hypoparathyroidism
Mouth and throat cancer
Neuroimaging
Paralysis
Parathyroidectomy
Pharynx
Pityriasis alba
Slipped disk
Stevens-Johnson syndrome
Streptococcal infections
Sympathectomy
Thyroid disorders
Thyroid gland
Thyroidectomy
Torticollis
Trachea
Tracheostomy
Vagus nerve
Whiplash
Whooping cough

NERVES
Agnosia
Alzheimer's disease
Anesthesia
Anesthesiology
Angelman syndrome
Avian influenza
Back pain
Bell's palsy
Biofeedback
Brain
Bulimia
Carpal tunnel syndrome
Cells

Cluster headaches
Concussion
Dyskinesia
Electromyography
Encephalitis
Epilepsy
Eye infections and disorders
Facial transplantation
Fibromyalgia
Guillain-Barré syndrome
Hearing
Herpes
Hirschsprung's disease
Huntington's disease
Leprosy
Leukodystrophy
Listeria infections
Local anesthesia
Lower extremities
Lumbar puncture
Lyme disease
Motor neuron diseases
Motor skill development
Multiple chemical sensitivity
    syndrome
Multiple sclerosis
Neonatal brachial plexus palsy
Nervous system
Neuroimaging
Neurology
Neurosis
Neurosurgery
Numbness and tingling
Palsy
Paralysis
Parkinson's disease
Physical rehabilitation
Poliomyelitis
Postherpetic neuralgia
Ptosis
Radiculopathy
Sarcoidosis
Sciatica
Seizures
Sense organs
Shock therapy
Skin
Slipped disk
Spinal cord disorders
Spinocerebellar ataxia
Sturge-Weber syndrome
Sympathectomy
Tics
Tinnitus
Touch
Tourette's syndrome
Tremors

Upper extremities
Vagotomy
Vasculitis

NERVOUS SYSTEM

Abscess drainage
Acupressure
Addiction
Adenoviruses
Adrenoleukodystrophy
Agnosia
Alcoholism
Altitude sickness
Alzheimer's disease
Amnesia
Amputation
Amyotrophic lateral sclerosis
Anesthesia
Anesthesiology
Aneurysms
Angelman syndrome
Anorexia nervosa
Anosmia
Anthrax
Antidepressants
Anxiety
Apgar score
Aphasia and dysphasia
Apnea
Aromatherapy
Ataxia
Atrophy
Attention-deficit disorder (ADD)
Auras
Avian influenza
Back pain
Balance disorders
Batten's disease
Behçet's disease
Beriberi
Biofeedback
Botulism
Brain
Brain damage
Brain disorders
Brain tumors
Brucellosis
Caffeine
Cells
Chagas' disease
Charcot-Marie-Tooth Disease
Chiari malformations
Chiropractic
Chronic wasting disease (CWD)
Cluster headaches
Cognitive development
Colon

Computed tomography (CT) scanning
Concussion
Congenital hypothyroidism
Creutzfeldt-Jakob disease (CJD)
Cutis marmorata telangiectatica
    congenita
Deafness
Defibrillation
Dementias
Developmental disorders
Developmental stages
Diabetes mellitus
Diphtheria
Disk removal
Dizziness and fainting
Down syndrome
Drowning
Dwarfism
Dyskinesia
Dyslexia
E. coli infection
Ear surgery
Ears
Ehrlichiosis
Electrical shock
Electroencephalography (EEG)
Electromyography
Encephalitis
Endocrinology
Enteroviruses
Epilepsy
Eyes
Facial transplantation
Fetal tissue transplantation
Fibromyalgia
Frontotemporal dementia (FTD)
Glands
Glasgow coma scale
Guillain-Barré syndrome
Hammertoe correction
Head and neck disorders
Headaches
Hearing tests
Heart transplantation
Hemiplegia
Hemolytic uremic syndrome
Histiocytosis
Huntington's disease
Hydrocephalus
Hypnosis
Hypothalamus
Intraventricular hemorrhage
Irritable bowel syndrome (IBS)
Kinesiology
Lead poisoning
Learning disabilities
Leprosy

Leptospirosis
Light therapy
Listeria infections
Local anesthesia
Lower extremities
Lumbar puncture
Lyme disease
Maple syrup urine disease (MSUD)
Measles
Memory loss
Ménière's disease
Meningitis
Mental retardation
Mental status exam
Mercury poisoning
Motion sickness
Motor neuron diseases
Motor skill development
Multiple chemical sensitivity
    syndrome
Multiple sclerosis
Mumps
Myasthenia gravis
Narcolepsy
Nausea and vomiting
Neurofibromatosis
Neuroimaging
Neurology
Neurosis
Neurosurgery
Niemann-Pick disease
Nuclear radiology
Numbness and tingling
Orthopedic surgery
Orthopedics
Overtraining syndrome
Palsy
Paralysis
Paraplegia
Parkinson's disease
Pharmacology
Phenylketonuria (PKU)
Physical rehabilitation
Pick's disease
Poisoning
Poliomyelitis
Porphyria
Precocious puberty
Preeclampsia and eclampsia
Prion diseases
Quadriplegia
Rabies
Radiculopathy
Restless legs syndrome
Reye's syndrome
Rocky Mountain spotted fever
Rubella

Sarcoidosis
Sciatica
Seasonal affective disorder
Seizures
Sense organs
Shingles
Shock therapy
Shunts
Skin
Sleep
Sleep disorders
Sleeping sickness
Sleepwalking
Slipped disk
Small intestine
Smell
Snakebites
Spina bifida
Spinal cord disorders
Spinocerebellar ataxia
Sports medicine
Staphylococcal infections
Strokes
Sturge-Weber syndrome
Stuttering
Sympathectomy
Synesthesia
Syphilis
Tardive dyskinesia
Taste
Tay-Sachs disease
Teeth
Tetanus
Thrombolytic therapy and TPA
Tics
Tinnitus
Touch
Tourette's syndrome
Toxoplasmosis
Tremors
Typhus
Upper extremities
Vagotomy
Vertigo
Vision
West Nile virus
Wilson's disease
Yoga

NOSE
Adenoids
Allergies
Anosmia
Antihistamines
Aromatherapy
Auras
Avian influenza

Cartilage
Casts and splints
Chickenpox
Childhood infectious diseases
Cold agglutinin disease
Common cold
Cornelia de Lange syndrome
Decongestants
Dengue fever
Epstein-Barr virus
Facial transplantation
Fifth disease
Hay fever
H1N1 influenza
Influenza
Methicillin-resistant staphylococcus
    aureus (MRSA) infection
Mold and mildew
Nasal polyp removal
Nasopharyngeal disorders
Otorhinolaryngology
Pharynx
Polyps
Pulmonary medicine
Respiration
Rhinitis
Rhinoplasty and submucous resection
Rhinoviruses
Rosacea
Rubinstein-Taybi syndrome
Sense organs
Sinusitis
Skin lesion removal
Smell
Sore throat
Stevens-Johnson syndrome
Taste
Tears and tear ducts
Vasculitis

PANCREAS
Abscess drainage
Alcoholism
Carbohydrates
Cholecystitis
Chyme
Diabetes mellitus
Digestion
Endocrine glands
Endocrinology
Endoscopic retrograde
    cholangiopancreatography (ERCP)
Fetal tissue transplantation
Food biochemistry
Gastroenterology
Gastrointestinal system
Glands

Hemochromatosis
Internal medicine
Malabsorption
Metabolism
Mumps
Pancreatitis
Polycystic kidney disease
Polycystic ovary syndrome
Transplantation

**PSYCHIC-EMOTIONAL
SYSTEM**
Acquired immunodeficiency
    syndrome (AIDS)
Addiction
Adrenoleukodystrophy
Alcoholism
Alzheimer's disease
Amnesia
Anesthesia
Anesthesiology
Angelman syndrome
Anorexia nervosa
Antianxiety drugs
Antidepressants
Antihistamines
Anxiety
Aphrodisiacs
Aromatherapy
Asperger's syndrome
Attention-deficit disorder (ADD)
Auras
Autism
Bariatric surgery
Biofeedback
Bipolar disorders
Body dysmorphic disorder
Bonding
Brain
Brain disorders
Bulimia
Chronic fatigue syndrome
Cognitive development
Colic
Death and dying
Dementias
Depression
Developmental disorders
Developmental stages
Dizziness and fainting
Down syndrome
Dyskinesia
Dyslexia
Eating disorders
Electroencephalography (EEG)
Encephalitis
Endocrinology

Factitious disorders
Failure to thrive
Fibromyalgia
Frontotemporal dementia (FTD)
Gender identity disorder
Gulf War syndrome
Headaches
Hormone therapy
Hormones
Hydrocephalus
Hypnosis
Hypochondriasis
Hypothalamus
Interpartner violence
Kinesiology
Klinefelter syndrome
Learning disabilities
Light therapy
Memory loss
Menopause
Mental retardation
Miscarriage
Morgellons disease
Motor skill development
Narcolepsy
Neurology
Neurosis
Neurosurgery
Obesity
Obsessive-compulsive disorder
Overtraining syndrome
Paranoia
Pharmacology
Phobias
Pick's disease
Postpartum depression
Post-traumatic stress disorder
Prader-Willi syndrome
Precocious puberty
Premenstrual syndrome (PMS)
Psychiatric disorders
Psychoanalysis
Psychosis
Rabies
Rape and sexual assault
Restless legs syndrome
Schizophrenia
Seasonal affective disorder
Separation anxiety
Sexual dysfunction
Sexuality
Shock therapy
Sleep
Sleep disorders
Sleeping sickness
Sleepwalking
Soiling

Speech disorders
Sperm banks
Steroid abuse
Strokes
Suicide
Synesthesia
Tics
Tinnitus
Toilet training
Tourette's syndrome
Weight loss and gain
West Nile virus
Wilson's disease
Yoga

REPRODUCTIVE SYSTEM
Abdomen
Abortion
Acquired immunodeficiency
    syndrome (AIDS)
Adrenoleukodystrophy
Amenorrhea
Amniocentesis
Anorexia nervosa
Assisted reproductive technologies
Avian influenza
Breast-feeding
Brucellosis
Candidiasis
Catheterization
Cervical procedures
Cesarean section
Childbirth
Childbirth complications
Chlamydia
Chorionic villus sampling
Computed tomography (CT) scanning
Conception
Congenital adrenal hyperplasia
Contraception
Culdocentesis
Cyst removal
Cystoscopy
Dysmenorrhea
Eating disorders
Ectopic pregnancy
Endocrine glands
Endocrinology
Endometrial biopsy
Endometriosis
Episiotomy
Erectile dysfunction
Fistula repair
Gamete intrafallopian transfer (GIFT)
Gender reassignment surgery
Genetic counseling
Gestational diabetes

Gigantism
Glands
Gonorrhea
Gynecology
Hermaphroditism and
    pseudohermaphroditism
Hernia
Herpes
Hormone therapy
Human papillomavirus (HPV)
Hydroceles
Hypospadias repair and urethroplasty
Hysterectomy
In vitro fertilization
Internal medicine
Klinefelter syndrome
Laparoscopy
Lead poisoning
Ligaments
Menopause
Menorrhagia
Menstruation
Miscarriage
Myomectomy
Obstetrics
Orchiectomy
Orchitis
Ovarian cysts
Pap test
Pelvic inflammatory disease (PID)
Penile implant surgery
Placenta
Polycystic ovary syndrome
Polyps
Precocious puberty
Preeclampsia and eclampsia
Pregnancy and gestation
Premature birth
Premenstrual syndrome (PMS)
Prostate cancer
Prostate enlargement
Prostate gland
Semen
Sexual differentiation
Sexual dysfunction
Sexuality
Sexually transmitted diseases (STDs)
Sperm banks
Sterilization
Steroid abuse
Stevens-Johnson syndrome
Stillbirth
Syphilis
Testicular surgery
Testicular torsion
Toxemia
Trichomoniasis

Tubal ligation
Turner syndrome
Ultrasonography
Urology
Uterus
Vas deferens
Vasectomy
Von Willebrand's disease

RESPIRATORY SYSTEM
Abscess drainage
Acidosis
Acquired immunodeficiency
    syndrome (AIDS)
Acute respiratory distress syndrome
    (ARDS)
Adenoviruses
Adrenoleukodystrophy
Altitude sickness
Amyotrophic lateral sclerosis
Anthrax
Antihistamines
Apgar score
Apnea
Asbestos exposure
Asphyxiation
Asthma
Avian influenza
Babesiosis
Bacterial infections
Bronchi
Bronchiolitis
Bronchitis
Cardiopulmonary resuscitation (CPR)
Chest
Childhood infectious diseases
Choking
Chronic obstructive pulmonary
    disease (COPD)
Cold agglutinin disease
Common cold
Computed tomography (CT) scanning
Coronaviruses
Coughing
Croup
Cystic fibrosis
Decongestants
Defibrillation
Diaphragm
Drowning
Dwarfism
Edema
Emphysema
Epiglottitis
Exercise physiology
Fetal surgery
Fluids and electrolytes

Food allergies
Fungal infections
Hantavirus
Hay fever
Head and neck disorders
Heart transplantation
Heimlich maneuver
Hiccups
H1N1 influenza
Hyperbaric oxygen therapy
Hyperventilation
Hypoxia
Influenza
Internal medicine
Kinesiology
Laryngectomy
Legionnaires' disease
Lung cancer
Lung surgery
Lungs
Measles
Mesothelioma
Methicillin-resistant staphylococcus
    aureus (MRSA) infection
Mold and mildew
Monkeypox
Multiple chemical sensitivity
    syndrome
Nasopharyngeal disorders
Niemann-Pick disease
Obesity
Otorhinolaryngology
Oxygen therapy
Pharynx
Plague
Plasma
Pneumocystis jirovecii
Pneumonia
Pneumothorax
Poisoning
Pulmonary diseases
Pulmonary edema
Pulmonary hypertension
Pulmonary medicine
Respiration
Resuscitation
Rheumatoid arthritis
Rhinitis
Rhinoviruses
Sarcoidosis
Severe acute respiratory syndrome
    (SARS)
Sinusitis
Sleep apnea
Smoking
Sore throat
Staphylococcal infections

Stevens-Johnson syndrome
Thoracic surgery
Thrombolytic therapy and TPA
Thrombosis and thrombus
Tonsillectomy and adenoid removal
Trachea
Tracheostomy
Transplantation
Tuberculosis
Tularemia
Tumor removal
Typhus
Vasculitis
Voice and vocal cord disorders
Whooping cough

SKIN
Abscess drainage
Acne
Acquired immunodeficiency
    syndrome (AIDS)
Acupressure
Adenoviruses
Adrenoleukodystrophy
Allergies
Amputation
Anesthesia
Anesthesiology
Angelman syndrome
Anorexia nervosa
Anthrax
Anxiety
Athlete's foot
Auras
Bacillus Calmette-Guérin (BCG)
Bariatric surgery
Batten's disease
Bedsores
Behçet's disease
Bites and stings
Blisters
Blood testing
Body dysmorphic disorder
Bruises
Burns and scalds
Candidiasis
Canker sores
Casts and splints
Cells
Chagas' disease
Chickenpox
Cleft lip and palate repair
Cold agglutinin disease
Cold sores
Collagen
Collodion baby
Corns and calluses

Cushing's syndrome
Cutis marmorata telangiectatica
    congenita
Cyanosis
Cyst removal
Dengue fever
Dermatitis
Dermatology
Dermatopathology
Ebola virus
Eczema
Edema
Electrical shock
Electrocauterization
Enteroviruses
Face lift and blepharoplasty
Facial transplantation
Fibrocystic breast condition
Fifth disease
Food allergies
Frostbite
Fungal infections
Gangrene
Glands
Gluten intolerance
Gulf War syndrome
Hair
Hair transplantation
Hand-foot-and-mouth disease
Heat exhaustion and heatstroke
Hematomas
Hemolytic disease of the newborn
Herpes
Histiocytosis
Hives
Hormone therapy
Host-defense mechanisms
Human papillomavirus (HPV)
Hyperhidrosis
Impetigo
Intravenous (IV) therapy
Jaundice
Kaposi's sarcoma
Kawasaki disease
Kwashiorkor
Laceration repair
Laser use in surgery
Leishmaniasis
Leprosy
Light therapy
Lower extremities
Lyme disease
Measles
Melanoma
Methicillin-resistant staphylococcus
    aureus (MRSA) infection
Mold and mildew

Moles
Monkeypox
Morgellons disease
Multiple chemical sensitivity
    syndrome
Nails
Necrotizing fasciitis
Neurofibromatosis
Numbness and tingling
Otoplasty
Pigmentation
Pinworms
Pityriasis alba
Pityriasis rosea
Polycystic ovary syndrome
Polydactyly and syndactyly
Porphyria
Psoriasis
Radiation sickness
Reiter's syndrome
Ringworm
Rocky Mountain spotted fever
Rosacea
Roseola
Rubella
Sarcoidosis
Scabies
Scarlet fever
Sense organs
Shingles
Skin cancer
Skin disorders
Skin lesion removal
Smallpox
Streptococcal infections
Sturge-Weber syndrome
Styes
Sweating
Tattoo removal
Tattoos and body piercing
Touch
Toxoplasmosis
Tularemia
Typhoid fever
Typhus
Umbilical cord
Upper extremities
Vasculitis
Vitiligo
Von Willebrand's disease
Williams syndrome
Wiskott-Aldrich syndrome

SPINE
Anesthesia
Anesthesiology
Ankylosing spondylitis

Atrophy
Back pain
Brain tumors
Brucellosis
Charcot-Marie-Tooth Disease
Chiari malformations
Chiropractic
Diaphragm
Disk removal
Fetal tissue transplantation
Head and neck disorders
Kinesiology
Laminectomy and spinal fusion
Lumbar puncture
Marfan syndrome
Meningitis
Mesenchymal stem cells
Methicillin-resistant staphylococcus
    aureus (MRSA) infection
Motor neuron diseases
Multiple sclerosis
Nervous system
Neuroimaging
Neurology
Neurosurgery
Orthopedic surgery
Orthopedics
Osteogenesis imperfecta
Osteoporosis
Paget's disease
Paralysis
Paraplegia
Physical rehabilitation
Poliomyelitis
Quadriplegia
Radiculopathy
Sciatica
Scoliosis
Slipped disk
Spina bifida
Spinal cord disorders
Spondylitis
Sports medicine
Stenosis
Sympathectomy
Whiplash
Williams syndrome

SPLEEN
Abscess drainage
Aspergillosis
Brucellosis
Cold agglutinin disease
Gaucher's disease
Hematology
Immune system
Internal medicine

Leptospirosis
Lymph
Lymphatic system
Malaria
Metabolism
Methicillin-resistant staphylococcus
  aureus (MRSA) infection
Mononucleosis
Niemann-Pick disease
Sarcoidosis
Sickle cell disease
Splenectomy
Thrombocytopenia
Transplantation
Typhoid fever

STOMACH
Abdomen
Abdominal disorders
Abscess drainage
Acid reflux disease
Adenoviruses
Allergies
Avian influenza
Bariatric surgery
Campylobacter infections
Chyme
Colitis
Digestion
Drowning
Eating disorders
Endoscopic retrograde
  cholangiopancreatography (ERCP)
Endoscopy
Esophagus
Food biochemistry
Food poisoning
Gastrectomy
Gastroenteritis
Gastroenterology
Gastrointestinal disorders
Gastrointestinal system
Gastrostomy
Hernia
Hernia repair
Internal medicine
Lactose intolerance
Malabsorption
Malnutrition
Metabolism
Motion sickness
Nausea and vomiting
Obesity
Peristalsis
Poisoning
Polyps
Pyloric stenosis

Radiation sickness
Ulcer surgery
Ulcers
Vagotomy
Weaning
Weight loss and gain

TEETH
Angelman syndrome
Bulimia
Cavities
Cornelia de Lange syndrome
Crowns and bridges
Dental diseases
Dentistry
Dentures
Eating disorders
Endodontic disease
Fluoride treatments
Fracture repair
Gastrointestinal system
Gingivitis
Gum disease
Jaw wiring
Lisping
Mouth and throat cancer
Oral and maxillofacial surgery
Orthodontics
Osteogenesis imperfecta
Periodontal surgery
Periodontitis
Prader-Willi syndrome
Rickets
Root canal treatment
Rubinstein-Taybi syndrome
Scurvy
Teething
Temporomandibular joint (TMJ)
  syndrome
Thumb sucking
Tooth extraction
Wisdom teeth

TENDONS
Ankylosing spondylitis
Carpal tunnel syndrome
Casts and splints
Collagen
Connective tissue
Exercise physiology
Ganglion removal
Hammertoe correction
Hemiplegia
Joints
Kneecap removal
Mesenchymal stem cells
Orthopedic surgery

Orthopedics
Osgood-Schlatter disease
Physical rehabilitation
Sports medicine
Tendinitis
Tendon disorders
Tendon repair

THROAT
Acid reflux disease
Acquired immunodeficiency
  syndrome (AIDS)
Adenoids
Antihistamines
Auras
Avian influenza
Catheterization
Choking
Croup
Decongestants
Diphtheria
Drowning
Eating disorders
Epiglottitis
Epstein-Barr virus
Esophagus
Fifth disease
Gastroenterology
Gastrointestinal system
Gonorrhea
Hay fever
Head and neck disorders
Heimlich maneuver
Hiccups
Histiocytosis
H1N1 influenza
Influenza
Laryngectomy
Laryngitis
Mononucleosis
Mouth and throat cancer
Nasopharyngeal disorders
Otorhinolaryngology
Pharyngitis
Pharynx
Polyps
Pulmonary medicine
Quinsy
Respiration
Rhinitis
Rhinoviruses
Smoking
Sore throat
Streptococcal infections
Tonsillectomy and adenoid removal
Tonsillitis
Tracheostomy

Tremors
Voice and vocal cord disorders
Whooping cough

URINARY SYSTEM
Abdomen
Abdominal disorders
Abscess drainage
Adenoviruses
Adrenalectomy
Avian influenza
Bed-wetting
Bladder cancer
Bladder removal
Candidiasis
Catheterization
Chlamydia
Cold agglutinin disease
Cystitis
Cystoscopy
Dialysis
Diuretics
E. coli infection
End-stage renal disease
Endoscopy
Fetal surgery
Fistula repair
Gonorrhea
Hematuria
Hemolytic uremic syndrome
Hermaphroditism and
    pseudohermaphroditism
Hormone therapy
Host-defense mechanisms
Hyperplasia
Hypertension
Incontinence
Internal medicine
Kidney cancer

Kidney disorders
Kidney transplantation
Kidneys
Laparoscopy
Leptospirosis
Lithotripsy
Nephrectomy
Nephrology
Plasma
Polyps
Prostate enlargement
Proteinuria
Pyelonephritis
Reiter's syndrome
Reye's syndrome
Schistosomiasis
Staphylococcal infections
Stevens-Johnson syndrome
Stone removal
Stones
Testicular cancer
Toilet training
Transplantation
Trichomoniasis
Ultrasonography
Uremia
Urethritis
Urinalysis
Urinary disorders
Urology

UTERUS
Abdomen
Abortion
Amniocentesis
Assisted reproductive technologies
Cervical procedures
Cesarean section
Childbirth

Childbirth complications
Chorionic villus sampling
Conception
Contraception
Dysmenorrhea
Electrocauterization
Embolization
Endocrinology
Endometrial biopsy
Endometriosis
Fistula repair
Gender reassignment surgery
Genetic counseling
Gynecology
Hormone therapy
Hyperplasia
Hysterectomy
In vitro fertilization
Internal medicine
Laparoscopy
Menopause
Menorrhagia
Menstruation
Miscarriage
Myomectomy
Obstetrics
Pap test
Pelvic inflammatory disease (PID)
Placenta
Polyps
Pregnancy and gestation
Premature birth
Reproductive system
Sexual differentiation
Sperm banks
Sterilization
Stillbirth
Tubal ligation
Ultrasonography

ENTRIES BY SPECIALTIES AND RELATED FIELDS

Eye infections and disorders
Fluoride treatments
Gangrene
Gastroenteritis
Genomics
Gingivitis
Gram staining
Impetigo
Infection
Insect-borne diseases
Laboratory tests
Legionnaires' disease
Leprosy
Leptospirosis
Listeria infections
Lyme disease
Mastitis
Methicillin-resistant staphylococcus
    aureus (MRSA) infection
Microbiology
Microscopy
Necrotizing fasciitis
Opportunistic infections
Osteomyelitis
Peritonitis
Plague
Salmonella infection
Sarcoidosis
Scarlet fever
Serology
Shigellosis
Staphylococcal infections
Streptococcal infections
Styes
Syphilis
Tetanus
Tuberculosis
Tularemia
Typhoid fever
Typhus
Urethritis
Whooping cough
Zoonoses

BIOCHEMISTRY
Acid-base chemistry
Acidosis
Amyotrophic lateral sclerosis
Antibodies
Antidepressants
Autopsy
Avian influenza
Bacteriology
Bulimia
Caffeine
Carbohydrates
Cholesterol

Collagen
Colon
Connective tissue
Corticosteroids
Digestion
Endocrine glands
Endocrinology
Enzyme therapy
Ergogenic aids
Fatty acid oxidation disorders
Fluids and electrolytes
Fluoride treatments
Food biochemistry
Food guide plate
Fructosemia
Galactosemia
Gaucher's disease
Genetic engineering
Genomics
Gigantism
Gingivitis
Glands
Glycogen storage diseases
Glycolysis
Gram staining
Gulf War syndrome
Histology
Hormones
Hyperadiposis
Hypothalamus
Insect-borne diseases
Leptin
Leukodystrophy
Lipids
Lumbar puncture
Macronutrients
Malabsorption
Malaria
Metabolic disorders
Metabolism
Nephrology
Niemann-Pick disease
Nutrition
Osteogenesis imperfecta
Ovaries
Pathology
Pharmacology
Phenylketonuria (PKU)
Pituitary gland
Plasma
Protein
Respiration
Retroviruses
Rhinoviruses
Sleep
Small intestine
Stem cells

Steroids
Thymus gland
Tourette's syndrome
Urinalysis
Wilson's disease

BIOTECHNOLOGY
Antibodies
Assisted reproductive technologies
Biological therapies
Bionics and biotechnology
Cloning
Computed tomography (CT) scanning
Defibrillation
Dialysis
Electrocardiography (ECG or EKG)
Electroencephalography (EEG)
Fatty acid oxidation disorders
Gene therapy
Genetic engineering
Genomics
Glycogen storage diseases
Huntington's disease
Hyperbaric oxygen therapy
Insect-borne diseases
Magnetic resonance imaging (MRI)
Malabsorption
Mesenchymal stem cells
Nephrology
Pacemaker implantation
Positron emission tomography (PET)
    scanning
Prostheses
Rhinoviruses
Severe combined immunodeficiency
    syndrome (SCID)
Sperm banks
Stem cells
Xenotransplantation

CARDIOLOGY
Acute respiratory distress syndrome
    (ARDS)
Aging: Extended care
Anemia
Aneurysms
Angina
Angiography
Angioplasty
Antihypertensives
Anxiety
Aortic aneurysm
Aortic stenosis
Arrhythmias
Arteriosclerosis
Aspergillosis
Atrial fibrillation

Biofeedback
Blood pressure
Blood vessels
Blue baby syndrome
Brucellosis
Bypass surgery
Cardiac arrest
Cardiac rehabilitation
Cardiac surgery
Cardiopulmonary resuscitation (CPR)
Carotid arteries
Catheterization
Chest
Circulation
Computed tomography (CT) scanning
Congenital heart disease
Coronary artery bypass graft
Critical care
Defibrillation
DiGeorge syndrome
Diphtheria
Diuretics
Dizziness and fainting
Echocardiography
Electrocardiography (ECG or EKG)
Electrocauterization
Embolism
Emergency medicine
End-stage renal disease
Endocarditis
Enteroviruses
Exercise physiology
Fetal surgery
Gigantism
Heart
Heart attack
Heart disease
Heart failure
Heart transplantation
Heart valve replacement
Hematology
Hemochromatosis
Hormone therapy
Hypercholesterolemia
Hypertension
Hypotension
Infarction
Internal medicine
Ischemia
Kawasaki disease
Kinesiology
Leptin
Lesions
Lyme disease
Marfan syndrome
Metabolic syndrome
Methicillin-resistant staphylococcus

aureus (MRSA) infection
Mitral valve prolapse
Mucopolysaccharidosis (MPS)
Muscles
Neonatology
Noninvasive tests
Nuclear medicine
Oxygen therapy
Pacemaker implantation
Palliative care
Palpitations
Paramedics
Plasma
Polycystic kidney disease
Prader-Willi syndrome
Progeria
Prostheses
Pulmonary edema
Pulmonary hypertension
Pulse rate
Rheumatic fever
Rubinstein-Taybi syndrome
Sarcoidosis
Single photon emission computed
   tomography (SPECT)
Spondylitis
Sports medicine
Staphylococcal infections
Stem cells
Stenosis
Stents
Systemic lupus erythematosus (SLE)
Thoracic surgery
Thrombolytic therapy and TPA
Thrombosis and thrombus
Transplantation
Ultrasonography
Uremia
Varicose veins
Vascular medicine
Vascular system
Vasculitis
Venous insufficiency
Williams syndrome

CRITICAL CARE
Acidosis
Aging: Extended care
Amputation
Anesthesia
Anesthesiology
Aneurysmectomy
Anthrax
Apgar score
Botulism
Burns and scalds
Carotid arteries

Catheterization
Chronic granulomatous disease
Club drugs
Concussion
Craniotomy
Defibrillation
Diuretics
Drowning
Echocardiography
Electrical shock
Electrocardiography (ECG or EKG)
Electrocauterization
Electroencephalography (EEG)
Embolization
Emergency medicine
Epidemics and pandemics
Grafts and grafting
Hantavirus
Heart attack
Heart transplantation
Heat exhaustion and heatstroke
Hydrocephalus
Hyperbaric oxygen therapy
Hyperthermia and hypothermia
Hypotension
Hypoxia
Infarction
Insect-borne diseases
Intravenous (IV) therapy
Ischemia
Lumbar puncture
Methicillin-resistant staphylococcus
   aureus (MRSA) infection
Necrotizing fasciitis
Neonatology
Nursing
Oncology
Osteopathic medicine
Oxygen therapy
Pain management
Paramedics
Peritonitis
Psychiatry
Pulmonary medicine
Pulse rate
Radiation sickness
Resuscitation
Safety issues for children
Safety issues for the elderly
Severe acute respiratory syndrome
   (SARS)
Shock
Stevens-Johnson syndrome
Streptococcal infections
Thrombolytic therapy and TPA
Toxic shock syndrome
Tracheostomy

Transfusion
Whooping cough
Wounds

CYTOLOGY
Acid-base chemistry
Bionics and biotechnology
Biopsy
Blood testing
Breast disorders
Cancer
Carcinoma
Cells
Cholesterol
Cytopathology
Dermatology
Dermatopathology
Epstein-Barr virus
Eye infections and disorders
Fluids and electrolytes
Food biochemistry
Gaucher's disease
Gene therapy
Genetic counseling
Genomics
Glycolysis
Gram staining
Healing
Hematology
Hirschsprung's disease
Histology
Hyperplasia
Immune system
Karyotyping
Laboratory tests
Lipids
Metabolism
Microscopy
Mutation
Oncology
Pathology
Pharmacology
Plasma
Rhinoviruses
Sarcoma
Serology
Stem cells

DENTISTRY
Aging: Extended care
Anesthesia
Anesthesiology
Canker sores
Cavities
Cerebral palsy
Cockayne Disease
Crowns and bridges

Dental diseases
Dentures
Eating disorders
Endodontic disease
Fluoride treatments
Forensic pathology
Fracture repair
Gastrointestinal system
Gingivitis
Gum disease
Head and neck disorders
Jaw wiring
Lisping
Local anesthesia
Mouth and throat cancer
Oral and maxillofacial surgery
Orthodontics
Osteogenesis imperfecta
Periodontal surgery
Periodontitis
Prader-Willi syndrome
Prostheses
Root canal treatment
Rubinstein-Taybi syndrome
Sense organs
Sjögren's syndrome
Teeth
Teething
Temporomandibular joint (TMJ) syndrome
Thumb sucking
Tooth extraction
Von Willebrand's disease
Wisdom teeth

DERMATOLOGY
Abscess drainage
Acne
Acquired immunodeficiency syndrome (AIDS)
Adrenoleukodystrophy
Allergies
Alopecia
Angelman syndrome
Anthrax
Anti-inflammatory drugs
Athlete's foot
Bedsores
Bile
Biopsy
Blisters
Body dysmorphic disorder
Burns and scalds
Carcinoma
Chickenpox
Chronic granulomatous disease
Coccidioidomycosis

Cockayne Disease
Collodion baby
Corns and calluses
Cryosurgery
Cutis marmorata telangiectatica congenita
Cyst removal
Dermatitis
Dermatopathology
Eczema
Electrocauterization
Enteroviruses
Facial transplantation
Fungal infections
Ganglion removal
Gangrene
Genetic engineering
Glands
Gluten intolerance
Grafts and grafting
Hair
Hair transplantation
Hand-foot-and-mouth disease
Healing
Herpes
Histology
Hives
Hyperhidrosis
Immunopathology
Impetigo
Laser use in surgery
Lesions
Light therapy
Local anesthesia
Lyme disease
Melanoma
Methicillin-resistant staphylococcus aureus (MRSA) infection
Moles
Monkeypox
Morgellons disease
Multiple chemical sensitivity syndrome
Nails
Necrotizing fasciitis
Neurofibromatosis
Pigmentation
Pinworms
Pityriasis alba
Pityriasis rosea
Plastic surgery
Podiatry
Polycystic ovary syndrome
Postherpetic neuralgia
Prostheses
Psoriasis
Puberty and adolescence

Reiter's syndrome
Ringworm
Rocky Mountain spotted fever
Rosacea
Sarcoidosis
Scabies
Scleroderma
Sense organs
Shingles
Skin
Skin cancer
Skin disorders
Skin lesion removal
Smallpox
Staphylococcal infections
Stevens-Johnson syndrome
Streptococcal infections
Stress
Sturge-Weber syndrome
Styes
Sweating
Systemic lupus erythematosus (SLE)
Tattoo removal
Tattoos and body piercing
Touch
Vasculitis
Vitiligo
Von Willebrand's disease
Wiskott-Aldrich syndrome

EMBRYOLOGY

Amniocentesis
Assisted reproductive technologies
Birth defects
Blue baby syndrome
Brain disorders
Chorionic villus sampling
Cloning
Conception
Down syndrome
Ectopic pregnancy
Fetal tissue transplantation
Gamete intrafallopian transfer (GIFT)
Genetic counseling
Genetic diseases
Genetic engineering
Genetic Imprinting
Genetics and inheritance
Genomics
Growth
Hermaphroditism and
    pseudohermaphroditism
In vitro fertilization
Karyotyping
Klinefelter syndrome
Meckel's diverticulum
Miscarriage

Mucopolysaccharidosis (MPS)
Multiple births
Neonatology
Obstetrics
Ovaries
Perinatology
Phenylketonuria (PKU)
Placenta
Pregnancy and gestation
Premature birth
Reproductive system
Rh factor
Sexual differentiation
Spina bifida
Stem cells
Syphilis
Teratogens
Ultrasonography
Uterus

EMERGENCY MEDICINE

Abdominal disorders
Abscess drainage
Acidosis
Adrenoleukodystrophy
Advance directives
Altitude sickness
Amputation
Anesthesia
Anesthesiology
Aneurysmectomy
Aneurysms
Angiography
Anthrax
Appendectomy
Appendicitis
Asphyxiation
Atrial fibrillation
Back pain
Bites and stings
Bleeding
Blurred vision
Botulism
Bruises
Burns and scalds
Cardiac arrest
Cardiology
Cardiopulmonary resuscitation (CPR)
Carotid arteries
Casts and splints
Catheterization
Cesarean section
Choking
Cholecystitis
Chronic granulomatous disease
Club drugs
Cold agglutinin disease

Computed tomography (CT) scanning
Concussion
Critical care
Croup
Defibrillation
Dizziness and fainting
Drowning
Echocardiography
Electrical shock
Electrocardiography (ECG or EKG)
Electrocauterization
Electroencephalography (EEG)
Embolization
Epiglottitis
First responder
Fracture and dislocation
Frostbite
Gangrene
Grafts and grafting
Head and neck disorders
Heart attack
Heart transplantation
Heat exhaustion and heatstroke
Heimlich maneuver
H1N1 influenza
Hyperbaric oxygen therapy
Hyperthermia and hypothermia
Hyperventilation
Hypotension
Hypoxia
Impetigo
Infarction
Influenza
Interpartner violence
Interstitial pulmonary fibrosis (IPF)
Intravenous (IV) therapy
Jaw wiring
Laceration repair
Local anesthesia
Lung surgery
Meningitis
Mental status exam
Monkeypox
Nail removal
Necrotizing fasciitis
Noninvasive tests
Nursing
Osteopathic medicine
Oxygen therapy
Pain management
Palliative medicine
Paramedics
Peritonitis
Physician assistants
Plague
Plastic surgery
Pleurisy

Pneumonia
Pneumothorax
Poisoning
Pulmonary medicine
Pulse rate
Pyelonephritis
Radiation sickness
Rape and sexual assault
Resuscitation
Reye's syndrome
Rocky Mountain spotted fever
Safety issues for children
Safety issues for the elderly
Severe acute respiratory syndrome
  (SARS)
Shock
Snakebites
Spinal cord disorders
Splenectomy
Sports medicine
Stevens-Johnson syndrome
Streptococcal infections
Strokes
Surgical technologists
Thrombolytic therapy and TPA
Toxic shock syndrome
Tracheostomy
Transfusion
Transplantation
Tularemia
Wounds

ENDOCRINOLOGY
Addison's disease
Adrenalectomy
Adrenoleukodystrophy
Amenorrhea
Anti-inflammatory drugs
Assisted reproductive technologies
Bariatric surgery
Carbohydrates
Computed tomography (CT) scanning
Congenital adrenal hyperplasia
Congenital hypothyroidism
Corticosteroids
Cushing's syndrome
Diabetes mellitus
Dwarfism
End-stage renal disease
Endocrine disorders
Endocrine glands
Ergogenic aids
Failure to thrive
Gamete intrafallopian transfer (GIFT)
Gender identity disorder
Gender reassignment surgery
Gestational diabetes

Gigantism
Glands
Glioma
Goiter
Growth
Gynecology
Gynecomastia
Hashimoto's thyroiditis
Hemochromatosis
Hermaphroditism and
  pseudohermaphroditism
Hormone therapy
Hormones
Hyperadiposis
Hyperparathyroidism and
  hypoparathyroidism
Hyperplasia
Hypertrophy
Hypoglycemia
Hypothalamus
Hysterectomy
Internal medicine
Klinefelter syndrome
Laboratory tests
Laparoscopy
Leptin
Liver
Melatonin
Menopause
Menstruation
Metabolic disorders
Metabolic syndrome
Nephrology
Neurology
Niemann-Pick disease
Nonalcoholic steatohepatitis (NASH)
Nuclear medicine
Obesity
Ovaries
Pancreas
Pancreatitis
Parathyroidectomy
Pharmacology
Pituitary gland
Plasma
Polycystic ovary syndrome
Precocious puberty
Prostate enlargement
Prostate gland
Puberty and adolescence
Pulse rate
Radiopharmaceuticals
Sexual differentiation
Sexual dysfunction
Sleep
Small intestine
Stem cells

Steroids
Systemic lupus erythematosus (SLE)
Testicular cancer
Thymus gland
Thyroid disorders
Thyroid gland
Thyroidectomy
Tumors
Turner syndrome
Vitamins and minerals
Vitiligo
Weight loss and gain
Weight loss medications
Williams syndrome

ENVIRONMENTAL HEALTH
Acidosis
Asbestos exposure
Asthma
Babesiosis
Blurred vision
Cholera
Cognitive development
Coronaviruses
Creutzfeldt-Jakob disease (CJD)
Drowning
Elephantiasis
Enteroviruses
Food poisoning
Frostbite
Gastroenteritis
Gulf War syndrome
Hantavirus
Hyperthermia and hypothermia
Insect-borne diseases
Lead poisoning
Legionnaires' disease
Lung cancer
Lungs
Mercury poisoning
Microbiology
Mold and mildew
Multiple chemical sensitivity
  syndrome
Occupational health
Parasitic diseases
Pigmentation
Plague
Poisoning
Pulmonary diseases
Pulmonary medicine
Roundworms
Schistosomiasis
Skin cancer
Sleeping sickness
Smallpox
Stress

Stress reduction
Trachoma
Tularemia
Typhoid fever
Typhus
West Nile virus
Yellow fever

EPIDEMIOLOGY

Acquired immunodeficiency
 syndrome (AIDS)
Amebiasis
Avian influenza
Bacillus Calmette-Guérin (BCG)
Bacterial infections
Bacteriology
Brucellosis
Candidiasis
Cerebral palsy
Chickenpox
Childhood infectious diseases
Cholera
Coronaviruses
Creutzfeldt-Jakob disease (CJD)
Diphtheria
E. coli infection
Ebola virus
Elephantiasis
Encephalitis
Epidemics and pandemics
Food poisoning
Forensic pathology
Gulf War syndrome
Hantavirus
Hepatitis
H1N1 influenza
Human papillomavirus (HPV)
Influenza
Insect-borne diseases
Laboratory tests
Legionnaires' disease
Leprosy
Leptospirosis
Lyme disease
Marburg virus
Mercury poisoning
Methicillin-resistant staphylococcus
 aureus (MRSA) infection
Microbiology
Multiple chemical sensitivity
 syndrome
Necrotizing fasciitis
Occupational health
Parasitic diseases
Phenylketonuria (PKU)
Plague
Pneumonia

Poisoning
Poliomyelitis
Prion diseases
Pulmonary diseases
Rabies
Rhinoviruses
Rocky Mountain spotted fever
Rotavirus
Roundworms
Screening
Severe acute respiratory syndrome
 (SARS)
Sexually transmitted diseases (STDs)
Sleeping sickness
Smallpox
Staphylococcal infections
Stress
Syphilis
Trichomoniasis
Tularemia
Typhoid fever
Typhus
Viral hemorrhagic fevers
Viral infections
West Nile virus
Yellow fever
Zoonoses

ETHICS

Abortion
Advance directives
Assisted reproductive technologies
Cloning
Defibrillation
Ergogenic aids
Facial transplantation
Fetal surgery
Fetal tissue transplantation
Gender identity disorder
Genetic engineering
Genomics
Gulf War syndrome
Longevity
Marijuana
Münchausen syndrome by proxy
Neurosis
Sperm banks
Stem cells
Xenotransplantation

EXERCISE PHYSIOLOGY

Acidosis
Ataxia
Biofeedback
Blood pressure
Bones and the skeleton
Cardiac rehabilitation

Carotid arteries
Defibrillation
Dehydration
Electrocardiography (ECG or EKG)
Ergogenic aids
Fascia
Glycolysis
Heart
Hemiplegia
Hypotension
Hypoxia
Juvenile rheumatoid arthritis
Kinesiology
Ligaments
Lungs
Massage
Metabolism
Motor skill development
Muscles
Osteoarthritis
Overtraining syndrome
Physical rehabilitation
Pulmonary medicine
Pulse rate
Respiration
Slipped disk
Sports medicine
Stenosis
Steroid abuse
Sweating
Tendinitis
Vascular system

FAMILY MEDICINE

Abdominal disorders
Abscess drainage
Acne
Advance directives
Alcoholism
Allergies
Amenorrhea
Amyotrophic lateral sclerosis
Anemia
Angelman syndrome
Angina
Anorexia nervosa
Anosmia
Antianxiety drugs
Antidepressants
Antihistamines
Antihypertensives
Anti-inflammatory drugs
Antioxidants
Aspergillosis
Ataxia
Atrophy
Attention-deficit disorder (ADD)

Autism
Bed-wetting
Bell's palsy
Beriberi
Biofeedback
Bleeding
Blisters
Blood pressure
Blurred vision
Body dysmorphic disorder
Bronchiolitis
Bronchitis
Bruises
Bulimia
Bunions
Burkitt's lymphoma
Caffeine
Candidiasis
Canker sores
Carotid arteries
Casts and splints
Cerebral palsy
Chagas' disease
Chickenpox
Childhood infectious diseases
Cholecystitis
Cholesterol
Chronic fatigue syndrome
Chronic granulomatous disease
Cirrhosis
Clostridium difficile infection
Coccidioidomycosis
Cold sores
Common cold
Conjunctivitis
Constipation
Corticosteroids
Coughing
Cryosurgery
Cushing's syndrome
Cytomegalovirus (CMV)
Death and dying
Decongestants
Deep vein thrombosis
Defibrillation
Dehydration
Dengue fever
Depression
Diabetes mellitus
Diarrhea and dysentery
Digestion
Diphtheria
Dizziness and fainting
E. coli infection
Earwax
Eating disorders
Echocardiography

Ehrlichiosis
Electrocauterization
Enterocolitis
Epiglottitis
Ergogenic aids
Exercise physiology
Factitious disorders
Failure to thrive
Fatigue
Fever
Fiber
Fifth disease
Fungal infections
Ganglion removal
Geriatric assessment
Giardiasis
Gigantism
Gynecology
Headaches
Healing
Heart disease
Heat exhaustion and heatstroke
Hemiplegia
Hemolytic uremic syndrome
Hemorrhoid banding and removal
Hemorrhoids
Herpes
Hiccups
Hirschsprung's disease
Hives
H1N1 influenza
Hormone therapy
Hyperadiposis
Hyperlipidemia
Hypertension
Hypertrophy
Hypoglycemia
Hypoxia
Impetigo
Incontinence
Infarction
Infection
Inflammation
Influenza
Interpartner violence
Intestinal disorders
Juvenile rheumatoid arthritis
Kawasaki disease
Keratitis
Kluver-Bucy syndrome
Kwashiorkor
Leishmaniasis
Leukodystrophy
Malabsorption
Maple syrup urine disease (MSUD)
Mastitis
Measles

Methicillin-resistant staphylococcus
    aureus (MRSA) infection
Mitral valve prolapse
Moles
Mononucleosis
Motion sickness
Mumps
Münchausen syndrome by proxy
Myringotomy
Nail removal
Nasal polyp removal
Nasopharyngeal disorders
Neurosis
Niemann-Pick disease
Nonalcoholic steatohepatitis (NASH)
Obesity
Orchitis
Osteopathic medicine
Otoplasty
Over-the-counter medications
Palliative medicine
Parasitic diseases
Pediatrics
Pharmacology
Physician assistants
Pick's disease
Pinworms
Pituitary gland
Pityriasis alba
Pityriasis rosea
Pleurisy
Pneumonia
Polycystic ovary syndrome
Polyps
Prader-Willi syndrome
Precocious puberty
Premenstrual syndrome (PMS)
Psychiatry
Ptosis
Puberty and adolescence
Pulse rate
Pyelonephritis
Raynaud's phenomenon
Reiter's syndrome
Rheumatic fever
Rhinitis
Ringworm
Rocky Mountain spotted fever
Roseola
Rubella
Safety issues for children
Safety issues for the elderly
Salmonella infection
Scabies
Scarlet fever
Sciatica
Sexuality

FORENSIC MEDICINE

GASTROENTEROLOGY

Taste
Toilet training
Ulcer surgery
Ulcerative colitis
Ulcers
Vagotomy
Vagus nerve
Vasculitis
Von Willebrand's disease
Weight loss and gain
Wilson's disease

GENERAL SURGERY
Abscess drainage
Achalasia
Adenoids
Adrenalectomy
Amputation
Anesthesia
Anesthesiology
Aneurysms
Appendectomy
Arthroplasty
Bariatric surgery
Biopsy
Bladder removal
Bone marrow transplantation
Brain tumors
Breast biopsy
Breast cancer
Breast disorders
Breast surgery
Bunions
Bypass surgery
Casts and splints
Catheterization
Cesarean section
Cholecystectomy
Chronic granulomatous disease
Cleft lip and palate repair
Coccidioidomycosis
Colon
Colonoscopy and sigmoidoscopy
Colorectal polyp removal
Colorectal surgery
Corneal transplantation
Cryosurgery
Culdocentesis
Cyst removal
Disk removal
Ear surgery
Electrocauterization
Endarterectomy
Eye infections and disorders
Eye surgery
Face lift and blepharoplasty
Fistula repair

Gallbladder cancer
Ganglion removal
Gastrectomy
Gender identity disorder
Gender reassignment surgery
Gigantism
Grafts and grafting
Hair transplantation
Hammertoe correction
Heart transplantation
Heart valve replacement
Heel spur removal
Hemorrhoid banding and removal
Hernia repair
Hydroceles
Hydrocephalus
Hypospadias repair and urethroplasty
Hypoxia
Hysterectomy
Infarction
Intravenous (IV) therapy
Kidney transplantation
Kneecap removal
Laceration repair
Laminectomy and spinal fusion
Laparoscopy
Laryngectomy
Lesions
Liposuction
Liver transplantation
Lumbar puncture
Lung surgery
Mastectomy and lumpectomy
Meckel's diverticulum
Mesothelioma
Methicillin-resistant staphylococcus
    aureus (MRSA) infection
Mouth and throat cancer
Nasal polyp removal
Nephrectomy
Neurosurgery
Oncology
Ophthalmology
Orthopedic surgery
Otoplasty
Pain
Parathyroidectomy
Penile implant surgery
Periodontal surgery
Peritonitis
Phlebitis
Physician assistants
Plasma
Plastic surgery
Polydactyly and syndactyly
Polyps
Prostate gland removal

Prostheses
Pulse rate
Pyloric stenosis
Rhinoplasty and submucous resection
Rotator cuff surgery
Sarcoma
Shunts
Skin lesion removal
Small intestine
Sphincterectomy
Splenectomy
Staphylococcal infections
Sterilization
Stone removal
Streptococcal infections
Surgical procedures
Surgical technologists
Sympathectomy
Tattoo removal
Tendon repair
Testicular cancer
Testicular surgery
Thoracic surgery
Thyroidectomy
Tonsillectomy and adenoid removal
Tonsillitis
Toxic shock syndrome
Trachea
Tracheostomy
Transfusion
Transplantation
Tumor removal
Ulcer surgery
Ulcerative colitis
Vagotomy
Varicose vein removal
Vasectomy
Xenotransplantation

GENETICS
Adrenoleukodystrophy
Agnosia
Amniocentesis
Angelman syndrome
Antibiotic resistance
Assisted reproductive technologies
Attention-deficit disorder (ADD)
Autism
Batten's disease
Bioinformatics
Biological therapies
Bionics and biotechnology
Birth defects
Bone marrow transplantation
Breast cancer
Charcot-Marie-Tooth Disease
Chemotherapy

Chorionic villus sampling
Chronic granulomatous disease
Cloning
Cockayne Disease
Cognitive development
Colorectal cancer
Congenital adrenal hyperplasia
Congenital disorders
Cornelia de Lange syndrome
Cystic fibrosis
Diabetes mellitus
DiGeorge syndrome
Down syndrome
Dwarfism
Embryology
Endocrinology
Enzyme therapy
Failure to thrive
Fetal surgery
Fragile X syndrome
Fructosemia
Galactosemia
Gaucher's disease
Gender identity disorder
Gene therapy
Genetic counseling
Genetic diseases
Genetic engineering
Genetic Imprinting
Genetics and inheritance
Genomics
Grafts and grafting
Hematology
Hemophilia
Hermaphroditism and
    pseudohermaphroditism
Huntington's disease
Hyperadiposis
Immunodeficiency disorders
Immunopathology
In vitro fertilization
Karyotyping
Klinefelter syndrome
Klippel-Trenaunay syndrome
Laboratory tests
Leptin
Leukodystrophy
Malabsorption
Maple syrup urine disease (MSUD)
Marfan syndrome
Mental retardation
Metabolic disorders
Motor skill development
Mucopolysaccharidosis (MPS)
Multiple births
Muscular dystrophy
Mutation

Neonatology
Nephrology
Neurofibromatosis
Neurology
Niemann-Pick disease
Obstetrics
Oncology
Osteogenesis imperfecta
Ovaries
Paget's disease
Pain
Pediatrics
Phenylketonuria (PKU)
Polycystic kidney disease
Polydactyly and syndactyly
Polyps
Porphyria
Prader-Willi syndrome
Precocious puberty
Reproductive system
Retroviruses
Rh factor
Rhinoviruses
Rubinstein-Taybi syndrome
Sarcoidosis
Sarcoma
Severe combined immunodeficiency
    syndrome (SCID)
Sexual differentiation
Sexuality
Sickle cell disease
Sperm banks
Spinocerebellar ataxia
Stem cells
Synesthesia
Tay-Sachs disease
Thalassemia
Tourette's syndrome
Transplantation
Tremors
Turner syndrome
Williams syndrome
Wiskott-Aldrich syndrome

**GERIATRICS AND
GERONTOLOGY**
Advance directives
Aging
Aging: Extended care
Alzheimer's disease
Arthroplasty
Assisted living facilities
Ataxia
Atrophy
Blindness
Blood pressure
Blurred vision

Bone disorders
Brain disorders
Cartilage
Cataracts
Chronic obstructive pulmonary
    disease (COPD)
Critical care
Deafness
Death and dying
Delirium
Dementias
Depression
Dyskinesia
Emergency medicine
End-stage renal disease
Eye infections and disorders
Eye surgery
Family medicine
Fatigue
Fiber
Frontal lobe syndrome
Geriatric assessment
Hip fracture repair
Hormone therapy
Hypotension
Incontinence
Interpartner violence
Joints
Light therapy
Longevity
Massage
Memory loss
Neuroscience
Nursing
Osteopathic medicine
Osteoporosis
Pain management
Palliative care
Paramedics
Parkinson's disease
Physician assistants
Pick's disease
Polymyalgia rheumatica
Psychiatry
Radiculopathy
Rheumatoid arthritis
Rheumatology
Safety issues for the elderly
Sleep disorders
Suicide
Temporal arteritis
Tremors
Vision disorders

GYNECOLOGY
Abdomen
Abortion

Acquired immunodeficiency
  syndrome (AIDS)
Amenorrhea
Assisted reproductive technologies
Biopsy
Bladder removal
Blurred vision
Breast biopsy
Breast cancer
Breast disorders
Breast-feeding
Cervical procedures
Cesarean section
Childbirth
Childbirth complications
Chlamydia
Conception
Contraception
Cryosurgery
Culdocentesis
Cyst removal
Cystitis
Cystoscopy
Dysmenorrhea
Ectopic pregnancy
Electrocauterization
Embolization
Endocrinology
Endometrial biopsy
Endometriosis
Endoscopy
Episiotomy
Fibrocystic breast condition
Gender reassignment surgery
Glands
Gonorrhea
Hermaphroditism and
  pseudohermaphroditism
Herpes
Hormone therapy
Human papillomavirus (HPV)
Hyperplasia
Hysterectomy
In vitro fertilization
Incontinence
Internal medicine
Laparoscopy
Leptin
Lesions
Mammography
Mastitis
Menopause
Menorrhagia
Menstruation
Miscarriage
Myomectomy
Obstetrics

Ovarian cysts
Ovaries
Pap test
Pelvic inflammatory disease (PID)
Polycystic ovary syndrome
Polyps
Postpartum depression
Preeclampsia and eclampsia
Pregnancy and gestation
Premenstrual syndrome (PMS)
Rape and sexual assault
Reiter's syndrome
Reproductive system
Sexual differentiation
Sexual dysfunction
Sexuality
Sexually transmitted diseases (STDs)
Sterilization
Syphilis
Toxic shock syndrome
Trichomoniasis
Tubal ligation
Turner syndrome
Ultrasonography
Urinary disorders
Urology
Uterus
Von Willebrand's disease

HEMATOLOGY
Acid-base chemistry
Acidosis
Acquired immunodeficiency
  syndrome (AIDS)
Anemia
Babesiosis
Biological therapies
Bleeding
Blood and blood disorders
Blood testing
Blood vessels
Bone grafting
Bone marrow transplantation
Bruises
Burkitt's lymphoma
Chronic fatigue syndrome
Circulation
Cold agglutinin disease
Connective tissue
Cyanosis
Cytology
Cytomegalovirus (CMV)
Cytopathology
Deep vein thrombosis
Dialysis
Disseminated intravascular
  coagulation (DIC)

Epidemics and pandemics
Epstein-Barr virus
Ergogenic aids
Fluids and electrolytes
Forensic pathology
Healing
Hemolytic disease of the newborn
Hemolytic uremic syndrome
Hemophilia
Histiocytosis
Histology
Hodgkin's disease
Hormone therapy
Host-defense mechanisms
Hypercholesterolemia
Hyperlipidemia
Hypoglycemia
Immune system
Immunopathology
Infection
Jaundice
Kidneys
Laboratory tests
Leukemia
Liver
Lymph
Lymphadenopathy and lymphoma
Lymphatic system
Nephrology
Niemann-Pick disease
Palliative care
Phlebotomy
Plasma
Rh factor
Septicemia
Serology
Sickle cell disease
Snakebites
Stem cells
Subdural hematoma
Thalassemia
Thrombocytopenia
Thrombolytic therapy and TPA
Thrombosis and thrombus
Transfusion
Uremia
Vascular medicine
Vascular system
Von Willebrand's disease

HISTOLOGY
Autopsy
Biopsy
Breast cancer
Breast disorders
Cancer
Carcinoma

Cells
Cold agglutinin disease
Colon
Cytology
Cytopathology
Dermatology
Dermatopathology
Endometrial biopsy
Eye infections and disorders
Fluids and electrolytes
Forensic pathology
Glioma
Healing
Laboratory tests
Microscopy
Nails
Necrotizing fasciitis
Pathology
Pityriasis alba
Rhinoviruses
Sarcoma
Small intestine
Smallpox
Tumor removal
Tumors

IMMUNOLOGY
Acquired immunodeficiency
    syndrome (AIDS)
Adenoids
Adenoviruses
Allergies
Ankylosing spondylitis
Antibiotics
Antibodies
Antihistamines
Aspergillosis
Asthma
Avian influenza
Bacillus Calmette-Guérin (BCG)
Bacterial infections
Biological therapies
Bionics and biotechnology
Bites and stings
Blood and blood disorders
Bone cancer
Bone grafting
Bone marrow transplantation
Cancer
Candidiasis
Carcinoma
Chickenpox
Childhood infectious diseases
Chronic fatigue syndrome
Chronic granulomatous disease
Cold agglutinin disease
Colorectal cancer

Coronaviruses
Corticosteroids
Crohn's disease
Cushing's syndrome
Cytology
Cytomegalovirus (CMV)
Dermatology
Dermatopathology
DiGeorge syndrome
Endocrinology
Epidemics and pandemics
Epstein-Barr virus
Fetal tissue transplantation
Food allergies
Fungal infections
Gluten intolerance
Grafts and grafting
Hay fever
Healing
Hematology
Histiocytosis
Hives
Homeopathy
Host-defense mechanisms
Human immunodeficiency virus
    (HIV)
Hypnosis
Immune system
Immunization and vaccination
Immunodeficiency disorders
Immunopathology
Juvenile rheumatoid arthritis
Kawasaki disease
Laboratory tests
Leprosy
Liver cancer
Lung cancer
Lymph
Lymphatic system
Malaria
Microbiology
Multiple chemical sensitivity
    syndrome
Multiple sclerosis
Myasthenia gravis
Nephritis
Noroviruses
Oncology
Opportunistic infections
Pancreas
Prostate cancer
Pulmonary diseases
Pulmonary medicine
Renal failure
Rheumatic fever
Rheumatoid arthritis
Rheumatology

Rhinitis
Rhinoviruses
Sarcoidosis
Scleroderma
Serology
Severe combined immunodeficiency
    syndrome (SCID)
Skin cancer
Small intestine
Smallpox
Stem cells
Stevens-Johnson syndrome
Stress
Stress reduction
Thalidomide
Thymus gland
Transfusion
Transplantation
Tularemia
Wiskott-Aldrich syndrome
Xenotransplantation

INTERNAL MEDICINE
Abdomen
Abdominal disorders
Acidosis
Acquired immunodeficiency
    syndrome (AIDS)
Adenoids
Alcoholism
Allergies
Alzheimer's disease
Amebiasis
Amyotrophic lateral sclerosis
Anemia
Angina
Anthrax
Antianxiety drugs
Antibodies
Anti-inflammatory drugs
Antioxidants
Anus
Anxiety
Aortic stenosis
Apnea
Arteriosclerosis
Arthritis
Aspergillosis
Ataxia
Auras
Babesiosis
Bacillus Calmette-Guérin (BCG)
Bacterial infections
Bariatric surgery
Bedsores
Behçet's disease
Bile

Rectum
Renal failure
Reye's syndrome
Rocky Mountain spotted fever
Sarcoidosis
Scarlet fever
Schistosomiasis
Sciatica
Septicemia
Severe acute respiratory syndrome (SARS)
Sexuality
Sexually transmitted diseases (STDs)
Shingles
Shock
Sinusitis
Sleep
Sleeping sickness
Small intestine
Sports medicine
Staphylococcal infections
Stevens-Johnson syndrome
Stones
Stress
Supplements
Syphilis
Tetanus
Thrombosis and thrombus
Toxic shock syndrome
Tremors
Tumors
Typhoid fever
Typhus
Ulcers
Ultrasonography
Urethritis
Viral infections
Vitamins and minerals
Weight loss medications
Wilson's disease
Wounds

MICROBIOLOGY
Acquired immunodeficiency syndrome (AIDS)
Amebiasis
Anthrax
Antibiotic resistance
Antibiotics
Antibodies
Aspergillosis
Autopsy
Bacillus Calmette-Guérin (BCG)
Bacterial infections
Bacteriology
Bionics and biotechnology
Brucellosis

Campylobacter infections
Chemotherapy
Chlamydia
Cholera
Chronic granulomatous disease
Coccidioidomycosis
Conjunctivitis
Creutzfeldt-Jakob disease (CJD)
Dengue fever
Diphtheria
E. coli infection
Enteroviruses
Epidemics and pandemics
Epstein-Barr virus
Fluoride treatments
Fungal infections
Gastroenteritis
Gastroenterology
Gastrointestinal disorders
Genomics
Gonorrhea
Gram staining
Hematuria
Human immunodeficiency virus (HIV)
Immune system
Immunization and vaccination
Impetigo
Insect-borne diseases
Laboratory tests
Leptospirosis
Methicillin-resistant staphylococcus aureus (MRSA) infection
Microscopy
Mold and mildew
Opportunistic infections
Pathology
Pelvic inflammatory disease (PID)
Peritonitis
Pharmacology
Plasma
Pneumocystis jirovecii
Protozoan diseases
Serology
Severe acute respiratory syndrome (SARS)
Sleeping sickness
Staphylococcal infections
Streptococcal infections
Syphilis
Toxic shock syndrome
Trichinosis
Tuberculosis
Urinalysis
Urology

NEONATOLOGY
Angelman syndrome

Apgar score
Apnea
Birth defects
Blue baby syndrome
Bonding
Breast disorders
Cesarean section
Childbirth
Childbirth complications
Cleft lip and palate
Cleft lip and palate repair
Collodion baby
Congenital disorders
Congenital heart disease
Cutis marmorata telangiectatica congenita
Cystic fibrosis
Disseminated intravascular coagulation (DIC)
E. coli infection
Embryology
Failure to thrive
Fetal surgery
Genetic diseases
Hemolytic disease of the newborn
Hydrocephalus
Intraventricular hemorrhage
Karyotyping
Malabsorption
Maple syrup urine disease (MSUD)
Motor skill development
Multiple births
Neonatal brachial plexus palsy
Nursing
Obstetrics
Pediatrics
Perinatology
Phenylketonuria (PKU)
Physician assistants
Premature birth
Pulse rate
Respiratory distress syndrome
Rh factor
Shunts
Spina bifida
Sudden infant death syndrome (SIDS)
Syphilis
Tay-Sachs disease
Transfusion
Trichomoniasis
Umbilical cord
Well-baby examinations

NEPHROLOGY
Abdomen
Addison's disease
Anemia

Aspergillosis
Chronic granulomatous disease
Diabetes mellitus
Dialysis
Diuretics
E. coli infection
Edema
End-stage renal disease
Ergogenic aids
Hematuria
Hemolytic uremic syndrome
Internal medicine
Kidney cancer
Kidney disorders
Kidney transplantation
Kidneys
Leptospirosis
Lesions
Lithotripsy
Nephrectomy
Nephritis
Palliative care
Polycystic kidney disease
Polyps
Preeclampsia and eclampsia
Proteinuria
Pyelonephritis
Renal failure
Sarcoidosis
Stenosis
Stone removal
Stones
Transplantation
Uremia
Urinalysis
Urinary disorders
Urinary system
Urology
Vasculitis
Williams syndrome

NEUROLOGY
Acquired immunodeficiency
  syndrome (AIDS)
Adrenoleukodystrophy
Aging: Extended care
Agnosia
Altitude sickness
Alzheimer's disease
Amnesia
Amyotrophic lateral sclerosis
Anesthesia
Anesthesiology
Aneurysms
Angelman syndrome
Anorexia nervosa
Anosmia

Antidepressants
Aphasia and dysphasia
Apnea
Ataxia
Atrophy
Attention-deficit disorder (ADD)
Audiology
Auras
Balance disorders
Batten's disease
Bell's palsy
Biofeedback
Blindsight
Botox
Brain
Brain damage
Brain disorders
Brain tumors
Brucellosis
Caffeine
Capgras syndrome
Carotid arteries
Carpal tunnel syndrome
Cerebral palsy
Charcot-Marie-Tooth Disease
Chiari malformations
Chiropractic
Chronic wasting disease (CWD)
Cluster headaches
Cockayne Disease
Cognitive enhancement
Concussion
Cornelia de Lange syndrome
Craniotomy
Creutzfeldt-Jakob disease (CJD)
Critical care
Cryosurgery
Cutis marmorata telangiectatica
  congenita
Delirium
Dementias
Developmental stages
Diabetes mellitus
Disk removal
Dizziness and fainting
Dyskinesia
Dyslexia
Ear infections and disorders
Ears
Electrical shock
Electroencephalography (EEG)
Electromyography
Embolism
Emergency medicine
Encephalitis
Enteroviruses
Epilepsy

Eye infections and disorders
Fascia
Fetal tissue transplantation
Frontal lobe syndrome
Frontotemporal dementia (FTD)
Gigantism
Glasgow coma scale
Glioma
Grafts and grafting
Guillain-Barré syndrome
Head and neck disorders
Headaches
Hearing
Hearing tests
Hematomas
Hemiplegia
Hemolytic disease of the newborn
Hiccups
Huntington's disease
Hydrocephalus
Hyperhidrosis
Hypothalamus
Hypoxia
Infarction
Intraventricular hemorrhage
Ischemia
Korsakoff's syndrome
Learning disabilities
Lesions
Leukodystrophy
Lower extremities
Lumbar puncture
Lyme disease
Marijuana
Melatonin
Memory loss
Meningitis
Mercury poisoning
Minimally conscious state
Morgellons disease
Motion sickness
Motor neuron diseases
Motor skill development
Multiple chemical sensitivity
  syndrome
Multiple sclerosis
Myasthenia gravis
Narcolepsy
Neonatal brachial plexus palsy
Nervous system
Neurofibromatosis
Neuropsychology
Neuroscience
Neurosis
Neurosurgery
Niemann-Pick disease
Numbness and tingling

Otorhinolaryngology
Pain
Palsy
Paralysis
Paraplegia
Parkinson's disease
Phenylketonuria (PKU)
Phrenology
Pick's disease
Poliomyelitis
Porphyria
Postherpetic neuralgia
Prader-Willi syndrome
Precocious puberty
Preeclampsia and eclampsia
Prion diseases
Psychiatry
Quadriplegia
Rabies
Radiculopathy
Restless legs syndrome
Reye's syndrome
Rubinstein-Taybi syndrome
Sarcoidosis
Sciatica
Seizures
Sense organs
Shingles
Shock therapy
Skin
Sleep
Sleep disorders
Sleeping sickness
Sleepwalking
Smell
Spinal cord disorders
Split-brain
Stem cells
Stenosis
Strokes
Sturge-Weber syndrome
Stuttering
Subdural hematoma
Sympathectomy
Synesthesia
Syphilis
Tardive dyskinesia
Taste
Tay-Sachs disease
Tetanus
Tics
Tinnitus
Torticollis
Touch
Tourette's syndrome
Transient ischemic attacks (TIAs)
Traumatic brain injury

Tremors
Upper extremities
Vagotomy
Vagus nerve
Vasculitis
Vertigo
Vision
Wernicke's aphasia
West Nile virus
Williams syndrome
Wilson's disease

NEUROPSYCHOLOGY
Capgras syndrome
Frontal lobe syndrome
Minimally conscious state
Neuroscience
Traumatic brain injury
Wernicke's aphasia
Williams syndrome

NEUROSCIENCE
Blindsight
Frontal lobe syndrome
Glasgow coma scale
Mirror neurons
Neuroethics
Neuropsychology
Phrenology
Split-brain
Traumatic brain injury
Wernicke's aphasia

NEUROSURGERY
Chiari malformations
Minimally conscious state
Wernicke's aphasia

NUCLEAR MEDICINE
Chemotherapy
Imaging and radiology
Magnetic resonance imaging (MRI)
Noninvasive tests
Nuclear radiology
Pneumocystis jirovecii
Positron emission tomography (PET)
  scanning
Radiation therapy
Single photon emission computed
  tomography (SPECT)

NURSING
Acidosis
Aging: Extended care
Alzheimer's disease
Ataxia
Atrophy

Bedsores
Cardiac rehabilitation
Carotid arteries
Casts and splints
Critical care
Diuretics
Drowning
Emergency medicine
Epidemics and pandemics
Eye infections and disorders
Fiber
Home care
H1N1 influenza
Hypoxia
Infarction
Influenza
Intravenous (IV) therapy
Methicillin-resistant staphylococcus
  aureus (MRSA) infection
Minimally conscious state
Palliative care
Pediatrics
Physician assistants
Polycystic ovary syndrome
Pulse rate
Radiculopathy
Surgical procedures
Surgical technologists
Well-baby examinations

NUTRITION
Aging: Extended care
Anorexia nervosa
Antioxidants
Bariatric surgery
Bedsores
Bell's palsy
Bile
Breast-feeding
Bulimia
Carbohydrates
Cardiac rehabilitation
Celiac sprue
Cholesterol
Colon
Crohn's disease
Cushing's syndrome
Dietary reference intakes (DRIs)
Digestion
Exercise physiology
Eye infections and disorders
Fatty acid oxidation disorders
Fiber
Food allergies
Food biochemistry
Food guide plate
Fructosemia

Galactosemia
Gastroenterology
Gastrointestinal system
Gestational diabetes
Gluten intolerance
Glycogen storage diseases
Hemolytic uremic syndrome
Hyperadiposis
Hypercholesterolemia
Irritable bowel syndrome (IBS)
Jaw wiring
Korsakoff's syndrome
Kwashiorkor
Lactose intolerance
Leptin
Leukodystrophy
Lipids
Macronutrients
Malabsorption
Malnutrition
Mastitis
Metabolic disorders
Metabolic syndrome
Metabolism
Nursing
Obesity
Osteoporosis
Phenylketonuria (PKU)
Phytochemicals
Pituitary gland
Plasma
Polycystic ovary syndrome
Protein
Rickets
Scurvy
Small intestine
Sports medicine
Supplements
Taste
Ulcer surgery
Ulcers
Vagotomy
Vitamin D deficiency
Vitamins and minerals
Weaning
Weight loss and gain
Weight loss medications

OBSTETRICS
Amniocentesis
Apgar score
Assisted reproductive technologies
Birth defects
Breast-feeding
Cerebral palsy
Cesarean section
Childbirth

Childbirth complications
Chorionic villus sampling
Conception
Congenital disorders
Contraception
Critical care
Cytomegalovirus (CMV)
Disseminated intravascular
  coagulation (DIC)
Down syndrome
Embryology
Emergency medicine
Endometrial biopsy
Endoscopy
Episiotomy
Family medicine
Fetal surgery
Gamete intrafallopian transfer (GIFT)
Genetic counseling
Genetic diseases
Gestational diabetes
Growth
Gynecology
Hirschsprung's disease
Incontinence
Intravenous (IV) therapy
Karyotyping
Listeria infections
Mastitis
Miscarriage
Multiple births
Neonatal brachial plexus palsy
Neonatology
Noninvasive tests
Ovaries
Perinatology
Pituitary gland
Placenta
Polycystic ovary syndrome
Postpartum depression
Preeclampsia and eclampsia
Pregnancy and gestation
Premature birth
Pyelonephritis
Reproductive system
Rh factor
Sexuality
Sperm banks
Stillbirth
Streptococcal infections
Teratogens
Toxemia
Trichomoniasis
Tubal ligation
Turner syndrome
Ultrasonography
Urology

Uterus

OCCUPATIONAL HEALTH
Acidosis
Agnosia
Altitude sickness
Angelman syndrome
Asbestos exposure
Asphyxiation
Ataxia
Bacillus Calmette-Guérin (BCG)
Biofeedback
Blurred vision
Brucellosis
Cardiac rehabilitation
Carpal tunnel syndrome
Charcot-Marie-Tooth Disease
Gulf War syndrome
Hearing tests
Leptospirosis
Leukodystrophy
Lung cancer
Mercury poisoning
Mesothelioma
Multiple chemical sensitivity
  syndrome
Nasopharyngeal disorders
Pneumonia
Prostheses
Pulmonary diseases
Pulmonary medicine
Radiation sickness
Skin disorders
Slipped disk
Spinocerebellar ataxia
Stress reduction
Tendinitis
Tendon disorders
Tendon repair

OCCUPATIONAL THERAPY
Home care
Minimally conscious state
Williams syndrome

ONCOLOGY
Acquired immunodeficiency
  syndrome (AIDS)
Aging: Extended care
Amputation
Anal cancer
Anemia
Antibodies
Antioxidants
Anus
Asbestos exposure
Assisted suicide

Cataract surgery
Cataracts
Cockayne Disease
Color blindness
Conjunctivitis
Eye infections and disorders
Eye surgery
Eyes
Glaucoma
Keratitis
Myopia
Ophthalmology
Pterygium/Pinguecula
Ptosis
Sarcoidosis
Sense organs
Spinocerebellar ataxia
Tears and tear ducts
Vision disorders
Williams syndrome

ORTHODONTICS
Bones and the skeleton
Dentistry
Jaw wiring
Periodontal surgery
Periodontitis
Teeth
Teething
Tooth extraction
Williams syndrome

ORTHOPEDICS
Amputation
Anti-inflammatory drugs
Arthritis
Arthroplasty
Arthroscopy
Ataxia
Atrophy
Bariatric surgery
Bone cancer
Bone disorders
Bone grafting
Bones and the skeleton
Bowlegs
Bunions
Cancer
Cartilage
Casts and splints
Cerebral palsy
Charcot-Marie-Tooth Disease
Chiropractic
Connective tissue
Craniosynostosis
Cutis marmorata telangiectatica
    congenita

Disk removal
Dwarfism
Endoscopy
Ergogenic aids
Ewing's sarcoma
Fascia
Feet
Flat feet
Foot disorders
Fracture and dislocation
Fracture repair
Growth
Hammertoe correction
Hammertoes
Heel spur removal
Hemiplegia
Hip fracture repair
Hip replacement
Hormone therapy
Joints
Juvenile rheumatoid arthritis
Kinesiology
Kneecap removal
Knock-knees
Kyphosis
Laminectomy and spinal fusion
Ligaments
Lower extremities
Marfan syndrome
Mesenchymal stem cells
Methicillin-resistant staphylococcus
    aureus (MRSA) infection
Motor skill development
Muscles
Necrosis
Neonatal brachial plexus palsy
Neurofibromatosis
Orthopedic surgery
Osgood-Schlatter disease
Osteoarthritis
Osteochondritis juvenilis
Osteogenesis imperfecta
Osteomyelitis
Osteonecrosis
Osteoporosis
Paget's disease
Physical rehabilitation
Pigeon toes
Podiatry
Prostheses
Radiculopathy
Reiter's syndrome
Rheumatology
Rickets
Rotator cuff surgery
Rubinstein-Taybi syndrome
Scoliosis

Slipped disk
Spondylitis
Sports medicine
Staphylococcal infections
Stenosis
Tendinitis
Tendon disorders
Tendon repair
Upper extremities
Whiplash

OSTEOPATHIC MEDICINE
Acidosis
Acquired immunodeficiency
    syndrome (AIDS)
Alternative medicine
Atrophy
Bones and the skeleton
Colon
Family medicine
Fascia
Ligaments
Muscles
Physical rehabilitation
Pituitary gland
Radiculopathy
Rickets
Slipped disk
Small intestine

OTOLARYNGOLOGY
Head and neck disorders
Ménière's disease
Vasculitis

OTORHINOLARYNGOLOGY
Acquired immunodeficiency
    syndrome (AIDS)
Adenoids
Allergies
Anosmia
Antihistamines
Anti-inflammatory drugs
Aromatherapy
Aspergillosis
Audiology
Cartilage
Cleft lip and palate
Cleft lip and palate repair
Cockayne Disease
Common cold
Croup
Cryosurgery
Decongestants
Ear infections and disorders
Ear surgery
Ears

Gaucher's disease
Gender identity disorder
Genetic diseases
Genetics and inheritance
Giardiasis
Glycogen storage diseases
Growth
Hand-foot-and-mouth disease
Hearing tests
Hemolytic uremic syndrome
Hirschsprung's disease
Hives
H1N1 influenza
Impetigo
Incontinence
Influenza
Interpartner violence
Intravenous (IV) therapy
Juvenile rheumatoid arthritis
Kawasaki disease
Klippel-Trenaunay syndrome
Kluver-Bucy syndrome
Knock-knees
Kwashiorkor
Lead poisoning
Learning disabilities
Leukodystrophy
Listeria infections
Malabsorption
Malnutrition
Maple syrup urine disease (MSUD)
Massage
Measles
Menstruation
Mercury poisoning
Metabolic disorders
Methicillin-resistant staphylococcus
    aureus (MRSA) infection
Mold and mildew
Mononucleosis
Motor skill development
Mucopolysaccharidosis (MPS)
Multiple births
Multiple sclerosis
Mumps
Münchausen syndrome by proxy
Muscular dystrophy
Nail removal
Neonatal brachial plexus palsy
Neonatology
Neuroscience
Niemann-Pick disease
Nonalcoholic steatohepatitis (NASH)
Nursing
Osgood-Schlatter disease
Osteogenesis imperfecta
Otoplasty

Otorhinolaryngology
Palliative medicine
Perinatology
Phenylketonuria (PKU)
Pigeon toes
Pinworms
Pituitary gland
Pityriasis alba
Poliomyelitis
Polycystic ovary syndrome
Polydactyly and syndactyly
Porphyria
Prader-Willi syndrome
Precocious puberty
Premature birth
Progeria
Puberty and adolescence
Pulse rate
Pyloric stenosis
Respiratory distress syndrome
Reye's syndrome
Rheumatic fever
Rhinitis
Rickets
Roseola
Rotavirus
Rubella
Rubinstein-Taybi syndrome
Safety issues for children
Salmonella infection
Scarlet fever
Seizures
Severe combined immunodeficiency
    syndrome (SCID)
Sexuality
Small intestine
Soiling
Sore throat
Steroids
Stevens-Johnson syndrome
Streptococcal infections
Sturge-Weber syndrome
Stuttering
Sudden infant death syndrome (SIDS)
Syphilis
Tay-Sachs disease
Teething
Testicular torsion
Thalassemia
Thumb sucking
Toilet training
Tonsillectomy and adenoid removal
Tonsillitis
Tonsils
Toxoplasmosis
Trachoma
Weaning

Well-baby examinations
Whooping cough
Wiskott-Aldrich syndrome

PERINATOLOGY
Amniocentesis
Assisted reproductive technologies
Birth defects
Breast-feeding
Cesarean section
Childbirth
Chorionic villus sampling
Congenital hypothyroidism
Embryology
Fatty acid oxidation disorders
Glycogen storage diseases
Hydrocephalus
Karyotyping
Metabolic disorders
Miscarriage
Motor skill development
Neonatal brachial plexus palsy
Neonatology
Nursing
Obstetrics
Pediatrics
Premature birth
Shunts
Spina bifida
Trichomoniasis
Umbilical cord
Uterus
Well-baby examinations

PHARMACOLOGY
Acid-base chemistry
Acidosis
Acquired immunodeficiency
    syndrome (AIDS)
Aging: Extended care
Allergies
Antianxiety drugs
Antibiotic resistance
Antibiotics
Antibodies
Antihistamines
Antihypertensives
Assisted suicide
Autism
Bacteriology
Blurred vision
Chemotherapy
Chronic granulomatous disease
Club drugs
Colon
Critical care
Digestion

Diuretics
Dyskinesia
Emergency medicine
Epidemics and pandemics
Ergogenic aids
Fluids and electrolytes
Food biochemistry
Genetic engineering
Genomics
Glycolysis
Homeopathy
Hormones
Hypercholesterolemia
Hypotension
Laboratory tests
Marijuana
Melatonin
Mesothelioma
Metabolism
Methicillin-resistant staphylococcus
   aureus (MRSA) infection
Narcotics
Neuropsychology
Neuroscience
Oncology
Over-the-counter medications
Pain management
Polycystic ovary syndrome
Prader-Willi syndrome
Psychiatry
Rheumatology
Sleep
Small intestine
Sports medicine
Steroids
Tardive dyskinesia
Thrombolytic therapy and TPA
Tremors

PHYSICAL THERAPY
Aging: Extended care
Amputation
Amyotrophic lateral sclerosis
Angelman syndrome
Arthritis
Ataxia
Atrophy
Biofeedback
Bowlegs
Burns and scalds
Cardiac rehabilitation
Casts and splints
Cerebral palsy
Charcot-Marie-Tooth Disease
Cornelia de Lange syndrome
Disk removal
Dyskinesia

Electromyography
Exercise physiology
Facial transplantation
Fascia
Grafts and grafting
Hemiplegia
Home care
Hydrotherapy
Kinesiology
Knock-knees
Leukodystrophy
Ligaments
Lower extremities
Massage
Minimally conscious state
Motor skill development
Muscles
Muscular dystrophy
Neonatal brachial plexus palsy
Neurology
Numbness and tingling
Orthopedic surgery
Orthopedics
Osteopathic medicine
Osteoporosis
Pain
Pain management
Palsy
Paralysis
Parkinson's disease
Physical rehabilitation
Pigeon toes
Plastic surgery
Prostheses
Pulse rate
Radiculopathy
Scoliosis
Slipped disk
Spinal cord disorders
Spinocerebellar ataxia
Sports medicine
Tendinitis
Tendon disorders
Torticollis
Upper extremities
Whiplash
Williams syndrome

PLASTIC SURGERY
Amputation
Bariatric surgery
Body dysmorphic disorder
Botox
Breast surgery
Burns and scalds
Cleft lip and palate
Cleft lip and palate repair

Craniosynostosis
Cryosurgery
Cyst removal
DiGeorge syndrome
Face lift and blepharoplasty
Facial transplantation
Gender reassignment surgery
Grafts and grafting
Hair transplantation
Healing
Jaw wiring
Laceration repair
Liposuction
Malignancy and metastasis
Mastectomy and lumpectomy
Mesenchymal stem cells
Moles
Necrotizing fasciitis
Neonatal brachial plexus palsy
Neurofibromatosis
Oral and maxillofacial surgery
Otoplasty
Otorhinolaryngology
Prostheses
Ptosis
Rhinoplasty and submucous resection
Skin
Skin lesion removal
Spina bifida
Sturge-Weber syndrome
Surgical procedures
Tattoos and body piercing
Varicose vein removal
Varicose veins
Vision

PODIATRY
Athlete's foot
Bones and the skeleton
Bunions
Cartilage
Cerebral palsy
Corns and calluses
Feet
Flat feet
Foot disorders
Gout
Hammertoe correction
Hammertoes
Heel spur removal
Joints
Lesions
Lower extremities
Methicillin-resistant staphylococcus
   aureus (MRSA) infection
Nail removal
Orthopedic surgery

Orthopedics
Polydactyly and syndactyly
Tendon disorders
Tendon repair

PREVENTIVE MEDICINE
Acidosis
Acupressure
Acupuncture
Alternative medicine
Anemia
Aneurysmectomy
Antibodies
Antihistamines
Antihypertensives
Aromatherapy
Assisted living facilities
Bacillus Calmette-Guérin (BCG)
Biofeedback
Blurred vision
Breast cancer
Brucellosis
Caffeine
Cardiac surgery
Cardiology
Cerebral palsy
Chemotherapy
Chiropractic
Cholesterol
Club drugs
Computed tomography (CT) scanning
Congenital hypothyroidism
Croup
Electrocardiography (ECG or EKG)
Endometrial biopsy
Exercise physiology
Family medicine
Fiber
Food guide plate
Genetic counseling
Genetic engineering
Hormone therapy
Host-defense mechanisms
Immune system
Immunization and vaccination
Insect-borne diseases
Lead poisoning
Mammography
Massage
Meditation
Melatonin
Mesothelioma
Noninvasive tests
Nursing
Nutrition
Occupational health
Osteopathic medicine

Over-the-counter medications
Oxygen therapy
Pharmacology
Phytochemicals
Polycystic ovary syndrome
Psychiatry
Rhinoviruses
Screening
Scurvy
Serology
Sleep
Slipped disk
Smallpox
Sports medicine
Stress reduction
Tendinitis
Vitamin D deficiency
Yoga

PROCTOLOGY
Acquired immunodeficiency
    syndrome (AIDS)
Anal cancer
Anus
Bladder removal
Chronic granulomatous disease
Colorectal cancer
Colorectal polyp removal
Colorectal surgery
Diverticulitis and diverticulosis
Endoscopy
Fistula repair
Hemorrhoid banding and removal
Hemorrhoids
Hirschsprung's disease
Internal medicine
Polyps
Prostate gland removal
Rectum
Reproductive system
Urology

PSYCHIATRY
Acquired immunodeficiency
    syndrome (AIDS)
Addiction
Adrenoleukodystrophy
Aging: Extended care
Alcoholism
Alzheimer's disease
Amnesia
Amyotrophic lateral sclerosis
Angelman syndrome
Anorexia nervosa
Antianxiety drugs
Antidepressants
Anxiety

Asperger's syndrome
Attention-deficit disorder (ADD)
Auras
Autism
Bariatric surgery
Bipolar disorders
Body dysmorphic disorder
Bonding
Brain
Brain damage
Brain disorders
Breast surgery
Bulimia
Chronic fatigue syndrome
Club drugs
Cognitive enhancement
Computed tomography (CT) scanning
Dementias
Depression
Developmental disorders
Developmental stages
Dyskinesia
Eating disorders
Electroencephalography (EEG)
Emergency medicine
Factitious disorders
Failure to thrive
Family medicine
Fatigue
Frontotemporal dementia (FTD)
Gender identity disorder
Gender reassignment surgery
Gynecology
Havening touch
Huntington's disease
Hypnosis
Hypochondriasis
Hypothalamus
Incontinence
Interpartner violence
Kluver-Bucy syndrome
Korsakoff's syndrome
Light therapy
Marijuana
Masturbation
Memory loss
Mental retardation
Mental status exam
Morgellons disease
Münchausen syndrome by proxy
Neuropsychology
Neuroscience
Neurosis
Neurosurgery
Obesity
Obsessive-compulsive disorder
Pain

Pain management
Paranoia
Penile implant surgery
Phobias
Phrenology
Pick's disease
Postpartum depression
Post-traumatic stress disorder
Prader-Willi syndrome
Premenstrual syndrome (PMS)
Psychiatric disorders
Psychoanalysis
Psychosis
Psychosomatic disorders
Rape and sexual assault
Restless legs syndrome
Schizophrenia
Seasonal affective disorder
Separation anxiety
Sexual dysfunction
Sexuality
Shock therapy
Single photon emission computed
    tomography (SPECT)
Sleep
Sleep disorders
Speech disorders
Split-brain
Steroid abuse
Stress
Stress reduction
Sudden infant death syndrome (SIDS)
Suicide
Synesthesia
Tardive dyskinesia
Tinnitus
Toilet training
Tourette's syndrome
Traumatic brain injury
Tremors

PSYCHOLOGY

Abuse of the elderly
Addiction
Aging
Aging: Extended care
Alcoholism
Amnesia
Amyotrophic lateral sclerosis
Angelman syndrome
Anorexia nervosa
Antidepressants
Anxiety
Aromatherapy
Asperger's syndrome
Attention-deficit disorder (ADD)
Auras

Bariatric surgery
Bed-wetting
Biofeedback
Bipolar disorders
Blindsight
Bonding
Brain
Brain damage
Bulimia
Capgras syndrome
Cardiac rehabilitation
Cerebral palsy
Cirrhosis
Club drugs
Cognitive development
Death and dying
Depression
Developmental disorders
Developmental stages
Dyslexia
Eating disorders
Electroencephalography (EEG)
Ergogenic aids
Facial transplantation
Factitious disorders
Failure to thrive
Family medicine
Forensic pathology
Frontal lobe syndrome
Gender identity disorder
Gender reassignment surgery
Genetic counseling
Gulf War syndrome
Gynecology
Huntington's disease
Hypnosis
Hypochondriasis
Hypothalamus
Interpartner violence
Juvenile rheumatoid arthritis
Kinesiology
Klinefelter syndrome
Kluver-Bucy syndrome
Korsakoff's syndrome
Learning disabilities
Light therapy
Marijuana
Memory loss
Mental retardation
Mental status exam
Mirror neurons
Miscarriage
Motor skill development
Münchausen syndrome by proxy
Neonatal brachial plexus palsy
Neuropsychology
Neurosis

Obesity
Obsessive-compulsive disorder
Occupational health
Overtraining syndrome
Pain management
Palliative care
Palliative medicine
Paranoia
Phobias
Phrenology
Pick's disease
Plastic surgery
Polycystic ovary syndrome
Postpartum depression
Post-traumatic stress disorder
Premenstrual syndrome (PMS)
Psychosomatic disorders
Puberty and adolescence
Restless legs syndrome
Separation anxiety
Sexual dysfunction
Sexuality
Sleep
Sleep disorders
Sleepwalking
Speech disorders
Split-brain
Sports medicine
Steroid abuse
Stress
Stress reduction
Sturge-Weber syndrome
Sudden infant death syndrome (SIDS)
Suicide
Synesthesia
Temporomandibular joint (TMJ)
    syndrome
Tics
Toilet training
Tourette's syndrome
Traumatic brain injury
Weight loss and gain
Wernicke's aphasia
Williams syndrome

PUBLIC HEALTH

Acquired immunodeficiency
    syndrome (AIDS)
Acute respiratory distress syndrome
    (ARDS)
Adenoviruses
Advance directives
Aging: Extended care
Alternative medicine
Amebiasis
Antibiotic resistance
Antibodies

Assisted living facilities
Babesiosis
Bacillus Calmette-Guérin (BCG)
Bacteriology
Blood testing
Brucellosis
Cerebral palsy
Chagas' disease
Chickenpox
Childhood infectious diseases
Cholera
Chronic obstructive pulmonary
    disease (COPD)
Club drugs
Common cold
Coronaviruses
Creutzfeldt-Jakob disease (CJD)
Dengue fever
Dermatology
Diarrhea and dysentery
E. coli infection
Ebola virus
Elephantiasis
Emergency medicine
Encephalitis
Epidemics and pandemics
Epidemiology
Food guide plate
Food poisoning
Forensic pathology
Gulf War syndrome
Hantavirus
H1N1 influenza
Human papillomavirus (HPV)
Immunization and vaccination
Influenza
Insect-borne diseases
Interpartner violence
Legionnaires' disease
Leishmaniasis
Leprosy
Leptospirosis
Macronutrients
Malaria
Malnutrition
Managed care
Marijuana
Measles
Meningitis
Methicillin-resistant staphylococcus
    aureus (MRSA) infection
Microbiology
Monkeypox
Multiple chemical sensitivity
    syndrome
Neurosis
Niemann-Pick disease

Nursing
Nutrition
Obesity
Occupational health
Osteopathic medicine
Parasitic diseases
Pharmacology
Physician assistants
Pinworms
Plague
Pneumonia
Poliomyelitis
Polycystic ovary syndrome
Prion diseases
Protozoan diseases
Psychiatry
Rabies
Radiation sickness
Rape and sexual assault
Retroviruses
Rhinoviruses
Roundworms
Salmonella infection
Schistosomiasis
Screening
Serology
Severe acute respiratory syndrome
    (SARS)
Sexually transmitted diseases (STDs)
Shigellosis
Sleeping sickness
Smallpox
Syphilis
Tapeworms
Tattoos and body piercing
Tetanus
Trichinosis
Trichomoniasis
Tuberculosis
Tularemia
Typhoid fever
Typhus
West Nile virus
Yellow fever
Zoonoses

PULMONARY MEDICINE

Acquired immunodeficiency
    syndrome (AIDS)
Acute respiratory distress syndrome
    (ARDS)
Adrenoleukodystrophy
Amyotrophic lateral sclerosis
Antihistamines
Apnea
Aspergillosis
Asthma

Bronchi
Bronchiolitis
Bronchitis
Catheterization
Chest
Chronic granulomatous disease
Chronic obstructive pulmonary
    disease (COPD)
Coccidioidomycosis
Cold agglutinin disease
Coronaviruses
Coughing
Critical care
Cyanosis
Cystic fibrosis
Diaphragm
Drowning
Edema
Emergency medicine
Emphysema
Endoscopy
Epidemics and pandemics
Fluids and electrolytes
Forensic pathology
Fungal infections
Hantavirus
Hyperbaric oxygen therapy
Hyperventilation
Hypoxia
Internal medicine
Interstitial pulmonary fibrosis (IPF)
Leptospirosis
Lesions
Lung cancer
Lung surgery
Lungs
Mesothelioma
Methicillin-resistant staphylococcus
    aureus (MRSA) infection
Mold and mildew
Occupational health
Oxygen therapy
Palliative care
Paramedics
Pediatrics
Pharynx
Pleurisy
Pneumocystis jirovecii
Pneumonia
Pneumothorax
Polyps
Prader-Willi syndrome
Pulmonary diseases
Pulmonary edema
Pulmonary hypertension
Respiration
Respiratory distress syndrome

Sarcoidosis
Severe acute respiratory syndrome (SARS)
Single photon emission computed tomography (SPECT)
Sleep apnea
Smoking
Stem cells
Stevens-Johnson syndrome
Thoracic surgery
Thrombolytic therapy and TPA
Trachea
Tuberculosis
Tumors
Vasculitis

RADIOLOGY
Achalasia
Angiography
Aspergillosis
Atrophy
Biopsy
Bone cancer
Brain tumors
Breast cancer
Cancer
Cartilage
Catheterization
Chronic granulomatous disease
Cold agglutinin disease
Computed tomography (CT) scanning
Critical care
Cushing's syndrome
Embolization
Emergency medicine
Endoscopic retrograde cholangiopancreatography (ERCP)
Ewing's sarcoma
Eye infections and disorders
Gallbladder cancer
Imaging and radiology
Joints
Liver cancer
Lung cancer
Magnetic resonance imaging (MRI)
Mammography
Mastectomy and lumpectomy
Meckel's diverticulum
Mesothelioma
Methicillin-resistant staphylococcus aureus (MRSA) infection
Mouth and throat cancer
Neonatal brachial plexus palsy
Noninvasive tests
Nuclear medicine
Nuclear radiology
Oncology

Palliative care
Palliative medicine
Pneumocystis jirovecii
Positron emission tomography (PET) scanning
Prostate cancer
Radiation sickness
Radiation therapy
Radiculopathy
Radiopharmaceuticals
Sarcoidosis
Single photon emission computed tomography (SPECT)
Stents
Testicular cancer
Ultrasonography

REHABILITATION
Neuropsychology
Traumatic brain injury

RHEUMATOLOGY
Aging: Extended care
Ankylosing spondylitis
Anti-inflammatory drugs
Arthritis
Arthroplasty
Arthroscopy
Atrophy
Behçet's disease
Bone disorders
Brucellosis
Bursitis
Cartilage
Cold agglutinin disease
Collagen
Connective tissue
Fibromyalgia
Gout
Hip replacement
Hydrotherapy
Inflammation
Joints
Ligaments
Lyme disease
Mesenchymal stem cells
Methicillin-resistant staphylococcus aureus (MRSA) infection
Orthopedic surgery
Orthopedics
Osteonecrosis
Paget's disease
Pain
Polymyalgia rheumatica
Radiculopathy
Rheumatoid arthritis
Rotator cuff surgery

Sarcoidosis
Scleroderma
Sjögren's syndrome
Sports medicine
Syphilis
Temporal arteritis
Vasculitis

SEROLOGY
Babesiosis
Blood and blood disorders
Blood testing
Chronic granulomatous disease
Cold agglutinin disease
Cytology
Cytopathology
Dialysis
Epidemics and pandemics
Fluids and electrolytes
Forensic pathology
Hematology
Hemophilia
Hodgkin's disease
Host-defense mechanisms
Hyperbaric oxygen therapy
Hyperlipidemia
Hypoglycemia
Immune system
Immunopathology
Laboratory tests
Leukemia
Lymph
Plasma
Rh factor
Rhinoviruses
Sarcoidosis
Septicemia
Snakebites
Transfusion
Tremors

SPEECH PATHOLOGY
Adenoids
Agnosia
Amyotrophic lateral sclerosis
Angelman syndrome
Aphasia and dysphasia
Ataxia
Audiology
Autism
Cerebral palsy
Cleft lip and palate
Deafness
Dyslexia
Ear surgery
Ears
Electroencephalography (EEG)

Urethritis
Urinalysis
Urinary disorders
Urinary system
Vas deferens
Vasectomy

VASCULAR MEDICINE
Acidosis
Amputation
Aneurysms
Angiography
Angioplasty
Antihypertensives
Anti-inflammatory drugs
Aortic aneurysm
Arteriosclerosis
Biofeedback
Bleeding
Blood pressure
Blood vessels
Bruises
Cardiac surgery
Cardiology
Carotid arteries
Cholesterol
Circulation
Claudication
Cold agglutinin disease
Computed tomography (CT) scanning
Congenital heart disease
Cutis marmorata telangiectatica
   congenita
Dehydration
Diabetes mellitus
Electrocauterization
Embolism
Embolization
End-stage renal disease
Endarterectomy
Endocarditis
Glands
Healing
Heart failure
Hematology
Histology
Hormone therapy
Hypercholesterolemia

Hyperlipidemia
Infarction
Ischemia
Klippel-Trenaunay syndrome
Lesions
Lipids
Lungs
Lymphadenopathy and lymphoma
Lymphatic system
Mitral valve prolapse
Necrotizing fasciitis
Osteochondritis juvenilis
Phlebitis
Plasma
Podiatry
Preeclampsia and eclampsia
Progeria
Pulse rate
Raynaud's phenomenon
Respiration
Shunts
Smoking
Stem cells
Stents
Strokes
Sturge-Weber syndrome
Thrombolytic therapy and TPA
Thrombosis and thrombus
Transfusion
Transient ischemic attacks (TIAs)
Ultrasonography
Varicose vein removal
Varicose veins
Vascular system
Venous insufficiency
Von Willebrand's disease

VIROLOGY
Avian influenza
Chickenpox
Childhood infectious diseases
Cold agglutinin disease
Common cold
Conjunctivitis
Coronaviruses
Creutzfeldt-Jakob disease (CJD)
Croup
Cytomegalovirus (CMV)

Dengue fever
Ebola virus
Encephalitis
Enteroviruses
Epidemics and pandemics
Epstein-Barr virus
Eye infections and disorders
Fever
Gastroenteritis
Hand-foot-and-mouth disease
Hantavirus
Hepatitis
Herpes
H1N1 influenza
Human immunodeficiency virus (HIV)
Human papillomavirus (HPV)
Infection
Influenza
Laboratory tests
Marburg virus
Measles
Microbiology
Microscopy
Monkeypox
Mononucleosis
Noroviruses
Opportunistic infections
Orchitis
Paget's disease
Parasitic diseases
Poliomyelitis
Pulmonary diseases
Rabies
Retroviruses
Rhinoviruses
Rotavirus
Sarcoidosis
Serology
Severe acute respiratory syndrome
   (SARS)
Sexually transmitted diseases (STDs)
Shingles
Smallpox
Viral hemorrhagic fevers
Viral infections
West Nile virus
Yellow fever
Zoonoses